GASTROINTESTINAL RADIOLOGY

GASTROINTESTINAL RADIOLOGY

A Pattern Approach

Second Edition

Ronald L. Eisenberg, M.D.

Professor and Chairman
Department of Radiology
Louisiana State University School of Medicine
Shreveport, Louisiana

J.B. LIPPINCOTT COMPANY
Philadelphia
Grand Rapids   New York   St. Louis   San Francisco
London   Sydney   Tokyo

The author and publisher have exerted every effort to ensure that drug selections and dosage set forth in this text are in accord with current recommendations and practice at the time of publication. However, in view of ongoing research, changes in government regulations, and the constant flow of information relating to drug therapy and drug reactions, the reader is urged to check the package insert for each drug for any change in indications and dosage and for added warnings and precautions. This is particularly important when the recommended agent is a new or infrequently employed drug.

Acquisitions Editor: Charles McCormick
Sponsoring Editor: DeLois Patterson
Manuscript Editor: Patrick O'Kane
Design and Production Coordinator: Caren Erlichman
Production Manager: Carol A. Florence
Indexer: Betty Herr Hallinger
Compositor: Tapsco, Inc.
Printer/Binder: Halliday Lithograph Corporation

Second Edition

6

Library of Congress Cataloging-in-Publication Data

Eisenberg, Ronald L.
  Gastrointestinal radiology.

  Includes bibliographies and index.
    1. Gastrointestinal system—Radiography—Atlases.
2. Gastrointestinal system—Diseases—Diagnosis.
I. Title. [DNLM: 1. Gastrointestinal System—
radiography. 2. Gastrointestinal System—radiography—atlases. WI 141 E36g]
RC804.R6E37 1989   616.3'0757   88-13036
ISBN 0-397-50943-X

*To Alex Margulis,
Teacher, Inspiration, Friend*

PREFACE

In the 7 years since the first edition of "Gastrointestinal Radiology: A Pattern Approach" was published, the number of gastrointestinal fluoroscopic procedures has been declining. Factors contributing to this decrease include the widespread availability of newer imaging techniques (ultrasound and computed tomography), competition from endoscopy, and the extensive use of effective histamine-blocking agents. Nevertheless, because of their relatively low cost, noninvasive nature, and high sensitivity for detecting severe or life-threatening diseases, it is probable that millions of gastrointestinal fluoroscopic studies will continue to be performed each year.

To reflect the significant impact of ultrasound and computed tomography on gastrointestinal radiology, numerous illustrations of these imaging modalities have been included in this second edition of the text and some examples of traditional contrast studies have been eliminated. For example, the value of ultrasound in examination of the gallbladder has been stressed, even though oral cholecystography is included both because it is becoming increasingly important in the nonsurgical therapy of gallstones and for the benefit of those radiologists whose referring clinicians still request this procedure for the initial diagnosis of gallbladder disease.

Regardless of the specific imaging modality utilized, the practicing radiologist is usually unaware of the underlying disease and is presented with a specific finding for which he or she must suggest a differential diagnosis. Therefore, the "pattern" approach remains a handy reference for the practicing radiologist and resident faced with the daily challenge of interpreting gastrointestinal examinations.

Ronald L. Eisenberg, M.D.

PREFACE
TO FIRST EDITION

With all the available books on gastrointestinal radiology, why should there be yet another one? Essentially all textbooks in gastrointestinal radiology (as well as other specialties in radiology) are disease-oriented, demonstrating and discussing all the radiographic manifestations of a specific disorder. Although this is an excellent approach for a large reference work, it is often of little value to the radiologist faced with the reality of daily film reading. The practicing radiologist is usually unaware of the underlying disease and is presented with a specific finding for which he or she must suggest a differential diagnosis and rational diagnostic approach. To address this problem, the gamut concept has been developed. Unfortunately, a book consisting only of gamuts is difficult and dull reading and still requires that a second textbook be consulted to aid in differentiating among the various diagnostic possibilities listed in the gamut. The "pattern" approach to gastrointestinal radiology presented here is an attempt to combine the best features of a list of gamuts and an extensive disease-oriented textbook. For each radiographic finding, an extensive gamut is presented, divided into subsections for convenient use. Textual material and a wealth of illustrations are then presented to aid the radiologist in arriving at a reasonable differential diagnosis.

I must stress that this book in no way intends to supplant the current excellent textbooks in gastrointestinal radiology. Rather, it is designed to complement these works by providing a handy reference for the practicing radiologist and resident faced with the daily challenge of interpreting gastrointestinal examinations.

Ronald L. Eisenberg, M.D.

ACKNOWLEDGMENTS

I want to offer special thanks to the following radiologists, who gave me free run of their extensive files and without whose case material this book could not have been compiled.

John R. Amberg, M.D.
Henry I. Goldberg, M.D.
Alexander R. Margulis, M.D.
Peter C. Meyers, M.D.
Hideyo Minagi, M.D.

The following colleagues have graciously permitted me to use radiographs from their unpublished cases.

Jose M. Alba, M.D.
Marvin S. Belasco, M.D.
Alan J. Davidson, M.D.
Michael Davis, M.D.
Herbert Y. Kressel, M.D.
Rajendra Kumar, M.D.
Marc S. Lapayowker, M.D.
Catherine V. Netchvolodoff, M.D.
Steven H. Ominsky, M.D.
Alphonse J. Palubinskas, M.D.

Sanford A. Rubin, M.D.
Melvin H. Schreiber, M.D.
McClure Wilson, M.D.
Justin J. Wolfson, M.D.

And, of course, I am grateful to the many physicians who have kindly allowed me to use their published material as illustrations in this book.

I would also like to express my thanks to Betty DiGrazia for the many hours she spent in the arduous task of typing and retyping the manuscript. I gratefully appreciate the efforts of James Kendrick of George Washington University, Howard Miller of M. D. Anderson Medical Center, and the Medical Communications Department at Louisiana State University School of Medicine in Shreveport for skillfully photographing the many illustrations. Thanks should also go to the radiology residents at LSU, who continuously had eagle eyes trained to find appropriate case material. Finally, I acknowledge the unceasing encouragement and support of the entire staff at J. B. Lippincott Company, who have made the immense technical problems of preparing a book as painless as possible.

CONTENTS

Part 1 ESOPHAGUS

1 Abnormalities of Esophageal Motility 3
2 Extrinsic Impressions on the Cervical
   Esophagus 26
3 Extrinsic Impressions on the Thoracic
   Esophagus 30
4 Esophageal Ulceration 46
5 Esophageal Narrowing 70
6 Esophageal Filling Defects 97
7 Esophageal Diverticula 117
8 Esophageal Varices 123
9 Esophagorespiratory Fistulas 129
10 Double-Barrel Esophagus 137
11 Diffuse Finely Nodular Lesions of the
    Esophagus 143

Part 2 DIAPHRAGM

12 Elevation of the Diaphragm 151
13 Diaphragmatic Hernias 159

Part 3 STOMACH

14 Gastric Ulcers 179
15 Superficial Gastric Erosions 201
16 Narrowing of the Stomach (Linitis
    Plastica Pattern) 205

17 Thickening of Gastric Folds 223
18 Filling Defects in the Stomach 238
19 Filling Defects in the Gastric Remnant 271
20 Gastric Outlet Obstruction 281
21 Gastric Dilatation Without Outlet
    Obstruction 291
22 Intrinsic/Extrinsic Masses of the Fundus 296
23 Widening of the Retrogastric Space 309
24 Gas in the Wall of the Stomach 312
25 Simultaneous Involvement of the
    Gastric Antrum and Duodenal Bulb 315

Part 4 DUODENUM

26 Postbulbar Ulceration of the Duodenum 323
27 Thickening of Duodenal Folds 329
28 Widening of the Duodenal Sweep 340
29 Extrinsic Pressure on the Duodenum 357
30 Duodenal Filling Defects 362
31 Duodenal Narrowing/Obstruction 387
32 Duodenal Dilatation (Superior Mesenteric
    Artery Syndrome) 401

Part 5 SMALL BOWEL

Introduction to Diseases of the Small
    Bowel 409
33 Small Bowel Obstruction 411

34 Adynamic Ileus 430
35 Dilatation with Normal Folds 441
36 Dilatation with Thickened Mucosal Folds 452
37 Regular Thickening of Small Bowel Folds 456
38 Generalized, Irregular, Distorted Small Bowel Folds 467
39 Solitary Filling Defects in the Jejunum and Ileum 482
40 Multiple Filling Defects in the Small Bowel 495
41 Sandlike Lucencies 506
42 Thickened Small Bowel Folds with Concomitant Involvement of the Stomach 513
43 Separation of Small Bowel Loops 517
44 Small Bowel Diverticula and Pseudodiverticula 529

Part 6   ILEOCECAL VALVE AND CECUM

45 Abnormalities of the Ileocecal Valve 543
46 Filling Defects in the Cecum 554
47 Coned Cecum 572

Part 7   COLON

48 Ulcerative Lesions of the Colon 585
49 Narrowing of the Colon 622
50 Single Filling Defects in the Colon 662
51 Multiple Filling Defects in the Colon 692
52 Large Bowel Obstruction 722
53 Toxic Megacolon 741
54 Thumbprinting of the Colon 746

55 Double Tracking in the Sigmoid Colon 756
56 Enlargement of the Retrorectal Space 760

Part 8   BILIARY SYSTEM

57 Nonvisualization of the Gallbladder 773
58 Alterations in Gallbladder Size 779
59 Displacement or Deformity of the Gallbladder 783
60 Filling Defects in an Opacified Gallbladder 787
61 Filling Defects in the Bile Ducts 805
62 Bile Duct Narrowing/Obstruction 818
63 Cystic Dilatation of the Bile Ducts 838
64 Enlargement of the Papilla of Vater 847
65 Gas in the Biliary System (Pancreaticobiliary Reflux) 852
66 Gas in the Portal Veins 858

Part 9   MISCELLANEOUS

67 Bull's-Eye Lesions in the Gastrointestinal Tract 865
68 Nondiaphragmatic Hernias 871
69 Gas in the Bowel Wall (Pneumatosis Intestinalis) 881
70 Pneumoperitoneum 892
71 Extraluminal Gas in the Upper Quadrants 903
72 Fistulas Involving the Small or Large Bowel 919
73 Abdominal Calcifications 936

Index 1017

PART ONE

ESOPHAGUS

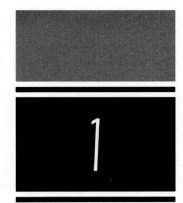

ABNORMALITIES OF ESOPHAGEAL MOTILITY

The esophagus is a muscular tube approximately 20 cm to 24 cm in length that begins at the level of the cricoid cartilage in the neck. The esophagus is lined predominantly by squamous epithelium, and its wall is composed of an outer longitudinal and an inner circular muscle layer. In the proximal one-third of the esophagus, there is mainly striated muscle; the distal two-thirds consist predominantly of smooth muscle. The point of demarcation between the striated and smooth muscle portions appears radiographically at about the level of the aortic knob.

There are two esophageal sphincters, areas that maintain a relatively high resting pressure compared with adjacent segments. The upper esophageal sphincter is about 1 cm to 3 cm in length and represents the zone of demarcation between the pharynx and esophagus. It is composed of the cricopharyngeus muscle proximally and intrinsic esophageal elements distally. The lower esophageal sphincter (1 cm to 4 cm in length) is located partially in both the thorax and the abdomen and straddles the diaphragmatic hiatus. It separates the positive intra-abdominal pressure from the esophagus, where pressure is negative with respect to the atmosphere.

The act of swallowing is a complex mechanism, mediated by several cranial nerves, that results in the well-ordered transport of a bolus from the mouth to the upper esophageal sphincter. Swallowing consists of posterior movement of the tongue, elevation of the soft palate with resultant closure of the nasopharynx, and closure of the respiratory pas-sage by contraction and elevation of the larynx, which abuts the epiglottis. Relaxation of the cricopharyngeus muscle (upper esophageal sphincter) normally occurs at the precise moment at which the bolus reaches the uppermost part of the esophagus.

There are three phases of normal esophageal peristaltic activity. Primary peristalsis is the major stripping wave that is initiated by the act of swallowing and that propels ingested material through the entire length of the esophagus into the stomach. The primary wave begins with an inhibitory impulse that passes down the esophagus and relaxes the lower esophageal sphincter before the bolus reaches it.

Secondary esophageal peristalsis consists of stripping waves similar to primary peristalsis but elicited by different stimuli. Rather than beginning with swallowing, as in primary peristalsis, the secondary peristaltic wave occurs in response to distention or irritation anywhere along the esophagus. It begins at the level of the focus of stimulation and propels esophageal contents distally. In effect, secondary peristalsis is a mechanism for ridding the esophagus of refluxed gastric contents or material left from a previous swallow.

The primary and secondary esophageal contraction waves depend on a complex control mechanism composed of a succession of reflex arcs, each of which must function without fault. Sensory receptors located in the mucosal, submucosal, and muscular layers of the esophagus send afferent impulses to the vagal nuclei in the medulla, from which motor impulses pass downward to the myenteric plexuses of Auerbach in the esophageal wall. Integration of segmental motility into an orderly peristaltic contraction is mediated by synaptic connections between the vagal fibers and ganglion cells in the myenteric plexus.

Tertiary contractions (nonperistaltic) are uncoordinated, nonpropulsive, segmental esophageal contractions, the function of which is unknown. Whether tertiary contractions are abnormal is a controversial question. They can be found in many asymptomatic persons and increase in incidence in patients of advanced age.

The three phases of esophageal peristalsis can be well demonstrated on barium swallow. During primary peristalsis, the upper end of the barium column assumes an inverted V-shaped configuration (Fig. 1-1). As the peristaltic wave progresses, the inverted V-shaped tail moves down the esophagus. If the barium column reaches the distal esophagus prior to relaxation of the lower esophageal sphincter, there can be a momentary delay before it enters the stomach. This results in the lower part of the barium column (adjacent to the closed sphincter) assuming a V-shaped configuration, with the proximal margin of the lower esophageal sphincter beginning at the point of the V (Fig. 1-2).

Secondary peristalsis has the same radiographic appearance as a primary contraction wave except that it arises in the body of the esophagus in response to local distention or irritation. The nonpropulsive tertiary waves are seen as annular or segmental contractions that simultaneously displace barium both orally and aborally from the site of contraction, resulting in a to-and-fro motion of the barium.

Disorders of esophageal motility can be conveniently divided according to the component of the process that is involved. There can be abnormalities of (1) striated muscle and the upper esophageal sphincter, (2) smooth muscle or innervation of the body of the esophagus, or (3) the lower esophageal sphincter.

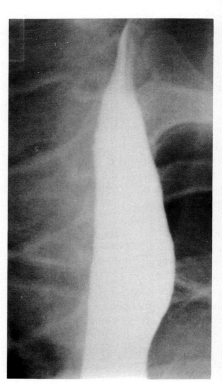

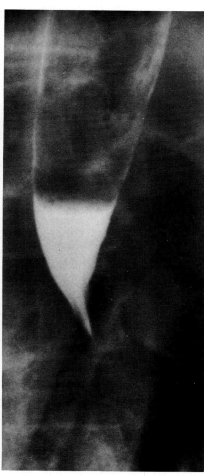

Fig. 1-1. Primary peristalsis. The upper end of the barium column has an inverted V-shaped configuration.

Fig. 1-2. Closed lower esophageal sphincter causing the V-shaped configuration of the lower part of the barium column.

1-1   1-2

ABNORMALITIES OF STRIATED MUSCLE AND THE UPPER ESOPHAGEAL SPHINCTER (CRICOPHARYNGEAL ACHALASIA)

Disease Entities

Normal variant
Minor, nonspecific neuromuscular dysfunction
Total laryngectomy (pseudodefect)
Radiation therapy
Primary muscle disorders
    Myasthenia gravis
    Myotonic dystrophy
    Polymyositis
    Dermatomyositis
    Amyotrophic lateral sclerosis
    Steroid myopathy
    Thyrotoxic myopathy
    Oculopharyngeal myopathy
Primary neural disorders
    Peripheral or cranial nerve palsy
    Cerebrovascular disease affecting the brain stem
    High unilateral cervical vagotomy
    Bulbar poliomyelitis
    Syringomyelia
    Huntington's chorea
    Familial dysautonomia (Riley-Day syndrome)
    Multiple sclerosis
    Diphtheria
    Tetanus

Cricopharyngeal achalasia is the failure of pharyngeal peristalsis to coordinate with relaxation of the upper esophageal sphincter. This condition, which occurs without mechanical obstruction or esophageal stenosis, is the result of any lesion that interferes with the complex neuromuscular activity in this region. When relaxation of the cricopharyngeus is incomplete, the characteristic radiographic appearance is that of a hemispherical or horizontal, shelflike posterior protrusion into the barium-filled pharyngoesophageal junction at approximately the C5-6 level (Fig. 1-3). Although the presence of this cricopharyngeus impression indicates the existence of some physiologic abnormality, lesser degrees of it may not be associated with clinical symptoms. More significant neuromuscular abnormalities can result in dysphagia by acting as obstructions to the passage of the bolus (Fig. 1-4). In severe disease, swallowing can result in an overflow of ingested material into the larynx and trachea and pulmonary complications of aspiration. This severe incoordination of pharyngeal peristalsis and upper esophageal sphincter function can appear on cinefluoroscopy as dilatation and atony of the pyriform sinuses, retention of barium in the valleculae, aspiration into the trachea, regurgitation into the nasopharynx, and apparent obstruction at the level of the cricopharyngeus muscle. When cricopharyngeal achalasia is accompanied by severe dysphagia, cricopharyngeal myotomy can relieve the obstruction created by the nonrelaxing cricopharyngeus muscle.

Cricopharyngeal achalasia has been suggested as an important factor in the development of posterior pharyngeal (Zenker's) diverticula. If relaxation of the cricopharyngeus is inadequate or if the upper esophageal sphincter closes too soon, the elevated intraluminal pressure created by an oncoming peristaltic wave may be responsible for mucosal protrusion through the anatomic weak spot between the oblique and transverse fibers of the cricopharyngeus (Killian's dehiscence), resulting in a Zenker's diverticulum.

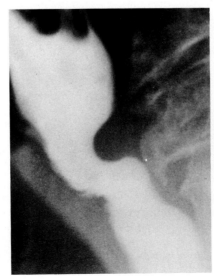 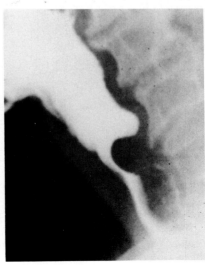

Fig. 1-3. Cricopharyngeal achalasia. A moderate posterior impression is visible on the esophagus of this 60-year-old man who had a cerebrovascular accident.

Fig. 1-4. Cricopharyngeal achalasia. There is a severe posterior impression on the esophagus.

1-3   1-4

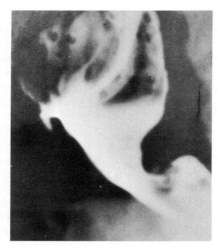

Fig. 1-5. Posterior cricopharyngeal impression following total laryngectomy for carcinoma.

TOTAL LARYNGECTOMY (PSEUDODEFECT)

An appearance identical to the posterior cricopharyngeal impression can be demonstrated in patients who have had a total laryngectomy for carcinoma (Fig. 1-5). The normal appearance of the neopharynx after total laryngectomy is a simple tube with smoothly conical borders. All laryngeal structures are absent, and the anatomic landmarks of the hypopharynx, including the pyriform sinuses and aryepiglottic folds, are removed. Only residual fibers of the cricopharyngeus muscle remain to indent the posterolateral surface of the neopharynx. Although total laryngectomy involves removal of the cricoid cartilage, which acts as the anterior fixation point of the cricopharyngeal muscle and should therefore theoretically lead to a patulous cricopharyngeus, the muscle bundles tend to bunch together when a nerve impulse reaches them, resulting in

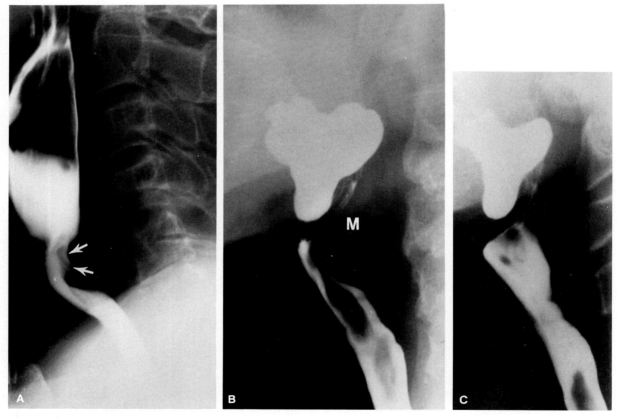

Fig. 1-6. Two patients with post-laryngectomy dysphagia. **(A)** On an examination 1 year after laryngectomy, a 2.8-cm mass indents the posterior neopharynx and causes some mucosal irregularity **(arrows)**. Biopsy showed recurrent tumor. **(B)** In another patient 3 months after laryngectomy, a 4-cm mass **(M)** indents the posterior neopharynx and narrows the lumen. **(C)** A second radiograph from the same study shows marked change in appearance indicating that the mass is muscular tissue, not a tumor. (Balfe DM, Koehler RE, Setzen M et al: Barium examination of the esophagus after total laryngectomy. Radiology 143:501–508, 1982)

a characteristic posterior impression. The radiologist must avoid the error of misdiagnosis of recurrent neoplasm in patients who have undergone total laryngectomy and demonstrate a prominent cricopharyngeal muscle defect (Fig. 1-6). This differential can usually be resolved at fluoroscopy because the benign cricopharyngeus impression tends to change in shape with swallowing. Clinically, patients with prominent posterior cricopharyngeal impressions following laryngectomy generally complain of dysphagia on the way down and dysphonia with esophageal speech on the way up. Because of the substantial incidence of cricopharyngeal problems postoperatively, some surgeons routinely perform a posterior cricopharyngeal myotomy at the time of laryngectomy.

RADIATION THERAPY

Cricopharyngeal incoordination and other functional abnormalities of the pharynx are commonly found in patients who have dysphagia after radiotherapy for malignancies of the pharynx. The combination of paresis of the pharyngeal constrictor muscles and delayed cricopharyngeal relaxation results in an inability to clear the pharynx. This results in hypopharyngeal retention of contrast material with reflux into the vestibule. Aspiration into the tracheobronchial tree is especially likely to occur because these patients seem to have a disturbed sensitivity in the vestibule and superior laryngeal aperture, which interferes with the reflex closure of the airways.

PRIMARY MUSCLE DISORDERS

Primary striated muscle disease can cause failure to develop a good pharyngeal peristaltic wave. Difficulty in swallowing in patients with myasthenia gravis is due to muscular fatigability resulting from the failure of neural transmission between the motor end-plate and muscle fibers. On the initial swallow of barium, peristalsis may appear normal. During repeated swallows, however, peristalsis in the upper esophagus becomes feeble or disappears completely. In patients with myasthenia gravis, peristalsis in the upper esophagus can be demonstrated to improve after the administration of neostigmine or Tensilon (edrophonium).

Myotonic dystrophy is an uncommon hereditary disease (autosomal dominant) in which an anatomic abnormality of the motor end-plate in striated muscle leads to atrophy and inability of the contracted muscle to relax (myotonia). Associated findings include swan neck, frontal baldness in men, testicular atrophy, cataracts, and a characteristic facial expression (myopathic facies). In addition to severely disturbed pharyngeal peristalsis, patients with myotonic dystrophy have reduced or absent resting pressure of the cricopharyngeus muscle. Because a major function of the upper esophageal sphincter is to prevent esophageal contents from refluxing into the pharynx, the diminished resting tone in patients with myotonic dystrophy permits easy regurgitation from the esophagus into the pharynx and leads to a high incidence of aspiration. Reflux across the cricopharyngeus results in the characteristic radiographic pattern of a continuous column of barium extending from the hypopharynx into the cervical esophagus (Fig. 1-7) even during the resting phase, when the patient is not swallowing.

Polymyositis and dermatomyositis are inflammatory degenerative diseases of striated muscle. Weakness and incoordination of the voluntary muscles of the soft palate, pharynx, and upper esophagus in patients with these conditions lead to dysphagia, regurgitation, and a propensity to develop aspiration pneumonia. Similarly, loss of motor neuron function in patients with amyotrophic lateral sclerosis (Lou Gehrig's disease) results in ineffective pharyngeal peristalsis. Other causes of the inability to develop a good pharyngeal wave and clear the barium meal from the pharynx include (1) myopathies secondary to steroids and abnormal thyroid function and (2) oculopharyngeal myopathy,

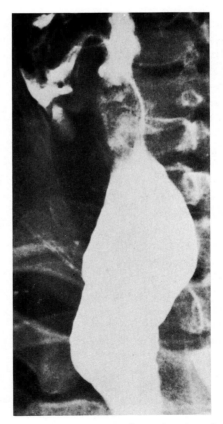

Fig. 1-7. Myotonic dystrophy. A continuous column of barium extends from the hypopharynx into the cervical esophagus, caused by reflux across the level of the cricopharyngeus muscle. (Seaman WB: Functional disorders of the pharyngoesophageal junction. Radiol Clin North Am 7:113–119, 1969)

an extremely rare disease (occurring as a dominant trait especially in families of French-Canadian ancestry) that presents relatively late in life with ptosis and dysphagia.

PRIMARY NEURAL DISORDERS

Diseases of the central and peripheral nervous systems can lead to profound motor incoordination of the pharynx and upper esophageal sphincter. This can be due to peripheral or central cranial nerve palsy or to cerebrovascular occlusive disease affecting the brain stem. A high unilateral cervical vagotomy during extensive head and neck surgery for resection of neoplastic disease can also result in incoordination of upper esophageal motility and sphincter function. Other neurologic causes include bulbar poliomyelitis, syringomyelia, Huntington's chorea, familial dysautonomia (Riley-Day syndrome), multiple sclerosis, diphtheria, and tetanus.

ABNORMALITIES OF SMOOTH MUSCLE AND INNERVATION OF THE BODY OF THE ESOPHAGUS

Disease Entities

Scleroderma
Other connective tissue disorders
    Systemic lupus erythematosus
    Rheumatoid arthritis
    Polymyositis
    Dermatomyositis
Disorders of myenteric plexus
    Achalasia
    Chagas' disease
    Metastases
Esophagitis
    Corrosive
    Reflux
    Infectious
    Radiation-induced
Alcoholic neuropathy
Diabetic neuropathy
Presbyesophagus
Anticholinergic medication
Myxedema
Amyloidosis
Muscular dystrophy

SCLERODERMA

Atony of the esophagus with failure of peristaltic activity can result from atrophy or cellular disruption of esophageal smooth muscle. In this disorder, the muscular layer of the esophagus is unable to respond to motor impulses transmitted by the vagus nerve.

This mechanism of disordered esophageal mo-

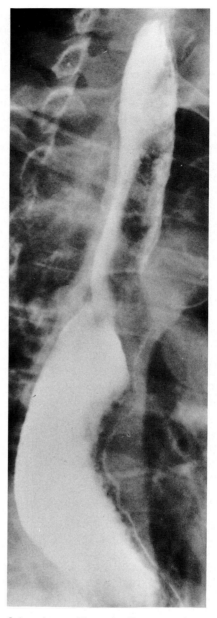

Fig. 1-8. *Scleroderma. There is dilatation of the esophagus with failure of peristaltic activity.*

tility is best illustrated by scleroderma (Fig. 1-8). The disease frequently (in up to 80% of cases) involves the esophagus, sometimes even before the characteristic skin changes become evident. In scleroderma, there is degeneration and atrophy of smooth muscle in the lower half to two-thirds of the esophagus with subsequent replacement of esophageal musculature by fibrosis. Neural elements, including ganglion cells, are normal.

The patient with diminished esophageal peristalsis due to scleroderma is often asymptomatic. Because the lower esophageal sphincter tone is severely decreased, eating or drinking in the sitting or erect position allows the bolus to be squirted well down the esophagus by the pharyngeal constrictors (striated muscle) and carried by gravity into the stomach. The incompetence of the lower esophageal sphincter, however, permits reflux of acid-pepsin gastric secretions into the distal esophagus. In about 40% of patients, this reflux leads to peptic esophagitis and stricture formation, resulting in heartburn and severe dysphagia.

Because the upper third of the esophagus is composed primarily of striated muscle infrequently affected by scleroderma, a barium swallow demonstrates a normal stripping wave that clears the upper esophagus but stops at about the level of the aortic arch. In early stages of scleroderma, some primary peristaltic activity and uncoordinated tertiary contractions can be observed in the lower two-thirds of the esophagus. However, these contractions are weak and infrequent and tend to disappear as the disease progresses. With the patient in the recumbent position, barium will remain for a long time in the dilated, atonic esophagus (Fig. 1-9). Multiple radiographs obtained several minutes apart can be effectively superimposed on each other. In contrast to the case in achalasia, however, when the patient with scleroderma is placed in the upright position, barium flows rapidly through the widely patent region of the lower esophageal sphincter (Fig. 1-10).

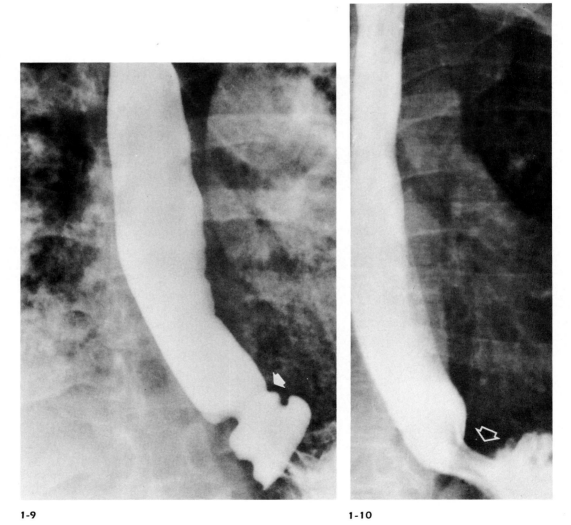

1-9   1-10

Fig. 1-9. Scleroderma. There is dilatation of the esophagus with almost no peristalsis to the level of the moderate hiatal hernia **(arrow)**. Severe pulmonary interstitial changes of scleroderma may be seen bilaterally in the lower lobes.

Fig. 1-10. Scleroderma. The esophagus is dilated and atonic, and the esophagogastric junction is patulous **(arrow)**.

OTHER CONNECTIVE TISSUE DISORDERS

A similar pattern of esophageal atony can be demonstrated in patients with other connective tissue diseases, such as systemic lupus erythematosus (Fig. 1-11), rheumatoid arthritis, polymyositis, or dermatomyositis (in which the proximal, striated muscle esophageal segment is also involved). Regardless of the underlying disease, almost all of these patients with esophageal dysfunction have Raynaud's phenomenon, suggesting that a vasospastic neurogenic abnormality may be responsible for the esophageal aperistalsis.

DISORDERS OF THE MYENTERIC PLEXUS

Failure of peristalsis and a markedly dilated esophagus are typical findings in patients with achalasia (Fig. 1-12). However, this appearance should cause no diagnostic difficulty, since patients with achalasia characteristically have a narrowed distal esophagus because of failure of relaxation of the lower esophageal sphincter (Fig. 1-13), in contrast to patients with scleroderma and other connective tissue disorders, who have a widely patent distal esophagus that frequently permits free gastroesophageal reflux. Destruction of ganglion cells in the myenteric plexus can lead to esophageal aperistalsis simulating achalasia. This can be caused by an inflammatory process, such as Chagas' disease, or by the invasion of tumor cells from a metastatic malignancy.

ESOPHAGITIS

In patients with esophagitis, whether secondary to corrosive agents, reflux, infection, or radiation injury, the earliest and most frequent radiographic abnormality is disordered esophageal motility (Fig. 1-14). Initially, there is failure of primary peristalsis to progress to the stomach, with interruption of the stripping wave in the region of the esophageal inflammation. Repetitive, nonperistaltic tertiary contractions often occur distal to the point of disruption of the primary wave. If the esophagitis is severe, complete aperistalsis can result.

ALCOHOLIC AND DIABETIC NEUROPATHIES

An esophageal motor abnormality can often be demonstrated in chronic alcoholics. It is characterized by selective deterioration of esophageal peristalsis, most pronounced in the distal portion, with preservation of sphincter function. The precise mechanism for this disordered motility, though unclear, probably represents a combination of alcoholic myopathy and neuropathy.

In diabetics, especially those with neuropathy of long duration, there is a marked diminution of amplitude of pharyngeal and peristaltic contractions as well as a decreased percentage of swallows followed by progressive peristalsis in the body of the esophagus. This results in a substantial delay in esophageal emptying when the patient is recumbent.

OTHER CAUSES

Presbyesophagus is an esophageal motor dysfunction associated with aging (Fig. 1-15). It is characterized by an inability to initiate and propagate primary peristalsis and by an increase in nonpropulsive tertiary contractions. Concomitant failure of the lower esophageal sphincter to relax produces moderate and even pronounced dilatation of the esophagus.

Anticholinergic agents, such as atropine and Pro-Banthine (propantheline), can cause aperistalsis and dilatation of the esophagus, which mimic the esophageal dysfunction seen in patients with scleroderma. Myxedema can produce a similar pattern. Symptoms of dysphagia and the radiographic appearance of a dilated esophagus with decreased

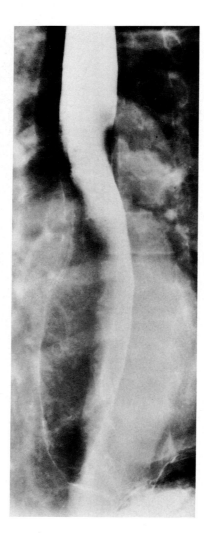

Fig. 1-11. *Systemic lupus erythematosus. Esophageal dilatation and atony simulate scleroderma.*

peristalsis are rarely the result of a massive deposition of amyloid in the muscular layers of the esophagus (Fig. 1-16) or a complication of muscular dystrophy.

FAILURE OF RELAXATION OF THE LOWER ESOPHAGEAL SPHINCTER (ACHALASIA PATTERN)

Disease Entities

Achalasia
Chagas' disease
Central and peripheral neuropathy
   Cerebrovascular accident
   Postvagotomy syndrome
   Diabetes mellitus

Chronic idiopathic intestinal pseudo-
   obstruction
Amyloidosis
Malignant lesions
   Destruction of myenteric plexus
   Metastases to midbrain vagal nuclei
   Direct involvement of vagus nerve
Stricture secondary to reflux esophagitis

ACHALASIA

Achalasia is a functional obstruction of the distal esophagus with proximal dilatation caused by incomplete relaxation of the lower esophageal sphincter combined with failure of normal peristalsis in the smooth muscle portion of the esophagus (Fig. 1-17). Failure of sphincter relaxation can be defined radiographically as barium retention above the lower esophageal sphincter for longer than 2.5

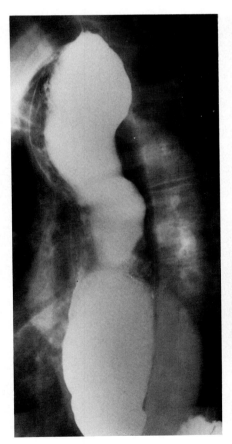
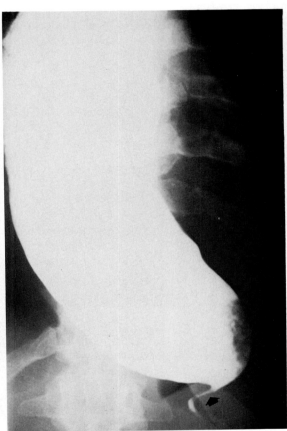
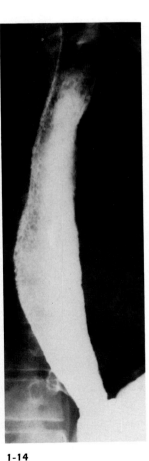

1-12   1-13   1-14

Fig. 1-12. Achalasia. There is esophageal dilatation and decreased peristalsis.

Fig. 1-13. Achalasia. Severe esophageal dilatation and aperistalsis are apparent. Note the narrowed distal esophagus **(arrow)**, which contrasts with the patulous esophagogastric junction in scleroderma.

Fig. 1-14. Candidiasis. Aperistalsis and esophageal dilatation are associated with diffuse ulceration.

sec after swallowing. Although the precise patho-genesis of achalasia is not known, the most accepted explanation is a defect in the cholinergic innerva-tion of the esophagus related to a paucity or absence of ganglion cells in the myenteric plexuses (Auer-bach) of the distal esophageal wall. This theory is supported by the demonstration in patients with achalasia of a denervation hypersensitivity response of the body of the esophagus to Mecholyl, a syn-thetic acetylcholine.

In addition to classic achalasia, generalized or localized interruption of the reflex arc controlling normal esophageal motility can also cause failure of relaxation of the lower esophageal sphincter. Thus, diseases of the medullary nuclei, an abnormality of the vagus nerve, or the absence or destruction of myenteric ganglion cells from any cause can pro-duce a similar radiographic pattern.

Most cases of classic achalasia occur in persons between the ages of 20 and 40. Dysphagia is pro-duced by ingestion of either solids or liquids and becomes worse during periods of emotional stress or when the patient is trying to eat rapidly. Regurgi-tation of retained material is common (it is often provoked by changes in position or by physical ex-ercise) and can result in aspiration and frequent

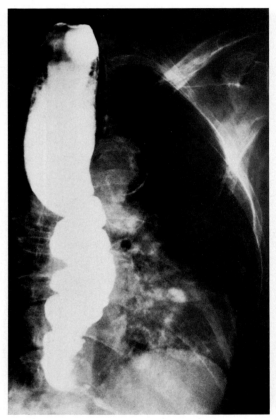 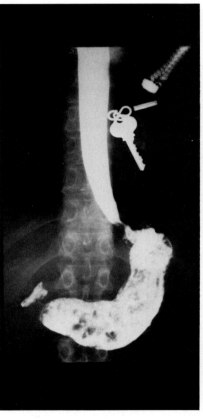 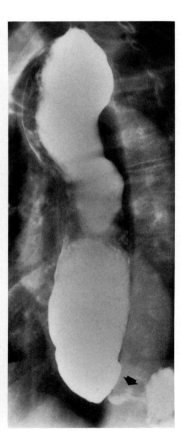

1-15   1-16   1-17

Fig. 1-15. Presbyesophagus. Esophageal dilatation is prominent. Tertiary contractions in-volve the lower esophagus. When there were no tertiary contractions, esophageal dilatation was relatively uniform. (Zboralske FF, Dodds WJ: Roentgenographic diagnosis of primary disorders of esophageal motility. Radiol Clin North Am 7:147–162, 1969)

Fig. 1-16. Amyloidosis. Dilatation and weak motor activity of the esophagus are associated with a considerable amount of material retained in the stomach. (Legge DA, Carlson HC, Wollaeger EE: Roentgenologic appearance of systemic amyloidosis involving gastrointestinal tract. AJR 110:406–412, 1970. Copyright 1970. Reproduced with permission)

Fig. 1-17. Achalasia. There is failure of relaxation of the region of the distal esophageal sphincter **(arrow)** with severe proximal dilatation.

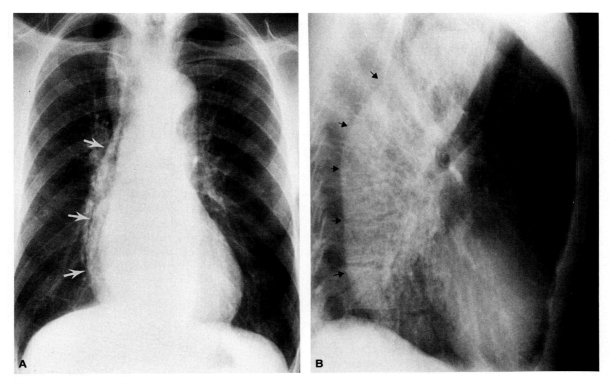

Fig. 1-18. Achalasia. **(A)** Frontal chest radiograph demonstrates the margin of the dilated, tortuous esophagus **(arrows)** parallel to the right border of the heart. **(B)** A lateral chest film shows a mixture of fluid and air density within the dilated esophagus **(arrows)**.

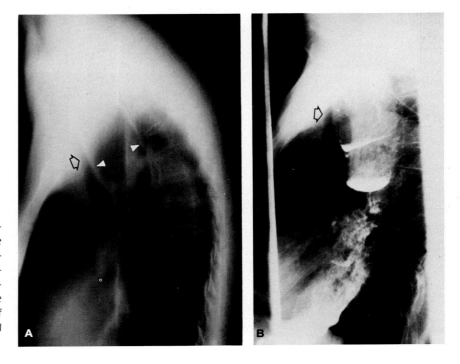

Fig. 1-19. Achalasia. **(A)** Lateral tomogram and **(B)** barium swallow show the trachea **(black arrow)** displaced and compressed by the dilated and tortuous esophagus **(white arrows)**. (Dominguez F, Hernandez–Ranz F, Boixeda D et al: Acute upper-airway obstruction in achalasia of the esophagus. Am J Gastroenterol 82:362–364, 1987)

attacks of pneumonia or, in combination with a reduction in food intake, can lead to significant
weight loss and nutritional deficiencies.

Radiographic Findings

Plain chest radiographs are frequently sufficient for
diagnosis of the achalasia pattern of failure of relaxation of the lower esophageal sphincter. Large
amounts of retained food and fluid can be seen in
the esophagus. Dilatation and tortuosity of the
esophagus can present as a widened mediastinum,
often with an air-fluid level, primarily on the right
side adjacent to the cardiac shadow (Fig. 1-18). Aspiration of material retained in and regurgitated from
the dilated esophagus frequently leads to chronic
interstitial pulmonary disease or intermittent epi-

sodes of acute pneumonia. A rare complication is
severe acute respiratory distress, caused by progressive distention of the esophagus with forward displacement, angulation over the sternum, and posterior compression of the trachea at the level of the
thoracic outlet (Fig. 1-19). The air bubble of the
gastric fundus on upright films is small or totally
absent.

After the ingestion of barium, the esophagus
usually demonstrates weak, nonpropulsive, dys-
rhythmic peristaltic waves (ripple like activity) that
are ineffective in propelling the bolus into the stomach. This disordered esophageal motility is not secondary to distal obstruction related to failure of relaxation of the lower esophageal sphincter; it can
antedate the radiographic appearance of distal narrowing and persists even after the narrowing has
been successfully overcome by surgery or balloon

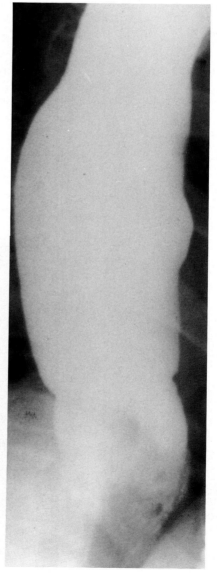

Fig. 1-20. Achalasia. Esophageal dilatation with multiple tertiary
contractions is apparent.

Fig. 1-21. Achalasia. There is marked esophageal dilatation and
elongation.

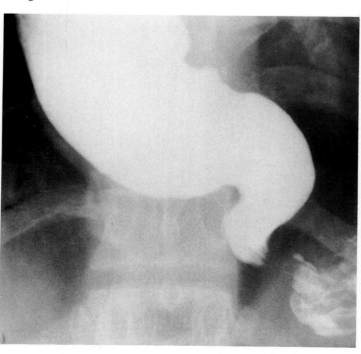

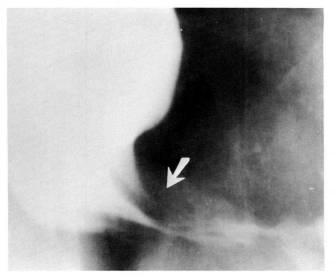

1-22

Fig. 1-22. Achalasia. Note the "rat-tail" narrowing of the distal esophageal segment **(arrow)**.

Fig. 1-23. Achalasia. There is characteristic narrowing of the distal esophageal segment ("beak" sign) **(arrow)**.

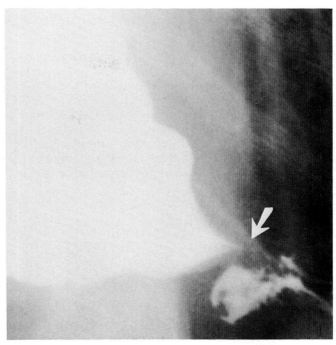

1-23

dilatation. In some cases, multiple tertiary contractions move the bolus up and down the esophagus in an uncoordinated fashion (hyperactive achalasia) (Fig. 1-20). As the disease progresses, marked esophageal distention, elongation, and tortuosity develop (Fig. 1-21).

The hallmark of the achalasia pattern is a gradually tapered, smooth, conical narrowing of the distal esophageal segment that extends some 1 cm to 3 cm in length ("rat-tail" or "beak" appearance) (Figs. 1-22, 1-23). Sequential radiographs, especially when the patient is in the erect position, demonstrate small spurts of barium entering the stomach through the narrowed distal segment (Fig. 1-24).

It is essential that the patient suspected of having achalasia be examined in the recumbent position. If the patient is in the erect position, gravity can simulate the effect of peristalsis and hide subtle abnormalities. The upright position is also necessary for the barium column to be high enough to provide adequate hydrostatic pressure to force even small amounts of contrast into the stomach. In patients with achalasia, complete emptying of the esophagus does not occur even in the erect position, a differential point from scleroderma, in which emptying is usually normal when the patient is upright.

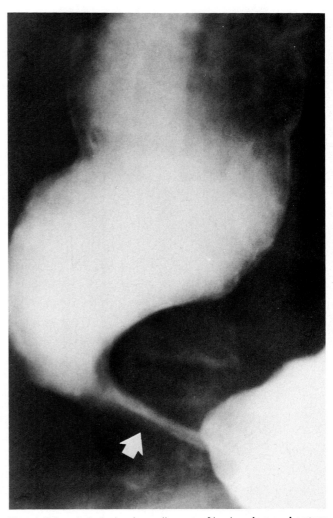

Fig. 1-24. Achalasia. A small spurt of barium **(arrow)** enters the stomach through the narrowed distal segment (jet effect).

CHAGAS' DISEASE

An achalasia pattern is often observed in patients with Chagas' disease, in which destruction of the myenteric plexuses is due to infection by the protozoan *Trypanosoma cruzi* (Fig. 1-25). Trypanosomiasis develops from the bite of an infected reduviid bug and the resultant contamination of the punctured skin by the insect's feces. These blood-sucking insects usually acquire the trypanosomes by feeding on the armadillo, the chief host for the organism. In addition to changes in the esophagus, Chagas' dis-

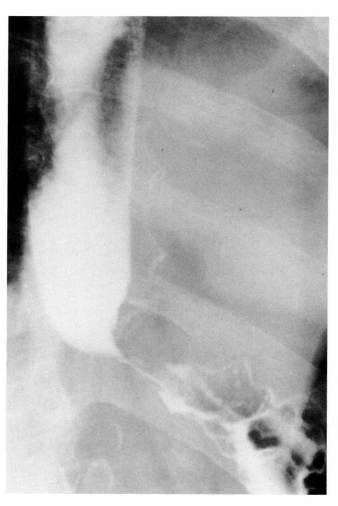

Fig. 1-26. Achalasia pattern (esophageal dilatation with distal narrowing) caused by the proximal extension of carcinoma of the fundus of the stomach.

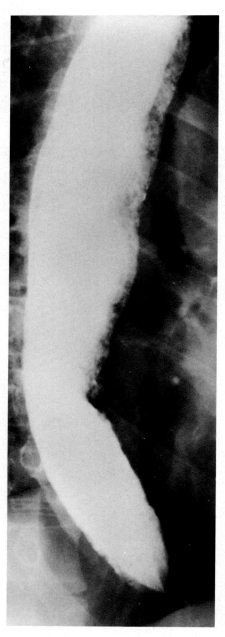

Fig. 1-25. Chagas' disease. There is esophageal dilatation and aperistalsis with a large amount of residual food.

ease can also result in megacolon with chronic constipation, dilatation of the ureters, acute or chronic myocarditis, and infestation of numerous body organs. The effects of Chagas' disease on the esophagus are most likely due to a neurotoxin that attacks and destroys ganglion cells in the myenteric plexuses of the affected organ.

CENTRAL AND PERIPHERAL NEUROPATHY

Central and peripheral neuropathy can result in the achalasia pattern. Brain stem abnormalities due to cerebrovascular accidents or infiltrating processes, such as amyloidosis or malignant lesions, can disrupt the reflex arc and result in failure of relaxation of the lower esophageal sphincter. A similar appearance can reflect a relatively infrequent postoperative complication of bilateral vagotomy. Dysphagia in patients who show this pattern typically occurs with the first ingestion of solid foods on the

7th to 14th postoperative day; the clinical symptoms and radiographic findings usually disappear spontaneously and completely within 2 months. An achalasia pattern can also occur in patients with diabetes, probably because of an arteritis of the vaso vasorum that interferes with the blood supply to the myenteric plexus. In patients with chronic idiopathic intestinal pseudo-obstruction, a radiographic appearance resembling achalasia has been reported as one of the manifestations of widespread congenital or acquired degeneration of innervation of the entire gut.

MALIGNANT LESIONS

Malignant lesions can produce an achalasia pattern by several mechanisms. Metastases to the midbrain or vagal nuclei, or direct extension of tumor to involve the vagus nerve, can result in failure of relaxation of the lower esophageal sphincter. A similar pattern can be produced by a carcinoma of the distal esophagus or a malignant lesion in the gastric cardia that invades the esophagus and destroys ganglion cells in the myenteric plexus (Fig. 1-26). Carcinoma-induced achalasia has also been reported in patients with gastrointestinal metastases (Fig. 1-27), with nongastrointestinal malignancies (hepatoma and carcinoma of the lung [Fig. 1-28], pancreas, and prostate), and with lymphoma of the distal esophagus. Successful removal of the tumor by surgery or

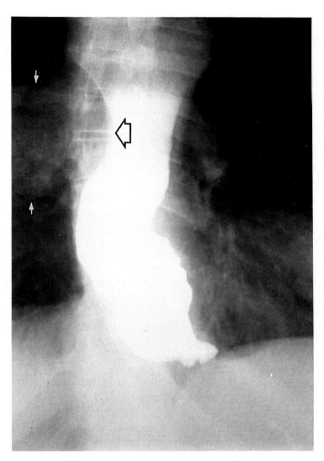

Fig. 1-28. *Secondary achalasia due to bronchogenic carcinoma. Note the large right hilar mass indenting the wall of the midesophagus* **(arrows)**. *(Feczko PJ, Halpert RD: Achalasia secondary to nongastrointestinal malignancies. Gastrointest Radiol 10:273–276, 1985)*

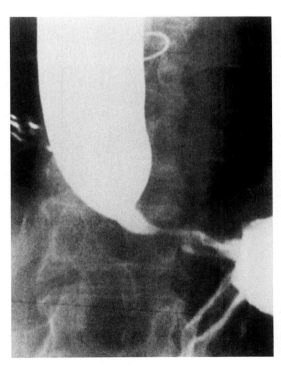

Fig. 1-27. *Secondary achalasia due to metastatic colon carcinoma. No peristalsis was present at fluoroscopic examination. (Agha FP: Secondary neoplasms of the esophagus. Gastrointest Radiol 12:187–193, 1987)*

irradiation (as in the case of lymphoma) can result in restoration of normal esophageal function.

ESOPHAGITIS

Stricture formation secondary to reflux esophagitis can simulate the narrowed distal esophagus of the achalasia pattern. However, patients with this condition usually have a demonstrable hiatal hernia and a long history of heartburn and regurgitation, facilitating the diagnosis.

DIFFERENTIATION BETWEEN BENIGN AND MALIGNANT CAUSES

Clinical and Radiographic Findings

The major problem in differential diagnosis is to distinguish between nonmalignant causes of the achalasia pattern and carcinoma of the distal esophagus or gastric cardia. This is made especially difficult because of the occurrence of esophageal carcinoma in about 5% to 10% of patients with long-standing achalasia. These squamous cell tumors usually develop in the middle third of the esophagus and are presumed to be induced by chronic irritation of the mucosa caused by constant stasis and the retention of food and fluid secretions. Patients with achalasia who develop carcinoma are generally younger than the average patient with esophageal malignancy. The lesions are often masked by large amounts of residual food and fluid in the esophagus that can obscure the mucosal pattern and produce confusing filling defects on barium examination.

Both clinical and radiographic features can aid in differentiating between benign and malignant causes of the achalasia pattern. Patients with classic benign achalasia are usually less than 40 years old and have symptoms of more than 1 year's duration; those with carcinoma of the esophagus or gastric cardia are generally older (average age, >60), and a majority have had symptoms for less than 6 months. Melena is unusual in achalasia but common in patients with carcinoma. Radiographically, there is persistence of the normal mucosal pattern in achalasia, in contrast to mucosal destruction or nodularity in carcinoma. The zone of transition in achalasia tapers gradually, unlike the sharply defined, more rapid transition zone between normal esophagus and neoplasm. Severe neuromuscular disturbance of the entire esophagus is common in achalasia but is rarely seen in patients with carcinoma. The distal segment in achalasia has some degree of pliability, in contrast to rigidity and lack of changeability in carcinoma. The presence of a mass in the gas-filled fundus, a deformity of fundal contour, irregular streaming of barium as it flows from the esophagus into the stomach, or an increase in the soft-tissue thickness between the fundus and the diaphragm suggests malignancy.

Pharmacologic Tests

Three pharmacologic tests can aid in establishing the diagnosis of idiopathic achalasia and distinguishing it from the "pseudoachalasia" caused by tumor infiltration of the distal esophagus. In the amyl nitrite test, radiographs are obtained before and immediately after the patient takes several deep inhalations from a freshly broken ampule of the drug. The smooth muscle relaxant effect of amyl nitrite causes a measurable increase of 2 mm or more in sphincter diameter in patients with idiopathic achalasia (Fig. 1-29), but has no effect on the narrowed lower esophageal sphincter segment in patients with malignant involvement. Contraindications to this test include hypertension, hypotension, and cardiac disease. Because amyl nitrite is a nonspecific smooth muscle relaxant that causes relaxation of vascular as well as gastrointestinal smooth muscle, the patient must be watched carefully for evidence of impending hypotensive syncope.

In the Mecholyl test, 5 mg to 10 mg of the parasympathomimetic drug is injected subcutaneously. In patients with achalasia, denervation hypersensitivity (Cannon's law) results in a substantial increase in peristaltic activity, though the waves are still ineffective in propelling barium into the stomach. The Mecholyl test is associated with numerous complications, including nausea and vomiting and severe chest pain, and should never be performed in a patient with a history of significant heart disease.

The Seidlitz test, though not infallible, can be helpful in differentiating achalasia from a malignant neoplasm or stricture and has the advantage of being far less uncomfortable for the patient than the Mecholyl test. The ingestion of Seidlitz powder or a carbonated beverage causes the rapid release of carbon dioxide in the esophagus. The resultant

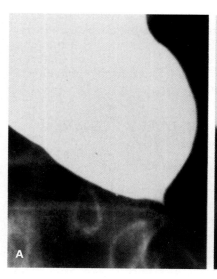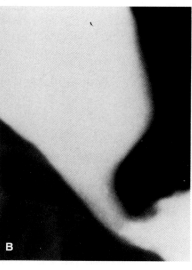

Fig. 1-29. Amyl nitrite test in idiopathic achalasia. **(A)** Initially, the lower esophageal sphincter segment has a bird-beaked configuration (maximum diameter 2 mm during transient sequences of barium flow). **(B)** After amyl nitrite, the lower esophageal sphincter diameter increased to 9 mm, and barium flowed freely into the stomach. (Dodds WJ, Stewart ET, Kishk SM et al: Radiologic amyl nitrite test for distinguishing pseudoachalasia from idiopathic achalasia. AJR 146:21–23, 1986. Copyright 1986. Reproduced with permission.)

acute increase in intraluminal esophageal pressure momentarily distends the contracted distal segment in the case of achalasia but has no effect on the fixed stenosis resulting from a malignant tumor or post-inflammatory fibrotic stricture.

TREATMENT OF ACHALASIA

Balloon dilatation or surgery can be used to treat achalasia. Balloon dilatation consists of the placement (under fluoroscopic control) of a pneumatic bougie so that its midportion is positioned at the narrowest level of the gastroesophageal junction (Fig. 1-30). With brisk, rapid dilatation, the radiopaque margin of the balloon is seen to expand the narrowed gastroesophageal segment to the desired degree of dilatation. This "bloodless myotomy" tears the circular muscle fibers of the lower esophageal sphincter in a graded manner, with the operator stopping just short of mucosal penetration. After the procedure, up to 75% of patients can eat a normal diet without dysphagia and have decreased retention of barium in the dilated esophagus.

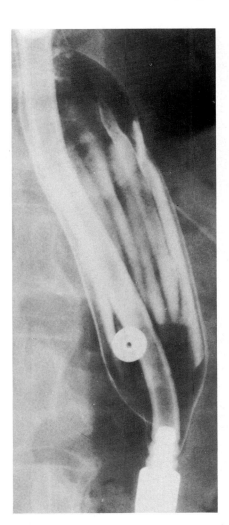

Fig. 1-30. *Pneumatic bougie for balloon dilatation of the esophagus in a patient with achalasia.*

The most serious, albeit uncommon, complication of balloon dilatation of the lower esophageal sphincter is esophageal rupture. It must be emphasized that esophageal perforation may not be radiographically detectable on a barium swallow obtained immediately after dilatation. Persistent or increasing symptoms in a patient who has undergone this procedure should suggest the possibility of delayed esophageal perforation and the need for a repeat radiographic evaluation.

Surgical therapy of achalasia (Heller myotomy) is designed to disrupt the lower esophageal sphincter from the outside of the esophagus. The operation involves incising the circular muscle fibers down to the mucosa and allowing the mucosa to protrude through. Heller myotomy results in a good clinical and radiographic remission in about 80% of cases. Unfortunately, disruption of the lower esophageal sphincter leads to a substantial incidence of gastroesophageal reflux, which can cause esophagitis and stricture.

TERTIARY CONTRACTIONS

Disease Entities

> Presbyesophagus
> Diffuse esophageal spasm
> Esophageal inflammation
>> Reflux esophagitis
>> Ingestion of corrosive agents
>> Infectious esophagitis (*e.g.,* candidiasis)
>> Radiation injury
> Nutcracker esophagus
> Hyperactive achalasia
> Neuromuscular disorders (*e.g.,* diabetes mellitus)
> Obstruction of the cardia
>> Malignant lesion
>> Distal esophageal stricture
>> Benign lesion
>> Postsurgical repair of hiatal hernia

Tertiary contractions are multiple, irregular, ring-like contractions that occur in the lower two-thirds of the esophagus. These nonpropulsive contractions appear and disappear rapidly, following each other from top to bottom with such speed that they appear to occur simultaneously. This phenomenon appears radiographically as asymmetric indentations of unequal width and depth along the esophagus, with pointed, rounded, or truncated projections between them (Fig. 1-31).

PRESBYESOPHAGUS

Nonpropulsive tertiary contractions are most commonly seen in patients with presbyesophagus, an esophageal motility disturbance associated with aging (Fig. 1-32). The cause of the disordered motor activity is probably interruption of the reflex arc, which in some cases may be the result of a minor cerebrovascular accident affecting the central nuclei. Most patients with presbyesophagus are asymptomatic; occasionally, a patient experiences moderate dysphagia when eating solid food. The radiographic appearance varies from occasional, mild, nonpropulsive contractions to frequent, strong, uncoordinated ones. Concomitant failure of relaxation of the lower esophageal sphincter can produce moderate dilatation of the esophagus.

DIFFUSE ESOPHAGEAL SPASM

Diffuse esophageal spasm is a controversial entity with a classic clinical triad of massive uncoordinated esophageal contractions, chest pain, and increased intraluminal pressure. Most patients, how-

ever, do not manifest all three components. Chest pain is characteristically intermittent and is usually substernal and moderate, though it can be colicky or mimic angina. Symptoms are frequently caused or aggravated by eating but can occur spontaneously and even awaken the patient at night.

Radiographically, peristalsis in the upper esophagus is initiated in response to some and occasionally all swallows, though the wave tends to break at about the level of the aortic arch. In the lower two-thirds of the esophagus, tertiary contractions of abnormally high amplitude can obliterate the lumen and cause compartmentalization of the barium column (Fig. 1-33). These segmental, nonpropulsive contractions can be accompanied by pain and result in barium being displaced both proximally and distally from the site of spasm, producing a corkscrew radiographic appearance of transient sacculations or pseudodiverticula ("rosary bead" esophagus) (Fig. 1-34).

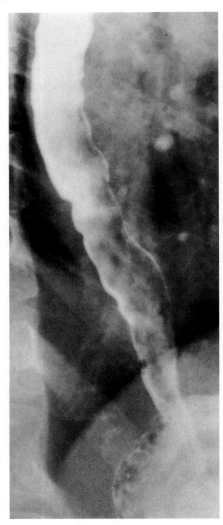 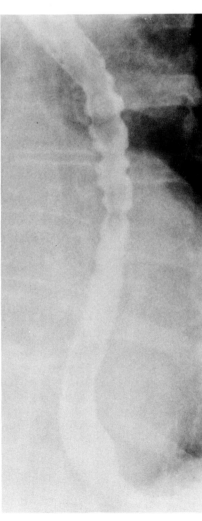

Fig. 1-31. Tertiary contractions.

Fig. 1-32. Presbyesophagus. Tertiary esophageal contractions are apparent in this elderly man.

1-31   1-32

ESOPHAGEAL INFLAMMATION

Reflux esophagitis causes continuous excitation of esophageal sensory receptors, and this can lead to the spillover of impulses to the motor ganglia in the myenteric plexus and result in uncoordinated contractions. These contractions range from mild fasciculations to severe segmental spasms that can be continuous and simulate a fixed stricture. In a similar manner, the ingestion of corrosive agents can act as an irritant and produce strong tertiary contractions. Nonpropulsive waves are also one of the manifestations of abnormal esophageal motility in patients with candida esophagitis (Fig. 1-35), amyloidosis (Fig. 1-36), or postirradiation inflammatory changes in the esophagus (Fig. 1-37).

NUTCRACKER ESOPHAGUS

Nutcracker esophagus is a recently described and relatively common esophageal motor disorder seen in some patients with otherwise unexplained chest pain or dysphagia. The nutcracker esophagus is primarily a manometric diagnosis made in the appropriate clinical setting and characterized by normal primary peristalsis with distal contractions of higher amplitude and increased duration. Some patients demonstrate tertiary contractions, though many have normal radiographic examinations.

OTHER CAUSES

Multiple tertiary contractions can occur during the early stages of achalasia (Fig. 1-38). In this "hyperactive" phase of the disease, uncoordinated muscular activity can cause the bolus to move up and down the esophagus with a to-and-fro motion.

Neuromuscular abnormalities, especially diabetes mellitus, can produce tertiary contractions of the esophagus (Fig. 1-39). This radiographic pattern has also been reported in patients with parkinsonism, amyotrophic lateral sclerosis, multiple sclerosis, thyrotoxic myopathy, and myotonic dystrophy.

Obstruction of the cardia by a malignant neoplasm can result in repetitive, prolonged, high-pressure esophageal contractions. This pattern of tertiary contractions can also be observed in patients who have distal esophageal strictures or benign neoplasms of the cardia, or who have undergone the surgical repair of a hiatal hernia.

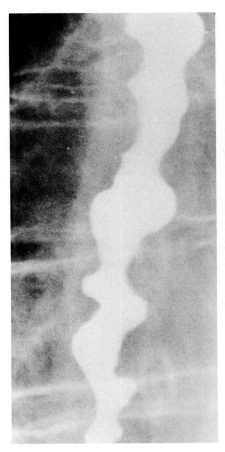

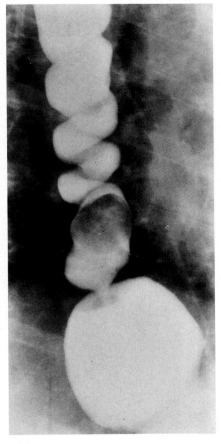

Fig. 1-33. Diffuse esophageal spasm. High amplitude contractions irregularly narrow the lumen of the esophagus.

Fig. 1-34. Diffuse esophageal spasm. Pronounced corkscrew pattern.

1-33

1-34

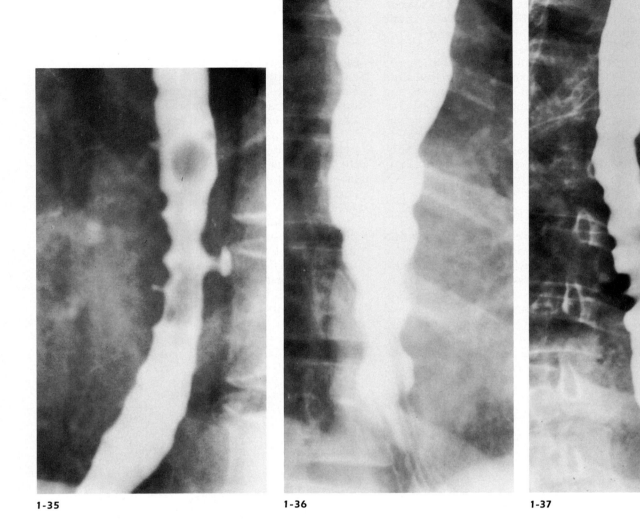

1-35   1-36   1-37

Fig. 1-35.   Candida esophagitis. Tertiary contractions are associated with a deep, penetrating ulcer.

Fig. 1-36.   Amyloidosis. Tertiary contractions are associated with diffuse deposition of amyloid within the wall of the esophagus.

Fig. 1-37.   Radiation injury. Tertiary contractions are secondary to esophageal motility disturbance due to radiation therapy for carcinoma of the lung. The disordered contractions begin at the upper margin of the treatment port. (Rogers LF, Goldstein HM: Roentgen manifestations of radiation injury to the gastrointestinal tract. Gastrointest Radiol 2:281–291, 1977)

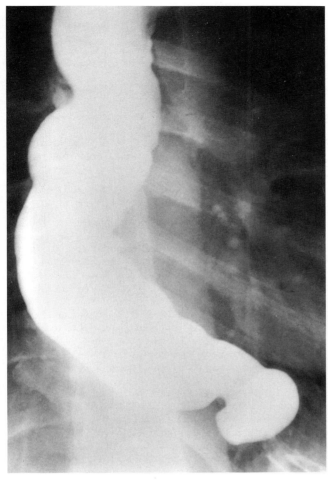

1-38

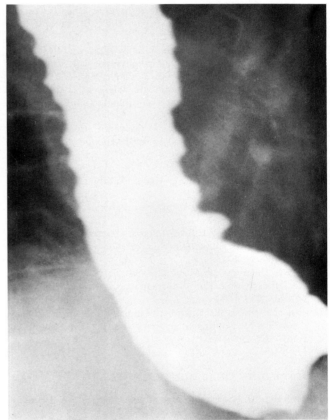

Fig. 1-38. Achalasia. Tertiary contractions are superimposed on a severely dilated esophagus.

Fig. 1-39. Diabetes mellitus. Note the diffuse tertiary contractions.

1-39

BIBLIOGRAPHY

Cricopharyngeal Achalasia

Balfe DM, Koehler RE, Setzen M et al: Barium examination of the esophagus after total laryngectomy. Radiology 143:501–508, 1982

Cohen S: Motor disorders of the esophagus. N Engl J Med 301:184–192, 1979

Curtis DJ, Cruess DF, Berg T: The cricopharyngeal muscle: A video recording review. AJR 142:492–500, 1984

Eckardt VF, Nix W, Kraus W et al: Esophageal motor function in patients with muscular dystrophy. Gastroenterology 90:628–635, 1986

Ekberg O: The cricopharyngeus revisited. Br J Radiol 59:875–879, 1986

Ekberg O, Lindgren S: Effect of cricopharyngeal myotomy on pharyngoesophageal function: Pre- and post-operative cineradiographic findings. Gastrointest Radiol 12:1–6, 1987

Ekberg O, Nylander G: Dysfunction of the cricopharyngeal muscle. Radiology 143:481–486, 1982

Ekberg O, Nylander G: Pharyngeal dysfunction after treatment for pharyngeal cancer with surgery and radiotherapy. Gastrointest Radiol 8:97–104, 1983

Horowitz M, McNeil JD, Maddern GJ et al: Abnormalities of gastric and esophageal emptying in polymyositis and dermatomyositis. Gastroenterology 90:434–439, 1986

Margulis AR, Koehler RE: Radiologic diagnosis of disordered esophageal motility: A unified physiologic approach. Radiol Clin North Am 14:429–439, 1976

Nowak TZ, Ionasescu V, Anuras S: Gastrointestinal manifestations of the muscular dystrophies. Gastroenterology 82:801–810, 1982

Seaman WB: Functional disorders of the pharyngo-esophageal junction: Achalasia and chalasia. Radiol Clin North Am 7:113–119, 1969

Seaman WB: Pathophysiology of the esophagus. Semin Roentgenol 16:214–227, 1981

Simpson AJ, Khilnani MT: Gastrointestinal manifestations of the muscular dystrophies. A review of roentgen findings. AJR 125:948–955, 1975

Torres WE, Clements JL, Austin GE et al: Cricopharyngeal muscle hypertrophy: Radiologic-anatomic correlation. AJR 141:927–930, 1984

Zboralske FF, Dodds WJ: Roentgenographic diagnosis of primary disorders of esophageal motility. Radiol Clin North Am 7:147–162, 1969

Abnormalities of Smooth Muscle

Anuras S, Shirazi SS: Colonic pseudo-obstruction. Am J Gastroenterology 79:525–532, 1984

Cohen S: Motor disorders of the esophagus. N Engl J Med 301:184–192, 1979

Horowitz M, McNeil JD, Maddern GJ et al: Abnormalities of gastric and esophageal emptying in polymyositis and dermatomyositis. Gastroenterology 90:434–439, 1986

Lepke RA, Libshitz HI: Radiation-induced injury of the esophagus. Radiology 148:375–378, 1983

Mandelstam P, Siegel CI, Lieber A et al: The swallowing disorder in patients with diabetic neuropathy–gastroenteropathy. Gastroenterology 56:1–12, 1969

Margulis AR, Koehler RE: Radiologic diagnosis of disordered esophageal motility: A unified physiologic approach. Radiol Clin North Am 14:429–439, 1976

Seaman WB: Pathophysiology of the esophagus. Semin Roentgenol 16:214–227, 1981

Simeone J, Burrell M, Toffler R et al: Aperistalsis and esophagitis. Radiology 123:9–14, 1977

Winship DH, Calfish GR, Zboralske FF et al: Deterioration of esophageal peristalsis in patients with alcoholic neuropathy. Gastroenterology 55:173–178, 1968

Achalasia Pattern

Agha FP: Secondary neoplasms of the esophagus. Gastrointest Radiol 12:187–193, 1987

Agha FP, Lee HH: The esophagus after endoscopic pneumatic balloon dilatation for achalasia. AJR 146:25–29, 1986

Davis JA, Kantrowitz PA, Chandler HL et al: Reversible achalasia due to reticulum-cell sarcoma. N Engl J Med 293:130–132, 1975

Dodds WJ, Stewart ET, Kishk SM et al: Radiologic amyl nitrite test for distinguishing pseudoachalasia from idiopathic achalasia. AJR 146:21–23, 1986

Dominguez F, Hernandez–Ranz F, Boixeda D et al: Acute upper-airway obstruction in achalasia of the esophagus. Am J Gastroenterol 82:362–364, 1987

Eaves R, Lambert J, Rees J et al: Achalasia secondary to carcinoma of prostate. Dig Dis Sci 28:278–284, 1983

Feczko PJ, Halpert RD: Achalasia secondary to nongastrointestinal malignancies. Gastrointest Radiol 10:273–276, 1985

Freeny PC, Marks WM: Adenocarcinoma of the gastroesophageal junction: Barium and CT examinations. AJR 138:1077–1084, 1982

Goldin NR, Burns TW, Ferrante WA: Secondary achalasia: Association with adenocarcinoma of the lungs and reversal with radiation therapy. Am J Gastroenterol 78:203–205, 1983

Reeder MM, Hamilton LC: Radiologic diagnosis of tropical diseases of the gastrointestinal tract. Radiol Clin North Am 7:57–81, 1969

Rogert LF: Transient post-vagotomy dysphagia: A distinct clinical and roentgenographic entity. AJR 125:956–960, 1975

Rohrmann CA, Ricci MT, Krishnamurthy S et al: Radiologic and histologic differentiation of neuromuscular disorders of the gastrointestinal tract: Visceral myopathy, visceral neuropathy and progressive systemic sclerosis. AJR 143:933–941, 1981

Simeone J, Burrell M, Toffler R: Esophageal aperistalsis secondary to metastatic invasion of the myenteric plexus. AJR 127:862–846, 1976

Stewart ET, Miller WN, Hogan WJ et al: Desirability of roentgen esophageal examination immediately after pneumatic dilatation for achalasia. Radiology 130:589–591, 1979

Vantrappen G, Hellemans J: Treatment of achalasia and related motor disorders. Gastrointest Radiol 79:144–154, 1980

Zegel HG, Kressel HY, Levine GM et al: Delayed esophageal perforation after pneumatic dilatation for the treatment of achalasia. Gastrointest Radiol 4:219–221, 1979

Tertiary Contractions

Bennett JR, Hendrix TR: Diffuse esophageal spasm: A disorder with more than one cause. Curr Clin Concepts 59:273–279, 1970

Cohen S: Motor disorders of the esophagus. N Engl J Med 301:184–192, 1979

Donner MW, Saba GP, Martinez CR: Diffuse disease of the esophagus: A practical approach. Semin Roentgenol 16:198–213, 1981

Margulis AR, Koehler RE: Radiologic diagnosis of disordered esophageal motility: A unified physiologic approach. Radiol Clin North Am 14:429–439, 1976

Ott DJ, Richter JE, Wu WC et al: Radiologic and manometric correlation in "Nutcracker esophagus." AJR 147:692–695, 1986

Ott DJ, Richter JE, Chen YM et al: Esophageal radiography and manometry: Correlation in 172 patients with dysphagia. AJR 149:307–311, 1987

Seaman WB: Pathophysiology of the esophagus: Semin Roentgenol 16:214–227, 1981

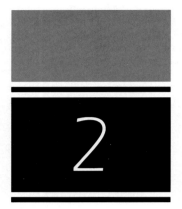

2

EXTRINSIC IMPRESSIONS ON THE CERVICAL ESOPHAGUS

Disease Entities

Cricopharyngeus muscle
Pharyngeal venous plexus (postcricoid impression)
Esophageal web
Anterior marginal osteophyte
Anterior herniation of intervertebral disk
Thyroid enlargement
Parathyroid enlargement
Ectopic gastric mucosa
Lymph node enlargement
Soft-tissue lesions
   Abscess
   Hematoma
Spinal lesions
   Neoplasm
   Inflammatory

CRICOPHARYNGEUS MUSCLE

Failure of the cricopharyngeus muscle to relax (cricopharyngeal achalasia) can produce a relatively constant posterior impression on the esophagus at about the C5-6 level (Fig. 2-1). A similar posterior impression on the barium-filled esophagus can often be observed after total laryngectomy, and some investigators have attributed this appearance to compensatory hyperactivity of the pharyngeal constrictor muscles.

PHARYNGEAL VENOUS PLEXUS

An anterior impression on the esophagus at about the C6 level can be caused by the prolapse of lax mucosal folds over the rich central submucosal pharyngeal venous plexus (Fig. 2-2). This "postcricoid impression" occurs as a small indentation just below the slight impression that may be produced by the posterior lamina of the cricoid cartilage. It sometimes has a weblike configuration or is so prominent that it suggests an intramural tumor. The appearance of the postcricoid impression may be seen to vary from swallow to swallow and even during a single swallow recorded on cine or videotape. The impression can frequently (in 70%–90% of adults) be demonstrated on careful study and is usually considered a normal finding.

ESOPHAGEAL WEB

Esophageal webs can present as extrinsic impressions on the barium-filled esophagus (see Fig. 2-1). Although they usually appear as thin, delicate membranes that sweep partially across the lumen, especially at the level of the pharyngoesophageal junction, esophageal webs can produce rounded, masslike impressions. They can be multiple and, since they tend to arise from the anterior wall, are best seen on lateral projection. Esophageal webs never appear on the posterior wall, an important differential distinction from the prominent cricopharyngeus impression, which always arises posteriorly.

ANTERIOR MARGINAL OSTEOPHYTE

Anterior marginal osteophytes of the cervical spine can produce smooth, regular indentations on the posterior wall of the cervical esophagus (Fig. 2-3). Profuse osteophytosis from vertebral margins in diffuse idiopathic skeletal hyperostosis (DISH, or Forrestier's disease) is especially likely to interfere with pharyngoesophageal function. These extrinsic impressions are best seen during complete filling of the esophageal segment and disappear during active contraction. Although usually asymptomatic, osteophytes impinging on the cervical esophagus may produce pain or difficulty in swallowing solids, the sensation of a foreign body, or a constant urge to clear the throat. When a posterior impression on the esophagus is seen at a midcervical intervertebral disk space level, the possibility of the presence of

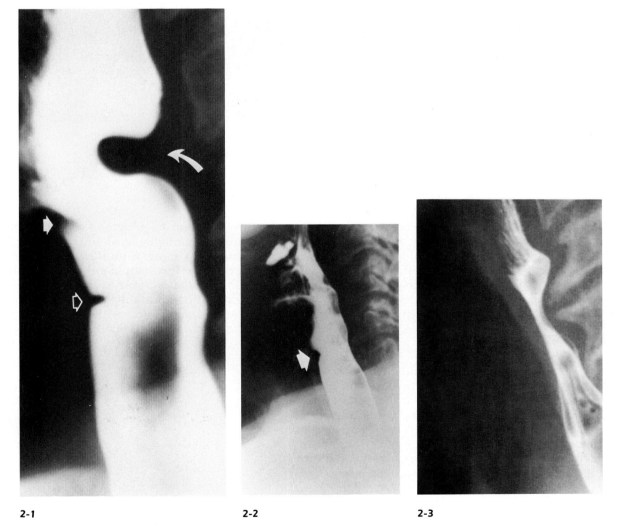

2-1   2-2   2-3

Fig. 2-1. Three impressions on the cervical esophagus: cricopharyngeal impression **(curved arrow)**, pharyngeal venous plexus **(short, closed arrow)**, and esophageal web **(short, open arrow)**. (Clements JL, Cox GW, Torres WE et al: Cervical esophageal webs: A roentgen-anatomic correlation. AJR 121:221–231, 1974. Copyright 1974. Reproduced with permission)

Fig. 2-2. Pharyngeal venous plexus. The anterior impression on the esophagus at about the C6 level **(arrow)** is due to the prolapse of lax mucosal folds over the rich central submucosal venous plexus.

Fig. 2-3. Anterior marginal osteophytes of the cervical spine. A smooth, regular indentation may be seen on the posterior wall at the level of an intervertebral disk space.

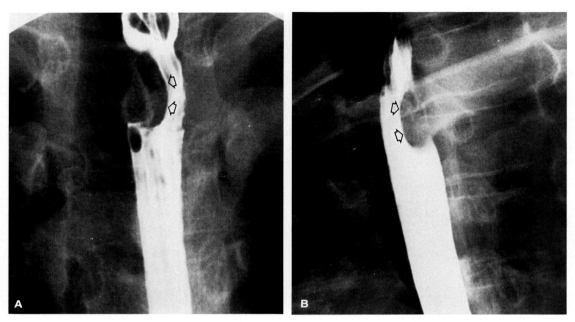

Fig. 2-4. *Herniated cervical intervertebral disk.* **(A)** *Frontal and* **(B)** *oblique views show a smooth extrinsic defect on the right posterolateral wall of the esophagus near the level of the first thoracic vertebra. (Picus D, McClennan BL, Balfe DM et al: "Discphagia": A case report. Gastrointest Radiol 9:5–7, 1984)*

anterior osteophytes must be closely evaluated. Rarely, a similar radiographic appearance is produced by anterior herniation of a cervical intervertebral disk (Fig. 2-4). Although this entity can cause dysphagia, it is almost always asymptomatic and is rarely recognized clinically.

THYROID ENLARGEMENT

Enlargement of the thyroid gland often causes compression and displacement of the cervical esophagus (Fig. 2-5). There is usually parallel displacement of the trachea, although, in some cases, a hypertrophic thyroid lobe can insinuate itself between the trachea and esophagus, displacing the trachea anteriorly and the esophagus posteriorly. A thyroid impression on the cervical esophagus can be caused by localized or generalized hypertrophy of the gland, inflammatory disease, or thyroid malignancy. Similarly, enlargement of a parathyroid gland can impinge upon the cervical esophagus. In a patient with symptoms of hyperparathyroidism due to a functioning parathyroid tumor, detection of an extrinsic impression on the cervical esophagus can be of great value in determining the site of the lesion.

ECTOPIC GASTRIC MUCOSA

Ectopic gastric mucosal rests in the upper esophagus can be detected endoscopically and pathologi-

cally in about 4% of patients. Unlike the acquired columnar metaplasia of Barrett's esophagus that extends proximally from the distal esophagus and is caused by reflux esophagitis, an isolated patch of ectopic gastric mucosa in the upper esophagus is a congenital condition that is almost always asymptomatic and associated with normal squamous mucosa distally. Rarely, isolated rests of gastric mucosa

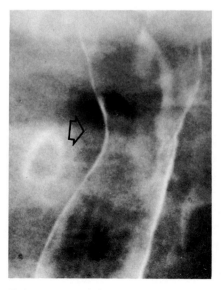

Fig. 2-5. *Enlargement of the thyroid gland. A smooth impression on the cervical esophagus is evident* **(arrow)**.

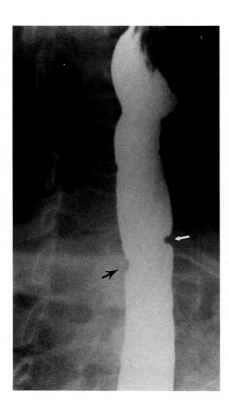

Fig. 2-6. *Ectopic gastric mucosa. Persistent ringlike narrowing* **(arrows)** *in the upper esophagus at the level of the thoracic inlet. (Williams SM, May C, Krause DW et al: Symptomatic congenital ectopic gastric mucosa in the upper esophagus. AJR 148:147–148, 1987. Copyright 1987. Reproduced with permission.)*

can cause a persistent ringlike narrowing that produces upper esophageal dysphagia (Fig. 2-6).

OTHER CAUSES

Cervical lymph node enlargement, due to either inflammation or malignancy, can cause an extrinsic impression on the adjacent esophagus. Similarly, abscesses or hematomas in the periesophageal soft tissues can produce indentations on the barium-filled esophagus. The combination of a posterior esophageal impression and vertebral bone destruction suggests the presence of a spinal neoplasm or osteomyelitis.

BIBLIOGRAPHY

Clements JL, Cox GW, Torres WE et al: Cervical esophageal webs: A roentgen-anatomic correlation. AJR 121:221–231, 1974

Ekberg O, Nylander G: Dysfunction of the cricopharyngeal muscle. Radiology 143:481–486, 1982

Picus D, McClennan BL, Balfe DM et al: ''Discphagia'': A case report. Gastrointest Radiol 9:5–7, 1984

Pitman RG, Fraser MG: The post-cricoid impression on the esophagus. Clin Radiol 16:34–39, 1965

Resnick D, Shaul SR, Robbins JM: Diffuse idiopathic skeletal hyperostosis (DISH) Forrestier's disease with extraspinal manifestations. Radiology 115:513–524, 1975

Williams SM, May C, Krause DW et al: Symptomatic congenital ectopic gastric mucosa in the upper esophagus. AJR 148:147–148, 1987

Yee C, Wong HY, Fewer HD et al: Two cases of dysphagia due to cervical spine osteophytes successfully treated surgically. Can Med Assoc J 132:810–812, 1985

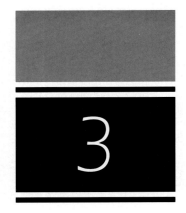

3

EXTRINSIC IMPRESSIONS ON THE THORACIC ESOPHAGUS

Normal structures
  Aortic knob
  Left main stem bronchus
  Left inferior pulmonary vein/confluence
    of left pulmonary veins
Vascular abnormalities
  Aortic lesions
    Right aortic arch
    Cervical aortic arch
    Double aortic arch
    Coarctation of the aorta
    Aortic aneurysm/tortuosity
  Nonaortic lesions
    Aberrant right subclavian artery
    Aberrant left pulmonary artery
    Anomalous pulmonary venous return
      (type III)
    Persistent truncus arteriosus
Cardiac enlargement
  Left atrium
  Left ventricle
Pericardial lesion
  Effusion
  Tumor
  Cyst
Mediastinal mass
  Tumor
  Duplication cyst
Pulmonary mass
  Tumor
  Bronchogenic cyst

Lymph node enlargement
Thoracic osteophyte
Paraesophageal hernia
Apical pleuropulmonary fibrosis (pseudo-
  impression)

During its course through the thorax, the esophagus runs through the posterior portion of the middle mediastinum and is in intimate contact with the aorta and its branches, the tracheobronchial tree, the heart, the lungs, and the interbronchial lymph nodes. Abnormalities in any of these or other structures in the middle or posterior portion of the mediastinum can compress or displace adjacent segments of the esophagus.

Esophageal deviation to one side of the chest usually results from an extrinsic mediastinal mass on the opposite side that is compressing and displacing the esophagus from its normal midline position. Less frequently, esophageal deviation may be caused by pulmonary, pleural, or mediastinal scarring with retraction of the esophagus toward the diseased hemithorax. Unless an obvious mass is observed radiographically, it can be difficult to determine whether the esophagus has been "pushed" or "pulled" from its normal position in the mediastinum. When the esophagus is displaced or pushed by an extrinsic mass in the mediastinum, the near wall of the esophagus (*i.e.,* the wall abutting the mass) is usually displaced more than the far wall, so that the esophagus tends to be narrower at this level than it is above or below the deviated segment (Fig. 3-1).

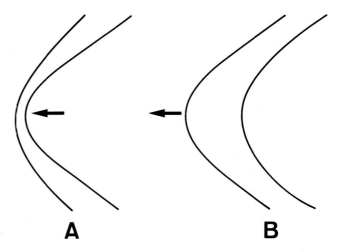

Fig. 3-1. Diagram of "pushed" vs "pulled" esophagus. **(A)** When the esophagus is displaced or pushed by an extrinsic mediastinal mass, it tends to be narrower at this level **(arrow)** than above or below the deviated segment. **(B)** When the esophagus is retracted or pulled by pleuropulmonary scarring and volume loss, however, it tends to be wider at this level **(arrow)** than above or below the deviated segment. (Levine MS, Gilchrist AM: Esophageal deviation: Pushed or pulled? AJR 149:513–514, 1987. Copyright 1987. Reproduced with permission.)

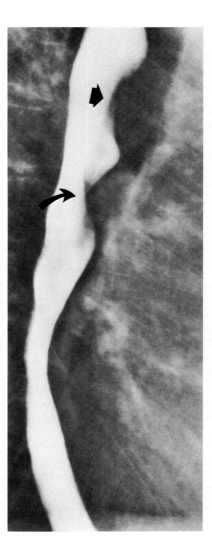

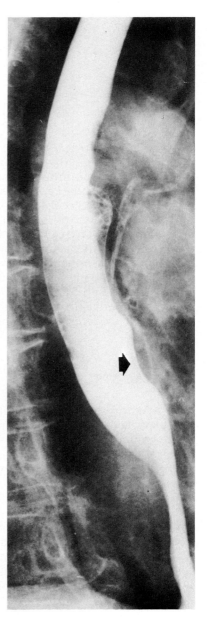

Fig. 3-2. Normal esophageal impressions caused by the aorta **(short arrow)** and left main stem bronchus **(long arrow)**.

Fig. 3-3. Normal pulmonary venous indentation **(arrow)** on the anterior left wall of the distal esophagus, best seen in a steep left posterior oblique projection. (Yeh HC, Wolf BS: A pulmonary venous indentation on the esophagus—A normal variant. Radiology 116:299–303, 1975)

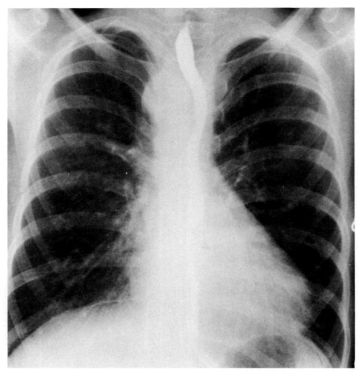

Fig. 3-4. *Right-sided aortic arch (pseudotruncus).*

Conversely, when the esophagus is retracted or pulled by pleuropulmonary scarring and volume loss, the near wall (*i.e.*, the wall abutting the diseased hemithorax) is also deviated more than the far wall, so that the esophagus tends to be wider at this level than it is above or below the deviated segment. The precise nature of esophageal deviation is important since esophageal retraction due to pleuropulmonary scarring can be noted and dismissed as an incidental finding, whereas esophageal displacement by a mediastinal mass may require further investigation to determine the nature and extent of the lesion.

NORMAL STRUCTURES

Two structures normally indent the anterior and lateral aspects of the thoracic esophagus (Fig. 3-2). The more cephalad normal impression, which is due to the transverse arch of the aorta (aortic knob), is more prominent as the aorta becomes increasingly dilated and tortuous with age. The more caudal impression is caused by the left main stem bronchus.

In about 10% of patients, the left inferior pulmonary vein or a common confluence of the left pulmonary veins near their insertion into the left atrium produces an extrinsic indentation on the anterior left wall of the esophagus about 4 cm to 5 cm below the carina (Fig. 3-3). This impression is best seen in a steep left posterior oblique horizontal position. The vascular nature of the indentation can be

confirmed by Valsalva and Müller maneuvers, in which the impression becomes smaller and more prominent, respectively.

VASCULAR ABNORMALITIES

RIGHT AORTIC ARCH

Vascular lesions of the aorta and its branches, as well as of the pulmonary arteries and veins, can cause extrinsic impressions on the thoracic esophagus. The most common aortic anomaly is a right-sided aortic arch (Fig. 3-4). This condition is easily detected on plain chest radiographs by the absence of the characteristic left aortic knob and its replacement by a slightly higher bulge on the right. The trachea is seen to deviate to the left, and the barium-filled esophagus is indented on the right.

When the aortic arch is right-sided, the descending aorta can run on either the right or the left. If it descends on the right, the brachiocephalic vessels can originate in one of three ways. With the mirror-image pattern, no vessels cross the mediastinum posterior to the esophagus, and, consequently, there is no esophageal indentation on the lateral projection. This anomaly is frequently associated with congenital heart disease, primarily tetralogy of Fallot.

The other two anomalies associated with a right-sided aortic arch and right descending aorta differ with respect to the origin of the left subclavian artery. In the more common type, the left subclavian artery arises as the most distal branch of the aorta (reverse of the aberrant right subclavian artery, which originates from a left aortic arch). In order to reach the left upper extremity, the left subclavian artery must course across the mediastinum posterior to the esophagus, producing a characteristic oblique posterior indentation on the esophagus (Fig. 3-5). Almost all patients with this anomaly have no associated congenital heart disease.

In the second type of anomaly, the left subclavian artery is atretic at its base and totally isolated from the aorta (isolated left subclavian artery). In this rare condition, the left subclavian artery receives blood from the left pulmonary artery, or from the aorta in a circuitous fashion through retrograde flow by way of the ipsilateral vertebral artery (congenital subclavian steal syndrome). The tenuous blood supply in patients with this condition often results in decreased pulses and ischemia of the left upper extremity.

A right aortic arch with left descending aorta is an uncommon anomaly. Because the aortic knob is on the right and the aorta descends on the left, the transverse portion must cross the mediastinum. This usually occurs posterior to the esophagus, resulting in a prominent posterior esophageal indentation that tends to be more transverse and much larger than that seen with an aberrant left subclavian artery.

CERVICAL AORTIC ARCH

A posterior impression on the esophagus associated with a pulsatile mass above the clavicle suggests the diagnosis of a cervical aortic arch (Fig. 3-6). The pulsatile mass may be mistaken for an aneurysm of the subclavian, carotid, or innominate artery. No

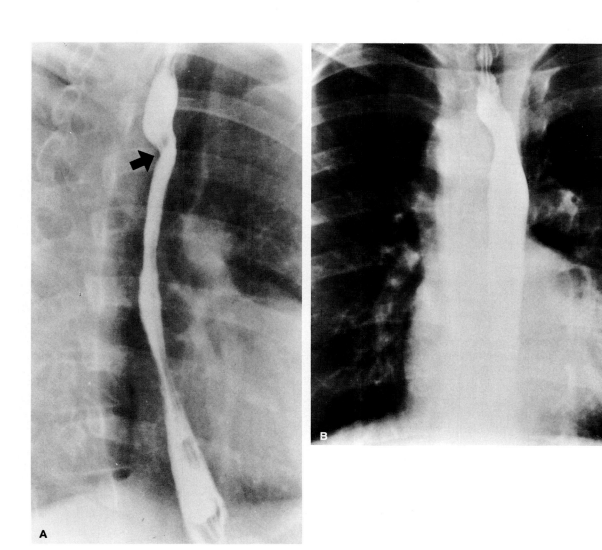

Fig. 3-5. Aberrant left subclavian artery with right aortic arch. **(A)** A posterior impression on the esophagus **(arrow)** is visible on the oblique view. **(B)** The right aortic arch **(arrow)** is evident on the frontal view.

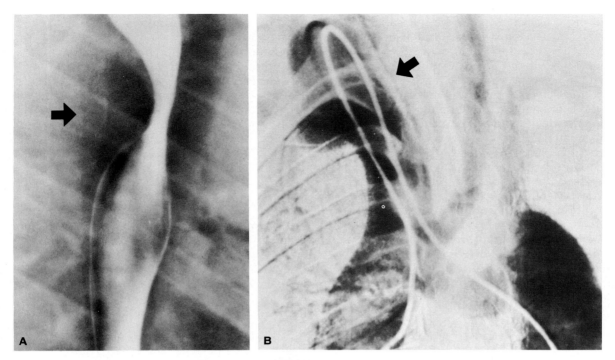

Fig. 3-6. Cervical aortic arch. **(A)** Posterior esophageal impression **(arrow)** caused by the retroesophageal course of the distal arch or the proximal descending aorta. **(B)** Subtraction film from an aortogram demonstrating the aortic arch extending into the neck **(arrow)**.

coexistent intracardiac congenital heart disease has been described in the few cases reported. The posterior esophageal impression is caused by the distal arch or proximal descending aorta as it courses in a retroesophageal position.

DOUBLE AORTIC ARCH

In most patients with a double aortic arch, the aorta ascends on the right, branches, and finally reunites on the left. The two limbs of the aorta completely encircle the trachea and esophagus, forming a ring. The anterior portion of the arch is usually smaller than the posterior part. When the aorta descends on the left (in about 75% of cases), the posterior arch is higher than the anterior arch; the reverse pattern is seen if the aorta descends on the right.

On plain chest radiographs, the two aortic limbs can appear as bulges on either side of the superior mediastinum, the right usually being larger and higher than the left. On barium swallow, a double aortic arch produces a characteristic reverse S-shaped indentation on the esophagus (Fig. 3-7). The upper curve of the S is produced by the larger posterior arch; the lower curve is related to the smaller anterior arch. Infrequently, a patient with a double aortic arch can have anterior and posterior esophageal indentations directly across from each other rather than in an S-shaped configuration.

The reverse S-shaped indentation of the esophagus is typical of all true vascular rings. For example,

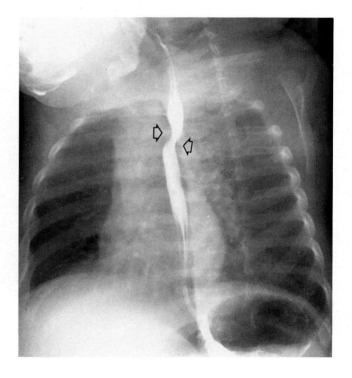

Fig. 3-7. Double aortic arch. Characteristic reverse S-shaped indentation on the esophagus **(arrows)**. As usual, the right (posterior) arch is higher and larger than the left (anterior) arch. (Swischuk LE: *Radiology of the Newborn and Young Infant.* Baltimore, Williams & Wilkins, 1980)

the vascular ring formed by an ascending right aortic arch, a left subclavian artery passing posteriorly to the esophagus, and a persistent ductus or ligamentum arteriosus extending from the left subclavian artery to the pulmonary artery produces a double impression on the esophagus essentially identical to that seen with a double aortic arch.

COARCTATION OF THE AORTA

Coarctation of the aorta can produce a characteristic "figure-3" sign on plain chest radiographs (Fig. 3-8*A*) and a reverse figure-3 or "figure-E" impression on the barium-filled esophagus (Fig. 3-8*B*). The more cephalad bulge represents dilatation of the proximal aorta and base of the left subclavian artery (prestenotic dilatation); the lower bulge reflects poststenotic aortic dilatation. Coarctation of the aorta usually occurs at or just distal to the level of the ductus arteriosus; much less frequently, the area of narrowing lies proximal to this point. In the latter type of coarctation, a ventricular septal defect and patent ductus arteriosus are always present so that blood can be delivered to the descending aorta from the pulmonary artery through the patent ductus.

Most patients with coarctation of the aorta do not develop symptoms until late childhood or early adulthood. Narrowing of the aorta causes systolic overloading and hypertrophy of the left ventricle. There is usually a substantial difference in blood pressure between the upper and lower extremities. The relative obstruction of aortic blood flow leads to the progressive development of collateral circulation, often seen radiographically as rib notching (usually involving the posterior fourth to eighth ribs), caused by pressure erosion by the dilated, pulsating collateral vessels (Fig. 3-8). Dilatation of mammary artery collaterals can produce retrosternal notching.

AORTIC ANEURYSM/TORTUOSITY

Elongation and unfolding of the descending thoracic aorta is frequently accompanied by a concomitant impression on the thoracic esophagus. Tortuosity of the epiphrenic segment of the aorta usually causes a sicklelike deformity with characteristic displacement of the esophagus anteriorly (Fig. 3-9*A*) and to the left (Fig. 3-9*B*). Localized aneurysmal dilatation of a segment of the thoracic aorta can also indent an adjacent portion of the esophagus.

ABERRANT RIGHT SUBCLAVIAN ARTERY

The most common nonaortic vascular lesion producing an impression on the barium-filled thoracic esophagus is an aberrant right subclavian artery. This artery, the last major vessel of the aortic arch, arises just distal to the left subclavian artery. In order to reach the right upper extremity, the aberrant right subclavian artery must course across the mediastinum behind the esophagus, and this produces a posterior esophageal indentation (Fig. 3-10). On the frontal view, the esophageal impression runs obliquely upward and to the right (Fig. 3-10). This appearance is so characteristic that no further radiographic investigation is required. An aberrant right subclavian artery rarely produces symptoms (other than occasional dysphagia), is usually an incidental finding during an upper gastrointestinal examination performed for other purposes, and is not associated with congenital heart disease.

ABERRANT LEFT PULMONARY ARTERY

Other nonaortic vascular impressions on the esophagus are rare. An aberrant left pulmonary artery arises from the right pulmonary artery and must cross the mediastinum to reach the left lung. As it courses between the trachea and esophagus, it produces a characteristic impression on the posterior aspect of the trachea just above the carina and a corresponding indentation on the anterior wall of the barium-filled esophagus (Figs. 3-11, 3-12).

ANOMALOUS PULMONARY VENOUS RETURN

In patients with anomalous pulmonary venous return, blood from the lungs returns to the right side of the heart (right atrium, coronary sinus, or systemic vein) rather than emptying normally into the left atrium. In almost all cases, the anomalous pulmonary veins unite to form a single vessel posterior to the heart before entering a cardiac chamber or systemic vein. In the type-III anomaly, the anomalous pulmonary vein travels with the esophagus through the diaphragm and inserts into a systemic vein or, more commonly, into the portal vein, usually producing an anterior indentation on the lower portion of the barium-filled esophagus (Fig. 3-13). It is important to note that this indentation occurs above the diaphragm but slightly below the expected site of left atrial indentation.

PERSISTENT TRUNCUS ARTERIOSUS

Persistent truncus arteriosus is a relatively uncommon anomaly that is due to the failure of the common truncus arteriosus to divide normally into the aorta and pulmonary artery. This results in a single vessel draining both ventricles and supplying the systemic, pulmonary, and coronary circulations. In one form of persistent truncus arteriosus, the pulmonary artery is absent and the lungs are supplied by collateral bronchial arteries. These dilated bronchial vessels, which can be quite large, produce dis-

Text continues on page 40

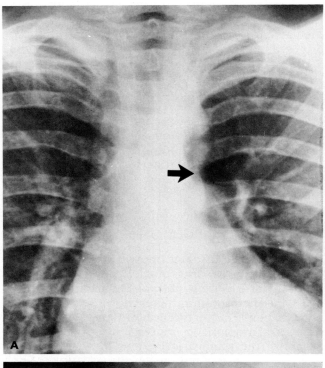

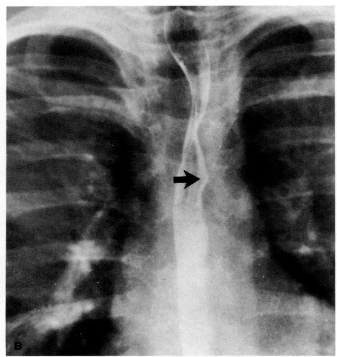

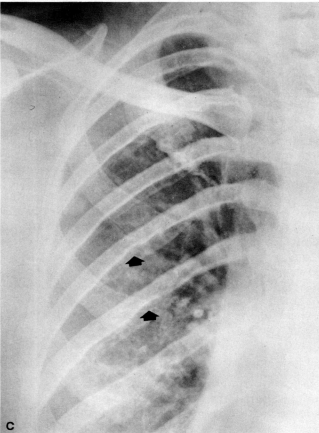

Fig. 3-8. Coarctation of the aorta. **(A)** Plain chest radiograph demonstrates the "figure-3" sign (the **arrow** points to the center of the 3). The upper bulge represents prestenotic dilatation, whereas the lower bulge represents poststenotic dilatation. **(B)** Barium swallow demonstrates the "reverse figure-3" sign (the **arrow** points to the center of the reverse figure-3). **(C)** Rib notching. There is notching of the posterior fourth through eighth ribs (the **arrows** point to two examples). (Swischuk LE: Plain Film Interpretation in Congenital Heart Disease. Baltimore, Williams & Wilkins, 1979)

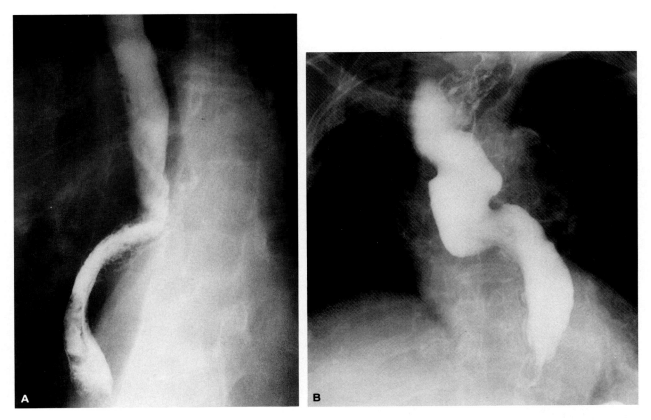

Fig. 3-9. Tortuosity of the descending thoracic aorta producing characteristic displacement of the esophagus **(A)** anteriorly and **(B)** to the left. Note the retraction of the upper esophagus to the right. This is caused by chronic inflammatory disease, which simulates an extrinsic mass arising from the opposite side.

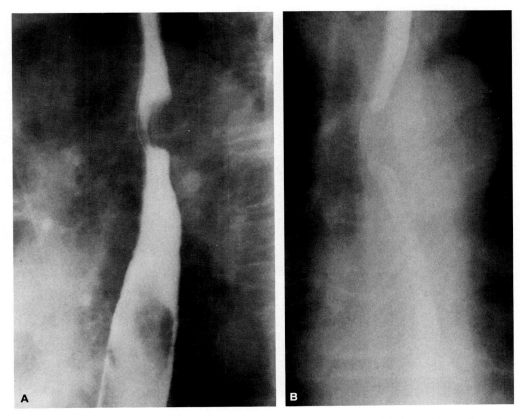

Fig. 3-10. Aberrant right subclavian artery. **(A)** Posterior esophageal indentation on lateral view. **(B)** Esophageal impression running obliquely upward and to the right on frontal view.

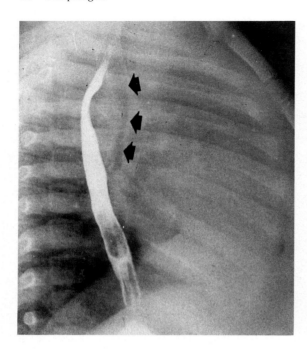

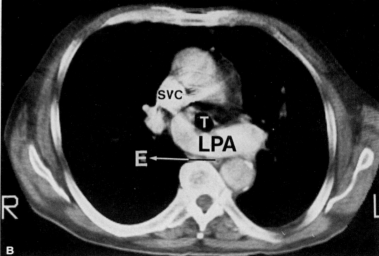

Fig. 3-11. Aberrant left pulmonary artery. The vessel crosses the mediastinum between the trachea **(arrows)** and the esophagus, producing impressions on the anterior aspect of the esophagus and the posterior margin of the trachea.

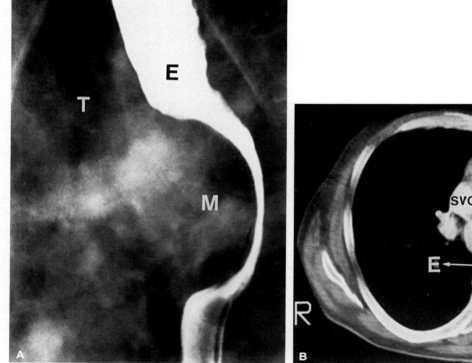

Fig. 3-12. Aberrant left pulmonary artery. **(A)** Lateral esophagram shows a smooth, ovoid soft-tissue mass **(M)** lying between the distal trachea **(T)** and midesophagus **(E)** and causing marked esophageal narrowing. **(B)** Dynamic CT scan of the thorax shows that the mass is in fact the proximal portion of a dilated left pulmonary artery **(LPA)**, which has an anomalous origin from the right pulmonary artery and courses between the trachea **(T)** and esophagus **(E)** toward the left hilum. **SVC** = superior vena cava. (Nguyen KT, Kosiuk J, Place C et al: Two unusual causes of dysphagia: A pictorial essay. J Can Assoc Radiol 38:42–44, 1987)

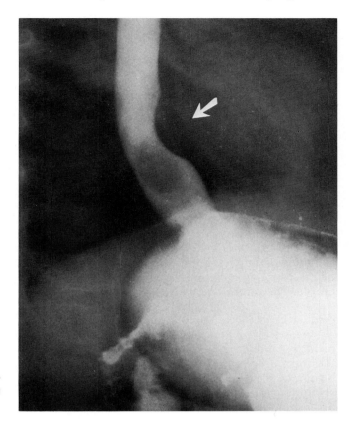

Fig. 3-13. Anomalous pulmonary venous return (type III). There is an anterior indentation on the lower border of the barium-filled esophagus **(arrow)**, slightly below the expected site of the left atrium.

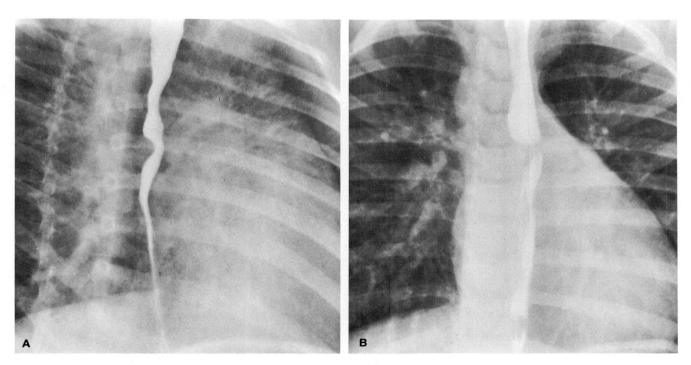

Fig. 3-14. Persistent truncus arteriosus. **(A)** Characteristic indentation on the posterior wall of the esophagus, which is somewhat lower than usually seen with an aberrant left subclavian artery. **(B)** Frontal view demonstrating a right-sided impression on the esophagus.

crete indentations on the posterior wall of the esophagus (Fig. 3-14) that are somewhat lower than those usually seen with aberrant left subclavian arteries.

CARDIAC ENLARGEMENT

LEFT ATRIUM

The left atrium is in direct contact with the anterior aspect of the esophagus. Enlargement of the left atrium, whether secondary to congenital heart disease, as in ventricular septal defect, patent ductus arteriosus, or double outlet right ventricle (Fig. 3-15), acquired mitral valve disease (Fig. 3-16), or left atrial tumor (Fig. 3-17), produces a characteristic anterior impression and posterior displacement of the esophagus beginning about 2 cm below the carina. The impression of an enlarged left atrium on the barium-filled esophagus is best seen in the lateral and right anterior oblique projections. On the posteroanterior view, enlargement of the left atrium produces some displacement of the esophagus to the right. Even minimal left atrial enlargement can be detected on barium swallow; however, it must be remembered that slight esophageal indentation at this level may also be seen in some normal persons. Therefore, this finding must be correlated with

clinical history and other radiographic signs of left atrial enlargement (e.g., posterior displacement of the left main stem bronchus, widening of the carina, bulging in the region of the left atrial appendage, "double density" on the frontal view).

LEFT VENTRICLE

Enlargement of the left ventricle also produces anterior indentation and posterior displacement of the esophagus (Fig. 3-18). Whether secondary to aortic valvular disease or to cardiac failure, the enlarged left ventricle causes an esophageal impression that is best appreciated on the lateral view. The indentation is situated at a level somewhat inferior to the impression caused by an enlarged left atrium.

OTHER CAUSES

PERICARDIAL LESIONS

Just as enlargement of specific heart chambers results in esophageal indentation, so can a lesion of the pericardium. Pericardial tumors and cysts can cause localized impressions on the anterior aspect of the barium-filled esophagus; pericardial effusions tend to produce broader impressions on the esophagus.

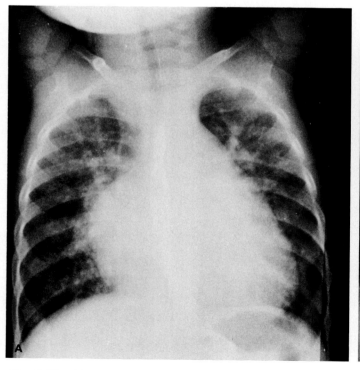
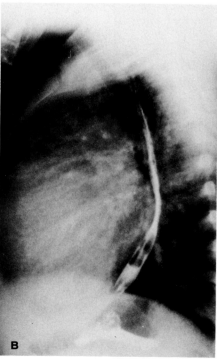

Fig. 3-15. Enlargement of the left atrium due to a double outlet right ventricle.

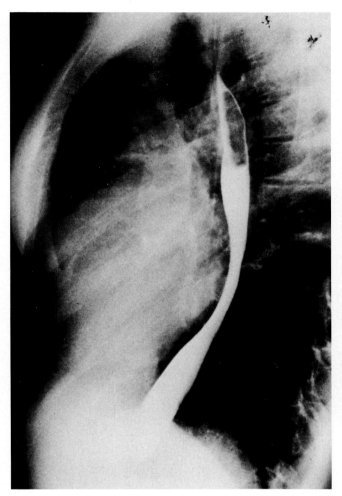

3-16

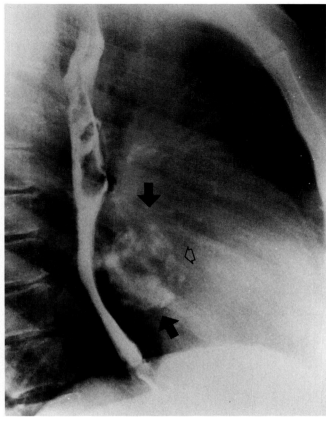

3-17

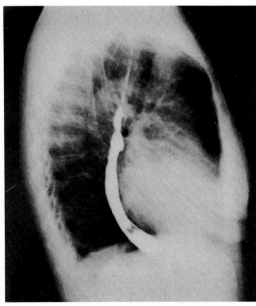

3-18

Fig. 3-16. Enlargement of the left atrium secondary to acquired mitral valve disease.

Fig. 3-17. Enlargement of the left atrium caused by a calcified left atrial tumor **(arrows)**.

Fig. 3-18. Enlarged left ventricle secondary to acquired aortic stenosis.

INTRATHORACIC MASSES

Any mass lesion adjacent to the esophagus that arises within the mediastinum (Fig. 3-19), lung (Fig. 3-20), trachea, or lymph nodes can impress the barium-filled esophagus. Depending on the size and position of the mass, there can be a focal (Fig. 3-21) or broad (Fig. 3-22) impression on the esophagus and displacement of the esophagus in any direction. The most common entities producing esophageal impressions by this mechanism are inflammatory and metastatic lesions involving lymph nodes in the carinal and subcarinal regions. Mediastinal extension of a pancreatic pseudocyst (Fig. 3-23) is an infrequent complication of pancreatitis that may occur late in the course of the disease and may have no associated biochemical abnormalities.

THORACIC OSTEOPHYTE

Thoracic osteophytosis, especially in association with diffuse idiopathic skeletal hyperostosis (DISH), can infrequently cause dysphagia by producing a posterior extrinsic impression on the thoracic esophagus (Fig. 3-24). Anterior marginal osteophytes much more commonly cause posterior compression of the esophagus in the cervical region.

PARAESOPHAGEAL HERNIA

The supradiaphragmatic portion of the stomach in a patient with a paraesophageal hernia can cause an impression on the distal esophagus as it courses toward the esophagogastric junction, which remains

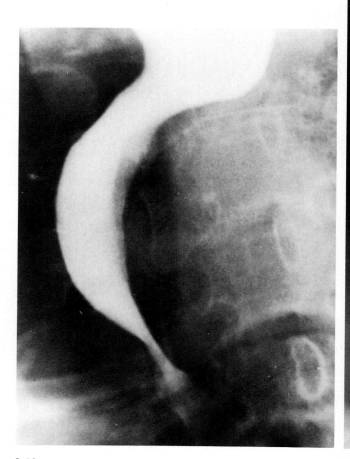

3-19

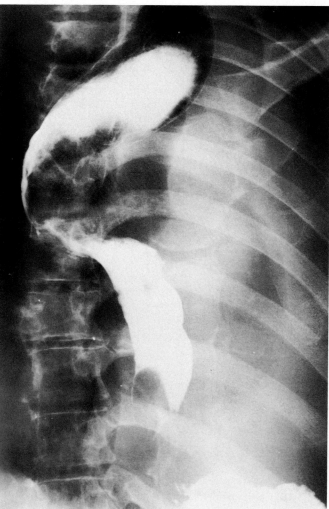

3-20

Fig. 3-19. Enlargement of a substernal thyroid causing an impression on the upper thoracic esophagus.

Fig. 3-20. Squamous carcinoma of the lung impressing and invading the midthoracic esophagus.

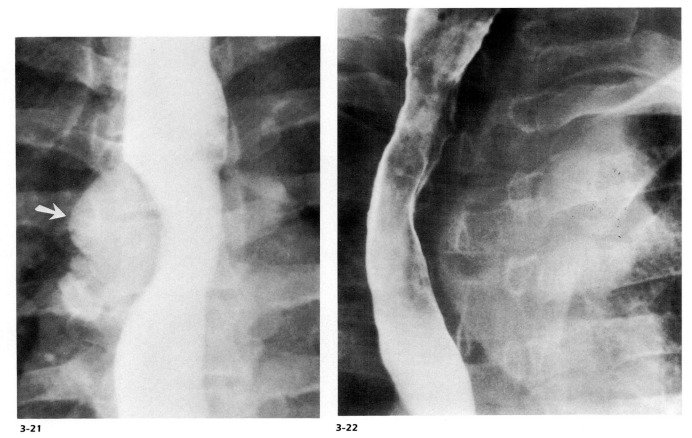

3-21   **3-22**

Fig. 3-21. Calcified mediastinal lymph nodes at the carinal level **(arrow)** causing a focal impression and displacement of the esophagus.

Fig. 3-22. Squamous carcinoma of the lung producing a broad impression on the upper thoracic esophagus.

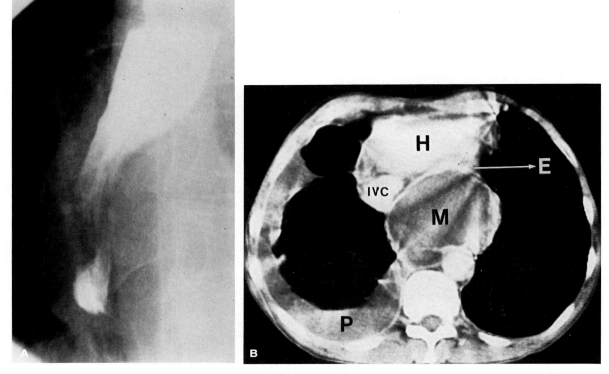

Fig. 3-23. Mediastinal pancreatic pseudocyst. **(A)** Barium swallow shows lateral displacement and obstruction of the distal esophagus, suggesting extrinsic compression. **(B)** CT scan shows marked displacement of the mediastinal structures by the mass **(M)**. **E** = esophagus; **H** = heart; **IVC** = inferior vena cava; **P** = pleural effusion. (Nguyen KT, Kosiuk J, Place C et al: Two unusual causes of dysphagia: A pictorial essay. J Can Assoc Radiol 38:42–44, 1987)

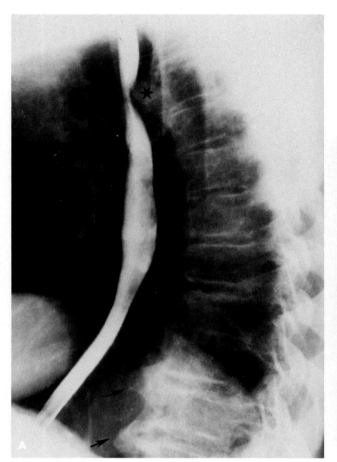

3-24

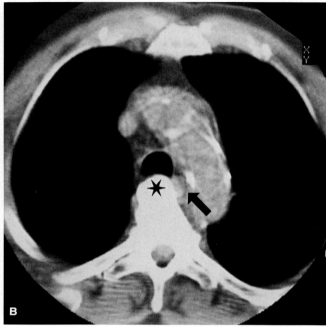

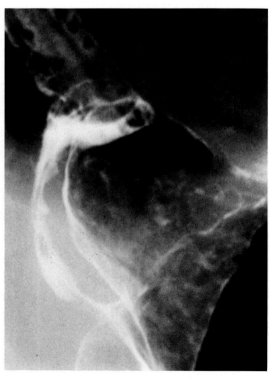

Fig. 3-24. Thoracic osteophyte. **(A)** Lateral view from a barium swallow shows a posterior extrinsic defect anterior to T4. Note the osteophytes and the flowing ossification anterior to the lower thoracic vertebral bodies **(arrow)** with preservation of the disk spaces. The anterior osteophyte of T4 **(✱)** is not optimally outlined on this view. **(B)** CT scan at the T4 level shows the large bony outgrowth **(✱)** compressing the collapsed esophagus **(arrow)** against the calcified aortic arch. Note the absence of a soft-tissue mass or aberrant vessel. This CT scan corresponds to the level of the defect seen on the barium swallow. (Willing S, El Gammal T: Thoracic osteophyte producing dysphagia in a case of diffuse idiopathic skeletal hypertrophy. Am J Gastroenterol 78:381–383, 1983)

Fig. 3-25. Paraesophageal hernia impressing the distal esophagus.

3-25

normally positioned below the diaphragm (Fig. 3-25). In this condition, the distal esophagus is usually displaced posteriorly and to the right, the extent of the impression depending on the amount of herniated stomach above the diaphragm.

APICAL PLEUROPULMONARY FIBROSIS

A "pseudoimpression" on the upper thoracic esophagus can be caused by apical pleuropulmonary fibrosis. This complication of chronic inflammatory disease, most commonly tuberculosis, produces retraction of the esophagus toward the side of the lesion (see Fig. 3-9*B*). The margin of the esophagus on which the traction is exerted assumes an asymmetric pseudodiverticular appearance.

BIBLIOGRAPHY

Levine MS, Gilchrist AM: Esophageal deviation: Pushed or pulled. AJR 149:513–514, 1987

Margulis AR, Burhenne HJ: Alimentary Tract Roentgenology. St. Louis, CV Mosby, 1983

Nguyen KT, Kosiuk J, Place C et al: Two unusual cases of dysphagia: A pictorial essay. J Can Assoc Radiol 38:42–44, 1987

Shuford WH, Sybers RG, Milledge RD et al: The cervical aortic arch. AJR 116:519–527, 1972.

Swischuck LE: Plain Film Interpretation in Congenital Heart Disease. Baltimore, Williams & Wilkins, 1979

Willing S, El Gammal T: Thoracic osteophyte producing dysphagia in a case of diffuse idiopathic skeletal hypertrophy. Am J Gastroenterol 78:381–383, 1983

Yeh HC, Wolf BS: A pulmonary venous indentation on the esophagus: A normal variant. Radiology 116:299–303, 1975

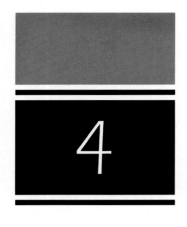

4 ESOPHAGEAL ULCERATION

Disease Entities

Reflux esophagitis
  Hiatal hernia
  Vomiting secondary to intra-abdominal disease
  Chalasia of infancy
  Pregnancy
  Scleroderma
  Medication
  Surgery
Barrett's esophagus
Infectious/granulomatous disorders
  Candidiasis
  Herpes simplex
  Cytomegalovirus
  Tuberculosis
  Crohn's disease
  Syphilis
  Histoplasmosis
  Acute alcoholic esophagitis
  Eosinophilic esophagitis
  Behcet's syndrome
  Epidermolysis bullosa
Malignant lesions
  Carcinoma
  Lymphoma
  Metastases
Corrosive esophagitis
Radiation injury

Drug-induced esophagitis
  Potassium chloride tablets
  Tetracycline
  Emepronium bromide
  Quinidine
  Ascorbic acid
  Ferrous sulfate
Sclerotherapy of esophageal varices
Intramural pseudodiverticulosis

REFLUX ESOPHAGITIS

The most common cause of esophageal ulceration is esophagitis due to reflux of gastric or duodenal contents into the esophagus (Fig. 4-1). In most cases, a combination of gastric acid and pepsin causes mucosal irritation of the esophagus. Reflux esophagitis can occur even in the absence of stomach acid because of regurgitation of alkaline bile and pancreatic juice, which act as corrosive irritants to the esophageal mucosa.

PREDISPOSING CONDITIONS

Reflux esophagitis occurs when the lower esophageal sphincter fails to act as an effective barrier to stomach contents entering the distal esophagus. Rather than a simple mechanical barrier, the lower esophageal sphincter is a complex, dynamic structure that responds to a variety of physical, humoral,

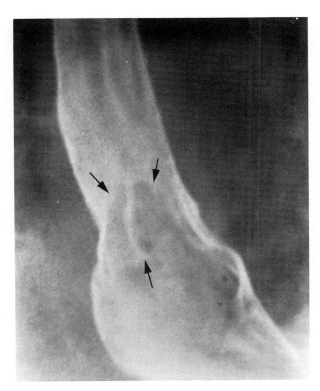

Fig. 4-1. *Reflux esophagitis. Linear ulcer surrounded by a lucent halo of edema* **(arrows)** *in the distal esophagus. (Goldstein HM, Bova JG: Esophagitis. In Taveras JM, Ferrucci JT (eds): Radiology: Diagnosis–Imaging–Intervention. Philadelphia, JB Lippincott, 1987)*

and neural stimuli to prevent reflux. Functional or structural changes at the gastroesophageal junction can disrupt the effectiveness of the barrier mechanism, thereby increasing the likelihood of reflux and the development of esophagitis and ulceration.

There is a higher than normal likelihood of gastroesophageal reflux in patients with sliding hiatal hernias. However, it must be emphasized that the competence of the lower esophageal sphincter is not dependent on its being situated above the diaphragm. In one endoscopic study, reflux esophagitis was observed in only 26% of patients with sliding hiatal hernias. Conversely, esophagitis is often encountered in patients in whom no hiatal hernia can be demonstrated. Reflux of acidic gastric contents into the esophagus can be caused by prolonged or repeated vomiting secondary to peptic ulcer, biliary colic, intestinal obstruction, acute alcoholic gastritis, pancreatitis, or migraine, or by vomiting following surgery or during pregnancy. Prolonged nasogastric intubation can decrease the competence of the lower esophageal sphincter, interfere with esophageal peristalsis, and facilitate gastroesophageal reflux and subsequent esophagitis.

Chalasia is a functional disturbance in which the lower esophageal sphincter fails to remain normally closed between swallows, thereby permitting regurgitation of large amounts of gastric contents

through it. Found during the immediate postnatal period, chalasia is a cause of vomiting in infants. However, as an infant matures, the development of neuromuscular control increases the competency of the lower esophageal sphincter, and free gastroesophageal reflux gradually disappears. Persistence of vomiting and reflux after several months suggests an abnormal sphincter or sliding hiatal hernia. Regurgitation and vomiting beginning after infancy are also abnormal and can result in nocturnal emesis, aspiration of gastric contents, and pulmonary complications.

A contrast esophagram demonstrates gastroesophageal reflux in most infants and children with chalasia. A more sensitive imaging technique for the detection of gastroesophageal reflux in children is the radionuclide "milk scan." After the child has ingested ^{99m}Tc sulfur colloid in a routine milk or formula feeding, sequential scanning can show gastroesophageal reflux of the isotope and tracheobronchial aspiration (Fig. 4-2). An additional value of this test is the ability to monitor patients for prolonged periods, because gastroesophageal reflux probably occurs intermittently and clearance from the upper airways may be rapid.

Up to half of pregnant women experience heartburn, usually during the third trimester. These women demonstrate a reduction in lower esophageal sphincter pressure that returns to normal levels after delivery. This reversible incompetence of the lower esophageal sphincter is probably of hormonal origin and appears to reflect a generalized smooth muscle response to female hormones.

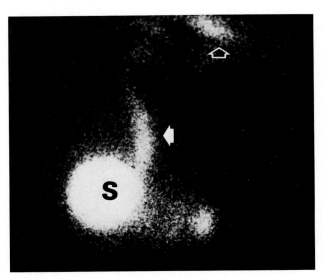

Fig. 4-2. *Chalasia. Radionuclide milk scan shows reflux of the isotope from the stomach* **(S)** *into the distal esophagus* **(closed arrow)***. The condition was so severe in this infant that increased isotope activity from reflux can even be seen in the mouth* **(open arrow)***. (Eisenberg RL: Diagnostic Imaging in Surgery. New York, McGraw–Hill, 1987)*

A patulous lower esophageal sphincter predisposing to reflux esophagitis is characteristically seen in patients with scleroderma (Fig. 4-3). Incompetence of the lower esophageal sphincter can also be related to drugs, such as anticholinergics, nitrites, beta-adrenergic agents, and some tranquilizers.

Surgical procedures in the region of the gastroesophageal junction can impair the normal function of the lower esophageal sphincter. Severing of the oblique muscles of the distal esophagus (Heller procedure for achalasia), total gastrectomy, and esophagocardiectomy can lead to reflux esophagitis. The disorder is particularly severe after vagotomy if the resulting stasis of gastric contents has not been relieved by a suitable drainage procedure.

CLINICAL SYMPTOMS

The symptoms of reflux esophagitis are due to gastric acid or alkaline bile and pancreatic juice irritating the distal esophageal mucosa. The most common symptom is heartburn, an uncomfortable burning sensation that starts below the sternum and tends to move up into the neck, waxing and waning in intensity. The retrosternal burning often occurs after eating and is aggravated by the ingestion of very hot or cold liquids, coffee, citrus juices, or alcoholic beverages. Reflux symptoms can be precipitated by any change in position that compresses the abdomen or increases intragastric pressure, such as bending or stooping, picking up objects from the floor, or lying flat after eating a large meal.

Regurgitation of gastric contents into the mouth is another classic symptom of reflux. This most frequently occurs during sleep and leads to the appearance of fluid on the pillow. The presence of gastric contents can cause a sour or metallic taste in the throat and mouth. Regurgitation implies severe reflux and often leads to aspiration and pulmonary complications.

Some patients with reflux have dysphagia. This does not reflect an organic stricture of the esophagus, since most patients with reflux esophagitis who have dysphagia have a normal intraluminal diameter. Hemorrhage related to esophagitis is usually a steady oozing of blood from the distal esophagus. Penetrating ulcers of the esophagus can cause brisk arterial bleeding.

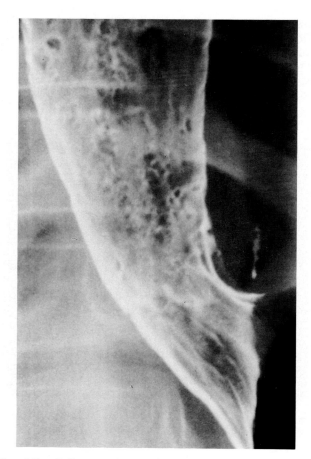

Fig. 4-3. *Reflux esophagitis in scleroderma. Note the patulous esophagogastric junction.*

RADIOGRAPHIC TECHNIQUES

A number of radiographic approaches have been suggested for demonstration of gastroesophageal reflux. One procedure is to increase intra-abdominal pressure by straight-leg raising or manual pressure on the abdomen with or without a Valsalva maneuver. Another approach is the water-siphon test, the significance of which is controversial. To perform this study, the physician pools barium in the cardia of the stomach (or in a hiatal hernia sac, if present) by turning the supine patient about 45° on his right side. The patient is then given several swallows of plain water. As the lower esophageal sphincter relaxes to allow passage of the water, barium may reflux from the stomach into the esophagus. Small amounts of reflux may be within normal limits. Reflux of barium of more than a few centimeters, however, is considered abnormal. At times, contrast can reflux as high as the aortic arch. Another method for demonstrating reflux is to have the patient change his position. As the patient turns from prone to supine or vice versa (either during fluoroscopy or for overhead views), reflux of barium from the stomach into the esophagus can often be detected.

It must be remembered that failure to demonstrate reflux radiographically does not exclude the possibility that a patient's esophagitis is related to reflux. As long as typical radiographic findings of reflux esophagitis are noted, there is little reason to persist in strenuous efforts to actually demonstrate retrograde flow of barium from the stomach into the esophagus. Conversely, demonstration of reflux in the absence of other radiographic findings in the distal esophagus does not permit the radiographic diagnosis of esophagitis. Whether or not reflux will lead to the development of esophagitis depends on such factors as the frequency with which the reflux occurs, the efficiency of secondary peristalsis in removing refluxed contents from the esophagus, and the acidity of the gastric contents. The presence or absence of a sliding hiatal hernia is of little practical significance, since reflux is not directly related to the presence of a hernia but rather is due to incompetence of the lower esophageal sphincter.

A radionuclide technique for demonstrating and measuring gastroesophageal reflux is to scan the lower esophagus and stomach after the oral administration of ^{99m}Tc DTPA (Fig. 4-4). If no spontaneous reflux of radionuclide from the stomach into the distal esophagus is observed, an abdominal binder is used to raise intragastric pressure. This radionuclide technique has been reported to have an accuracy rate of about 90% in demonstrating gastroesophageal reflux.

RADIOGRAPHIC FINDINGS

Compared with direct esophagoscopy, the barium swallow has been considered a relatively insensitive procedure for demonstrating early esophageal changes consistent with reflux esophagitis. As the severity of esophageal inflammation increases, the sensitivity and accuracy of the barium swallow improve.

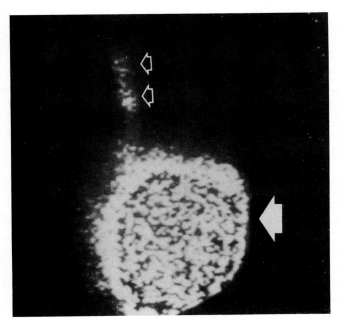

Fig. 4-4. Gastroesophageal reflux. Note the reflux of radionuclide into the esophagus **(small, open arrows)** from the stomach **(large, solid arrow)** following the oral administration of ^{99m}Tc DTPA.

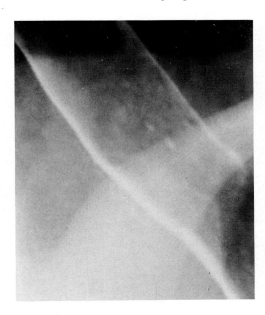

Fig. 4-5. Reflux esophagitis. Superficial ulcerations or erosions appear as streaks or dots of contrast superimposed on the flat mucosa of the distal esophagus.

The earliest radiographic findings in reflux esophagitis are detectable on double-contrast studies. They consist of superficial ulcerations or erosions that appear as streaks or dots of barium superimposed on the flat mucosa of the distal esophagus (Fig. 4-5). These ulcers often have a linear configuration and may be associated with fine radiating folds and slight retraction of the esophageal wall (Fig. 4-6). In single-contrast studies of patients with esophagitis, the outer borders of the barium-filled esophagus are not sharply seen, but rather have a hazy, serrated appearance with shallow, irregular protrusions that are indicative of erosions of varying length and depth (Fig. 4-7). This marginal serration must be distinguished from the fine, regular transverse folds (feline esophagus, so named because it is characteristic of the distal third of the esophagus of the cat) that were originally described as a normal variant on double-contrast studies but are now considered a transient motility phenomenon seen with increased frequency in patients with gastroesophageal reflux (Fig. 4-8). These folds are transient in nature, are often seen on only one of a number of spot films during a given examination, and are probably caused by contraction of longitudinal fibers of the muscularis mucosae. Fixed transverse folds in the esophagus, producing a series of horizontal, relatively parallel collections of barium in a "stepladder" arrangement, have been reported to reflect longitudinal scarring from reflux esophagitis. Unlike the delicate feline folds that are transient and extend completely across the esophagus without interruption, the fixed transverse folds in chronic esophagitis are wider and fewer, and do not extend completely across the esophagus. Fixed transverse

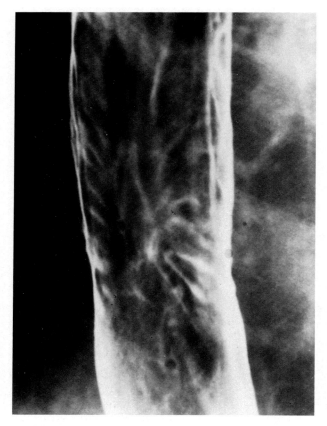

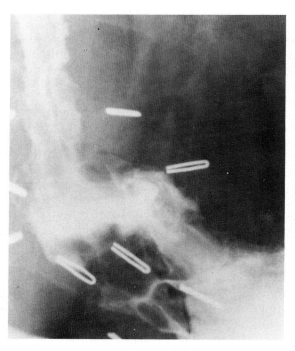

Fig. 4-6. Reflux esophagitis. Numerous radiating folds surround a distal esophageal ulceration. (Goldstein HM, Bova JG: Esophagitis. In Taveras JM, Ferrucci JT (eds): Radiology: Diagnosis–Imaging–Intervention. Philadelphia, JB Lippincott, 1987)

Fig. 4-7. Esophagitis following a failed Nissen procedure for a hiatal hernia and gastroesophageal reflux. The margins of the distal esophagus appear hazy and serrated.

folds are persistent throughout the entire examination and are almost invariably associated with other evidence of scarring from reflux esophagitis. In some cases the folds are associated with longitudinally oriented, linear ulcers which may predispose to longitudinal scarring of the esophagus. The fixed transverse folds must be distinguished from the broad transverse bands that are a transient phenomenon in patients with nonpropulsive, tertiary esophageal contractions.

In esophagitis there is a smudgy, irregular pattern of residual barium in contrast to the fine, sharply demarcated longitudinal folds of the collapsed esophagus in normal persons. In more severe disease, obvious erosions can be seen extending even into the midesophagus. Widening and coarsening of edematous longitudinal folds can simulate filling defects.

In addition to diffuse erosion, reflux esophagitis can result in large penetrating ulcers (marginal ulcers) in the region of the junction between the esophagus and stomach or hiatal hernia sac (Fig.

4-9), or in the hiatal hernia sac itself (Fig. 4-10). In about 15% of patients, a marginal ulcer penetrates through the wall of the esophagus into adjacent vital structures. Free perforation, though uncommon, is associated with such complications as peritonitis, subphrenic abscess, mediastinitis, pericarditis, and empyema. Marginal ulcers have a radiographic appearance similar to gastric ulcers due to chronic peptic disease. A nichelike projection is surrounded by intramural inflammation (ulcer collar), often with much local esophageal spasm and narrowing. Healing of a large or penetrating esophageal ulcer can result in stricture formation (Fig. 4-11).

BARRETT'S ESOPHAGUS

Barrett's esophagus is a condition in which the normal stratified squamous lining of the lower esophagus is replaced by columnar epithelium similar to that of the stomach. This process is presumed to

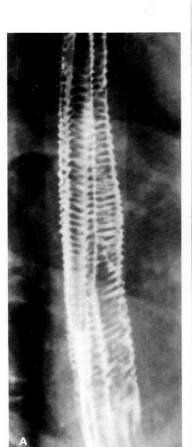

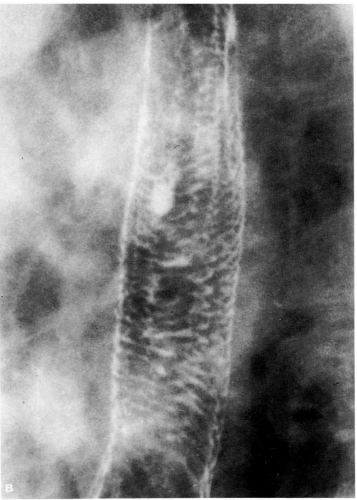

4-8

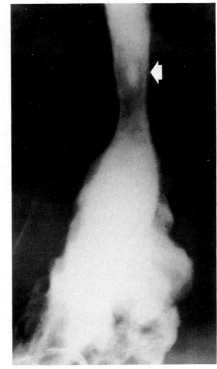

4-9

Fig. 4-8. Feline esophagus. Two examples of prominent transverse esophageal folds. ([**A**] Bova JG, Goldstein HM: The esophagus, examination technique and anatomy. In Taveras JM, Ferrucci JT (eds): Radiology: Diagnosis–Imaging–Intervention. Philadelphia, JB Lippincott, 1987; [**B**] Gohel VK, Edell SL, Laufer I et al: Transverse folds in the human esophagus. Radiology 128:303–308, 1978)

Fig. 4-9. Large, penetrating ulcer **(arrow)** in reflux esophagitis.

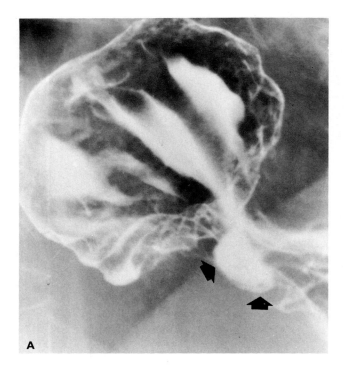

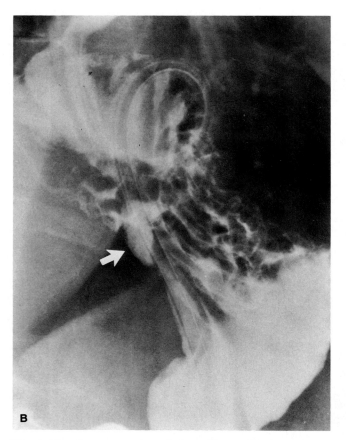

Fig. 4-10. Two examples of ulcers **(arrows)** in large hiatal hernia sacs.

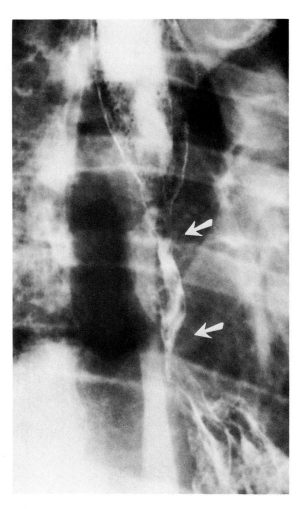

Fig. 4-11. Stricture **(arrows)** following healing of reflux esophagitis.

occur as a complication of reflux esophagitis, especially in view of the frequency with which the syndrome is associated with a sliding hiatal hernia and demonstrable gastroesophageal reflux.

RADIOGRAPHIC FINDINGS

Esophageal ulceration in Barrett's esophagus can occur anywhere along the columnar epithelium and tends to develop at a distance from the cardia, even as high as the aortic arch (Fig. 4-12). Unlike the shallow ulceration usually caused by reflux esophagitis in the squamous epithelium, the Barrett's ulcer tends to be deep and penetrating and identical to peptic gastric ulceration (Fig. 4-13). Stricture formation usually accompanies the ulceration. Not infrequently, no ulceration is evident and only a smooth, tapered stricture is seen.

The presence of a delicate reticular pattern of multiple barium-filled grooves or crevices in the esophagus adjacent to a stricture and extending dis-

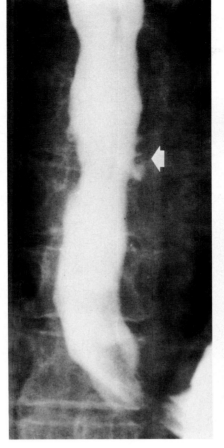

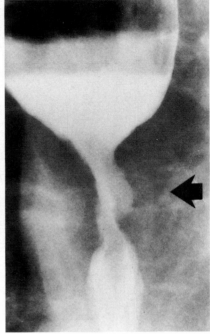

Fig. 4-12. Barrett's esophagus. Ulcerations **(arrow)** have developed at a distance from the esophagogastric junction.

Fig. 4-13. Barrett's esophagus. Note the deep ulcer **(arrow)** with stricture formation.

Fig. 4-14. Barrett's esophagus. Double-contrast view of the midesophagus in a patient with midsternal discomfort shows an irregular nodular mucosal pattern. (Torres WE: Radiology of the esophagus. In Gedgaudas–McClees RK [ed]: Handbook of Gastrointestinal Imaging. New York, Churchill Livingstone, 1987)

4-12

4-13

tally a short but variable distance from it or within an area of columnar epithelium has been suggested as a specific radiographic indication of the villous metaplasia of the specialized columnar epithelium of Barrett's esophagus (Figs. 4-14, 4-15). However, this reticular pattern is apparently nonspecific and has also been reported in such conditions as candidal and viral esophagitis, superficial spreading carcinoma (Fig. 4-16), and areae gastricae in a small hiatal hernia.

A sliding hiatal heria with gastroesophageal reflux is commonly demonstrated in patients with Barrett's esophagus. In most cases, however, the Barrett's ulcer is separated from the hiatal hernia by a variable length of normal-appearing esophagus (Fig. 4-17), in contrast to reflux esophagitis, in which the distal esophagus is abnormal down to the level of the hernia.

Radionuclide examination with intravenous pertechnetate can be used to demonstrate a Barrett's esophagus. Because this radionuclide is actively taken up by the gastric type of mucosa, continuous concentration of the isotope in the distal esophagus to a level that corresponds approximately to that of the ulcer or stricture is indicative of a Barrett's esophagus and may obviate the need for mucosal biopsy (Fig. 4-18).

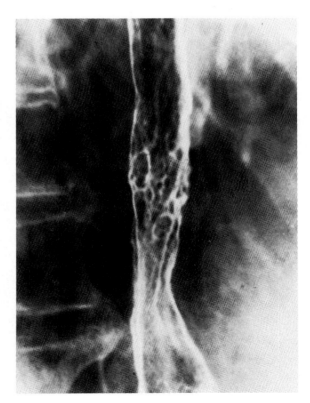

4-14

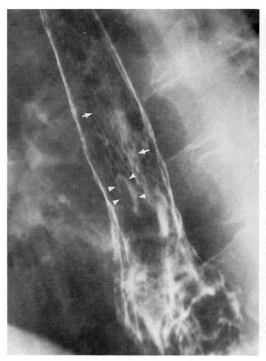

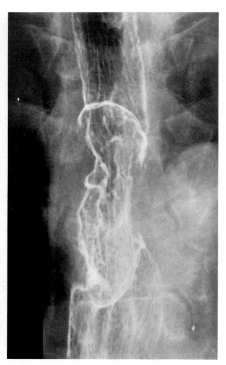

4-15

4-16

Fig. 4-15. Reticular pattern in Barrett's esophagus. Reticular pattern **(arrows)** in columnar epithelium with esophagitis proximal to a large ulcer niche **(arrowheads)**. (Vincent ME, Robbins AH, Spechler SJ et al: The reticular pattern as a radiographic sign of the Barrett esophagus: An assessment. Radiology 153:333–335, 1984)

Fig. 4-16. Reticular pattern in squamous carcinoma. The mucosa both proximal and distal to this tumor shows a fine linear reticular pattern, which may represent lymphedema or submucosal infiltration of the tumor. (Vincent ME, Robbins AH, Spechler SJ et al: The reticular pattern as a radiographic sign of the Barrett esophagus: An assessment. Radiology 153:333–335, 1984)

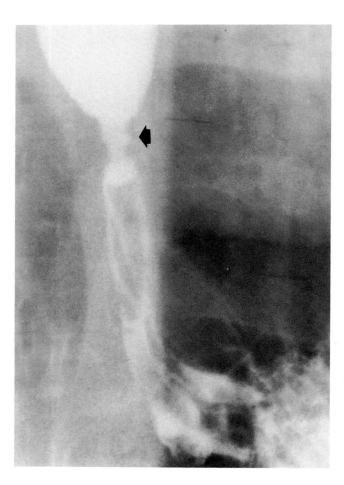

Fig. 4-17. Barrett's esophagus. Several centimeters of relatively normal-appearing, nondilated esophagus separate the Barrett's ulcer **(arrow)** from the hiatal hernia sac.

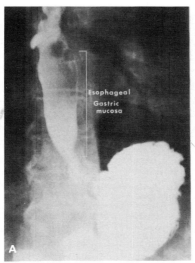
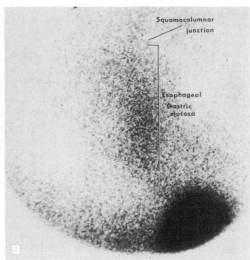

Fig. 4-18. Barrett's esophagus. **(A)** Barium swallow. **(B)** ^{99m}Tc pertechnetate scintigram. The uptake of isotope extends above the esophagogastric junction to a level comparable to the esophageal stricture and ulcer on the radiograph. (Berquist TH, Nolan NG, Stephens DH et al: Radioisotope scintigraphy in diagnosis of Barrett's esophagus. AJR 123:401–411, 1975. Copyright 1975. Reproduced with permission)

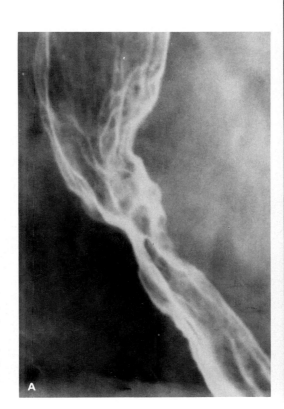
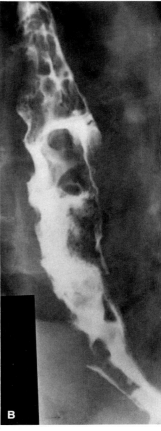

Fig. 4-19. Adenocarcinoma in Barrett's esophagus. **(A)** Irregular, infiltrating stricture. **(B)** Varicoid appearance due to submucosal spread of tumor. (Levine MS, Caroline D, Thompson JJ et al: Adenocarcinoma of the esophagus: Relationship to Barrett mucosa. Radiology 150:305–309, 1984)

In addition to postinflammatory stricture, Barrett's esophagus has an unusually high propensity for developing malignancy in the columnar-lined portion. In one series, adenocarcinoma, which is usually very rare in the esophagus, developed in 10% of patients with Barrett's esophagus. Radiographically, adenocarcinoma arising in Barrett's esophagus may have a polypoid, ulcerating, infiltrating, or varicoid appearance that is indistinguishable from squamous cell carcinoma (Fig. 4-19). Unlike squamous cell carcinoma of the esophagus, however, in the majority of cases the adenocarcinoma arising in Barrett's esophagus spreads distally to involve the gastric cardia or fundus.

CANDIDA ESOPHAGITIS

The most common infectious disease of the esophagus is candidiasis, caused by the usually harmless fungus *Candida albicans*. *Candida* is found in the mouth, throat, sputum, and feces of many normal children and adults. Acute infection by *Candida* develops when there is an immunologic imbalance between the host and the normal body flora. Esophageal candidiasis occurs most frequently in patients with leukemia or lymphoma and in patients receiving radiation therapy, chemotherapy, corticosteroids, or other immunosuppressive agents. Chronic debilitating diseases predisposing to the development of esophageal candidiasis include diabetes mellitus, systemic lupus erythematosus, multiple myeloma, primary hypoparathyroidism, and renal failure. In a recent study, candidal infestation of the oral cavity and the esophagus was the most common gastrointestinal infection encountered in patients with AIDS (Fig. 4-20). More than 75% of these patients will develop oroesophageal candidiasis during the course of the disease. Esophageal candidiasis can be found in otherwise healthy adults who have received antibiotics (especially tetracycline) for upper respiratory infection. It has been suggested that the fungi overgrow in this case because they do not have to compete for nutritive substances with the normal bacterial flora that have been destroyed by the antibiotics. Esophageal candidiasis has been reported as a complication of stasis secondary to functional or mechanical obstruction. On rare occasions, candidal infection may occur in patients who are in apparently good health and have no predisposing disease.

The symptoms of esophageal candidiasis can be acute or insidious. In acute disease, adynophagia (pain associated with swallowing) is usually intense and is localized to the upper retrosternal area, often radiating into the back. Chest pain may precede dysphagia and be so severe that a myocardial infarction is suggested. It is important to remember that esophageal candidiasis can occur with minimal or absent oral involvement (thrush). If it is promptly treated, complete recovery can be rapid. If the organism enters the circulation through ruptured esophageal vessels, systemic invasion can lead to the dissemination of *Candida* to other organs and often to a fatal outcome.

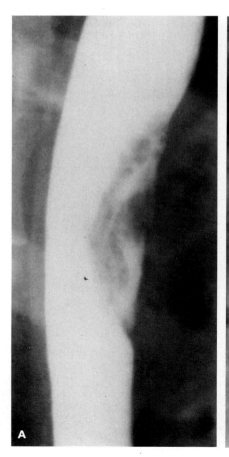
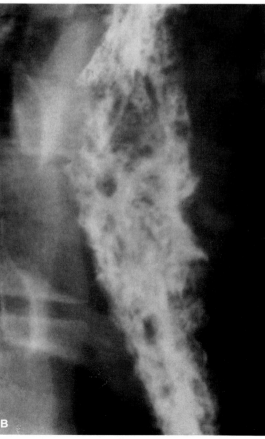

Fig. 4-20. *Candida* esophagitis in AIDS. **(A)** Ulcerating, nodular mass involving the anterior wall of the esophagus. Because the fixed nature of the lesion suggested a neoplasm, endoscopic biopsy was performed that revealed *Candida* infestation. After 5 weeks of treatment with amphotericin B and 5-fluorocytosine, repeat endoscopy showed resolution of esophageal ulceration. **(B)** Barium swallow 3 weeks later when the patient complained of odynophagia shows severe mucosal ulceration and nodularity of the entire esophagus. (Farman J, Tavitian A, Rosenthal LE et al: Focal esophageal candidiasis in acquired immunodeficiency syndrome (AIDS). Gastrointest Radiol 11:213–217, 1986)

RADIOGRAPHIC FINDINGS

The radiographic changes in candidiasis frequently involve the entire thoracic esophagus, though the upper half is often relatively spared. Early in the course of disease, an esophagram generally shows only abnormal motility and a slightly dilated, virtually atonic esophagus. The earliest morphologic changes are small, marginal filling defects (simulating tiny air bubbles) with fine serrations along the outer border. As the disease progresses, an irregular cobblestone pattern is produced that reflects either submucosal edema in combination with ulceration or small pseudomembranous plaques composed of fungi and debris that cover the ulcerated esophageal mucosa (Fig. 4-21). The nodular appearance of the esophageal surface can also be due to the direct seeding of *Candida* colonies on the mucosa. The classic radiographic appearance of esophageal candidiasis is a shaggy marginal contour caused by deep ulcerations and sloughing of the mucosa (Fig. 4-22). Ulcerations are multiple and of varying size (Fig. 4-23); the intervening esophageal contour is nodular, with irregular round and oval defects that can resemble varices. The overlying pseudomembrane occasionally partially separates from the

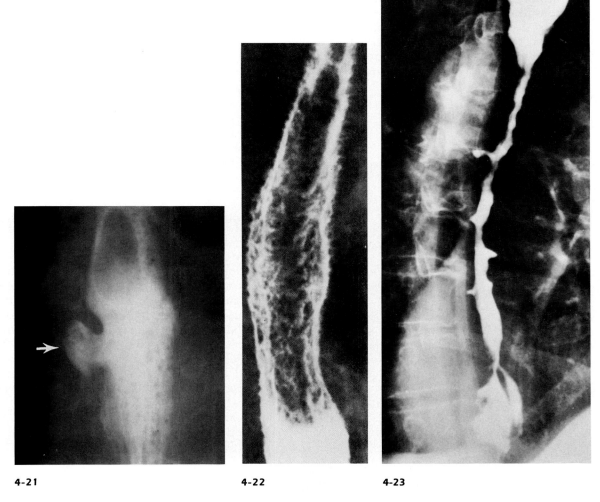

4-21   4-22   4-23

Fig. 4-21. Candidiasis. A nodular cobblestone pattern is seen in combination with large, discrete ulceration.

Fig. 4-22. *Candida* esophagitis. Multiple ulcers and nodular plaques produce the grossly irregular contour of a shaggy esophagus. This manifestation of far-advanced candidiasis is now infrequent because of earlier and better treatment of the disease.

Fig. 4-23. Candidiasis. Diffuse transverse ulcerations are evident with irregular esophageal narrowing. (Ott DJ, Gelfand DW: Esophageal stricture secondary to candidiasis. Gastrointest Radiol 2:323–325, 1978)

esophageal wall, permitting barium to penetrate under it and form a double track paralleling the esophageal lumen.

In patients with AIDS, candidiasis may present as a single large esophageal ulcer rather than the multiplicity of small ulcers seen in patients with other underlying disorders (Fig. 4-24). The remainder of the esophagus typically appears normal on radiographic examination, though endoscopic examination usually shows diffuse superficial involvement of the entire esophagus. Recognition of this unusual focal esophageal lesion in AIDS is essential to prevent the incorrect diagnosis of esophageal carcinoma.

In patients with a hematologic malignancy, chronic debilitating disease, or AIDS, or in patients who have recently undergone a course of antibiotic or chemotherapy, the development of dysphagia and retrosternal pain should strongly suggest the diagnosis of esophageal candidiasis. A barium swallow usually confirms the diagnosis; only if the radiographic findings are not diagnostic is esophagoscopy indicated.

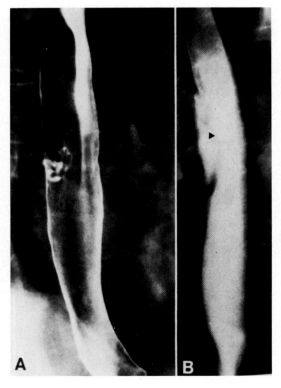

Fig. 4-24. Focal candidiasis in AIDS. **(A)** Initial double-contrast examination of the esophagus shows an oval-shaped ulcer with a lobulated distal margin. **(B)** Single-contrast examination 1 month later after a short course of amphotericin B again demonstrates an oval-shaped ulcer. (Bier SJ, Keller RJ, Krivisky BA et al: Esophageal monoliasis: A new radiographic presentation. Am J Gastroenterol 80:734–737, 1985)

HERPETIC ESOPHAGITIS

A clinical and radiographic pattern indistinguishable from *Candida* esophagitis can be caused by herpes simplex infection (Fig. 4-25). Herpetic esophagitis predominantly affects patients with disseminated malignancy or abnormal immune systems. Occasionally, herpes esophagitis may occur in otherwise healthy patients presenting with odynophagia, dysphagia, or gastrointestinal bleeding.

Double-contrast radiographic studies may demonstrate multiple discrete ulcers, plaquelike defects without ulceration, or a combination of ulcers and plaques in the mid or occasionally distal esophagus. When plaquelike defects are identified, the findings may be indistinguishable radiographically from *Candida* esophagitis (Fig. 4-26). However, the presence of discrete, superficial ulcers on an otherwise normal background mucosa should suggest the diagnosis of herpetic esophagitis (Fig. 4-27), because the ulceration in candidiasis almost always occurs on a background of diffuse plaque formation. Because the viral inflammation is usually self-limited, a response to antifungal therapy cannot be considered proof that the characteristic radiographic changes are the result of *Candida* infection. For the diagnosis of herpetic esophagitis to be made, esophagoscopy with biopsy and cytology is required.

CYTOMEGALOVIRUS ESOPHAGITIS

Cytomegalovirus is a herpesvirus that is widely distributed in nature. In the normal adult host, infection is usually subclinical. However, the organism is a major cause of morbidity in immunocompromised patients, including those with disseminated malignancy and organ transplantation, and most recently in patients with AIDS (Fig. 4-28). Esophageal involvement may produce a diffuse or segmental ulcerative esophagitis, primarily affecting the distal half of the esophagus with extension into the gastric fundus. Occasionally, a focal giant esophageal ulcer may develop, most likely related to ischemic necrosis of the bowel wall due to a viral-induced vasculitis.

TUBERCULOUS ESOPHAGITIS

Tuberculosis of the esophagus is rare and almost invariably secondary to terminal disease in the lungs. Tuberculous involvement of the esophagus can result from the swallowing of infected sputum, direct extension from laryngeal or pharyngeal lesions, or contiguous extension from caseous hilar lymph nodes or infected vertebrae; it also can be part of generalized, disseminated miliary disease.

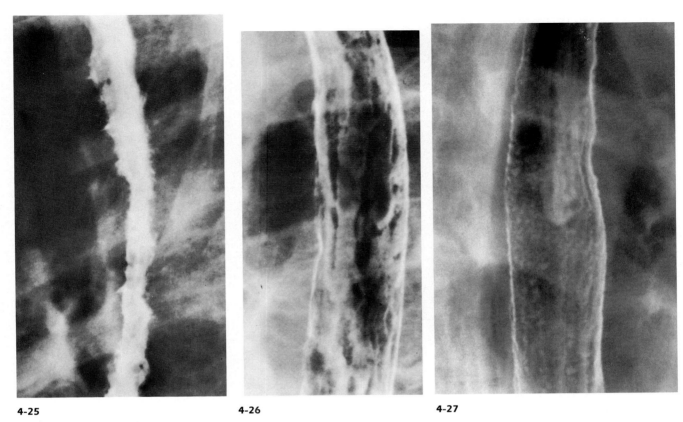

4-25   4-26   4-27

Fig. 4-25. Herpetic esophagitis. The diffuse irregularity and ulceration are indistinguishable from *Candida* esophagitis.

Fig. 4-26. Herpetic esophagitis. Fine ulcerations are superimposed on a pattern of thickened folds and plaquelike defects.

Fig. 4-27. Herpetic esophagitis. Numerous discrete, superficial ulcers in the midesophagus. (DeGaeta L, Levine MS, Guglielmi GE et al: Herpes esophagitis in an otherwise healthy patient. AJR 144:1205–1206, 1985. Copyright 1985. Reproduced with permission.)

The most common manifestation of tuberculosis of the esophagus is single or multiple ulcers (Fig. 4-29). An intense fibrotic response often causes narrowing of the esophageal lumen. Numerous miliary granulomas in the mucosal layer occasionally give the appearance of multiple nodules. Sinuses and fistulous tracts are common; their presence in a patient with severe pulmonary tuberculosis who has a midesophageal ulcer or stricture in the region of the tracheal bifurcation should suggest a tuberculous etiology.

CROHN'S ESOPHAGITIS

The esophagus is the rarest site of Crohn's disease involvement in the gastrointestinal tract. When the esophagus is involved, the patient almost always has concomitant ileocolic disease. As elsewhere in the gastrointestinal tract, the earliest radiographic sign of esophageal Crohn's disease is the presence of aphthous ulcers, which appear as punctate, slitlike, or ringlike collections of barium surrounded by a faint radiolucent halo (Fig. 4-30). With further esophageal involvement, the size and number of the ulcers may increase, producing a localized or diffuse esophagitis. As these ulcers enlarge, they often assume a linear or serpiginous configuration. Eventually, the esophagus may be diffusely involved by deep, irregular areas of ulceration. Severe esophagitis may also be manifested by thickened, nodular, or varicoid folds, pseudomembrane formation, and rarely a diffusely cobblestoned mucosal pattern. The transmural nature of the disease may be reflected by the development of multiple transverse or, more commonly, longitudinal intramural fistulous tracts similar to those found in granulomatous colitis (Fig. 4-31). In advanced cases, esophageal perforation may lead to the formation of esophagorespiratory, esophagomediastinal, or esophagogastric fistulas.

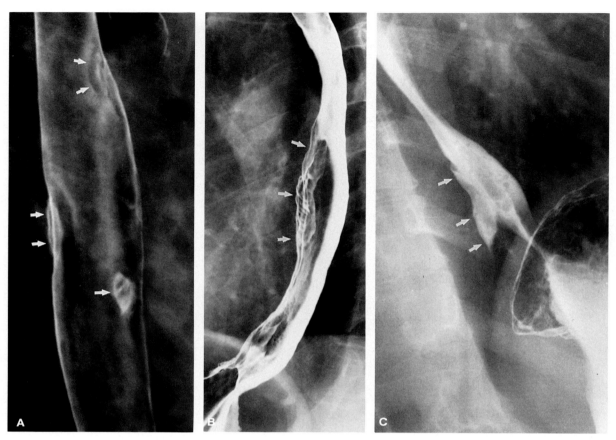

Fig. 4-28. Cytomegalovirus esophagitis in three different patients. **(A)** Four discrete ulcers **(arrows)**. **(B)** Inflammatory mucosal changes involving a short segment of the distal esophagus **(arrows)**. **(C)** Deep focal ulcer in the distal esophagus. (Balthazar EJ, Megibow AJ, Hulnick DH: Cytomegalovirus esophagitis and gastritis in AIDS. AJR 144:1201–1204, 1985. Copyright 1985. Reproduced with permission.)

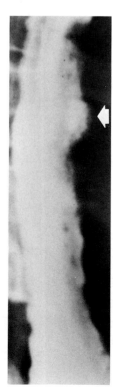

Fig. 4-29. Tuberculosis. A large, midesophageal ulcer **(arrow)** with surrounding inflammatory edema mimics carcinoma. Note the generalized irregularity which represents diffuse ulcerative disease.

OTHER INFECTIOUS/GRANULOMATOUS/ INFLAMMATORY CAUSES OF ESOPHAGITIS

One of the many appearances of syphilis involving the esophagus is fine mucosal irregularity or frank esophageal ulceration. An ulcerated midesophageal mass due to lymph node erosion can be seen in patients with mediastinal histoplasmosis. Acute alcohol ingestion may produce a severe erosive esophagitis with multiple superficial ulcers in the mid and distal portions (Fig. 4-32). It is unclear whether this appearance reflects chemical irritation by alcohol or a combination of increased gastroesophageal reflux and associated motor dysfunction that commonly occurs in alcohol intoxication and results in impaired clearance of refluxed material from the esophagus. Marked clinical improvement occurs 1 to 2 weeks after alcohol is withdrawn. Nodularity and fine superficial ulcerations have been described in a single case of esophagitis with peripheral and submucosal eosinophilia resembling eosinophilic gastroenteritis (Fig. 4-33). A rare manifestation of Behcet's syndrome is single or multiple esophageal ulcers, which may be complicated by perforation or severe luminal stenosis (see Fig.

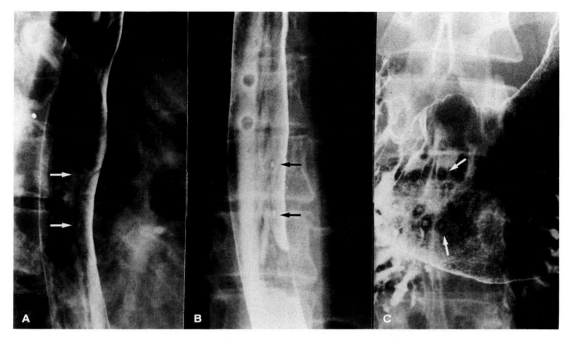

Fig. 4-30. Crohn's esophagitis. **(A, B)** Two aphthous ulcers in the middle third of the esophagus **(arrows)**. They consist of a small central collection of barium with a diameter of 2–3 mm, surrounded by a radiolucent halo of 2 mm. **(C)** In the same patient, numerous aphthous ulcers are also present in the horizontal segment of the stomach **(arrows)**. (Degryse HRM, DeSchepper AMAP: Aphthoid esophageal ulcers in Crohn's disease of ileum and colon. Gastrointest Radiol 9:197–201, 1984)

Fig. 4-31. Crohn's esophagitis. Long intramural sinus tract **(arrows)**. (Ghahremani GG, Gore RM, Breuer RI et al: Esophageal manifestations of Crohn's disease. Gastrointest Radiol 7: 199–203, 1982)

Fig. 4-32. Acute alcoholic esophagitis. Multiple superficial ulcers in the mid and distal portions in a patient with hematemesis, odynophagia, and dysphagia following an alcoholic episode.

Fig. 4-33. Eosinophilic esophagitis. Fine, superficial ulcerations are visible with diffuse nodularity. (Picus D, Frank PH: Eosinophilic esophagitis. AJR 136:1001–1003, 1981. Copyright 1981. Reproduced with permission)

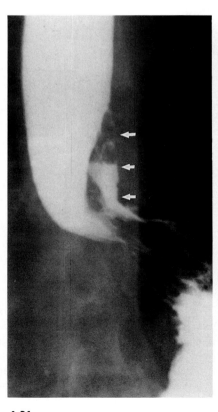 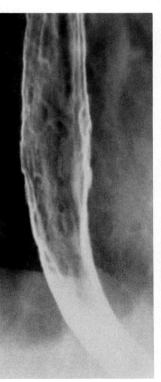 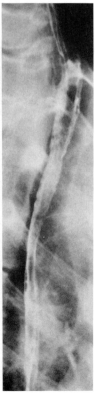

4-31 4-32 4-33

5-42). Ulceration can rarely be seen in association with more characteristic strictures in epidermolysis bullosa (Fig. 4-34).

CARCINOMA OF THE ESOPHAGUS

Carcinoma of the esophagus (95% squamous cell) is frequently associated with some degree of mucosal ulceration (Fig. 4-35). An ulcerating carcinoma typically appears as a crater surrounded by a bulging

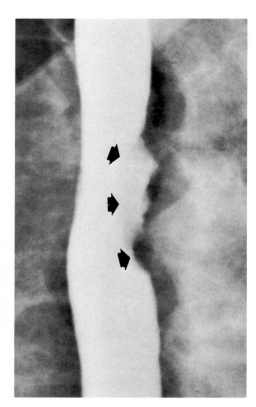

Fig. 4-35. *Squamous carcinoma of the esophagus. Note the eccentric, ulcerated mass* **(arrows)**.

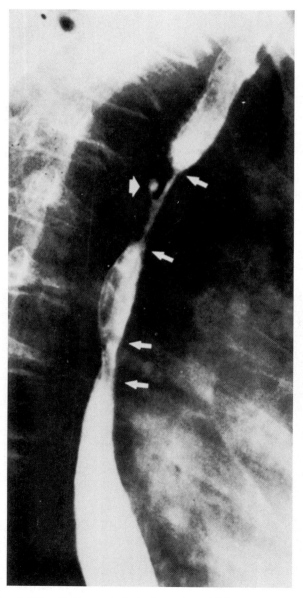

Fig. 4-34. *Epidermolysis bullosa. In addition to the two strictures* **(thin arrows)**, *there is an ulcer* **(broad arrow)** *that projects posteriorly from the midportion of the upper stricture. (Agha FP, Francis IR, Ellis CN: Esophageal involvement in epidermolysis bullosa dystrophica: Clinical and roentgenographic manifestations. Gastrointest Radiol 8:111–117, 1983)*

mass projecting into the esophageal lumen (Fig. 4-36). When examined in profile, the underside of the oval ulcer niche is often found to be bordered by a clear ridge extending from its upper to its lower limits, an excellent sign of malignancy. The ulcerated surface is rigid and remains unchanged by the passage of barium or primary peristaltic waves (Fig. 4-37). The wall opposite the niche may be normal but often demonstrates irregularity and lack of pliability, indicating mucosal destruction from an infiltrating tumor. In the relatively uncommon primary ulcerative esophageal carcinoma, ulceration of virtually all of an eccentric, flat mass produces a meniscoid appearance analagous to the Carman sign seen with gastric malignancy (Figs. 4-38, 4-39). Ulceration in a polypoid mass or an area of irregular narrowing is an infrequent manifestation of lymphoma of the esophagus. Progressive metastatic enlargement of mediastinal lymph nodes may cause erosion and even mucosal ulceration of the esophagus.

CORROSIVE ESOPHAGITIS

The ingestion of corrosive agents causes acute and chronic inflammatory changes that are most commonly seen in the lower two-thirds of the esophagus (Fig. 4-40). The most severe corrosive injuries are caused by alkali (lye, dishwasher detergents, washing soda) that penetrate the layers of the esophagus and cause a severe liquefying necrosis. Ingestion of acids (sulfuric, nitric, hydrochloric) is less likely to produce severe damage because of coagulation of the superficial layers, which forms a firm eschar limiting penetration to the deeper layers. The harmful effect of ingested acid is also partially neutralized by the alkaline *p*H of the esophagus.

Mucosal ulceration always occurs following the ingestion of corrosive materials. Superficial penetration of the toxic agent results in only minimal ulceration with mild erythema or mucosal edema. Deeper penetration into the submucosal and mus-

cular layers causes sloughing of destroyed tissue and deep ulceration. In such cases, the resultant granulation tissue with numerous fibroblasts leads to the deposition of collagen, fibrous scarring, and gradual narrowing of the esophagus (Fig. 4-40).

RADIATION INJURY

Esophagitis can be an undesirable side-effect of mediastinal radiation therapy, especially if combined with chemotherapy. Doses of radiation of greater

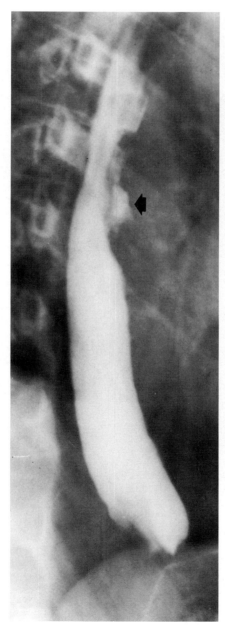

4-36

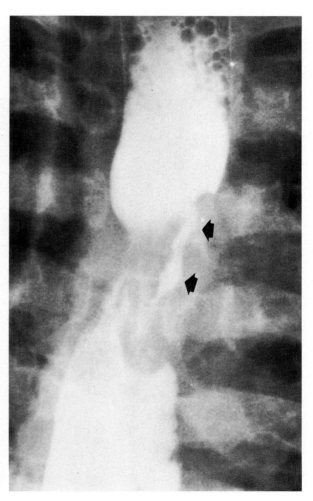

4-37

Fig. 4-36. *Squamous carcinoma of the esophagus. On profile view, the lesion appears as an ulcer crater* **(arrow)** *surrounded by a bulging mass projecting into the esophageal lumen.*

Fig. 4-37. *Squamous carcinoma of the esophagus. Note the long ulceration* **(arrows)** *in the large, rigid lesion.*

than 4500 rad frequently lead to severe esophagitis with irreversible stricture formation. Similar complications can occur with doses of less than 2000 rads of mediastinal radiation in patients who simultaneously or sequentially receive Adriamycin (doxorubicin) or actinomycin D (Fig. 4-41). With each course of chemotherapy, there are recurrent episodes of esophagitis (recall phenomenon). The radiographic appearance of esophagitis in these patients is indistinguishable from that of *Candida* esophagitis, a far more common condition in patients undergoing chemotherapy and radiation therapy for malignant disease. The correct diagnosis

should be suggested whenever a patient who develops esophagitis after radiation therapy and administration of Adriamycin (doxorubicin) has no clinical evidence of oral or pharyngeal candidiasis and does not respond to treatment with appropriate antifungal agents.

DRUG-INDUCED ESOPHAGITIS

Drug-induced ulceration of the esophagus is caused by a direct irritant effect of the medication due to

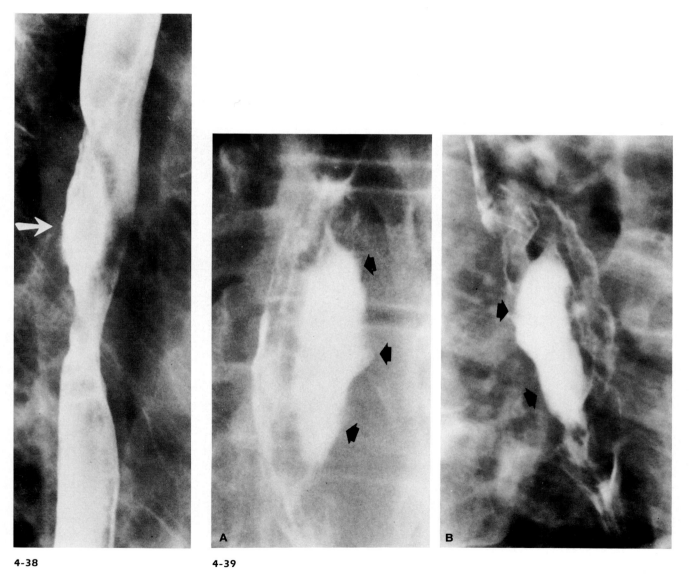

4-38   4-39

Fig. 4-38. Primary ulcerative carcinoma. An esophagram demonstrates a typical meniscoid ulcer **(arrow)** surrounded by a rim of neoplastic tissue. (Gloyna RE, Zornoza J, Goldstein HM: Primary ulcerative carcinoma of the esophagus. AJR 129:599–600, 1977. Copyright 1977. Reproduced with permission)

Fig. 4-39. Primary ulcerative carcinoma. Characteristic meniscoid ulceration **(arrows)** surrounded by a tumor mass is seen in **(A)** frontal and **(B)** lateral projections.

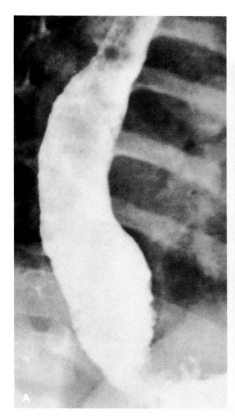

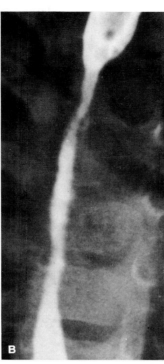

Fig. 4-40. Caustic esophagitis. **(A)** Dilated, boggy esophagus with ulceration 8 days after the ingestion of a corrosive agent. **(B)** Stricture formation is evident on an esophagram performed 3 months after the caustic injury.

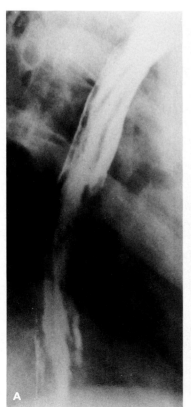

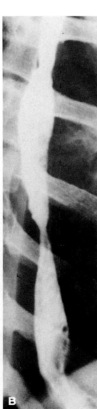

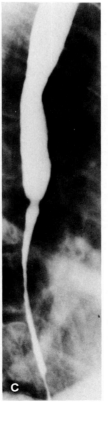

Fig. 4-41. Esophagitis induced by combined radiation and Adriamycin (doxorubicin). **(A))** Barium esophagram performed 10 days after the onset of symptoms demonstrates a dilated esophagus with thickened mucosal folds. Peristaltic activity was diminished at fluoroscopy. **(B)** Esophagram 16 days after the onset of symptoms demonstrates a narrowed esophagus with markedly irregular mucosa and formation of a stricture in the distal half. No peristalsis was evident at fluoroscopy. **(C)** High-grade stenosis involving about 9 cm of the distal esophagus with significant obstruction was found on follow-up examination 2 months after the onset of symptoms. The lumen of the stricture is irregular. The transition from the proximal esophagus, although abrupt, appears benign and is characterized by concentric narrowing. (Boal DKB, Newburger PE, Teele RL: Esophagitis induced by combined radiation and adriamycin. AJR 132:567–570, 1979. Copyright 1979. Reproduced with permission)

prolonged contact with the esophageal mucosa. Slow clearance of the medication due to the large size of the tablet or delayed esophageal transit time is a contributing factor, though most patients with drug-induced esophagitis have no intrinsic esophageal disease. A typical scenario is a patient who ingested medication, particularly with little or no water, immediately before going to bed. A relative obstruction, such as an esophageal stricture or marked left atrial enlargement, may also lead to a drug remaining in prolonged contact with the mucosal surface of the esophagus.

The most common drugs causing esophageal ulceration include potassium chloride in tablet form, tetracycline, emepronium bromide (an anticholinergic agent commonly used in the treatment of urinary frequency and nocturia), quinidine, ascorbic acid, and ferrous sulfate. All of these drugs are apparently weak caustic agents that are innocuous when they pass rapidly through the esophagus.

The clinical presentation of drug-induced esophagitis is the sudden or rapid onset of dysphagia, retrosternal pain, or odynophagia 1 to 12 hours after ingestion of the medication. Radiographically, solitary or multiple shallow ulcers are seen on one wall or may be distributed circumferentially in the proximal esophagus (Fig. 4-42). The predilection for involvement of the aortic segment of the esophagus may be due to its being the transition zone between skeletal and smooth muscle and thus subject to discoordinate peristaltic activity that permits prolonged mucosal contact with ingested medication.

SCLEROTHERAPY OF ESOPHAGEAL VARICES

Inflammatory changes characteristic of an acute esophagitis frequently develop following sclerotherapy of esophageal varices. The ulcerations may be focal or diffuse, vary in size, shape, and depth, and are the most frequent cause of postsclerotherapy rebleeding (Fig. 4-43). The degree of ulceration is directly related to the amount of sclerosant solution used, the number of injections, and the number of columns of varices injected. Superficial ulcerations heal with no sequelae or minor mucosal irregular-

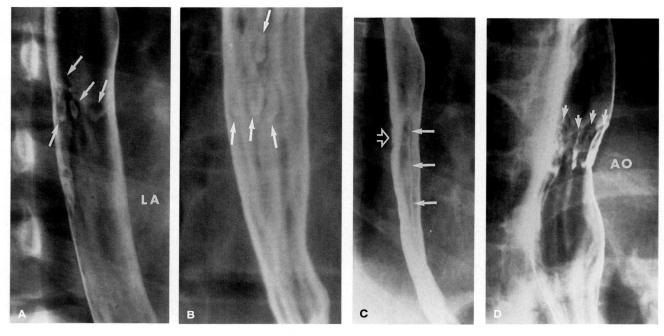

Fig. 4-42. *Medication-induced esophagitis.* **(A)** *Several discrete ulcers* **(arrows)** *with lucent halos of edema located above the level of the left atrium* **(LA)** *in a young woman who experienced sudden chest pain and odynophagia after taking aspirin regularly for 8 days for headaches.* **(B)** *Cluster of ovoid ulcerations* **(arrows)** *with surrounding edema in the midesophagus of a young man with severe odynophagia after nine vitamin and mineral tablets daily for 3 months.* **(C)** *Focal ulcer in profile* **(open arrow)** *and a long, linear ulceration* **(arrows)** *related to doxycycline therapy.* **(D)** *Several focal and linear ulcers* **(arrows)** *coalescing in the proximal thoracic esophagus at the level of the aortic arch* **(AO)** *related to the ingestion of penicillin tablets for pharyngitis.* (Bova JG, Dutton NE, Goldstein HM et al: Medication-induced esophagitis: Diagnosis by double-contrast esophagography. AJR 148:731–732, 1987. Copyright 1987. Reproduced with permission.)

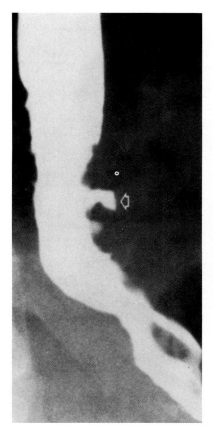

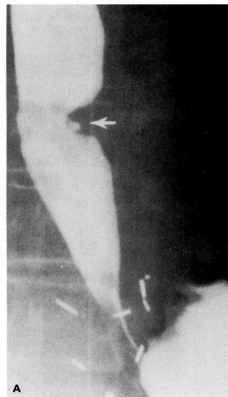

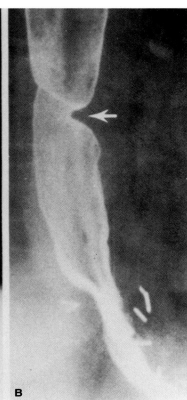

4-43

4-44

Fig. 4-43. Variceal sclerotherapy. Barium esophagram performed 2 weeks following two courses of endoscopic injection sclerotherapy shows diffuse ulceration in the distal third of the esophagus and one intramural sinus tract **(arrow)**. (Agha FP: The esophagus after endoscopic injection sclerotherapy: Acute and chronic changes. Radiology 153:37–42, 1984)

Fig. 4-44. Variceal sclerotherapy. **(A)** Initial esophagram obtained 1 week after endoscopic injection sclerotherapy shows a localized deep ulcer surrounded by mucosal edema **(arrow)** in the distal third of the esophagus. The patient had previously undergone the Sequira operation and fundoplication. **(B)** Repeat esophagram obtained 3 months later because of progressive dysphagia shows the development of a circumferential stricture **(arrow)** at the site of previous ulceration. (Agha FP: The esophagus after endoscopic injection sclerotherapy: Acute and chronic changes. Radiology 153:37–42, 1984)

Fig. 4-45. Intramural esophageal pseudodiverticulosis. Innumerable outpouchings representing dilated esophageal glands simulate the appearance of multiple esophageal ulcerations.

Fig. 4-46. Intramural esophageal pseudodiverticulosis. The multiple outpouchings mimic the pattern of Rokitansky-Aschoff sinuses in the gallbladder.

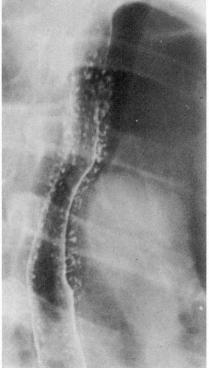

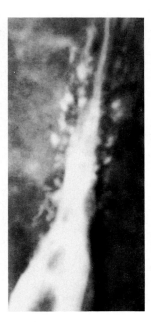

4-45

4-46

ities. Deeper ulcers usually lead to luminal narrowing and stricture formation (Fig. 4-44).

INTRAMURAL ESOPHAGEAL PSEUDODIVERTICULOSIS

Intramural esophageal pseudodiverticulosis can simulate multiple esophageal ulcers (Fig. 4-45). Patients with this disease typically present with mild or moderate dysphagia that is intermittent or slowly progressive and usually of long duration. A proximal esophageal stricture is frequently seen. Radiographically, innumerable pinhead-sized outpouchings project from the lumen and end at the same level. The pseudodiverticula represent dilated esophageal glands that are radiographically similar to the Rokitansky-Aschoff sinuses in the gallbladder (Fig. 4-46) and probably result from a diffuse inflammatory process in the esophagus. Although *Candida albicans* is often cultured from the esophagus in patients with intramural pseudodiverticulosis, the presence of the fungus appears to be a secondary phenomenon rather than an etiologic factor.

BIBLIOGRAPHY

Agha FP: The esophagus after endoscopic injection sclerotherapy: Acute and chronic changes. Radiology 153:37–42, 1984

Agha FP: Barrett carcinoma of the esophagus: Clinical and radiographic analysis of 34 cases. AJR 145:41–46, 1985

Agha FP, Lee HH, Nostrand TT: Herpetic esophagitis: A diagnostic challenge in immunocompromised patients. Am J Gastroenterol 81:246–253, 1986

Agha FP, Wilson JAP, Nostrand TT: Medication-induced esophagitis. Gastrointest Radiol 11:7–11, 1986

Balthazar EJ, Megibow AJ, Hulnick et al: Cytomegalovirus esophagitis in AIDS: Radiographic features in 16 patients. AJR 149:919–923, 1987

Berquist HT, Nolan NG, Stephens DH et al: Radioisotope scintigraphy in the diagnosis of Barrett esophagus. AJR 123:401–411, 1975

Bier SJ, Keller RJ, Krivisky BA et al: Esophageal moniliasis: A new radiographic presentation. Am J Gastroenterol 80:734–737, 1985

Boal DKB, Newburger PE, Teel RL: Esophagitis induced by combined radiation and Adriamycin. AJR 132:567–570, 1979

Bova JG, Dutton NE, Goldstein HM et al: Medication-induced esophagitis: Diagnosis by double-contrast esophagography. AJR 148:731–732, 1987

Castillo S, Aburashed A, Kimmelman J et al: Diffuse intramural esophageal pseudodiverticulosis: New cases and review. Gastroenterology 71:541–545, 1977

Chen YM, Gelfand DW, Ott DJ et al: Barrett esophagus as an extension of severe esophagitis: Analysis of radiologic signs in 29 cases. AJR 145:275–281, 1985

Cleveland RH, Kushner DC, Schwartz AN: Gastroesophageal reflux in children: Results of a standardized fluoroscopic approach. AJR 141:53–56, 1983

Creteur V, Laufer I, Kressel HY et al: Drug-induced esophagitis detected by double-contrast radiography. Radiology 147:365–368, 1983

Crummy AB: The water test in the evaluation of gastroesophageal reflux: Its correlation with pyrosis. Radiology 78:501–504, 1966

De Gaeta L, Levine MS, Guglielmi GE et al: Herpes esophagitis in an otherwise healthy patient. AJR 144:1205–1206, 1985

Degryse HRM, De Schepper AMAP: Aphthoid esophageal ulcers in Crohn's disease of ileum and colon. Gastrointest Radiol 9:197–201, 1984

Farman J, Tavitian A, Rosenthal LE et al: Focal esophageal candidiasis in acquired immunodeficiency syndrome (AIDS). Gastrointest Radiol 11:213–217, 1986

Feczko PJ, Halpert RD, Zonca M: Radiographic abnormalities in eosinophilic esophagitis. Gastrointest Radiol 10:321–324, 1985

Franken EA: Caustic damage of the gastrointestinal tract: Roentgen features. AJR 118:77–85, 1973

Ghahremani GG, Gore RM, Breuer RI et al: Esophageal manifestations of Crohn's disease. Gastrointest Radiol 7:199–203, 1982

Gloyna RE, Zornoza J, Goldstein HM: Primary ulcerative carcinoma of the esophagus. AJR 129:599–600, 1977

Halpert RD, Feczko PJ, Chason DP: Barrett's esophagus: Radiological and clinical considerations. J Can Assoc Radiol 35:120–123, 1984

Heyman S, Kirkpatrick JA, Winter HS et al: An improved radionuclide method for diagnosis of gastroesophageal reflux and aspiration in children (milk scan). Radiology 131:479–482, 1987

Hishikawa Y, Tanaka S, Miura T: Esophageal ulceration induced by intracavitary irradiation for esophageal carcinoma. AJR 143:269–273, 1984

Ito J, Kobayashi S, Kasugai P: Tuberculosis of the esophagus. Am J Gastroenterol 65:454–456, 1976

Jenkins DW, Fisk DE, Byrd RB: Mediastinal histoplasmosis with esophageal abscess. Gastroenterology 70:190–211, 1976

Kressel HY, Glick SN, Laufer I et al: Radiologic features of esophagitis. Gastrointest Radiol 6:103–108, 1981

Levine MS: Crohn's disease of the upper gastrointestinal tract. Radiol Clin North Am 25:79–91, 1987

Levine MS, Goldstein HM: Fixed transverse folds in the esophagus: A sign of reflux esophagitis. AJR 143:275–278, 1984

Levine MS, Laufer I, Kressel HY et al: Herpes esophagitis. AJR 136:863–866, 1981

Levine MS, Moolten DN, Herlinger H et al: Esophageal intramural pseudodiverticulosis: A re-evaluation. AJR 147:1165–1170, 1986

Lewicki AM, Moore JP: Esophageal moniliasis: A review of common and less frequent characteristics. AJR 125:218–225, 1975

Megibow AJ, Balthazar EJ, Hulnick DH: Radiology of non-neoplastic gastrointestinal disorders in acquired immune difficiency syndrome. Semin Roentgenol 22:31–41, 1987

Mori S, Yoshihira A, Kawamura H et al: Esophageal involvement in Behcet's disease. Am J Gastroenterol 78:548–553, 1983

Muhletaler CA, Gerlock AJ, de Soto L et al: Acid corrosive esophagitis: Radiographic findings. AJR 134:1137–1140, 1980

O'Riordan D, Levine MS, Laufer I: Acute alcoholic esophagitis. J Can Assoc Radiol 37:54–55, 1986

Shapir J, DuBrow R, Frank P: Barrett oesophagus: Analysis of 19 cases. Br J Radiol 58:491–493, 1985

St. Onge G, Bezahler GH: Giant esophageal ulcer associated with cytomegalovirus. Gastroenterology 83:127–130, 1982

Stone J, Friedberg SA: Obstructive syphilitic esophagitis. JAMA 177:711, 1961

Teixidor HS, Honig CL, Norsoph E et al: Cytomegalovirus infection of the alimentary canal: Radiologic findings with pathologic correlation. Radiology 163:317–323, 1987

Williams SM, Harned RK, Kaplin P et al: Work in progress: Transverse striations of the esophagus: Association with gastroesophageal reflux. Radiology 146:25–27, 1983

Williford ME, Thompson WM, Hamilton JD et al: Esophageal tuberculosis: Findings on barium swallow and computed tomography. Gastrointest Radiol 8:119–122, 1983

Vincent ME, Robbins AH, Spechler SJ et al: The reticular pattern as a radiographic sign of the Barrett's esophagus: An assessment. Radiology 153:333–335, 1984

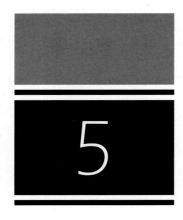

5

ESOPHAGEAL NARROWING

Disease Entities

Congenital conditions
  Esophageal web
  Lower esophageal ring (Schatzki ring)
  Cartilaginous esophageal ring
  Congenital stricture
Neoplastic lesions
  Carcinoma of the esophagus
  Carcinoma of the stomach
  Direct spread from adjacent malignancy
  Hematogenous/lymphangitic metastases
  Lymphoma
  Benign tumors
Reflux esophagitis
Corrosive esophagitis
Barrett's esophagus
Postsurgical stricture (*e.g.,* after hiatal hernia
    repair, gastric surgery)
Post-nasogastric intubation stricture
Infectious/inflammatory esophagitis
  Candidiasis
  Tuberculosis
  Syphilis
  Histoplasmosis
  Crohn's disease
  Eosinophilic esophagitis
  Behcet's syndrome
Radiation injury
Epidermolysis bullosa
Benign mucous membrane pemphigoid

Graft-vs-host disease
Sclerotherapy of esophageal varices
Motility disorders
  Achalasia pattern
  Esophageal spasm
Intramural esophageal pseudodiverticulosis
Mallory-Weiss syndrome

ESOPHAGEAL WEB

Congenital esophageal webs are smooth, thin, delicate membranes covered with normal-appearing mucosa (Fig. 5-1). Most congenital esophageal webs are situated in the cervical esophagus within 2 cm of the pharyngoesophageal junction. The typical transverse web arises from the anterior wall of the esophagus (never from the posterior wall) and is best seen in the lateral projection. It forms a right angle with the wall of the esophagus and protrudes into the esophageal lumen. A rarer circumferential type of web appears as a symmetric annular radiolucent band that concentrically narrows the barium-filled esophagus (Fig. 5-2). Webs are occasionally found in the distal esophagus (Fig. 5-3*A*), possibly representing a complication of gastroesophageal reflux. Multiple webs may develop anywhere in the esophagus (Fig. 5-3*B*). Esophageal webs can usually be seen only when the barium-filled esophagus is maximally distended. Because rapid peristalsis permits cervical esophageal webs to be visible for only a fraction

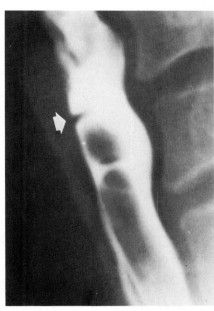

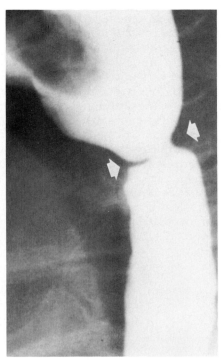

Fig. 5-1. Esophageal web. A smooth, thin membrane covered with normal-appearing mucosa protrudes into the esophageal lumen **(arrow)**.

Fig. 5-2. Circumferential esophageal web **(arrows)**.

5-1

5-2

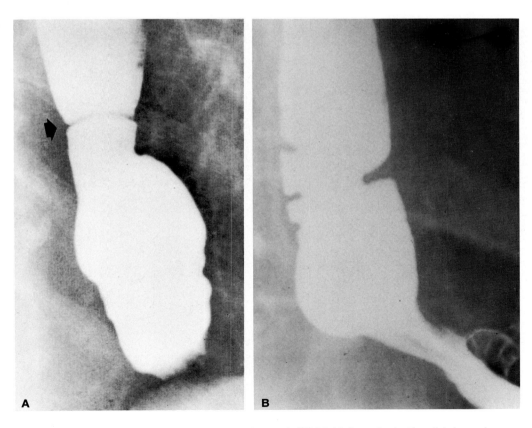

A

B

Fig. 5-3. **(A)** Single distal esophageal web **(arrow)**. **(B)** Multiple webs in the distal esophagus.

of a second, cinefluorography is often required for radiographic demonstration.

An esophageal web is usually an incidental finding of no clinical importance. Because it is not associated with any lack of distensibility, a transverse web only rarely occludes enough of the esophageal lumen to cause dysphagia. In contrast, circumferential webs can cause intermittent dysphagia because of constriction of the esophageal lumen. At times, the web itself is not visible, but a liquid bolus of barium can be demonstrated to squirt in a jet through the opening in the web (Fig. 5-4). The width of the jet immediately below the level of the web indicates the size of the orifice. This jet phenomenon occasionally simulates a long, smooth stenotic lesion.

The Plummer-Vinson syndrome is a controversial entity in which esophageal webs have been reported in combination with dysphagia, iron deficiency anemia, and mucosal lesions of the mouth, pharynx, and esophagus. The condition has been associated with a disturbance in iron metabolism, predominantly in middle-aged women. A correlation between the Plummer-Vinson syndrome and cancer has been suggested. In recent years, the validity of the Plummer-Vinson syndrome has been challenged because of the relative infrequency with which many of the component signs and symptoms have occurred together. Most authors consider that the discovery of an esophageal web in this "syndrome" merely represents a coincidental scar or adhesion from one of the variety of disease pro-

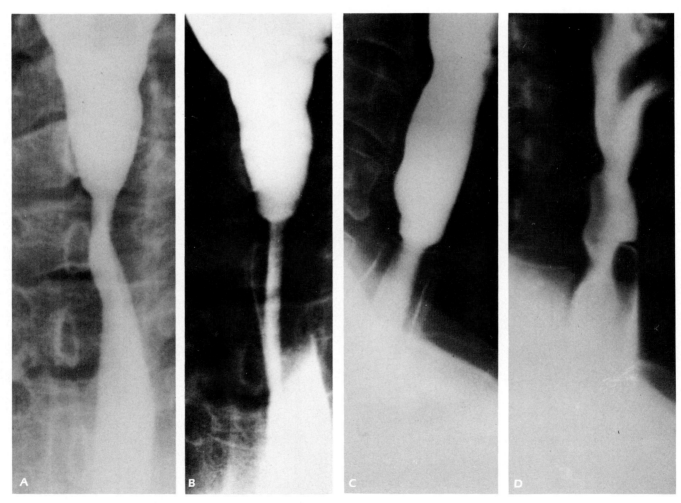

Fig. 5-4. Jet phenomenon of esophageal web. **(A)** A frontal projection demonstrates an abruptly narrowed barium column simulating a long stenosing lesion in the upper esophagus. **(B)** The double-contrast effect below the web indicates the width of the jet and the normal caliber of the esophagus below the web. **(C)** The lateral projection better illustrates the annular constriction of the esophagus produced by the web. **(D)** Further opacification of the esophagus more graphically delineates the web. (Shauffer IA, Phillips HE, Sequeira J: The jet phenomenon: A manifestation of esophageal web. AJR 129:747–748, 1977. Copyright 1977. Reproduced with permission.)

cesses with which esophageal webs have occasionally been associated.

LOWER ESOPHAGEAL RING

The lower esophageal ring (Schatzki ring) is a smooth, concentric narrowing several centimeters above the diaphragm that marks the junction between the esophageal and gastric mucosae (Fig. 5-5). The ring is present constantly and does not change in position. However, it is only visible when the esophagus above and below is filled sufficiently to dilate to a width greater than that of the ring (Fig. 5-6). If the luminal opening in the Schatzki ring is greater than 12 or 13 mm, symptoms of obstruction are unlikely. Rings with a narrowed luminal opening are prone to cause long-standing symptoms of intermittent dysphagia, particularly when large chunks of solid material are ingested. These symptoms can occasionally be reproduced if the patient swallows a barium capsule, radiopaque tablet, or marshmallow, any of which may temporarily become lodged in the esophagus just above the lower esophageal ring. Sudden, total esophageal obstruction can sometimes be caused by impaction of a large piece of meat.

The lower esophageal ring has long been considered a transverse mucosal fold of noninflammatory origin. Recent reports demonstrate transformation of the esophagogastric junction both from a normal distal esophagus to a lower esophageal ring and from a lower esophageal ring to a distal esophageal stricture in patients with reflux esophagitis (Fig. 5-7). This suggests that some mucosal rings may be part of the spectrum of reflux esophagitis and represent thin, annular peptic strictures (Fig. 5-8).

CARTILAGINOUS RING (TRACHEOBRONCHIAL REST)

A cartilaginous ring consisting of tracheobronchial rests is an unusual cause of distal esophageal obstruction (Fig. 5-9). This anomaly probably results from sequestration of tracheal cartilage in the primitive esophagus before the two tubes have completely separated from each other. Because the cartilage is usually found in the distal esophagus, it is presumed that these cells were carried down the esophagus during the normal process of growth. Most cases of cartilaginous rings appear in infancy or early childhood with recurrent vomiting, failure to thrive, and aspiration pneumonia. Several adults, all of whom had long histories of dysphagia or other esophageal symptoms, have been described with this disorder. Characteristic radiographic findings are linear tracks of barium, representing ducts of tracheobronchial glands, that extend from the area of narrowing.

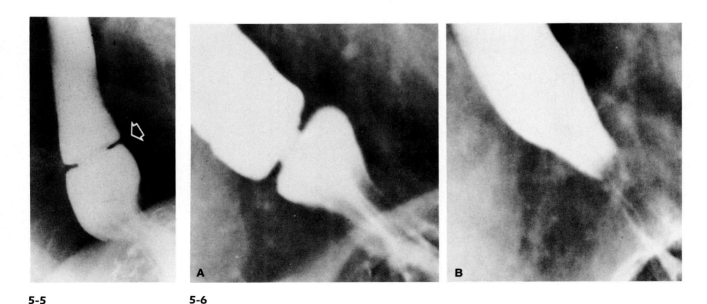

5-5   **5-6**

Fig. 5-5. Lower esophageal ring (Schatzki ring) **(arrow)**. Smooth, concentric narrowing of the distal esophagus marks the junction between the esophageal and gastric mucosae.

Fig. 5-6. Lower esophageal ring. **(A)** Typical appearance in the filled esophagus. **(B)** The ring is not visible in the partially collapsed esophagus.

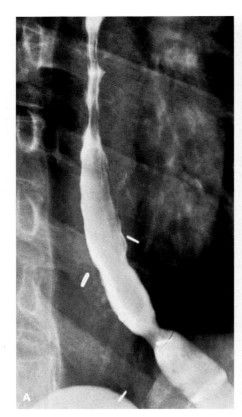
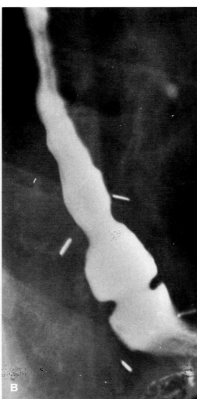

Fig. 5-7. Progression of lower esophageal ring. **(A)** A 7-mm wide, 10-mm long stricture **(arrows)** replaces a 22-mm mucosal ring **(B)** demonstrated 5 years earlier. (Chen YM, Gelfand DW, Ott DJ et al: Natural progression of the lower esophageal mucosal ring. Gastrointest Radiol 12:93–98, 1987)

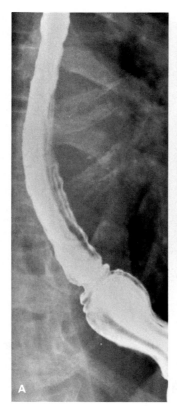
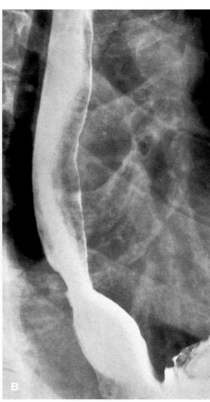

Fig. 5-8. Progression of lower esophageal ring. Two mucosal rings, 14 and 21 mm in diameter **(A)**, associated with severe esophagitis, transformed over 2 years to a 12-mm wide, 25-mm long stricture **(B)** with an ulcer at the esophagogastric junction. (Chen YM, Gelfand DW, Ott DJ et al: Natural progression of the lower esophageal mucosal ring. Gastrointest Radiol 12:93–98, 1987)

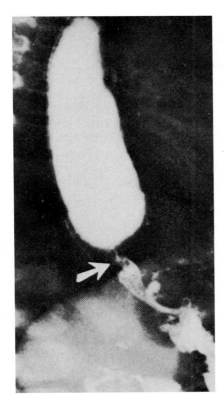

Fig. 5-9. Cartilaginous ring of tracheobronchial rests. Note the lower esophageal stricture **(arrow)** with proximal dilatation. (Rose JS, Kassner EG, Jurgens KH et al: Congenital oesophageal strictures due to cartilaginous rings. Br J Radiol 48:16–18, 1975)

CONGENITAL STRICTURE

A congenital stricture of the esophagus is an uncommon lesion that represents an incomplete occlusion. It appears as a smooth fusiform narrowing of the esophageal lumen and causes a variable degree of obstruction and proximal dilatation. In the newborn, such a stricture is almost invariably of congenital origin; in the older infant or child, it may be impossible to distinguish between a congenital stricture and one of acquired origin caused by the swallowing of caustic material.

CARCINOMA OF THE ESOPHAGUS

Infiltrating carcinoma of the esophagus can extend under the esophageal mucosa and narrow the esophagus even in the absence of luminal proliferation. Unfortunately, symptoms of esophageal carcinoma tend to appear late in the course of the disease, so that the tumor is often in an advanced stage when first detected radiographically. Most carcinomas of the esophagus are of the squamous cell type. Excluding tumors of the gastric cardia that spread upward to involve the distal esophagus, about half of all esophageal carcinomas occur in the

middle third. Of the remainder, slightly more occur in the lower than in the upper third. The incidence of carcinoma of the esophagus is far higher in men than in women, and the disease is more prevalent in blacks than in whites.

ETIOLOGIC FACTORS

Numerous etiologic factors have been suggested in the development of carcinoma of the esophagus. In the United States, there is a definite association between excessive alcohol intake, smoking, and esophageal carcinoma. Heavy use of alcohol and tobacco also significantly increases the risk of developing squamous carcinoma of the head and neck. Indeed, awareness of the not infrequent coexistence of tumors in these two sites may permit detection of small and potentially curable cancers of the esopha-

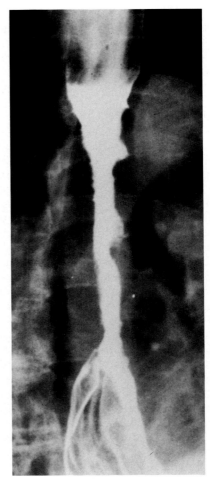

Fig. 5-10. Adenocarcinoma in Barrett's esophagus. Extensive, infiltrative, 16-cm long lesion involves the thoracic esophagus. There is significant luminal narrowing and mucosal irregularity. Note the associated hiatal hernia. (Agha FP: Barrett's carcinoma of the esophagus: Clinical and radiographic analysis of 34 cases. AJR 145:41–46, 1985. Copyright 1985. Reproduced with permission.)

gus in patients with known carcinoma of the head and neck. In Iran, China, and Russia, countries in which hot tea is a major beverage, carcinoma of the esophagus is very common and may be due to tissue damage secondary to raised intraesophageal temperature. Carcinoma of the esophagus occurs with significantly higher incidence than normal in patients with lye strictures, frequently developing at an unusually early age. The long-term stasis of esophageal contents in patients with untreated achalasia is also associated with a higher than normal incidence of carcinoma. Most of these lesions, however, occur in the midesophagus rather than in the distal portion. A relationship between hiatal hernia, reflux esophagitis, and carcinoma has been suggested. This is difficult to prove conclusively, since gastrointestinal reflux is so common in the general population. Patients with Barrett's esophagus have a definitely higher than normal risk of developing adenocarcinoma (up to a 10% incidence) (Fig. 5-10). Rare disorders that have been linked to the development of esophageal cancer include the Plummer-Vinson syndrome (sideropenic dysphagia) and tylosis, a genetically transmitted disease characterized by thickened skin of the hands and feet.

CLINICAL SYMPTOMS

Progressive dysphagia is the most common clinical presentation of carcinoma of the esophagus. In persons over 40 years of age, dysphagia must be assumed to be due to cancer until proven otherwise. Early in the disease, dysphagia is noted only with solid food; eventually, even fluids are regurgitated. Mild substernal pain or fullness may be an early sign of carcinoma of the esophagus. Persistent or severe discomfort, however, is usually due to extension of the tumor to the mediastinum and is therefore an unfavorable sign. Because the esophagus has no limiting serosa, direct extension of the tumor at the time of initial diagnosis is common and contributes to the dismal prognosis in this disease. Many patients with esophageal carcinoma have weight loss, which is closely related to the duration and severity of the esophageal obstruction. Hoarseness can occur if the recurrent laryngeal nerve is involved; anemia may be produced by slow, chronic blood loss. Pulmonary complications, such as aspiration pneumonia and esophagorespiratory fistula, are not infrequent (Fig. 5-11).

RADIOGRAPHIC FINDINGS

The earliest radiographic appearance of infiltrating carcinoma of the esophagus is a flat, plaquelike lesion, occasionally with central ulceration, that involves one wall of the esophagus (Fig. 5-12). At this stage, there is minimal reduction in the caliber of the lumen, and the lesion is seen to best advantage on double-contrast views of the distended esophagus. Unless the patient is carefully examined in various projections, this early and often curable form of esophageal carcinoma can be missed. As the infiltrating cancer progresses, luminal irregularities indicating mucosal destruction are noted (Fig. 5-13). Advanced lesions encircle the lumen completely, causing annular constrictions with overhanging margins, luminal narrowing, and, often, some degree of obstruction (Fig. 5-14). The lumen through the stenotic area is irregular, and mucosal folds are absent or severely ulcerated. Proximal dilatation of the esophagus is seen in obstructing carcinoma but is usually less pronounced than in achalasia. Because multiple synchronous foci of carcinoma of the esophagus sometimes occur, albeit rarely, a careful and complete examination of the remainder of the esophagus is essential, even when one obvious lesion has been demonstrated. High esophageal carcinoma usually causes difficulty in swallowing with frequent aspiration into the trachea. Carcinoma of the cervical portion of the esophagus can cause forward displacement of the tracheal air shadow on lateral view and the suggestion of a prevertebral mass. Upper thoracic lesions produce widening (>3–4 mm) of the retrotracheal soft-tissue stripe (Fig. 5-15).

Computed tomography (CT) is currently the single most accurate preoperative staging method for evaluating the patient with carcinoma of the esophagus (Fig. 5-16). It can provide information on tumor size, extension, and resectability previously available only at thoracotomy. The major CT findings of carcinoma of the esophagus are a soft-tissue mass and focal wall thickening with an eccentric or irregular lumen. Evidence of the spread of tumor includes the obliteration of the fat planes between the esophagus and adjacent structures (left atrium, aorta, trachea), the formation of a sinus tract or fistula to the tracheobronchial tree, and evidence of metastatic disease that primarily appears as enlargement of mediastinal, retrocrural, left gastric, or celiac lymph nodes, or as low-density masses in the liver. The major limitation of CT in demonstrating tumor invasion into adjacent structures is the lack of adequate mediastinal and abdominal fat planes around the esophagus that may be encountered in these often severely cachectic patients.

TREATMENT AND PROGNOSIS

Because the nature of esophageal cancer brings the patient to medical attention relatively late in the course of the disease, the long-term survival rate is low. An exception is "early esophageal cancer," which is defined histologically as cancer limited to the mucosa or submucosa without lymph node metastases; it is a readily curable lesion with reported 5-year survival rates approaching 90%. Most cases of

Text continues on page 79

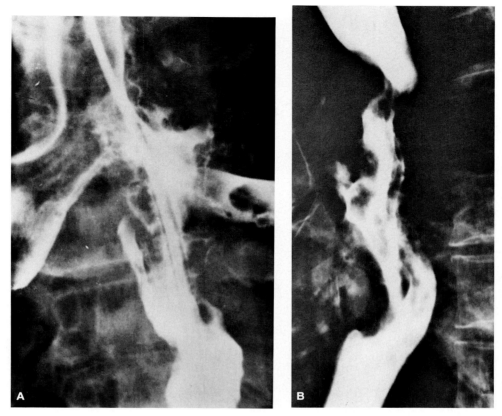

Fig. 5-11. **(A)** Esophagorespiratory fistula as a complication of squamous carcinoma of the esophagus. **(B)** Esophagram showing the extensive malignant lesion.

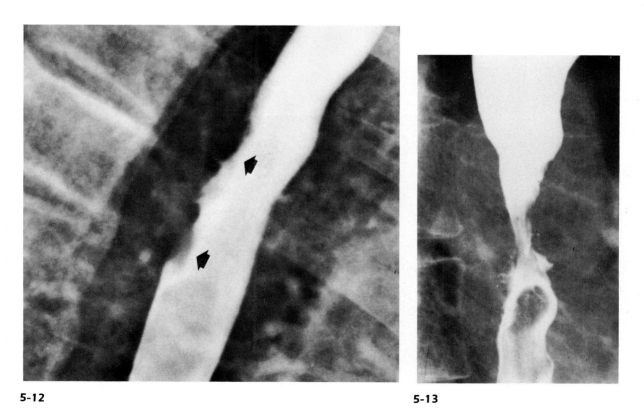

5-12

5-13

Fig. 5-12. Early squamous carcinoma of the esophagus. A flat, plaquelike lesion **(arrows)** involves the posterior wall of the esophagus.

Fig. 5-13. Ulcerating squamous carcinoma of the esophagus.

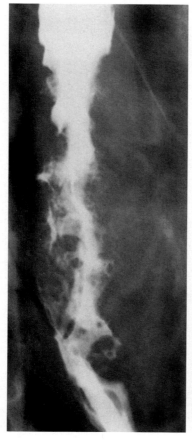

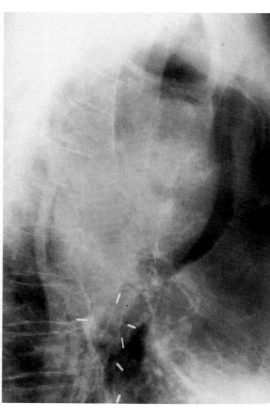

5-14

5-15

Fig. 5-14. Squamous carcinoma. Irregular narrowing of an extensive segment of the thoracic portion of the esophagus.

Fig. 5-15. Squamous carcinoma. Massive widening of the retrotracheal soft tissues causes anterior bowing of the tracheal air shadow.

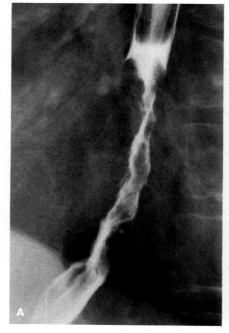

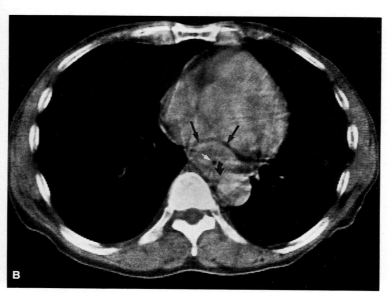

Fig. 5-16. CT staging of esophageal carcinoma. **(A)** Esophagram demonstrates an infiltrating lesion causing irregular narrowing of the distal esophagus. **(B)** CT scan shows the circumferential mass of the bulky carcinoma **(straight black arrows)** filling the lumen **(white arrow)**. Obliteration of the fat plane adjacent to the aorta **(curved arrow)** indicates mediastinal invasion. (Eisenberg RL: Diagnostic Imaging in Surgery. New York, McGraw–Hill, 1987)

early esophageal cancer have been detected in China or in other areas where the high incidence of esophageal malignancy has led to mass screening of asymptomatic patients to detect these lesions at the earliest possible stage. In contrast, symptomatic patients with esophageal carcinoma usually develop dysphagia only after the tumor has invaded periesophageal lymphatics or other mediastinal structures and is thus unresectable at the time of presentation.

In some patients with carcinoma of the esophagus, a radical resection can be performed and reconstruction achieved with the stomach (Fig. 5-17), right or left colon, or jejunum pulled up through the intrathoracic, retrosternal, or antethoracic subcutaneous tissue. Unfortunately, tumor frequently recurs at the anastomotic site (Fig. 5-18). In many cases, only palliative treatment can be offered. The easiest method of restoring oral intake to these patients with esophageal cancer is by passing an indwelling tube through the lesion. A simple gastrostomy or jejunostomy can be performed to supply nutrition to the patient. Radiation therapy is often used either in conjunction with a radical operation or as palliative therapy in patients in whom surgery cannot be performed. Squamous cell carcinoma of the esophagus responds to radiation therapy in a majority of patients; indeed, radiation therapy has been reported to be curative in up to 10% of cases (Fig. 5-19).

Fluoroscopically guided balloon dilatation can be used to treat malignant or postinflammatory strictures of the esophagus (Fig. 5-20). This technique uses radially directed forces rather than the longitudinal sheer forces generated during bouginage, so that the risk of both perforation and rupture of the esophagus is substantially less (especially if

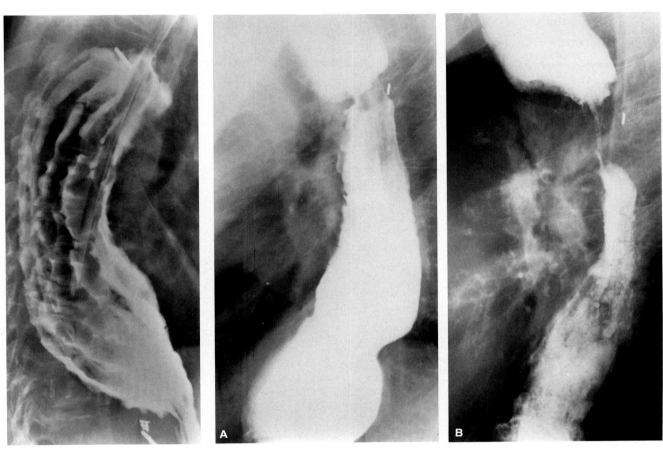

5-17   **5-18**

Fig. 5-17. Gastric pull-through following the radical resection of a large esophageal carcinoma. A surgical clip indicates the site of anastomosis with the remaining esophagus.

Fig. 5-18. Recurrent esophageal carcinoma at the anastomotic site. **(A)** Baseline barium swallow following surgical resection. There is mild narrowing, but the mucosal pattern at the anastomotic site (surgical clip) appears normal. **(B)** Ten months later, irregular, high-grade stenosis and the surrounding mass reflect tumor recurrence.

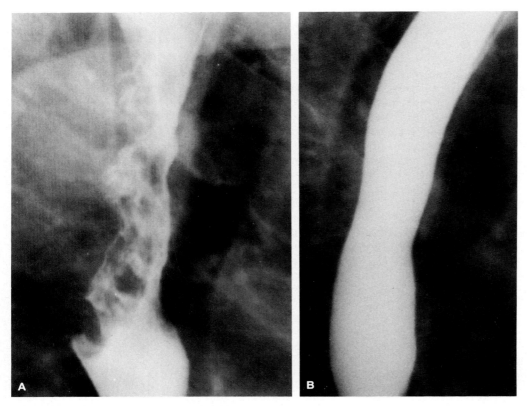

Fig. 5-19. Effect of radiation therapy on squamous carcinoma of the esophagus. **(A)** Original malignant lesion in the midthoracic esophagus. **(B)** Essentially normal esophagram in the same patient 9 years after radiation therapy.

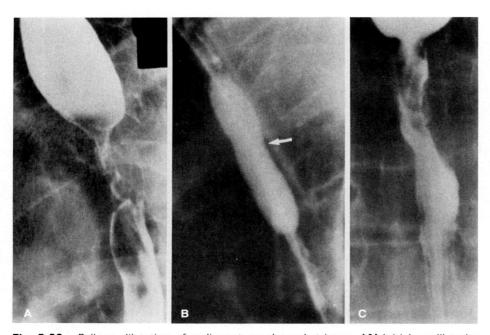

Fig. 5-20. Balloon dilatation of malignant esophageal stricture. **(A)** Initial predilatation radiograph demonstrates an irregular malignant stricture representing carcinoma of the upper thoracic esophagus. **(B)** A 15-mm, 4-cm balloon was positioned fluoroscopically in the center of the stricture. A small narrowing **(arrow)** is seen on the radiograph after 1 minute of inflation. **(C)** Frontal radiograph after dilatation demonstrates a lumen diameter of approximately 1.5 times the initial size. This increased size allowed the patient to eat solid foods, drink liquids, and perform home bougienage. The patient lived symptom free for 7 months after the procedure. (Dawson SL, Mueller PR, Ferrucci JT et al: Severe esophageal strictures: Indications for balloon catheter dilatation. Radiology 153:631–635, 1984)

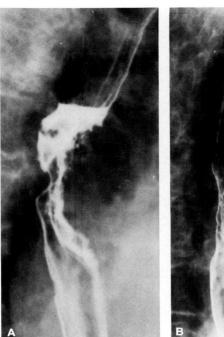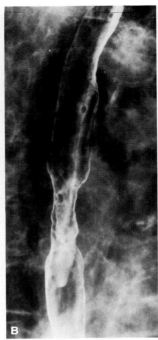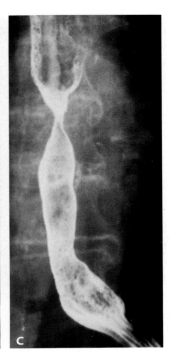

Fig. 5-21. Laser therapy of esophageal malignancy. **(A)** Initial radiograph before laser treatment of esophageal carcinoma. **(B)** Four days after laser treatment, there is successful dilatation of the midesophageal lesion. **(C)** Repeat examination 4½ months later shows subsequent regrowth of tumor that has a more strictured appearance and less bulky neoplastic components than the original lesion. (Wolf EL, Frager J, Brandt LJ et al: Radiographic appearance of the esophagus and stomach after laser treatment of obstructing carcinoma. AJR 146:519–522, 1986. Copyright 1986. Reproduced with permission.)

the lumen is less than 12 mm in diameter). Although infrequent, esophageal rupture may occur after balloon dilatation, and the patient should be instructed to return to the hospital if chest pain or fever develops following the procedure.

High-energy laser therapy that destroys neoplastic tissue by tumor ablation is now being used increasingly as a palliative endoscopic technique to treat malignant obstructions of the esophagus and esophagogastric junction in patients who have advanced disease or are poor surgical risks (Fig. 5-21). Rapid symptomatic and radiographic improvement usually lasts about 3 to 6 months, and the procedure may be repeated whenever necessary as symptoms recur. The most common complications after laser treatment are perforation and tracheoesophageal fistula, which have been reported in 2% to 15% of patients.

CARCINOMA OF THE STOMACH

About 12% of adenocarcinomas of the stomach arising near the cardia invade the lower esophagus at an early stage and cause symptoms of esophageal ob-

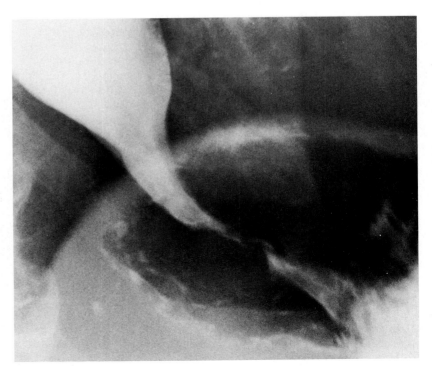

Fig. 5-22. Adenocarcinoma of the stomach invading the distal esophagus.

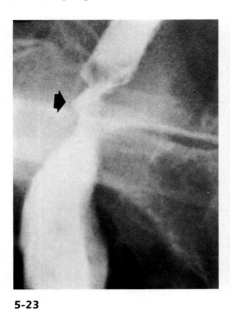

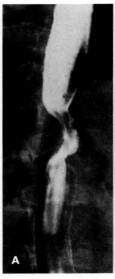

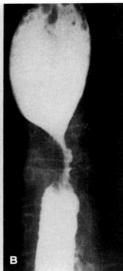

Fig. 5-23. Metastatic carcinoma invading the esophagus. The direct extension of carcinoma of the thyroid causes constriction and relative obstruction of the lower cervical esophagus **(arrow)**.

Fig. 5-24. Metastatic breast carcinoma. **(A)** Initial radiograph shows a short circumferential stricture in the midesophagus. **(B)** Progressive narrowing of the lumen 9 months later. Note the irregular mucosal contour and eccentric nature of the stricture. (Agha FP: Secondary neoplasms of the esophagus. Gastrointest Radiol 12:187–193, 1987)

5-23

5-24

struction. This process can produce an irregularly narrowed, sometimes ulcerated lesion simulating carcinoma of the distal esophagus (Fig. 5-22). A careful examination of the cardia is necessary to demonstrate the gastric origin of the tumor. Narrowing of the distal esophagus secondary to gastric carcinoma may be due not only to direct extension of tumor but also to destruction of cells in the myenteric plexus, which produces an achalasia-like pattern.

METASTATIC LESIONS

Other malignant lesions can spread to the esophagus and produce luminal narrowing. In the cervical region, direct extension from carcinoma of the larynx or thyroid can constrict the esophagus and cause relative obstruction (Fig. 5-23). Narrowing of the thoracic esophagus by tumor-containing lymph nodes or blood-borne metastases most commonly results from a primary site in either the breast (Fig. 5-24) or lung. This lesion typically appears radiographically as a symmetric stricture with smooth borders. Although concentric narrowing due to metastatic malignancy characteristically affects a short segment of the esophagus, long segmental stenosis occasionally occurs with metastatic carcinoma of the breast or diffuse mediastinal involvement by mesothelioma (Fig. 5-25). Irregular, ulcerated narrowing of the esophagus due to metastatic disease may also occur (Fig. 5-26).

LYMPHOMA

Transcardial extension of gastric lymphoma to involve the distal esophagus has been described in 2% to 10% of cases (Fig. 5-27). This typically presents as

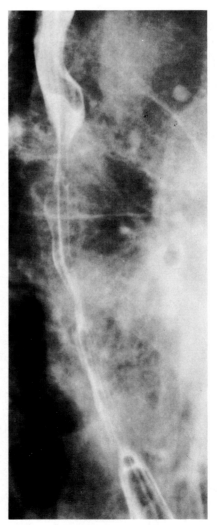

Fig. 5-25. Mesothelioma. Diffuse mediastinal involvement causes long, segmental stenosis of the esophagus.

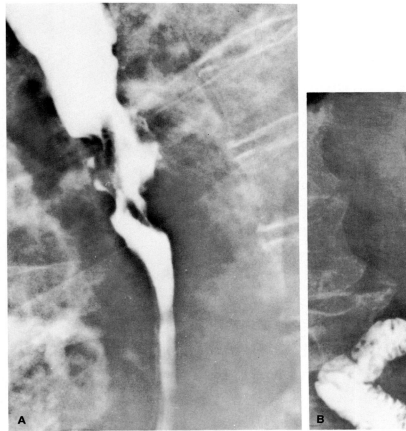
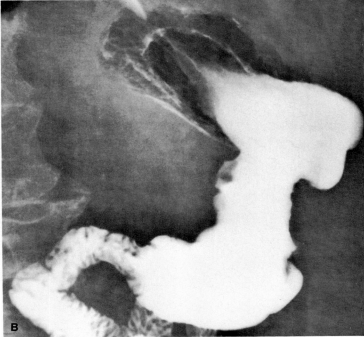

Fig. 5-26. Metastases to the esophagus from carcinoma of the stomach. **(A)** Irregular, ulcerated mass in the midesophagus. **(B)** Primary adenocarcinoma of the body of the stomach.

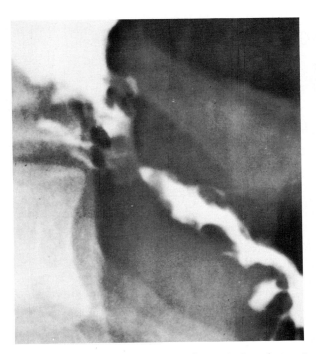

Fig. 5-27. Transcardial extension of gastric lymphoma to involve the distal esophagus.

nodularity and nonobstructive narrowing and may be indistinguishable from distal esophageal involvement by gastric adenocarcinoma. Esophageal narrowing can also be caused by enlarged masses of lymphomatous nodes. Primary esophageal lymphoma is rare (Fig. 5-28).

BENIGN TUMORS

Benign tumors, primarily leiomyomas, are submucosal intramural masses that can appear to eccentrically narrow the esophageal lumen.

REFLUX ESOPHAGITIS

Distal esophageal narrowing is a severe complication of gastroesophageal reflux and peptic esophagitis (Fig. 5-29). The narrowing may be reversible if it is due to the intense spasm and inflammatory reaction that accompany a marginal ulcer at the gastroesophageal junction. A fixed, relatively obstructing stricture of the distal esophagus may be due to fibrotic healing of a localized marginal ulcer or to diffuse reflux esophagitis (Fig. 5-30). Strictures sec-

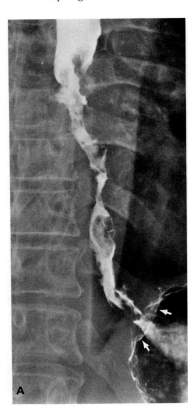
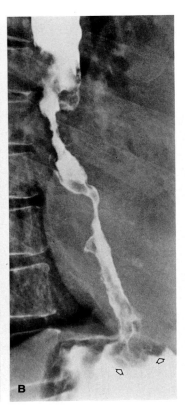

Fig. 5-28. Primary esophageal lymphoma. **(A)** Frontal and **(B)** lateral views show the diffuse destructive process involving much of the thoracic esophagus. Note the extension of the lesion to the fundus of the stomach **(arrows)**.

ondary to reflux esophagitis tend to be asymmetric, funnel-shaped, or broad-based, with no demonstrable mucosal pattern. An associated hiatal hernia is frequently detected (Fig. 5-31); however, the absence of a hernia in no way eliminates the possibility that a distal esophageal stricture is due to reflux esophagitis.

CORROSIVE ESOPHAGITIS

A major complication of the ingestion of corrosive agents is the development of an esophageal stricture as the intense mucosal and intramural inflammation heals (Fig. 5-32). Strictures can appear as soon as 2 weeks after the ingestion of a caustic substance. Corrosive strictures tend to be long lesions involving large portions of the thoracic esophagus, sometimes extending the entire distance between the aortic knob and the diaphragm (Fig. 5-33).

BARRETT'S ESOPHAGUS

In Barrett's esophagus, a variable length of the distal esophagus is lined by a gastric type of epithelium that is more susceptible to ulceration and inflammation than is the normal esophagus. Cyclic ulceration and healing leads to scarring and progressive stricture formation at the squamocolumnar junction (Fig. 5-34). Although classically described as occur-

ring in the midesophagus, more recent studies have indicated that the strictures in Barrett's esophagus are more common in the lower esophagus. The Barrett's stricture tends to be short and tight, typically causing eccentric narrowing of the lumen in contrast to the smooth, symmetric, and circumferential luminal narrowing in conventional peptic strictures. A specific sign of Barrett's esophagus is the ascending or migrating stricture, in which there is progressive upward extension of both the squamocolumnar junction and the level of the stricture on serial examinations (Fig. 5-35).

Luminal narrowing in Barrett's esophagus may also be due to the development of adenocarcinoma of the esophagus. This most commonly produces an irregular infiltrating-stenosing appearance involving an unusually long vertical segment of the thoracic esophagus (see Fig. 5-10). Varicoid, polypoid, and ulcerative lesions may also develop (see Fig. 4-19).

POSTSURGICAL/POSTINTUBATION STRICTURES

Strictures near the esophagogastric junction may occur after surgical repair of a hiatal hernia (Fig. 5-36). Reflux of bile from the small bowel into the stomach after gastric surgery can cause severe esophagitis and stricture formation if concomitant gastroesophageal reflux permits the bile to come in

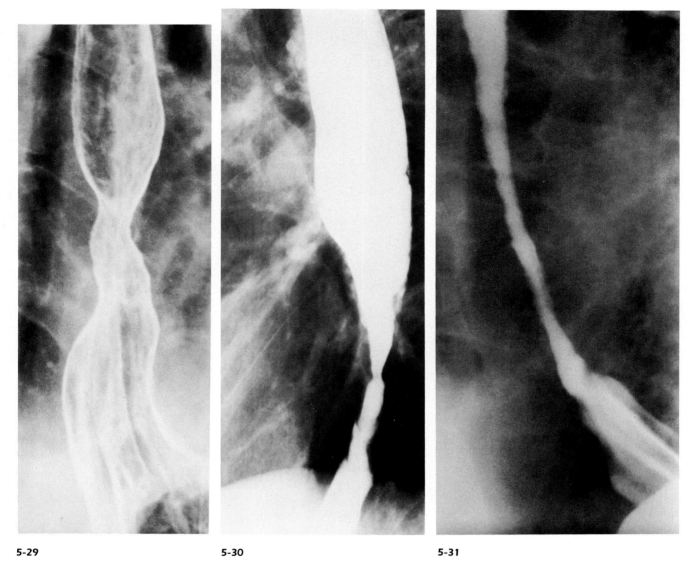

5-29   5-30   5-31

Fig. 5-29. Reflux stricture. Smooth narrowing of the distal esophagus extends to the level of the hiatal hernia.

Fig. 5-30. Esophageal stricture secondary to reflux esophagitis.

Fig. 5-31. Long esophageal stricture, due to reflux esophagitis, with an associated hiatal hernia.

contact with the sensitive mucosa of the distal esophagus. Prolonged nasogastric intubation produces a form of severe peptic esophagitis. The presence of a nasogastric tube renders the lower esophageal sphincter incompetent and interferes with esophageal peristalsis. Thus, gastroesophageal reflux occurs frequently, and the refluxed material is cleared poorly from the esophagus. The resulting severe esophagitis can lead to the rapid development of a long, tapered stricture in the distal esophagus, often within several days of intubation (Fig. 5-37).

INFECTIOUS/GRANULOMATOUS ESOPHAGITIS

Strictures can develop during the healing phase of infectious and inflammatory processes involving the esophagus. In candidal infestation of the esophagus, compromise of luminal diameter can occur both from edema of the mucosa and from the presence of an overlying pseudomembrane. As the disease spreads through the esophageal wall, a long segment of the esophagus may become constricted (Fig. 5-38). The proximal and distal margins of the

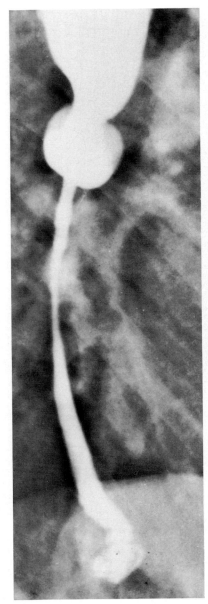

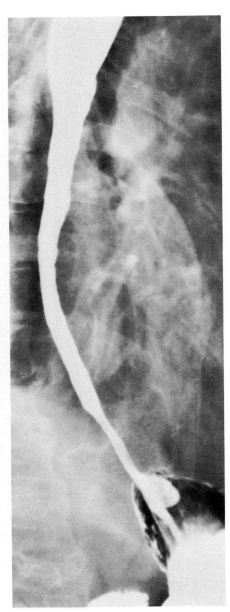

5-32   5-33

Fig. 5-32. Corrosive stricture resulting from the ingestion of lye.

Fig. 5-33. Extensive caustic stricture due to lye ingestion, involving almost the entire thoracic esophagus.

stricture are usually tapered, though there is occasionally asymmetry and an abrupt change in diameter simulating an infiltrating esophageal neoplasm.

Stricture formation is common during the healing phase of esophageal inflammation due to granulomatous diseases such as tuberculosis, syphilis, and histoplasmosis. Severe luminal narrowing also has been described in patients with Crohn's disease of the esophagus (Fig. 5-39), herpes simplex infestation (Fig. 5-40), eosinophilic esophagitis (Fig. 5-41), and Behcet's syndrome (Fig. 5-42).

RADIATION INJURY

Although the esophagus is generally considered to be a relatively radioresistant structure, radiation-induced changes may occur within the radiotherapy portal, especially in patients who have intracavitary radiation or who simultaneously or sequentially receive chemotherapy. Marked thickening of the submucosal and muscular layers due to edema and fibrosis can result in a stricture that has a benign appearance with tapered margins and relatively smooth mucosal surfaces.

Esophageal stricture within the field of irradiation is a relatively infrequent long-term complication of mediastinal radiation therapy. Marked thickening of the submucosal and muscular layers due to edema and fibrosis can result in a stricture that has a benign appearance, with tapered margins and relatively smooth mucosal surfaces (Fig. 5-43). The narrowing may be due in part to radiation changes involving surrounding mediastinal structures.

Radiation-induced carcinoma of the esophagus

Text continues on page 90

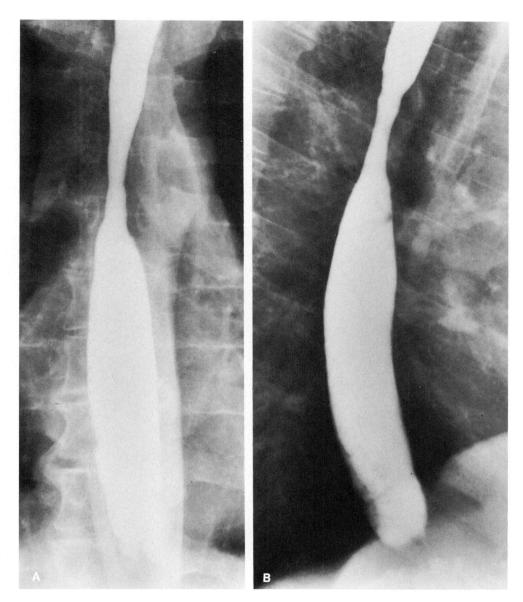

Fig. 5-34. Barrett's stricture. **(A)** Frontal and **(B)** lateral projections demonstrate a smooth upper thoracic esophageal stricture.

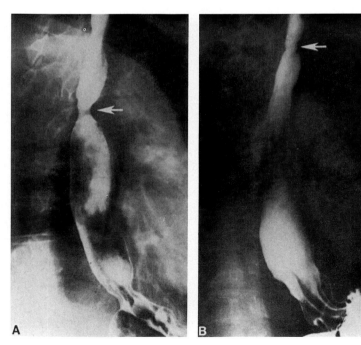

Fig. 5-35. Ascending stricture in Barrett's esophagus. **(A)** Initial esophagram shows a midesophageal stricture **(arrow)**. **(B)** Two years later, there is evidence for 4-cm proximal migration of the stricture **(arrow)**. (Agha FP: Radiologic diagnosis of Barrett's esophagus: Critical analysis of 65 cases. Gastrointest Radiol 11:123–130, 1986).

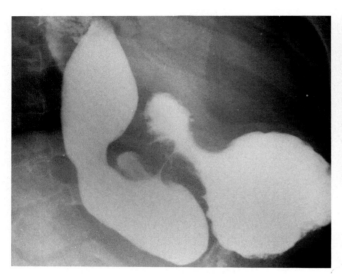

5-36

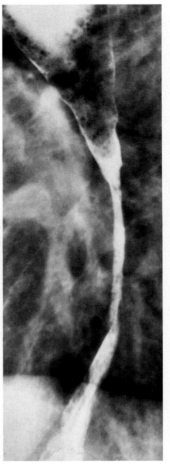

5-37

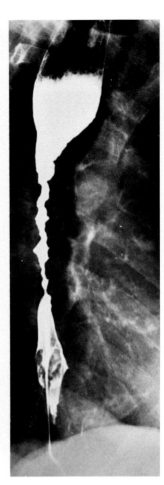

5-38

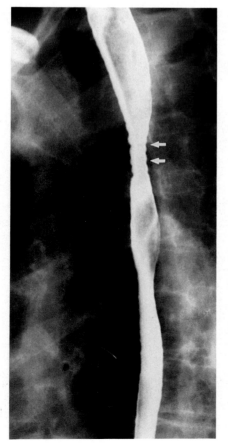

5-39

Fig. 5-36. Postoperative esophageal stricture. There is severe narrowing near the esophagogastric junction and a large residual pouch, which developed 2 weeks after the surgical repair of a hiatal hernia.

Fig. 5-37. Stricture due to prolonged nasogastric intubation. The severe esophagitis associated with the nasogastric intubation led to the development of a long stricture within 2 weeks.

Fig. 5-38. Candidiasis. There is irregular narrowing of the distal two thirds of the esophagus with multiple transverse ulcerations. (Ott DJ, Gelfand DW: Esophageal strictures secondary to candidiasis. Gastrointest Radiol 2:323–325, 1978)

Fig. 5-39. Crohn's disease. Note the long area of narrowing in the midesophagus.

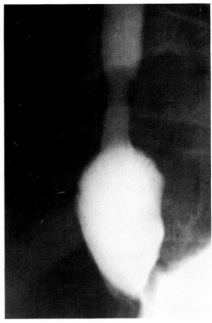

Fig. 5-40. Herpes simplex. A short, smooth stricture is visible in the distal esophagus.

Fig. 5-41. Eosinophilic esophagitis. Tapered stricture of the upper third of the esophagus with some marginal irregularity producing a "corrugated" appearance. A mild motility disturbance was also demonstrated by manometry. (Feczko PJ, Halpert RD, Zonca M: Radiographic abnormalities in eosinophilic esophagitis. Gastrointest Radiol 10:321–324, 1985)

Fig. 5-42. Behcet's syndrome. **(A)** Rigidity and irregularity of the esophageal wall producing a 15-cm area of stenosis from the upper to the lower esophagus. **(B)** Four months later, the degree of stenosis has progressed. (Mori S, Yoshihira A, Kawamura H et al: Esophageal involvement in Behcet's disease. Am J Gastroenterol 78:548–553, 1983)

5-40

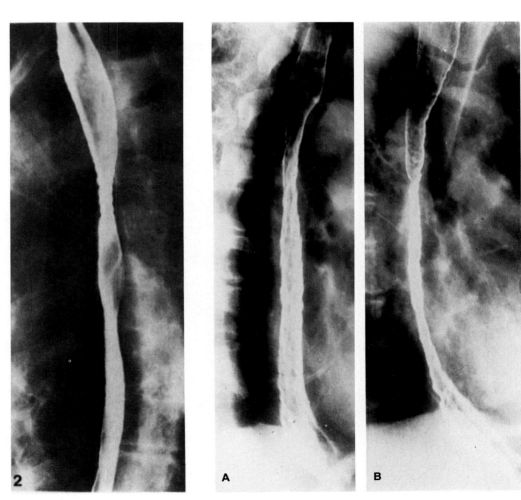

5-41   **5-42**

is rare. A major factor is that most patients with malignant disorders who undergo radiotherapy have advanced disease and rarely live long enough to develop irradiation-induced malignancy. The typical scenario is acute radiation esophagitis that progresses to chronic fibrotic stricturing, with the development of an ulcerating esophageal cancer after a prolonged latent period (Fig. 5-44).

EPIDERMOLYSIS BULLOSA

Epidermolysis bullosa is a rare hereditary disorder in which the skin blisters spontaneously or with minimal trauma. Subepidermal blisters characteristically affect the mucous membranes, giving rise to buccal contractures and feeding difficulties in infancy and childhood. Esophageal blebs tend to occur at sites of maximal trauma by ingested material, primarily the most proximal and distal esophagus as well as the level of the carina. The bullae may resolve, or they may ulcerate and bleed. Postinflammatory scarring may produce single or multiple strictures of variable length that most commonly involve the upper third of the esophagus (Fig. 5-45). The stricture typically has an abrupt transition from normal to abnormal mucosa at its proximal margin, whereas gradual tapering with smooth

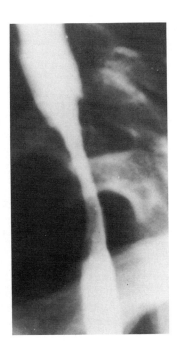

Fig. 5-43. *Radiation-induced stricture. The stricture, which developed after the administration of 6000 rad to the mediastinum for treatment of metastatic disease, has a benign appearance, with tapered margins and smooth mucosal surfaces.*

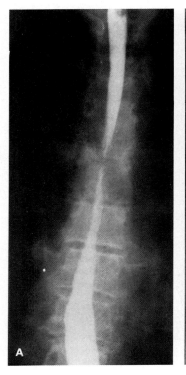
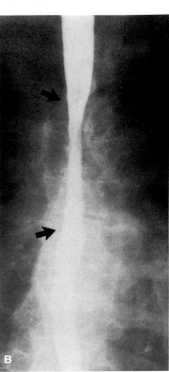
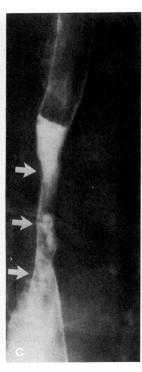

Fig. 5-44. Radiation-induced carcinoma of the esophagus. **(A)** An esophagram after the patient underwent mediastinal radiotherapy with 5000 rad shows severe radiation esophagitis causing mucosal ulcerations and narrowing of the radiated midesophagus. **(B)** Six months later, the formation of a long fibrotic stricture **(black arrows)** required dilatation by repeat bougienage. **(C)** Ten years later, an ulcerated esophageal carcinoma **(white arrows)** involved the previously radiated segment. (O'Connell EW, Seaman WB, Ghahremani GG: Radiation-induced esophageal carcinoma. Gastrointest Radiol 9:287–291, 1984)

or scarred mucosa is seen distally. Transverse and circumferential webs may also occur. Complete occlusion of the lumen of the esophagus may develop due to diffuse bullous and ulcerative lesions of the esophagus, long stenotic lesions (see Fig. 4-34), and multiple areas of stricture formation. Dysphagia is reversible when caused by bullae or webs, but is permanent when due to cicatrizing strictures.

BENIGN MUCOUS MEMBRANE PEMPHIGOID

Benign mucous membrane pemphigoid is a chronic blistering disease which, in contrast to other forms of pemphigus, particularly involves the mucous membranes of the mouth and conjunctiva, runs a chronic course, and tends to produce scarring. Symptoms of dysphagia usually precede radiographic findings by several months or years. When the pharynx and esophagus are affected, the earliest radiographic abnormalities are diffuse nonspecific inflammatory changes of mucosal edema, areas of inconstant narrowing and spasm, and superficial ulceration secondary to eruption of bullae. Postinflammatory scarring leads to adhesions that radio-graphically simulate esophageal webs (Fig. 5-46). Recurrent episodes of the disease produce smooth strictures that may be single or multiple, most commonly involve the upper esophagus, and are of variable lengths.

GRAFT-VS-HOST DISEASE

Chronic graft-vs-host disease (GVHD) is an important late complication of allogenic bone marrow transplantation in which donor lymphocytes damage host tissues. This immunologic disorder may cause esophageal mucosal destruction that produces symptoms months to years after successful marrow transplantation. Radiographic findings include thin, eccentric webs (Fig. 5-47), somewhat thicker ringlike narrowings in the cricopharyngeal region, and longer tapering strictures (Fig. 5-48) in the proximal and midesophagus. The radiographic appearance bears a striking resemblance to epidermolysis bullosa and benign mucous membrane pemphigoid, autoimmune diseases associated with esophageal mucosal desquamation similar to the lesions of chronic GVHD.

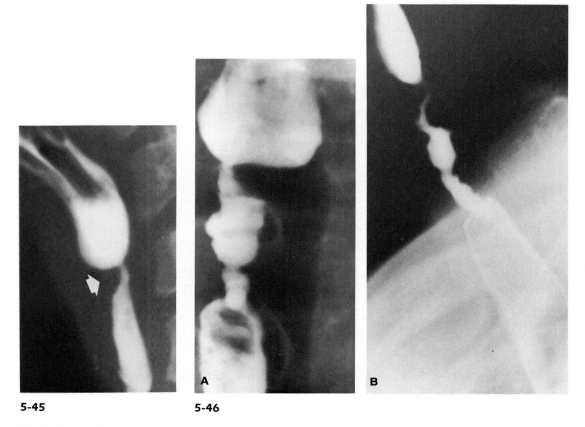

5-45   **5-46**

Fig. 5-45. Epidermolysis bullosa. A stenotic web **(arrow)** results from the healing of subepidermal blisters involving the mucous membranes.

Fig. 5-46. Benign mucous membrane pemphigoid. Postinflammatory scarring causes a long, irregular area of narrowing suggestive of a malignant process.

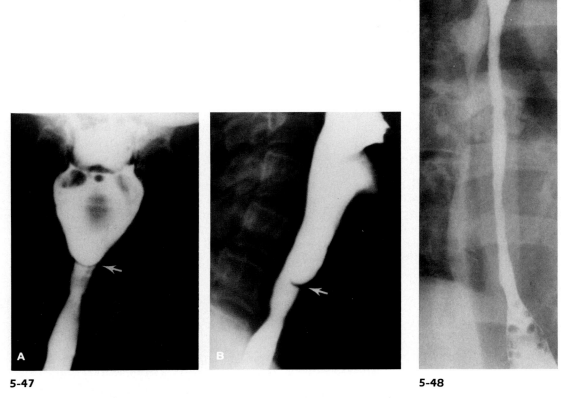

5-47   **5-48**

Fig. 5-47.   Graft-versus-host disease. **(A)** Frontal and **(B)** lateral views of the hypopharynx and upper esophagus 5 months following bone marrow transplantation show a thin web **(arrows)** in the upper esophagus. Below the web is an area of ringlike narrowing that did not distend. At endoscopy, the web was a thin, filmy membrane confluent with a desquamative process involving the upper esophagus. (McDonald GB, Sullivan KM, Plumley TF: Radiographic features of esophageal involvement in chronic graft-vs-host disease. AJR 142:501–506, 1984. Copyright 1984. Reproduced with permission)

Fig. 5-48.   Graft-versus-host disease. Two years after bone marrow transplantation and immunosuppressive therapy, there is a long stricture of the mid and lower esophagus. (McDonald GB, Sullivan KM, Plumley TF: Radiographic features of esophageal involvement in chronic graft-vs-host disease. AJR 142:501–506, 1984. Copyright 1984. Reproduced with permission)

SCLEROTHERAPY OF ESOPHAGEAL VARICES

Endoscopic sclerotherapy has become widely used to treat patients with portal hypertension and esophageal varices, either during acute variceal bleeding or as an elective long-term therapy. After the varices are injected with sclerosing agents, the initial thrombosis of the varix is followed by progressive scarring. Radiographically, fixed, noncollapsible, rather rigid-appearing filling defects in the barium column lead to complete fixation and lack of distensibility of the esophagus. The stenotic zone may be asymmetric and even have overhanging edges, mimicking carcinoma (Fig. 5-49). If the overlying mucosa becomes denuded, an ulceration may develop which may penetrate the mucosa and submucosa and undermine the muscularis, occasionally

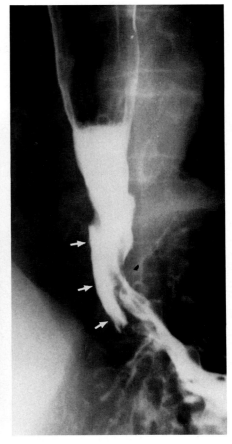

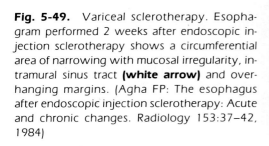

Fig. 5-49. Variceal sclerotherapy. Esophagram performed 2 weeks after endoscopic injection sclerotherapy shows a circumferential area of narrowing with mucosal irregularity, intramural sinus tract **(white arrow)** and overhanging margins. (Agha FP: The esophagus after endoscopic injection sclerotherapy: Acute and chronic changes. Radiology 153:37–42, 1984)

Fig. 5-50. Variceal sclerotherapy. Ulceration with subintimal dissection **(white arrows)**, which extends both proximally and distally from a fixed nodular contour defect on the opposite wall **(black arrow)**. There is resultant narrowing of the distal esophagus. (Bridges R, Runyon BA, Hamlin JA et al: Sclerotherapy induced pseudo-carcinoma. J Can Assoc Radiol 35:199–201, 1984)

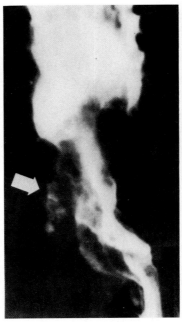

5-49   **5-50**

extending to dissect longitudinally into the intramural portions of the esophagus (Fig. 5-50).

MOTILITY DISORDERS

Severe narrowing of the distal esophagus with proximal dilatation is characteristic of the failure of relaxation of the lower esophageal sphincter in patients with achalasia (Fig. 5-51). In diffuse esophageal spasm, prolonged, strong contractions can cause marked narrowing of the esophageal lumen simulating the appearance of a fixed stricture.

INTRAMURAL ESOPHAGEAL PSEUDODIVERTICULOSIS

A smooth stricture of the esophagus is found in about 90% of patients with intramural esophageal pseudodiverticulosis (Fig. 5-52). In about two-thirds of cases, it is located in the upper third of the esophagus. Dilatation of the stricture generally results in amelioration of symptoms of dysphagia.

In a recent report, the most common pattern of intramural esophageal pseudodiverticulosis was segmental disease with isolated involvement of the distal esophagus. Most patients had ten or fewer pseudodiverticula and distal esophageal strictures typical of peptic disease. This suggests that in some patients pseudodiverticula represents a sequela of chronic esophagitis, especially due to reflux.

MALLORY-WEISS SYNDROME

One case of conical narrowing of the esophagus has been described in association with the Mallory-Weiss syndrome (Fig. 5-53). In this patient, an intermediate degree of gastroesophageal mucosal injury and bleeding produced large mounds of adherent intraluminal thrombus, which caused esophageal obstruction.

DIFFERENTIATION BETWEEN BENIGN AND MALIGNANT CAUSES

In the patient with esophageal narrowing, the critical differential diagnosis is between carcinoma and a nonmalignant lesion. As a general rule, malignant neoplasms produce discrete, irregular, and fixed strictures, often with sharply demarcated filling defects with overhanging edges that bulge toward the

Fig. 5-51. Achalasia. Failure of relaxation of the lower esophageal sphincter produces distal narrowing **(arrow)** and severe proximal dilatation.

Fig. 5-52. Intramural esophageal pseudodiverticulosis. A stricture in the upper thoracic esophagus **(arrow)** is associated with diffuse filling of esophageal glands mimicking multiple ulcerations.

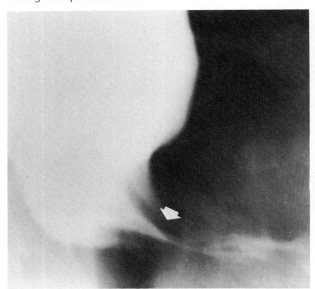

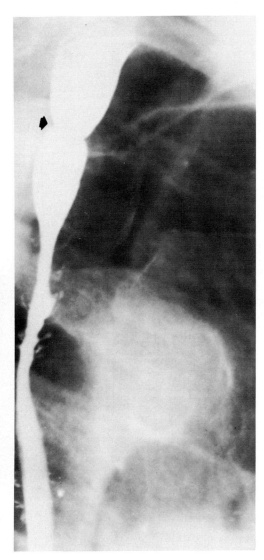

5-51

5-52

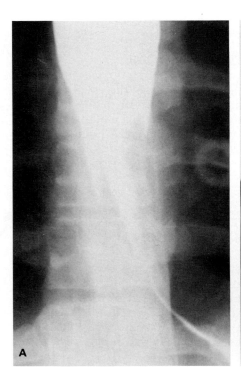

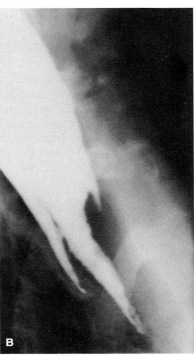

A

B

Fig. 5-53. Mallory-Weiss syndrome. Large mounds of adherent thrombus produce marked narrowing of the distal esophagus. (Curtin MJ, Milligan FD: Mallory-Weiss syndrome with esophageal obstruction secondary to adherent intraluminal thrombus. AJR 129:508–510, 1977. Copyright 1977. Reproduced with permission)

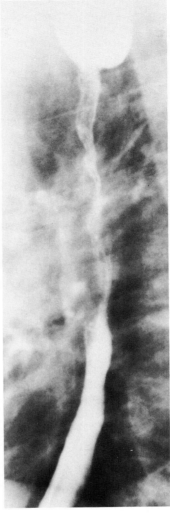

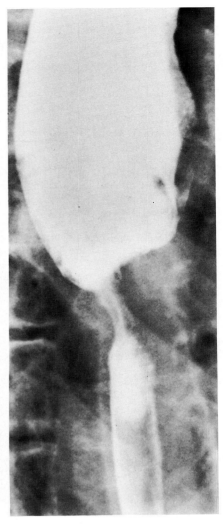

Fig. 5-54. Malignant stricture (squamous carcinoma). Note that the stricture is long, irregular, and eccentric.

Fig. 5-55. Malignant stricture (squamous carcinoma). The marked asymmetry and eccentricity of the stricture favors a malignant etiology.

5-54　　　　　　　　　**5-55**

lumen (Fig. 5-54). Associated ulceration is frequent and often has an irregular configuration. At times, however, esophageal narrowing due to malignancy can appear relatively smooth with tapering margins and closely simulate a benign lesion. Asymmetry or eccentricity of the stricture favors a malignant etiology (Fig. 5-55). Unless the clinical history and radiographic appearance are typical of a benign process and the patient improves on medical therapy, esophagoscopy and biopsy are necessary for an unequivocal diagnosis to be made.

BIBLIOGRAPHY

Agha FP: Barrett carcinoma of the esophagus: Clinical and radiographic analysis of 34 cases. AJR 145:41–46, 1985

Agha FP: Candidiasis-induced esophageal strictures. Gastrointest Radiol 9:283–286, 1984

Agha FP: Radiologic diagnosis of Barrett's esophagus: Critical analysis of 65 cases. Gastrointest Radiol 11:123–130, 1986

Agha FP, Francis IR, Ellis CN: Esophageal involvement in epidermolysis bullosa dystrophica: Clinical and roentgenographic manifestations. Gastrointest Radiol 8:111–117, 1983

Agha FP, Raji MR: Esophageal involvement in pemphigoid: Clinical and roentgen manifestations. Gastrointest Radiol 7:109–112, 1982

Al-Kutoubi MA, Eliot C: Oesophageal involvement in benign mucous membrane pemphigoid. Clin Radiol 35:131–135, 1984

Chen YM, Gelfand DW, Ott DJ et al: Natural progression of the lower esophageal mucosal ring. Gastrointest Radiol 12:93–98, 1987

Clements JL, Cox GW, Torres WE et al: Cervical esophageal webs—A roentgen-anatomic correlation. AJR 121:221–231, 1974

Curtin MJ, Milligan FD: Mallory–Weiss syndrome with esophageal obstruction secondary to adherent intraluminal thrombus. AJR 129:508–510, 1977

Dawson SL, Mueller PR, Ferrucci JT et al: Severe esophageal strictures: Indications for balloon catheter dilatation. Radiology 153:631–635, 1984

Donner MW, Saba GP, Martinez CR: Diffuse diseases of the esophagus: A practical approach. Semin Roentgenol 16:198–213, 1981

Feczko PJ, Halpert RD, Zonca M: Radiographic abnormalities in eosinophilic esophagitis. Gastrointest Radiol 10:321–324, 1985

Fisher MS: Metastasis to the esophagus. Gastrointest Radiol 1:249–251, 1976

Franken EA: Caustic damage of the gastrointestinal tract: Roentgen features. AJR 118:77–85, 1973

Ghahremani GG, Gore RM, Breuer RI et al: Esophageal manifestations of Crohn's disease. Gastrointest Radiol 7:199–203, 1982

Goldstein HM, Zornoza J: Association of squamous cell carcinoma of the head and neck with cancer of the esophagus. AJR 131:791–794, 1978

Goldstein HM, Zornoza J, Hopens T: Intrinsic diseases of the adult esophagus: Benign and malignant tumors. Semin Roentgenol 16:183–197, 1981

Halpert RD, Feczko PJ, Chason DP: Barrett's esophagus: Radiological and clinical considerations. J Can Assoc Radiol 35:120–123, 1984

Halvorsen RA, Thompson WM: Computed tomography staging of gastrointestinal malignancies. Part I. Esophagus and stomach. Invest Radiol 22:2–16, 1987

Han SY, Mihas AA: Circumferential web of the upper esophagus. Gastrointest Radiol 3:7–9, 1978

Hishikawa Y, Tanaka S, Miura T: Esophageal ulceration induced by intracavitary irradiation for esophageal carcinoma. AJR 143:269–273, 1984

Hutton CF: Plummer–Vinson syndrome. Br J Radiol 29:81–85, 1956

Koehler RE, Moss AA, Margulis AR: Early radiographic manifestations of carcinoma of the esophagus. Radiology 119:1–5, 1976

Lansing PB, Ferrante WA, Ochsner JL: Carcinoma of the esophagus at the site of lye stricture. Am J Surg 118:108–111, 1973

Laufer I: Radiology of esophagitis. Radiol Clin North Am 20:687–699, 1982

Levine MS: Crohn's disease of the upper gastrointestinal tract. Radiol Clin North Am 25:79–91, 1987

Levine MS, Dillon EC, Saul SH et al: Early esophageal cancer. AJR 146:507–512, 1986

Levine MS, Langer J, Laufer I et al: Radiation therapy of esophageal carcinoma: Correlation of clinical and radiographic findings. Gastrointest Radiol 12:99–105, 1987

Levine MS, Moolten DN, Herlinger H et al: Esophageal intramural pseudodiverticulosis: A reevaluation. AJR 147:1165–1170, 1986

Martel W: Radiologic features of esophagogastritis secondary to extremely caustic agents. Radiology 103:31–36, 1972

Mauro MA, Parker LA, Hartley WS et al: Epidermalysis bullosa: Radiographic findings in 16 cases. AJR 149:925–927, 1987

McDonald GB, Sullivan KM, Plumley TF: Radiographic features of esophageal involvement in chronic graft-vs.-host disease. AJR 142:501–506, 1984

Nosher JL, Campbell WL, Seaman WB: The clinical significance of cervical esophageal and hypopharyngeal webs. Radiology 117:45–47, 1975

O'Connell EW, Seaman WB, Ghahremani GG: Radiation-induced esophageal carcinoma. Gastrointest Radiol 9:287–291, 1984

Ott DJ, Chen YM, Wu WC et al: Radiographic and endoscopic sensitivity in detecting lower esophageal mucosal ring. AJR 147:261–265, 1986

Ott DJ, Gelfand DW: Esophageal stricture secondary to candidiasis. Gastrointest Radiol 2:323–325, 1978

Parnell DD, Johnson SAM: Tylosis palmaris et plantaris: Its occurrence with internal malignancy. Arch Dermatol 100:7–9, 1969

Picus D, Frank PH: Eosinophilic esophagitis. AJR 136:1001–1003, 1981

Rose JS, Kassner EG, Jurgens KH et al: Congenital oesophageal strictures due to cartilaginous rings. Br J Radiol 48:16–18, 1975

Rosengren JE, Goldstein HM: Radiologic demonstration of multiple foci of malignancy in the esophagus. Gastrointest Radiol 3:11–13, 1978

Schatzki R, Gary JE: The lower esophageal ring. AJR 75:246–261, 1956

Shauffer IA, Phillips HE, Sequeira J: The jet phenomenon: A manifestation of esophageal web. AJR 129:747–748, 1977

Starck E, Paolucci V, Herzer M et al: Esophageal stenosis: Treatment with balloon catheters. Radiology 153:637–640, 1984

Weaver JW, Kaude JV, Hamlin DJ: Webs of the lower esophagus: A complication of gastroesophageal reflux? AJR 142:289–292, 1984

Williford ME, Rice RP, Kelvin FM et al: Revascularized jejunal graft replacing the cervical esophagus: Radiographic evaluation. AJR 145:533–536, 1985

Williford ME, Thompson WM, Hamilton JD et al: Esophageal tuberculosis: Findings on barium swallow and computed tomography. Gastrointest Radiol 8:119–122, 1983

Wolf EL, Frager J, Brandt LJ et al: Radiographic appearance of the esophagus and stomach after laser treatment of obstructing carcinoma. AJR 146:519–522, 1986

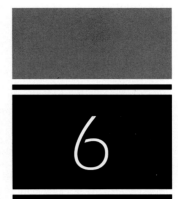

ESOPHAGEAL FILLING DEFECTS

Disease Entities

Neoplastic lesions
  Benign tumors
    Spindle cell tumor (*e.g.,* leiomyoma)
    Fibrovascular polyp
    Squamous papilloma
    Inflammatory esophagogastric polyp
    Adenomatous polyp
  Tumors of intermediate malignant potential
    Villous adenoma
  Malignant tumors
    Carcinoma of the esophagus
    Gastric carcinoma with upward extension
    Metastases
    Leiomyosarcoma
    Spindle cell squamous carcinoma
    Melanoma
    Lymphoma
    Kaposi's sarcoma
    Verrucous squamous cell carcinoma
Lymph node enlargement (extrinsic lesions)
  Malignant lesion
  Granulomatous process
Infectious/Granulomatous/Inflammatory
    esophagitis
  Candidiasis
  Herpetic esophagitis
  Reflux esophagitis
  Crohn's disease
  Eosinophilic esophagitis

Varices
Duplication cyst
Foreign bodies/air bubbles
Intramural hematoma
Hirsute esophagus
Prolapsed gastric folds

SPINDLE CELL TUMOR

Leiomyoma is the most common benign tumor of the esophagus (Fig. 6-1). Like the other benign spindle cell tumors of the esophagus, most leiomyomas are asymptomatic and are discovered during radiographic examination for nonesophageal complaints or incidentally at autopsy. In the few patients with symptoms, dysphagia and substernal pain are common complaints. Leiomyomas are most frequently found in the lower third of the esophagus. The vast majority are located intramurally and have little, if any, tendency to undergo malignant transformation. Unlike gastric leiomyomas, tumors of this cell type in the esophagus rarely ulcerate or bleed. Multiple tumors are occasionally present (Fig. 6-2).

When viewed in profile, an esophageal leiomyoma appears radiographically as a smooth, rounded intramural defect in the barium column (Fig. 6-3). The characteristic half-moon or crescent-shaped mass is sharply demarcated from adjacent portions of the esophageal wall. The superior and inferior margins of the tumor form a right or slightly obtuse angle with the wall of the esophagus. There is no evidence of infiltration, ulceration, or undercutting at the tumor margin. When examined *en face*, a

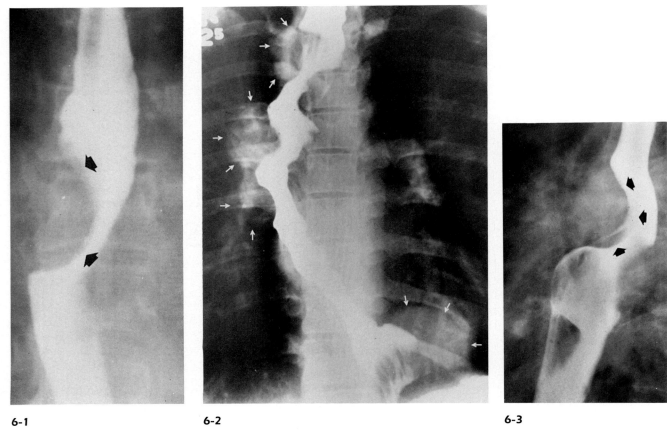

6-1   6-2   6-3

Fig. 6-1. Leiomyoma. A smooth, rounded intramural defect is evident in the barium column
(arrows).

Fig. 6-2. Multiple esophageal leiomyomas. Several smoothly rounded filling defects in the
barium column conform to the companion soft-tissue masses **(arrows)**. The masses
move freely during swallowing, indicating a lack of adhesions or mediastinal infiltration.
(Shaffer HA: Multiple leiomyomas of the esophagus. Radiology 118:29–34, 1976)

Fig. 6-3. Leiomyoma. Note the smooth, rounded intramural defect in the barium column
(arrows).

leiomyoma appears as a round or lobulated filling
defect sharply outlined by the barium flowing
around each side. Esophageal motility is normal
and dilatation above the tumor infrequent. An
esophageal leiomyoma may have a large extramural
component that is visible as it projects into the mediastinum and is outlined against adjacent lung.
Rarely, leiomyomas of the distal esophagus contain
enough calcium to be visible radiographically (Fig.
6-4). Because tumoral calcification has not been
described in any other esophageal lesion, the presence of amorphous calcification in a retrocardiac
esophageal mass is diagnostic of a leiomyoma.

Other benign spindle cell submucosal tumors
are extremely rare. These include lipomas (Fig. 6-5),
fibrolipomas (Fig. 6-6), myxofibromas, hemangiomas, lymphangiomas, schwannomas (Fig. 6-7), and
granular cell tumors (Fig. 6-8).

FIBROVASCULAR POLYP

Fibrovascular polyps, though rare, are the second
most common type of solid benign tumor of the
esophagus. They consist of varying amounts of fibrovascular tissue, adipose cells, and stroma that arise
in the mucosa or submucosa and are covered by
epidermoid epithelium, which can become secondarily eroded and bleed. Fibrovascular polyps can
grow to a huge size without being suspected. Dysphagia is the most common symptom. Pain varies
from severe epigastric distress to mild substernal
and epigastric discomfort. Very large tumors can
compress the trachea and cause respiratory distress.
Occasionally, pedunculated fibrovascular polyps
present catastrophically by being regurgitated into
the mouth, causing asphyxiation and death.

Fibrovascular polyps appear radiographically

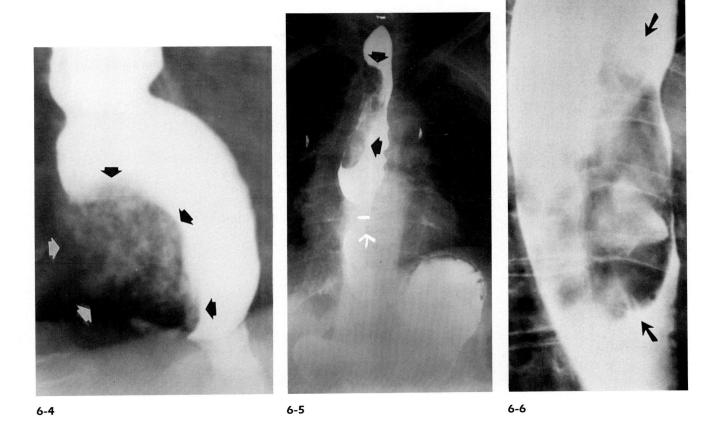

6-4   6-5   6-6

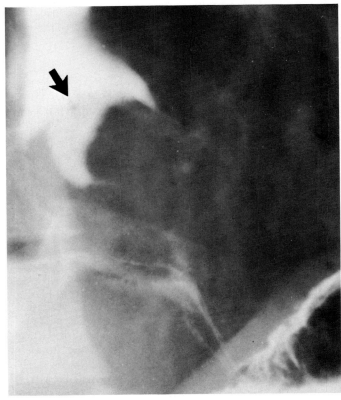

6-7

Fig. 6-4. Leiomyoma of the distal esophagus. Note the amorphous calcifications in the smoothly lobulated intramural tumor **(arrows)**. (Ghahremani GG, Meyers MA, Port RB: Calcified primary tumors of the gastrointestinal tract. Gastrointest Radiol 2:331–339, 1978)

Fig. 6-5. Lipoma. A sausage-shaped mass **(arrows)** is visible in the upper thoracic esophagus.

Fig. 6-6. Fibrolipoma **(arrows)**.

Fig. 6-7. Schwannoma **(arrow)**.

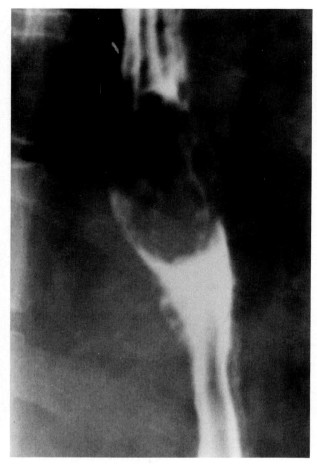

Fig. 6-8. *Granular cell tumor. Well-circumscribed filling defect with normal surrounding mucosa. (Mauro MA, Jaques PF: Granular cell tumors of the esophagus and common bile duct. J Can Assoc Radiol 32:254–256, 1981)*

as large intraluminal filling defects (Fig. 6-9). They are oval-shaped or elongated, sausage-like masses with a smooth or mildly lobulated surface. At fluoroscopy, barium can be observed to flow around the intraluminal tumor and completely surround it. A large fibrovascular polyp can cause local widening of the esophagus but not the complete obstruction or wall rigidity that may be seen with an esophageal carcinoma.

OTHER BENIGN LESIONS

Squamous papillomas consist of a papillary structure lined with normal squamous epithelium. They are usually too small to be detected radiographically but occasionally present as large, movable, soft-appearing papillary intraluminal tumors (Fig. 6-10).

An inflammatory esophagogastric polyp is a round, firm lesion seen at or just below the esophagogastric junction. It contains squamous or gastric epithelium with inflammatory changes and has an inflamed, prominent fold leading up to it from the

gastric fundus (Fig. 6-11). The inflammatory polyp and thickened gastric fold complex probably represent a stage in the evolution of chronic esophagitis, with the polyp reflecting thickening of the proximal aspect of an inflamed sentinel fold.

Benign adenomatous polyps are rare lesions that can present as intraluminal filling defects in the esophagus (Fig. 6-12).

VILLOUS ADENOMA

Villous adenomas, tumors of intermediate malignant potential, can appear as filling defects in the esophagus (Fig. 6-13). As with tumors of this cell type elsewhere in the bowel, barium characteristically fills the frondlike interstices of the lesion.

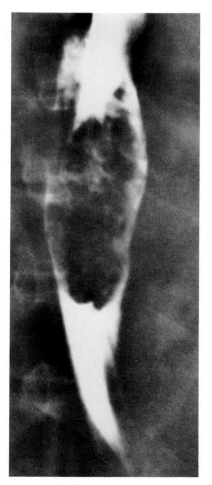

Fig. 6-9. *Fibrovascular polyp. Note the bulky, sausage-shaped mass with a mildly lobulated surface.*

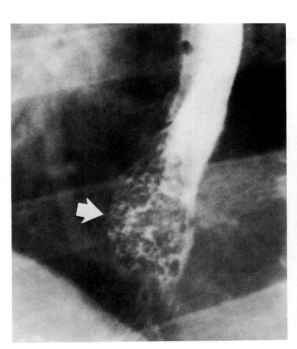

6-10

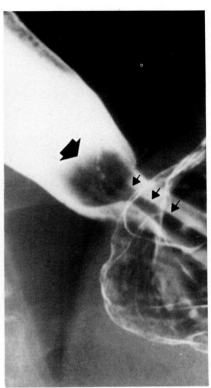

6-11

Fig. 6-10. Giant papilloma. There is a large, bubbly-appearing collection of tumor **(arrow)** in the distal esophagus. (Walker JH: Giant papilloma of the thoracic esophagus. AJR 131:519–520, 1978. Copyright 1978. Reproduced with permission)

Fig. 6-11. Inflammatory esophagogastric polyp. Distal esophageal filling defect **(large arrow)** in continuity with a thickened gastric fold **(small arrows).**

Fig. 6-12. Benign adenomatous polyp **(arrow).**

Fig. 6-13. Villous adenoma. Pathologic examination confirmed that the tumor **(arrow)** arose from the gastric mucosa at the esophagogastric junction. (Miller JH, Gisvold JJ, Weiland LH et al: Upper gastrointestinal tract: Villous tumors. AJR 134:933–936, 1980. Copyright 1980. Reproduced with permission)

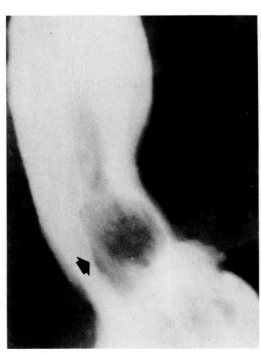

6-12

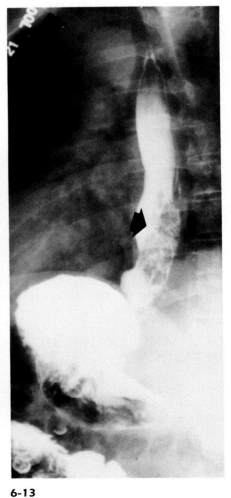

6-13

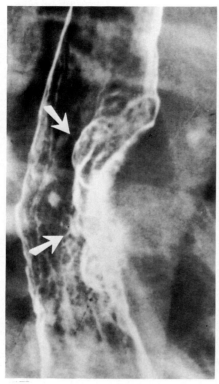

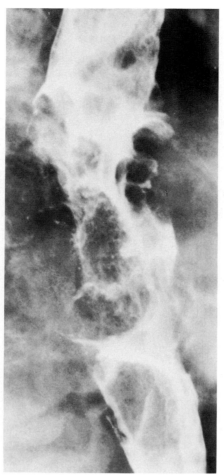

6-14   6-15

Fig. 6-14. Squamous carcinoma of the esophagus. Note the localized polypoid mass with ulceration **(arrows)**.

Fig. 6-15. Squamous carcinoma of the esophagus. A bulky, irregular filling defect with destruction of mucosal folds may be seen.

CARCINOMA OF THE ESOPHAGUS

Carcinoma of the esophagus can present as a localized polypoid mass, often with deep ulceration and a fungating appearance (Fig. 6-14). This bulky filling defect is found predominantly in the lower end of the esophagus. Esophageal carcinoma more frequently appears as a clearly defined, irregular filling defect, with destruction of mucosal folds, overhanging margins, and an abrupt transition to adjacent normal tissue (Fig. 6-15).

CARCINOMA OF THE STOMACH/ METASTASES

Lower esophageal filling defects, usually with irregular surfaces, can be seen in patients with carcinoma of the gastric cardia extending upward into the distal esophagus. A very rare manifestation of hematogenous metastases to the esophagus is the appearance of single or multiple filling defects in the barium column. Lymphatic metastases can rarely produce single or multiple polypoid lesions

that have a smooth surface but may develop central ulceration (Fig. 6-16).

SARCOMA

Leiomyosarcomas of the esophagus are very rare. Though usually bulky and ulcerated (Fig. 6-17), a leiomyosarcoma occasionally appears radiographically as a smooth, rounded esophageal filling defect with regular outlines, closely simulating a benign tumor.

Spindle cell squamous carcinoma is now the generally accepted term to describe the rare malignant esophageal tumor consisting of polypoid carcinoma with spindle cell components. The sarcomatous component of the squamous cell carcinoma appears to originate from mesenchymal metaplasia of squamous cells. A distinction was previously made between "carcinosarcoma," composed of nests of squamous epithelium surrounded by interlacing bundles of spindle-shaped cells with numerous mitoses, and "pseudosarcoma," consisting entirely of oval and spindle-shaped cells without squamous ele-

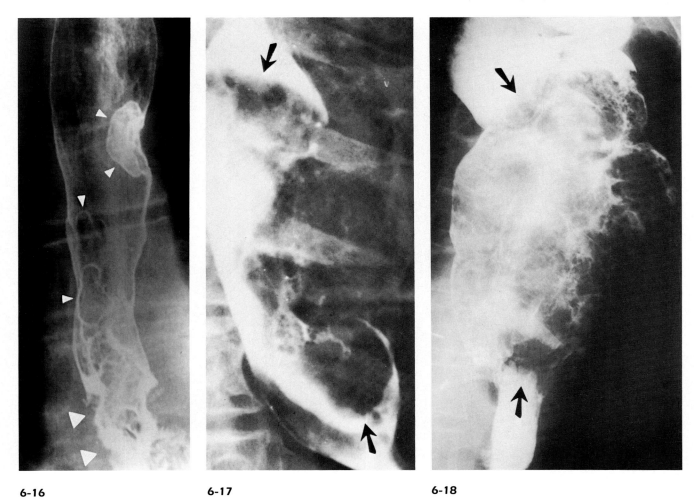

6-16   6-17   6-18

Fig. 6-16. Lymphatic metastases. Multiple polypoid masses in the midesophagus **(small arrowheads)** representing discontinuous lymphatic spread from carcinoma involving the eso phagogastric region **(large arrowheads)**. (Steiner H, Lammer J, Hackl A: Lymphatic metastases of the esophagus. Gastrointest Radiol 9:1–4, 1984)

Fig. 6-17. Leiomyosarcoma. The bulky, ulcerated mass involves more than half of the thoracic esophagus **(arrows)**.

Fig. 6-18. Carcinosarcoma. The bulky, intraluminal, polypoid mass **(arrows)** has produced a large defect in the barium-filled esophagus.

ments, to imply that these large lesions metastasize rarely or late and have better survival rates than squamous cell carcinoma. However, recent studies have demonstrated that despite the unusual histologic features, the prognosis is equally grim. Regardless of terminology, these lesions appear radiographically as bulky, intraluminal polypoid masses that usually occur in the lower half of the esophagus and produce large defects when the esophagus is filled with barium (Fig. 6-18). The surface may be smooth, lobulated, or scalloped, and this may create a "cupola effect" (Fig. 6-19). There may be mucosal ulcerations of variable size and a pedicle. Although

the mass is large and bulky, there is relatively little obstruction to the flow of contrast material.

MELANOMA

Melanocytes in the basal cell layer of the esophageal epithelium may give rise to malignant melanoma. Metastatic melanoma also occasionally involves the esophagus. Esophageal melanoma usually appears radiographically as a smooth polypoid filling defect but can present as a multilobulated esophageal mass (Fig. 6-20).

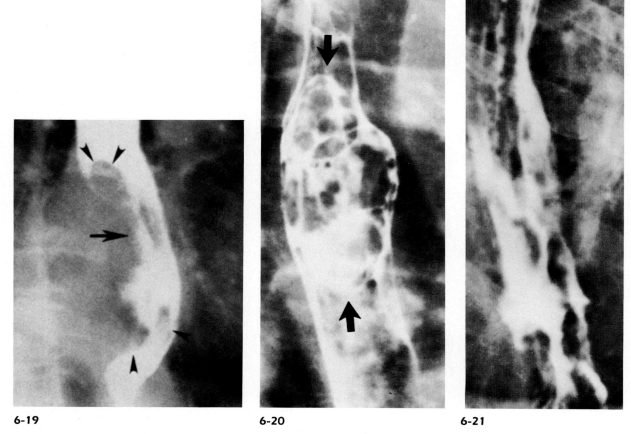

6-19   6-20   6-21

Fig. 6-19. Cupola effect in spindle cell squamous carcinoma. Elongated polypoid intraluminal mass with linear ulceration **(arrow)** occupies the lower half of the thoracic esophagus. Note the cupola effect along the superior aspect of the tumor **(arrowheads)**. (Agha FP, Keren DF: Spindle cell squamous carcinoma of the esophagus: A tumor with biphasic morphology. AJR 145:541–545, 1985. Copyright 1985. Reproduced with permission.)

Fig. 6-20. Metastatic melanoma. This multilobulated esophageal filling defect **(arrows)** arose several years after the patient had scratched a dark mole off his skin.

Fig. 6-21. Lymphoma. Submucosal lymphomatous infiltration in the thoracic esophagus causes an appearance simulating varices. (Carnovale RL, Goldstein HM, Zornoza J et al: Radiologic manifestations of esophageal lymphoma. AJR 128:751–754, 1977. Copyright 1977. Reproduced with permission)

LYMPHOMA

Radiographic demonstration of lymphoma involving the esophagus is rare. In almost all cases, the esophagus is affected secondarily as a result of extrinsic lymph node compression. In the extremely rare case of direct involvement of the esophagus by lymphoma, the radiographic appearance depends on the activity of the tumor. If the lymphoma grows inward toward the lumen, it can appear as a large filling defect, often with ulceration. If the tumor remains confined to the submucosa, the resulting long, nonulcerated intramural lesion may closely resemble esophageal varices (Fig. 6-21). Infrequently, multiple tiny submucosal nodules may produce a pattern of diffuse nodularity.

KAPOSI'S SARCOMA

Kaposi's sarcoma is now considered a systemic, multifocal, steadily progressive tumor of the reticuloendothelial system. Visceral involvement is thought to be an expression of the multicentric potential of this systemic neoplasm rather than a representation of metastatic dissemination. Infrequent esophageal involvement appears as nonspecific single or multiple polypoid filling defects.

VERRUCOUS CARCINOMA

Verrucous tumors can occur on any stratified squamous mucosa or modified skin. They have been recognized in the mouth, nose, larynx, and genital organs. Verrucous squamous cell carcinoma involving the esophagus is a slowly progressing lesion that presents radiographically as a large filling defect with a smooth surface and benign appearance (Fig. 6-22). This exophytic, papillary, or warty tumor rarely metastasizes and has a far better prognosis than typical squamous cell carcinoma of the esophagus.

LYMPH NODE ENLARGEMENT

Lymph node enlargement can produce an extrinsic impression on the esophagus simulating an intramural lesion (Fig. 6-23). This appearance is usually caused by a metastatic malignant tumor or by a granulomatous process, most commonly tuberculosis, but is occasionally due to syphilis, sarcoidosis, histoplasmosis, or Crohn's disease.

INFECTIOUS/GRANULOMATOUS ESOPHAGITIS

Candidiasis may present as multiple round and oval nodular defects in the barium-filled esophagus. The plaquelike lesions tend to be longitudinally oriented and appear as linear or irregular filling defects with intervening segments of normal mucosa (Fig. 6-24). This pattern may be due to mucosal edema, formation of a pseudomembrane, or seeding of actual colonies of *Candida albicans* on the surface of the esophageal mucosa. In most cases of esophageal candidiasis, the associated ulceration and shaggy contour of the wall of the esophagus should suggest the proper diagnosis. A similar appearance with multiple diffuse, small, nodular filling defects has been described in herpetic esophagitis (Fig. 6-25). In patients with reflux esophagitis, pseudomembrane formation may produce irregular or linear plaquelike lesions mimicking candidiasis or a single longitudinal plaque radiographically indistinguishable from carcinoma arising in Barrett's esophagus. Crohn's disease involving the esophagus may produce multiple nodular filling defects (cobblestone

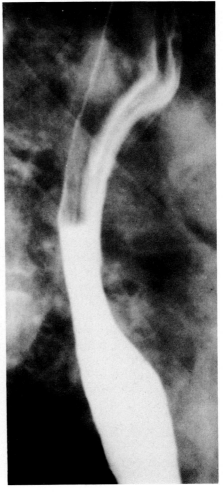

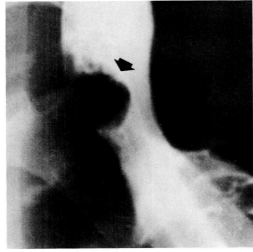

Fig. 6-22. Verrucous squamous cell carcinoma. The smooth-surfaced filling defect in the distal esophagus **(arrow)** has a benign appearance.

Fig. 6-23. Subcarinal lymph node enlargement (sarcoidosis) producing an extrinsic impression that simulates an intramural mass.

6-22

6-23

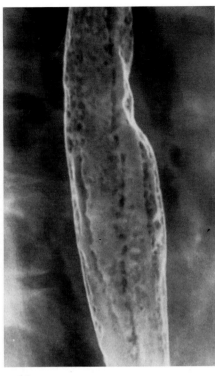

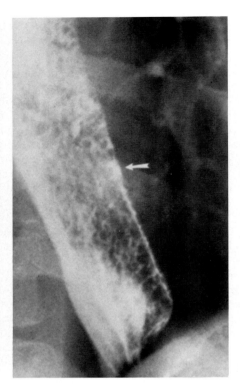

6-24   6-25

Fig. 6-24. Candidiasis. Numerous plaquelike defects in the mid and distal esophagus. Note the characteristic appearance of the plaques with discrete margins and predominantly longitudinal orientation. (Levine MS, Macones AJ, Laufer I: *Candida* esophagitis: Accuracy of radiographic diagnosis. Radiology 154:581–587, 1985)

Fig. 6-25. Herpetic esophagitis. Diffuse, small nodular filling defects throughout the esophagus. Note the one focally penetrating ulcer **(arrow)**. (Agha FP, Lee HH, Nostrant TT: Herpetic esophagitis: A diagnostic challenge in immunocompromised patients. (Am J Gastroenterol 81:246–253, 1986)

pattern) or filiform polyps identical to those commonly seen in the colon (Fig. 6-26). Single or multiple polypoid lesions are a rare manifestation of eosinophilic esophagitis (Fig. 6-27).

VARICES

Esophageal varices appear radiographically as serpiginous submucosal masses representing dilated venous structures (Fig. 6-28). Varices can usually be easily differentiated from other esophageal filling defects because their size and appearance change with variations in intrathoracic pressure (see Chapter 8). Rarely, an isolated varix may appear as a solitary submucosal mass in the esophagus. Effacement of the lesion by gaseous distention of the esophagus should suggest its vascular origin (Fig. 6-29). However, if the varix is thrombosed it is unaffected by changes in patient position or degree of esophageal distention and is indistinguishable from a submucosal neoplasm (Fig. 6-30).

DUPLICATION CYST

A duplication cyst can produce an eccentric impression on the barium-filled esophagus simulating an intramural or mediastinal mass (Fig. 6-31). Du-

plications occur less commonly in the esophagus than in other portions of the gastrointestinal tract. These cystic structures are closely attached to the normal esophagus and are covered by muscle that is lined with gastric or enteric epithelium. As a duplication dilates with retained material, it may compress the esophagus and produce dysphagia. Cough, cyanosis, and respiratory distress may occur. Although contrast material infrequently fills a duplication (Fig. 6-32), in most cases there is no connection between the duplication and the esophageal lumen.

FOREIGN BODIES

A wide spectrum of foreign bodies can become impacted in the esophagus. Pieces of chicken bone (Fig. 6-33) or fishbones (Fig. 6-34) may be swallowed accidentally. If large enough, they will become impacted, predominantly in the cervical esophagus at or just above the level of the thoracic inlet. Metallic objects such as pins, coins (Fig. 6-35), and small toys (Fig. 6-36) are swallowed frequently by infants and young children. It is essential that a suspected foreign body be evaluated on two views in order for the physician to be certain that the dense object projected over the esophagus truly lies within it (Fig. 6-37). Most metals are very radiopaque and

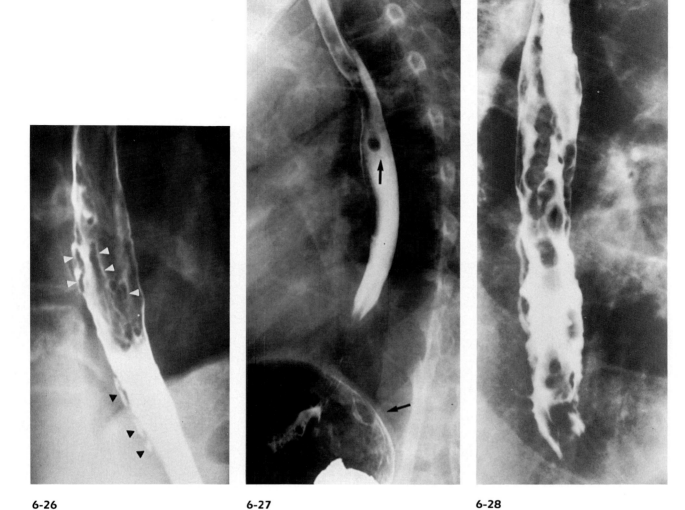

6-26   6-27   6-28

Fig. 6-26. Crohn's esophagitis. Filiform polyps **(white arrowheads)** are associated with mucosal nodularity, deep ulcers, and intramural sinus tracts **(black arrowheads)**. (Cockey BM, Jones B, Bayless TM et al: Filiform polyps of the esophagus with inflammatory bowel disease. AJR 144:1207–1208, 1985. Copyright 1985. Reproduced with permission.)

Fig. 6-27. Eosinophilic esophagitis. Small polyp in the midesophagus **(upper arrow)** as well as a polyp in the fundus of the stomach **(lower arrow)** in a young woman with abdominal pain and malabsorption. Endoscopy demonstrated multiple polyps throughout the upper gastrointestinal tract. (Feczko PJ, Halpert RD, Zonca M: Radiographic abnormalities in eosinophilic esophagitis. Gastrointest Radiol 10:321–324, 1985)

Fig. 6-28. Esophageal varices. Serpiginous submucosal masses represent dilated venous structures.

easily visualized on radiographs or during fluoroscopy. Objects made of aluminum and some light alloys may be impossible to detect radiographically, because the density of these metals is almost equal to that of soft tissue.

The presence of nonopaque foreign bodies in the esophagus, especially pieces of poorly chewed meat, can be demonstrated only after the ingestion of barium (Fig. 6-38). Such foreign bodies usually become impacted in the distal esophagus just above the level of the diaphragm and are often associated with a distal stricture (Fig. 6-39). These intraluminal filling defects usually have a nonhomogeneous surface that is either marbled or spotted and may resemble a completely obstructing carcinoma. Impactions may also be due to strictures in the cervical portion of the esophagus (Fig. 6-40).

Complications of ingested foreign bodies in the esophagus include penetration of the esophageal wall, which can lead to a periesophageal abscess or

Text continues on page 113

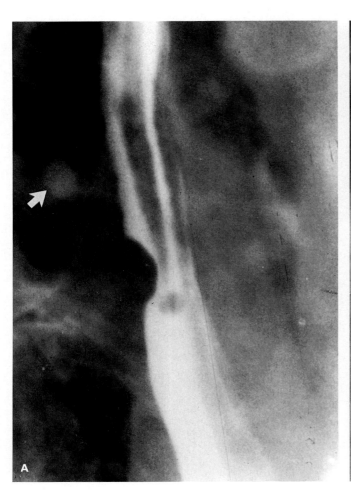 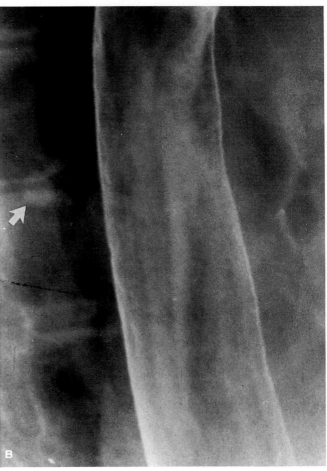

Fig. 6-29. Isolated esophageal varix. **(A)** Single-contrast view of the esophagus with partial distention shows a smooth submucosal lesion in the midesophagus. Note the relation of the lesion to the calcified granuloma **(arrow)** in the lung. **(B)** Double-contrast radiograph shows complete obliteration of the lesion when the esophagus is maximally distended. Again note the calcified granuloma **(arrow)** in the adjacent lung. Although this isolated varix mimics a submucosal mass in the nondistended esophagus, its effacement with increasing esophageal distention suggests its vascular origin. (Trenkner SW, Levine MS, Laufer I et al: Idiopathic esophageal varix. AJR 141:43–44, 1983. Copyright 1983. Reproduced with permission.)

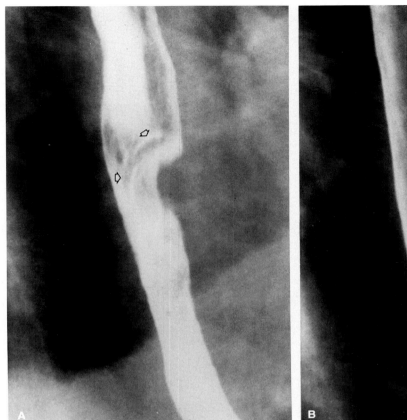
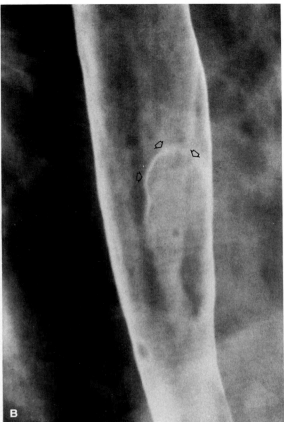

6-30

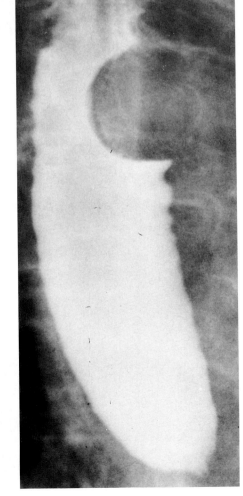

Fig. 6-30. Isolated esophageal varix. **(A)** View of the esophagus with partial distention demonstrates a submucosal mass in the midesophagus **(arrows)**. **(B)** With greater gaseous distention of the esophagus, the lesion shows no evidence of effacement **(arrows)**. In this case, the unchanging radiographic appearance with esophageal distention resulted from variceal thrombosis. (Trenkner SW, Levine MS, Laufer I et al: Idiopathic esophageal varix. AJR 141:43–44, 1983. Copyright 1983. Reproduced with permission.)

Fig. 6-31. Duplication cyst. Eccentric compression on the barium-filled esophagus simulates an intramural mass.

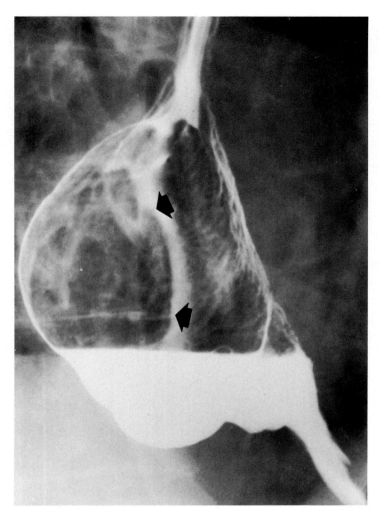

Fig. 6-32. Esophageal duplication with postsurgical communication with the esophageal lumen. **Arrows** point to the duplication cyst.

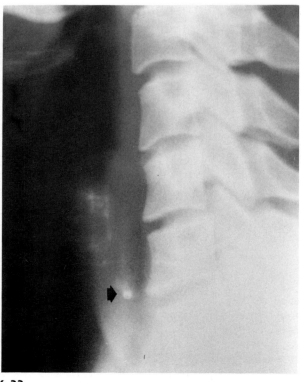

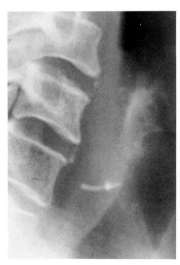

Fig. 6-33. Cornish game-hen bone **(arrow)** impacted in the lower cervical esophagus.

Fig. 6-34. Fishbone impacted in the lower cervical esophagus.

6-33

6-34

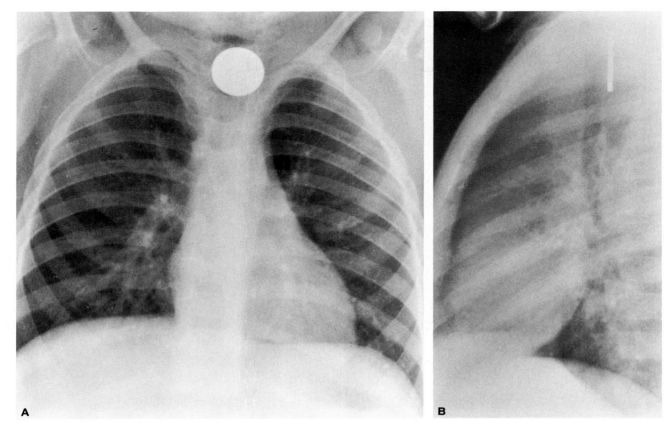

Fig. 6-35. Metallic coin impacted in the esophagus. **(A)** Frontal and **(B)** lateral projections.

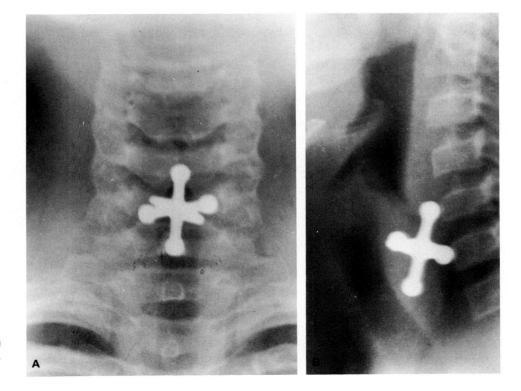

Fig. 6-36. Metallic jack impacted in the esophagus. **(A)** Frontal and **(B)** lateral projections.

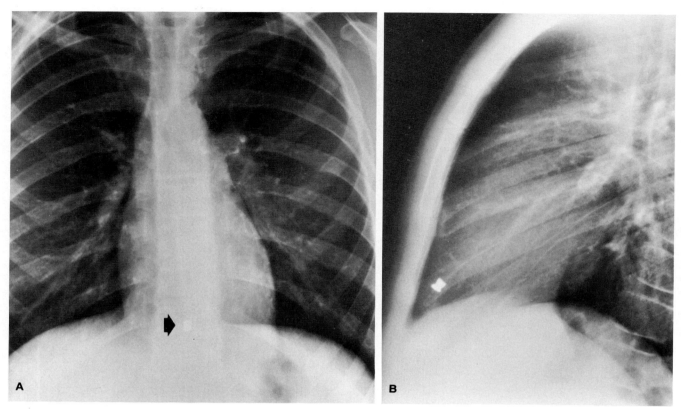

Fig. 6-37. Bullet in the right atrium of a child simulating an esophageal foreign body. **(A)** The frontal view reveals the metallic density **(arrow)** to be situated at the level of the distal esophagus. **(B)** The lateral view clearly demonstrates the anterior, intracardiac location of the bullet. The child was shot in the neck, and the bullet travelled through the jugular vein and superior vena cava to the heart.

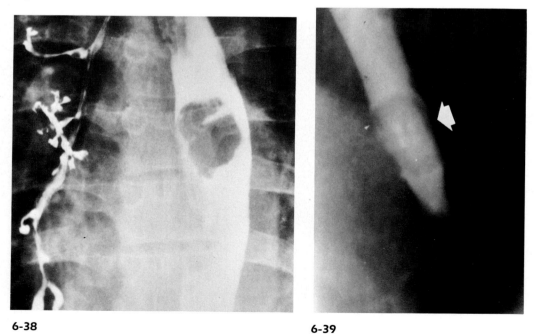

6-38   6-39

Fig. 6-38. Meat impaction. A large bolus of a hot dog is trapped in the midesophagus of a patient with quadriplegia. Barium in the bronchial tree is due to aspiration.

Fig. 6-39. Button **(arrow)** impacted in the distal esophagus just above the level of the diaphragm. The nonopaque plastic button appears as a filling defect in the barium column, with small amounts of contrast showing the four holes in it.

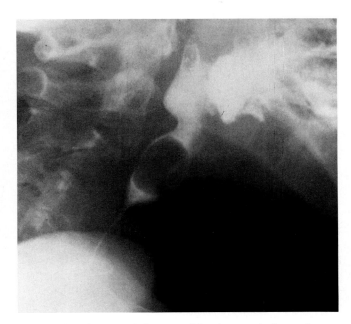

Fig. 6-40. Cherry pit impacted in the cervical esophagus proximal to a caustic stricture.

diffuse mediastinitis. In children, stridor or recurrent pneumonia can be caused by an esophageal foreign body not known to have been ingested.

A variety of interventive techniques have been used to relieve an acute food impaction in the distal esophagus. These include topical proteolytic enzymes, intravenous glucagon, extraction with a Foley catheter, and the oral administration of tartaric acid and sodium bicarbonate to produce carbon dioxide that distends the esophagus and propels the meat into the stomach (Fig. 6-41). In some cases, however, endoscopic removal of the impacted food is required. Metallic foreign bodies can sometimes be removed from the esophagus by means of a magnet inserted into the end of an orogastric tube.

INTRAMURAL HEMATOMA

Submucosal bleeding and intramural dissection of the esophageal wall giving rise to an intramural hematoma has been described as resulting from emetics, after ingestion of a foreign body and endoscopic instrumentation, following remote trauma, in patients with impaired hemostasis (hemophilia, thrombocytopenia), in patients receiving anticoagulant therapy, and as an unusual complication of

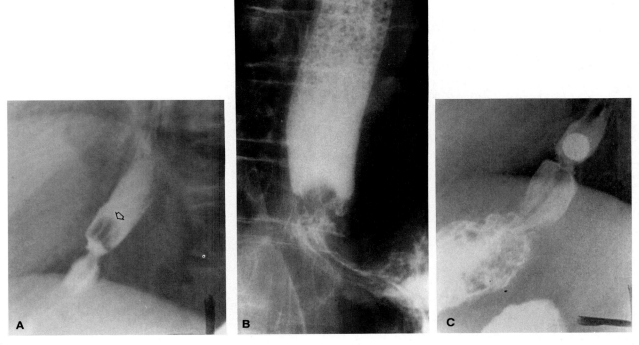

Fig. 6-41. Treatment of acute esophageal food impaction. **(A)** Initial barium swallow shows meat **(arrow)** lodged above an esophageal narrowing. **(B)** Following the oral administration of tartaric acid and sodium bicarbonate, a radiograph taken during expulsion of the meat shows it passing the site of obstruction. **(C)** Esophagram with a barium pill after passage of the meat shows that a stenotic Schatzki ring was the cause of the stenosis. (Rice BT, Spiegel PK, Dombrowski PJ: Acute esophageal food impaction treated by gas-forming agents. Radiology 146:299–301, 1983)

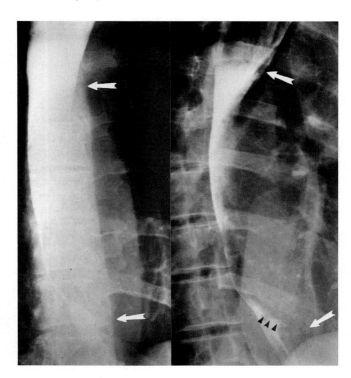

Fig. 6-42. Intramural hematoma following variceal sclerotherapy. Right anterior oblique view shows a large filling defect on the left lateroventral wall in the lower two-thirds of the esophagus **(between large arrows)**. The combination of regular lining, smooth surface, and sharp transition **(arrowheads)** of the filling defect indicates a submucosal rather than an extrinsic mass. (van Steenbergen W, Fevery J, Broeckaert L et al: Intramural hematoma of the esophagus: Unusual complication of variceal sclerotherapy. Gastrointest Radiol 9:293–295, 1984)

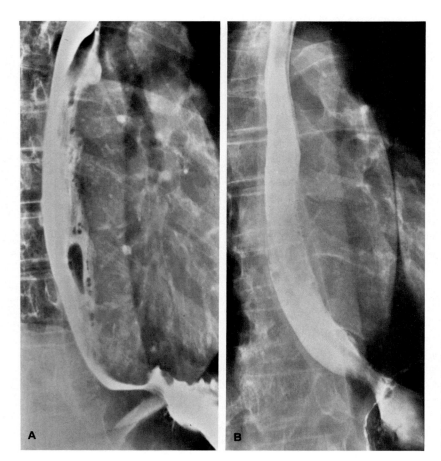

Fig. 6-43. Intramural hematoma. **(A)** Large sausage-shaped submucosal mass with partial obliteration of the esophageal lumen. **(B)** Following 5 days of conservative therapy, a repeat barium swallow shows a normal esophagus. (Dallemand S, Amorosa JK, Morris DW et al: Intramural hematomas of the esophagus. Gastrointest Radiol 8:7–9, 1983)

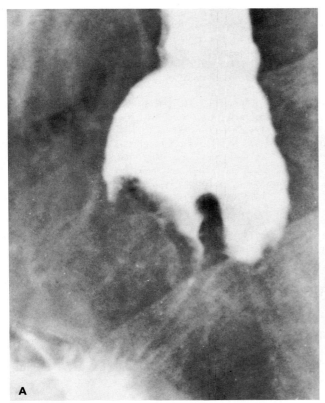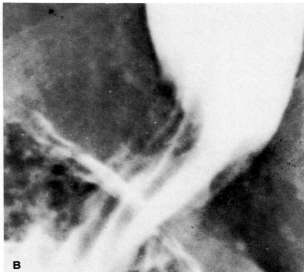

Fig. 6-44. Prolapse of gastric mucosal folds. **(A)** Irregular filling defect in the distal esophagus. **(B)** After reduction of the prolapse, the distal esophagus appears normal.

sclerotherapy for esophageal varices. Patients with intramural esophageal hematoma present with the sudden onset of dysphagia, odynophagia, and hematemesis. This is in contrast to patients with Mallory–Weiss lacerations, who present with signs of upper gastrointestinal bleeding with or without pain, and patients with Boerhaave's syndrome, who present with excruciating pain in the thorax or upper abdomen, signs of circulatory collapse, and often subcutaneous or mediastinal emphysema. Radiographically, an intramural hematoma typically produces a soft, elongated filling defect with smooth borders (Fig. 6-42). If there is no delayed rupture, the hematoma may completely resolve without surgical intervention (Fig. 6-43A, B).

HIRSUTE ESOPHAGUS

In one type of reconstructive surgery of the pharynx and esophagus, skin flaps are mobilized and rotated to reconstruct a "skin tube esophagus" to restore anatomic continuity of the gastrointestinal tract. The inner surface of this tube may bear hair follicles, which usually atrophy in 6 to 12 months. In rare instances, excessive amounts of hair continue to grow and cause the clinical triad of progressive dysphagia, hair spitting, and choking spells due to large masses of hair. The multiple hair follicles pro-

duce numerous rounded filling defects in the barium column, whereas a mass of hair appears as a large polypoid filling defect that changes its position in several projections (see Fig. 11-10). Periodic endoscopic "hair cuts" may be required.

PROLAPSED GASTRIC FOLDS

Prolapse of gastric mucosal folds can produce an irregular filling defect in the distal esophagus (Fig. 6-44A). Serial films demonstrate reduction of the prolapse, return of the gastric folds below the diaphragm, and a normal distal esophagus (Fig. 6-44B).

BIBLIOGRAPHY

Agha FP, Keren DF: Spindle-cell squamous carcinoma of the esophagus: A tumor with biphasic morphology. AJR 145:541–545, 1985

Agha FP, Weatherbee L, Sams JS: Verrucous carcinoma of the esophagus. Am J Gastroenterol 79:844–849, 1984

Agha FP, Wimbish KJ: Hirsute esophagus: Clinical and roentgen features. Gastrointest Radiol 9:297–300, 1984

Anderson MF, Harell GS: Secondary esophageal tumors. AJR 135:1243–1246, 1980

Bleshman MH, Banner MP, Johnson RC et al: The inflammatory esophagogastric polyp and fold. Radiology 128:589–593, 1978

Boulafendis D, Damiani M, Sie E et al: Primary malignant melanoma of the esophagus in a young adult. Am J Gastroenterol 80:417–420, 1985

Carnovale RL, Goldstein HM, Zornoza J et al: Radiologic manifestations of esophageal lymphoma. AJR 138:751–754, 1977

Carter MM, Kulkarni MV: Giant fibrovascular polyp of the esophagus. Gastrointest Radiol 9:301–303, 1984

Cho SR, Henry DA, Schneider V et al: Polypoid carcinoma of the esophagus: A distinct radiological and histopathological entity. Am J Gastroenterol 78:476–480, 1983

Cockey BM, Jones B, Bayless TM et al: Filiform polyps of the esophagus with inflammatory bowel disease. AJR 144:1207–1208, 1985

Dallemand S, Amorosa JK, Morris DW et al: Intramural hematomas of the esophagus. Gastrointest Radiol 8:7–9, 1983

Feczko PJ, Halpert RD, Zonca M: Radiographic abnormalities in eosinophilic esophagitis. Gastrointest Radiol 10:321–324, 1985

Ghahremani GG, Meyers MA, Port RB: Calcified primary tumors of the gastrointestinal tract. Gastrointest Radiol 2:331–339, 1978

Goldstein HM, Zornoza J, Hopens T: Intrinsic diseases of the adult esophagus: Benign and malignant tumors. Semin Roentgenol 16:183–197, 1981

Govoni AF: Hemangiomas of the esophagus. Gastrointest Radiol 7:113–117, 1982

Jang GC, Clouse ME, Fleischner FG: Fibrovascular polyp: A benign intraluminal tumor of the esophagus. Radiology 92:1196–1200, 1969

Kuhlman JE, Fishman EK, Wang KP et al: Esophageal duplication cyst: CT and transesophageal needle aspiration. AJR 145:531–532, 1985

Levine MS, Cajade, Herlinger H et al: Pseudomembranes in reflux esophagitis. Radiology 159:43–45, 1986

Levine MS, Macones AJ Jr, Laufer I: Candida esophagitis: Accuracy of radiographic diagnosis. Radiology 154:581–587, 1985

Mauro MA, Jaques PF: Granular-cell tumors of the esophagus and common bile duct. J Can Assoc Radiol 32:254–256, 1981

Meyers C, Durkin MG, Love L: Radiographic findings in herpetic esophagitis. Radiology 119:21–22, 1976

Minielly JA, Harrison EG, Fontana RS et al: Verrucous squamous cell carcinoma of the esophagus. Cancer 20:2078–2087, 1967

Parnell S, Pepperom MA, Antoniola DA et al: Squamous cell papilloma of the esophagus. Gastroenterology 74:910–913, 1978

Rice BT, Spiegel PK, Dombrowski PJ: Acute esophageal food impaction treated by gas-forming agents. Radiology 146:299–301, 1983

Rose HS, Balthazar EJ, Megibow AJ et al: Alimentary tract involvement in Kaposi sarcoma: Radiographic and endoscopic findings in 25 homosexual men. AJR 139:661–666, 1982

Rubesin S, Herlinger H, Sigal H: Granular cell tumors of the esophagus. Gastrointest Radiol 10:11–15, 1985

Shaffer HA: Multiple leiomyomas of the esophagus. Radiology 118:29–34, 1976

Smith PC, Swischuk LE, Fagan CJ: An elusive and often unsuspected cause of stridor or pneumonia (the esophageal foreign body). AJR 122:80–89, 1974

Steiner H, Lammer J, Hackl A: Lymphatic metastases to the esophagus. Gastrointest Radiol 9:1–4, 1984

Styles RA, Gibb SP, Tarshis A et al: Esophagogastric polyps: Radiographic and endoscopic findings. Radiology 154:307–311, 1985

Trenkner SW, Levine MS, Laufer I et al: Idiopathic esophageal varix. AJR 141:43–44, 1983

Trenkner SW, Maglinte DDT, Lehman GA et al: Esophageal food impaction: Treatment with glucagon. Radiology 149:401–403, 1983

Van Steenbergen W, Fevery J, Broeckaert L et al: Intramural hematoma of the esophagus: Unusual complication of variceal sclerotherapy. Gastrointest Radiol 9:293–295, 1984

Volle E, Hanel D, Beyer P et al: Ingested foreign bodies: Removal by magnet. Radiology 160:407–409, 1986

Walker JH: Giant papilloma of the thoracic esophagus. AJR 131:519–520, 1978

Whitaker JA, Deffenbough LD, Cooke AR: Esophageal duplication cyst. Am J Gastroenterol 73:329–332, 1980

ESOPHAGEAL DIVERTICULA

Disease Entities

Cervical diverticula
  Zenker's (pharyngoesophageal)
  Traction (from surgery, infection)
  Lateral
Midesophageal diverticula
  Traction (interbronchial)
  Pulsion (interaorticobronchial)
Epiphrenic diverticula
Intramural esophageal pseudodiverticulosis

Esophageal diverticula are common lesions that are best divided according to the sites at which they occur. Their walls can contain all esophageal layers (traction) or be composed only of mucosa and submucosa herniating through the muscularis (pulsion). Almost all are acquired lesions.

ZENKER'S DIVERTICULA

A Zenker's diverticulum arises in the upper esophagus, its neck lying in the midline of the posterior wall at the pharyngoesophageal junction (approximately the C5-6 level). The development of a Zenker's diverticulum is apparently related to the premature contraction or other motor incoordination of the cricopharyngeus muscle, which produces increased intraluminal pressure and a pulsion diverticulum at a point of anatomic weakness between the oblique and circular fibers of the muscle. Although many of these diverticula are asymptomatic, they may cause the insidious development of throat irritation with excessive mucus or the sensation during swallowing of the presence of a foreign body. A gurgling in the throat can be noted when liquids are swallowed. As the diverticulum enlarges, dysphagia becomes more marked, and regurgitation of food and mucus may occur after meals and at night. Drugs can also accumulate in a huge Zenker's diverticulum, leading to a loss of bioavailability. Pulmonary complications secondary to aspiration pneumonia are not uncommon. A Zenker's diverticulum occasionally enlarges to such an extent that it compresses the esophagus at the level of the thoracic inlet and produces esophageal obstruction.

On plain radiographs of the neck, a Zenker's diverticulum may appear as a widening of the retrotracheal soft-tissue space, often with an air-fluid level (Fig. 7-1). Oral contrast is necessary to differentiate this appearance from a retrotracheal abscess. A Zenker's diverticulum presents as a saccular outpouching protruding from the esophageal lumen and connected to it by a relatively narrow neck (Fig. 7-2). Because the diverticulum arises from the posterior wall of the esophagus, it is best visualized at barium swallow in the lateral projection, though slight obliquity sometimes may be necessary. As the sac enlarges, it extends downward and posteriorly, displacing the cervical esophagus anteriorly and often causing marked narrowing of the adjacent esophageal lumen (Fig. 7-3). Barium and

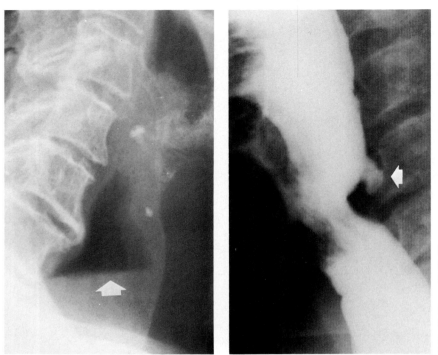

7-1

7-2

Fig. 7-1. Air-fluid level **(arrows)** in the retrotracheal soft-tissue space representing a Zenker's diverticulum.

Fig. 7-2. Small Zenker's diverticulum. The saccular outpouching **(arrow)** arises just proximal to the posterior cricopharyngeus impression.

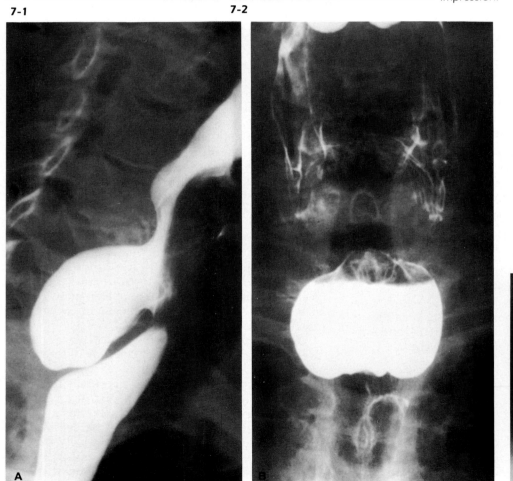

A

B

7-3

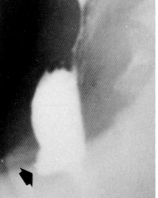

7-4

Fig. 7-3. **(A)** Oblique and **(B)** frontal views of a large Zenker's diverticulum almost occluding the esophageal lumen.

Fig. 7-4. Traction diverticulum **(arrow)** in the cervical esophagus caused by postoperative scarring following total laryngectomy.

food may be retained in a Zenker's diverticulum for hours or even days after they have been ingested.

CERVICAL TRACTION DIVERTICULA

Traction diverticula may also occur in the cervical esophagus. In this region, they can be the result of fibrous healing of an inflammatory process in the neck or be secondary to postsurgical changes (*e.g.,* laryngectomy; Fig. 7-4).

LATERAL DIVERTICULA

Diverticula in the cervical region have been described that emerge in a lateral or anterolateral direction through a weak area in the anterolateral aspect of the pharyngoesophageal junction just below the transverse portion of the cricopharyngeus muscle (Fig. 7-5). Although these lateral cervical diverticula have been found more frequently among patients with dysphagia than in asymptomatic volunteers, the presence of other functional and morphodynamic abnormalities in most of these patients makes it difficult to assess whether these lateral diverticula are symptomatic or have any causal relationship to the patient's dysphagia.

THORACIC DIVERTICULA

Diverticula of the thoracic portion of the esophagus are primarily found in the middle third opposite the bifurcation of the trachea in the region of the hilum of the lung. These interbronchial diverticula are almost invariably traction diverticula that develop in response to the pull of fibrous adhesions following

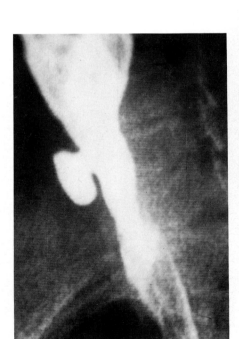
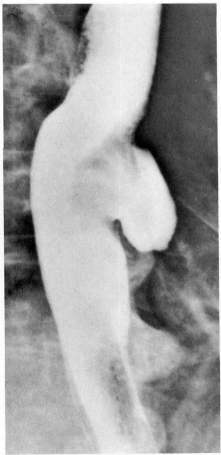
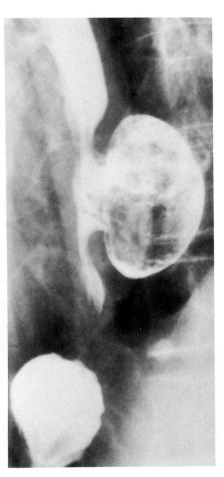

7-5 **7-6** **7-7**

Fig. 7-5. Lateral cervical diverticulum. (Ekberg O, Nylander G: Lateral diverticula from the pharyngoesophageal junction area. Radiology 146:117–122, 1983)

Fig. 7-6. Traction diverticulum of the midthoracic esophagus.

Fig. 7-7. Epiphrenic diverticulum.

infection of the mediastinal lymph nodes. Associated symptoms are rare, though mediastinal abscess or esophagorespiratory fistula may occur. Barium swallow demonstrates a diverticular collection of contrast that may have a funnel, cone, tent, or fusiform shape and is usually best visualized in the left anterior oblique projection (Fig. 7-6). Calcified mediastinal nodes from healed granulomatous disease (especially tuberculosis) are often seen adjacent to the diverticulum.

Much less frequently, midesophageal diverticula may be of the pulsion type. These interaortico-bronchial diverticula arise in a relatively weak area on the left anterolateral wall of the esophagus between the inferior border of the aortic arch and the upper external margin of the left main bronchus. Because of its position, an interaorticobronchial diverticulum can be seen only in the right anterior oblique projection, in which it is separated from superimposition on the esophageal lumen.

EPIPHRENIC DIVERTICULA

Epiphrenic diverticula are usually of the pulsion type and occur in the distal 10 cm of the esophagus (Fig. 7-7). These diverticula appear to be associated with motor abnormalities of the esophagus and are probably related to incoordination of esophageal peristalsis and sphincter relaxation, resulting in the lower esophageal segment being subjected to increased intraluminal pressure. An epiphrenic diverticulum is rarely symptomatic, though it may produce symptoms because of its large size and the retention of food within it. Radiographically, an epiphrenic diverticulum tends to have a broad and short neck. If small, it can simulate an esophageal ulcer, though the normal appearance of the mucosal pattern of the adjacent esophagus usually permits differentiation between these two entities.

CARCINOMA DEVELOPING IN DIVERTICULA

Pulsion diverticula in the cervical or distal esophagus are usually smooth in contour. Irregularity of a diverticulum in either of these regions should suggest the possibility of infection or malignancy (Fig. 7-8). If prior radiographs are available for comparison, the interval development of an irregular mar-

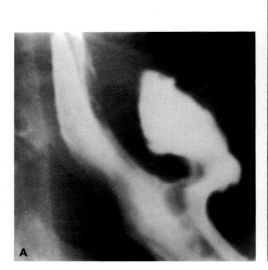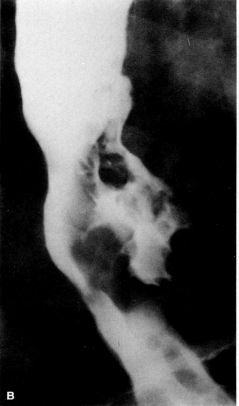

Fig. 7-8. *Carcinoma arising in an epiphrenic diverticulum.* **(A)** The initial esophagram demonstrates a mild irregularity of the diverticulum that was not appreciated at the time of the examination. **(B)** Six months later, the large, ulcerating carcinoma of the esophagus is obvious.

gin in a previously smooth diverticulum is an ominous sign.

INTRAMURAL ESOPHAGEAL PSEUDODIVERTICULOSIS

Intramural esophageal pseudodiverticulosis can simulate diverticular involvement of the esophagus. In this extremely rare disorder, numerous small (1–3 mm), flask-shaped outpouchings in longitudinal rows parallel to the long axis of the esophagus represent dilated ducts coming from submucosal glands (Fig. 7-9). Because the necks of the pseudodiverticula are 1 mm or less in diameter, incomplete filling may erroneously suggest lack of communication with the esophageal lumen. Thin, low-density barium seems to enter these structures more readily than the high-density barium used for double-contrast studies. About 90% of reported pa-

tients have associated smooth strictures, most frequently in the upper third of the esophagus. Because these are not true diverticula of the muscular esophageal wall, the term pseudodiverticulosis is most correct. The radiographic appearance of multiple ulcerlike projections has been likened to a chain of beads and to the Rokitansky–Aschoff sinuses of the gallbladder. *Candida albicans* can be cultured from about half the patients with intramural pseudodiverticulosis, though there is no evidence to suggest the fungus as a causative agent.

In a recent report, the most common pattern of intramural esophageal pseudodiverticulosis was segmental disease with isolated involvement of the distal esophagus. Most patients in this study had ten or fewer pseudodiverticula and distal esophageal strictures typical of peptic disease (Fig. 7-10). This suggests that in some patients pseudodiverticulosis represents a sequela of chronic esophagitis, particularly reflux esophagitis. The reason so very few of

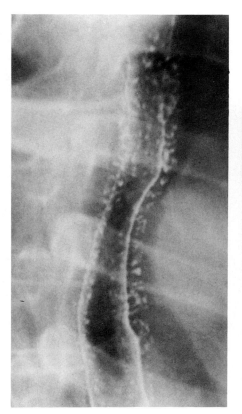

7-9

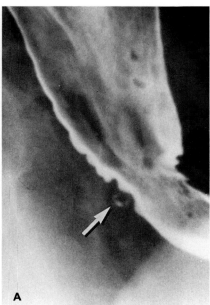

A

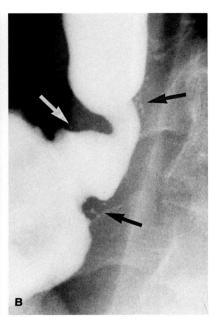

B

7-10

Fig. 7-9. Intramural esophageal pseudodiverticulosis. The numerous diverticular outpouchings represent dilated ducts coming from submucosal glands in the wall of the esophagus.

Fig. 7-10. Localized pseudodiverticulosis. **(A)** Double-contrast and **(B)** single-contrast esophagrams in different patients demonstrate peptic strictures with localized pseudodiverticulosis **(arrows)** in the region of stricture. Most of the pseudodiverticula do not appear to communicate with the esophageal lumen. (Levine MS, Moolten DN, Herlinger H et al: Esophageal intramural pseudodiverticulosis: A reevaluation. AJR 147:1165–1170, 1986. Copyright 1986. Reproduced with permission.)

the patients with chronic esophagitis develop this condition is unclear.

BIBLIOGRAPHY

Baron SH: Zenker's diverticulum as a cause for loss of drug availability: A "new" complication. Am J Gastroenterol 77:152–153, 1982

Bruggeman LL, Seaman WB: Epiphrenic diverticula: An analysis of 80 cases. AJR 119:266–276, 1973

Bruhlmann WF, Zollikofer CL, Maranta E et al: Intramural pseudodiverticulosis of the esophagus: Report of seven cases and literature review. Gastrointest Radiol 6:199–208, 1981

Cho SR, Sanders MM, Turner MA et al: Esophageal intramural pseudodiverticulosis. Gastrointest Radiol 6:9–16, 1981

Ekberg O, Nylander G: Lateral diverticula from the pharyngoesophageal junction area. Radiology 146:117–122, 1983

Levine MS, Moolten DN, Herlinger H et al: Esophageal intramural pseudodiverticulosis: A reevaluation. AJR 147:1165–1170, 1986

Saldana JA, Cone RO, Hopens TA et al: Carcinoma arising in an epiphrenic esophageal diverticulum. Gastrointest Radiol 7:15–18, 1982

Shirazi KK, Daffner RH, Gaede JT: Ulcer occurring in Zenker's diverticulum. Gastrointest Radiol 2:117–118, 1977

Wychulis RA, Gunnlaugsson HG, Clagett OT: Carcinoma occurring in pharyngoesophageal diverticulum. Surgery 66:976–979, 1969

ESOPHAGEAL VARICES

8

Disease Entities

Portal hypertension
  Hepatic cirrhosis
  Carcinoma of the pancreas
  Pancreatitis
  Retroperitoneal inflammatory disease
  High-viscosity-slow-flow states (*e.g.*, poly-
    cythemia)
Noncirrhotic liver disease
  Metastatic carcinoma
  Carcinoma of the liver
  Congestive heart failure
Idiopathic
Superior vena cava obstruction
  Mediastinal tumors (e.g., bronchogenic
    carcinoma)
  Chronic fibrosing mediastinitis
  Retrosternal goiter
  Thymoma

ETIOLOGY

Esophageal varices, dilated veins in the subepithelial connective tissue, are most commonly a result
of portal hypertension (Fig. 8-1). Increased pressure
in the portal venous system is usually secondary to
cirrhosis of the liver. Other causes of portal hypertension include obstruction of the portal or splenic
veins by carcinoma of the pancreas, pancreatitis,

inflammatory disease of the retroperitoneum, and
high-viscosity-slow-flow states (*e.g.*, polycythemia),
which predispose to intravascular thrombosis. In
patients with portal hypertension, much of the portal blood cannot flow along its normal pathway
through the liver to the inferior vena cava and then
on to the heart. Instead, it must go by a circuitous
collateral route through the coronary vein, across
the esophagogastric hiatus, and into the periesophageal plexus before reaching the azygos and hemiazygos systems, superior vena cava, and right
atrium. The periesophageal plexus communicates
with veins in the submucosa of the esophagus and
gastric cardia. Increased blood flow through these
veins causes the development of esophageal (and
gastric) varices.

Esophageal varices are infrequently demonstrated in the absence of portal hypertension. They
have been observed in patients with noncirrhotic
liver disease such as metastatic carcinoma, carcinoma of the liver, and congestive heart failure.
"Idiopathic" varices may develop as a result of congenital weakness in the venous channels of the
esophagus. "Downhill" varices are produced when
venous blood from the head and neck cannot reach
the heart because of an obstruction of the superior
vena cava (Fig. 8-2). This is usually secondary to
progressive and prolonged compression of the superior vena cava by tumors or inflammatory disease in
the mediastinum. In this situation, blood flows
"downhill" through the azygos–hemiazygos system,
the periesophageal plexus, and the coronary veins
before eventually entering the portal vein, through

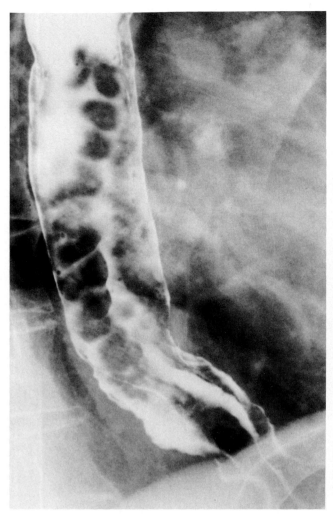

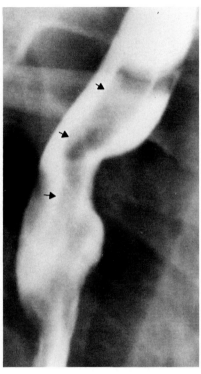

8-1   8-2

Fig. 8-1. Esophageal varices seen as a line of round filling defects representing dilated veins in the subepithelial connective tissue.

Fig. 8-2. "Downhill" varices **(arrows)** in a patient with carcinomatous obstruction of the superior vena cava.

which it flows to the inferior vena cava and right atrium. In patients with carcinomatous obstruction of the superior vena cava, the dilated submucosal veins tend to the confined to the upper esophagus. In patients with chronic venous obstruction due to mediastinal fibrosis, varices can involve the entire esophagus. Concomitant enlargement of intercostal vein collaterals occasionally causes rib notching.

CLINICAL SYMPTOMS

Bleeding, the major complication of esophageal varices, is nearly as likely to occur in small varices as in larger and more extensive lesions. Immediate death from exsanguination occurs in about 10% to 15% of patients with variceal bleeding. The diag-

nosis of esophageal varices in patients with cirrhotic liver disease implies significant portal venous hypertension and is an ominous sign. Up to 90% of the deaths from liver disease in patients with cirrhosis occur within 2 years of the diagnosis of varices.

RADIOGRAPHIC TECHNIQUES

The radiographic demonstration of esophageal varices requires precise technique. The object of the fluoroscopic examination is to line the esophageal mucosa with a very thin layer of barium so as to enhance the characteristic serpiginous appearance of the varices. Multiple radiographs must be taken during the resting stage following a swallow of barium. Complete filling of the esophagus with barium may obscure varices; powerful contractions of the esophagus may squeeze blood out of the varices and make them impossible to detect.

The examination for esophageal varices must include radiographs with the patient in a horizontal position. In this position, the transit of barium is slowed, mucosal coating is prolonged, and distention of varices is enhanced.

Varices related to portal hypertension are most commonly demonstrated in the lower third of the esophagus. When they are voluminous and extensive, varices can be seen in any projection. Early varices are generally situated on the right anterolateral wall of the distal segment of the esophagus and are therefore most easily identified in the left anterior oblique projection.

Numerous techniques have been suggested to enhance visualization of small esophageal varices.

One maneuver is to obtain radiographs with the patient in deep, blocked inspiration. This lowers the position of the diaphragm and better demonstrates the distal esophagus. In addition, forced inspiration causes ballooning of the varices, making them easier to detect.

Pharmacologic agents have been used to better demonstrate small varices that cannot be identified on conventional studies. The use of 30 mg of Pro-Banthine (probantheline bromide) intramuscularly or intravenously several minutes before the administration of thick barium causes relaxation of the musculature of the distal esophagus and permits varices to fill better and remain dilated. However, the use of this anticholinergic drug is contraindicated in patients with a history of glaucoma, previous myocardial infarction, or urinary tract obstruction. Although some authors have employed

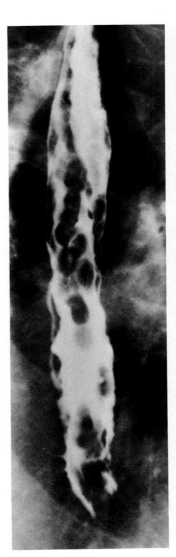
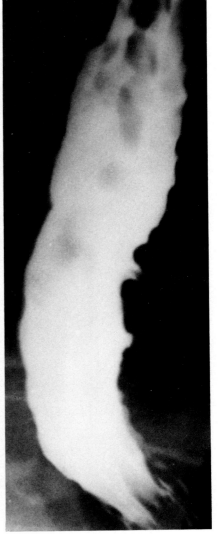

Fig. 8-3. Esophageal varices. Note the diffuse round and oval filling defects resembling the beads of a rosary.

Fig. 8-4. Esophageal varices. There is moderate thickening of folds and irregularity of the esophageal outline.

8-3 8-4

glucagon to better demonstrate varices, the esophagus, unlike the rest of the gut, appears to be relatively insensitive to this drug.

RADIOGRAPHIC FINDINGS

The characteristic radiographic appearance of esophageal varices is serpiginous thickening of folds, which appear as round or oval filling defects resembling the beads of a rosary (Fig. 8-3). Initially, there is only mild thickening of folds and irregularity of the esophageal outline (Fig. 8-4). Distention with barium hides these thickened folds and causes the esophageal border to have an irregularly

notched (worm-eaten) appearance (Fig. 8-5). Once the typical tortuous, ribbonlike defects are visible, the radiographic diagnosis of esophageal varices is usually easy to make (Fig. 8-6). In patients with severe portal hypertension, varices can be demonstrated throughout the entire thoracic esophagus (Fig. 8-7).

An isolated varix may mimic the radiographic appearance of a submucosal esophageal mass. If the examination is performed with the patient in both the upright and recumbent positions with variable esophageal distention, the demonstration of effacement or obliteration of the lesion is indicative of its vascular origin (see Fig. 6-29). However, an isolated thrombosed varix will be unaffected by changes in

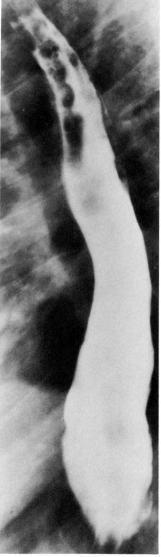

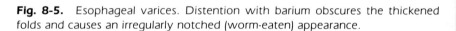

Fig. 8-5. Esophageal varices. Distention with barium obscures the thickened folds and causes an irregularly notched (worm-eaten) appearance.

Fig. 8-6. Esophageal varices (Banti's syndrome).

Fig. 8-7. Esophageal varices. The varices extend to the level of the aortic arch in this patient with severe portal hypertension.

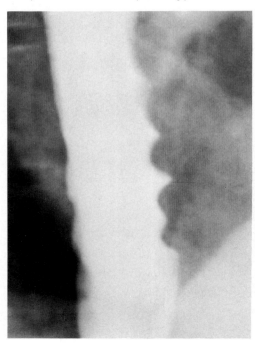

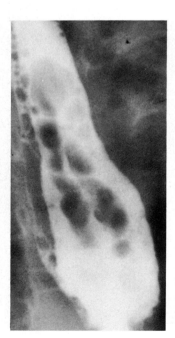

8-5   8-6   8-7

patient position or the degree of esophageal distention (see Fig. 6-30).

DISORDERS SIMULATING VARICES

Several other disorders can simulate the radiographic appearance of esophageal varices. When varices are small, the thickening of mucosal folds and wall irregularity caused by them can be almost indistinguishable from mild chronic esophagitis. When varices are very large, irregular, and arrayed in a chaotic pattern, they may be confused with the varicoid form of esophageal carcinoma (Figs. 8-8, 8-9). Varices can be successfully differentiated from carcinoma in these cases by the demonstration of pliability of the walls of the esophagus, change in

appearance when the esophagus is contracted and distended, and preservation of peristalsis. Rarely, lymphoma presents as a large intramural submucosal tumor with nodular folds closely resembling esophageal varices (Fig. 8-10).

SCLEROTHERAPY OF ESOPHAGEAL VARICES

Sclerotherapy of esophageal varices is now widely accepted as an effective nonsurgical treatment modality in the management of variceal hemorrhage. The procedure significantly reduces the risk of rebleeding, although its effect on long-term survival is uncertain. It is particularly useful in patients with

Fig. 8-8. Varicoid carcinoma.

Fig. 8-9. Varicoid carcinoma.

Fig. 8-10. Lymphoma presenting as thick, nodular folds that mimic esophageal varices.

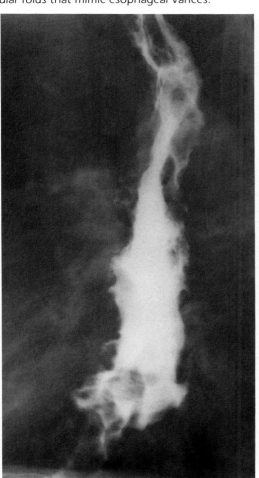

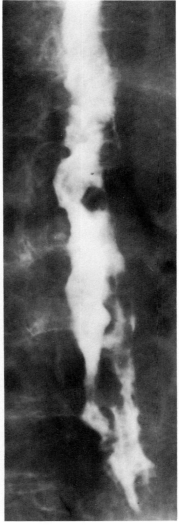

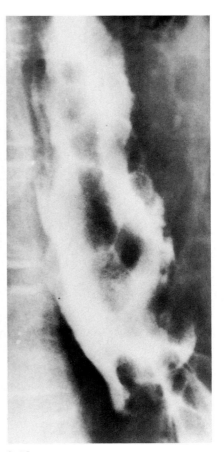

8-8

8-9

8-10

severe or advanced liver disease in whom portal-systemic shunt surgery cannot be performed. Sclerotherapy produces venous thrombosis accompanied by a necrotizing inflammation of the esophageal veins and subsequent fibrosis. The spectrum of radiographic findings following variceal sclerotherapy includes esophageal dysmotility, mucosal ulceration (see Fig. 4-43), luminal narrowing and obstruction (see Fig. 4-44), filling defects due to intramural hematoma (see Fig. 6-42), sinuses, fistulas, esophageal dissection, and perforation.

BIBLIOGRAPHY

Agha FP: The esophagus after endoscopic injection sclerotherapy: Acute and chronic changes. Radiology 153:37–42, 1984

Cockerill EM, Miller RE, Chernish SM et al: Optimal visualization of esophageal varices. AJR 126:512–523, 1976

Felson B, Lessure AP: "Downhill" varices of the esophagus. Dis Chest 46:740–746, 1964

Glanz S, Koser MW, Dallemand S et al: Upper esophageal varices: Report of three cases and review of the literature. Am J Gastroenterol 77:194–198, 1982

Nelson SW: The roentgenologic diagnosis of esophageal varices. AJR 77:599–611, 1957

Trenkner SW, Levine MS, Laufer I et al: Idiopathic esophageal varix. AJR 141:43–44, 1983

Van Steenbergen W, Fevery J, Broeckaert L et al: Intramural hematoma of the esophagus: Unusual complication of variceal sclerotherapy. Gastrointest Radiol 9:293–295, 1984

Yates CW, LeVine MA, Jensen KM: Varicoid carcinoma of the esophagus. Radiology 122:605–608, 1977

ESOPHAGORESPIRATORY FISTULAS

9

Disease Entities

Congenital disorders
Malignancies
  Carcinoma of the esophagus
  Carcinoma of the lung
Trauma
  Instrumentation
  Surgery
  Foreign body
Corrosive esophagitis
Inflammatory disease
  Tuberculosis
  Syphilis
  Histoplasmosis
  Actinomycosis
  Crohn's disease
  Behcet's syndrome
Perforated diverticulum
Pulmonary sequestration or cyst
Spontaneous esophageal rupture

CONGENITAL TRACHEOESOPHAGEAL FISTULAS

Congenital tracheoesophageal (TE) fistulas result from failure of a satisfactory esophageal lumen to develop completely separate from the trachea. In embryologic development, the trachea and upper alimentary tract have a common origin from the caudal end of the embryonic pharynx. By the second intrauterine month, however, these two structures have divided. The esophagus assumes a dorsal position, and the trachea and lung buds lie ventrally. Failure of complete separation leads to development of a TE fistula.

TYPE-III FISTULAS

The most common type of TE fistula, type III (85%–90%), consists of an upper segment ending in a blind pouch at the level of the bifurcation of the trachea or slightly above it and a lower segment attached to the trachea by a short fistulous tract. After one or two normal swallows, the newborn infant with this condition has ingested fluids returned through the nose and mouth. The child coughs, struggles, becomes cyanotic, and may even stop breathing. Radiographic demonstration of looping of a small esophageal feeding tube indicates that the proximal esophagus ends in a blind pouch. Plain radiographs of the abdomen demonstrate the presence of air in the bowel that has freely entered the stomach through the fistulous connection between the trachea and distal esophagus. The combination of air in the stomach and a blind proximal esophageal pouch is pathognomonic of type-III TE fistulas. Contrast material is rarely required for diagnosis. When used, contrast should be introduced through a catheter (to control the amount of contrast and avoid overflow) and radiographs obtained with the child in an upright position (Fig. 9-1).

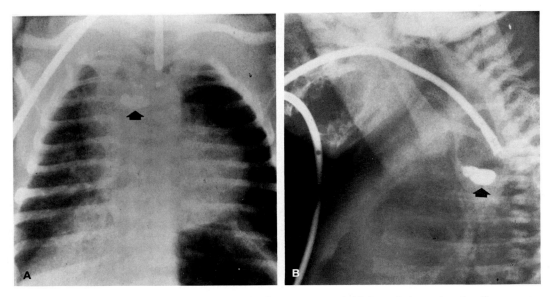

Fig. 9-1. Tracheoesophageal fistula (type III). Contrast material injected through a feeding tube demonstrates occlusion of the proximal esophageal pouch **(arrows)** in **(A)** frontal and **(B)** lateral projections. Note the air in the stomach. (Eisenberg RL: Diagnostic Imaging in Surgery. New York, McGraw–Hill, 1987)

TYPE-I FISTULAS

In the next most common type of esophageal anomaly, type I, both the upper and the lower segments of the esophagus are blind pouches. The symptomatology is identical to that of infants with type-III lesions, and the two disorders can be differentiated only by plain abdominal radiographs, which demonstrate absence of air below the diaphragm in the type-I lesion (Fig. 9-2) and air within the stomach in the type-III lesion (see Fig. 9-1).

TYPE-II FISTULAS

In the type-II form of TE fistula, the upper esophageal segment communicates with the trachea while the lower segment ends in a blind pouch. Infants with this anomaly have excessive amounts of pharyngeal secretions and may suffer severe choking if feeding is continued after the first swallow. Because there is no connection between the trachea and the stomach, there is no radiographic evidence of gas within the abdomen. Oral administration of contrast in this condition immediately outlines the tracheobronchial tree.

TYPE-IV FISTULAS

There are two forms of type-IV TE fistula. In one, the upper and lower esophageal segments end in

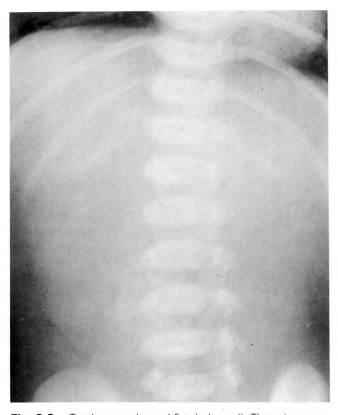

Fig. 9-2. Tracheoesophageal fistula (type I). There is no gas in the abdomen.

blind pouches, both of which are connected to the tracheobronchial tree. In this case, gas is seen in the stomach, and oral contrast material outlines both fistulas as well as the bronchial tree. In the other form of type-IV fistula (H fistula), both the trachea and the esophagus are intact. These two structures are connected by a single fistulous tract that can be found at any level from the cricoid to the tracheal bifurcation (Fig. 9-3). The H fistula may not be identified in infancy and, if it is small and only occasionally causes emptying of material into the lungs, is compatible with survival into adulthood. Because the fistula usually has a sharp downward course from the trachea to the esophagus, it sometimes is not demonstrated by oral contrast studies.

ASSOCIATED CONGENITAL MALFORMATIONS

Esophageal atresia and TE fistula are associated with congenital malformations involving other systems. These include skeletal anomalies (usually minor, affecting vertebrae and ribs), cardiovascular anomalies (atrial and ventricular septal defects, tetralogy of Fallot), and gastrointestinal anomalies (duodenal and anal atresia).

ACQUIRED TRACHEOESOPHAGEAL FISTULAS

About 50% of acquired esophagorespiratory fistulas are due to malignancy in the mediastinum. Almost all of the rest are secondary to infectious processes or trauma.

MALIGNANT LESIONS

A major complication of esophageal carcinoma is involvement of contiguous organs, primarily fistulization between the esophagus and the respiratory tract (Fig. 9-4). Fistulization is usually a late complication and often a terminal event. An esophagorespiratory fistula can also be a complication of erosion into the esophagus by carcinoma of the lung arising near or metastasizing to the middle mediastinum (Fig. 9-5) or by mediastinal metastases from other primary sites (Fig. 9-6). Fistulas between the esophagus and airway may develop following radiation therapy (Fig. 9-7), presumably due to lysis of tumor with subsequent erosion or to extension of a radiation-induced ulcer. Regardless of therapy, the overall prognosis of malignant esophagorespiratory fistulas is dismal. About 80% of patients with this

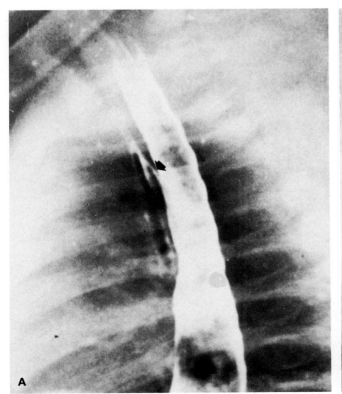
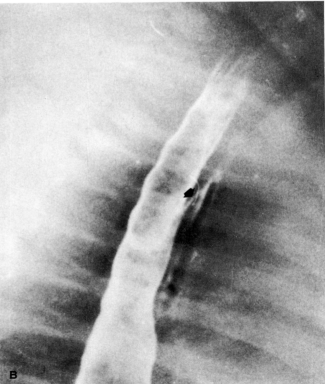

Fig. 9-3. Tracheoesophageal fistula (type IV, or H fistula). Note the sharp downward course from the trachea to the esophagus **(arrows)** in two patients with this type of congenital fistula.

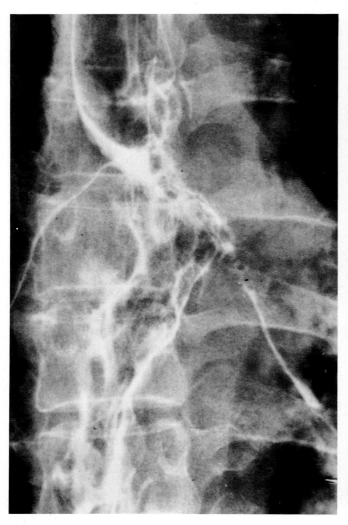

9-4

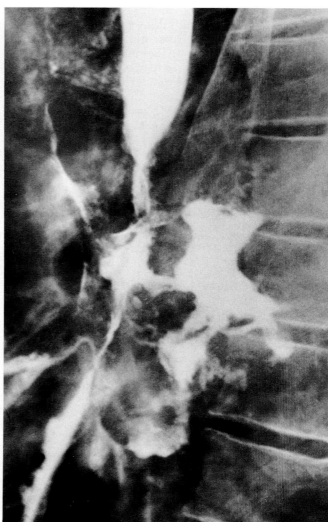

9-5

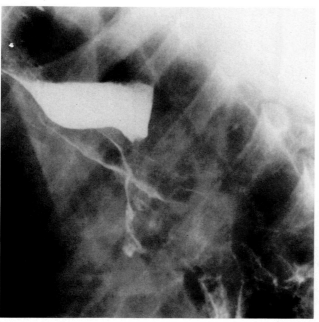

9-6

Fig. 9-4. Esophagorespiratory fistula due to squamous carcinoma of the esophagus.

Fig. 9-5. Esophagorespiratory fistula secondary to squamous carcinoma of the lung.

Fig. 9-6. Esophagorespiratory fistula caused by mediastinal metastases from adenocarcinoma of the cervix.

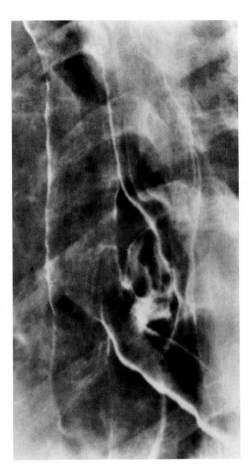

Fig. 9-7. Radiation-induced fistula between the esophagus and the left main stem bronchus. The fistula developed 3 months after radiotherapy and combination chemotherapy for adenocarcinoma of the lung. (Lepke RA, Libshitz HI: Radiation-induced injury of the esophagus. Radiology 148:375–378, 1983)

tegrity of the esophagus; there is a higher than normal rate of postdilatation perforation in patients with caustic strictures, recent esophageal or periesophageal surgery, and malignant tumors (Fig. 9-9). Blunt or penetrating trauma to the chest, especially after crush injury, can result in esophageal perforation and fistulization. There is a relationship between the traumatic agent and the site of communication between the esophagus and the respiratory tract. Fistulas caused by instrumentation of esophageal strictures or ingested foreign bodies tend to communicate with either the right or the left main stem bronchus. Those caused by compression injury tend to communicate with the trachea.

Traumatic perforation of the thoracic esophagus leads to excruciating chest, back, or epigastric pain accompanied by dysphagia and respiratory dis-

complication die within 3 months; only a few survive more than 1 year. The cause of death in these patients is either pulmonary infection due to repeated aspiration pneumonias, or uncontrollable hemorrhage.

ESOPHAGEAL INSTRUMENTATION/ VOMITING/TRAUMA

Fistulous communication between the esophagus and the trachea can be the result of esophageal instrumentation and perforation. This is most common after esophagoscopy but may also occur after dilatation of strictures by bouginage with direct vision, the use of weighted mercury nasogastric bougies (especially the Sengstaken-Blakemore tube for tamponade), pneumatic dilatation for the treatment of achalasia, or even insertion of a nasogastric tube (Fig. 9-8). The incidence of instrumental perforation depends to some extent on the underlying in-

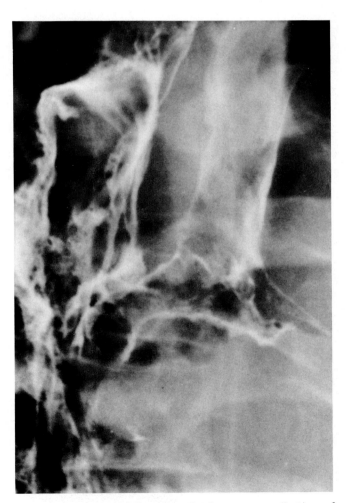

Fig. 9-8. Esophagorespiratory fistula as a complication of nasogastric tube placement in a patient with squamous carcinoma of the esophagus.

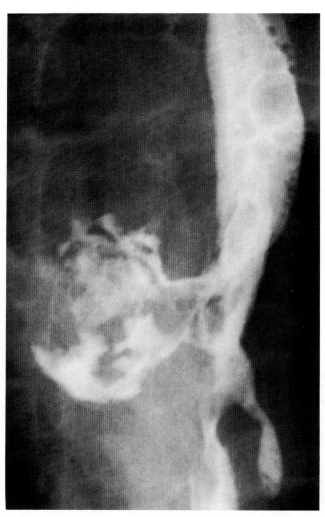

Fig. 9-9. Esophageal rupture following esophagoscopy in a patient with squamous carcinoma of the esophagus.

tress. Chest radiographs demonstrate air dissecting within the mediastinum and soft tissues, often with pleural effusion or hydropneumothorax. The introduction of an oral contrast agent may demonstrate the site of perforation and the extent of fistulization.

Esophageal rupture caused by severe vomiting appears clinically as epigastric pain radiating to the shoulder blades in a patient who appears gravely ill with pallor, sweatiness, tachycardia, and often shock. This disorder most frequently occurs in males and usually follows heavy drinking and a large meal (Boerhaave's syndrome) (Fig. 9-10). However, since this postemetic rupture usually occurs near the esophagogastric junction, it does not generally lead to development of an esophago-respiratory fistula.

CORROSIVE ESOPHAGITIS

Another form of traumatic insult to the esophagus is the ingestion of corrosive agents, especially alkali such as lye. Deep penetration of these toxic agents and necrosis through the entire wall of the esophagus can cause perforation, mediastinal inflammation, and fistulization, which may lead to a communication between the esophagus and respiratory tract (Fig. 9-11).

INFECTIOUS/GRANULOMATOUS/INFLAMMATORY ESOPHAGITIS

Fistulous communication between the esophagus and respiratory tract may be due to a variety of infectious processes. Mediastinal lymph nodes that undergo caseation or necrosis may rupture into the esophagus and tracheobronchial tree. In addition, any ulcerative lesion in the midesophagus or upper

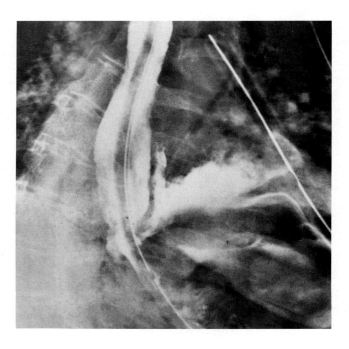

Fig. 9-10. Boerhaave's syndrome. Esophageal rupture occurred as a complication of severe vomiting in an elderly alcoholic.

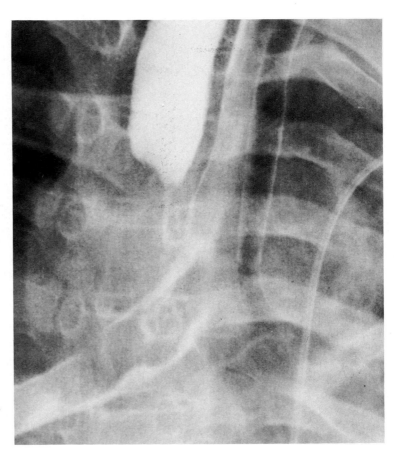

Fig. 9-11. Caustic esophagorespiratory fistula. The fistula developed in a patient who had ingested lye 1 month previously.

esophagus can extend through the wall and penetrate into the trachea or bronchus, causing an esophagorespiratory fistula.

In the early literature, tuberculosis and syphilis were reported as relatively common causes of esophagorespiratory fistulas. However, the esophagus is one of the organs least likely to be involved by tuberculosis. There is almost always evidence of the disease elsewhere, primarily in the lungs. In addition to its more common manifestations, such as ulceration and fibrotic narrowing, tuberculosis may result in sinuses or fistulous tracts.

Syphilis of the esophagus is a rare lesion. Inflammation of mediastinal lymph nodes in this disease may secondarily involve the esophagus. This process can cause extensive compression, resulting in esophageal obstruction, or necrosis and perforation, leading to a fistulous connection with the respiratory tract. The relentless pounding of a syphilitic aortic aneurysm can weaken the walls of the adjacent esophagus and trachea and lead to a communication between them.

Although histoplasmosis does not primarily affect the esophagus, the disease frequently causes a granulomatous inflammatory process involving mediastinal lymph nodes. Infrequently, this can lead to ulceration and fistulization between the esophagus and trachea.

Actinomycosis, though uncommonly involving the esophagus, can spread to that organ from adjacent foci by direct penetration or by hematogenous spread from a distant site. Radiographically, actinomycosis produces nonspecific ulceration, inflammation, and, not infrequently, an esophagorespiratory fistula. Fistulization between the esophagus and the respiratory tract is a rare complication of Crohn's disease and Behcet's syndrome (Fig. 9-12) involving the esophagus.

OTHER CAUSES

Rarely, traction diverticula of the midesophagus perforate, causing the development of a mediastinal abscess or esophagorespiratory fistula (Fig. 9-13). These diverticula, which arise opposite the bifurcation of the trachea or near the left main stem bronchus, are generally related to fixation and traction exerted by the healing of inflamed lymph nodes (tuberculosis, histoplasmosis) adherent to the esophagus. On occasion, vertebral disease is the underlying factor.

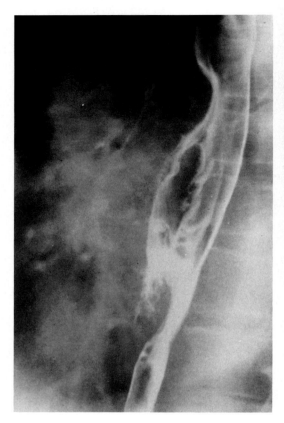

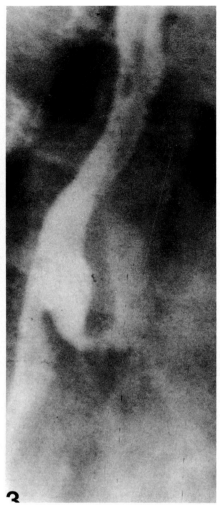

Fig. 9-12. Behcet's syndrome. Esophagorespiratory fistula from the midportion of the esophagus to the right lower lobe bronchus. (Mori S, Yoshihira A, Kawamura H et al: Esophageal involvement in Behcet's disease. Am J Gastroenterol 78:548–553, 1983)

Fig. 9-13. Esophagorespiratory fistula secondary to ruptured traction diverticulum. There is a short, fistulous tract extending from the diverticulum to the left main stem bronchus. (Balthazar EJ: Esophagobronchial fistula secondary to ruptured traction diverticulum. Gastrointest Radiol 2:119–121, 1977)

9-12   9-13

Fistulization can occur between the esophagus and a pulmonary cyst or sequestered portion of the lung. Sequestration of the lung is a congenital pulmonary malformation in which a portion of pulmonary tissue is detached from the remainder of the normal lung and receives its blood supply from a systemic artery. Mediastinal cysts, especially if infected, can invade or erode the esophagus and trachea, causing esophagorespiratory fistulas similar to those secondary to mediastinal tumors.

On rare occasions, "spontaneous" fistulas occur between the esophagus and respiratory tract. In patients with this disorder, no evidence of preexisting or concomitant disease can be demonstrated.

BIBLIOGRAPHY

Balthazar EJ: Esophagobronchial fistula secondary to ruptured traction diverticulum. Gastrointest Radiol 2:119–121, 1977

Cameron DC: Non-malignant oesophago-bronchial fistulae in the adult: Case reports and review of the literature. Australas Radiol 27:143–153, 1983

Coleman FP: Acquired non-malignant esophagorespiratory fistula. Am J Surg 93:321–328, 1957

Ghahremani GG, Gore RM, Breuer RI et al: Esophageal manifestations of Crohn's disease. Gastrointest Radiol 7:199–203, 1982

Lepke RA, Libshitz HI: Radiation-induced injury of the esophagus. Radiology 148:375–378, 1983

Martini N, Goodner JT, D'Angio GJ: Tracheoesophageal fistula due to cancer. J Thorac Cardiovasc Surg 59:319–324, 1970

Mori S, Yoshihira A, Kawamura H et al: Esophageal involvement in Behcet's disease. Am J Gastroenterol 78:548–553, 1983

Nelson RJ, Benfield JR: Benign esophagobronchial fistula. Arch Surg 100:685–688, 1970

Silverman FN: Caffey's Pediatric X-ray Diagnosis: An Integrated Imaging Approach. 8th edition; pp 1810–1820. Chicago, Year Book Medical Publishers, 1985

Spalding AR, Burney DP, Richie RE: Acquired benign bronchoesophageal fistulas in the adult. Ann Thorac Surg 28:378–383, 1979

DOUBLE-BARREL ESOPHAGUS

10

Disease Entities

Dissecting intramural hematoma
  Emetogenic injury
  Trauma
  Instrumentation
  Ingestion of a foreign body
  Spontaneous (bleeding diathesis)
Intramural abscess
Intraluminal diverticulum
Esophageal duplication

The term double-barrel esophagus refers to the radiographic appearance of an intramural dissecting channel opacified by barium that is separated by an intervening lucent line (mucosal stripe) from the normal esophageal lumen (Fig. 10-1). The radiographic pattern is strikingly similar to the typical findings in dissecting aneurysm of the aorta (Fig. 10-2), the esophageal mucosal stripe of the former being the equivalent of the undermined aortic intima of the latter.

INTRAMURAL HEMATOMA

EMETOGENIC INJURY

Vomiting consists of a complex series of movements controlled by the vagus nerve. The diaphragm descends to a deep inspiratory position as the expiratory muscles contract. As the glottis closes, the pyloric part of the stomach contracts while the body, cardia, and esophagus dilate. Compression of the flaccid stomach by raised intra-abdominal pressure due to the descent of the diaphragm and the contraction of abdominal wall muscles causes evacuation of stomach contents. Repeated vomiting at short intervals can impair neuromuscular coordination and produce muscular fatigue. If the cardia fails to open as the abdominal muscles vigorously contract, tears are likely to result.

The severity of emetogenic injury varies from a relatively minor mucosal laceration to complete rupture of the wall of the esophagus. Superficial mucosal lacerations result in little or no significant hemorrhage. In patients with severe vomiting, whether from dietary or alcoholic indiscretion or from any other cause, the sudden development of severe epigastric pain should suggest an esophageal perforation (Boerhaave's syndrome). In this condition, plain chest radiographs must be carefully examined for evidence of pneumomediastinum or cervical emphysema as well as for pleural changes at the left base. Contrast studies may demonstrate extravasation through a transmural perforation (Fig. 10-3).

The Mallory-Weiss syndrome is characterized by upper gastrointestinal bleeding due to superficial mucosal lacerations or fissures near the esophagogastric junction that are caused by an increase in intraluminal and intramural pressure gradients. Most lacerations occur in the gastric mucosa or extend across the esophagogastric junction. In about 10% of cases, only the esophageal mucosa is involved (Fig. 10-4).

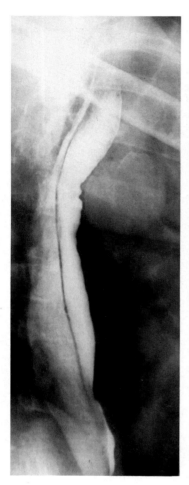

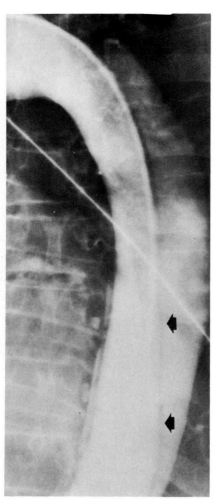

Fig. 10-1. Submucosal dissection of the esophagus following instrumentation. Characteristic double-barrel appearance of an intramural dissecting channel opacified by water-soluble contrast that is separated by an intervening lucent line **(mucosal stripe)** from the normal esophageal lumen filled with higher density barium. (Foley MJ, Ghahremani GG, Rogers LF: Reappraisal of contrast media used to detect upper gastrointestinal perforations. Radiology 144:231–237, 1982)

Fig. 10-2. Dissection of the aorta. Note the similarity of the undermined aortic intima **(arrows)** to the esophageal mucosal stripe.

10-1   10-2

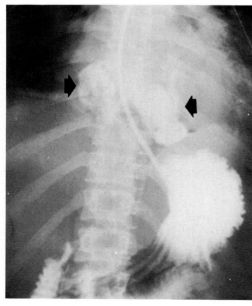

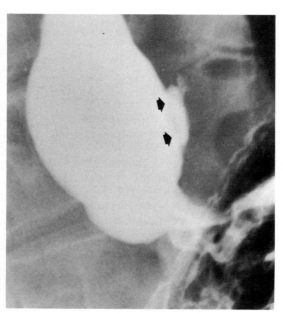

10-3   10-4

Fig. 10-3. Boerhaave's syndrome. An esophagram demonstrates the extravasation of contrast **(arrows)** through a transmural perforation.

Fig. 10-4. Mallory-Weiss tear confined to the esophageal mucosa **(arrows)**.

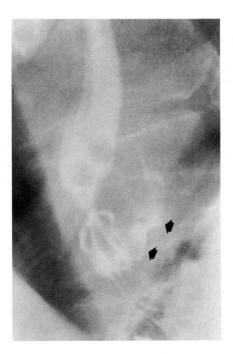

Fig. 10-5. Mallory-Weiss tear **(arrows)**.

Mallory-Weiss tears usually occur in men over the age of 50 who have a history of alcohol excess. They present clinically with repeated vomiting followed by hematemesis. The syndrome occasionally develops without vomiting; coughing, defecation, and lifting of heavy loads have been implicated as causative factors.

Unlike the situation with complete esophageal perforation, radiographic findings are very rarely seen in patients with the Mallory–Weiss syndrome. An esophagram may sometimes demonstrate barium penetration into the wall of the esophagus (Fig. 10-5).

Between the two extremes, emetogenic injury infrequently causes an intermediate laceration with bleeding into the wall of the esophagus and dissection of the esophageal wall in the submucosal plane. Unless spontaneously decompressed into the lumen or externally by rupture, the ensuing hematoma within the esophagus may be extensive.

RADIOGRAPHIC FINDINGS

An intramural esophageal hematoma that is not connected to the lumen produces compression and

Fig. 10-6. Intramural esophageal hematoma. **(A)** An esophagram with Gastrografin demonstrates two midesophageal strictures **(white arrows)**. Distal to the lower stricture are two columns of contrast material separated by a radiolucent stripe **(black arrows)**. The smaller, posterior column represents the intramural collection of contrast material. **(B)** A follow-up esophagram shows the complete resolution of the intramural hematoma. Only strictures are demonstrated. (Bradley JL, Han SY: Intramural hematoma (incomplete perforation) of the esophagus associated with esophageal dilatation. Radiology 130:59–62, 1979)

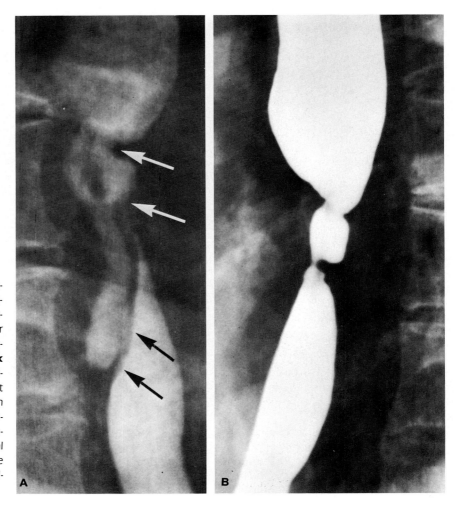

displacement of the barium-filled esophagus. Its appearance is similar to that seen in arteriographic studies of dissecting aortic aneurysms. If the hematoma has decompressed into the lumen, barium examination reveals contrast filling the false intramural channel as well as the true lumen of the esophagus (Fig. 10-6). The close approximation of the intraluminal and intramural collections of barium and the relatively rapid emptying of the intramural channel should permit differentiation from complete rupture of the esophagus, in which contrast material enters the mediastinum and is retained in periesophageal tissues.

Water-soluble iodinated agents should be used in the initial radiographic evaluation of suspected perforations of the gastrointestinal tract. Experimental and clinical data have shown that these media are rapidly absorbed following extravasation, do not exacerbate inflammation in an already contaminated mediastinum or peritoneum, and usually do not induce significant changes in the exposed tissues. However, deleterious systemic effects due to the hypertonicity of these iodinated compounds (electrolyte imbalance, significant fluid shifts from the vascular compartment, pulmonary edema if aspirated, or intestinal necrosis in some cases of obstructive bowel) may develop following both oral and rectal administration in infants and debilitated elderly patients. The use of barium sulfate is generally discouraged, since peritoneal contamination with barium and fecal material can result in significant complications such as foreign-body granulomas and peritoneal adhesions. Nevertheless, small tears, fistulas, and penetrating ulcers may not be detectable on water-soluble contrast studies, and thus negative or equivocal findings do not exclude perforation. In such cases, immediate re-examination with barium sulfate is a safe and simple method for detecting small perforations and improving radiographic accuracy.

TRAUMA/INSTRUMENTATION

Intramural hematomas may occur following trauma or instrumentation. The incidence of esophageal perforation during esophagoscopy has been estimated at 0.25% with a mortality rate of 0.06%. The rate of perforation associated with esophageal dilatation using mercury bougies is about 0.5%; with pneumatic dilators, it is even higher. Perforation can be complete or be incomplete and confined to

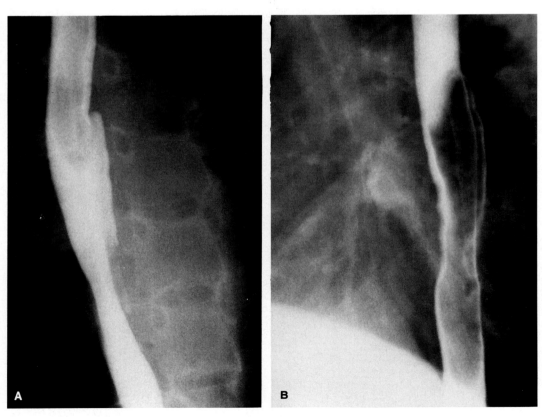

Fig. 10-7. Food laceration of the esophagus. **(A)** Single-contrast and **(B)** double-contrast esophagrams of a young man demonstrate a deep linear tear with extravasation of barium into the submucosa that developed after he ate hard taco shells. (Hunter TB, Protell RL, Horsley WW: Food laceration of the esophagus: The taco tear. AJR 140:503–504, 1983. Copyright 1983. Reproduced with permission.)

the mucosa. In the latter instance, a submucosal hematoma can produce dissection of the esophageal wall resulting in a double-barrel esophagus, with the true and false lumens separated by a radiolucent mucosal stripe.

Dissecting intramural hematomas of the esophagus can occur after the ingestion of sharp foreign bodies (Fig. 10-7). Intramural hemorrhage related to a bleeding diathesis may also develop without trauma. This has been described as a complication of anticoagulant therapy and in a patient with renal failure.

INTRAMURAL ABSCESS

When damage to the esophageal wall by foreign bodies or instrumental trauma involves only the mucosa, leaving the muscular layer intact, infected materials from the mouth may cross this mucosal breech and gain access to the submucosa. As the inflammatory process progresses, a dissection of the mucosa from the esophageal musculature may permit infectious contents to extend into the intramural space and form an intramural abscess. After esophagoscopy, persistent pain in the neck with

dysphagia and elevation of temperature suggests the possibility of esophageal rupture. If plain radiographs of the chest and neck show no evidence of the subcutaneous emphysema that is usually seen with complete perforation of the esophagus, an intramural dissection with abscess formation must be considered. The radiographic appearance of a double-barrel esophagus in this condition is indistinguishable from that of an intramural hematoma.

INTRALUMINAL DIVERTICULUM

An intraluminal diverticulum is a pocketlike structure, open proximally and closed distally, that is attached to the inner wall of the esophagus (Fig. 10-8). Its wall is formed by a thin membrane covered on both sides by esophageal mucosa. Intraluminal diverticula are probably related to chronic esophageal inflammation. Increased intraluminal pressure, possibly caused by esophageal constriction due to mucosal edema and spasm, may permit the development of a small mucosal outpouching through a congenital or acquired weakness of the supporting structures of the esophageal wall. Mucosal scarring and adhesions may lead to the

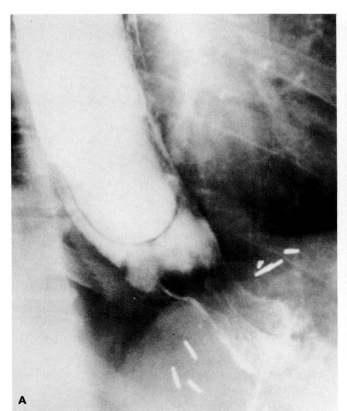
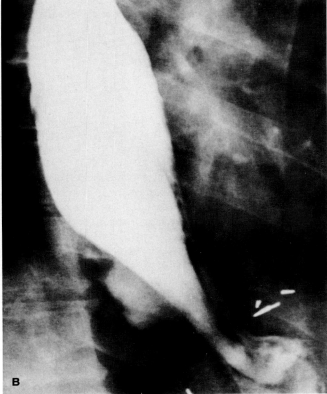

A   **B**

Fig. 10-8. Intraluminal diverticulum of the esophagus. **(A)** An esophagram reveals the thin membrane that forms the wall of the diverticular sac. **(B)** A subsequent film demonstrates prolapse of the elongated diverticulum through the esophagogastric junction and into the proximal stomach. (Schreiber MH, Davis M: Intraluminal diverticulum of the esophagus. AJR 129:595–597, 1977. Copyright 1977. Reproduced with permission)

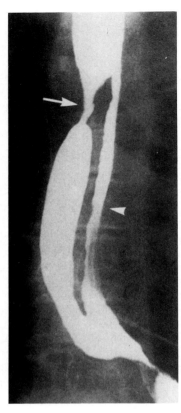

Fig. 10-9. *Communicating esophageal diverticulum. Long tubular structure* **(arrowhead)** *arising from the posterolateral aspect of the distal esophagus. There is a stricture* **(arrow)** *in the midportion of the true esophagus. (Kwok–Liu JPY, Tuttle RJ: Duplication of the esophagus. J Can Assoc Radiol 33:281–282, 1982)*

be a transient artifactual phenomenon mimicking an intraluminal diverticulum. This appearance is most likely produced by the interface of the barium bolus with viscous retained secretions or air and may be enhanced in the presence of an esophageal motility disorder.

ESOPHAGEAL DUPLICATION

An esophageal duplication can produce a double-barrel appearance if there is a communication between this tubular congenital anomaly and the esophageal lumen (Fig. 10-9).

BIBLIOGRAPHY

Boerhaave H: Atrocis, nec descripti prius, morbi historia. Secondum medicae artis leges conscripta. Luguni Batavorium, 1724

Bradley JL, Han SY: Intramural hematoma (incomplete perforation) of the esophagus associated with esophageal dilatation. Radiology 130:59–62, 1979

Butler ML: Radiolgic diagnosis of Mallory–Weiss syndrome. Br J Radiol 46:553–554, 1973

Carr JC: The Mallory–Weiss syndrome. Clin Radiol 24:107–112, 1973

Cho SR, Henry DA, Shaw CI et al: Vanishing intraluminal diverticulum of the esophagus. Gastrointest Radiol 7:315–317, 1982

Foley, MJ, Ghahremani GG, Rogers LF: Reappraisal of contrast media used to detect upper gastrointestinal perforations. Radiology 144:231–237, 1982

Hunter TB, Protell RL, Horsley WW: Food laceration of the esophagus: The taco tear. AJR 140:503–504, 1983

Joffe N, Millan BG: Postemetic dissecting intramural hematoma of the esophagus. Radiology 95:379–380, 1970

Kwok-Liu JPY, Tuttle RJ: Duplication of the esophagus. J Can Assoc Radiol 33:281–232, 1982

Love L, Berkow AE: Trauma to the esophagus. Gastrointest Radiol 2:305–321, 1978

Lowman RM, Goldman R, Stern H: The roentgen aspects of intramural dissection of the esophagus: The mucosal stripe sign. Radiology 93:1329–1331, 1969

Maglinte DDT, Edwards MC: Spontaneous closure of esophageal tear in Boerhaave's syndrome. Gastrointest Radiol 4:223–225, 1979

Phillips LG, Cunningham J: Esophageal perforation. Radiol Clin North Am 22:607–613, 1984

Schreiber MH, Davis M: Intraluminal diverticulum of the esophagus. AJR 129:595–597, 1977

Thompson NW, Ernst CB, Fry WJ: The spectrum of emetogenic injury to the esophagus and stomach. Am J Surg 113:13–26, 1967

formation of a weblike structure that balloons into a diverticulum. If this pulsion diverticulum is restrained by the muscular wall of the esophagus, it can only grow into the lumen, carrying a layer of esophageal mucosa before it. This process results in a thin radiolucent line separating barium in the intraluminal diverticulum from barium in the remainder of the esophageal lumen, creating a double-barrel appearance. An intraluminal diverticulum can also be caused by downward ballooning of a congenital partial esophageal web under certain conditions of intraluminal pressure and flexibility of the web.

In some patients, an intraluminal collection of barium surrounded by a fine radiolucent line may

DIFFUSE FINELY NODULAR LESIONS OF THE ESOPHAGUS

Disease Entities

Glycogenic acanthosis
Esophagitis
  Reflux
  Corrosive
  Eosinophilic
  Radiation-induced
  Candidal
  Herpetic
  Barrett's
  Tuberculous
Superficial spreading esophageal carcinoma
Acanthosis nigricans
Leukoplakia
Hirsute esophagus
Bullous pemphigoid
Ectopic sebaceous glands
Papillomatosis
Lymphoma
Multiple hamartoma syndrome (Cowden
    disease)

GLYCOGENIC ACANTHOSIS

Glycogenic acanthosis of the esophagus is a common benign entity characterized by multifocal plaques of hyperplastic squamous epithelium with abundant intracellular glycogen deposits. It appears to be an age-related progressive phenomenon that may represent a degenerative or reactive process involving the squamous esophageal epithelium. Radiographically, the individual nodules are round or oval and range from 1 to 4 mm in diameter, though they are usually uniform in size in each patient (Fig. 11-1A). On occasion, a few larger nodules or, rarely, plaques as large as 1 cm may be seen on a diffuse background of smaller uniformly sized nodules (Fig. 11-1B). When the esophagus is slightly collapsed, the nodules may appear to be arranged in a linear pattern along the longitudinal folds (Fig. 11-2A). Vertically contiguous nodules may produce slightly thickened longitudinal folds with scalloped contours and uniformly spaced, barium-filled transverse grooves representing crevices between adjacent nodules (Fig. 11-2B). Glycogenic acanthosis should be considered a normal variant. Endoscopy is required only when the appearance is atypical or the clinical suspicion of esophageal disease is high.

ESOPHAGITIS

A pattern of diffuse granularity and nodularity of the esophageal mucosa can be seen on double-contrast examinations in an early stage of reflux (Fig. 11-3), corrosive (Fig. 11-4), eosinophilic, and radiation-induced esophagitis. A similar pattern of subtle marginal filling defects due to small pseudomembranous plaques that can be mistaken for tiny air bubbles is the earliest morphologic abnormality in candidal esophagitis (Fig. 11-5). As the disease progresses, there is increasing variability in nodule

143

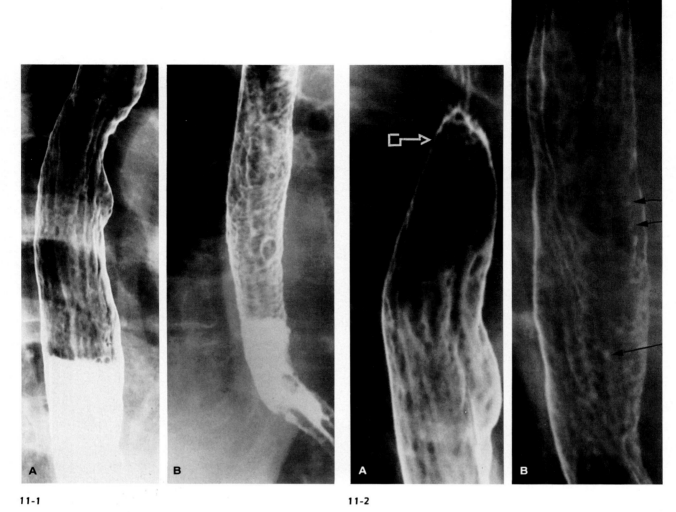

11-1   11-2

Fig. 11-1. Glycogenic acanthosis. **(A)** Multiple small esophageal nodules. Note the prominent longitudinal folds representing coexistent reflux esophagitis. **(B)** Markedly nodular or
cobblestone mucosal pattern in an elderly woman. (Ghahremani GG, Rushovich AM: Glycogenic acanthosis of the esophagus: Radiographic and pathologic features. Gastrointest Radiol
9:93–98, 1984)

Fig. 11-2. Glycogenic acanthosis. **(A)** Linear pattern of nodules along longitudinal folds.
Peristaltic contraction of the proximal part of the esophagus demonstrates incorporation of the
nodules by transverse esophageal folds **(arrow)**. The lucent areas between intersecting folds
are more rounded than usually seen with transverse fold contraction. **(B)** Punctate collections
of barium in pits between nodules simulate erosions **(arrows)**. Note the linear distribution of
the collections, which disappeared with further distention. (Glick SN, Teplick SK, Goldstein J:
Glycogenic acanthosis of the esophagus. AJR 139:683–188, 1982. Copyright 1982. Reproduced with permission.)

size and a tendency for irregular nongeometric
shapes (Fig. 11-6). Multiple finely nodular lesions
may also develop in herpetic esophagitis and the
villous type of Barrett's esophagus; these lesions
may also be a manifestation of numerous miliary
granulomas in patients with tuberculous involvement of the esophagus.

SUPERFICIAL SPREADING
ESOPHAGEAL CARCINOMA

Superficial spreading esophageal carcinoma, if its
invasion is limited to the submucosal layer, may
appear radiographically as a granular pattern (Fig.
11-7). Impaired distensibility of the wall of the

esophagus in addition to multiple finely nodular filling defects suggests the diagnosis of superficial spreading esophageal carcinoma.

ACANTHOSIS NIGRICANS

Acanthosis nigricans is a premalignant skin disorder characterized by papillomatosis, pigmentation, and hyperkeratosis. When it involves the esophagus, multiple verrucous proliferations throughout the mucosa similar to the skin changes may produce the radiographic appearance of finely nodular filling defects (Fig. 11-8). Acanthosis nigricans has been associated with a higher than normal incidence of malignant tumors, usually in the stomach or elsewhere in the abdomen.

LEUKOPLAKIA

Esophageal involvement by leukoplakia is the subject of controversy since a number of investigators doubt its occurrence. The term refers to small round foci of epithelial hyperplasia that appear on esophagoscopy as tiny white patches. They can occasionally be seen radiographically as small, superficial nodular filling defects with somewhat poorly defined borders (Fig. 11-9). Peristalsis is not impaired. Prominent lesions of leukoplakia are re-

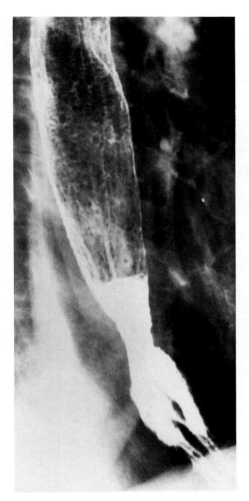
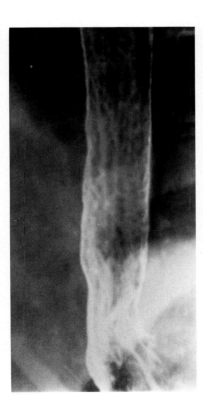
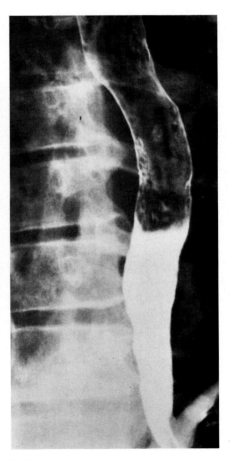

11-3 **11-4** **11-5**

Fig. 11-3. Reflux esophagitis. Note the diffuse granular appearance.

Fig. 11-4. Corrosive esophagitis following lye ingestion.

Fig. 11-5. Candidiasis. Filling defects representing small pseudomembranous plaques simulate tiny air bubbles.

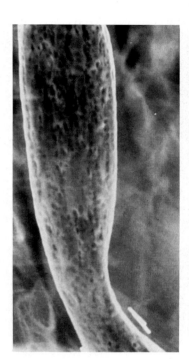 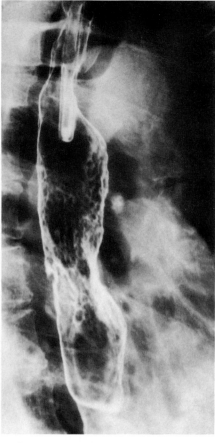 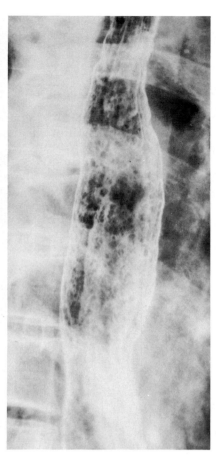

11-6 **11-7** **11-8**

Fig. 11-6. Candidal esophagitis. Numerous plaquelike defects in the mid and distal esophagus. Note that the plaques have discrete margins and a predominantly longitudinal orientation.

Fig. 11-7. Superficial spreading esophageal carcinoma with dense, granular lesions in the midesophagus. A nasogastric tube used for air insufflation is seen at the level of the aortic knob. (Itai J, Kogure P, Okujama J et al: Diffuse finely nodular lesions of the esophagus. AJR 128:563–566, 1977. Copyright 1977. Reproduced with permission)

Fig. 11-8. Acanthosis nigricans. Innumerable elevations are seen without evidence of serration of the esophageal margins. (Itai J, Kogure P, Okujama J et al: Diffuse finely nodular lesions of the esophagus. AJR 128:563–566, 1977. Copyright 1977. Reproduced with permission)

ported to most commonly involve the middle third of the esophagus.

HIRSUTE ESOPHAGUS

Numerous round filling defects representing hair follicles may occasionally be seen on the rough surface of the "skin tube esophagus" that is created to restore anatomic continuity of the gastrointestinal tract during reconstructive surgery of the pharynx and esophagus (Fig. 11-10). Exuberant hair growth and masses of hair within the pseudoesophagus may produce the clinical triad of progressive dysphagia, hair spitting, and choking spells due to large masses of hair.

MISCELLANEOUS DISORDERS

Extremely rare causes of the pattern of diffuse finely nodular lesions of the esophagus include bullous pemphigoid, ectopic sebaceous glands, esophageal papillomatosis, lymphoma, and the multiple hamartoma syndrome (Cowden disease).

Fig. 11-9. Leukoplakia. Small, superficial nodular filling defects with somewhat poorly defined borders are visible. (Itai J, Kogure P, Okujama J et al: Diffuse finely nodular lesions of the esophagus. AJR 128:563–566, 1977. Copyright 1977. Reproduced with permission)

Fig. 11-10. Hirsute esophagus. Numerous small round filling defects in the endopharyngoesophagus. A large polypoid filling defect **(arrows)** is due to a mass of hair. (Agha FP, Wimbish KJ: Hirsute esophagus: Clinical and roentgen features. Gastrointest Radiol 9:297–300, 1984)

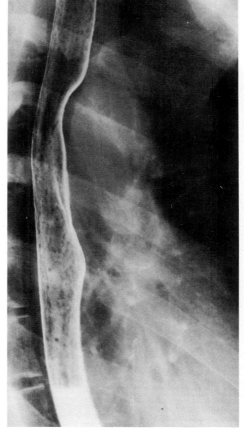

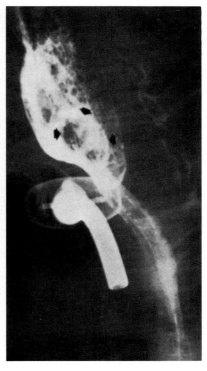

11-9   **11-10**

ARTIFACTS

A variety of artifacts may produce a transient appearance simulating diffuse finely nodular lesions of the esophagus. These include air bubbles, lung markings seen through the esophagus, and lucencies between contracted transverse and longitudinal folds.

BIBLIOGRAPHY

Agha FP: Radiologic diagnosis of Barrett's esophagus: Critical analysis of 65 cases. Gastrointest Radiol 11:123–130, 1986

Agha FP, Wimbish KJ: Hirsute esophagus: Clinical and roentgen features. Gastrointest Radiol 9:297–300, 1984

Darani M, Villi F: Multiple squamous papillomas of esophagus diagnosed by endoscopy. JAMA 236:2655, 1976

Ghahremani GG, Rushovich AM: Glycogenic acanthosis of the esophagus: Radiographic and pathologic features. Gastrointest Radiol 9:93–98, 1984

Glick SN, Teplick SK, Goldstein J et al: Glycogenic acanthosis of the esophagus. AJR 139:683–688, 1982

Graziani L, Bearzi I, Romagnoli A et al: Significance of diffuse granularity and nodularity of the esophageal mucosa at double-contrast radiography. Gastrointest Radiol 10:1–6, 1985

Hauser H, Ody B, Plojoux O et al: Radiological findings in multiple hamartoma syndrome (Cowden disease). Radiology 137:317–324, 1980

Itai Y, Kogure T, Okuyama Y et al: Diffuse fine nodular lesions of the esophagus. AJR 128:563–566, 1977

Itai Y, Kogure T, Okuyama Y et al: Radiological manifestations of esophageal involvement in acanthosis nigricans. Br J Radiol 49:592–593, 1976

Itai Y, Kogure T, Okuyama Y et al: Superficial esophageal carcinoma. Radiology 126:597–601, 1978

Levine MS, Sunshine AG, Reynolds JC et al: Diffuse nodularity in esophageal lymphoma. AJR 145:1218–1220, 1985

Ott DJ, Gelfand DW, Wu WC: Reflux esophagitis: Radiographic and endoscopic correlation. Radiology 130:583–588, 1979

Ramakhshnan T, Brinker JE: Ectopic sebaceous glands in the esophagus. Gastrointest Endosc 24:293–294, 1978

Sharon P, Greene M, Rachemilewitz D: Esophageal involvement in bullous pemphigoid. Gastrointest Endosc 24:122–123, 1978

PART TWO

DIAPHRAGM

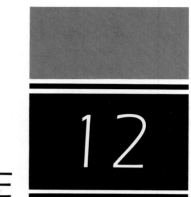

ELEVATION OF THE DIAPHRAGM

Disease Entities

Eventration of the diaphragm
Paralysis of the diaphragm
  Surgical damage to the phrenic nerve
  Tumors
    Bronchogenic carcinoma
    Metastatic malignancy
  Neurologic disorders
    Myelitis
    Encephalitis
    Herpes zoster
    Poliomyelitis
    Tetanus antitoxin
    Diphtheria
  Trauma
    Wounds/accidents
    Brachial plexus block
    Birth injury
  Mechanical causes
    Substernal thyroid
    Aortic aneurysm
  Infections
    Tuberculosis
    Pneumonia
    Empyema
    Adhesive pleurisy
  Idiopathic
Increased intra-abdominal volume
  Ascites
  Obesity
  Pregnancy

Infradiaphragmatic abdominal infection
  Subphrenic abscess
  Hepatic abscess
  Cholecystitis
  Pancreatitis
  Peritonitis
Intra-abdominal masses
  Cyst
  Tumor
  Aortic aneurysm
Supradiaphragmatic pulmonary processes
  Chest wall injury
  Atelectasis
  Pulmonary embolus
  Infrapulmonic effusion (pseudodiaphragmatic contour)

The diaphragm is a muscular structure separating the thoracic and abdominal cavities. It is attached to the xiphoid process and lower costal cartilages anteriorly, the ribs laterally, and the ribs and upper three lumbar vertebrae posteriorly. The diaphragm has a central membranous portion (central tendon) in which there is no muscle. The muscles of the diaphragm arch upward toward the central tendon to form a smooth, dome-shaped appearance on both sides.

The height of the diaphragm varies considerably with the phase of respiration. On full inspiration, the diaphragm is usually at about the level of the tenth posterior intercostal space. In expiration, it may appear two or three intercostal spaces higher.

151

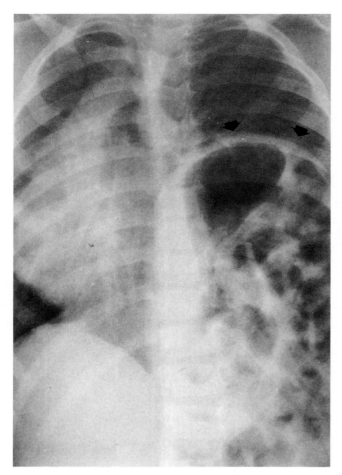

Fig. 12-1. Total eventration of the left hemidiaphragm of a child. The dome of the left hemidiaphragm is at the level of the sixth posterior rib **(arrows)**.

The position of the diaphragm in children and young adults is somewhat higher than in full-grown adults; in the aged, the diaphragm is usually lower in position. The level of the diaphragm rises as a patient moves from an upright to a supine position. The dome of the diaphragm tends to be about half an interspace higher on the right than on the left. However, in about 10% of patients, the hemidiaphragms are at the same height or the left is higher than the right.

Diseases causing failure of normal diaphragmatic movement may occur at five levels. In *central* disease, there may be failure of the respiratory centers, resulting in diminished or absent respiratory drive. Damage to the *upper motor neuron* may occur after high transection of the cord following trauma or be due to transverse or ascending myelitis. Damage to the *lower motor neuron* (phrenic nerve) most commonly occurs due to inadvertent surgical transection, malignant involvement, or a variety of intrinsic neurologic diseases. At the *diaphragmatic* level, there may be an abnormality of nerve conduction at the neuromuscular junction, degenerative change in the muscle itself (dystrophy or myositis), or total or partial congenital hypoplasia (eventration) of the diaphragm. At the *paradiaphragmatic* level, pleural effusion, collapse of the lung, or a subphrenic abscess may cause diminished diaphragmatic movement.

EVENTRATION OF THE DIAPHRAGM

Eventration of the diaphragm is a congenital abnormality in which one hemidiaphragm (very rarely both) is hypoplastic, consisting of a thin, membranous sheet attached peripherally to normal muscle at points of origin from the rib cage. The peripheral musculature and phrenic innervation are intact. Because the thinned, weakened musculature is inadequate to restrain the abdominal viscera, the diaphragm rises to a more cephalad position than normal. Total eventration occurs almost exclusively on the left (Fig. 12-1) and usually in a male. If only a portion of the diaphragm is weakened, a localized bulge may be seen. This usually involves the anteromedial portion of the right hemidiaphragm, through which a portion of the right lobe of the liver bulges (Fig. 12-2). Partial eventration can also occur elsewhere, particularly posteriorly, where it may contain portions of the stomach, spleen, and kidney (Fig. 12-3). Upward displacement of the kidney can produce a rounded mass simulating a neoplasm (Fig. 12-4*A*, *B*). In this situation, excretory urography clearly demonstrates the nature of the lesion (Fig. 12-4*C*).

Eventration of the diaphragm is usually asymptomatic and an incidental radiographic finding. Infrequently, nonspecific dyspepsia, epigastric discomfort or burning, and eructation can occur. Cardiopulmonary distress is uncommon in adults,

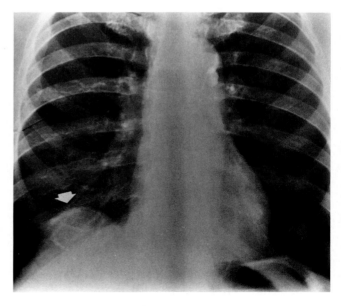

Fig. 12-2. Partial eventration of the right hemidiaphragm **(arrow)**.

though cardiovascular embarrassment can be a result of eventration of the diaphragm in neonates.

Radiographically, eventration appears as localized bulging or generalized elevation of the diaphragm (Fig. 12-5). At fluoroscopy, movement of the diaphragm may be normal or diminished; absent respiratory excursion on the affected side may be noted. The cardiomediastinal structures may be displaced toward the contralateral side. Paradoxical diaphragmatic motion is occasionally demonstrated, though it is much more commonly seen in patients with paralysis of the diaphragm. In rare instances, localized bulging of the diaphragm can be caused by tumors, cysts, or inflammatory lesions of the diaphragm. Differentiation of these rare entities from simple localized eventration is usually impossible without a strongly suggestive clinical history or an interval change from prior radiographs.

PARALYSIS OF THE DIAPHRAGM

Elevation of one or both leaves of the diaphragm can be caused by paralysis resulting from any process that interferes with the normal function of the phrenic nerve. Paralysis of the right hemidiaphragm is suspected if it is more than two rib spaces higher than the left hemidiaphragm; paralysis of the left hemidiaphragm may be indicated if it is more than one rib space higher than the right hemidiaphragm. Diaphragmatic paralysis may be due to inadvertent surgical transection of the phrenic nerve, involvement of the nerve by primary bronchogenic carcinoma (Fig. 12-6) or metastatic malignancy in the mediastinum, or a variety of intrinsic neurologic diseases. Diaphragmatic paralysis can be caused by injury to the phrenic nerve as a result of trauma to the thoracic cage or cervical spine or as a consequence of damage during brachial plexus block or forceps delivery, in which injury to the phrenic nerve may be accompanied by an associated brachial palsy or Erb's paralysis. Pressure on the phrenic nerve from a substernal thyroid or aortic aneurysm can cause diaphragmatic paralysis on a mechanical basis. Infectious processes involving the lung and mediastinum, such as tuberculosis and acute, nonnecrotizing, nonorganizing pneumonia, can result in temporary or permanent diaphrag-

Text continues on page 156

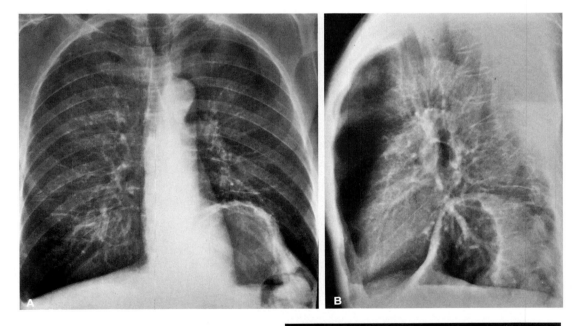

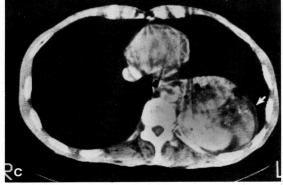

Fig. 12-3. Partial eventration of the left hemidiaphragm. **(A)** Frontal and **(B)** lateral radiographs of the chest and **(C)** a CT scan show that the eventration contains portions of the air-filled fundus of the stomach, spleen (with calcifications), and left kidney (enhanced by contrast material). Note the intact rim of the diaphragm **(arrow)**. (Tarver RD, Godwin JD, Putman CE: The diaphragm. Radiol Clin North Am 22:615–631, 1984)

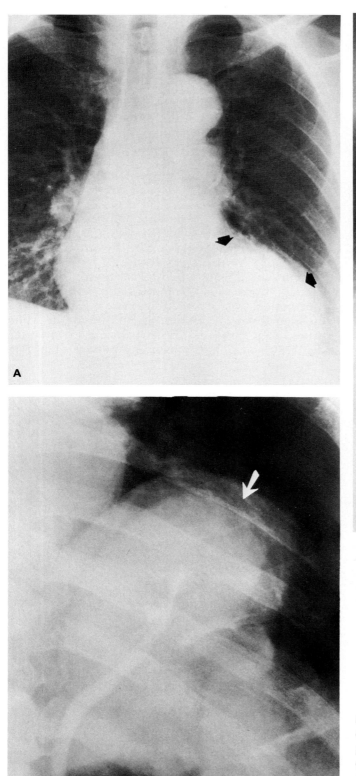

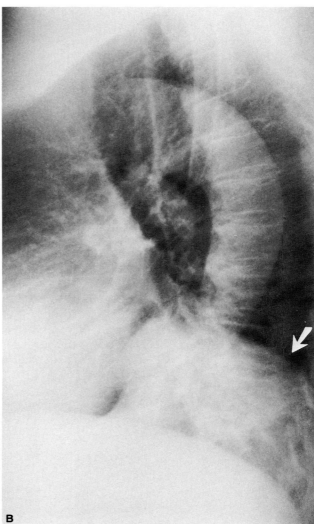

Fig. 12-4. (A) Frontal and (B) lateral radiographs of the chest demonstrate a rounded mass simulating a neoplasm posteriorly at the left base **(arrows)**. (C) An excretory urogram clearly shows that the mass represents upward displacement of a normal kidney **(arrow)** in a patient with local eventration of the left hemidiaphragm.

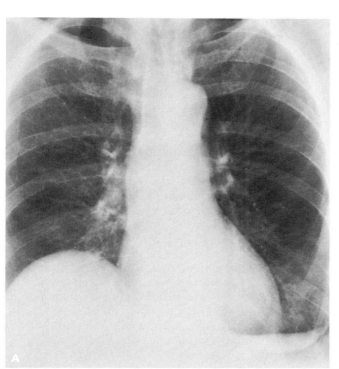

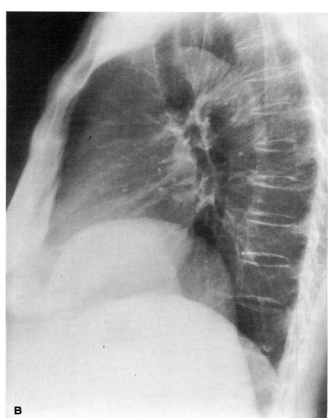

Fig. 12-5. Eventration of the right hemidiaphragm viewed on **(A)** frontal and **(B)** lateral projections.

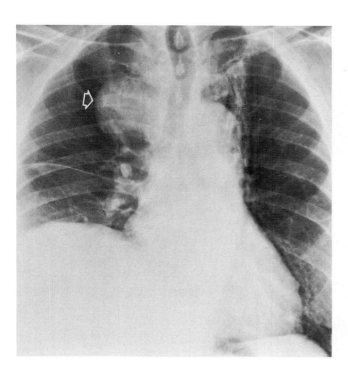

Fig. 12-6. Paralysis of the right hemidiaphragm due to involvement of the phrenic nerve by primary bronchogenic carcinoma **(arrow)**.

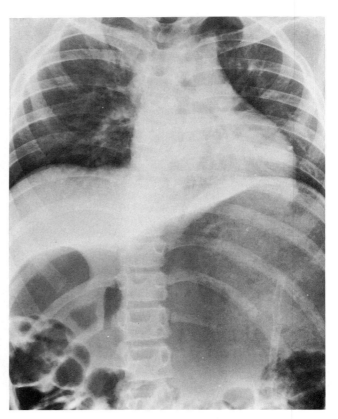

Fig. 12-7. Diffuse elevation of both leaves of the diaphragm caused by severe, acute gastric dilatation.

matic paralysis. In some cases, there is no obvious cause for the loss of diaphragmatic motion, and the paralysis must be termed idiopathic.

A radiographic hallmark of diaphragmatic paralysis is paradoxical motion of the diaphragm in response to the "sniff" test. Under fluoroscopic observation of the diaphragm, the patient is instructed to close his mouth, relax his abdomen, and inhale rapidly. This rapid inspiration causes a quick, downward thrust of a normal leaf of the diaphragm. The paralyzed diaphragm, in contrast, tends to ascend with inspiration because of the increased intra-abdominal pressure. Although small amounts of unilateral paradoxical excursion of the diaphragm on sniffing are not infrequent, a marked degree of paradoxical motion is a valuable aid in discriminating between paralysis of the diaphragm and limited diaphragmatic motion secondary to intrathoracic or intra-abdominal inflammatory disease.

Stimulation of the phrenic nerve by applying an electrical impulse to the neck during fluoroscopy or real-time ultrasound (sonoscopy) of the diaphragm has been reported to allow more precise functional evaluation than fluoroscopy or sonoscopy alone. Following phrenic nerve stimulation, some patients may show partial but diminished diaphragmatic contractions, suggesting that the nerve has undergone neuropraxia rather than more severe damage. In cases of traumatic high cervical quadriplegia, this technique can be of value in the critical determination whether the diaphragmatic paralysis is secondary to phrenic nerve injury or to an upper motor neuron lesion.

OTHER CAUSES OF ELEVATION OF THE DIAPHRAGM

Diffuse elevation of the diaphragm can be caused by ascites, obesity, pregnancy, or any other process in which the intra-abdominal volume is increased (Fig. 12-7). In these instances, intact innervation and musculature permits some diaphragmatic movement, albeit possibly decreased.

Intra-abdominal inflammatory disease can lead to elevation of one or both leaves of the diaphragm, with severe limitation of diaphragmatic motion. This appearance is especially marked in patients with subphrenic abscesses, in whom there is associated blunting of the costophrenic angle and often subphrenic collections of gas. The limitation of diaphragmatic motion in patients with intra-abdominal inflammation is probably related to an attempt to avoid the pain associated with deep inspiration. The degree of limitation of movement is related to the severity of the disease process and its location in relation to the diaphragm. Thus, an abscess in the pelvis has far less effect on the position and motion of the diaphragm than does acute cholecystitis or a subphrenic abscess.

Intra-abdominal masses arising in the upper quadrants can also cause diaphragmatic elevation. Localized or generalized bulging of the diaphragm may be due to a cyst or tumor in the liver (Fig. 12-8), spleen, kidney, adrenal, or pancreas. One case of left hemidiaphragmatic elevation has been reported to be secondary to a large suprarenal abdominal aortic aneurysm (Fig. 12-9).

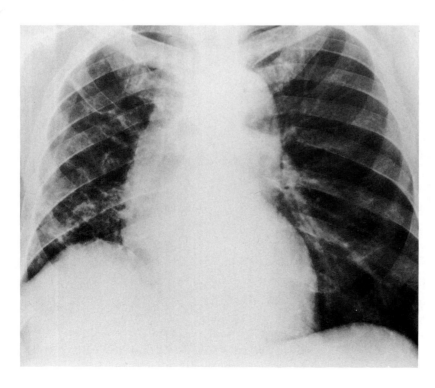

Fig. 12-8. Elevation of the right hemidiaphragm caused by a huge gumma of the liver.

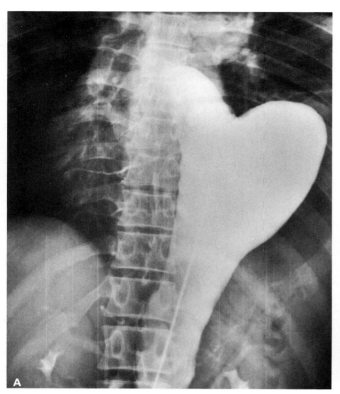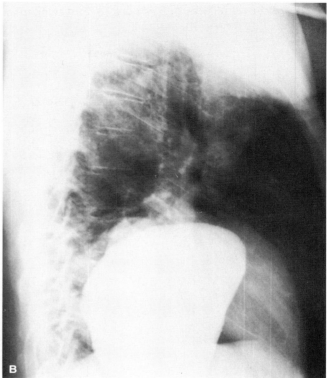

Fig. 12-9. Elevation of the left hemidiaphragm due to an abdominal aortic aneurysm. **(A)** Frontal and **(B)** lateral projections reveal the opacified, saccular abdominal aortic aneurysm elevating the left hemidiaphragm. (Phillips G, Gordon D: Abdominal aortic aneurysm: Unusual cause for left hemidiaphragmatic elevation. AJR 136:1221–1223, 1981. Copyright 1981. Reproduced with permission)

Acute intrathoracic processes can also cause elevation of the diaphragm due to splinting of the diaphragm secondary to chest wall injury, atelectasis, or pulmonary embolus. An infrapulmonic effusion can closely simulate an elevated diaphragm. Pleural effusions initially form inferior to the lung. With increasing amounts of fluid, spillover into the costophrenic sulci produces the classic radiographic sign of blunting of the costophrenic angles. For unclear reasons, fluid can continue to accumulate in an infrapulmonary location without spilling into the costophrenic sulci or extending up along the chest wall. This produces a radiographic pattern (pseudodiaphragmatic contour) that mimics diaphragmatic elevation on the erect film.

On the posteroanterior projection, the peak of the pseudodiaphragmatic contour is lateral to that of the normal hemidiaphragm (Fig. 12-10) and situated near the junction of the middle and lateral thirds, rather than near the center. In addition, the pseudodiaphragmatic contour slopes down rapidly toward the lateral costophrenic recess. On lateral projection, the ascending portion of the pseudodiaphragmatic contour rises abruptly in almost a straight line to the region of the major fissure, rather than assuming a normal, more rounded configuration. At fluoroscopy, the patient with an infrapulmonic effusion demonstrates no impairment of diaphragmatic excursion during respiration. Tilting

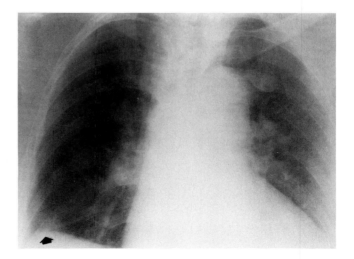

Fig. 12-10. Pseudodiaphragmatic contour (subpulmonic effusion). The peak of the right hemidiaphragm **(arrow)** is situated more laterally than normal.

the patient to one side causes fluid to spill over into the lateral costophrenic sulcus.

BIBLIOGRAPHY

Alexander C: Diaphragm movements and the diagnosis of diaphragmatic paralysis. Clin Radiol 17:79–83, 1966

Campbell JA: The diaphragm in roentgenology of the chest. Radiol Clin North Am 1:395–410, 1963

Laxdall OE, McDougall HA, Mellin GW: Congenital eventration of the diaphragm. N Engl J Med 250:401–408, 1954

Lundius B: Intrathoracic kidney. AJR 125:678–681, 1975

Lundstrom CH, Allen PR: Bilateral congenital eventration of the diaphragm. AJR 97:216–217, 1966

McCauley RGK, Labib KB: Diaphragmatic paralysis evaluated by phrenic nerve stimulation during fluoroscopy or real-time ultrasound. Radiology 153:33–36, 1984

Phillips G, Gordon DG: Abdominal aortic aneurysm: Unusual cause for left hemidiaphragmatic elevation. AJR 136:1221–1223, 1981

Riley EA: Idiopathic diaphragmatic paralysis. Am J Med 32:404–415, 1962

Tarver RD, Godwin JD, Putman CE: The diaphragm. Radiol Clin North Am 22:615–631, 1984

Thomas T: Nonparalytic eventration of the diaphragm. J Thorac Cardiovasc Surg 55:586–593, 1968

DIAPHRAGMATIC HERNIAS

13

Disease Entities

  Hiatal
  Paraesophageal
  Foramen of Morgagni
  Foramen of Bochdalek
  Traumatic
  Intrapericardial

HIATAL HERNIA

Hiatal hernias are probably the most common problem confronting the gastroenterologist and the abnormality most frequently detected on upper gastrointestinal examination. The spectrum of hiatal hernia is broad, ranging from large esophagogastric hernias (Fig. 13-1) in which much of the stomach lies within the thoracic cavity and there is a predisposition to volvulus (Fig. 13-2) to small hernias that emerge above the diaphragm only under certain circumstances (related to changes in intra-abdominal or intrathoracic pressure) and easily slide back into the abdomen through the hiatus (Fig. 13-3).

The clinical significance of hiatal hernia is extremely controversial, and a full discussion is beyond the scope of this book. The classic symptoms associated with hiatal hernia—heartburn, regurgitation, pain, and dysphagia—are due to gastric or duodenal contents coming in contact with the sensitive esophageal mucosa (gastroesophageal reflux). Although gastroesophageal reflux and hiatal hernia coexist in many patients, reflux often occurs in the absence of a radiographically demonstrable hernia. Many small hiatal hernias are not associated with either reflux or clinical symptoms. Therefore, it is generally agreed that the critical determinant of symptomatology in patients with a hiatal hernia is the presence of gastroesophageal reflux, not the hiatal hernia itself.

The major complications of hiatal hernia and gastroesophageal reflux are esophagitis, esophageal ulcer, and stenosis of the esophagus secondary to fibrotic healing of the inflammatory process (Fig. 13-4). Ulceration within the hernia sac can occur (Fig. 13-5). Massive upper gastrointestinal hemorrhage is a rare complication, most likely due to concomitant gastric or duodenal ulcer or esophageal varices. Free perforation of an esophageal ulcer is rare, though penetration into adjacent structures is not uncommon. In patients with large hiatal hernias, volvulus of the stomach with strangulation can be a life-threatening complication (Fig. 13-6).

Large hiatal hernias, especially in elderly and obese patients, can cause compromised lung excursion and respiratory distress. Retention of food or refluxed gastric contents predisposes to pulmonary aspiration. Compression of the heart by a large hiatal hernia can reduce coronary blood flow sufficiently to cause syncope, tachycardia, angina, dyspnea, and cyanosis.

Hiatal hernias are extremely common and may even be physiologic in later life. As a person ages, normal loss of fat tissue and decreased elasticity of

Text continues on page 162

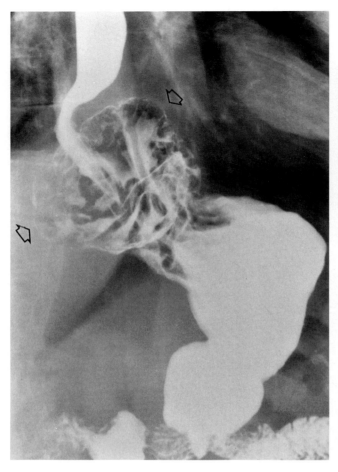

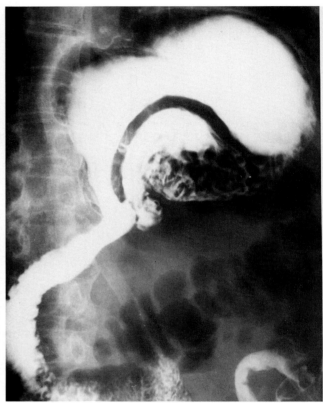

13-1

13-2

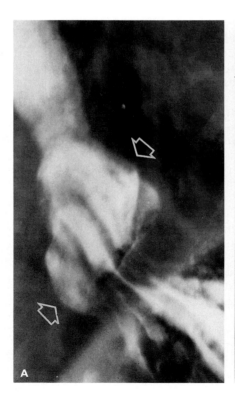

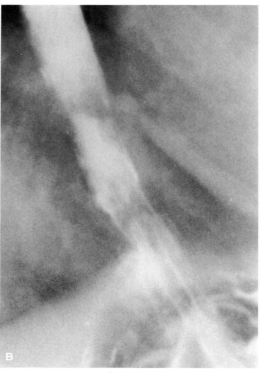

13-3

Fig. 13-1. Large hiatal hernia **(arrows)**.

Fig. 13-2. Large hiatal hernia with organoaxial gastric volvulus.

Fig. 13-3. Sliding hiatal hernia. **(A)** Moderate hiatal hernia visible above the left hemidiaphragm. **(B)** Reduction of the hiatal hernia. The marginal irregularity and thickened folds in the esophagus suggest esophagitis.

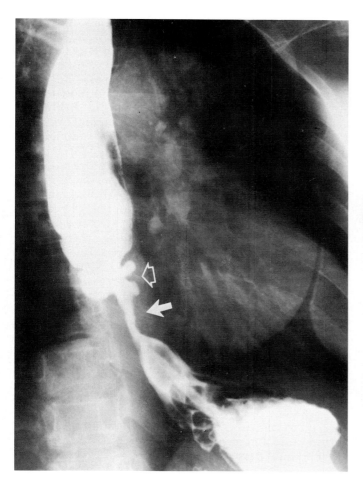

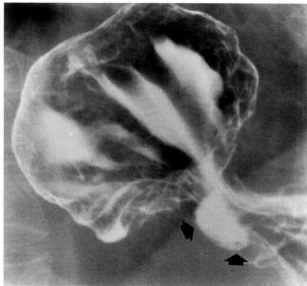

13-4   **13-5**

Fig. 13-4. Stricture of the distal esophagus **(solid arrow)** with proximal esophageal ulceration **(open arrow)** and a hiatal hernia.

Fig. 13-5. Penetrating ulcer **(arrows)** in a large hiatal hernia sac.

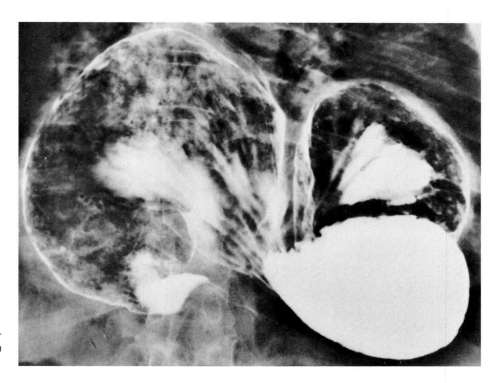

Fig. 13-6. Volvulus of the stomach trapped in a large hiatal hernia sac.

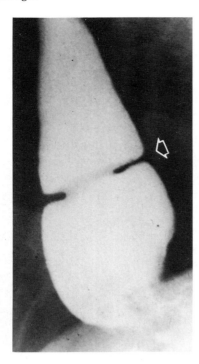

Fig. 13-7. Lower esophageal ring (Schatzki ring). The ring **(arrow)** indicates the transition zone between the esophageal and the gastric mucosae.

connective tissue of the dome of the diaphragm result in relaxation and displacement of the muscular tissue of the hiatus. In adult patients with symptoms suggesting an esophageal disorder, up to 75% have a radiographically detectable hiatal hernia. Even when there are no symptoms, a hiatal hernia can be demonstrated in at least 10% of all adults over the age of 50.

RADIOGRAPHIC FINDINGS

It is difficult to determine precise radiographic criteria for the presence of a hiatal hernia. This is especially true with regard to the small, sliding hernias that comprise about 90% of all radiographically demonstrable lesions. For determination of whether a hiatal hernia is present, the exact levels of the diaphragmatic opening and the junction between the esophagus and stomach must be precisely located. The site of the diaphragmatic opening is difficult to determine radiographically. Radiopaque clips placed on the edge of the esophageal hiatus at endoscopy can be seen well above, at, or below the dome of the diaphragm on radiographic examination. The junction between the esophagus and stomach also cannot be readily defined radiographically.

An exception is the lower esophageal ring (Schatzki ring) which indicates the transition zone between esophageal and gastric mucosae (Fig. 13-7). The detection of a lower esophageal ring implies that the esophagogastric junction is above the diaphragm, thereby denoting the existence of a hiatal hernia.

Plain chest radiographs may be sufficient for diagnosis of a large hiatal hernia (Fig. 13-8), which appears as a soft-tissue mass in the posterior mediastinum and often contains a prominent air-fluid level (Fig. 13-9). Demonstration of a small hiatal hernia, however, is difficult if a lower esophageal ring cannot be detected. A bolus of swallowed barium usually hesitates briefly at the lower end of the esophagus before filling a somewhat flared portion of the esophagus (vestibule) just proximal to the stomach. This site of hesitation represents the uppermost portion of an area of high resting pressure ("A" ring) that appears radiographically as an indentation separating the tubular esophagus above from the slightly dilated vestibule (phrenic ampulla) below (Fig. 13-10). The vestibule leads into the cardiac portion of the stomach, usually forming an acute angle (angle of His) as it crosses the diaphragm. The presence of a second indentation above the diaphragm ("B" ring) is usually considered to represent the site of transition between the vestibule and gastric cardia, implying the existence of a hiatal hernia (Fig. 13-11).

Several other radiographic findings have been used to aid in the diagnosis of small hiatal hernias. The presence of obvious gastric folds, more than four or five folds, a mucosal notch, and a supradiaphragmatic pouch without peristalsis and not in a line with the body of the esophagus have all been suggested as factors indicating that a hernia is present. Nevertheless, the diagnosis of most small hiatal hernias remains equivocal.

PARAESOPHAGEAL HERNIA

A paraesophageal hernia is progressive herniation of the stomach anterior to the esophagus, usually through a widened esophageal hiatus but occasionally through a separate adjacent gap in the diaphragm (Fig. 13-12). Unlike the situation with a hiatal hernia, the terminal esophagus in the patient with a paraesophageal hernia remains in its normal position, and the esophagogastric junction is situated below the diaphragm (Fig. 13-13). True paraesophageal hernias are uncommon, appearing in only 5% of all patients operated on for hiatal hernia. Initially, only the fundus of the stomach is situated above the diaphragm. As herniation progresses, increasing amounts of the greater curvature roll into the hernia sac, inverting the stomach so that the greater curvature lies uppermost. At times, spleen, omentum, transverse colon, or small bowel may accompany the herniated stomach into the thorax.

Infrequently, acquired paraesophageal hernias

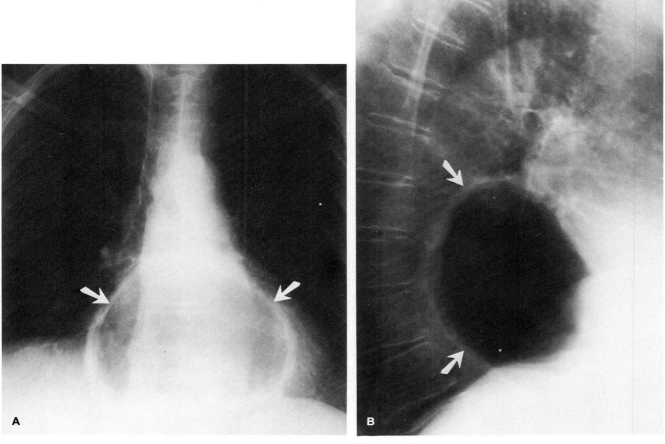

Fig. 13-8. Huge, air-filled hiatal hernia appearing as a mediastinal mass **(arrows)**.

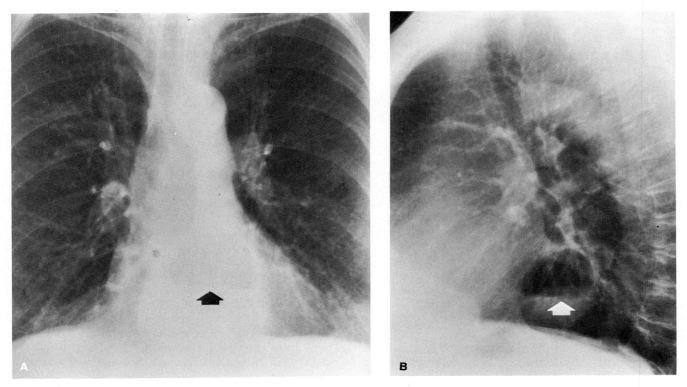

Fig. 13-9. Air-fluid level **(arrows)** in a hiatal hernia seen on plain chest radiographs.

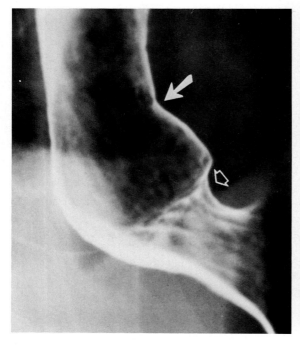

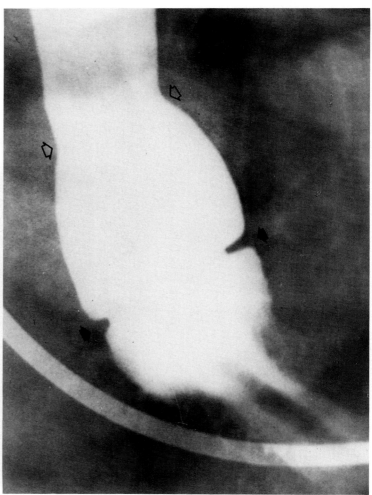

13-10   13-11

Fig. 13-10. "A" ring. An indentation **(solid arrow)** separates the tubular esophagus above from the dilated vestibule below. The **open arrow** marks the level of the junction between the esophageal and the gastric mucosae.

Fig. 13-11. "B" ring. The presence of a second indentation **(solid arrows)** below the "A" ring **(open arrows)** implies the existence of a hiatal hernia.

develop following hiatal hernia repair. Regardless of the type of surgical procedure done, the distal end of the esophagus and the cardia are firmly anchored below the diaphragm, whereas the free part of the fundus of the stomach lies against the old hiatus, which has been sutured closed. Re-expansion of the hiatus around the esophagus may permit the fundus to slide through the opening and become a paraesophageal hernia. Acquired paraesophageal hernias can even develop through a diaphragmatic opening created for admission of the surgeon's fingers (Fig. 13-14).

Many patients with paraesophageal hernias are asymptomatic, even if the condition has progressed to herniation of the entire stomach into the thorax. Not infrequently, paraesophageal hernias are first identified on routine chest radiographs when an air-fluid level is detected behind the cardiac silhouette (Fig. 13-15). Patients can present with vague symptoms of postprandial indigestion, substernal fullness, nausea, occasional retching, and, if the hernia is large, dyspnea after meals. Unlike sliding hiatal hernias, paraesophageal hernias are associated with normal functioning of the gastroesophageal junction, and reflux esophagitis does not occur.

Although paraesophageal hernias usually have a relatively long, benign clinical course, they occasionally have serious complications. Asymptomatic anemia can be caused by blood loss from hemorrhagic gastritis of the herniated fundus; this complication is presumably related to enlarged rugal folds that are edematous because of venous and lym-

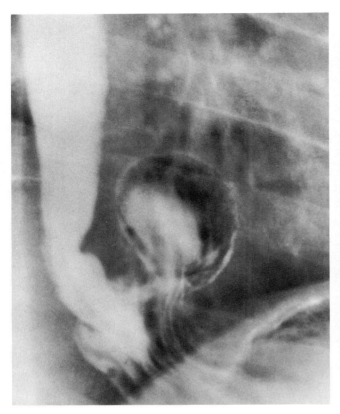

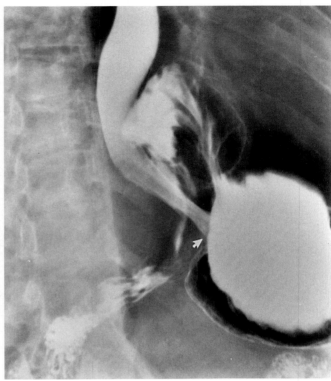

13-12   **13-13**

Fig. 13-12. Paraesophageal hernia.

Fig. 13-13. Paraesophageal hernia. Note that the esophagogastric junction **(arrow)** remains below the level of the left hemidiaphragm. There is an associated gastric volvulus with a portion of the stomach located within the hernia sac.

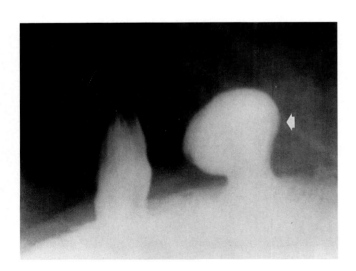

Fig. 13-14. Paraesophageal hernia through an opening in the left hemidiaphragm that had been created for admission of the surgeon's fingers during a previous hiatal hernia repair. (Hoyt T, Kyaw MM: Acquired paraesophageal and disparaesophageal hernias. AJR 121:248–251, 1974. Copyright 1974. Reproduced with permission)

phatic obstruction and therefore prone to erosion. Patients with paraesophageal hernias frequently develop gastric ulcers at the point at which the herniated stomach crosses the crus of the diaphragm. The most serious complication of large paraesophageal hernias is gastric volvulus. If not promptly recognized and relieved by insertion of a nasogastric tube or by surgical repair, gastric volvulus can rapidly progress to incarceration and strangulation of the stomach. Because of the risk of serious complications and the ineffectiveness of medical treatment, paraesophageal hernias are frequently considered for surgical repair.

OTHER DIAPHRAGMATIC HERNIAS

Diaphragmatic hernias through orifices other than the esophageal hiatus are due to congenital abnormalities in the formation of the diaphragm. Many small diaphragmatic hernias contain only omentum. Larger lesions usually include parts of the stomach, transverse colon, and greater omentum.

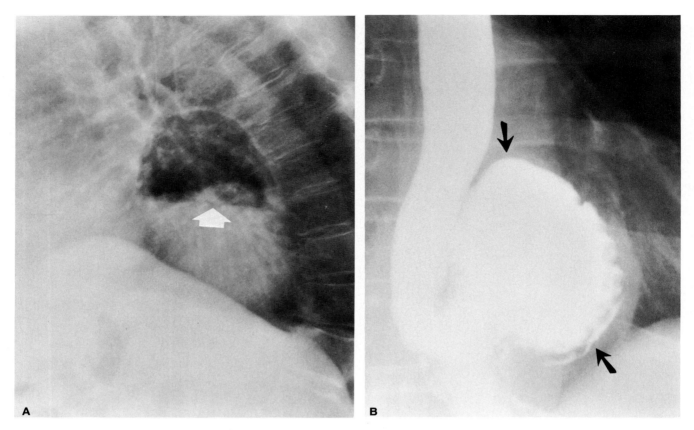

Fig. 13-15.   Paraesophageal hernia. **(A)** A lateral plain chest radiograph reveals an air-fluid level **(arrow)** behind the cardiac silhouette. **(B)** A barium swallow clearly shows the paraesophageal hernia **(arrows)**.

In most cases, these abdominal structures are not fixed within a diaphragmatic hernia and can be withdrawn with ease. Infrequently, the small bowel, cecum, liver, or pancreas can be found in a diaphragmatic hernia.

The symptoms caused by large diaphragmatic hernias depend on the size of the hernia, the viscera that have herniated, and whether the herniated structures are fixed or capable of sliding back and forth between the abdomen and the thorax. Because the stomach is usually situated within large diaphragmatic hernias, some degree of postprandial distress is common. Symptoms of intermittent partial bowel obstruction are frequent, and, if there is interference with the blood supply of the portion of intestine that is within the hernia sac, strangulation and gangrenous necrosis may result.

Large diaphragmatic hernias can produce pressure on the heart and a shift of mediastinal structures that result in intermittent episodes of syncope, vertigo, tachycardia, palpitations, and cyanosis, all aggravated by physical effort, eating, and change of position. The hernia can cause decreased aeration of the ipsilateral lung and lead to respiratory complaints, such as dyspnea, cyanosis, and irritating

cough, that are most marked after exercise. Superimposed pneumonia often develops. Large hernias can even irritate the phrenic nerve, resulting in spasm of the diaphragm and severe left chest pain, which can be referred to the left shoulder and arm and be indistinguishable from angina pectoris.

FORAMEN OF MORGAGNI HERNIA

Herniations through the anteromedial foramina of Morgagni can occur on either side of the attachment of the diaphragm to the sternum. Morgagni hernias typically present in adults and are often associated with obesity, trauma, or other causes of increased intra-abdominal pressure. They are more common on the right, possibly because the pericardial attachment to the diaphragm is more extensive on the left. Herniation through the foramen of Morgagni typically presents radiographically as a large, smoothly marginated soft-tissue mass in the right cardiophrenic angle (Fig. 13-16A). On lateral view, the anterior position of the hernia is evident. When a loop of gas-filled bowel (especially transverse

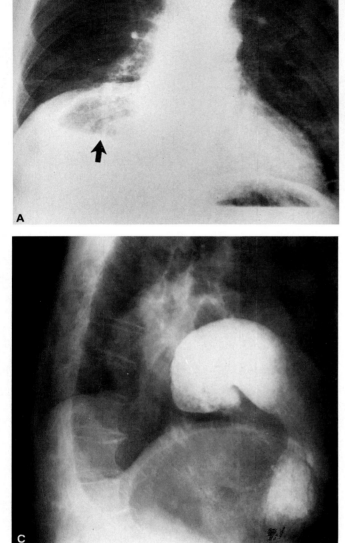

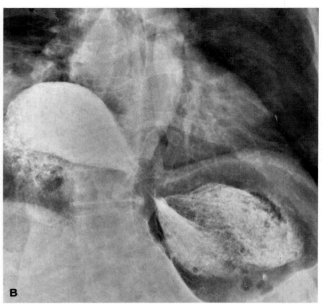

Fig. 13-16. Herniation through the anteromedial foramen of Morgagni. **(A)** A chest radiograph demonstrates a soft-tissue mass in the right cardiophrenic angle. In this view, the gas within the mass **(arrow)** is in the inverted gastric antrum. The gas on the left is in the fundus. **(B)** Frontal and **(C)** lateral views with barium show typical herniation of the stomach through the right foramen of Morgagni with volvulus. The anterior position of the hernia is clearly visible on the lateral view. (Rennell CL: Foramen of Morgagni hernia with volvulus of the stomach. AJR 117:248–250, 1973. Copyright 1973. Reproduced with permission)

colon) is seen within the soft-tissue mass, the proper diagnosis is easy to make. However, if the hernia contains only omentum and no gas-filled bowel, it may be impossible on plain chest radiographs to distinguish a hernia through the foramen of Morgagni from a pericardial cyst (Fig. 13-17), pulmonary hamartoma (Fig. 13-18), or epicardial fat pad. In this situation, a contrast examination is required (Fig. 13-16*B*, *C*).

FORAMEN OF BOCHDALEK HERNIA

Herniations through the posterolateral foramina of Bochdalek more commonly occur on the left than on the right, presumably because of some degree of

protection of the right dome of the diaphragm by the liver. About 75% of patients with this type of hernia have symptoms, primarily vague, intermittent abdominal pain with occasional chest pain, cardiovascular symptoms, and dyspnea. Incarceration of intestine within a Bochdalek hernia results in acute, sharp substernal pain radiating to the left upper quadrant or back, as well as the typical symptoms of intestinal obstruction. In addition to bowel, Bochdalek hernias can contain omentum, stomach, kidney, spleen, liver, or pancreas. A lateral chest radiograph demonstrates a posterior mass and blunted costophrenic angle, often with a small effusion. When a gas-filled intestinal loop is revealed within the posterior mass, the diagnosis of herniation through the foramen of Bochdalek is estab-

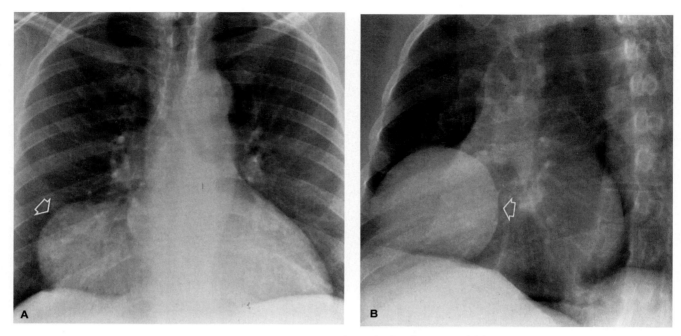

Fig. 13-17. Pericardial cyst **(arrows)** mimicking herniation through the foramen of Morgagni. **(A)** Frontal and **(B)** oblique views.

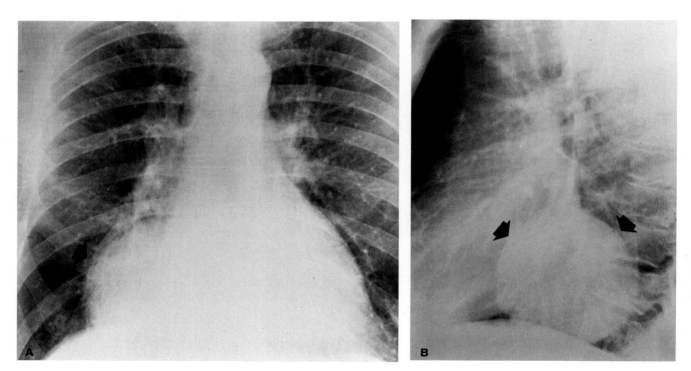

Fig. 13-18. Hamartoma of the lung **(arrows)** mimicking herniation through the foramen of Morgagni. **(A)** Frontal and **(B)** lateral views.

lished (Fig. 13-19). Intestinal contrast studies are occasionally required to detect small hernias.

Most congenital diaphragmatic hernias occur through the left foramen of Bochdalek (Fig. 13-20). In contrast to foramen of Morgagni hernias, these posterolateral hernias do not have a hernial sac, because the abdominal contents enter the thorax before the space between the septum transversum and pleuroperitoneal membrane is closed. In the newborn, large congenital hernias are extremely serious and frequently lead to severe cyanosis, asphyxia, and rapid death. Symptoms of respiratory distress arise soon after birth, because the hernia causes hypoplasia, displacement, and collapse of adjacent lung and a shift of the mediastinal structures to the contralateral side. Most children with large congenital hernias die soon after birth or live only a few years. A few survive to adult life, though most have incapacitating gastrointestinal, pulmonary, or cardiovascular complaints. Infrequently, a large congenital hernia is essentially asymptomatic until late adolescence or early adulthood (Fig. 13-21), when acute symptoms are produced by unusual physical effort or by obstruction of incarcerated stomach or intestine within the hernia sac (Fig. 13-22).

The chest radiograph of a large congenital diaphragmatic hernia is usually pathognomonic (Fig. 13-23); contrast studies are rarely required. Typically, there are multiple radiolucencies within the chest due to gas-filled loops of bowel, and this can

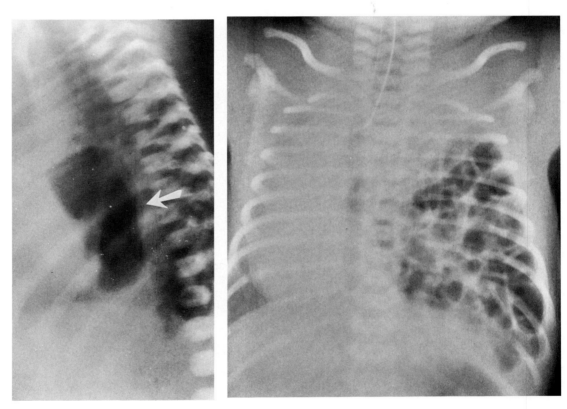

13-19　　　　　　**13-20**

Fig. 13-19.　Herniation through the foramen of Bochdalek. A gas-filled loop of bowel **(arrow)** is visible posteriorly in the thoracic cavity.

Fig. 13-20.　Congenital Bochdalek hernia. Frontal radiograph in a newborn infant with severe respiratory distress shows shift of the mediastinum to the right caused by bowel herniated into the left hemithorax. At surgery, a Bochdalek was repaired, but postoperatively the patient died because of severely hypoplastic lungs. (Tarver RD, Godwin JD, Putman CE: The diaphragm. Radiol Clin North Am 22:615–631, 1984)

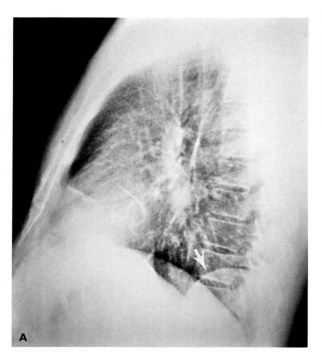

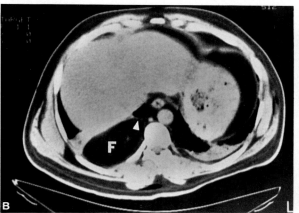

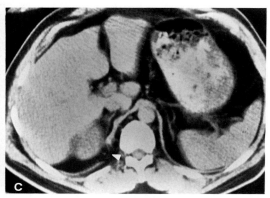

Fig. 13-21. Adult Bochdalek hernia. **(A)** Lateral radiograph demonstrates a posterior mass abutting the right hemidiaphragm **(arrow)**. **(B)** CT scan demonstrates herniated fat in the posterior right hemithorax **(F)**. Retrocrural air **(arrow)** abuts the mass, establishing that it is intrathoracic. **(C)** CT scan 6 cm below level in **B** shows the defect in the diaphragm **(arrow)** that was the cause of the hernia. (Tarver RD, Godwin JD, Putman CE: The diaphragm. Radiol Clin North Am 22:615–631, 1984)

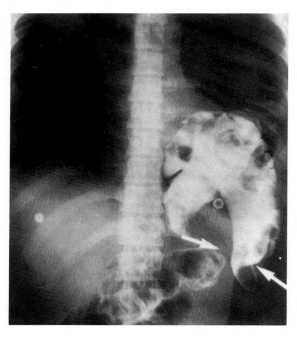

Fig. 13-22. Adult Bochdalek hernia. Barium enema examination shows the splenic flexure of the colon in an unexpectedly high position. Note that the limbs of the flexure are approximated posterolaterally at the L1 vertebral level **(arrows)**, suggesting that the flexure has traversed a diaphragmatic foramen and that it lies in a supradiaphragmatic, intrathoracic position. (Weinshelbaum AM, Weinshelbaum EI: Incarcerated adult Bochdalek splenic infarction. Gastrointest Radiol 7:287–289, 1982)

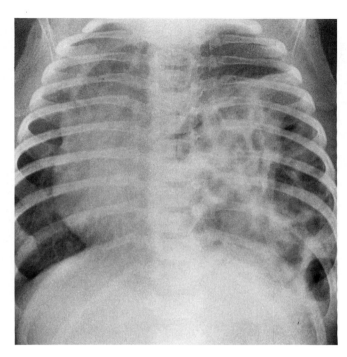

Fig. 13-23. Congenital diaphragmatic hernia. A plain chest radiograph demonstrates multiple radiolucencies in the chest due to gas-filled loops of bowel. Contrast examination is not required for diagnosis.

sometimes simulate the appearance of cystic adenomatoid malformation of the lung. In contrast to this latter condition, however, patients with large congenital diaphragmatic hernias generally have a relative absence of gas-containing bowel loops in the abdomen and an abnormally small abdominal girth. In the unusual case of congenital herniation through the right foramen of Bochdalek, only the liver may herniate into the chest, and the classic sign of intrathoracic intestinal gas is absent. The diagnosis of this condition can be extremely difficult and is based on the paradoxical findings of right pleural effusion, displacement of the heart and mediastinal structures to the left, and the presence of bowel gas high in the right upper quadrant. Large congenital diaphragmatic hernias may not be obviously present at birth but instead develop within the first few days or month of life. A relationship between delayed-onset right diaphragmatic hernias and group B streptococcal infections in newborns may be due to the severe infection adversely affecting an inborn weakness of the diaphragm.

TRAUMATIC DIAPHRAGMATIC HERNIA

Traumatic diaphragmatic hernias most commonly follow direct laceration by a knife, bullet, or other penetrating object (Fig. 13-24). They can also occur

as a result of a marked increase in intra-abdominal pressure and should be suspected in any patient with a history of blunt abdominal trauma who develops vague upper abdominal symptoms. Traumatic hernias occur much more frequently (90-95% of the time) on the left than on the right, both because of an embryologic point of weakness in the left hemidiaphragm and because of the protecting effect of the liver on the right. Stomach, colon, omentum, spleen, or small bowel can be found above the diaphragm. The early clinical course tends to be dominated by accompanying injuries, so that signs of visceral herniation are delayed. Symptoms of postprandial fullness, cramps, nausea, vomiting, chest pain, dyspnea, bowel obstruction, or strangulation may not develop until many years after the traumatic episode. In addition, the hernia may not arise immediately after injury but may follow an additional violent effort or blow that causes the previous scar to weaken. The association of an old traumatic diaphragmatic hernia with bleeding in the chest can result in the development of adhesions that cause fixation of abdominal viscera within the thorax. A potentially fatal complication is the spill of septic bowel contents or highly irritating gastric juice into the pleural cavity. This catastrophic event may be misdiagnosed as coronary occlusion or pulmonary embolism if no history of prior herniation is available.

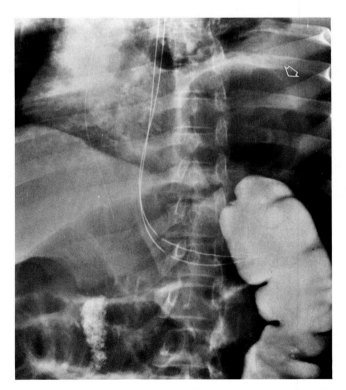

Fig. 13-24. Post-traumatic diaphragmatic hernia. Herniation of a portion of the splenic flexure **(arrow)** with obstruction to the retrograde flow of barium.

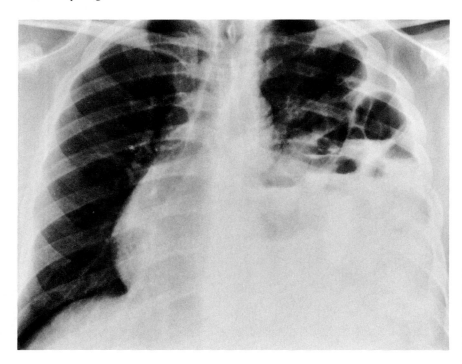

Fig. 13-25. Post-traumatic diaphragmatic hernia due to a motor vehicle accident. A plain frontal radiograph of the chest reveals herniated bowel contents above the expected level of the left hemidiaphragm.

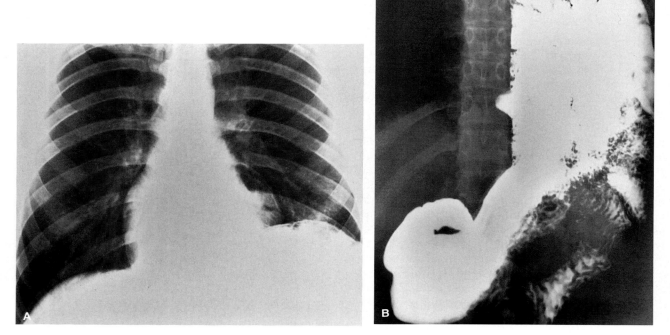

Fig. 13-26. Post-traumatic diaphragmatic hernia. **(A)** The radiographic appearance on frontal projection simulates eventration or diaphragmatic paralysis. **(B)** Administration of barium clearly demonstrates herniation of bowel contents into the chest.

Plain radiographs of the chest usually demonstrate herniated bowel contents above the expected level of the diaphragm (Fig. 13-25). Often, the diaphragm itself cannot be delineated. The radiographic appearance can simulate eventration or diaphragmatic paralysis, since the herniated viscera can parallel the diaphragm on both frontal and lateral projections (Fig. 13-26). This apparent elevation tends to change in shape with altered patient position, strongly suggesting the presence of a hernia. Administration of barium by mouth or by rectum may be required to demonstrate the relationship of the gastrointestinal tract to the diaphragm (Fig. 13-26). A major differential point is the constriction of the afferent and efferent loops of bowel as they traverse a laceration in the diaphragm, in contrast to the wide separation of loops that is typically seen with eventration or paralysis of the diaphragm.

INTRAPERICARDIAL HERNIA

Intrapericardial diaphragmatic hernias (peritoneal-pericardial) are extremely rare. They can be either congenital (Fig. 13-27) or post-traumatic (Fig. 13-28) and can contain (in decreasing order of frequency) omentum, colon, small bowel, liver, or stomach. Although patients with intrapericardial diaphragmatic hernias may be asymptomatic for long periods, most eventually present with either cardiorespiratory (angina, shortness of breath, cardiac tamponade) or gastrointestinal (cramping abdominal pain, constipation, abdominal distention) complaints. Radiographically, gas-filled loops of bowel can be seen lying alongside the heart (see Fig. 13-27). On multiple projections, including decubitus views, the herniated loops can be seen to remain in conformity with the heart border.

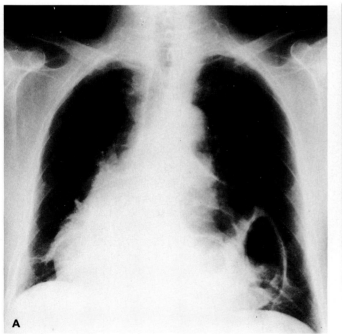 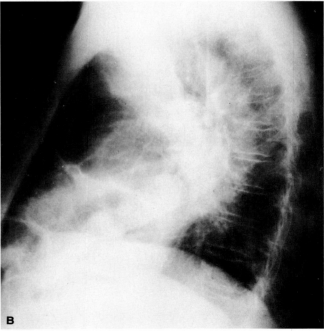

Fig. 13-27. Congenital intrapericardial hernia in an asymptomatic elderly man. **(A)** Frontal and **(B)** lateral views show loops of bowel in the chest conforming to the left pericardial border. (Wallace DB: Intrapericardial diaphragmatic hernia. Radiology 122:596, 1977)

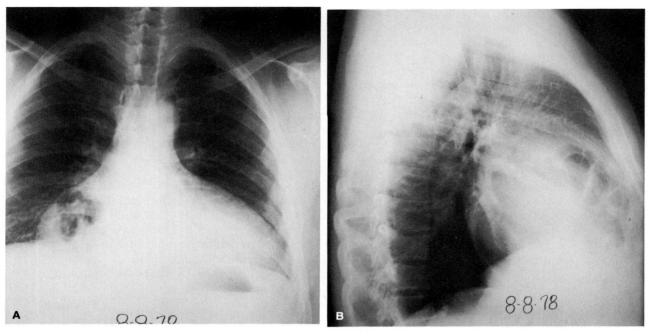

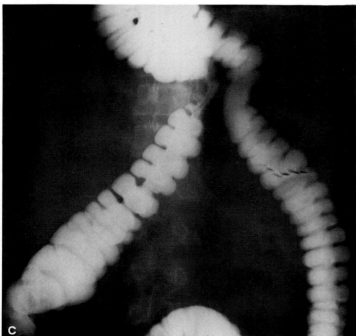

Fig. 13-28. Traumatic intrapericardial diaphragmatic hernia. **(A)** Plain frontal and **(B)** lateral chest radiographs demonstrate a collection of bowel gas superimposed on a widened cardiac silhouette. The location of the bowel gas corresponds to what one might anticipate in a hernia through the foramen of Morgagni. Note the smooth, sloping, unlobulated margins of the mediastinal shadow. **(C)** A barium enema examination confirms the presence of bowel in the thorax. A portion of the transverse colon is projected above the diaphragm into the mediastinum. (Fagan CJ, Schreiber MH, Amparo EG et al: Traumatic diaphragmatic hernia into the pericardium: Verification of diagnosis by computed tomography. J Comput Assist Tomogr 3:405–408, 1979)

BIBLIOGRAPHY

Ahrend T, Thompson B: Hernia of the foramen of Bochdalek in the adult. Am J Surg 122:612–615, 1971

Ball T, McCrory R, Smith JO et al: Traumatic diaphragmatic hernia: Errors in diagnosis. AJR 138:633–637, 1982

Fagan CJ, Schrieber MH, Amparo EG et al: Traumatic diaphragmatic hernia into the pericardium: Verification of diagnosis by computed tomography. J Comput Assist Tomogr 3:405–408, 1979

Friedland GW: Historical review of the changing concepts of lower esophageal anatomy. AJR 131:373–388, 1978

Govoni AF, Whalen JP, Kazam E: Hiatal hernia: A relook. Radio-Graphics 3:612–644, 1983

Hill LD: Incarcerated paraesophageal hernia: A surgical emergency. Am J Surg 126:286–291, 1973

Hood R: Traumatic diaphragmatic hernia. Ann Thorac Surg 12:311–324, 1971

Hoyt T, Kyaw MM: Acquired paraesophageal and disparaesophageal hernias: Complications of hiatal hernia repair. AJR 121:248–251, 1974

Linsman JF: Gastroesophageal reflux elicited while drinking water (water siphonage test): Its clinical correlation with pyrosis. AJR 94:325–332, 1965

McCarten KM, Rosenberg HK, Borden S et al: Delayed appearance of right diaphragmatic hernia associated with group B streptococcal infection in newborns. Radiology 139:385–389, 1981

Ott DJ, Gelfand DW, Wu WC et al: Esophagogastric region and its rings. AJR 142:281–287, 1984

Panicek DM, Benson CB, Gottlieb RH: The diaphragm: Anatomic, pathologic, and radiologic considerations. Radiographics 8:385–425, 1988

Rennell CL: Foramen of Morgagni hernia with volvulus of the stomach. AJR 117:248–250, 1973

Tarver RD, Godwin JD, Putman CE: The diaphragm. Radiol Clin North Am 22:615–631, 1984

Wallace DB: Intrapericardial diaphragmatic hernia. Radiology 122:596, 1977

Weinshelbaum AM, Weinshelbaum EI: Incarcerated adult Bochdalek hernia with splenic infarction. Gastrointest Radiol 7:287–289, 1982

Wolf BS: Sliding hiatal hernia: The need for redefinition. AJR 117:231–247, 1973

PART THREE

STOMACH

GASTRIC ULCERS

14

The detection of gastric ulcers and the decision as to whether these represent benign or malignant processes are major parts of the upper gastrointestinal examination. It is estimated that 90% to 95% of gastric ulcers can be revealed by expert radiographic study. This requires demonstration of the ulcer crater in both profile and *en face* views. The latter is particularly helpful in evaluating the surrounding gastric mucosa to differentiate between benign and malignant ulcers.

Certain technical factors preclude demonstration of a small percentage of gastric ulcers. The ulcer can be shallow or filled with residual mucus, blood, food, or necrotic tissue that prevents barium from filling it. Similarly, the margins of an ulcer can be so edematous that barium cannot enter it; a small ulcer can be obscured by large rugal folds. Scattered radiation in obese patients can impair image quality and detail, especially on lateral views. In contrast, false-positive ulcerlike patterns can be caused by barium trapped between gastric folds. These "non-ulcers" are most commonly noted along the greater curvature and the upper body and antrum of the lesser curvature. Careful technique with graded compression and distention of the stomach usually permits obliteration of these non-ulcers.

The classic appearance of a gastric ulcer on profile view is a conical or button-shaped projection from the gastric lumen (Fig. 14-1). On the *en face* view, the ulcer appears as a round or oval collection of barium that is denser than the barium or air-bar-

ium mixture covering the surrounding gastric mucosa (Fig. 14-2).

On double-contrast studies, an ulcer crater on the dependent wall can collect a pool of barium as on single-contrast studies. If the ulcer crater is very shallow, however, it can be coated by only a thin layer of barium, resulting in a ring shadow (Fig. 14-3A). Turning the patient may permit barium to flow across the surface of the ulcer and fill the crater (Fig. 14-3B). The walls of an ulcer crater on the nondependent wall of the stomach may remain coated with barium even after contrast has flowed out of the crater. The significance of the resulting ring shadow can be confirmed by demonstration of the ulcer in a profile view or by turning the patient so that the ulcer is in the dependent position and fills with barium.

SIGNS OF BENIGN GASTRIC ULCERS

The traditional sign of a benign gastric ulcer on profile view is penetration—the clear projection of the ulcer outside of the normal barium-filled gastric lumen due to the ulcer representing an excavation in the wall of the stomach (Fig. 14-4). Three other features seen on profile view are additional evidence for benignity of a gastric ulcer: the Hampton line, an ulcer collar, and an ulcer mound. These signs are related to undermining of the mucosa due to the relative resistance to peptic digestion of the

Text continues on page 182

179

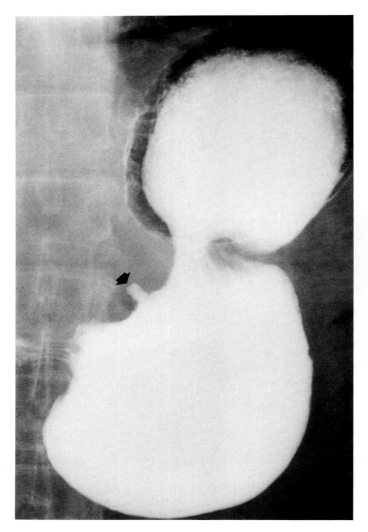

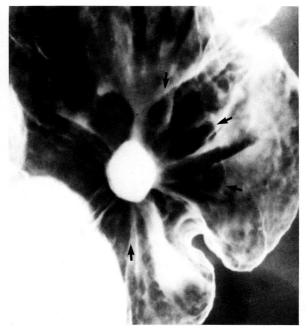

14-1

14-2

Fig. 14-1.   Benign gastric ulcer **(arrow)** projecting from the lumen of the stomach.

Fig. 14-2.   Benign gastric ulcer. On an *en face* view, there are prominent radiating folds that extend directly to the ulcer. The lucency around the ulcer **(arrows)** reflects inflammatory mass effect. (Margulis AR, Burhenne HJ (eds): Alimentary Tract Radiology. St. Louis, CV Mosby, 1983)

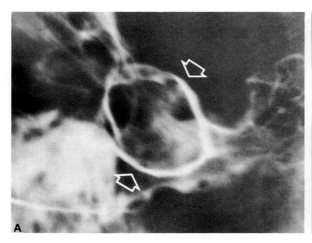

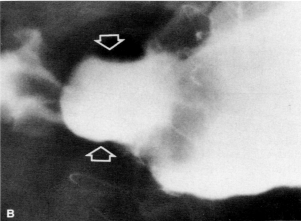

Fig. 14-3.   Ring sign of gastric ulcer. **(A)** A thin layer of barium coats the margin of the ulcer crater **(arrows)**. **(B)** Turning the patient permits barium to flow across the surface of the ulcer and fill the crater **(arrows)**. Note the smooth mucosal folds radiating to the edge of this benign gastric ulcer.

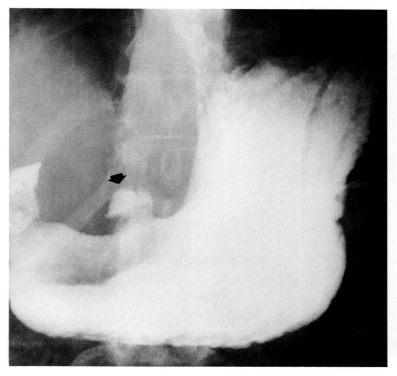

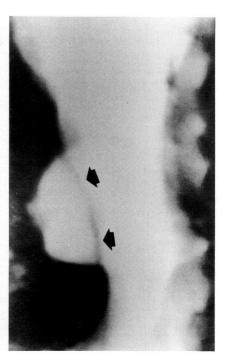

14-4

14-5

Fig. 14-4. Penetration of a benign gastric ulcer. The crater **(arrow)** clearly projects beyond the expected confines of the inner margin of the stomach.

Fig. 14-5. Hampton line of a benign gastric ulcer. A thin, sharply demarcated, lucent line with parallel straight margins **(arrows)** is situated at the base of the ulcer crater.

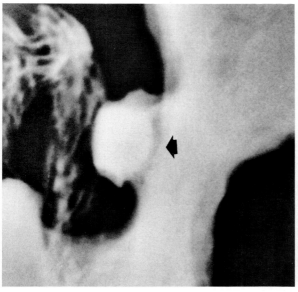

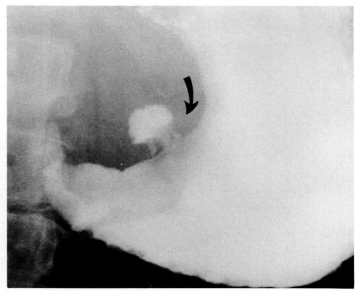

14-6

14-7

Fig. 14-6. Ulcer collar of a benign gastric ulcer. The lucent collar **(arrow)** separates the ulcer crater from the gastric lumen.

Fig. 14-7. Ulcer mound of a benign gastric ulcer **(arrow)**. Note the smooth margin of the gastric wall surrounding the mound.

mucosal layer compared to the submucosa. This results in the more resistant mucosa appearing to overhang the more rapidly destroyed submucosa. With minimal edema of the overhanging mucosa, a perfect profile view may demonstrate a thin, sharply demarcated lucent line (Hampton line) with parallel straight margins at the base of the crater (Fig. 14-5). An increased amount of mucosal edema due to inflammatory exudate results in a larger, lucent ulcer collar separating the ulcer from the gastric lumen (Fig. 14-6). If this collar is irregular or more prominent on one side than the other, malignancy must be suspected. An ulcer mound is produced by extensive mucosal edema and lack of distensibility of the gastric wall (Fig. 14-7). Unlike the Hampton line or ulcer collar, the ulcer mound can extend considerably beyond the limits of the ulcer itself. If the mound is large, the niche may not project beyond the contour of the stomach when viewed in profile. This appearance can simulate a neoplasm. The benignancy of this process is suggested by the central location of the ulcer within the mound; the smooth, sharply delineated, gently sloping, and symmetrically convex tissue around the ulcer; and the smooth, obtuse angle at which the margins of the mound join the adjacent normal gastric wall.

Extensive edema of the overhanging mucosa can almost occlude the orifice of some benign ulcer craters, creating a "crescent" sign (Fig. 14-8). This configuration of trapped barium in a benign ulcer was first reported in connection with oral cholecystographic contrast material trapped deep within a large undermined crater, the entrance to which was

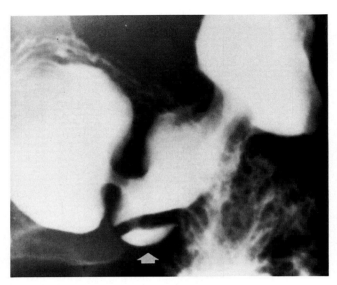

Fig. 14-9. Antral diverticulum **(arrow)** simulating the crescent sign of a benign gastric ulcer.

partially obstructed by markedly edematous overhanging mucosa. A somewhat similar appearance can be caused by a rare antral diverticulum simulating an ulcer crater (Fig. 14-9). Conversely, benign ulcers occasionally mimic diverticula arising from the lumen of the stomach (Fig. 14-10).

RADIATION OF MUCOSAL FOLDS

Radiation of mucosal folds to the edge of the crater is usually considered pathognomic of a benign gastric ulcer. The appearance can be demonstrated on single- (Fig. 14-11*A*) or double-contrast (Fig. 14-11*B*) examinations. However, radiating folds can be identified in both malignant and benign ulcers, and the character of the folds must therefore be carefully assessed. If the folds are smooth, slender, and appear to extend into the edge of the crater, the ulcer is most likely benign (Fig. 14-12). In contrast, irregular folds that merge into a mound of polypoid tissue around the crater suggest malignancy (Fig. 14-13). If there is extensive edema about the ulcer, *en face* views demonstrate a wide, lucent band that symmetrically surrounds the ulcer (halo defect). Radiation of mucosal folds to the margin of the halo indicates benignancy. Even if there are no radiating folds, the smooth contour of the surrounding edematous tissue suggests a benign ulcer, as opposed to the nodularity associated with a malignant ulcer. The halo defect caused by benign edematous tissue has a somewhat hazy and indistinct border, in contrast to the sharp demarcation and abrupt transition of the junction between neoplastic tissue and the normal gastric wall.

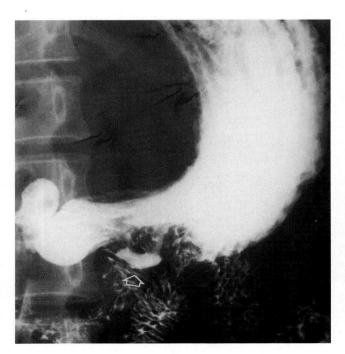

Fig. 14-8. Crescent sign **(arrow)** of a benign gastric ulcer.

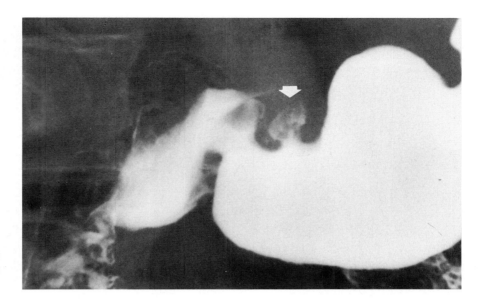

Fig. 14-10. Benign lesser curvature ulcer with an appearance mimicking a diverticulum **(arrow)**.

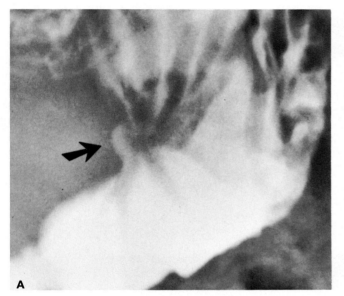

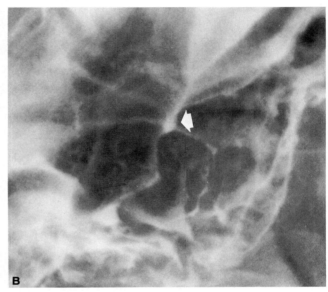

Fig. 14-11. Two examples of radiation of mucosal folds to the edge of benign gastric ulcer craters **(arrows)**. **(A)** Single-contrast and **(B)** double-contrast examinations.

SIZE, SHAPE, NUMBER, AND LOCATION

The size, shape, number, and location of gastric ulcers have in the past been suggested as criteria for distinguishing between benign and malignant lesions. For the most part, however, these "signs" have proved to be of no practical value.

Gastric ulcers can be of any size. Although large gastric ulcers used to be considered malignant by virtue of their size alone, it is now generally accepted that the size of an ulcer bears no relationship to the presence of malignancy (Fig. 14-14). Similarly, the contour of the ulcer base is of little diagnostic value. Although a benign ulcer tends to have a smooth base, it can be irregular if blood, mucus, or necrotic or exogenous debris is lodged within it (Fig. 14-15). With the increasing use of double-contrast techniques, linear (Fig. 14-16), rod-shaped, rectangular, and flame-shaped ulcers have been described in addition to the classic appearance of an ulcer crater as a circular collection of barium.

Although multiplicity of gastric ulcers has been suggested as a sign of benignancy (Fig. 14-17), the demonstration of synchronous gastric ulcers is of little value in distinguishing benign from malignant ulcers. The frequency of multiple gastric ulcers on single-contrast barium studies has ranged up to 12.5%; an even higher incidence has been reported with double-contrast techniques (Fig. 14-18). In one study, 20% of patients with multiple ulcers had a

Text continues on page 186

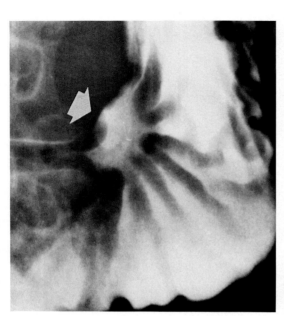

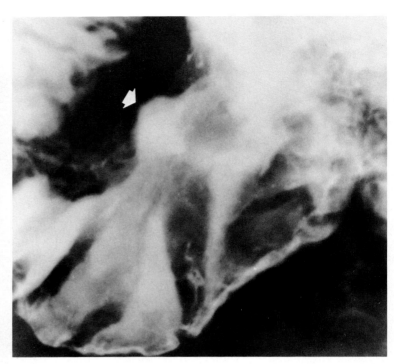

14-12 **14-13**

Fig. 14-12. Radiating folds in a benign gastric ulcer. The small, slender folds extending to the edge of the crater **(arrow)** indicate the benign nature of the ulcer.

Fig. 14-13. Malignant gastric ulcer. Thick folds radiate to an irregular mound of tissue around the ulcer **(arrow)**.

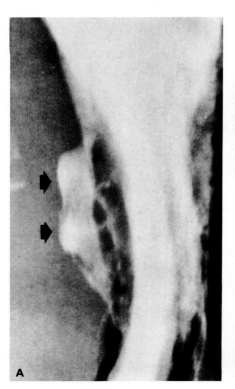

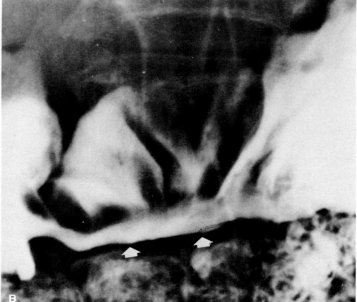

Fig. 14-14. Long ulcers **(arrows)** of **(A)** the body and **(B)** the antrum. Both ulcers were histologically benign.

Fig. 14-15. Irregular filling defect (blood clot) in a benign ulcer **(arrow)** on the lesser curvature of the stomach.

Fig. 14-16. Linear ulcer **(arrow)** in the gastric antrum.

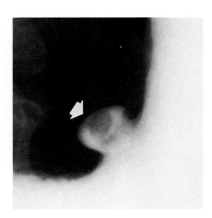

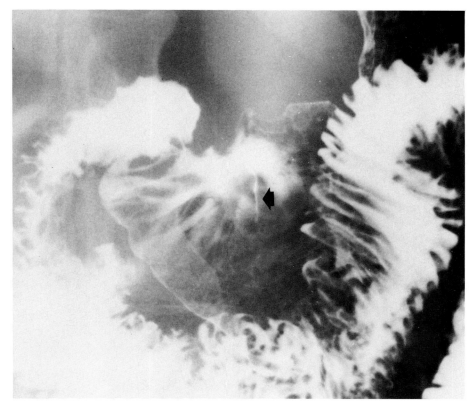

14-15   **14-16**

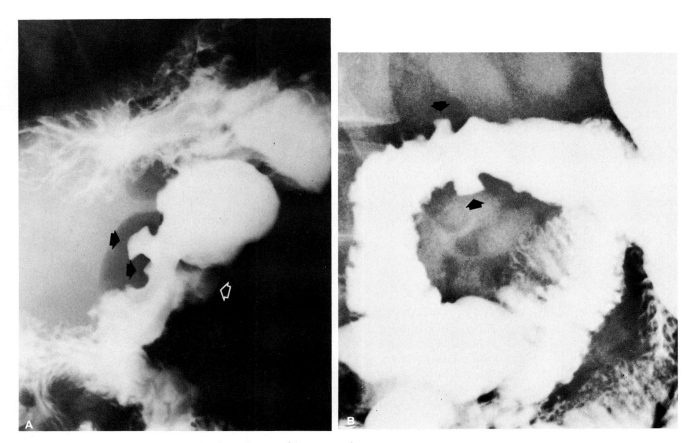

Fig. 14-17. Multiple benign gastric ulcers **(arrows)** in two patients.

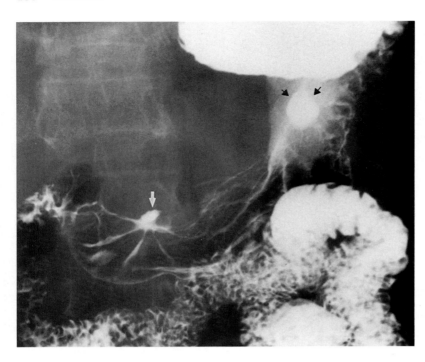

Fig. 14-18. Multiple benign gastric ulcers. Characteristic radiating folds extend to the large ulcer seen *en face* **(black arrows)** and to the smaller ulcer seen in profile **(white arrow)**.

malignant lesion. Therefore, each gastric ulcer must be individually evaluated according to classic radiographic criteria for the possibility of malignancy.

Except for the gastric fundus above the level of the cardia, where essentially all ulcers are malignant, the location of an ulcer has no significance with respect to whether an ulcer is benign or malignant. Although benign gastric ulcers are most commonly found along the lesser curvature of the stomach or on its posterior wall, they can be found almost anywhere. In young patients, ulcers tend to occur in the distal part of the stomach; in older persons, ulcers are more frequently seen high on the lesser curvature.

BENIGN ULCERS ON THE GREATER CURVATURE

Benign greater curvature ulcers can cause diagnostic difficulty, since they sometimes do not demonstrate the same characteristic radiographic features of benignancy that are seen on profile views of lesser curvature ulcers. Indeed, a benign greater curvature ulcer typically demonstrates features that would suggest malignancy if the ulcer were situated on the lesser curvature. Benign ulcers on the greater curvature frequently have an apparent intraluminal location rather than clearly penetrating

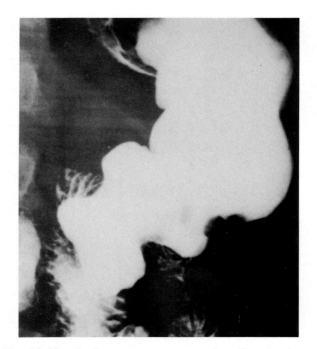

Fig. 14-19. Benign greater curvature ulcer. The ulcer has an apparent intraluminal location, shouldered edges, and a scalloped border proximal to it, all of which would suggest a malignant lesion if the ulcer were on the lesser curvature. (Zboralske FF, Stargardter FL, Harrell GS: Profile roentgenographic features of benign gastric curvature ulcers. Radiology 127:63–67, 1978)

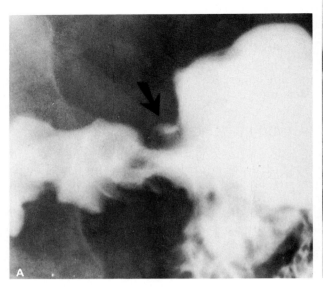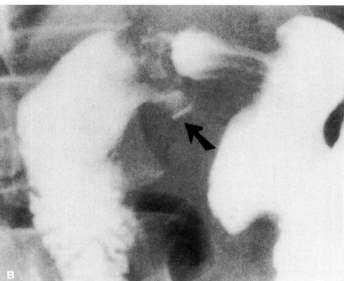

Fig. 14-20. Ellipse sign. Two benign gastric ulcers are seen as persistent barium collections **(arrows)** running parallel to the lumen. (Eisenberg RL, Hedgcock MW: The ellipse sign: An aid in the diagnosis of acute ulcers. J Can Assoc Radiol 30:26–29, 1979)

beyond the expected limit of the wall of the stomach (Fig. 14-19). Spasm of the circular muscles of the portion of the gastric wall surrounding the ulcer causes the more mobile greater curvature to be pulled toward the relatively fixed lesser curvature, producing an indentation (incisura) along the greater curvature. Since the ulcer is at the base of the incisura, it projects into the gastric lumen and may simulate an ulcerated mass. In addition, a scalloped or nodular gastric contour suggesting a malignant lesion can be seen adjacent to a benign greater curvature ulcer, probably due to spasm of the surrounding circular muscles.

ELLIPSE SIGN

At times, it may be difficult to decide whether a persistent collection of barium represents an acute ulceration or a nonulcerating deformity. If the barium collection has an elliptic configuration, the orientation of the long axis of the ellipse can be an indicator of the nature of the pathologic process (ellipse sign). If the long axis is parallel to the lumen, the collection represents an acute ulceration (Fig. 14-20). If the long axis is perpendicular to the lumen, the collection represents a deformity without acute ulceration (Fig. 14-21). Both ulcer

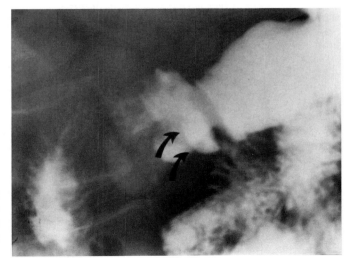

Fig. 14-21. Ellipse sign. The long axis of the bizarre barium collection **(arrows)** is perpendicular to the lumen in this post-ulcer deformity. (Eisenberg RL, Hedgcock MW: The ellipse sign: An aid in the diagnosis of acute ulcers. J Can Assoc Radiol 30:26–29, 1979)

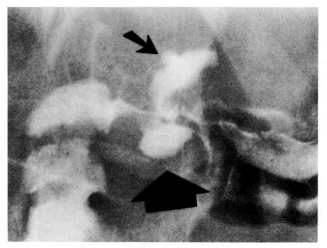

Fig. 14-22. *Ellipse sign. The upper collection of barium* **(small arrow)** *running perpendicular to the lumen represents a nonulcerating deformity. The lower collection* **(large arrow)** *parallel to the lumen was found at endoscopy to be an acute ulcer. (Eisenberg RL, Hedgcock MW: The ellipse sign: An aid in the diagnosis of acute ulcers. J Can Assoc Radiol 30:26–29, 1979)*

and deformity can coexist in the same area (Fig. 14-22).

HEALING

The vast majority of gastric ulcers (more than 95%) are benign and heal completely with medical therapy. Most benign ulcers diminish to one-half or less of their original size within 3 weeks and show complete healing within 6 weeks. Complete healing does not necessarily mean that the stomach returns to an absolutely normal radiographic appearance; bizarre deformities can result (Fig. 14-23). As healing proceeds, the surrounding ulcer mound subsides, and the ulcer crater decreases in size and depth. Retraction and stiffening of the wall of the stomach can lead to residual deformity or stenosis. On double-contrast studies, a gastric ulcer scar characteristically appears as a collection of folds converging toward the site of the healed ulcer (Fig. 14-24*A*). A central pit or depression can often be seen (Fig. 14-24*B*). Evidence of a mass, rigidity, or a distorted mucosal pattern, however, suggests an underlying malignancy.

Some benign ulcers do not heal completely within 6 weeks and may not heal even after a longer period of medical management. This may be due to the base of the ulcer containing poorly vascularized fibrous tissue, which does not favor complete healing. Although such lesions may be clearly benign, the significant danger of hemorrhage or perforation

with recurrent ulceration can be an indication for surgery.

Many malignant ulcers show significant healing. Nevertheless, although rare exceptions have been reported, complete radiographic healing is generally considered a sign of the benign nature of a gastric ulcer.

ROLE OF ENDOSCOPY

The role of endoscopy in evaluating patients with gastric ulcers is controversial. Several studies have shown that double-contrast upper gastrointestinal studies are virtually 100% accurate if the radiographic appearance of a gastric ulcer is unequivocally benign. Therefore, typically benign ulcers can be followed radiographically until completely healed, without any need for endoscopic intervention. At present, endoscopy is indicated only when the radiographic findings are not typical of a benign ulcer, if healing of the ulcer does not progress at the expected rate, or if the mucosa surrounding a healed ulcer crater has a nodular surface or any other feature suggestive of an underlying early gastric cancer.

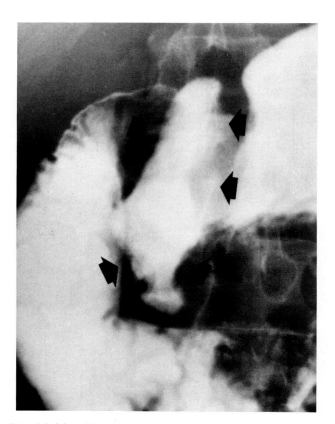

Fig. 14-23. *Bizarre deformity representing the healing stage of a huge gastric ulcer. (Eisenberg RL, Hedgcock MW: The ellipse sign: An aid in the diagnosis of acute ulcers. J Can Assoc Radiol 30:26–29, 1979)*

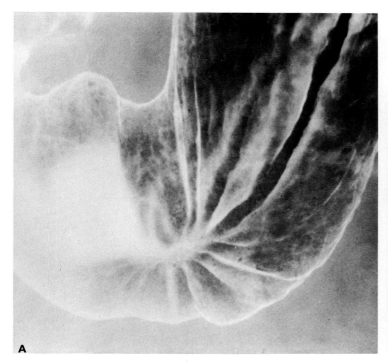

Fig. 14-24. Healing of gastric ulcer. **(A)** Conversions of folds toward the site of previous ulcer. **(B)** In this patient, the folds converge to a residual central depression **(arrow)**.

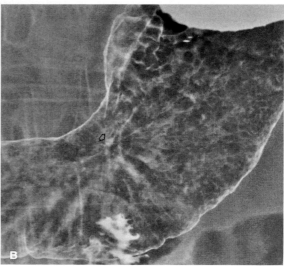

SIGNS OF MALIGNANT GASTRIC ULCERS

Carman's meniscus sign is diagnostic of a specific type of ulcerated neoplasm. When examined in profile with compression, the ulcer is seen to have a semicircular (meniscoid) configuration (Fig. 14-25). The combination of this characteristic type of barium-filled ulcer and a radiolucent shadow of the elevated ridge of neoplastic tissue surrounding it is called the Kirklin complex (Fig. 14-26). The inner margin of the barium trapped in the ulcer is usually irregular. It is always *convex* toward the lumen, in contrast to the crescent sign of a benign gastric ulcer, in which the inner margin is *concave* toward the lumen (see Fig. 14-8). The base (outer margin) of the barium collection trapped within this malignant neoplasm is almost always located where the normal gastric wall would be expected to be. This is because the underlying tumor has relatively little intraluminal mass, except for the elevated rim of tissue at the periphery of the lesion.

An abrupt transition between the normal mucosa and the abnormal tissue surrounding a gastric ulcer is characteristic of a neoplastic lesion (Fig. 14-27), in contrast to the diffuse and almost imperceptible transition between the mound of edema surrounding a benign ulcer and the normal gastric mucosa. Neoplastic tissue surrounding a malignant

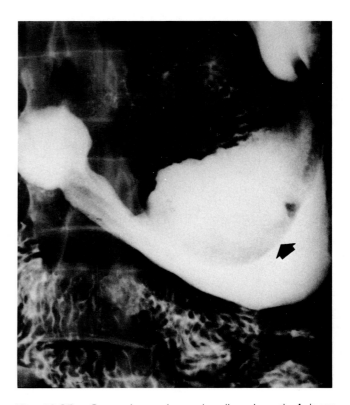

Fig. 14-25. Carman's meniscus sign (lymphoma). A huge ulcer is present with a semicircular configuration and an inner margin convex toward the lumen **(arrow)**.

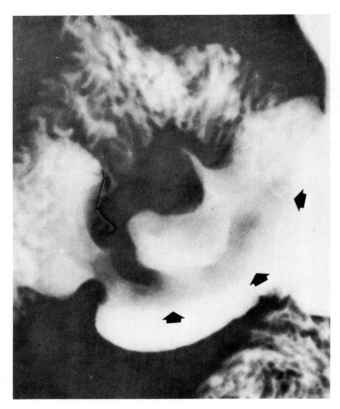

Fig. 14-26. Kirklin complex (adenocarcinoma of the stomach). Note the combination of a Carman-type ulcer and the radiolucent shadow of the elevated ridge of neoplastic tissue that surrounds it **(arrows)**.

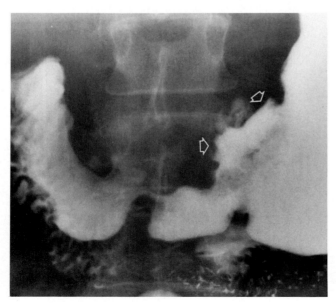

Fig. 14-27. Malignant gastric ulcer. There is an abrupt transition between the normal mucosa and the abnormal tissue surrounding the irregular gastric ulcer **(arrows)**.

ulcer is usually nodular, unlike the edematous mound about a benign ulcer, which has a smooth contour. There is distortion or obliteration of the normal areae gastricae surrounding the ulcer. Nodularity, clubbing, effusion, or amputation of radiating folds also suggest a malignant lesion. A malignant ulcer does not penetrate beyond the normal gastric lumen but remains within it, because the ulcer merely represents a necrotic area within an intramural or intraluminal mass.

ETIOLOGY OF GASTRIC ULCERS

Disease Entities

Benign
    Peptic ulcer disease
    Gastritis
    Granulomatous disease
    Benign tumors (e.g., leiomyoma)
    Radiation-induced ulcer
    Pseudolymphoma
    Suture line ulceration
    Hepatic arterial infusion chemotherapy
Malignant
    Carcinoma
    Lymphoma
    Leiomyosarcoma
    Metastases (e.g., melanoma)
    Carcinoid tumor
Marginal ulceration

BENIGN CAUSES

The overwhelming majority of gastric ulcers are a manifestation of peptic ulcer disease (Fig. 14-28). However, gastric ulceration can also be a complication or primary manifestation of other benign disorders involving the stomach. Localized or diffuse nonmalignant ulcers can be the result of inflammatory disease, such as any form of gastritis (Fig. 14-29) or granulomatous infiltration of the stomach. Benign gastric tumors, especially leiomyomas, can present as ulcerated masses (Fig. 14-30). All of these disease entities are more extensively discussed in other sections.

Radiation Injury

Radiation-induced ulcers can be a complication of a dose of more than 4500 rads to the high para-aortic or upper abdominal area. These ulcers, which can occur any time between 1 month and 6 years after treatment (median time, 5 months), closely resemble peptic ulcers radiographically (Fig. 14-31). Unlike peptic ulceration, however, the pain associated with a radiation-induced ulcer is often unrelenting and has no relationship to meals. A high incidence of perforation and hemorrhage has been reported.

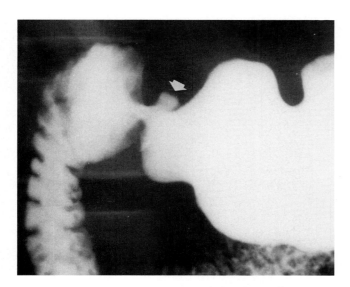

Fig. 14-28. Benign pyloric channel ulcer **(arrow)**.

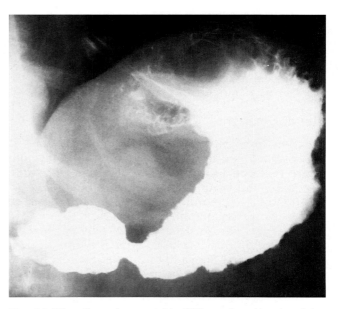

Fig. 14-29. Corrosive gastritis. Diffuse ulceration involving the body and antrum is due to the ingestion of hydrochloric acid.

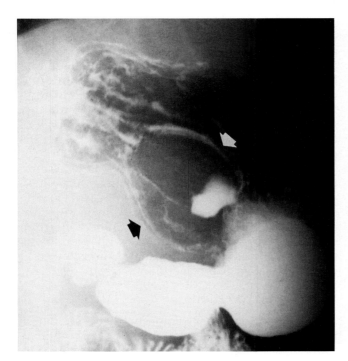

Fig. 14-30. Ulcerated leiomyoma of the body of the stomach **(arrows)**.

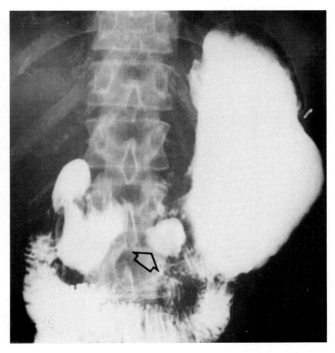

Fig. 14-31. Radiation-induced benign gastric ulcer **(arrow)**. Six months previously, the patient had received 5000 rad to the epigastrium. (Rogers LF, Goldstein HM: Roentgen manifestations of radiation injury to the gastrointestinal tract. Gastrointest Radiol 2:281–291, 1977)

Despite intense medical therapy, healing of radiation-induced gastric ulcers is minimal, presumably because of the degree of vascular damage rather than to any failure of regeneration of the epithelium itself. Serial examinations usually demonstrate progressive gastric deformity.

Pseudolymphoma

Pseudolymphoma (gastric lymphoid hyperplasia) of the stomach is a benign proliferation of lymphoid tissue that can clinically and histologically simulate malignant lymphoma. Although the etiology of this condition remains obscure, it is considered to represent a nonspecific late reaction to chronic peptic ulcer disease. It is unclear why certain patients develop this marked, atypical lymphoreticular response; an abnormal immunologic reaction to mucosal ulceration has been suggested as a contributing factor. In addition to gastric involvement, pseudolymphoma has been described in the small bowel, frequently in association with ulcers.

Most patients with pseudolymphoma have a long history of gastrointestinal complaints, usually without a palpable abdominal mass. This is in contrast to the short and devastating course that is typical of gastric carcinoma and some malignant lymphomas.

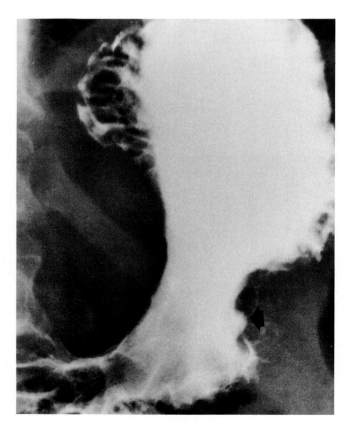

Fig. 14-32. *Pseudolymphoma. Greater curvature ulcer **(arrow)** surrounded by a soft-tissue mass and associated with regional enlargement of rugal folds.*

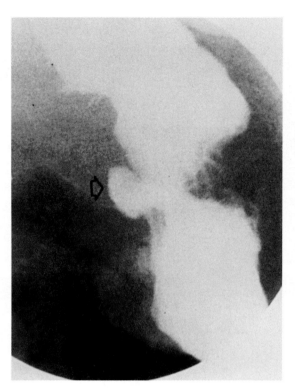

Fig. 14-33. *Suture line ulceration: Large benign-appearing ulcer niche **(arrow)** on the lesser curvature at the level of an intact gastric partition. (Nunes JR, van Sonnenberg E, Pressman JH et al: Suture line ulceration: A complication of gastric partitioning. Gastrointest Radiol 9:315–317, 1984)*

A large ulcer surrounded by a mass and associated with regional or generalized enlargement of the rugal folds is characteristic of pseudolymphoma (Fig. 14-32). The ulcer is usually well defined and looks benign, though it may be poorly defined and irregular and simulate a malignant lesion. Additional gastric or duodenal ulcers are commonly seen. Other manifestations of pseudolymphoma of the stomach include tumor masses and enlarged gastric rugal folds without ulceration.

Histologically, pseudolymphoma is characterized by proliferation of lymphoid tissue, usually in an irregular or nodular pattern, with varying amounts of fibrous tissue. Because in many cases malignant lymphoma cannot be excluded on frozen section or biopsy, most patients with pseudolymphoma of the stomach are usually subjected to at least a partial gastric resection.

Suture Line Ulceration

A benign-appearing ulceration on the lesser curvature may develop at the suture line as a complication of gastric partitioning for morbid obesity (Fig. 14-33). The patient typically complains of severe chronic epigastric pain weeks to months after operation. At endoscopy, suture material is seen in or adjacent to the ulcer crater. Suture line ulceration most likely is due to local ischemia or abscess formation. Suture ulcers from nonabsorbable material have also been described following other types of gastric surgery.

Hepatic Arterial Infusion Chemotherapy

Ulceration of the stomach with bleeding and complaints of pain, nausea, and vomiting can be a complication of the infusion of chemotherapeutic agents through a catheter in the hepatic artery. Intra-arterial chemotherapy is more effective than systemic chemotherapy since it achieves a greater drug level within the tumor and less, though still significant, toxicity than does systemic infusion of the drug. Gastrointestinal complications are more likely to occur if the intra-arterial catheter becomes displaced into the left gastric or the gastroduodenal artery, though the toxic effects commonly occur even if the position of the catheter is maintained in the common or proper hepatic artery. Both aphthous ulcers and frank gastric ulcers may occur (Fig. 14-34). Other radiographic findings include thickening of gastric (and duodenal) folds and decreased distensibility of the antrum. The gastrointestinal complications are reversible if they are recognized early and the chemotherapeutic infusions are discontinued promptly.

MALIGNANT CAUSES

CARCINOMA

Approximately 90% to 95% of malignant gastric tumors are carcinomas. Carcinoma of the stomach has a dismal prognosis because symptoms are rarely

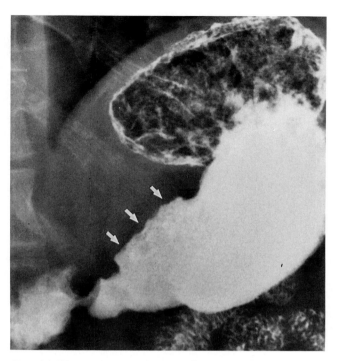

Fig. 14-35. *Adenocarcinoma of the gastric antrum. The long, plaquelike ulceration along the lesser curvature* **(arrows)** *represents a malignant ulcer. Note the somewhat irregular margins of the ulcer, in contrast to the smooth borders of a benign gastric ulcer.*

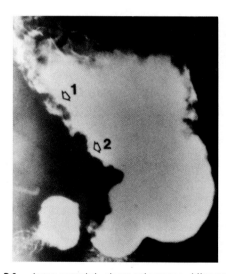

Fig. 14-34. *Intra-arterial chemotherapy. Ulcerations and spiculations* **(2)** *combined with thickened gastric folds* **(1)** *secondary to gastrointestinal toxicity associated with the intra-arterial infusion of 5-fluorouracil. (Mann FA, Kubal WS, Ruzicka FF et al: Radiographic manifestations of gastrointestinal toxicity associated with intra-arterial 5 fluorouracil infusion. RadioGraphics 2:329–339, 1982)*

noted until the disease is far advanced. There are enormous differences in the incidence of gastric carcinoma throughout the world; the prevalence of the disease in Japan, Chile, and Iceland is about 30 times greater than that in the United States. For an unknown reason, the incidence of the disease in this country has been decreasing.

Several conditions appear to predispose persons to the development of carcinoma of the stomach. Gastric atrophy, achlorhydria and hypochlorhydria, and pernicious anemia are all associated with a higher than normal likelihood of developing stomach cancer. Nutritional habits, chemicals, and living conditions, as well as racial and geographic factors, have been implicated in the pathogenesis of carcinoma of the stomach. The questions of whether gastric cancer arises within an adenoma and, if so, how frequently are still controversial.

The most common symptoms of gastric carcinoma are pain and weight loss. The pain is frequently only a mild or vague discomfort, often similar to that associated with peptic ulcer disease. Although gross hematemesis is unusual, occult bleeding is extremely common. Dysphagia can occur if the disease involves the fundus of the stomach near the esophagogastric junction.

Ulceration can develop in any gastric carcinoma. The radiographic appearance of malignant ulceration runs the gamut from shallow erosions in relatively superficial mucosal lesions (Fig. 14-35) to

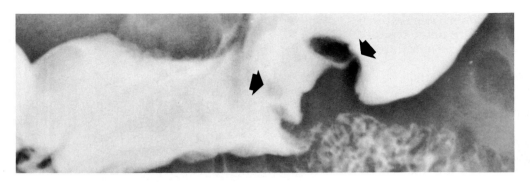

Fig. 14-36. Adenocarcinoma of the stomach. A huge ulcer is evident in a fungating polypoid mass **(arrows)**.

huge excavations within fungating polypoid masses (Fig. 14-36).

LYMPHOMA

Lymphoma constitutes about 2% of all gastric neoplasms. Although the stomach can be involved primarily, it is more commonly affected secondarily in patients with diffuse disease. Gastric lymphoma is often associated with a vague and nondescript abdominal pain that is indistinguishable from that due to peptic ulcer disease or carcinoma. Weight loss is common, as are nausea and vomiting. Hematemesis and melena occur in about 20% of patients, though massive gastrointestinal bleeding is relatively uncommon.

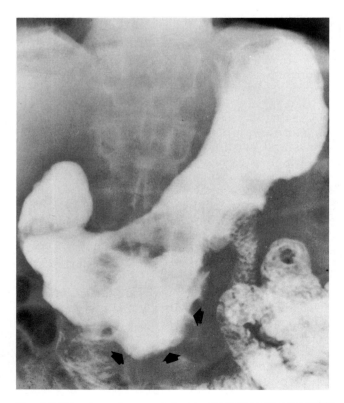

Fig. 14-37. Lymphoma. A huge, irregular ulcer is visible **(arrows)** in a neoplastic gastric mass.

The presence of a large ulcerated mass is one of the major manifestations of gastric lymphoma (Fig. 14-37). When relatively small, lymphomatous ulcers in the stomach are often surrounded by a tumor mass and are indistinguishable from other malignant gastric lesions. Multiplicity of malignant ulcers suggests lymphoma as the diagnosis. An aneurysmal appearance of a single, huge ulcer (the diameter of which exceeds that of the adjacent gastric lumen) is characteristic of lymphoma (Fig. 14-38). The combination of a large ulcer and extraluminal mass can produce a bizarre configuration resembling extravasation of barium. In many cases, it is difficult to differentiate lymphoma from carcinoma of the stomach. Findings suggestive of lymphoma are relative flexibility of the gastric wall, enlargement of the spleen, and associated prominence of retrogastric and other regional lymph nodes that can cause extrinsic impressions on the barium-filled stomach.

Gastric lymphoma can demonstrate a spectrum of responses to chemotherapy. An ulcerated mass may decrease dramatically to resemble a benign gastric ulcer (Fig. 14-39) or a healed ulcer scar (Fig. 14-40). At times, a lymphomatous lesion may heal completely without scarring. Conversely, after chemotherapy a nonulcerating gastric lymphoma may develop ulceration with occult gastrointestinal bleeding.

SARCOMA

Leiomyosarcomas are rare intramural tumors that are prone to develop large central ulcerations (Fig. 14-41). They are often radiographically indistinguishable from their benign spindle cell counterparts. Neurogenic sarcoma, fibrosarcoma, and liposarcoma are extremely rare causes of ulcerated gastric masses.

METASTATIC MALIGNANCY

Single or multiple ulcerated masses can be caused by hematogenous metastases to the stomach. These "bull's-eye" lesions, with central and relatively large ulcerations that arise as the metastases out-

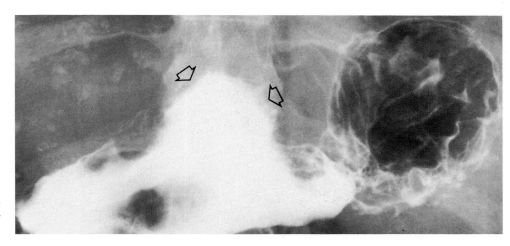

Fig. 14-38. Lymphoma. Note the bizarre, huge gastric ulcer **(arrows)**.

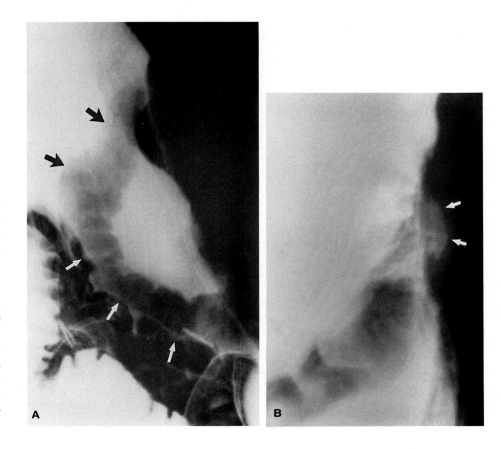

Fig. 14-39. Lymphoma healing to benign-appearing ulcer. **(A)** Large ulcerated lymphomatous mass **(arrows)** on the anterior wall of the stomach. **(B)** One month after completion of chemotherapy, there is a benign-appearing ulcer **(arrows)** with radiating folds on the anterior wall at the site of the previous lymphomatous mass. (Fox ER, Laufer I, Levine MS: Response of gastric lymphoma to chemotherapy: Radiographic appearance. AJR 142:711–714, 1984. Copyright 1984. Reproduced with permission.)

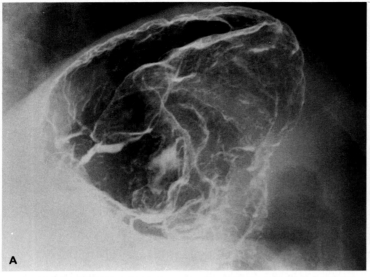

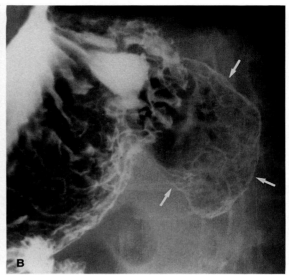

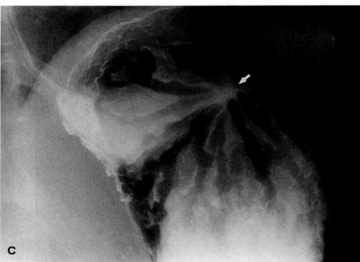

Fig. 14-40. Lymphoma healing to benign-appearing ulcer scar. **(A)** Large lobulated mass involves the gastric fundus along the greater curvature. **(B)** Forty days after completion of chemotherapy, there is a large extraluminal collection of barium and air **(arrows)** that represents excavation of the lymphomatous lesion in the gastric fundus. **(C)** One month later, the excavation has healed, leaving prominent folds radiating to a benign-appearing ulcer scar **(arrow)**. (Fox ER, Laufer I, Levine MS: Response of gastric lymphoma to chemotherapy: Radiographic appearance. AJR 142:711–714, 1984. Copyright 1984. Reproduced with permission.)

grow their blood supply, are most commonly seen in patients with malignant melanoma (Fig. 14-42). A similar appearance can be due to metastases from carcinoma of the breast (Fig. 14-43) or lung. Breast cancer can also produce radiographic changes resembling small or even large ulcer craters (pseudoulcerations) that are apparently due to redundancy of the mucosa associated with marked submucosal infiltration by tumor cells. Direct extension of metastases from adjacent organs can result in malignant gastric ulcerations (Fig. 14-44).

CARCINOID TUMOR

Gastrointestinal carcinoid tumors develop from the Kulchitsky cells found in the crypts of Lieberkuhn. These cells originate in the precursor neuroectodermal cells which have migrated from the neural crest during the developmental process. Although carcinoid tumors rarely occur in the stomach, they often

are ulcerated (see Fig. 18-22). Solitary intramural tumors develop ulcerations due to compression with thinning and ischemia of the overlying mucosa, tumor infiltration with necrotic changes, and associated hyperacidity due to the histamine production. An unusual radiographic presentation is a large penetrating gastric ulcer accompanied by a thick and irregular ulcer mound suggesting underlying malignancy (Fig. 14-45). Although gastric carcinoid tumors metastasize in up to one-third of cases, the lesions typically grow slowly and long survivals are seen even in the presence of regional or hepatic dissemination.

MARGINAL ULCERATION

Marginal ulceration is a postoperative complication of gastric surgery performed for the treatment of peptic ulcer disease (Fig. 14-46). The marginal ulcer

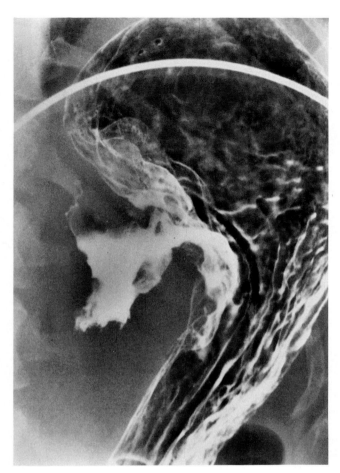

Fig. 14-41. Leiomyosarcoma. Submucosal mass on the lesser curvature with a large and irregular ulceration. (Nauert EC, Zornoza J, Ordonez N: Gastric leiomyosarcomas. AJR 139:291–297, 1982)

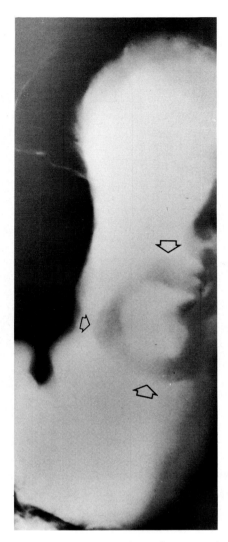

Fig. 14-43. Ulcerated metastasis to the stomach **(arrows)** from carcinoma of the breast.

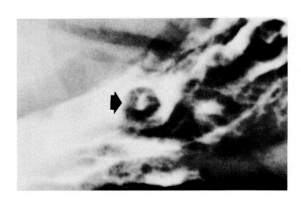

Fig. 14-42. Melanoma metastatic to the stomach **(arrow)** producing a bull's-eye pattern.

is not a recurrent one but represents a new ulceration that is usually situated in the jejunum within the first few centimeters of the anastomosis (Fig. 14-47). Marginal ulcers are rarely found on the gastric side of the anastomosis; indeed, development of postoperative ulceration at this site should suggest the possibility of gastric stump malignancy.

Although marginal ulcers can develop within a few weeks of surgery, most become symptomatic only within 2 to 4 years of partial gastrectomy. Bleeding is the most common presenting symptom. Typical ulcer pain is frequent, though often situated slightly more to the left than the original ulcer pain.

The likelihood of a person developing a postoperative marginal ulcer depends on several factors. In almost all cases, the site of the original ulcer for which surgery was performed is the duodenum. Marginal ulcers are much less frequent following surgery for gastric ulcers. The combination of vagotomy and hemigastrectomy (removal of essen-

Text continues on page 200

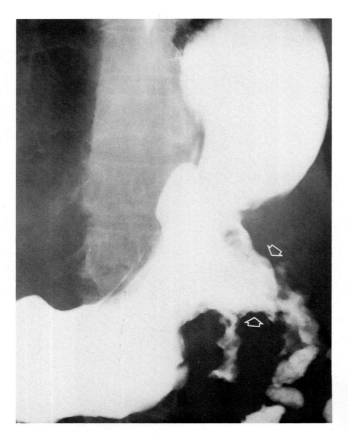

Fig. 14-44. Huge malignant ulcer **(arrows)** on the greater curvature representing direct invasion by carcinoma of the pancreas.

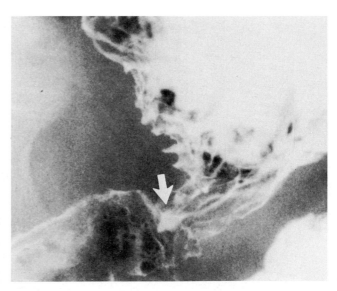

Fig. 14-46. Marginal ulceration **(arrow)** following Billroth-I anastomosis.

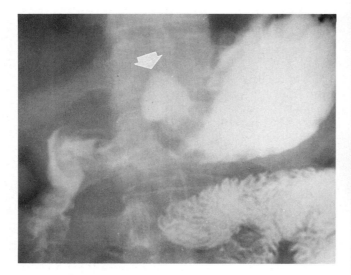

Fig. 14-45. Carcinoid tumor. Large penetrating gastric ulcer **(arrow)** on the lesser curvature of the stomach with an associated adjacent mass. (Balthazar EJ, Megibow A, Bryk D et al: Gastric carcinoid tumors: Radiographic features in eight cases. AJR 139:1123–1127, 1982. Copyright 1982. Reproduced with permission.)

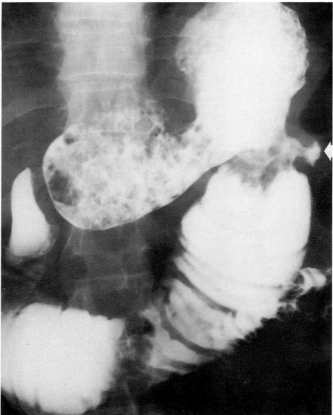

Fig. 14-47. Marginal ulceration **(arrow)** following gastrojejunostomy. The ulcer appears in the jejunum within the first few centimeters of the anastomosis.

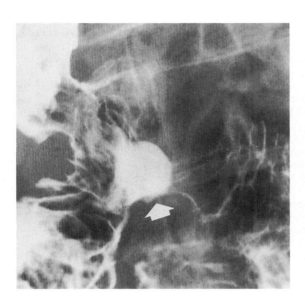

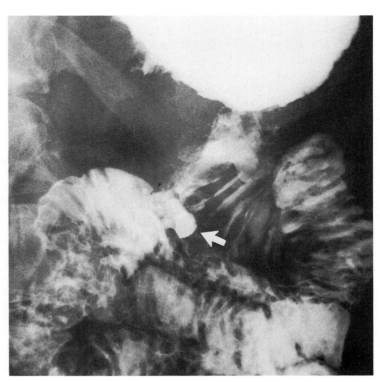

14-48

14-49

Fig. 14-48. Deep marginal ulcer **(arrow)** following Billroth-II anastomosis.

Fig. 14-49. Marginal ulcer with conical configuration **(arrow)** following Billroth-II anastomosis.

Fig. 14-50. Marginal ulcer **(arrow)** following Billroth-II anastomosis. Marked edema of jejunal folds at the anastomotic site suggests recurrent ulcer disease. There is also narrowing of the stoma with relative separation of the jejunal and gastric segments.

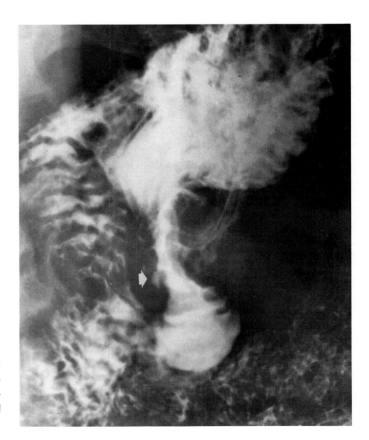

tially all of the acid-producing cells of the gastric antrum) is associated with the lowest rate of marginal ulceration, about 2%, far less than the 6% to 8% recurrence rate after vagotomy and drainage procedure alone.

Up to half of marginal ulcers are not detected radiographically. Frequently, these ulcerations are too superficial or shallow to be demonstrated. Overlapping jejunal mucosal folds can hide an ulcer; conversely, barium trapped between converging gastric or jejunal folds about the anastomotic site can simulate an ulcer niche. At times, it is difficult to distinguish an acute ulcer from postsurgical deformity at the anastomotic site.

Anastomotic ulcers often penetrate deeply (Fig. 14-48) and have a tent-shaped or conical configuration (Fig. 14-49). Enlargement of such an ulcer can cause penetration into adjacent structures. Secondary signs of marginal ulceration suggest the proper diagnosis in up to 80% of cases. These signs include edema of the duodenal or jejunal folds at the anastomotic site (Fig. 14-50), and flattening and rigidity of the jejunum adjacent to the ulcer. Narrowing and thickening of the stoma with edema surrounding the anastomotic site can efface the adjacent jejunum and produce wide separation of jejunal and gastric segments. As with all complications of surgery for peptic disease, a baseline postoperative study is essential for discrimination of narrowing of the lumen or effacement of the mucosal pattern near the anastomosis due to the spasm or edema of ulcer disease from a similar appearance produced by distortion caused by operative manipulation.

BIBLIOGRAPHY

Balthazar EJ, Megibow A, Bryk D et al: Gastric carcinoid tumors: Radiographic features in eight cases. AJR 139:1123–1127, 1982

Bloch C: Roentgen features of Hodgkin's disease of the stomach. AJR 99:175–181, 1967

Bonfield RE, Martel W: The problem of differentiating benign antral ulcers from intramural tumors. Radiology 106:25–27, 1973

Carman RD: A new roentgen-ray sign of ulcerating gastric cancer. JAMA 77:990–1002, 1921

Chiles JT, Platz CE: The radiographic manifestations of pseudolymphoma of the stomach. Radiology 116:551–556, 1975

Cockrell CH, Cho SR, Messmer JM et al: Intramural gastric diverticulum: A report of three cases. Br J Radiol 57:285–288, 1984

Eisenberg RJ, Hedgcock MW: The ellipse sign: An aid in the diagnosis of acute ulcers. J Can Assoc Radiol 30:26–29, 1979

Fox ER, Laufer I, Levine MS et al: Response of gastric lymphoma to chemotherapy: Radiographic appearance. AJR 142:711–714, 1984

Gelfand DW, Ott DJ: Gastric ulcer scars. Radiology 140:37–43, 1981

Goldstein HM, Rogers LF, Fletcher GH et al: Radiological manifestations of radiation-induced injury to the normal upper gastrointestinal tract. Radiology 117:135–140, 1975

Han SY, Witten DM: Benign gastric ulcer with "crescent" (quarter moon) sign. Radiology 113:573–575, 1974

Joffe N: Metastatic involvement of the stomach secondary to breast carcinoma. AJR 123:512–521, 1975

Kagan AR, Steckel RJ: Gastric ulcer in a young man with apparent healing. AJR 128:831–834, 1977

Levine MS, Creteur V, Kressel HY et al: Benign gastric ulcers: Diagnosis and follow-up with double-contrast radiography. Radiology 164:9–13, 1987

Mann FA, Kubal WS, Ruzicka FF et al: Radiographic manifestations of gastrointestinal toxicity associated with intraarterial 5-fluorouracil infusion. RadioGraphics 2:329–339, 1982

Megibow AJ, Balthazar EJ, Hulnick DH: Radiology of nonneoplastic gastrointestinal disorders in acquired immune deficiency syndrome. Semin Roentgenol 22:31–41, 1987

Nauert TC, Zornoza J, Ordonez N: Gastric leiomyosarcomas. AJR 139:291–297, 1982

Nelson SW: The discovery of gastric ulcers and the differential diagnosis between benignancy and malignancy. Radiol Clin North Am 7:5–25, 1969

Nunes JR, vanSonnenberg E, Pressman JH et al: Suture line ulceration: A complication of gastric partitioning. Gastrointest Radiol 9:315–317, 1984

Orr RK, Lininger JR, Lawrence W: Gastric pseudolymphoma: A challenging clinical problem. Ann Surg 200:185–194, 1984

Perez CA, Dorfman RF: Benign lymphoid hyperplasia of the stomach and duodenum. Radiology 87:505–510, 1966

Rogers LF, Goldstein HM: Roentgen manifestations of radiation injury to the gastrointestinal tract. Gastrointest Radiol 2:281–291, 1977

Rubin SA, Davis M: "Bull's eye" or "target" lesions of the stomach secondary to carcinoma of the lung. Am J Gastroenterol 80:67–69, 1985

Sato T, Sakai Y, Ishiguro S et al: Radiologic manifestations of early gastric lymphoma. AJR 146:513–517, 1986

Schirmer BD, Jones RS: Peptic ulcer disease. Invest Radiol 22:437–446, 1987

Sherrick DW, Hodgson JR, Dockerty MB: The roentgenologic diagnosis of primary gastric lymphoma. Radiology 84:925–932, 1965

Taxin, RN, Livingston PA, Seaman WB: Multiple gastric ulcers: A radiographic sign of benignancy? Radiology 114:23–27, 1975

Thompson G, Somers S, Stevenson GW: Benign gastric ulcer: A reliable radiologic diagnosis? AJR 141:331–333, 1983

Wolf BS: Observations on roentgen features of benign and malignant gastric ulcers. Semin Roentgen 6:140–150, 1971

Zboralske FF, Stargardter FL, Harell GS: Profile roentgenographic features of benign greater curvature ulcers. Radiology 127:63–67, 1978

SUPERFICIAL GASTRIC EROSIONS

Disease Entities

Alcohol
Anti-inflammatory agents (*e.g.*, aspirin, steroids)
Analgesics
Crohn's disease
Herpetic gastritis
Syphilitic gastritis
Cytomegalovirus gastritis
Candidiasis
Idiopathic

Superficial gastric erosions are defects in the epithelium of the stomach that do not penetrate beyond the muscularis mucosae (Fig. 15-1). Because they are very small and shallow, superficial gastric erosions have rarely been demonstrated on conventional upper gastrointestinal series. With the increasing use of air-contrast techniques, however, more than half of the superficial gastric erosions noted endoscopically can also be demonstrated radiographically.

CLINICAL SYMPTOMS

About 10% to 20% of patients with superficial gastric erosions present with gastrointestinal hemorrhage. These patients should undergo endoscopy as the primary diagnostic procedure, since the pres-

ence of large amounts of blood in the stomach precludes good mucosal coating and a satisfactory double-contrast study. Once bleeding has subsided, however, a double-contrast examination may reveal the erosions or an adherent blood clot.

If they do not have gastrointestinal bleeding, associated ulcers, or tumors, most patients with superficial gastric erosions complain of dyspepsia or epigastric pain often indistinguishable from peptic ulcer disease. The relationship of the erosions to the patient's symptoms is unclear.

RADIOGRAPHIC FINDINGS

The classic radiographic appearance of a superficial gastric erosion is a tiny fleck of barium, which represents the erosion, surrounded by a radiolucent halo, which represents a mound of edematous mucosa (Fig. 15-2). The resultant target lesions are usually multiple, though a solitary erosion is occasionally demonstrated. The number of erosions is usually underestimated on radiographic examination, probably because of difficulty in performing a double-contrast study of the anterior wall of the stomach. Superficial gastric erosions can also appear as flat epithelial defects without surrounding reaction that coat with barium and are represented by reproducible linear streaks or dots of contrast. These incomplete erosions, which are thought to be strongly suggestive of gastritis induced by aspirin or other nonsteroidal anti-inflammatory drugs (NSAIDs), are rarely aligned on rugal folds and are

Text continues on page 204

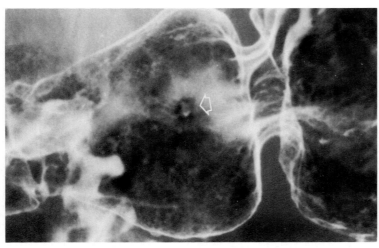

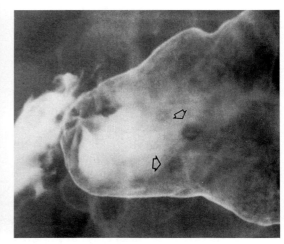

15-1

15-2

Fig. 15-1. Superficial gastric erosions in a patient with gastritis. The collection of barium represents a shallow erosion surrounded by a radiolucent halo **(arrow)**.

Fig. 15-2. Superficial gastric erosions. Radiolucent halos of edema surround the small, barium-filled erosions.

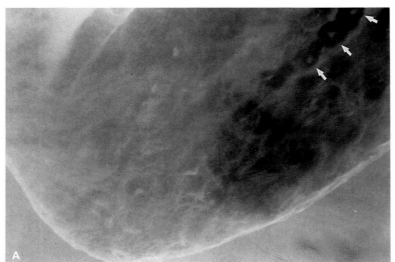

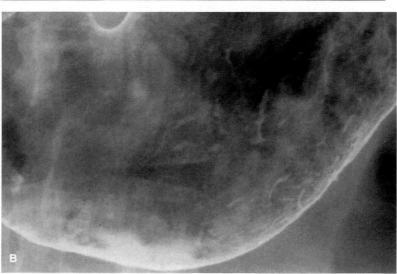

Fig. 15-3. Superficial gastric erosions due to **(A)** aspirin and **(B)** indomethacin. The incomplete linear and serpiginous erosions are predominantly located near the greater curvature. In **A,** typical superficial gastric erosions can also be seen more proximally in the stomach, aligned on rugal folds **(arrows)**. (Levine MS, Verstandig A, Laufer I: Serpiginous gastric erosions caused by aspirin and other nonsteroidal anti-inflammatory drugs. AJR 146:31–34, 1986. Copyright 1986. Reproduced with permission.)

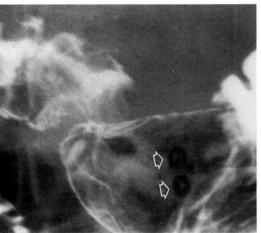

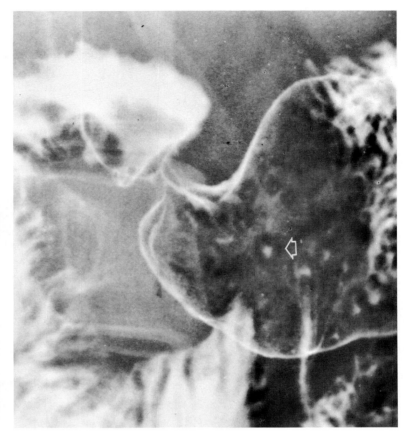

15-4   **15-5**

Fig. 15-4. Aphthoid ulcerations **(arrows)** due to acute alcohol abuse.

Fig. 15-5. Aphthoid ulcer in Crohn's disease **(arrow)**. The radiographic appearance is indistinguishable from that of other types of superficial gastric erosions.

Fig. 15-6. Aphthoid ulcerations in gastric candidiasis. Coned view demonstrates numerous aphthoid ulcers **(arrowheads)**. The black ring represents the slightly raised, inflammatory edge surrounding the shallow, barium-filled depression. (Cronan J, Burrell M, Trepeta R: Aphthoid ulcerations in gastric candidiasis. Radiology 134:607–611, 1980)

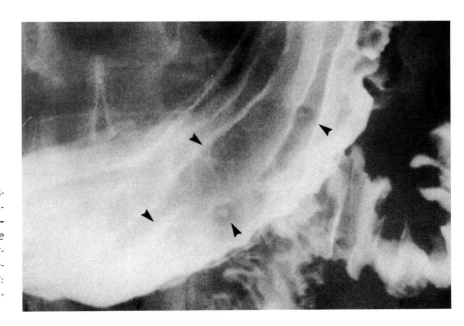

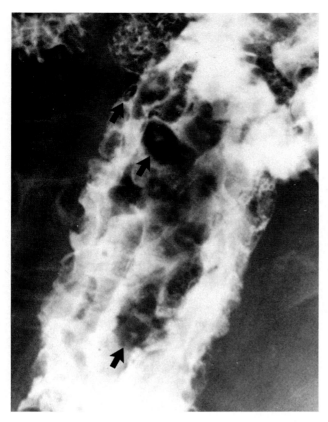

Fig. 15-7. Lymphoma. Thickened nodular gastric folds **(arrows)** with tiny stellate ulcers. (Scholz FJ: Gastritis. In Taveras JM, Ferrucci JT (eds): Radiology: Diagnosis, Imaging, Intervention. Philadelphia, JB Lippincott, 1987)

more difficult to demonstrate radiographically since the surrounding mucosa is normal (Fig. 15-3). Aspirin- and NSAID-induced ulcers are often located on the greater curvature of the body or antrum of the stomach. It has been postulated that these ulcers result from localized mucosal injury as the dissolving tablets collect by gravity in the most dependent part of the stomach.

ETIOLOGY

In about half the patients, superficial gastric erosions have no known predisposing cause. Specific etiologic factors include alcohol (Fig. 15-4), anti-inflammatory agents (aspirin, steroids, phenylbutazone, indomethacin), analgesics, and emotional stress. Aphthoid ulcers in the stomach in patients with Crohn's disease are indistinguishable radiographically from superficial gastric erosions (Fig. 15-5) and are similar to the erosions seen in the colon in the early stages of Crohn's disease. They probably represent early, asymptomatic Crohn's disease in the stomach, which can progress to deeper ulcers, scarring, and stenosis. Biopsies of the aphthoid gastric ulcers of Crohn's disease reveal them to be noncaseating granulomas, unlike mucosal biopsies of superficial gastric erosions which usually show only a nonspecific chronic inflammatory reaction. Similar aphthoid erosions have been described in herpetic, syphilitic, and cytomegalovirus gastritis and as the earliest radiographically detectable changes in patients with gastric candidiasis, (Fig. 15-6). Lymphoma may mimic erosive gastritis with tiny ulcerations in nodular folds (Fig. 15-7).

BIBLIOGRAPHY

Ariyama J, Wehlin L, Lindstrom CG et al: Gastroduodenal erosions in Crohn's disease. Gastrointest Radiol 5:121–125, 1980

Cronan J, Burrell M, Trepata R: Aphthoid ulcerations in gastric candidiasis. Radiology 134:607–611, 1980

Gallagher CG, Lennon JR, Crowe JP: Chronic erosive gastritis: A clinical study. Am J Gastroenterol 82:302–306, 1987

Laufer I, Costopoulos L: Early lesions of Crohn's disease. AJR 130:307–311, 1978

Laufer I, Hamilton J, Mullens JE: Demonstration of superficial gastric erosions by double contrast radiography. Gastroenterology 68:387–391, 1975

Levine MS, Verstandig A, Laufer I: Serpiginous gastric erosions caused by aspirin and other nonsteroidal antiinflammatory drugs. AJR 146:31–34, 1986

McLean AM, Paul RE, Philipps E et al: Chronic erosive gastritis: Clinical and radiological features. J Can Assoc Radiol 33:158–162, 1982

Poplack W, Paul RE, Goldsmith M et al: Demonstration of erosive gastritis by the double-contrast technique. Radiology 117:519–521, 1975

Sperling HV, Reed WG: Herpetic gastritis. Am J Dig Dis 22:1033–1034, 1977

NARROWING OF THE STOMACH (LINITIS PLASTICA PATTERN)

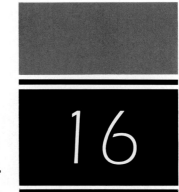

Disease Entities

Malignant neoplasms
  Carcinoma
  Lymphoma (Hodgkin's disease)
  Metastases
    Direct extension from carcinoma of the pancreas and transverse colon
    Omental cakes
    Hematogenous metastases (*e.g.,* carcinoma of the breast)
Gastric ulcer disease
Granulomatous infiltration
  Crohn's disease
  Sarcoidosis
  Syphilis
  Tuberculosis
  Histoplasmosis
  Actinomycosis
Eosinophilic gastritis
Polyarteritis nodosa
Other gastritis
  Infections
    Phlegmonous gastritis
    Strongyloidiasis
    Cytomegalovirus
  Corrosive agents
  Gastric irradiation
  Gastric freezing
  Iron intoxication
  Hepatic arterial infusion chemotherapy
  Stenosing antral gastritis
Amyloidosis
Pseudolymphoma
Intramural gastric hematoma
Extrinsic masses impressing stomach
Gastric restrictive surgery for morbid obesity
Perigastric adhesions

CARCINOMA

Linitis plastica (leather bottle stomach) refers to any condition in which marked thickening of the gastric wall causes the stomach to appear as a narrowed, rigid tube. By far the most common cause of this radiographic pattern is scirrhous carcinoma of the stomach (Fig. 16-1). Tumor invasion of the gastric wall stimulates a desmoplastic response, which produces diffuse thickening and fixation of the stomach wall (Fig. 16-2). The involved stomach is contracted into a tubular structure without normal pliability. At fluoroscopy, peristalsis does not pass through the tumor site. Extension of tumor growth into the mucosa can produce nodular or irregular mucosal folds. Although scirrhous carcinoma can arise anywhere in the stomach, it usually begins near the pylorus and progresses slowly upward, the fundus being the area least involved (Fig. 16-3). The infiltration does not end abruptly but merges gradually into normal tissue. The duodenal bulb is often

Text continues on page 209

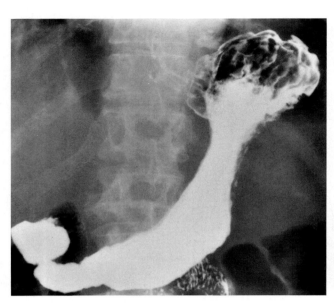

16-1

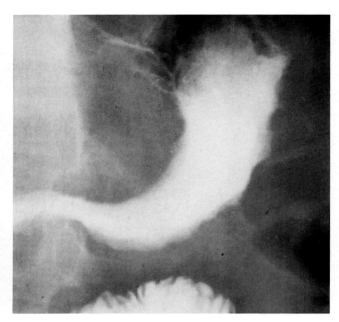

16-2

Fig. 16-1. Scirrhous carcinoma of the stomach.

Fig. 16-2. Scirrhous carcinoma of the stomach. An intense desmoplastic reaction causes nodular thickening and fixation of the gastric wall.

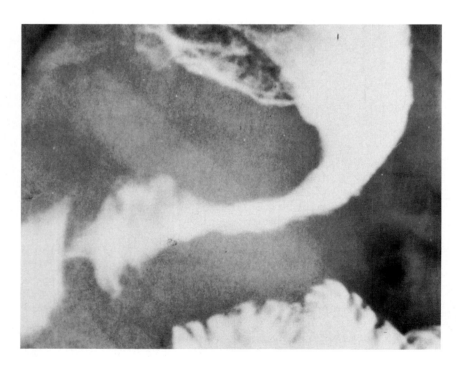

Fig. 16-3. Scirrhous carcinoma of the stomach. Generalized luminal narrowing tends to spare the fundus.

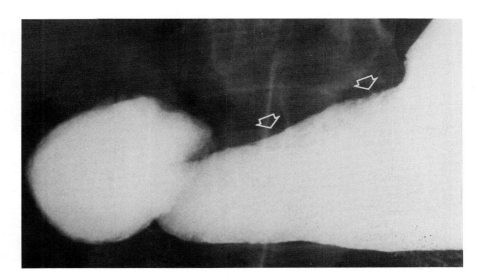

Fig. 16-4. Early adenocarcinoma of the stomach. A plaquelike lesion infiltrates the lesser curvature of the antrum **(arrows)**.

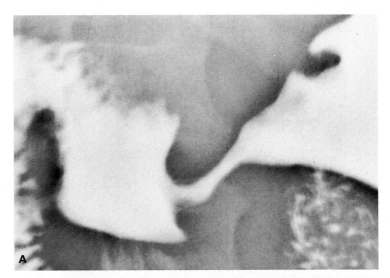

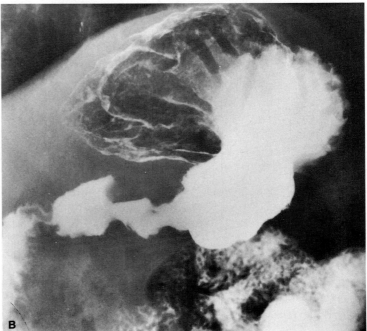

Fig. 16-5. Two patients with constricting adenocarcinomas of the antrum of the stomach.

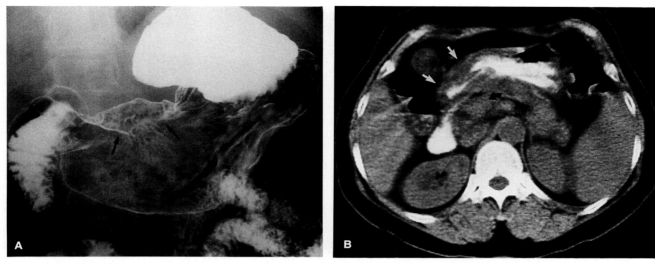

Fig. 16-6. CT staging of gastric carcinoma. **(A)** Double-contrast study demonstrates a large lesser curvature mass **(arrows)**. **(B)** CT scan shows narrowing of the antrum by the gastric carcinoma **(white arrows)** and adjacent nodal metastases **(curved arrow)**. (Eisenberg RL: Diagnostic Imaging in Surgery. New York, McGraw–Hill, 1987)

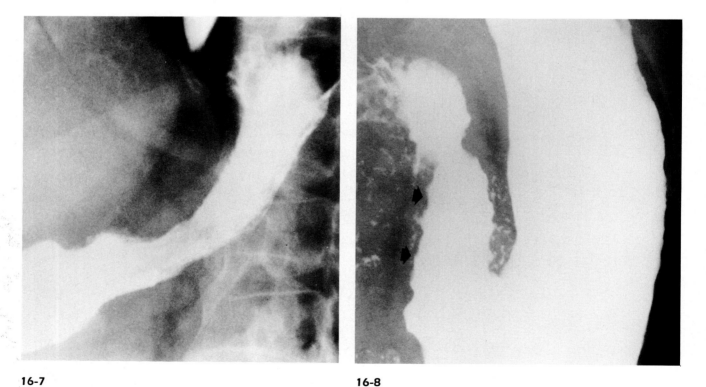

16-7   16-8

Fig. 16-7. Gastric lymphoma. A severe desmoplastic reaction produces a radiographic pattern that mimics scirrhous carcinoma.

Fig. 16-8. Gastric lymphoma. Infiltrative Hodgkin's disease causes irregular narrowing of the distal antrum **(arrows)**.

dilated and tends to remain filled because of rapid emptying of the rigid, pipelike stomach.

Another major manifestation of gastric carcinoma is narrowing of a segment of the stomach. At an early stage, gastric malignancy can appear as a plaquelike infiltrative lesion along one curvature (Fig. 16-4). Advanced carcinoma can encircle a segment of stomach and cause a constricting lesion similar to that produced by annular carcinoma of the colon (Fig. 16-5).

Computed tomography (CT) is the imaging modality of choice for preoperative staging and treatment planning of gastric carcinoma as well as for assessing the response to therapy and detecting recurrence. Carcinoma of the stomach may appear as concentric (Fig. 16-6A) or focal (Fig. 16-6B) thickening of the gastric wall or as an intraluminal mass. Obliteration of the perigastric fat planes is a reliable indicator of the extragastric spread of tumor. Computed tomography can demonstrate direct tumor extension to intra-abdominal organs and distant metastases to lymph nodes (Fig. 16-6B), liver, ovary, adrenals, kidneys, and peritoneum.

LYMPHOMA

Invasion of the gastric wall by an infiltrative type of lymphoma (especially the Hodgkin's type) can cause a severe desmoplastic reaction and a radiographic appearance that mimics scirrhous carcinoma (Fig. 16-7). Thickening of the gastric wall narrows the lumen, especially in the antral region (Fig. 16-8). The overlying mucosal pattern is often effaced and indistinct, though without discrete ulceration. Unlike the rigidity and fixation of scirrhous carcinoma, residual peristalsis and flexibility of the stomach wall are often preserved in Hodgkin's disease.

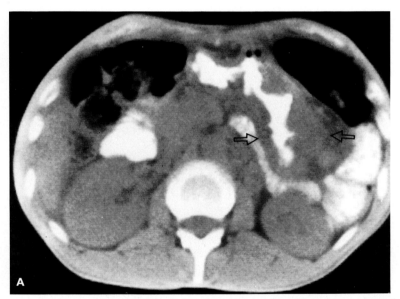

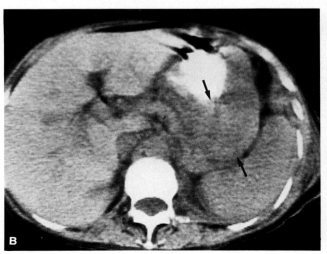

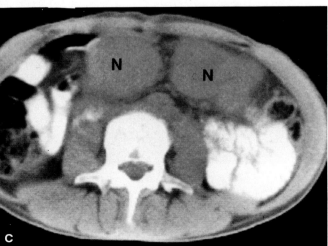

Fig. 16-9. Lymphoma of the stomach. **(A)** CT scan shows a circumferential intramural mass **(arrows)** causing gross distortion of the contrast-filled gastric lumen. **(B)** Focal masslike thickening of the gastric wall **(arrows)**. **(C)** The presence of large mesenteric **(N)** and periaortic nodes suggests the correct histologic diagnosis. (A & C, from Mauro MA, Koehler RE: Alimentary tract. In Lee JKT, Sagel SS, Stanley RJ (eds): Computed Body Tomography. New York, Raven, 1983)

On CT scanning, gastric lymphoma tends to produce bulky masses and a lobulated inner contour of the gastric wall representing thickened gastric rugae. However, gastric lymphoma may also produce smooth, concentric wall thickening or a focal mass simulating adenocarcinoma of the stomach (Fig. 16-9). The demonstration of other signs of lymphoma (splenomegaly, diffuse retroperitoneal and mesenteric lymphadenopathy), when present, suggests the correct histologic diagnosis.

METASTATIC LESIONS

Carcinoma of the pancreas is the major extragastric malignancy that produces a linitis plastica pattern. Circumferential narrowing of the stomach due to direct extension of tumor (Fig. 16-10) or metastases to perigastric nodes (Fig. 16-11) can result in an appearance indistinguishable from primary gastric carcinoma. A similar pattern can be caused by carcinoma of the transverse colon spreading to the stomach by way of the gastrocolic ligament, or by omental "cakes," bulky metastases to the greater omentum that most often result from widespread intraperitoneal seeding of pelvic or gastrointestinal malignancies (Fig. 16-12). Hematogenous metastases, primarily from poorly differentiated carcinoma of the breast, can diffusely infiltrate the wall of the stomach with highly cellular deposits and produce a linitis plastica appearance (Fig. 16-13). The changes may involve the entire stomach or be more limited. At an early stage, the mucosa is often intact; a spiculated or nodular mucosal pattern can develop. Because the linitis plastica pattern in patients with metastatic lesions rarely occurs in the absence of far-advanced carcinoma with multiple sites of metastatic disease, the proper diagnosis is usually evident.

BENIGN CAUSES

GASTRIC ULCER DISEASE

Although the contracted, rigid pattern of linitis plastica of the stomach is almost always the result of malignant disease, benign processes can produce a radiographically indistinguishable appearance. Antral narrowing and rigidity can be caused by the

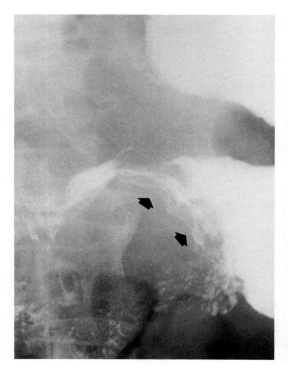

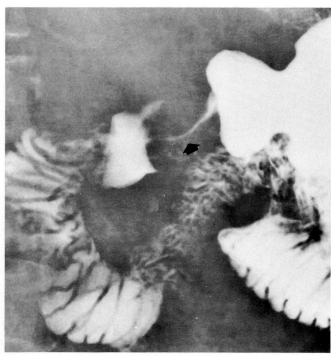

16-10

16-11

Fig. 16-10. Direct extension of carcinoma of the pancreas causing severe narrowing of the distal antrum **(arrows)**.

Fig. 16-11. Circumferential narrowing of the distal stomach **(arrow)** secondary to pancreatic carcinoma metastatic to perigastric lymph nodes.

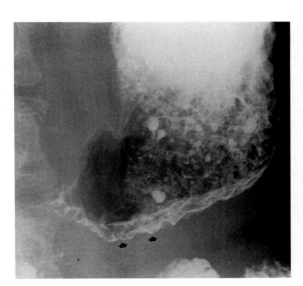

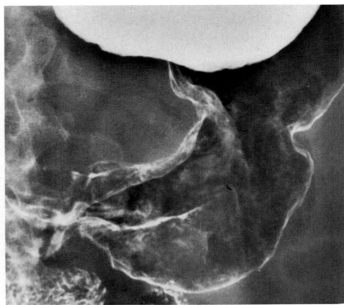

16-12 **16-13**

Fig. 16-12. Omental ''cakes.'' Flattening and nodularity of the greater curvature of the stomach **(arrows)** with circumferential narrowing of the antrum is due to encasement by omental metastases from ovarian carcinoma. (Rubesin SE, Levine MS, Glick SN: Gastric involvement by omental cakes: Radiographic findings. Gastrointest Radiol 11:223–228, 1986)

Fig. 16-13. Scirrhous metastatic carcinoma of the breast infiltrating the wall of the stomach and narrowing the gastric lumen.

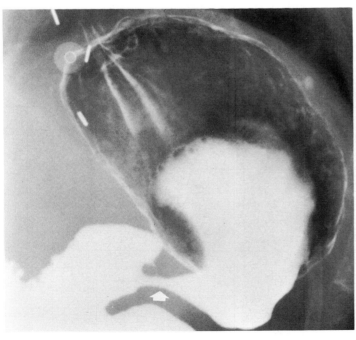

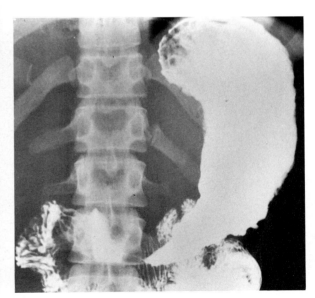

16-14 **16-15**

Fig. 16-14. Peptic ulcer disease causing antral narrowing and rigidity **(arrow)**. Note the vagotomy clips.

Fig. 16-15. Crohn's disease. Smooth, tubular narrowing of the antrum producing the ''ram's horn'' sign. (Farman J, Faegenburg D, Dalemand S et al: Crohn's disease of the stomach: The ''ram's horn'' sign. AJR 123:242–251, 1975. Copyright 1975. Reproduced with permission)

intense spasm associated with a distal gastric ulcer (Fig. 16-14). Indeed, the ulcer sometimes cannot even be seen because of the lack of antral distensibility. In contrast to the linitis plastica pattern produced by malignant lesions, peptic-induced rigidity should not persist in the case of benign ulcers, most of which heal with adequate antacid therapy. An unusual cause of narrowing of a short segment of the stomach is the "geriatric" ulcer. Whereas gastric ulcers in young patients are relatively infre-

quent in the proximal half of the stomach, ulcers in elderly patients are particularly prone to arise high on the posterior wall of the stomach. As fibrous healing progresses, a typical "hourglass" deformity may result.

CROHN'S DISEASE

Crohn's disease involving the stomach can result in a smooth, tubular antrum that is poorly distensible

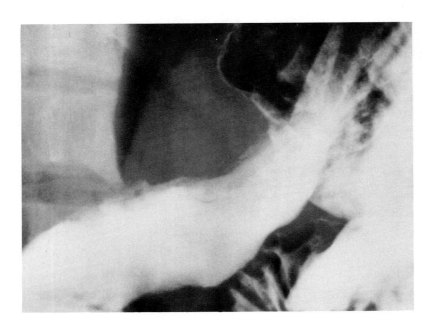

Fig. 16-16. Crohn's disease. Diffuse narrowing of the antrum, duodenal bulb, and proximal sweep simulates the radiographic appearance of a partial gastrectomy and Billroth-I anastomosis (pseudo-Billroth-I pattern).

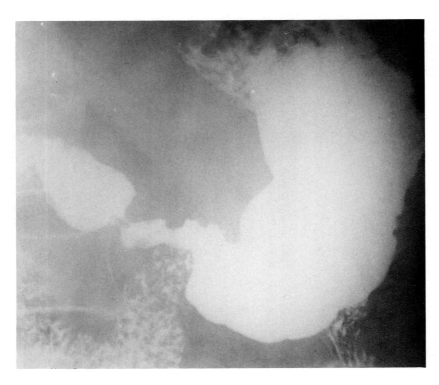

Fig. 16-17. Sarcoidosis. There is irregular narrowing of the distal antrum.

and exhibits sluggish peristalsis. The narrowed antrum flares out into a normal gastric body and fundus, giving the appearance of a ram's horn (Fig. 16-15). Because the adjacent duodenal bulb and proximal sweep are almost always also involved, the diffuse narrowing can mimic the radiographic appearance in a patient who has undergone partial gastrectomy and Billroth-I anastomosis (pseudo-Billroth-I pattern) (Fig. 16-16). In addition to antral narrowing, there can be cobblestoning of antral folds with fissures and ulceration. Gastric outlet obstruction is not uncommon. The diagnosis of Crohn's disease causing the linitis plastica pattern can be made with confidence only if characteristic signs of coexistent extragastric disease can be detected in the small or large bowel.

SARCOIDOSIS

About 10% of patients with sarcoidosis have evidence of stomach involvement on gastroscopic biopsy. Although most of these patients are asymptomatic, some have a clinical picture of epigastric pain, weight loss, and gastric hypochlorhydria that closely simulates carcinoma of the stomach. Localized sarcoid granulomas can produce discrete mass defects. Diffuse lesions cause severe mural thickening and luminal narrowing, predominantly in the antrum, which mimic Crohn's disease and the radiographic pattern of linitis plastica (Fig. 16-17). Ulcerations or erosions can lead to acute upper gastrointestinal hemorrhage.

SYPHILIS

Tertiary syphilis involving the stomach is now an exceedingly rare disease. Although discrete, nodular, gummalike lesions can occur, diffuse involvement of the stomach is more common. Swelling and thickening of the gastric wall can result in mural rigidity and narrowing of the lumen indistinguishable from scirrhous carcinoma. As with most infiltrative granulomatous diseases of the stomach, syphilis has a predilection for involving the antrum. Narrowing of the lumen produces a tubular deformity or funnel-shaped defect in which the apex of the funnel is at or near the pylorus (Fig. 16-18). The defect is often concentric, symmetric, and smooth,

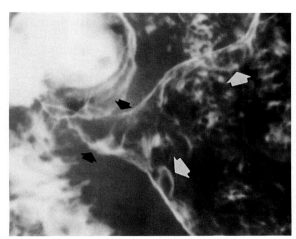

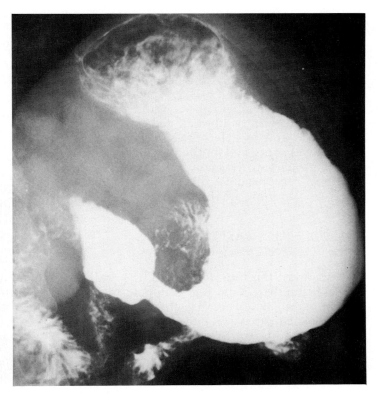

16-18   **16-19**

Fig. 16-18. Syphilis of the stomach. Diffuse thickening of the gastric wall results in narrowing of the antrum **(black arrows)** and scattered gummatous polyps **(white arrows)**. (Eisenberg RL: Diagnostic Imaging in Internal Medicine, New York, McGraw–Hill, 1986)

Fig. 16-19. Tuberculosis of the stomach. Fibrotic healing produces narrowing and rigidity of the distal antrum.

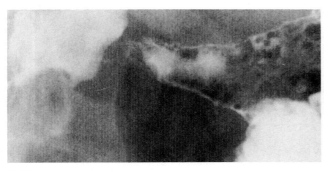
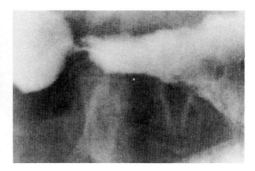

16-20   **16-21**

Fig. 16-20. *Eosinophilic gastritis. Diffuse infiltration of predominantly mature eosinophils thickens the muscular layer and narrows the lumen of the stomach.*

Fig. 16-21. *Polyarteritis nodosa. Moderately irregular narrowing of the antrum is due to ischemia and inflammation.*

though large, shallow antral ulcerations can occur. Severe involvement of the midportion of the stomach can produce an hourglass pattern of narrowing.

TUBERCULOSIS

Primary tuberculosis of the stomach is unusual; involvement of the stomach secondary to tuberculosis elsewhere is exceedingly rare. The most common symptoms are ulcerlike epigastric distress, vomiting suggesting pyloric obstruction, loss of weight and strength, fever, and hemorrhage. Diffuse inflammation or fibrotic healing causes rigidity of the distal stomach and a linitis plastica pattern (Fig. 16-19). Ulcerations and fistulas between the antrum and small bowel can simulate the radiographic appearance of gastric involvement by Crohn's disease. In extremely rare instances, histoplasmosis and actinomycosis also infiltrate the wall of the stomach.

EOSINOPHILIC GASTRITIS AND POLYARTERITIS NODOSA

Thickening of the muscle layer of the wall of the stomach due to edema and a diffuse infiltrate of predominantly mature eosinophils can produce the linitis plastica pattern in persons with eosinophilic gastritis (Fig. 16-20). Extensive disease can irregularly narrow the distal antrum and cause some degree of gastric outlet obstruction. If the subserosal layer of the stomach is also involved, eosinophilic ascites or pleural effusion can occur. Although eosinophilic gastritis can simulate a more aggressive process, it is essentially a benign condition that is self-limited, and it often completely returns to normal after steroid therapy. In the patient with the linitis plastica pattern, associated peripheral eosinophilia and a history of abdominal distress following the ingestion of specific foods should suggest the diagnosis of eosinophilic gastritis, especially if there is also relatively long contiguous spread of disease into the small bowel (eosinophilic gastroenteritis).

A radiographic appearance identical to eosinophilic gastroenteritis may be due to polyarteritis nodosa (Fig. 16-21). In this condition, irregular narrowing of the antrum secondary to ischemia and inflammation can coexist with thickening of folds in the small bowel.

INFECTION

Phlegmonous gastritis is an extremely rare condition in which bacterial invasion causes thickening of the wall of the stomach associated with discolored mucosa and an edematous submucosa. Bacteria can be seen enmeshed in a fibrinopurulent exudate on histologic sections of the stomach wall. Most cases of phlegmonous gastritis are due to alpha-hemolytic streptococci, though pneumococci, staphylococci, *Escherichia coli*, and, rarely, *Proteus vulgaris* and *Clostridium welchii* can also be the causative organisms. Although the exact mechanism is unclear, infections of the gastric wall appear to arise from direct invasion of the gastric mucosa, hematogenous spread from a septic focus (*e.g.*, endocarditis), or lymphatic spread from a contiguous process (*e.g.*, cholecystitis). The duodenum and esophagus are usually spared.

Clinically, the patient with phlegmonous gastritis is usually a woman over the age of 40 who presents with symptoms of acute abdominal catastrophe (abrupt onset of midepigastric pain, nausea, and vomiting). Purulent emesis, an extremely rare occurrence, is pathognomonic of phlegmonous gastritis. Many patients with this condition have signs of peritoneal irritation (muscle guarding, rebound tenderness on palpation) as well as fever, chills, severe prostration, and hiccups (due to diaphragmatic irritation). The abdominal pain may disappear if the patient assumes a sitting position (Dienenger's sign), a finding that has been suggested as specific for diffuse phlegmonous gastritis. Immediate surgery with vigorous antimicrobial therapy has somewhat reduced the previous 100% mortality rate following medical treatment of the disease.

Phlegmonous gastritis usually causes diffuse thickening of the wall of the stomach with effaced mucosa and a linitis plastica pattern often indistinguishable from infiltrating carcinoma (Fig. 16-22). Radiographic differentiation between these two entities is possible only if bubbles of gas can be demonstrated in the wall of the stomach. This signifies the development of emphysematous gastritis, an extremely lethal form of bacterial invasion of the stomach wall.

In addition to bacteria, the parasite *Strongyloides stercoralis* can infest the wall of the stomach and duodenum. Nodular intramural defects secondary to granuloma formation can be identified during early stages of the disease. In advanced cases, severe inflammatory changes and diffuse fibrosis can cause mural rigidity and the linitis plastica pattern. At times, narrowing of the gastric outlet can be so advanced as to delay gastric emptying.

CYTOMEGALOVIRUS

In patients with AIDS, cytomegalovirus gastritis may produce a circumferentially narrowed antrum deformed by numerous large nodular contour defects (Fig. 16-23). Endoscopy reveals severe swelling of gastric rugae, usually with multiple superficial ulcerations. Narrowing and rigidity of the gastric antrum may also be due to cryptosporidiosis, a parasitic disease of the gastrointestinal tract that causes a cholera-like diarrhea in patients with AIDS (Fig. 16-24).

CORROSIVE AGENTS

The ingestion of corrosive agents, primarily concentrated acids, causes a coagulative necrosis of the stomach that has a predilection to involve the antrum. The acute inflammatory reaction heals by fibrosis and scarring, which results in stricturing of the antrum within several weeks of the initial injury (Fig. 16-25). In patients who have rigidity and narrowing of the stomach without a history of corrosive ingestion, the clinical symptoms of weight loss and early satiety, combined with the radiographic pat-

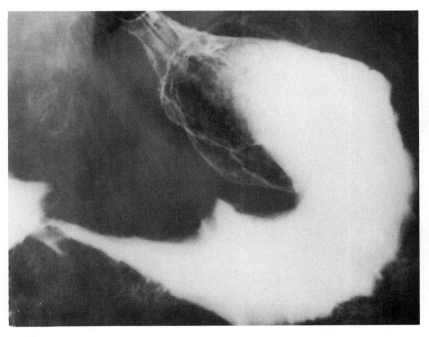

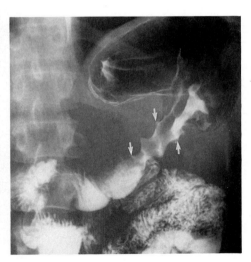

16-22

16-23

Fig. 16-22. Phlegmonous gastritis. There is irregular narrowing of the antrum and distal body of the stomach with effacement of mucosal folds along the lesser curvature and marked thickening of folds along the greater curvature. (Turner MA, Beachley MC, Stanley B: Phlegmonous gastritis. AJR 133:527–528, 1979. Copyright 1979. Reproduced with permission)

Fig. 16-23. Cytomegalovirus gastritis. Broad nodular contour defects associated with narrowing of the distal stomach and limited distensibility **(arrows)** in a patient with AIDS. (Balthazar EJ, Megibow AJ, Hulnick DH: Cytomegalovirus esophagitis and gastritis in AIDS. AJR 144:1201–1204, 1985. Copyright 1985. Reprinted with permission)

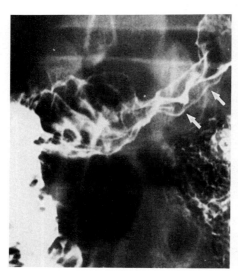

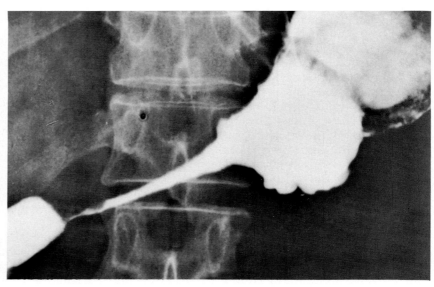

16-24   **16-25**

Fig. 16-24. Cryptosporidiosis gastritis. Contraction of the gastric antrum in a patient with AIDS. (Berk RN, Wall SD, McArdle CB et al: Cryptosporidiosis of the stomach and small intestine in patients with AIDS. AJR 143:549–554, 1984. Copyright 1984. Reproduced with permission)

Fig. 16-25. Corrosive stricture of the antrum following the ingestion of hydrochloric acid.

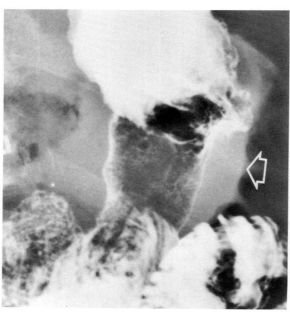

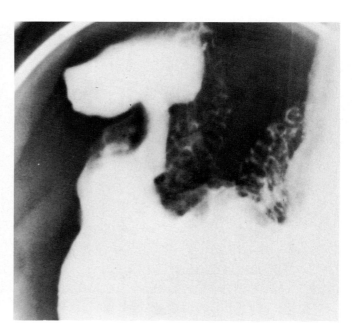

16-26   **16-27**

Fig. 16-26. Luminal narrowing and severe thickening of the wall of the stomach **(arrow)** following radiation therapy.

Fig. 16-27. Stricture of the antrum, which developed 1 year after the patient had received 5000 rads to the epigastrium. Note the irregular mucosal surface along the lesser curvature. (Rogers LF, Goldstein HM: Roentgen manifestations of radiation injury to the gastrointestinal tract. Gastrointest Radiol 2:281–291, 1977)

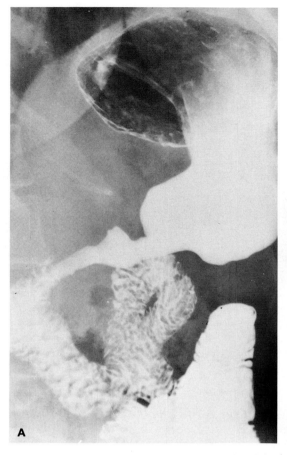

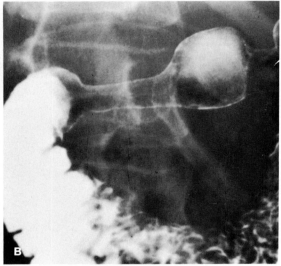

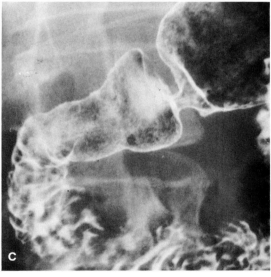

Fig. 16-28. Gastroduodenal changes during hepatic arterial infusion chemotherapy. **(A)** The distal stomach and duodenum are distorted and narrowed, with small ulcerations in the duodenum. **(B)** Distention is limited and mucosa effaced in the duodenal bulb during intra-arterial chemotherapy. **(C)** With a medical ulcer regimen and the cessation of chemotherapy, the duodenal mucosa and configuration approach normal. (Hall DA, Clouse ME, Gramm HF: Gastroduodenal ulceration after hepatic arterial infusion chemotherapy. AJR 136:1216–1218, 1981. Copyright 1981. Reproduced with permission)

tern of linitis plastica, can be impossible to distinguish from gastric malignancy.

GASTRIC IRRADIATION/FREEZING

Linitis plastica can be caused by thickening of the wall of the stomach secondary to gastritis due to physical agents. Radiation injury to the stomach can develop in patients who receive more than 4500

rads to the upper abdomen (Fig. 16-26). The relatively low incidence of this complication is not due to decreased radiosensitivity of the stomach compared to other parts of the bowel, but rather reflects the infrequency with which the stomach is included in the more common lower abdominal and pelvic treatment fields. Radiation injury to the stomach results in acute gastritis, with or without ulceration, followed by a reduction in the parietal cell population and hypochlorhydria or achlorhydria of several months' duration. This reduction in acid secretion was the rationale for the previous use of gastric irradiation in patients who were suffering from intractable peptic ulcer disease and in whom surgery was contraindicated. Healing of acute radiation injury by excessive fibrous scarring can produce varying degrees of fixed luminal narrowing and mural rigidity (Fig. 16-27).

Gastric freezing was formerly used to treat peptic ulcer disease, though the value of this technique has never been established. Gastric freezing causes hemorrhagic necrosis of the stomach mucosa, usually followed by rapid restoration of normal structure and function. Fibrotic changes during the healing phase occasionally cause mural thickening and persistent narrowing of the lumen of the stomach.

IRON INTOXICATION

The ingestion of ferrous sulfate can produce acute iron toxicity, with clinical symptoms of nausea, vomiting, bloody diarrhea, acidosis, shock, coma, and eventually death. This predominantly occurs in children, who are attracted by brightly colored iron-containing tablets. Iron has an intense corrosive action on the gastric mucosa, which becomes acutely congested and covered with thick layers of mucus. Superficial necrosis and petechial hemorrhages are common. If the child survives, stricture

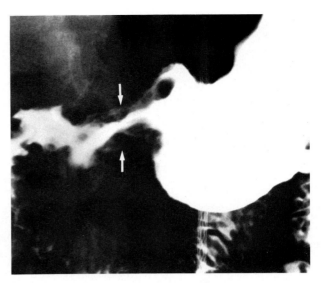

Fig. 16-30. Amyloidosis. Localized irregular circumferential infiltration of the antrum **(arrows)**. At surgery, the lesion was ulcerated and resembled infiltrating carcinoma. (Balthazar EJ: Miscellaneous disorders of the stomach. In Taveras JM, Ferrucci JT (eds): Radiology: Diagnosis—Imaging—Intervention. Philadelphia, JB Lippincott, 1987)

of the stomach, primarily the antrum, may develop within 10 days to 6 weeks of the ingestion of the iron tablets.

HEPATIC ARTERIAL INFUSION CHEMOTHERAPY

Narrowing and rigidity of the antrum and body of the stomach can be a complication of infusion of chemotherapeutic agents through a catheter in the hepatic artery (Fig. 16-28*A, B*). Far higher doses of these medications can be delivered to metastatic and primary hepatic tumors by direct arterial infusion than by the intravenous route. The complication of gastroduodenal ulceration and narrowing may be related to leakage of the chemotherapeutic agent directly into the blood supply of nonhepatic organs. The radiographic pattern tends to return to normal after chemotherapy is discontinued (Fig. 16-28*C*).

STENOSING ANTRAL GASTRITIS

The stenosing form of antral gastritis can cause narrowing of the distal stomach due to submucosal fibrosis resulting from the inflammatory process. Initially, the mucosal folds are prominent and fixed. With advanced disease, the folds can become obliterated, and the deformity is indistinguishable from infiltrating carcinoma. Damage to the intramural

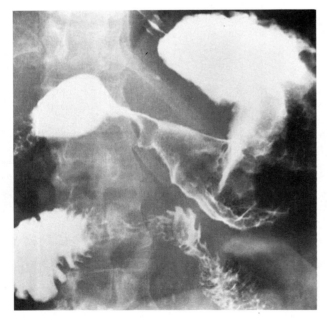

Fig. 16-29. Amyloidosis. Narrowing of the antrum with effacement of the mucosal pattern caused by submucosal deposits of amyloid. (Carlson HC, Breen JF: Amyloidosis and plasma cell dyscrasias. Gastrointestinal involvement. Semin Roentgenol 21:128–138, 1986)

neural plexus may further contribute to the reflex spasm. Although the term antral gastritis is generally used to describe this condition, involvement of the remainder of the stomach can usually be demonstrated at gastroscopy. The preponderance of antral involvement is probably related to the comparatively intense motor and secretory activity of this segment.

AMYLOIDOSIS

In systemic amyloidosis, there is diffuse tissue deposition of an amorphous, eosinophilic, extracellular protein-polysaccharide complex. This process can affect blood vessels, connective tissue, muscles, skin, mucous membranes, and the parenchyma of many organs. Amyloid infiltration causes marked thickening and rigidity of the wall of the stomach, especially in the antrum (Fig. 16-29), leading to luminal narrowing and the radiographic pattern of linitis plastica (Fig. 16-30).

PSEUDOLYMPHOMA

A constricting lesion of the body or antrum of the stomach, usually involving large segments of the organ, is one manifestation of pseudolymphoma (Fig. 16-31). The linitis plastica pattern in this disorder is almost invariably associated with a large

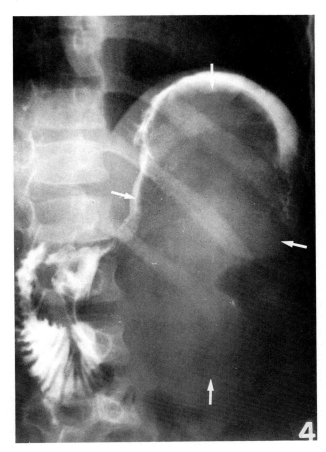

Fig. 16-32. Intramural gastric hematoma. Huge submucosal mass **(arrows)** occupies virtually the entire stomach and causes extreme narrowing of the gastric lumen. Repeat examination 2 weeks later showed resolution of the hematoma. (Balthazar EJ: Miscellaneous disorders of the stomach. In Taveras JM, Ferrucci JT (eds): Radiology: Diagnosis—Imaging —Intervention. Philadelphia, JB Lippincott, 1987)

gastric ulcer crater. Pseudolymphoma is a benign condition that probably represents a reaction to chronic peptic ulcer disease and mimics lymphoma clinically and histologically.

INTRAMURAL GASTRIC HEMATOMA

Intramural gastric hematoma is a relatively rare condition that may develop as a complication of trauma or as an inherited or acquired bleeding diathesis. Radiographically, an intramural gastric hematoma typically produces a large, localized, smooth-surfaced submucosal mass simulating a mesenchymal tumor. The lesion tends to involve the fundus of the stomach, though occasionally a massive hematoma may involve the entire stomach and produce severe narrowing of the gastric lumen (Fig. 16-32).

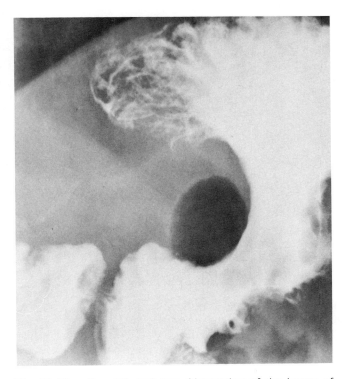

Fig. 16-31. Pseudolymphoma. Narrowing of the lumen of the stomach is associated with thickening of rugal folds.

EXOGASTRIC MASSES

A large exogastric mass can cause extrinsic pressure on the stomach and appear to narrow the barium-filled lumen. This is most commonly seen in patients with severe hepatomegaly (Fig. 16-33) but can also be identified in patients with pancreatic pseudocysts (Fig. 16-34) or enlargement of other upper abdominal organs.

GASTRIC RESTRICTIVE SURGERY FOR MORBID OBESITY

Gastric restrictive operations attempt to limit gastric capacity and restrict gastric outflow, thus provoking early satiety, causing the patient to curtail oral intake, and resulting in weight control. A variety of gastroplasty (gastric partition) procedures

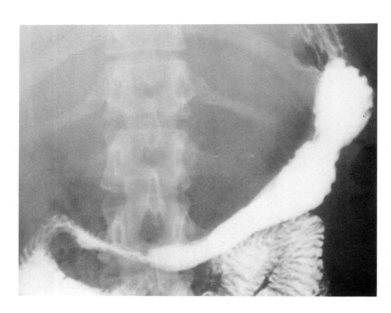

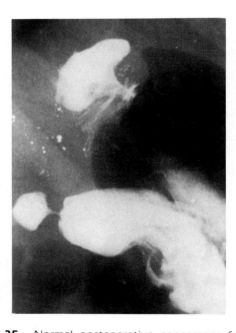

Fig. 16-33. Narrowing of the lumen of the stomach secondary to extrinsic impression by a huge liver (echinococcal cystic disease).

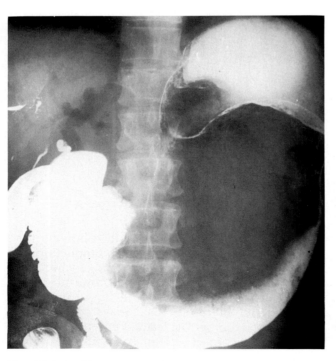

Fig. 16-34. Huge pancreatic pseudocyst impressing the stomach and almost obliterating the lumen.

Fig. 16-35. Normal postoperative appearance following Gomez gastroplasty. The proximal fundic pouch has an elliptical configuration and communicates through a 12-mm stoma to the distal gastric segment. (Agha FP, Harris HH, Boustany MM: Gastroplasty for morbid obesity: Roentgen evaluation and spectrum of complications. Gastrointest Radiol 7:217–223, 1982)

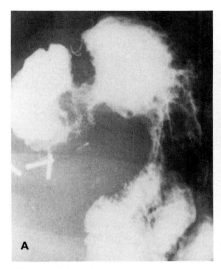
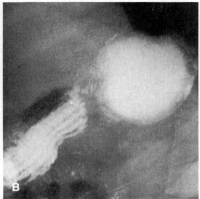
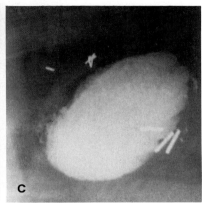

Fig. 16-36. Complications of gastroplasty. **(A)** Stomal dilatation. **(B)** Stomal stenosis with distention of the proximal pouch. **(C)** Complete obstruction of the stoma with marked distention of the proximal pouch. (Agha FP, Harris HH, Boustany MM: Gastroplasty for morbid obesity: Roentgen evaluation and spectrum of complications. Gastrointest Radiol 7:217–223, 1982)

have been developed that divide the stomach into a small proximal reservoir (50–75 ml) and a large distal segment with a small connecting channel (Fig. 16-35). Complications of gastric restrictive procedures can occur in the early and late postoperative periods. Leakage, perforation, and abscess formation are usually early complications; pouch dilatation, channel widening, and ulceration are usually late occurrences. Staple-line disruption, channel stenosis, and obstruction of the distal gastric or afferent limb can occur at any time.

The radiographic evaluation of a patient following gastric restrictive surgery includes an assessment of the size and shape of the proximal pouch and the width of the outlet channel (Fig. 16-36). Enlargement or change in shape of the proximal gastric pouch should suggest an underlying abnormality such as stenosis of the stoma, which can even lead to complete obstruction. The ideal channel size to allow for adequate food intake and control weight loss is in the range of 10 to 12 mm, though some patients tolerate channels of smaller diameter without developing symptoms of outlet obstruction. Staple-line dehiscence can lead to widening of the channel (Fig. 16-37A), and in complete dehiscence it is almost impossible to radiographically recognize that there has been an operative procedure involving the stomach (Fig. 16-37B).

Fig. 16-37. Complications of gastroplasty. **(A)** Incomplete staple-line dehiscence. **(B)** Complete staple-line dehiscence. In this patient, it is impossible to determine if any gastroplasty was performed. (Agha FP, Harris HH, Boustany MM: Gastroplasty for morbid obesity: Roentgen evaluation and spectrum of complications. Gastrointest Radiol 7:217–223, 1982)

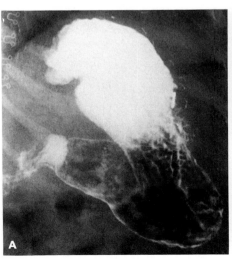
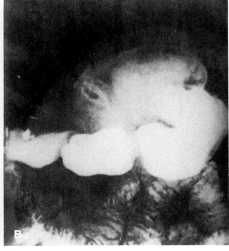

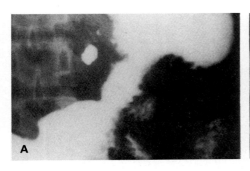 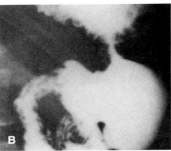

Fig. 16-38. Perigastric adhesions. Two views show circumferential narrowing of the body of the stomach causing partial obstruction. (Schwartz GE, Sclafani SJA: Post-traumatic gastric stenosis due to perigastric adhesions. Radiology 154:14, 1985)

PERIGASTRIC ADHESIONS

Gastric narrowing and deformity secondary to post-surgical or post-traumatic perigastric adhesions is a rare entity. Radiographically, it produces circumferential narrowing of the antrum or body of the stomach that may mimic scirrhous carcinoma or a metastatic process (Fig. 16-38). Demonstration of mucosal integrity, lack of interval change, and absence of mass effect, infiltration, peristaltic abnormality, or localized fixation can aid in distinguishing this benign lesion from a malignant one.

BIBLIOGRAPHY

Agha FP, Harris HH, Boustany MM: Gastroplasty for morbid obesity: Roentgen evaluation and spectrum of complications. Gastrointest Radiol 7:217–223, 1982

Balthazar EJ, Megibow AJ, Hulnick DH: Cytomegalovirus esophagitis and gastritis in AIDS. AJR 144:1201–1204, 1985

Berk RN, Wall SD, McArdle CB et al: Cryptosporidiosis of the stomach and small intestine in patients with AIDS. AJR 143:549–554, 1984

Carlson HC, Breen JF: Amyloidosis and plasma cell dyscrasias: Gastrointestinal involvement. Semin Roentgenol 21:128–138, 1986

Franken EA: Caustic damage of the gastrointestinal tract: Roentgen features. AJR 118:77–85, 1973

Geffen A, Feldman F: Antral deformity due to perigastric adhesions or bands simulating carcinoma of the stomach. Radiology 77:237–247, 1961

Goldstein HM, Rogers LF, Fletcher GH et al: Radiological manifestations of radiation-induced injury to the normal upper gastrointestinal tract. Radiology 117:135–140, 1975

Gonzalez G, Kennedy T: Crohn's disease of the stomach. Radiology 113:27–29, 1974

Hall DA, Clouse ME, Gramm HF: Gastroduodenal ulceration after hepatic arterial infusion chemotherapy. AJR 136:1216–1218, 1981

Halvorsen RA, Thompson WM: Computed tomographic staging of gastrointestinal tract malignancies. Part I. Esophagus and stomach. Invest Radiol 22:2–16, 1987

Joffe N: Metastatic involvement of the stomach secondary to breast carcinoma. AJR 123:512–521, 1975

Martel W, Abell MR, Allan TNK: Lymphoreticular hyperplasia of the stomach (pseudolymphoma). AJR 127:261–265, 1976

McLaughlin JS, Van Eck W, Thayer W et al: Gastric sarcoidosis. Ann Surg 153:283–288, 1961

Messinger NH, Bobroff LM, Beneventano T: Lymphosarcoma of the stomach. AJR 117:281–286, 1973

Nicks AJ, Hughes F: Polyarteritis nodosa "mimicking" eosinophilic gastroenteritis. Radiology 116:53–54, 1975

Rubesin SE, Levine MS, Glick SN: Gastric involvement by omental cakes: Radiographic findings. Gastrointest Radiol 11:223–228, 1986

Smith C, Gardiner R, Kubicka RA: Radiology of gastric restrictive surgery. RadioGraphics 5:193–216, 1985

Turner MA, Beachley MC, Stanley D: Phlegmonous gastritis. AJR 133:527–528, 1979

Vuthibhagdee A, Harris NF: Antral stricture as a delayed complication of iron intoxication. Radiology 103:163–164, 1972

Wehnut WD, Olmsted WW, Neiman HL et al: Eosinophilic gastritis. Radiology 120:85–89, 1976

THICKENING OF GASTRIC FOLDS

17

Disease Entities

Normal variant
Gastritis
  Alcoholic
  Hypertrophic
  Antral
  Corrosive
  Infectious
  Postradiation
  Postfreezing
Peptic ulcer disease
Zollinger-Ellison syndrome
Menetrier's disease
Lymphoma
Pseudolymphoma
Carcinoma
Varices
Infiltrative processes
  Eosinophilic gastritis
  Crohn's disease
  Sarcoidosis
  Tuberculosis
  Syphilis
  Amyloidosis
Adjacent pancreatic disease
  Acute pancreatitis
  Extension of carcinoma of the pancreas

The gastric mucosa is normally thrown into numerous longitudinal folds or rugae that run predominantly in the direction of the long axis of the stomach. Folds in the vicinity of the lesser curvature run lengthwise in parallel fashion and form the magenstrasse that permits the rapid transport of fluid toward the duodenum. Gastric folds are not only composed of epithelium but also contain the lamina propria, the muscularis mucosae, and varying amounts of the submucosa. Therefore, edema of the mucosa or submucosa, as well as infiltration by neoplastic or inflammatory cells or vascular engorgement, can result in the radiographic pattern of thickened gastric folds.

There is much variability in the normal radiographic appearance of gastric folds. Folds in the fundus tend to be thicker and more tortuous than those in the distal part of the stomach. Antral folds measuring more than 5 mm in width are generally considered abnormal; folds of the same size in the fundus would probably be within normal limits. When the stomach is filled, the mucosa may be stretched evenly and smoothly and appear thinned. Conversely, when the stomach is partially empty or partially contracted, the gastric rugae are more prominent. Thus, in many patients, apparent thickening of the mucosal folds, especially in the fundus and proximal body to the stomach, merely represents a normal variant rather than a true pathologic process.

GASTRITIS

ALCOHOLIC

Many inflammatory diseases involving the stomach can result in the radiographic appearance of thick-

223

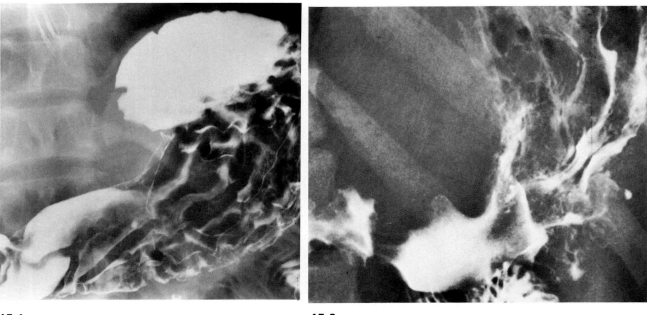

17-1   17-2

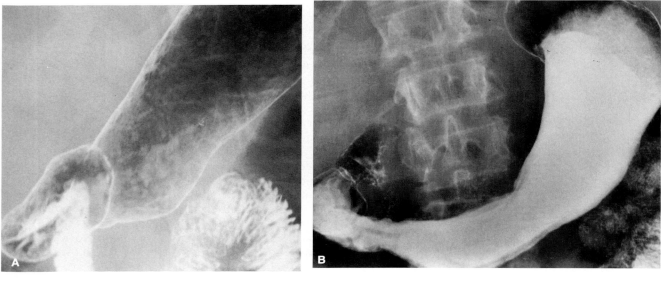

17-3

Fig. 17-1.   *Alcoholic gastritis. Diffuse thickening of gastric rugal folds.*

Fig. 17-2.   *Alcoholic gastritis. Bizarre, large folds simulate a malignant process.*

Fig. 17-3.   *Chronic atrophic gastritis.* **(A)** *Relative absence of folds in a patient with a long drinking history.* **(B)** *Tubular stomach with a striking decrease in the usually prominent rugal folds in a patient with megaloblastic anemia.*

ened rugal folds. Overindulgence in alcoholic beverages is the most common cause of acute exogenous gastritis. The radiographic appearance of thickened gastric folds (Fig. 17-1) parallels the pathologic observation of hyperemic engorged rugae, which usually subside completely after withdrawal of alcohol. Bizarre rugal thickening occasionally mimics malignant disease (Fig. 17-2). In patients with long drinking histories, chronic gastritis and a relative absence of folds is frequently seen (Fig. 17-3*A*), though this can be related to such factors as cirrhosis, age, malnutrition, medication, and other systemic disease (Fig. 17-3*B*) in addition to the alcohol itself.

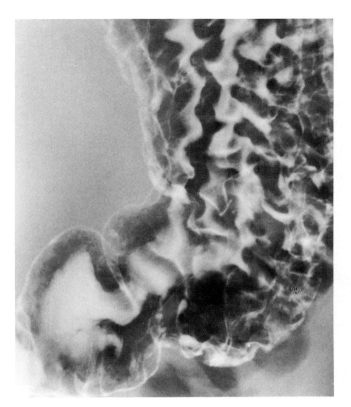

Fig. 17-4. Hypertrophic gastritis in a patient with high acid output and peptic ulcer disease.

HYPERTROPHIC

Hypertrophic gastritis is thickening of the mucosa due to localized or diffuse hyperplasia of surface epithelial cells (Fig. 17-4). This is a controversial entity that appears to be related to chronic inflammation of the gastric mucosa in which there is thickening, without destruction, of glandular elements. The pathogenesis is not clear, though many investigators have considered hypertrophic gastritis to be a functional lesion possibly related to transient edema, neuromuscular disturbances, or high acid output.

Radiographically, hypertrophic gastritis produces thickening of rugal folds that is usually associated with increased secretions. Prominent areae gastricae up to 4 to 5 mm in diameter (normal, 1–2 mm) may be seen throughout the stomach (Fig. 17-5). These prominent areae gastricae appear angular or polygonal, rather than their normal round or oval shape. Because an association between prominence and enlargement of areae gastricae and the presence of peptic ulcer disease has been demonstrated, the radiographic detection of hypertrophic gastritis mandates a thorough investigation of the stomach and duodenum for peptic ulcer.

ANTRAL

Antral gastritis is a cause of thickening of mucosal folds localized to the antrum (Fig. 17-6). This is a controversial entity that most likely reflects one end of the spectrum of peptic ulcer disease. Isolated antral gastritis appears without fold thickening or acute ulceration in the duodenal bulb. The term antral gastritis is actually a misnomer, since, in most cases, there is gastroscopic evidence of disease elsewhere in the stomach that is not radiographically detectable.

In addition to fold thickening, some authors have used the term antral gastritis to refer to tran-

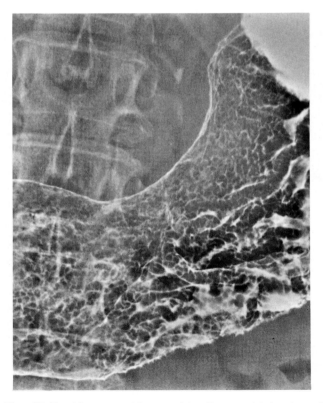

Fig. 17-5. Hypertrophic gastritis. Coarse thickening of areae gastricae throughout the stomach.

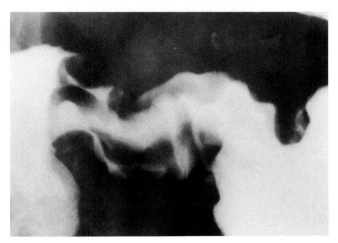

Fig. 17-6. Antral gastritis. Thickening of gastric rugal folds is confined to the antrum.

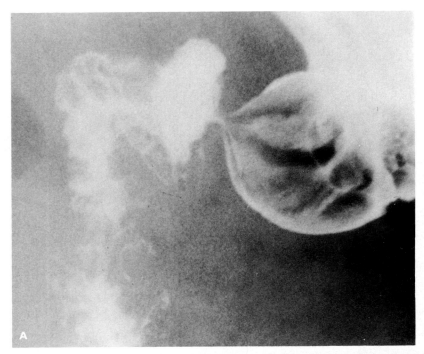

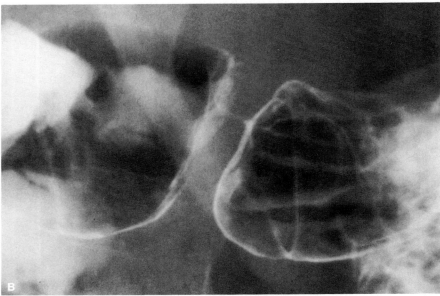

Fig. 17-7. Antral gastritis. **(A)** Prominent flattening of the prepyloric shoulders. **(B)** In a normal patient, there is full, symmetric distention of both the greater and lesser curvatures in the prepyloric region.

sient antral spasm and lack of normal distention on single-contrast examination. Normal patients have full, symmetric distention of both the greater and the lesser curvatures of the stomach in the prepyloric region. In antral gastritis, there is flattening and narrowing of the antrum with loss of one (generally the lesser curvature) or both of the prepyloric shoulders (Fig. 17-7). The antral deformity usually persists throughout the examination, but even transient asymmetry is reported to represent significant superficial mucosal disease. Additional radiographic findings in antral gastritis include transient or persistent mucosal crenulation (a wrinkled or irregularly corrugated appearance of the antrum)

and antral spasm (Fig. 17-8). Patients with antral gastritis usually have epigastric pain, frequently of long duration, that has little relation to eating and is not completely relieved by antacids. The radiographic findings of antral gastritis may persist even when the patient is clinically well and tend to increase when symptoms recur.

CORROSIVE

The ingestion of corrosive agents results in a severe form of acute gastritis characterized by intense mucosal edema and inflammation. Radiographically,

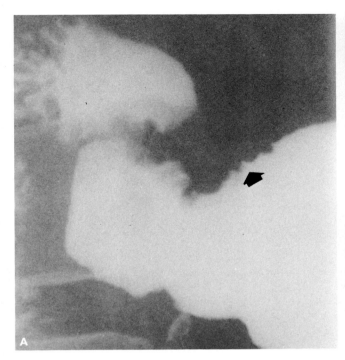
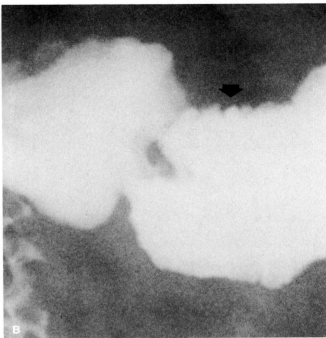

Fig. 17-8. Two patients with antral gastritis, which is seen as the flattening of the prepyloric shoulder of the lesser curvature with the corrugated appearance of mucosal crenulation **(arrows)**.

thickened gastric folds are associated with mucosal ulcerations, atony, and rigidity (Fig. 17-9). A fixed, open pylorus is usually seen, probably due to extensive damage to the muscular layer. The presence of gas in the wall of the stomach after the ingestion of

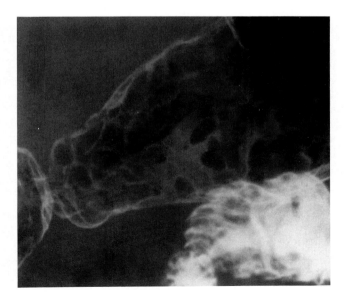

Fig. 17-9. Corrosive gastritis. Multiple polypoid filling defects in the body and antrum of the stomach represent thickened, inflamed mucosa surrounded by denuded and necrotic areas. (Johns TT, Thoeni RF: Severe corrosive gastritis related to Drano: An unusual case. Gastrointest Radiol 8:25–28, 1983)

corrosive agents is an ominous sign; free gastric perforation may occur.

Caustic ingestion occurs primarily in children and young adults. Most cases in children are accidental; those in young adults are usually associated with suicide attempts. Accidental ingestion of caustic materials in adults most often occurs in alcoholics and psychotics.

Strong corrosives descend down the lesser curvature along the magenstrasse and accumulate in the antrum. Once a caustic agent reaches the distal antrum, it produces a tetanic contraction of the pylorus that prevents the noxious substance from passing further down the gastrointestinal tract. Because the bulk of the corrosive agent is thus concentrated in the lower part of the gastric body and antrum of the stomach, the resultant injury is most severe in these areas.

Acids generally produce more severe gastric damage than do ingested alkali. This is presumably due to partial neutralization of alkaline agents by the gastric acidity. Highly concentrated alkali, however, especially in liquid form, are also capable of causing severe damage to the wall of the stomach.

INFECTIOUS

In infectious gastritis, bacterial invasion of the stomach wall or bacterial toxins (*e.g.,* botulism, diphtheria, dysentery, typhoid fever) result in hyperemia of the mucosa, edema, exudation, and a layering of fibrinous material on the mucosa that pro-

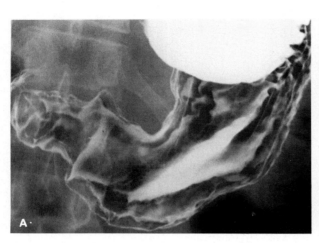 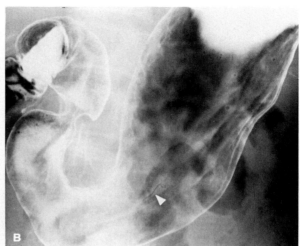

Fig. 17-10. Anisakiasis. **(A)** Diffuse fold thickening due to mucosal edema involves over three-quarters of the gastric wall from the antrum to the body. **(B)** An arrow points to the thin outline of the larva itself. (Kusuhara P, Watanabe K, Fukuda M: Radiographic study of acute gastric anisakiasis. Gastrointest Radiol 9:305–309, 1984)

duces the radiographic appearance of thickened gastric folds. Involvement by gas-forming organisms can produce the characteristic pattern of gas within the wall of the stomach.

An unusual infestation of the stomach is acute anisakiasis, a form of visceral larva migrans ac-

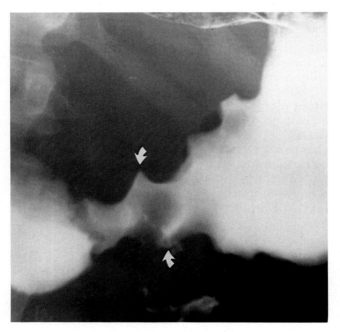

Fig. 17-11. Cytomegalovirus gastritis. Broad nodular contour defects associated with narrowing of the distal stomach and limited distensibility **(arrows).** Endoscopy revealed severe swelling of gastric rugae with multiple superficial ulcerations. (Balthazar EJ, Megibow AJ, Hulnick DH: Cytomegalovirus esophagitis and gastritis in AIDS. AJR 144:1201–1204, 1985. Copyright 1985. Reprinted with permission)

quired by the ingestion of raw or poorly cooked fish containing *Anisakis* larvae. This ascaris-like nematode spends its larval stage within tiny crustaceans that are eaten by such salt-water fish as herring, cod, and mackerel. Marine mammals, such as the whale and dolphin, are its final hosts. When humans break the natural chain and consume infected fish, the *Anisakis* worms penetrate the mucosa of the gastrointestinal tract and cause symptoms of acute, cramping abdominal pain within 4 hr to 6 hr of ingestion. The disease is self-limited, because the worms cannot grow in humans and die within a few weeks.

In the appropriate clinical setting, the presence of localized or generalized coarse, broad gastric folds due to mucosal edema is suggestive of, though not specific for, the diagnosis of anisakiasis (Fig. 17-10*A*). A definitive radiologic diagnosis requires the demonstration of a threadlike filling defect about 30 mm in length that represents the larva itself (Fig. 17-10*B*). The worms can appear serpiginous, circular, or ringlike and can change their shape during the examination.

In patients with AIDS, infection with cytomegalovirus may cause a diffuse gastritis with lack of distensibility and large nodular rugal folds representing edema (Fig. 17-11). This appearance must be distinguished from the discrete nodules of Kaposi's sarcoma, which are seen against a background of normal mucosa.

POSTRADIATION/POSTFREEZING

Thickening of gastric folds can be seen after radiation or freezing therapy for gastric ulcer disease. Although a decrease in gastric secretion can be achieved by these techniques, they are rarely performed since less hazardous medical therapy has become available.

PEPTIC ULCER DISEASE AND THE ZOLLINGER-ELLISON SYNDROME

Hypersecretion of acid in patients with peptic ulcer disease or the Zollinger-Ellison syndrome is one of the most common causes of diffuse thickening of gastric folds (Fig. 17-12). In the body and fundus of the stomach (not the antrum), there appears to be a close correlation between the degree of enlargement of gastric folds and the level of acid secretions. In the Zollinger-Ellison syndrome, great glandular length and encroachment of fundal-type mucosa into the antrum produce characteristic increased rugosity and gastric secretions. Localized thickening of mucosal folds due to inflammatory edema can be seen surrounding an acute ulcer crater. The presence of thickened gastric folds radiating toward the crater is a traditional radiographic sign of a benign gastric ulcer (Fig. 17-13).

Hypersecretory states result in large amounts of retained gastric fluid despite fasting and lack of any organic obstruction. This is especially prominent in the Zollinger-Ellison syndrome, in which the gastric mucosa responds maximally to the stimulus of the gastrinlike hormone produced by the ulcerogenic tumor or its metastases.

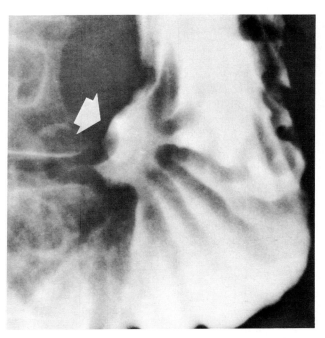

Fig. 17-13. Benign gastric ulcer. Thickened gastric folds radiate toward the crater **(arrow)**.

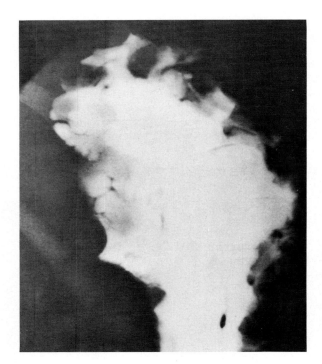

Fig. 17-14. Menetrier's disease. Characteristic rugal fold thickening is confined to the proximal stomach.

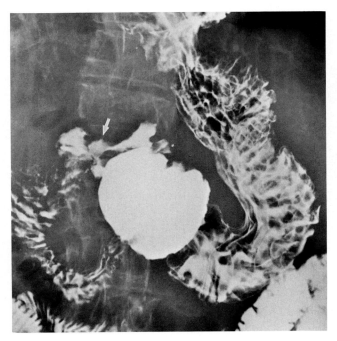

Fig. 17-12. Zollinger–Ellison syndrome. Diffuse thickening of the gastric folds. Note the large ulcer **(arrow)** in a markedly deformed duodenal bulb.

MENETRIER'S DISEASE

Menetrier's disease (giant hypertrophic gastritis) is an uncommon disorder that is characterized by massive enlargement of rugal folds due to hyperpla-

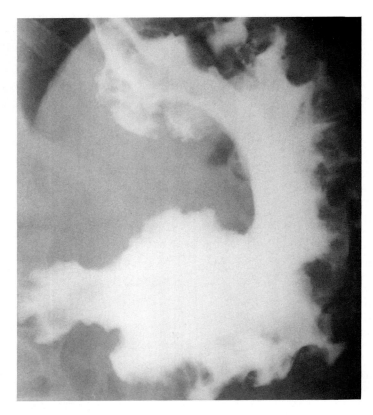

Fig. 17-15. *Menetrier's disease. Generalized rugal fold thickening involves the entire stomach.*

sia and hypertrophy of the gastric glands. There is usually hyposecretion of acid and excessive secretion of gastric mucus that can be associated with protein loss into the lumen of the stomach. The thickened gastric rugae become contorted and folded on each other in a convolutional pattern suggestive of the gyri and sulci of the brain. Enlarged rugal folds are particularly prominent along the greater curvature. Although the disorder is classically described as a lesion of the fundus and body (Fig. 17-14), involvement of the entire stomach can occur (Fig. 17-15). The disease can be diffuse or localized, and the transition between normal and pathologic folds is usually abrupt.

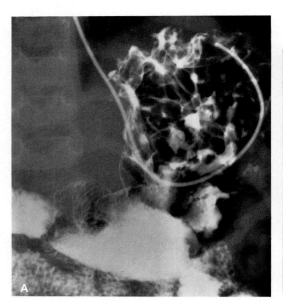
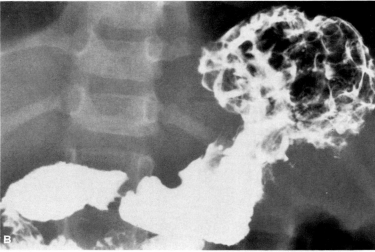

Fig. 17-16. *Pediatric hypertrophic gastropathy.* **(A)** *Enlarged folds in the fundus and body.* **(B)** *As in the previous case, there is rugal hypertrophy in the proximal portions of the stomach with the distal portions spared. (Marks MP, Lanza MV, Kahlstrom EJ et al: Pediatric hypertrophic gastropathy. AJR 147:1031–1032, 1986. Copyright 1986. Reproduced with permission)*

Menetrier's disease is classified as one of the protein-losing enteropathies. In some patients, altered mucosal permeability leads to protein loss into the lumen of the stomach, resulting in hypoproteinemia and edema. Although acid secretion is reduced in this condition, most patients tend to have chronic, vague gastrointestinal symptoms such as epigastric pain, vomiting, and bleeding.

The radiographic *sine qua non* of Menetrier's disease is the demonstration of enlarged rugal folds. Typically, the folds are thick, tortuous, and angular, with no uniformity of pattern or direction. When seen on end, the folds may closely simulate polypoid filling defects. Lines of barium can be seen perpendicular to the stomach because of spicules of contrast trapped by apposed giant rugal folds. Even if the thickened gastric folds are not well seen, a rough estimate of their height may be made by measurement of the length of these barium lines.

The excessive amounts of gastric mucus in Menetrier's disease can cause the enlarged rugal folds to have a peculiar mottled or reticular appearance. The thick layer of mucus can effectively fill the narrow crypts and furrows between enlarged rugae, thereby preventing barium from entering these spaces and impairing radiographic demonstration of the thickened folds. Patients with Menetrier's disease usually have increased thickness of the gastric wall, as measured by the distance between the faintly lucent serosal line of the greater curvature and the intraluminal barium column. Peristalsis is frequently strikingly sluggish; motility is often delayed.

Several case reports have demonstrated coexistence of Menetrier's disease and adenocarcinoma of the stomach. This suggests the possibility that Menetrier's disease may have a malignant potential and indicates a need for close follow-up of patients with this condition.

A similar but even more uncommon entity of protein-losing enteropathy and hypertrophic gastric rugae has been described in children and termed "pediatric hypertrophic gastropathy" (Fig. 17-16*A*). The children present with hypoalbuminemia in the absence of discernible liver disease, proteinuria, or malnutrition. There is often a prodromal history of viral respiratory or gastrointestinal tract infection. Radiographs show involvement of the proximal stomach and sparing of the antral region (Fig. 17-16*B*), as often happens in adult cases. However,

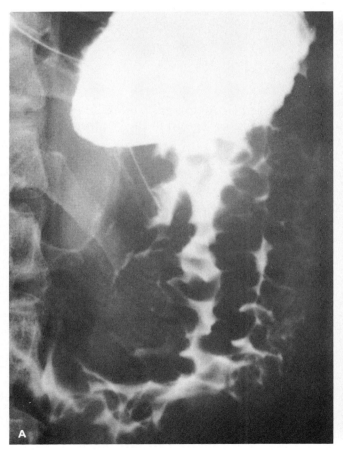

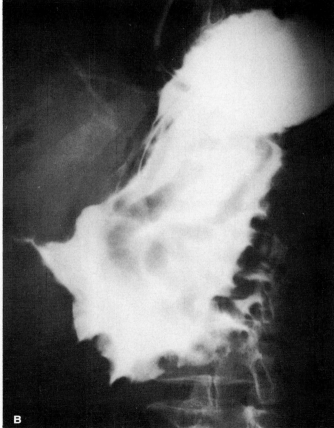

Fig. 17-17. Lymphoma. There is diffuse thickening, distortion, and nodularity of gastric folds.

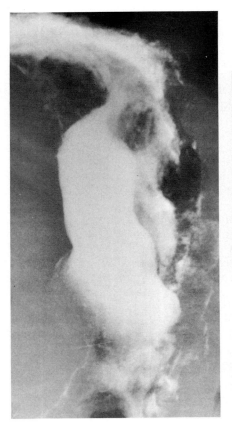

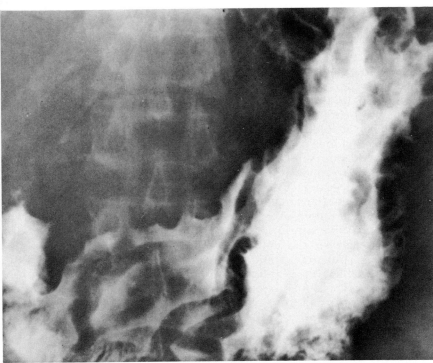

17-18   **17-19**

Fig. 17-18. Lymphoma. Diffuse thickening of folds is associated with a huge gastric ulcer.

Fig. 17-19. Lymphoma. Bizarre thickening of folds is most prominent in the antrum.

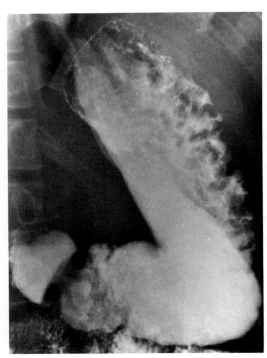

Fig. 17-20. Menetrier's disease. Fold thickening involves the greater curvature of the fundus and body and spares the lesser curvature and antrum.

the pediatric disease follows a more benign course, usually resolving spontaneously after weeks or months.

LYMPHOMA

One appearance of lymphoma of the stomach is thickening, distortion, and nodularity of gastric rugal folds (Fig. 17-17). This pattern of fold enlargement is often found in proximity to a polypoid mass or an ulcerated lesion (Fig. 17-18). Although lymphoma can in most cases be distinguished radiographically from Menetrier's disease, a biopsy is sometimes required. If the enlarged rugal folds predominantly involve the distal portion of the stomach and the lesser curvature, if there is associated ulceration, or if there is some loss of pliability of the gastric wall, lymphoma is more likely (Fig. 17-19). An extrinsic impression by enlarged retrogastric and other regional lymph nodes or an enlarged spleen also suggests this diagnosis. However, if the process stops at the incisura and spares the lesser curvature, if there is no ulceration or true rigidity, or if excess mucus can be demonstrated, Menetrier's disease is the probable diagnosis (Fig. 17-20). Diffuse fold thickening can also be seen in patients

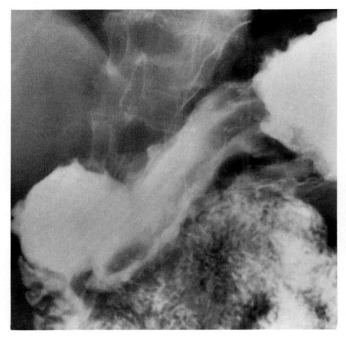

17-21

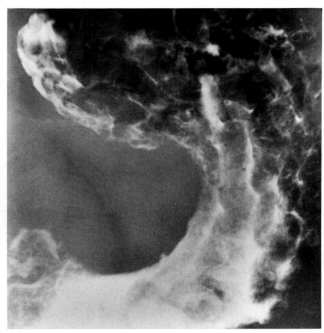

17-22

Fig. 17-21. Leukemic infiltrate of the wall of the stomach causing thickened gastric folds.

Fig. 17-22. Pseudolymphoma. There is thickening of rugal folds in the midportion of the stomach in this patient, who had a long history of peptic ulcer disease.

with leukemic infiltration of the stomach wall (Fig. 17-21).

PSEUDOLYMPHOMA

Enlargement of gastric folds is one of the manifestations of pseudolymphoma, a benign proliferation of lymphoid tissue that can be mistaken histologically for malignant lymphoma (Fig. 17-22). The thickened rugal folds in this condition are usually associated with a large gastric ulcer.

CARCINOMA

Although carcinoma of the stomach tends to produce either discrete filling defects or generalized narrowing of the stomach with marked loss of pliability, the disease occasionally presents a radiographic pattern of enlarged, tortuous, and coarse gastric folds simulating lymphoma (Fig. 17-23). Unlike most cases of diffuse infiltrating adenocarcinoma, this form of the disease shows preservation of a relatively normal gastric volume, pliability, and peristaltic activity. Biopsy is necessary to distinguish this appearance from lymphoma. Punctate

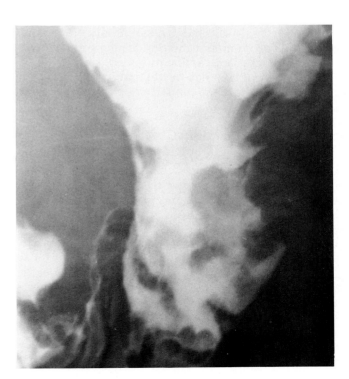

Fig. 17-23. Adenocarcinoma of the stomach. Enlarged, tortuous, and coarse rugal folds simulate lymphoma.

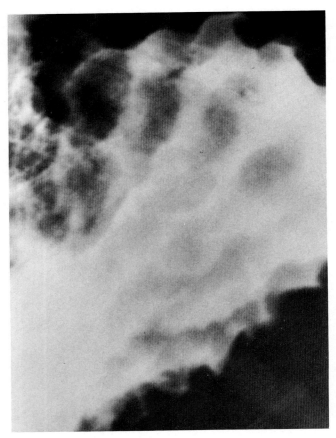

Fig. 17-24. Fundal gastric varices. Multiple smooth, lobulated filling defects represent the dilated venous structures.

calcifications are occasionally seen within the thickened, rigid wall and are essentially diagnostic of colloid carcinoma or mucinous adenocarcinoma of the stomach. The calcifications are suggestive of psammoma bodies, may be related to the high calcium content of mucin, and are not seen in association with lymphoma.

GASTRIC VARICES

Gastric varices can appear as prominent mucosal folds. Usually associated with esophageal varices, varices in the fundus represent dilated peripheral branches of the short gastric and left gastric veins due to portal hypertension. The presence of gastric varices without esophageal varices is a very specific sign of isolated splenic vein occlusion. This is most commonly secondary to pancreatitis or pancreatic carcinoma, though it can be caused by retroperitoneal lesions or hyperviscosity states such as polycythemia. Obstruction of the splenic vein forces the large amount of blood normally carried by the splenic artery to the spleen to find a different route to the vena cava. Blood is shunted through the short gastric veins in their course from the splenic hilum over the fundus of the stomach to anastomose with

branches of the coronary vein and distal esophageal plexus. If the portal vein is patent, blood can return to the liver through the coronary vein, and no esophageal varices are produced.

Radiographically, fundal gastric varices appear as multiple smooth, lobulated filling defects projecting between curvilinear, crescentic collections of barium (Fig. 17-24). They are best demonstrated by barium swallow with small amounts of barium or by air-contrast techniques, since they may be completely effaced or obscured if the fundus is filled with barium. Associated enlargement of the spleen can produce an extrinsic pressure defect on the greater curvature of the stomach.

Gastric varices can usually be readily differentiated from other causes of thickened folds in the fundus of the stomach. The considerable changeability in the size and shape of varices effectively eliminates the possibility of a neoplastic process. Extension along the lesser curvature makes Menetrier's disease unlikely. Additional evidence for gastric varices includes the presence of concomitant esophageal varices and an appropriate clinical history. At times, however, it can be impossible to distinguish gastric varices radiographically from Menetrier's disease or a malignant lesion; gastroscopy is then required for diagnosis.

Gastric varices occurring at sites other than the fundus are unusual and may pose a diagnostic dilemma. Varices of the antrum and body of the stomach can be produced by obstruction of the splenic vein proximal to a patent coronary vein, resulting in collateral flow to the liver through a dilated, tortuous gastroepiploic vein (Fig. 17-25). The enlarged mucosal folds, which occur primarily along the greater curvature, can be differentiated from a malignant lesion because of their pliability and variation in size and shape in response to external compression, change in position, and degree of distention of the stomach.

INFILTRATIVE PROCESSES

A variety of infiltrative processes can result in the radiographic pattern of thickened gastric folds. During the acute phase of eosinophilic gastritis, diffuse infiltration by eosinophilic leukocytes causes enlargement of rugal folds. This thickening of folds is usually limited to the distal half of the stomach, but can involve the entire organ (Fig. 17-26). Increased mucosal permeability may cause the loss of protein and red blood cells into the gastric lumen. If this occurs, there is generally an associated increase in the eosinophil count in the peripheral blood and intolerance to specific foods.

Granulomatous processes, such as Crohn's disease, sarcoidosis, tuberculosis, and syphilis, can produce a pattern of rugal enlargement before the more characteristic antral narrowing and rigidity

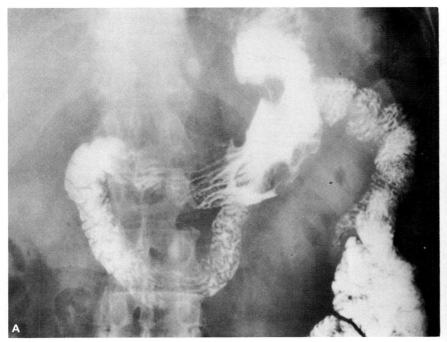

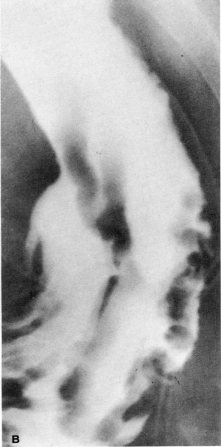

Fig. 17-25. Nonfundic gastric varices. **(A)** Giant "folds" in the body of the stomach, particularly along the greater curvature, produce lobulated filling defects. There is no evidence of fundic varices or splenomegaly. **(B)** Fluoroscopic pressure spot-film reveals discrete varices as the cause of the enlarged rugae. (Sos T, Meyers MA, Baltaxe HA: Nonfundic gastric varices. Radiology 105:579–580, 1972)

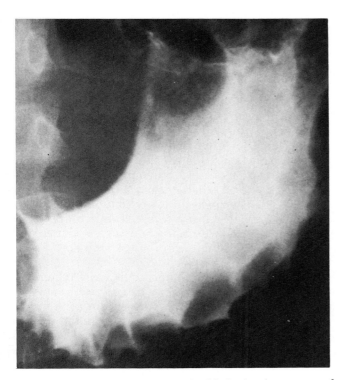

Fig. 17-26. Eosinophilic gastritis. Marked enlargement of rugal folds is caused by diffuse infiltration of eosinophilic leukocytes.

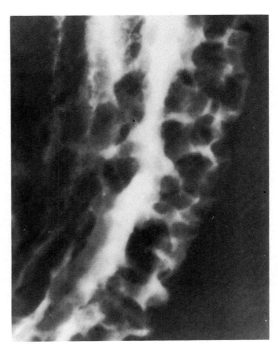

Fig. 17-27. Amyloidosis. Huge, nodular folds are caused by diffuse infiltration of the stomach by amyloid.

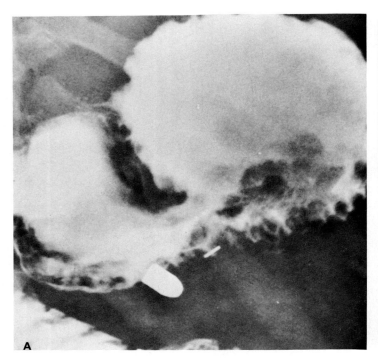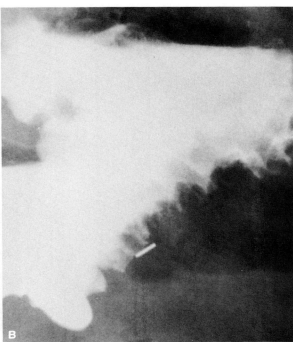

Fig. 17-28. Two films demonstrating a pseudocyst of the body and tail of the pancreas following a gunshot wound. Adjacent inflammatory changes and edema produce irregular thickening of folds along the greater curvature of the stomach.

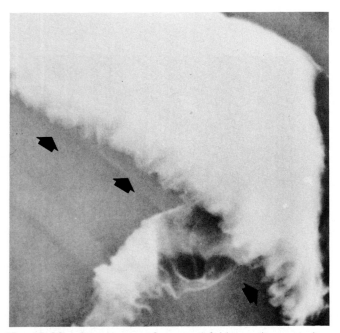

Fig. 17-29. Prominence of mucosal folds on the posterior wall of the stomach **(arrows)** and a large retrogastric mass in a patient with acute pancreatitis.

develop. Infiltration of the stomach wall by amyloid can also result in thickening of the gastric rugal folds (Fig. 17-27).

ADJACENT PANCREATIC DISEASE

Thickened gastric folds are a manifestation of adjacent pancreatitis, often with pseudocyst formation (Fig. 17-28). Selective prominence of nodular, serpentine mucosal folds on the posterior wall and lesser curvature of the stomach has been reported as a frequent and reliable sign of acute pancreatitis (Fig. 17-29). The rugal folds in the fundus and body along the greater curvature are normally more prominent than those on the lesser curvature and posterior wall of the barium-filled stomach. Selective enlargement of folds along the lesser curvature and posterior wall in patients with acute pancreatitis is presumably due either to activated enzymes producing mural irritation with spasm of the muscular layer or to a severe perigastric inflammatory response (fibrosis, adhesions). The radiographic pattern of thickened rugal folds does not become evident until a few days after clinical onset of the disease and returns to normal when the patient's clinical symptoms improve. The presence of prominent folds appears to correlate well with the intensity of the inflammatory process in the pancreas and is not seen in patients with mild forms of the disease.

Direct metastatic extension of carcinoma of the pancreas to the stomach can also produce a radiographic pattern of thickened gastric folds predominantly involving the greater curvature.

BIBLIOGRAPHY

Balthazar EJ: Effects of acute and chronic pancreatitis on the stomach: Patterns of radiographic involvement. Am J Gastroenterol 72:568–580, 1979

Balthazar EJ, Davidian MM: Hyperrugosity in gastric carcinoma: Radiographic, endoscopic and pathologic features. AJR 136:531–535, 1981

Balthazar EJ, Henderson M: Prominent folds on the posterior wall and lesser curvature of the stomach: A sign of acute pancreatitis. Radiology 110:319–321, 1974

Bateson EM: Duodenal and antral varices. Br J Radiol 42:744–747, 1969

Feinberg SB, Tully TE: Secondary gastric mural abnormalities simulating primary disease in isolated chronic left subphrenic abscess and isolated chronic pancreatitis. AJR 122:413–418, 1974

Hunter TB, Bjelland JC: Gastrointestinal complications of leukemia and its treatment. AJR 142:513–518, 1984

Jacobs DS: Primary gastric malignant lymphoma and pseudolymphoma. Am J Clin Pathol 40:379–394, 1963

Johns TT, Thoeni RF: Severe corrosive gastritis related to Drano: An unusual case. Gastrointest Radiol 8:25–28, 1983

Klein NC, Hargrove RL, Sleisenger MH et al: Eosinophilic gastroenteritis. Medicine 49:299–319, 1970

Kusuhara T, Watanabe K, Fukuda M: Radiographic study of acute gastric anisakiasis. Gastrointest Radiol 9:305–309, 1984

Legge DA, Carlson HC, Judd ES: Roentgenologic features of regional enteritis of the upper gastrointestinal tract. AJR 110:355–360, 1970

Marks MP, Lanza MV, Kahlstoma EJ et al: Pediatric hypertrophic gastropathy. AJR 147:1031–1034, 1986

Marshak RH, Lindner AE, Maklansky D: Lymphoreticular disorders of the gastrointestinal tract. Roentgenographic features. Gastrointest Radiol 4:103–120, 1979

Marshak RH, Wolf BS, Cohen N et al: Protein-losing disorders of the gastrointestinal tract: Roentgen features. Radiology 77:893–905, 1961

McIlrath DC, Hallenbeck GA: A review of gastric freezing. JAMA 190:715–718, 1964

Megibow AJ, Balthazar EJ, Hulnick DH: Radiology of nonneoplastic gastrointestinal disorders in acquired immune deficiency syndrome. Semin Roentgenol 22:31–41, 1987

Menuch LS: Gastric lymphoma, a radiolgic diagnosis. Gastrointest Radiol 1:159–161, 1976

Muhletaler CA, Gerlock AJ, de Soto L et al: Gastroduodenal lesions of ingested acids: Radiographic findings. AJR 135:1247–1252, 1980

Muhletaler CA, Gerlock AJ, Goncharenko V et al: Gastric varices secondary to splenic vein occlusion: Radiographic diagnosis and clinical significance. Radiology 132:593–598, 1979

Nakata H, Takeda K, Nakayama T: Radiological diagnosis of acute gastric anisakiasis. Radiology 135:49–53, 1980

Olmsted WW, Cooper PH, Madewell JE: Involvement of the gastric antrum in Menetrier's disease. AJR 126:524–529, 1976

Orr RK, Lininger JR, Lawrence W: Gastric pseudolymphoma: A challenging clinical problem. Ann Surg 200:185–194, 1984

Press AJ: Practical significance of gastric rugal folds. AJR 125:172–183, 1975

Reese DF, Hodgson JR, Dockerty MB: Giant hypertrophy of the gastric mucosa (Menetrier's disease): A correlation of the roentgenographic, pathologic and clinical findings. AJR 88:619–626, 1962

Sato T, Sakai Y, Ishiguro S et al: Radiologic manifestations of early gastric lymphoma. AJR 146:513–517, 1986

Smookler BH: Gastric varices: Characteristics and clinical significance. Gastroenterology 31:581–587, 1956

Sos T, Meyers MA, Baltaxe HA: Nonfundic gastric varices. Radiology 105:579–580, 1972

18

FILLING DEFECTS IN THE STOMACH

Disease Entities

Areae gastricae
Neoplasms
  Benign tumors
    Hyperplastic polyp
    Adenomatous polyp
    Hamartoma
      Peutz-Jeghers syndrome
      Cowden's disease
      Ruvalcaba–Myhre–Smith syndrome
    Spindle cell tumor
  Tumors of variable malignant potential
    Villous adenoma
    Carcinoid tumor
  Malignant tumors
    Carcinoma
    Lymphoma
    Metastases
    Sarcoma
    Plasmacytoma
Extrinsic cystic or inflammatory masses
Ectopic pancreas
Thickened folds simulating nodules
  Menetrier's disease
  Gastric varices
  Crohn's disease
  Sarcoidosis
  Tuberculosis
Eosinophilic gastritis
Hypertrophied antral-pyloric fold

Bezoar
Foreign body
Blood clots/intramural hematoma
Peptic ulcer (surrounding edematous mass; incisura)
Double pylorus
Eosinophilic granuloma (inflammatory fibroid polyp)
Arterial impression
Gastric duplication cyst
Pseudolymphoma
Intragastric gallstone
Tumefactive extramedullary hematopoiesis
Amyloidoma
Candidiasis
Postoperative defect
  Suture granuloma
  Fundoplication
Jejunogastric intussusception
Gastric varices
Anisakis larva
Prolapsed esophageal mucosa

AREAE GASTRICAE

Areae gastricae are normal anatomic features of the gastric mucosa. On double-contrast studies, they produce a fine reticular pattern surrounded by barium-filled grooves, resulting in a radiographic appearance that simulates multiple filling defects (Fig. 18-1).

Areae gastricae are rarely demonstrated on conventional barium upper gastrointestinal series but are seen in a majority of properly performed double-contrast studies. Although most commonly identified in the antrum distal to the incisura angularis, areae gastricae not infrequently can be demonstrated proximally. Technical considerations are extremely important in demonstrating areae gastricae. The barium must be of high density and low viscosity, and the stomach must be well distended. The use of hypotonic agents (glucagon) and antifoaming substances aids in the production of a technically optimal examination. The amount and consistency of gastric mucus also determines whether areae gastricae can be demonstrated radiographically. A thick, tenacious coat of mucus may fill in the grooves so that barium cannot penetrate them. Therefore, inability to demonstrate areae gastricae may reflect an enhanced protective capability of the gastric mucus layer. Conversely, patients in whom areae gastricae are clearly seen in the antrum may have a thinner mucus layer and consequently a greater incidence of ulcer disease.

The radiographic appearance of enlarged (≥4 mm) and coarsened areae gastricae in the proximal body and fundus of the stomach has been reported to correlate closely with the endoscopic pattern of hypertrophic mucosa that is considered an indication of a hypersecretory gastropathy (Fig. 18-2). The etiology appears to be not organic disease but rather intense stimulation of fundal mucosal growth and function, probably caused by vagal hyperactivity. This increased vagal stimulation of the parietal, chief, and mucus neck cells causes the fundal glands to produce acid, pepsin, and mucus and is frequently associated with peptic ulcer.

BENIGN TUMORS

With the increased use of the double-contrast technique, gastric polyps are being detected more frequently. In two large series, polyps were demonstrated in about 1.7% of upper gastrointestinal examinations. Although most gastric polyps are

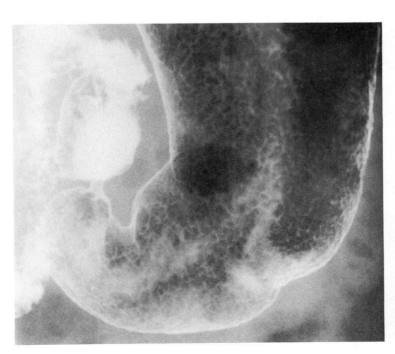

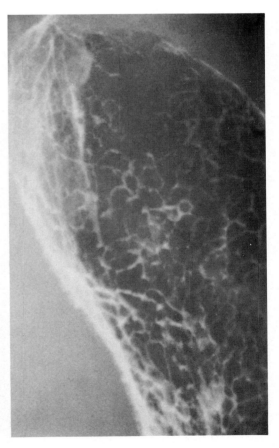

18-1

18-2

Fig. 18-1. Areae gastricae. A normal, fine reticular pattern is seen on double-contrast examination.

Fig. 18-2. Coarsened areae gastricae. The patient had high acid secretion and peptic ulcer disease.

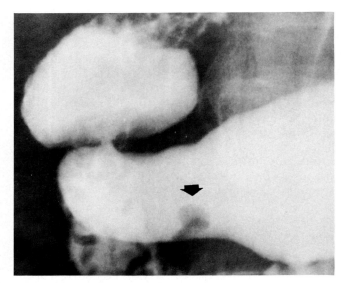

Fig. 18-3. Hyperplastic polyp. Note the small, sharply defined filling defect with a smooth contour **(arrow)**. A short stalk connects the head of the polyp to the stomach wall.

HYPERPLASTIC POLYP

Hyperplastic polyps are the most common causes of discrete filling defects in the stomach. These polyps are not true neoplasms, but result from excessive regeneration of superficial epithelium as a response to inflammatory destruction of the mucosa of the stomach in an area of chronic gastritis. They are typically asymptomatic, small and smooth-surfaced, often multiple, and randomly distributed throughout the stomach. The polyps are composed of hyperplastic glands that are often cystic and are lined by a single layer of mature mucus cells with abundant cytoplasm and small, basally located nuclei. Mitoses are rare, except in areas of surface inflammation. The stroma shows varying degrees of inflammation and granulation tissue. Although malignant transformation virtually never occurs, hyperplastic polyps can be associated with an independent, coexisting carcinoma elsewhere in the stomach.

ADENOMATOUS POLYP

Adenomas are true neoplasms that are composed of dysplastic glands and are capable of continued growth. They have a definite tendency toward malignant transformation, and the reported incidence of this complication increases with the size of the polyp (average, about 40%). Most adenomas are relatively large with an irregular, lobulated surface and deep fissures extending down to the base. They can be sessile or pedunculated. The majority are single lesions situated in the antrum. Histologically,

asymptomatic and discovered as incidental findings, some can bleed and produce hematemesis or melena. On rare occasions, a gastric polyp may prolapse through the pylorus and cause gastric outlet obstruction. The vast majority of epithelial polyps of the stomach can be divided into two groups: hyperplastic (regenerative) polyps and adenomas.

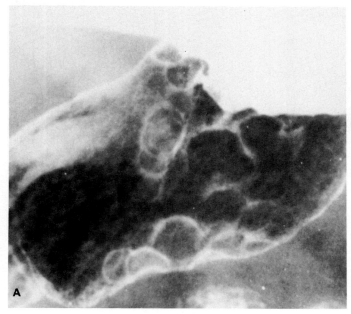

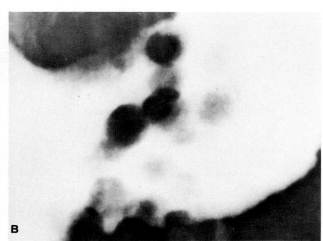

Fig. 18-4. Hyperplastic polyps. Multiple smooth filling defects of similar size are seen on **(A)** double-contrast and **(B)** filled views.

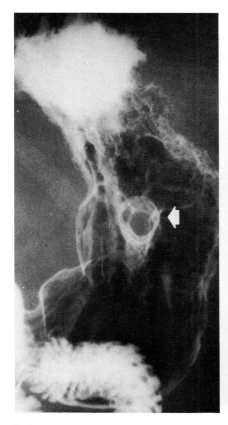

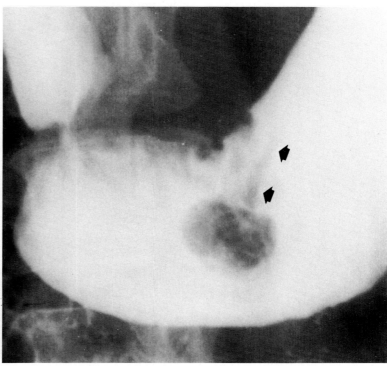

18-5   18-6

Fig. 18-5. Adenomatous polyp **(arrow)**.

Fig. 18-6. Adenomatous polyp. A long, thin pedicle **(arrows)** extends from the head of the polyp to the stomach wall.

adenomas have a papillary configuration with frequent mitoses in pseudostratified and poorly differentiated component cells. Inflammatory changes are not a prominent feature.

Radiographic Findings of Hyperplastic and Adenomatous Polyps

It has long been considered that the radiographic appearances of hyperplastic and adenomatous gastric polyps are distinct and reflect their pathologic characteristics. According to this concept, the hyperplastic polyp is typically a small (average, 1 cm), sharply defined filling defect with a smooth contour and no evidence of contrast in it (Fig. 18-3). When multiple, as is frequently the case, they all tend to be of about the same size (Fig. 18-4). Conversely, the adenomatous polyp has been thought to usually be a large (>2 cm) sessile lesion with an irregular surface (Fig. 18-5). Contrast material entering deep fissures and furrows in the polyp tends to produce a papillary or villous appearance. Adenomatous polyps are usually single and are most commonly

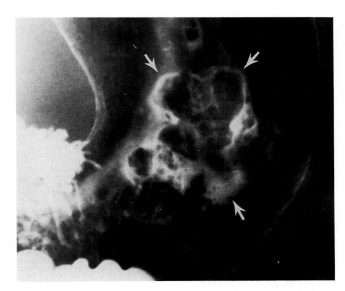

Fig. 18-7. Large hyperplastic gastric polyps. Coned view shows a conglomerate mass measuring over 4 cm in diameter in the body of the stomach. The size and broad-based configuration of this lesion raised the question of malignancy. (Smith HJ, Lee EL: Large hyperplastic polyps of the stomach. Gastrointest Radiol 8:19–23, 1983)

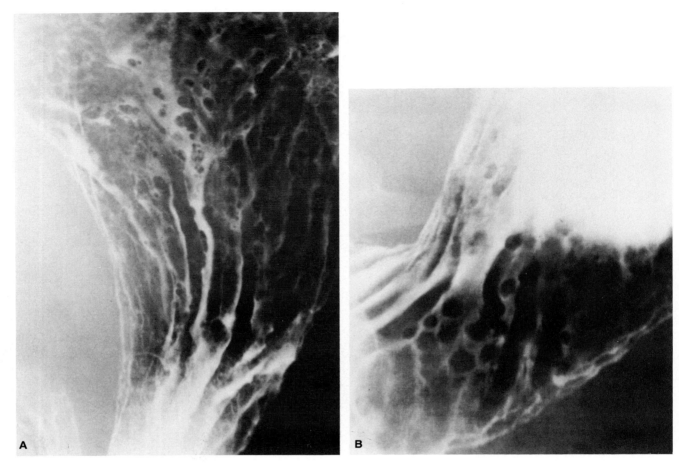

Fig. 18-8. Gastric polyposis associated with familial polyposis of the colon. (Denzler TB, Harned RK, Pergram CJ: Gastric polyps in familial polyposis coli. Radiology 130:63–66, 1979)

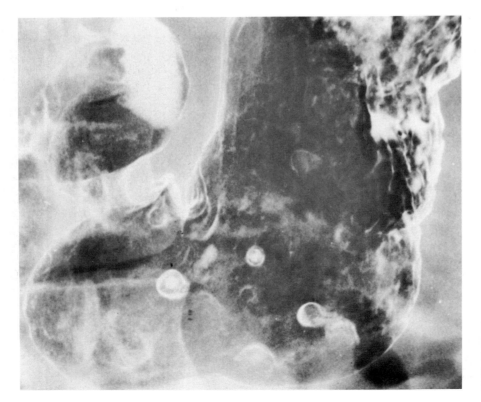

Fig. 18-9. Peutz-Jeghers syndrome. Note the multiple hamartomas of the stomach. The patient had small bowel polyps and mucocutaneous pigmentation.

found in the antrum. Active peristalsis in the stomach may permit a gastric polyp to develop a fairly long pedicle. This appears as a narrow, stalklike defect extending from the head of the polyp to the stomach wall (Fig. 18-6).

Unfortunately, more recent studies have demonstrated that the radiographic appearance may not be a reliable criterion for distinguishing between hyperplastic and adenomatous polyps. Reports of large hyperplastic polyps are not uncommon, and simple hyperplastic polyps may show lobulated or irregular contours suggestive of gastric adenoma or even frank malignancy (Fig. 18-7). On rare occasions, hyperplastic polyps demonstrate substantial growth within a relatively short time.

Although gastric adenomas can develop into carcinoma, usually this happens only with large lesions. Multiple small polyps in older patients are almost certainly hyperplastic. Therefore, it is currently recommended that endoscopy with biopsy and polypectomy is required only in patients with solitary gastric polyps or polyps larger than 2 cm in order to provide precise histologic identification. Surgery should be reserved for patients with obvious atypia or carcinoma.

Both hyperplastic and adenomatous polyps tend to develop in patients with chronic atrophic gastritis, a condition known to be associated with a high incidence of carcinoma. Thus, even though a gastric polyp is proved to be benign, the entire stomach must be carefully examined for the possibility of a coexisting carcinoma.

There is a higher than normal incidence of adenomatous and hyperplastic gastric polyps in patients with familial polyposis of the colon (Fig. 18-8). Gastric polyposis also occurs in the Cronkhite-Canada syndrome (colon polyposis, nail and hair changes), in which enlarged rugal folds and whiskering (multiple tiny projections due to barium trapped between nodular excrescences of rugae) have also been described.

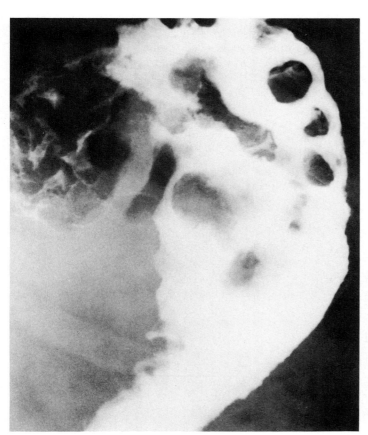

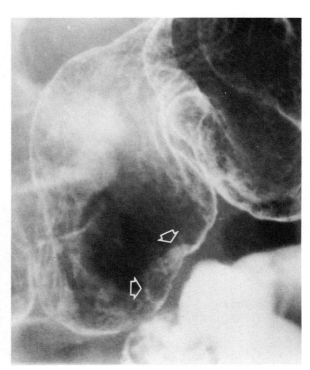

18-10   18-11

Fig. 18-10. Cowden's disease. Note the multiple gastric hamartomas. The patient had characteristic circumoral papillomatosis and nodular gingival hyperplasia. (Hauser H, Ody B, Plojoux O et al: Radiological findings in multiple hamartoma syndrome (Cowden disease). Radiology 137:317–323, 1980)

Fig. 18-11. Leiomyoma of the stomach. A small nodule **(arrows)** is seen on double-contrast examination.

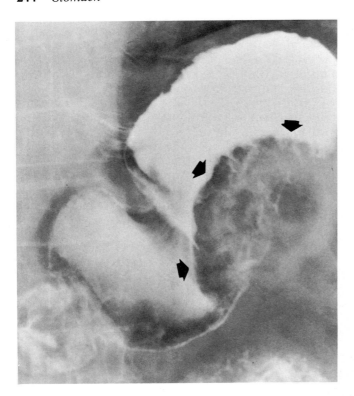

Fig. 18-12. Large leiomyoma involving the greater curvature of the stomach **(arrows)**.

HAMARTOMAS

Multiple gastric polyps can develop in patients with the Peutz-Jeghers syndrome (Fig. 18-9). The polyps, which are hamartomas with essentially no malignant potential, are composed of normal constituents of the mucosa arranged in a different manner. The true nature of the gastric filling defects in this condition is usually evident when other manifestations of the Peutz-Jeghers syndrome (small bowel polyps, mucocutaneous pigmentation) are present. In Cowden's disease (multiple hamartoma syndrome), hamartomas in the stomach and other parts of the gastrointestinal tract can be associated with the characteristic circumoral papillomatosis and nodular gingival hyperplasia (Fig. 18-10). In the Ruvalcaba–Myhre–Smith syndrome, hamartomas in the stomach and other parts of the gastrointestinal tract are associated with macrocephaly and hyperpigmented genital macules.

SPINDLE CELL TUMOR

Spindle cell tumors constitute the overwhelming majority of benign submucosal gastric neoplasms. These lesions vary in size from tiny nodules (Fig. 18-11), often discovered incidentally at laparotomy or autopsy, to bulky tumors with large intraluminal

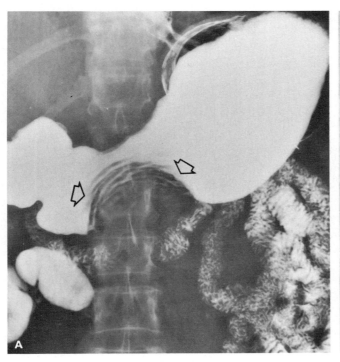

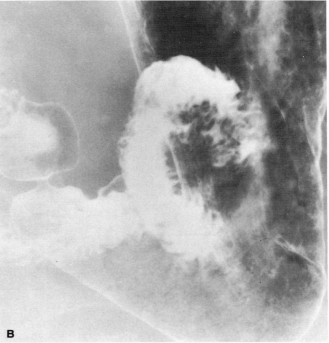

Fig. 18-13. Pseudomass **(arrows)**. **(A)** On the filled, supine film, the large "mass" simulates a spindle cell tumor on the greater curvature. **(B)** On the double-contrast view with the patient in a different position, the "mass" has disappeared. It therefore clearly represented a transient, extrinsic compression by a contiguous structure.

components that can be associated with hemorrhage, obstruction, or perforation (Fig. 18-12). Some spindle cell tumors have extensive exogastric components that can mimic extrinsic compression of the stomach by normal or enlarged liver, spleen, pancreas, or kidney. It is therefore essential that an apparent mass be identified on several projections with the patient in various positions so that the physician may be certain that the mass represents a true lesion and not merely extrinsic compression by a contiguous structure (Fig. 18-13). It may be extremely difficult to distinguish radiographically between benign spindle cell tumors and their malignant counterparts. Although large, markedly irregular filling defects with prominent ulcerations suggest malignancy, a radiographically benign tumor can be histologically malignant.

Leiomyoma is the most common spindle cell tumor of the stomach. Usually single rather than multiple, leiomyomas are composed of well-differentiated smooth muscle cells forming criss-crossing bundles that separate a richly vascularized collagen tissue. Small intramural tumor nodules cause cir-

cumscribed, rounded filling defects that closely resemble sessile gastric polyps. Leiomyomas can be extremely large and predominantly located in intraluminal (Fig. 18-14), intramural (Fig. 18-15), or extramural (Fig. 18-16) locations. Because of their tendency toward central necrosis and ulceration, bleeding is common as the tumor grows. Hematemesis or melena are frequent symptoms. Up to 5% of gastric leiomyomas demonstrate coarse calcification simulating uterine fibroids. Multiplicity of tumors suggests malignancy, though evidence of metastases is often the only radiographic indication that the lesion is not benign.

Lipomas, hemangiomas, fibromas, and neurogenic tumors, all of which can be radiographically indistinguishable from leiomyomas, are far less common submucosal gastric neoplasms. Lipomas are usually single and of moderate size (Fig. 18-17). They occur primarily in the antrum and tend to develop toward the lumen of the stomach and become pedunculated. Deep ulceration frequently occurs. Due to their pliability, gastric lipomas change shape in response to peristalsis and produce compressible

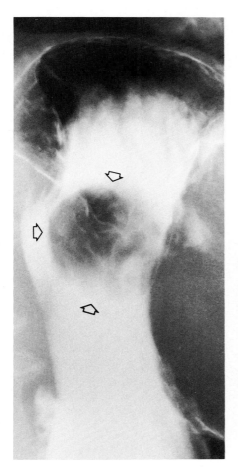

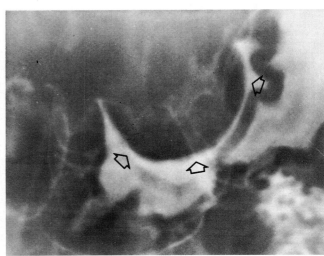

18-14   18-15

Fig. 18-14. Leiomyoma presenting as an intraluminal gastric mass **(arrows)**.

Fig. 18-15. Leiomyoma presenting as an intramural gastric mass **(arrows)**.

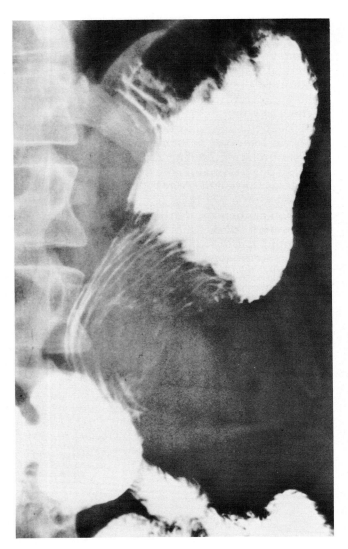

Fig. 18-16. Leiomyoma with a large exophytic component simulating an extrinsic mass.

nodular defects. Their fatty nature can be easily documented on computed tomography (Fig. 18-18 *A*, *B*), especially after the oral administration of dilute water-soluble material to reduce the artifacts due to air in the stomach so that the low-density mass may be more clearly imaged (Fig. 18-18*C*). Gastric hemangiomas are very rare and require the identification of characteristic phleboliths for preoperative diagnosis (Fig. 18-19). Fibromas are firm, elastic tumors consisting of fibroblasts grouped together in dense, intricate bundles. These very slow growing tumors are usually found in the antrum. Neurogenic tumors include neurolemmomas (Fig. 18-20) and neurofibromas and are sometimes a manifestation of von Recklinghausen's disease. Granular cell tumors are uncommon lesions of probable Schwann cell origin that may be associated with small asymptomatic masses in the skin, subcutaneous tissue, or mouth.

TUMORS OF VARIABLE MALIGNANT POTENTIAL

VILLOUS ADENOMA

Villous adenomas of the stomach are rare lesions that histologically and radiographically resemble colon tumors of the same type. Retention of contrast material among the villous projections results in a fine lacework of radiodense particles interspersed throughout the sessile mucosal lesion, producing a soap-bubble or frondlike appearance (Fig. 18-21). Often multiple, villous adenomas of the stomach are soft, pliable, and nonobstructing. As with this type of tumor in the colon, villous adenomas of the stomach have a substantial incidence of malignancy. In one large series of 16 villous adenomas of the stomach, all had evidence of *in situ* or invasive carcinoma.

CARCINOID TUMOR

Gastric carcinoid tumors arise from precursor neuroectodermal cells and most commonly present as sharply circumscribed, broad-based filling defects that are often ulcerated and may be located anywhere in the stomach (Fig. 18-22). Another radiographic manifestation is multiple sessile gastric polyps that are rarely pedunculated and usually do

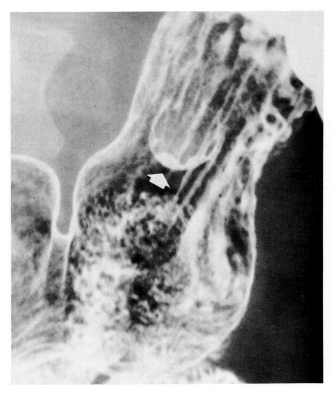

Fig. 18-17. Lipoma. A smooth, polypoid mass may be seen in the body of the stomach **(arrow)**.

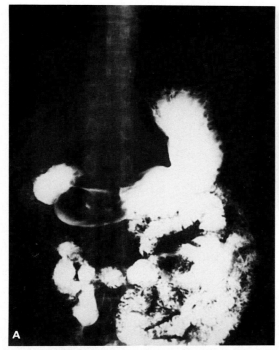

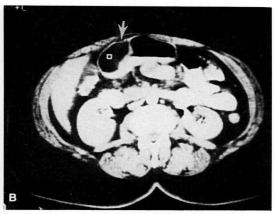

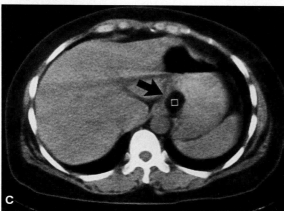

Fig. 18-18. Gastric lipoma. **(A)** Upper gastrointestinal series shows a round, smooth, large, fixed filling defect in the antrum with a persistent central collection of barium. The mass was soft to compression and caused no obstruction. **(B)** CT scan shows a submucosal antral mass **(arrow)**. The attenuation value (−100 HU) indicated that it was composed of fat. **(C)** CT scan shows an oval, sharply marginated, uniform fatty mass (attenuation value −100 HU) in the contrast-filled fornix of the stomach. (**[A,B]** Maderal F, Hunter F, Fuselier G et al: Gastric lipomas: An update of clinical presentation, diagnosis, and treatment. Am J Gastroenterol 79:964–967, 1984; **[C]** Imoto T, Nobe T, Koga M et al: Computed tomography of gastric lipomas. Gastrointest Radiol 8:129–131, 1983)

not ulcerate. A few cases have been reported of polypoid intraluminal tumors with irregular ulcerations and infiltration of the wall that produces an appearance indistinguishable from gastric adenocarcinoma. The reported incidence of metastases is 15% to 35%, but the lesions grow slowly and long survivals are seen even in the presence of regional or hepatic dissemination. Evidence of local invasion is common with tumors larger than 2 to 3 cm.

MALIGNANT TUMORS

POLYPOID CARCINOMA

The origin of polypoid carcinomas of the stomach is controversial. In most cases, they probably arise *de novo*, though malignant degeneration of an originally benign adenomatous polyp can occur. Patients with polypoid carcinoma of the stomach are frequently asymptomatic. The major clinical presentations are epigastric pain and unexplained anemia. Polypoid carcinoma develops more frequently in patients with atrophic gastritis and pernicious anemia than in the general population.

The radiographic distinction between benign and malignant gastric polyps can be extremely difficult. Lesions of less than 1 cm in diameter are usually benign. Polyps larger than 2 cm, particularly sessile ones, are more likely to be malignant, though many are benign. Irregularity and ulceration suggest malignancy (Fig. 18-23). Demonstration of a stalk, pliability of the wall of the stomach, normal-appearing gastric folds extending to the tumor, and unimpaired peristalsis are signs of benignancy. Mottled, granular calcific deposits in association with a gastric mass suggest a mucinous adenocarcinoma of the stomach (Fig. 18-24).

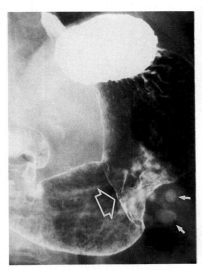

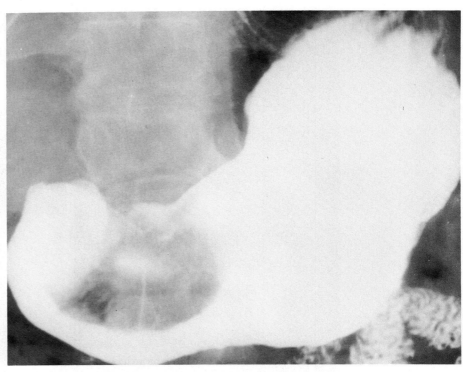

18-19   18-20

Fig. 18-19. Gastric hemangioma. Large mass **(open arrow)** involving the distal body of the stomach associated with characteristic phleboliths **(closed arrows)**. (Simms SM: Gastric hemangioma associated with phleboliths. Gastrointest Radiol 10:51–53, 1985)

Fig. 18-20. Neurolemmoma. The antral mass is large and smooth with central ulceration.

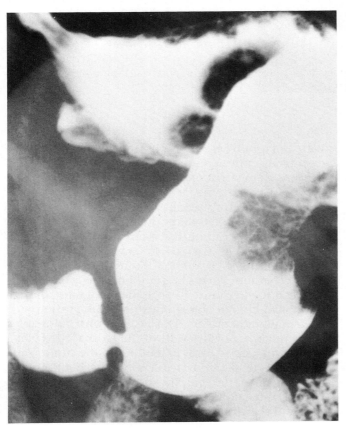

Fig. 18-21. Villous adenoma. Barium entering the interstices of the tumor creates a frondlike appearance. (Miller JH, Gisvold JJ, Weiland LH: Upper gastrointestinal tract: Villous tumors. AJR 134:933–936, 1980. Copyright 1980. Reproduced with permission)

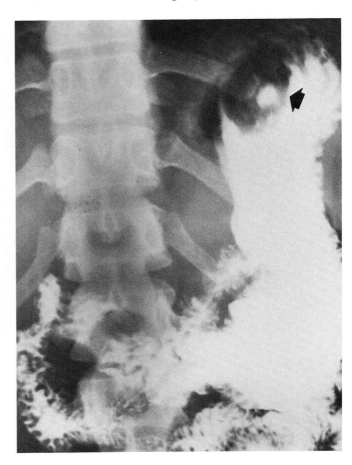

Fig. 18-22. Gastric carcinoid tumor. Ulcerated submucosal mass in the fundus **(arrow)** that is radiographically indistinguishable from leiomyoma. (Balthazar EJ, Megibow A, Bryk D et al: Gastric carcinoid tumors: Radiographic features in eight cases. AJR 139:1123–1127, 1982 Copyright 1982. Reproduced with permission.)

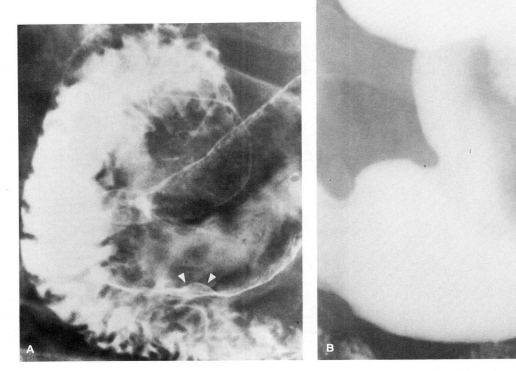

Fig. 18-23. Adenocarcinoma of the stomach. **(A)** Tiny malignant mass **(arrowheads)** on the greater curvature. **(B)** Large ulcerated polypoid mass in the body of the stomach.

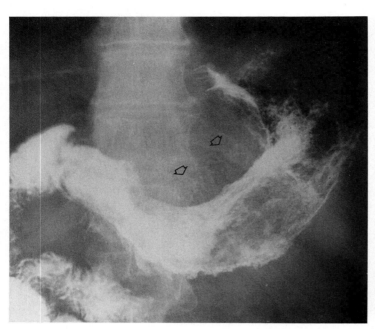

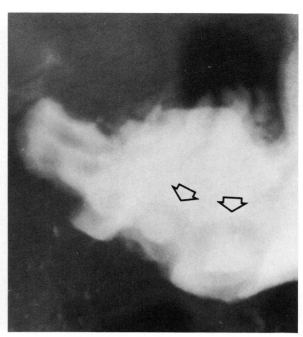

18-24

18-25

Fig. 18-24. Mucinous adenocarcinoma. Numerous granular calcifications are present in the thickened gastric wall **(arrows)**. (Ghahremani GG, Meyers MA, Port RB: Calcified primary tumors of the gastrointestinal tract. Gastrointestinal Radiol 2:331–339, 1978)

Fig. 18-25. Lymphoma. Multiple ulcerated, polypoid gastric masses are visible **(arrows)**.

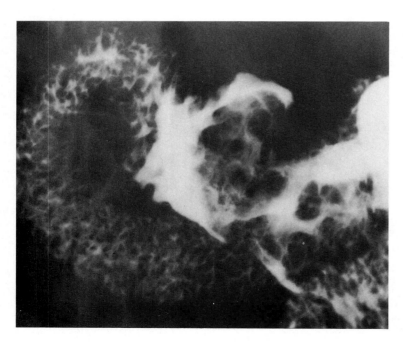

Fig. 18-26. Lymphoma. Multiple polypoid filling defects with generalized thickening of folds involve the antrum and duodenal bulb.

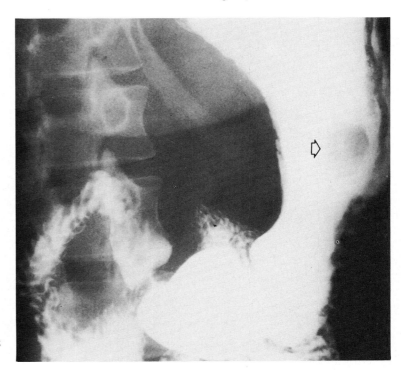

Fig. 18-27. Burkitt's lymphoma. A solitary mass **(arrow)** is evident in the body of the stomach.

LYMPHOMA

As elsewhere in the bowel, lymphoma of the stomach is a great imitator of both benign and malignant disease. One manifestation of gastric lymphoma is a large, bulky polypoid lesion, usually irregular and ulcerated, that can be difficult to differentiate from gastric carcinoma. A radiographic finding favoring the diagnosis of lymphoma is the presence of multiple ulcerating, polypoid tumors (Fig. 18-25). These polyps can be combined with thickened folds (infiltrative form of lymphoma) (Fig. 18-26) or separated by a normal-appearing mucosal pattern, unlike the atrophic mucosal background that is seen with multiple carcinomatous polyps in patients with pernicious anemia. Filling defects in the stomach are unusual manifestations of Burkitt's lymphoma (Fig. 18-27).

METASTASES

Hematogenous metastases infrequently involve the stomach and produce single (Fig. 18-28) or multiple (Fig. 18-29) gastric filling defects. Abdominal symptoms tend to be relatively nonspecific or entirely absent. Anorexia, nausea, vomiting, and epigastric distress are the most common complaints, but these symptoms are frequently attributed to other gastric disorders or to the side-effects of chemotherapeutic drugs. On rare occasions, gastric hemorrhage or outlet obstruction develops.

Metastatic melanoma is the most common hematogenous metastasis to cause single or multiple filling defects in the barium-filled stomach. These lesions are usually ulcerated or umbilicated and have a bull's-eye appearance (Fig. 18-30). Gastric metastases from malignant melanoma are almost invariably associated with the common metastases of this tumor to the small bowel.

Rarely, single or multiple discrete filling defects, with or without associated ulceration, can be demonstrated in patients with metastases to the stomach from carcinoma of the breast (Fig. 18-31). Much more commonly, gastric involvement by this primary tumor produces narrowing of the stomach and a linitis plastica pattern. Direct invasion of the stomach by carcinoma of the pancreas or transverse colon (by way of the gastrocolic ligament) typically causes a filling defect (often irregular) along the greater curvature (Fig. 18-32). A similar pattern can be produced by so-called omental "cakes," bulky metastases to the greater omentum that most often result from widespread intraperitoneal seeding of pelvic or gastrointestinal malignancies (Fig. 18-33).

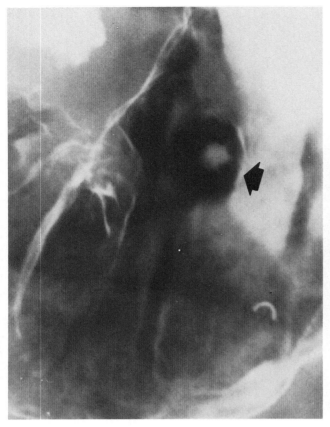

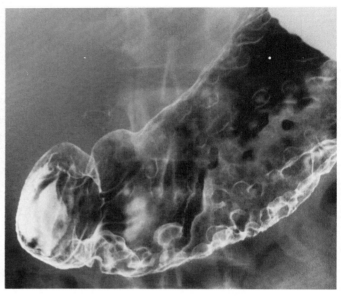

18-28   18-29

Fig. 18-28. Undifferentiated carcinoma metastatic to the stomach. Note the ulcerated filling defect **(arrow)**.

Fig. 18-29. Bronchogenic carcinoma metastatic to the stomach. Multiple filling defects, several of which contain central ulceration.

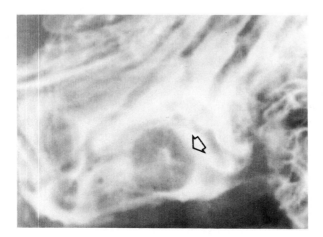

Fig. 18-30. Metastatic melanoma. Note the large, ulcerated filling defect with a bull's-eye appearance **(arrow)**. Several smaller, nodular lesions can also be seen.

Spread of carcinoma of the body or tail of the pancreas can also extend around the stomach and invade the lesser curvature (Fig. 18-34).

SARCOMA

Sarcomas are rare malignant tumors of the stomach. Most are leiomyosarcomas, large, bulky tumors most often found in the body of the stomach. Although originally arising in an intramural location, leiomyosarcomas often present as intraluminal (Fig. 18-35), occasionally pedunculated masses. They frequently undergo extensive central necrosis, causing ulceration and gastrointestinal bleeding. Leiomyosarcomas are usually single lesions but infrequently are multiple. Extensive spread into surrounding tissues is common (as are metastases to

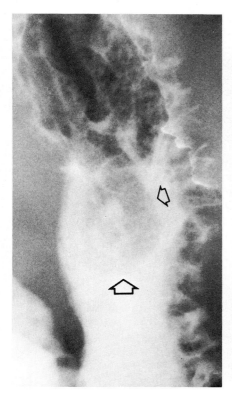

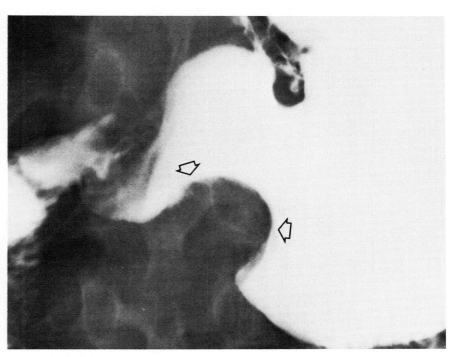

18-31   **18-32**

Fig. 18-31. Metastatic breast carcinoma. There is a filling defect with central ulceration **(arrows)** in the body of the stomach.

Fig. 18-32. Metastatic adenocarcinoma of the pancreas. A smooth mass **(arrows)** is visible along the greater curvature of the antrum.

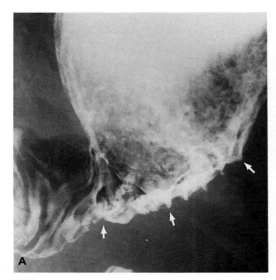

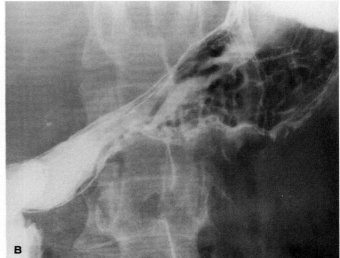

Fig. 18-33. Omental "cakes." **(A)** Nodularity and tethered spiculated mucosal folds on the greater curvature of the stomach **(arrows)** caused by direct extension of omental metastases from breast carcinoma. (Antral narrowing seen on this film was a transient finding due to gastric peristalsis.) **(B)** Mass effect and nodularity of the greater curvature due to omental metastases from cecal carcinoma. (Rubesin SE, Levine MS, Glick SN: Gastric involvement by omental cakes: Radiographic findings. Gastrointest Radiol 11:223–228, 1986)

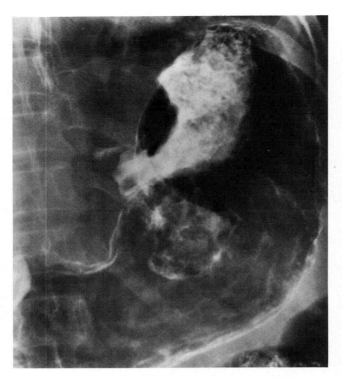

Fig. 18-34. Metastatic adenocarcinoma of the body and tail of the pancreas. The irregular, ulcerated mass predominantly involves the lesser curvature of the stomach.

the liver, omentum, and retroperitoneum), and the resulting large exogastric component may suggest an extrinsic lesion (Fig. 18-36). It is frequently difficult to radiographically differentiate leiomyosarcoma from leiomyoma, its benign spindle cell counterpart. The presence of a large exogastric mass suggests the presence of malignancy.

Computed tomography may demonstrate either the primary intragastric lesion or the large extraluminal component of a leiomyosarcoma (Fig. 18-37). Characteristic findings in tumors of this histologic type are small foci of calcification and well-defined, low-density areas within the mass, representing either areas of necrosis and liquefaction or a cystic component to the tumor. Unlike gastric adenocarcinoma or lymphoma, leiomyosarcomas of the stomach commonly metastasize to the liver and lung; spread to regional lymph nodes is unusual.

Rare sarcomas of the stomach include liposarcoma (Fig. 18-38) and leiomyoblastoma. Leiomyoblastomas are low-grade malignancies that arise from a distinct smooth muscle cell (leiomyoblast) (Fig. 18-39). These intramural masses have a tendency to grow into the lumen as they enlarge. Except for their marked predilection to arise in the antrum rather than in the body or fundus of the stomach, gastric leiomyoblastomas are radiographically essentially identical to other sarcomas.

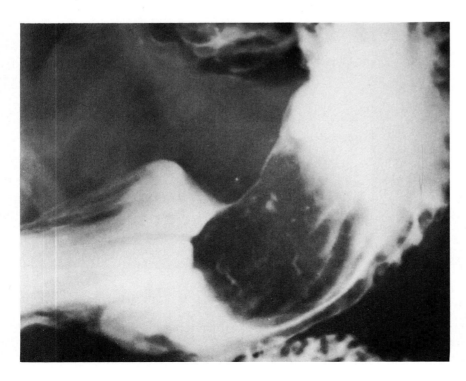

Fig. 18-35. Leiomyosarcoma. The bulky tumor, which arises in the body of the stomach, contains some central ulceration.

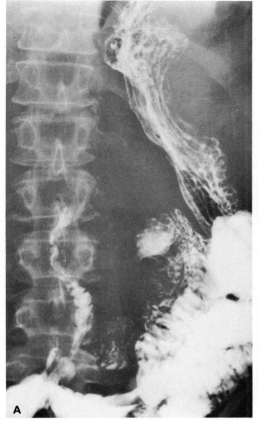
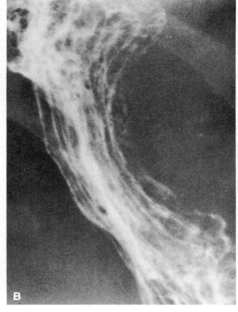
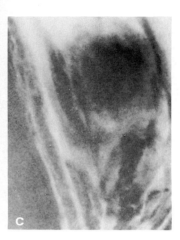

Fig. 18-36. Leiomyosarcoma. **(A)** Full and **(B)** coned-down views demonstrate the large exogastric component of the lesion. The liver is enormously enlarged. **(C)** The *en face* view demonstrates the intramural portion of the mass, suggesting a tumor of the spindle cell type.

In patients with AIDS, Kaposi's sarcoma can produce multiple different-sized submucosal nodules, most of which show no umbilications or ulcerations (Fig. 18-40). Multiple coalescing nodules infiltrating the submucosa can cause thickening and irregularity of rugal folds and even lead to circumferential narrowing of the lumen.

PLASMACYTOMA

Isolated plasmacytoma is a rare lesion of the intestinal tract that involves the stomach and small bowel much more often than the colon or esophagus. At times, the plasma cell neoplasm involving the stomach may be a manifestation of multiple myeloma. Depending on the site of involvement, a plasmacytoma may cause symptoms of gastric ulcer or outlet obstruction. Most patients are over age 50, and men predominate.

The radiographic findings of plasmacytoma of the stomach are varied and may simulate carcinoma, lymphoma, solitary or multiple polypoid lesions of any histologic type (Fig. 18-41), or inflammatory stricture. Radiation is often the treatment used for primary extramedullary plasmacytoma, with careful follow-up to ensure that the lesion is not a precursor of multiple myeloma.

EXTRINSIC CYSTIC OR INFLAMMATORY MASSES

Cystic and inflammatory masses arising outside the stomach can cause extrinsic impressions mimicking intramural or intraluminal gastric lesions. Cysts of the liver (Fig. 18-42), spleen, kidney, or adrenal and upper abdominal abscesses (Fig. 18-43) can produce this radiographic appearance.

ECTOPIC PANCREAS

Aberrant pancreatic tissue (ectopic pancreas) can be found in many areas of the gastrointestinal tract but is most common on the distal greater curvature of the gastric antrum within 3 cm to 6 cm of the pylorus (Fig. 18-44). About half of patients with ectopic pancreas are symptomatic and complain of vague abdominal pain, nausea, and occasional vom-

Text continues on page 259

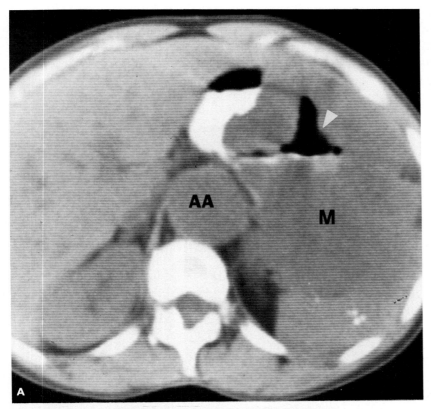

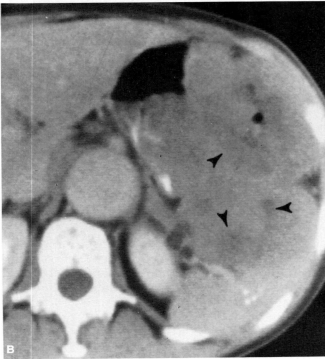

Fig. 18-37. Leiomyosarcoma. **(A)** CT scan shows a large mass **(M)** that is primarily exogastric. There is contrast material in the distorted gastric lumen as well as in an excavation **(arrowhead)** within the tumor. An abdominal aortic aneurysm **(AA)** is also present. **(B)** Following the administration of intravenous contrast material, low-density areas **(arrowheads)** characteristic of leiomyosarcoma are evident within the mass. (Mauro MA, Koehler RE: Alimentary tract. In Lee JKT, Sagel SS, Stanley RJ (eds): Computed Body Tomography, New York, Raven, 1983)

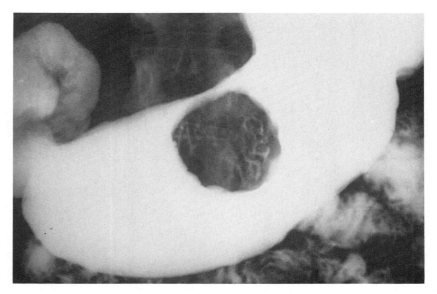

18-38

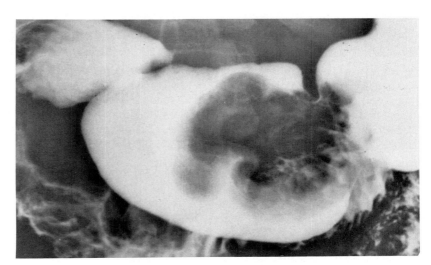

18-39

Fig. 18-38. Liposarcoma. The mildly irregular antral filling defect is extremely radiolucent, probably reflecting its fatty composition.

Fig. 18-39. Leiomyoblastoma. The antral mass is huge and irregular.

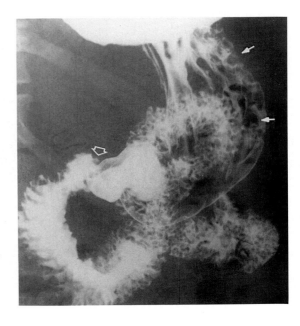

Fig. 18-40. Kaposi's sarcoma in a young homosexual male with AIDS. Multiple nodules are evident in the body of the stomach **(closed arrows)** and duodenal bulb **(open arrow)**, and there is narrowing of the lumen of the transverse duodenum. (Wall FD, Ominsky S, Altman DF et al: Multifocal abnormalities of the gastrointestinal tract in AIDS. AJR 146:1–5, 1986)

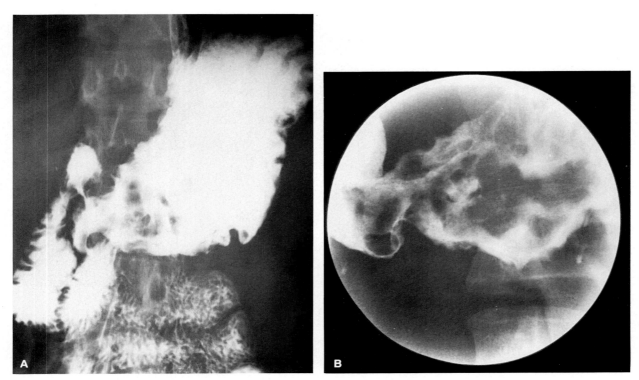

Fig. 18-41.   Gastric plasmacytoma. **(A)** Full and **(B)** coned views of a single-contrast upper gastrointestinal series demonstrate markedly thickened folds with ulcerations that appeared endoscopically as multiple ulcerated polypoid lesions. Two years after the examination the patient had not developed any other lesions or evidence of multiple myeloma. (Carlson HC, Breen JF: Amyloidosis and plasma cell dyscrasias: Gastrointestinal involvement. Semin Roentgenol 21:128–138, 1986)

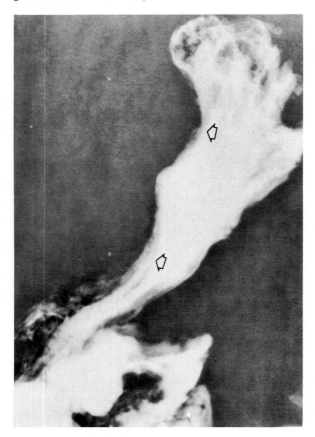

Fig. 18-42.   Polycystic liver. The two large, extrinsic impressions **(arrows)** on the anterior aspect of the stomach mimic intramural lesions.

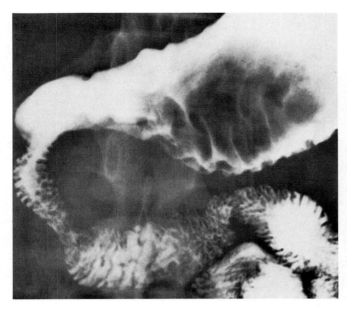

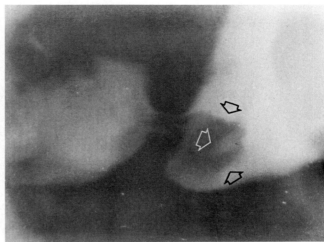

18-43

18-44

Fig. 18-43. Pancreatic abscess. The large retrogastric inflammatory process causes edema and effacement of rugal folds. Radiographically, the abscess appears as a discrete mass in the body and antrum of the stomach.

Fig. 18-44. Ectopic pancreas. There is a filling defect in the distal antrum **(black open arrows)** with a central collection of barium **(white open arrow)**.

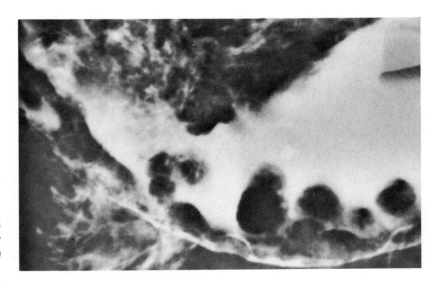

Fig. 18-45. Multiple nodular filling defects suggesting polyps. The filling defects are due to enlarged gastric folds, which are viewed on end in this patient with alcoholic gastritis.

iting. Bleeding can occur if the overlying mucosa becomes ulcerated. Radiographically, ectopic pancreas appears as a smooth submucosal mass, rarely more than 2 cm in diameter, that often has a central dimple or umbilication representing the orifice of the duct associated with the aberrant pancreatic tissue.

ENLARGED GASTRIC FOLDS

Enlarged gastric folds, when viewed on end, can produce a radiographic pattern of multiple nodular filling defects suggesting polyps (Fig. 18-45). This appearance can be seen in patients with Menetrier's disease (Fig. 18-46) or gastric varices (Fig. 18-47), as

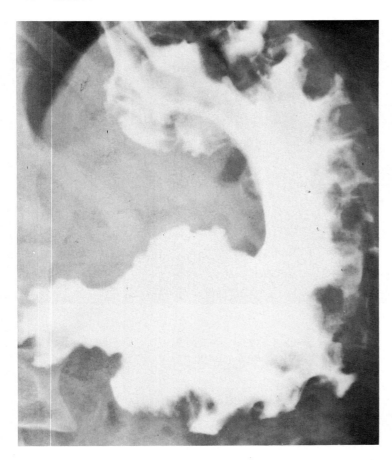

Fig. 18-46. Menetrier's disease. Diffuse thickening of rugal folds simulates the appearance of multiple polypoid filling defects.

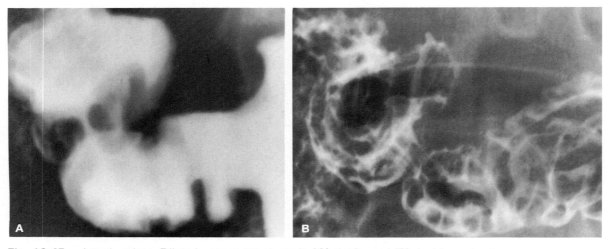

Fig. 18-47. Antral varices. Dilated venous structures in **(A)** single- and **(B)** double-contrast views simulate multiple polypoid filling defects.

well as in persons with thickened rugal folds due to granulomatous infiltration (Crohn's disease, sarcoidosis, tuberculosis) or eosinophilic gastritis.

HYPERTROPHIED ANTRAL-PYLORIC FOLD

A short, fixed, solitary prominent fold in the gastric antrum that extends across the pylorus into the duodenal bulb and is best seen with antral distention (Fig. 18-48) has been recently reported in about 3% of double-contrast upper gastrointestinal examinations. Although the clinical significance of this fold is undetermined, endoscopic examination suggests it is a manifestation of chronic gastritis. This appearance must be distinguished from transpyloric herniation of antral mucosa (antral prolapse), which is transient, appears more prominent when the antrum is contracted, and usually disappears during antral diastole. In addition, antral mucosal prolapse is usually associated with generalized antral fold thickening, expands the pylorus, and generally appears as submucosal filling defects on both the superior and inferior aspects of the base of the duodenal bulb. The characteristic location of the prominent mucosal fold with extension across a nondistorted pylorus to the base of the bulb is distinctive and should permit differentiation of a hypertrophied antral-pyloric fold from a true gastric or duodenal submucosal mass or a gastric mucosal neoplasm.

BEZOAR

A bezoar is an intragastric mass composed of accumulated ingested material (Fig. 18-49). Phytobezoars, which are composed of undigested vegetable material, have classically been associated with the eating of unripe persimmons, a fruit containing substances that coagulate on contact with gastric acid to produce a stickly gelatinous material, which then traps seeds, skin, and other foodstuffs. Numerous other substances that can apparently form bezoars include glue (especially in persons making model airplanes), tar, paraffin, shellac, asphalt, bismuth carbonate, magnesium carbonate, laundry starch, and wood fibers.

Trichobezoars (hairballs) occur predominantly in females, especially those with schizophrenia or other mental instability. The accumulated matted mass of hair can enlarge to occupy the entire volume of the stomach, often assuming the shape of the organ. A small percentage of bezoars are composed of both hair and vegetable matter and are termed trichophytobezoars.

Symptoms of gastric bezoars result from the mechanical presence of the foreign body. They include cramplike epigastric pain and a sense of dragging, fullness, lump, or heaviness in the upper abdomen. The incidence of associated peptic ulcers is high, especially with the more abrasive phytobezoars. When bezoars are large, symptoms of pyloric

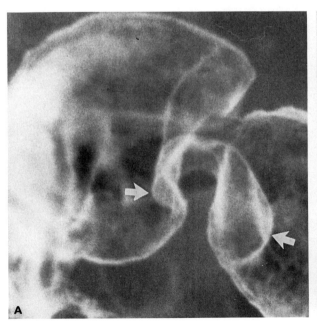
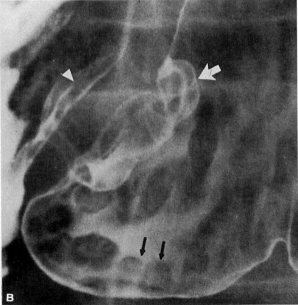

Fig. 18-48. Hypertrophied antral-pyloric fold. **(A)** Hypertrophied fold **(arrows)** on the greater curvature aspect of the pylorus. **(B)** In another patient, a nodular fold **(white arrow)** simulates a plaquelike mass on the lesser curvature of the antrum. Note the characteristic extension into the duodenal bulb **(arrowhead)**. Nodular erosions are also present in the antrum **(black arrows)**. (Glick SN, Cavanaugh B, Teplick SK: The hypertrophied antral-pyloric fold. AJR 145:547–549, 1985. Copyright 1985. Reproduced with permission.)

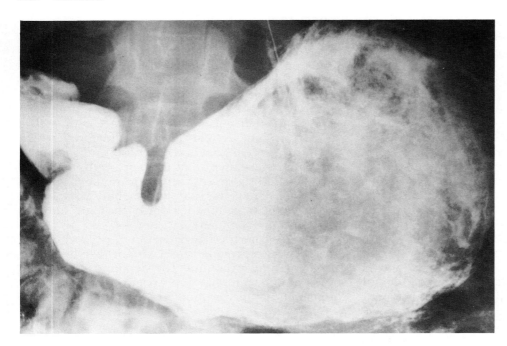

Fig. 18-49. Bezoar. The large intragastric filling defect is composed of accumulated ingested material.

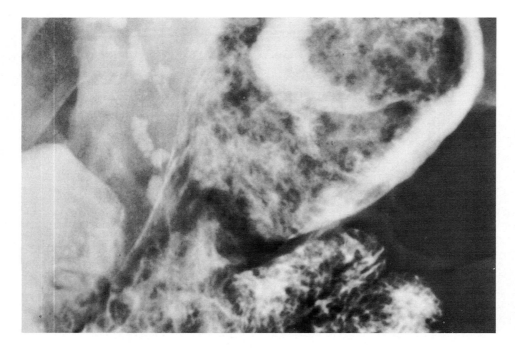

Fig. 18-50. Bezoar. Infiltration of contrast into the interstices of the mass results in a characteristic mottled appearance.

obstruction can clinically simulate symptoms of a gastric carcinoma.

Plain abdominal radiographs often show the bezoar as a soft-tissue mass floating in the stomach at the air-fluid interface. On barium studies, contrast coating of the mass and infiltration into the interstices result in a characteristic mottled or streaked appearance (Fig. 18-50). The filling defect is occasionally completely smooth, simulating an enormous gas bubble that is freely movable within the stomach (Fig. 18-51).

FOREIGN BODY/INTRAMURAL HEMATOMA

Foreign bodies can present as lucent filling defects within the barium-filled stomach. This appearance can be produced by a variety of ingested substances including food, pills, and nondigestable material. In patients with esophageal or gastric bleeding, blood clots can appear as single or multiple filling defects in the stomach. Hemorrhage into the wall of the stomach secondary to a bleeding diathesis, anticoagulant therapy, or trauma can present as a large intramural gastric mass (Fig. 18-52), which most commonly involves the fundus.

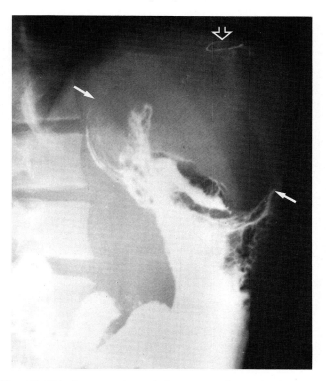

Fig. 18-52. Intramural gastric hematoma. Large fundal mass **(closed arrows)** that developed in a patient on anticoagulant therapy because of mitral and aortic valve replacement. Note the surgical wires in the lower sternum indicative of previous sternotomy **(open arrow)**. Follow-up examination after 6 weeks of conservative management showed complete resolution. (Balthazar EJ: Miscellaneous disorders of the stomach. In Taveras JM, Ferruci JT (eds): Radiology: Diagnosis–Imaging–Intervention. Philadelphia, JB Lippincott, 1987)

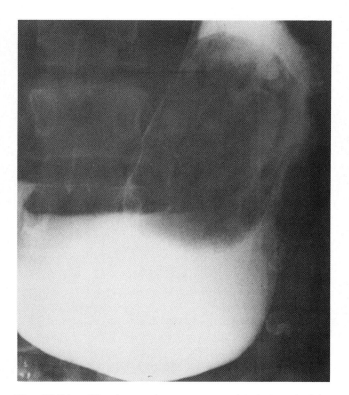

Fig. 18-51. Glue bezoar in a young model-airplane builder. The smooth mass simulates an enormous gas bubble.

BENIGN GASTRIC ULCER

A benign gastric ulcer surrounded by a large mound of edema can mimic the discrete filling defect produced by an ulcerated intramural tumor (Fig. 18-53). Thickened folds in the vicinity of the ulcerated lesion, especially if they radiate toward it, suggest peptic disease (Fig. 18-54). Even if classic radiating folds are not evident, point-like projections from the ulcer crater representing termination of radiating folds probably have similar significance. Follow-up examination usually shows rapid healing of the ulcer and diminished size of the filling defect due to the edematous ulcer mound.

A large incisura on the greater curvature can simulate a discrete filling defect in the stomach (Fig. 18-55). The true nature of this "mass" is evident once the lesser curvature ulcer inciting the incisura formation has been identified.

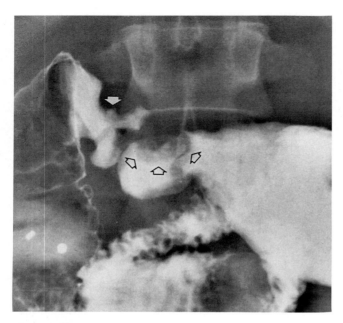

Fig. 18-53. *Prepyloric antral ulcer. Extensive edema surrounding the benign ulcer simulates a discrete filling defect* **(open arrows)**. *Note the associated ulceration* **(solid arrow)** *and deformity of the duodenal bulb.*

DOUBLE PYLORUS

Double pylorus is a form of gastroduodenal fistula that consists of a short accessory channel connecting the lesser curvature of the prepyloric antrum to the superior aspect of the duodenal bulb (Fig. 18-56). This phenomenon is almost invariably associated with acute or chronic peptic disease. An ulcer crater can usually be demonstrated within or immediately adjacent to the accessory channel. The formation of a second channel often results in the reduction of ulcer pain, presumably due to improvement of gastric emptying. The two pyloric channels are separated by a bridge or septum of normal mucosa that appears radiographically as a round lucency simulating a discrete filling defect (Fig. 18-57).

EOSINOPHILIC GRANULOMA

Eosinophilic granuloma of the stomach, most commonly located in the gastric antrum, usually appears radiographically as a sharply defined, smooth-bordered, round or oval filling defect (Fig.

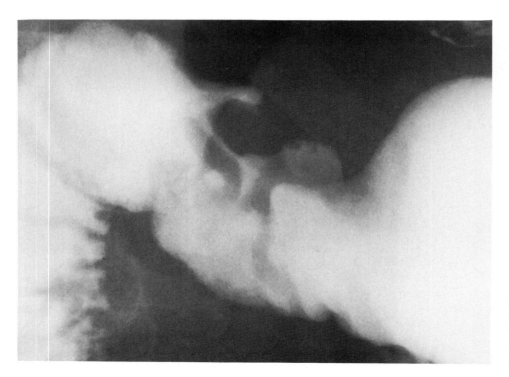

Fig. 18-54. *Prepyloric antral ulcer simulating a discrete mass. The thickened folds radiating toward the lesion suggest peptic ulcer disease.*

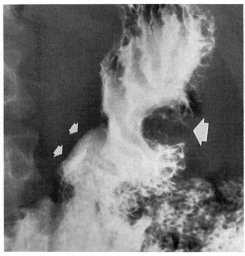 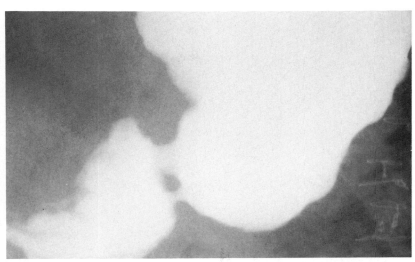

18-55   18-56

Fig. 18-55.   Large incisura simulating a filling defect on the greater curvature **(large arrow)**. The incisura is incited by a long ulcer **(small arrows)** on the lesser curvature.

Fig. 18-56.   Double pylorus.

Fig. 18-57.   Double pylorus. The true pylorus and the accessory channel along the lesser curvature are separated by a bridge, or septum, that produces the appearance of a discrete lucent filling defect **(arrow)**.

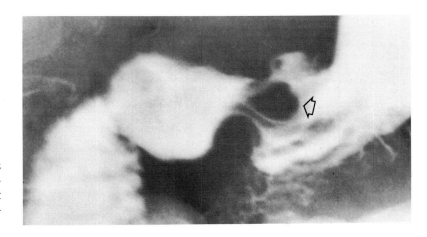

18-58). It is unrelated to the lesion of the same name in bone and lung. Eosinophilic granuloma of the stomach is a benign polypoid process containing a nonspecific inflammatory infiltrate. Because the histologic appearance of the lesion suggests that it is a special type of granulation and connective tissue response, it has also been labeled inflammatory fibroid polyp. Although the polyp is infiltrated by varying numbers of eosinophils, it differs from eosinophilic gastritis in that it is not associated with any food allergy or peripheral eosinophilia. Most eosinophilic granulomas of the stomach are solitary and sessile; a few are pedunculated. Patients with eosinophilic granuloma of the stomach are usually asymptomatic, though some have pain occasionally

accompanied by nausea and vomiting. Intermittent pyloric obstruction by the polyp or bleeding secondary to erosion of the overlying mucosa can occur in this disorder.

ARTERIAL IMPRESSION

The splenic artery frequently produces a contour defect on the posteromedial aspect of the stomach, particularly in elderly patients. When the artery is tortuous or aneurysmal, the impression is prominent and may simulate a gastric neoplasm (Fig. 18-59). The proximal portion of the splenic artery

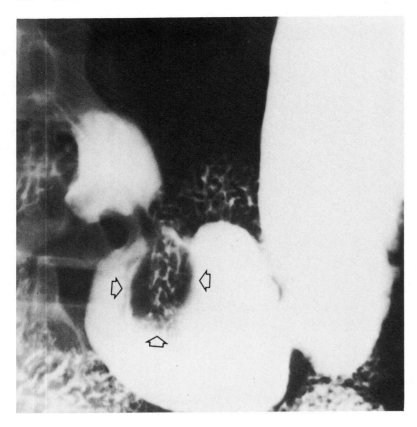

Fig. 18-58. Eosinophilic granuloma. A sharply defined, smooth-bordered oval filling defect may be seen in the gastric antrum **(arrows)**.

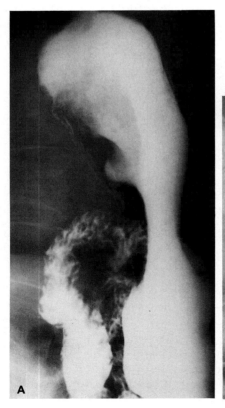

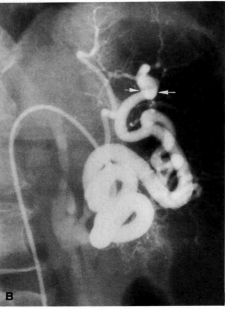

Fig. 18-59. Arterial impression. **(A)** Lateral view of the stomach shows a broad multilobular defect on the posterior wall. Barium between adjacent defects simulates an ulcer. **(B)** Arteriogram shows that the splenic artery is extremely tortuous and indents the contour of the gas-filled stomach. There is also a small aneurysm **(arrows)**. (Childress MH, Cho KY, Newlin N et al: Arterial impressions on the stomach. AJR 132:769–772, 1979. Copyright 1979. Reproduced with permission.)

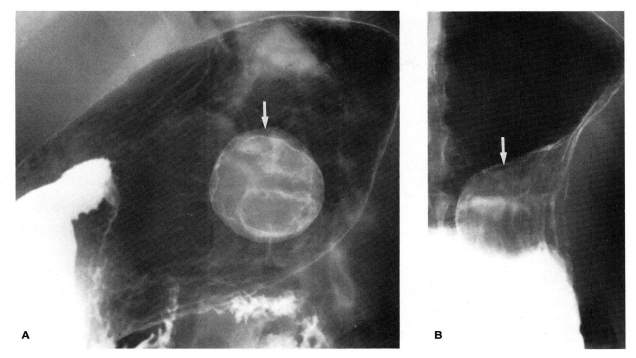

Fig. 18-60. Gastric duplication cyst. **(A)** *En face* and **(B)** profile views show the typical intramural fluid-filled mass with a smooth surface covered by normal gastric mucosa. (Balthazar EJ: Miscellaneous disorders of the stomach. In Taveras JM, Ferruci JT [eds]: Radiology: Diagnosis–Imaging–Intervention. Philadelphia, JB Lippincott, 1987)

may involve the stomach near the incisura, whereas the more distal segment of the artery often produces a defect near the cardia. The impression on the stomach is almost always broad and shallow, characteristic of an extrinsic rather than an intramural lesion. The overlying gastric mucosa is invariably intact. Calcification of the splenic artery can indicate the position of the vessel. Gastric impressions can also be produced by tortuosity or aneurysm of the abdominal aorta.

GASTRIC DUPLICATION CYST

Gastric duplications are very rare lesions that contain all layers of the gastric wall. They vary in size and can be tubular, fusiform, or spherical. Gastric duplications are most commonly found along the greater curvature and rarely communicate with the lumen of the stomach.

In the majority of patients, the diagnosis of gastric duplication cyst is made during infancy because of an abdominal mass, vomiting, failure to thrive, or anemia. Less commonly, patients may be asymptomatic, and the congenital lesion remains unrecognized until it causes upper abdominal pain, an epigastric mass, or obstructive symptoms, or until it is noted as an incidental finding on an upper gastrointestinal series. Peptic ulceration in communicating

duplications causes bleeding that can present as hematemesis, melena, or unexplained anemia. Perforation of a gastric duplication is a serious complication that can result in severe peritonitis.

On barium examination, a gastric duplication cyst usually appears as an extrinsic or intramural mass in a characteristic location along the greater curvature of the stomach (Fig. 18-60). Contrast material is rarely seen to fill the duplication by way of a communication between it and the gastric lumen (Fig. 18-61). A CT scan can demonstrate the relationship of the mass to the gastric wall and reveal the nonenhancing homogeneous or fluid/debris contents of the cyst or its filling with small amounts of barium or gas (Fig. 18-62).

PSEUDOLYMPHOMA

Pseudolymphoma can cause a tumorlike gastric mass that often demonstrates superficial or large, central ulceration. This disorder represents benign, reactive proliferation of lymphoid tissue clinically and histologically simulating lymphoma.

INTRAGASTRIC GALLSTONE

An extremely rare cause of filling defects in the stomach is intragastric gallstones. A gallstone may

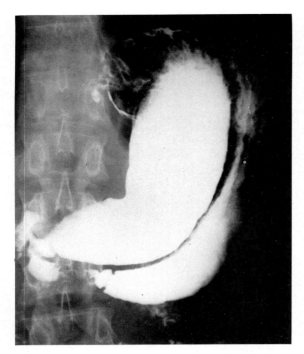

Fig. 18-61. *Communicating gastric duplication cyst. Both lumens are clearly visualized during an upper gastrointestinal examination. (Balthazar EJ: Miscellaneous disorders of the stomach. In Taveras JM, Ferruci JT (eds): Radiology: Diagnosis–Imaging–Intervention. Philadelphia, JB Lippincott, 1987)*

pass from the duodenum into the stomach either by retrograde flow from the duodenum following cholecystoduodenal fistula or directly through a cholecystogastric fistula. Like other foreign bodies in the stomach, intragastric gallstones can cause mucosal irritation leading to ulceration, bleeding, perforation, and even gastric outlet obstruction.

TUMEFACTIVE EXTRAMEDULLARY HEMATOPOIESIS

Tumefactive extramedullary hematopoiesis of the stomach very rarely produces a submucosal gastric mass (Fig. 18-63). Extramedullary hematopoiesis develops when normal blood-forming sites cannot maintain a rate of red-blood-cell formation sufficient for body demand, as in patients with leukemia, myelofibrosis, severe anemia, polycythemia, Hodgkin's disease, and chronic poisoning with marrow-toxic substances. Extramedullary hematopoietic collections, usually microscopic, are most commonly found in the liver, spleen, and lymph nodes. Infrequently, extramedullary hematopoiesis can form significant tumor masses involving multiple organs, including the upper gastrointestinal tract. In patients with chronic myelogenous leukemia, tumefactive extramedullary hematopoiesis of the stomach may be indistinguishable from a gastric polypoid mass secondary to leukemic infiltrate.

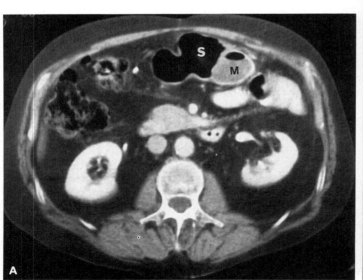

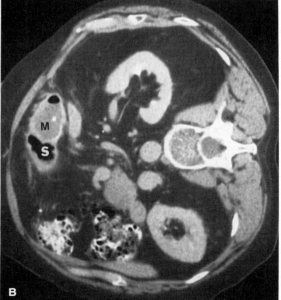

Fig. 18-62. *Gastric duplication cyst.* **(A)** *With the patient scanned in the routine supine position, the mass* **(M)** *is seen associated with the gastric wall* **(S**, *stomach). There is a gas–fluid level within the cyst, which has a smooth, thin, and symmetric wall.* **(B)** *CT scan obtained in the lateral decubitus position confirms the location of the mass* **(M)** *within the stomach* **(S)** *wall. Note that the gas–fluid level has changed position and that there is a fleck of barium within the cyst. (Hulnick DH, Balthazar EJ: Gastric duplication cyst: GI series and CT correlation. Gastrointest Radiol 12:106–108, 1987)*

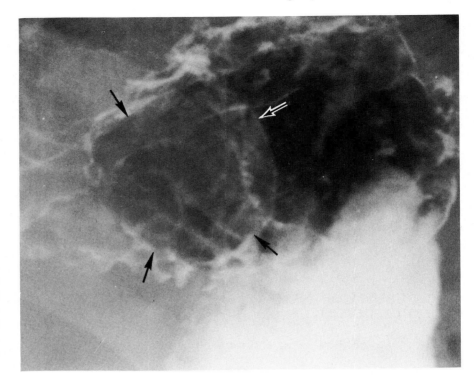

Fig. 18-63. Tumefactive extramedullary hematopoiesis. There is a sharply marginated smooth-walled gastric mass adjacent to the esophagogastric junction. (Gomes AS, Harell GS: Tumefactive extramedullary hematopoiesis of the stomach. Gastrointest Radiol 1:163–165, 1976)

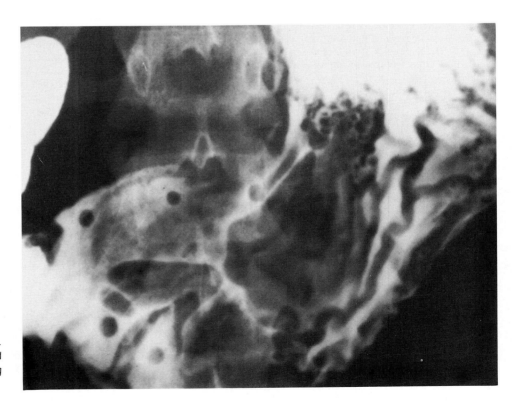

Fig. 18-64. Amyloidosis. Submucosal masses of amyloid appear as multiple lucent filling defects simulating air bubbles.

AMYLOIDOSIS

A gastric filling defect, often with ulceration, can be produced by localized deposition of amyloid within the wall of the stomach. Although amyloidosis is usually associated with diffuse involvement of the gastrointestinal tract, isolated amyloidomas of the stomach can occur (Fig. 18-64).

CANDIDIASIS

Candidal infection in an immunosuppressed patient has been reported to cause multiple scattered, nodular filling defects in the stomach. Central ulcerations or depressions in the lesions tend to produce a bull's-eye appearance.

OTHER CAUSES OF GASTRIC FILLING DEFECTS

Several causes of filling defects in the stomach are discussed specifically in other sections. These include postoperative defects such as suture granuloma and fundoplication, jejunogastric intussusception, gastric varices, the *Anisakis* larva, and prolapsed esophageal mucosa.

BIBLIOGRAPHY

Balfe DM, Koehler RE, Karstaedt N et al: Computed tomography of gastric neoplasms. Radiology 140:431–436, 1981

Balthazar EJ, Megibow A, Bryk D et al: Gastric carcinoid tumors: Radiographic features in eight cases. AJR 139:1123–1127, 1982

Braxton M, Jacobson G: Intragastric gallstone. AJR 78:631–632, 1957

Carlson HC, Breen JF: Amyloidosis and plasma cell dyscrasias: Gastrointestinal involvement. Semin Raentgenol 21:128–138, 1986

Childress MH, Cho KJ, Newlin N et al: Arterial impressions on the stomach. AJR 132:769–772, 1979

Chiles JT, Platz CE: The radiographic manifestations of pseudolymphoma of the stomach. Radiology 116:551–556, 1975

Dastur KJ, Ward JF: Amyloidoma of the stomach. Gastrointest Radiol 5:17–20, 1980

Dunnick NR, Harell GS, Parker BR: Multiple "bull's-eye" lesions in gastric lymphoma. AJR 126:965–969, 1976

Einhorn RI, Grace ND, Banks PA: The clinical significance and natural history of the double pylorus. Dig Dis Sci 29:213–218, 1984

Faegenburg D, Farman J, Dallemand S et al: Leiomyoblastoma of the stomach: Report of nine cases. Radiology 117:297–300, 1975

Feczko PJ, Halpert RD, Ackerman LV: Gastric polyps: Radiological evaluation and clinical significance. Radiology 155:581–584, 1985

Foster MA, Kilcoyne RF: Ruvalcaba–Myhre–Smith syndrome: A new consideration in the differential diagnosis of intestinal polyposis. Gastrointest Radiol 11:349–350, 1986

Glick SN, Cavanaugh B, Teplick SK: The hypertrophied antral-pyloric fold. AJR 145:547–549, 1985

Gomes AS, Harell GS: Tumefactive extramedullary hematopoiesis of the stomach. Gastrointest Radiol 1:163–165, 1976

Hulnick DH, Balthazar EJ: Gastric duplication cyst: GI series and CT correlation. Gastrointest Radiol 12:106–108, 1987

Imoto T, Nobe T, Koga M et al: Computed tomography of gastric lipomas. Gastrointest Radiol 8:129–131, 1983

Joffe N: Metastatic involvement of the stomach secondary to breast carcinoma. AJR 123:512–521, 1975

Kavlie H, White TT: Leiomyomas of the upper gastrointestinal tract. Surgery 71:842–848, 1972

Kilcheski T, Kressel HY, Laufer I et al: The radiographic appearance of the stomach in Cronkhite–Canada syndrome. Radiology 141:57–60, 1981

Maderal F, Hunter F, Fuselier G et al: Gastric lipomas: An update of clinical presentation, diagnosis, and treatment. Am J Gastroenterol 79:964–967, 1984

Meltzer AD, Ostrum BJ, Isard HJ: Villous tumors of the stomach and duodenum: Report of three cases. Radiology 78:511–513, 1966

Meyers MA, McSweeny J: Secondary neoplasms of the bowel. Radiology 105:1–11, 1972

Nauert TC, Zornoza J, Ordonez N: Gastric leiomyosarcomas. AJR 139:291–297, 1982

Op den Orth JO, Dekker W: Gastric adenomas. Radiology 141:289–293, 1981

Perez CA, Dorfman RF: Benign lymphoid hyperplasia of the stomach and duodenum. Radiology 87:505–510, 1966

Pomerantz H, Margolin HN: Metastases to the gastrointestinal tract from malignant melanoma. AJR 88:712–717, 1962

Privett JTJ, Davies ER, Roylance J: The radiological features of gastric lymphoma. Clin Radiol 28:457–463, 1977

Radin DR, Zelner R, Ray MJ et al: Multiple granular cell tumors of the skin and gastrointestinal tract. AJR 147:1305–1307, 1986

Rappaport AS: Gastroduodenal fistulae and double pyloric canal. Gastrointest Radiol 2:341–346, 1978

Rose HS, Balthazar EJ, Megibow AJ et al: Alimentary tract involvement in Kaposi sarcoma: Radiographic and endoscopic findings in 25 homosexual men. AJR 139:661–666, 1982

Rubesin SE, Levine MS, Glick SN: Gastric involvement by omental cakes: Radiographic findings. Gastrointest Radiol 11:223–228, 1986

Rubin SA, Davis M: "Bull's eye" or "target" lesions of the stomach secondary to carcinoma of the lung. Am J Gastroenterol 80:67–69, 1985

Sherrick DW, Hodgson JR, Dockerty MB: The roentgenologic diagnosis of primary gastric lymphoma. Radiology 84:925–932, 1965

Simms SM: Gastric hemangioma associated with phleboliths. Gastrointest Radiol 10:51–53, 1985

Smith HJ, Lee EL: Large hyperplastic polyps of the stomach. Gastrointest Radiol 8:19–23, 1983

Thoeni RF, Gedgaudas RK: Ectopic pancreas: Usual and unusual features. Gastrointest Radiol 5:37–42, 1980

Tim LO, Banks S, Marks IN et al: Benign lymphoid hyperplasia of the gastric antrum: Another cause of "état mammelonné." Br J Radiol 50:29–31, 1977

Watanabe H, Magota S, Shiiba Ş et al: Coarse areae gastricae in the proximal body and fundus: A sign of gastric hypersecretion. Radiology 146:303–306, 1983

Wright FW, Matthews JM: Hemophilic pseudotumor of the stomach. Radiology 98:547–549, 1971

FILLING DEFECTS IN THE GASTRIC REMNANT

19

Disease Entities

Surgical deformity
Suture granuloma
Bezoar
Carcinoma
    Gastric stump carcinoma
    Recurrent carcinoma
Gastric stump lymphoma
Hyperplastic polyps and bile (alkaline) reflux
      gastritis
Jejunogastric intussusception

Partial resection of the stomach is most commonly performed for peptic ulcer disease. Although the 1.5% mortality rate that is associated with partial gastric resection and vagotomy is somewhat higher than that for vagotomy with a drainage procedure alone, the rate of recurrent ulcers of less than 2% after vagotomy and hemigastrectomy is far less than the rate of 6% to 8% after vagotomy and a drainage procedure. Resection of a portion of the stomach can also be performed as surgical therapy for gastric malignancy.

SURGICAL DEFORMITY

Anastomosis after partial gastrectomy can be either a gastroduodenostomy (Billroth I) or gastrojejunostomy (Billroth II). In both of these procedures, the cut end of the stomach is usually partially oversewn to minimize problems associated with a large gastric stoma. The oversewn area produces a typical deformity or plication defect on subsequent contrast examinations. One example is the characteristic plication defect associated with the Hofmeister type of anastomosis, a procedure developed to minimize the problems associated with a large gastric stoma (Fig. 19-1). With this technique, the open end of the gastric stump is closed, with a line of sutures extending from the lesser curvature for one-half to two-thirds of the distance to the greater curvature, and the anastomosis then performed. The resulting filling defect corresponds to the closure line of the invaginated cut surface of the stomach. It is frequently apparent on initial postoperative studies and can decrease in size or disappear on subsequent examinations.

Surgical deformities, especially in patients undergoing partial gastric resection for malignancy, can closely simulate neoplastic processes. Therefore, it is essential that a baseline upper gastrointestinal series be obtained soon after partial gastric resection. Filling defects and extrinsic impressions demonstrated within the first few months of surgery clearly represent surgical deformities rather than discrete lesions. In contrast, subsequent development of a new filling defect or distortion of the region of the anastomosis should be viewed with concern and be considered an indication for gastroscopy.

Another surgery-induced filling defect in the gastric remnant is a suture granuloma (Fig. 19-2).

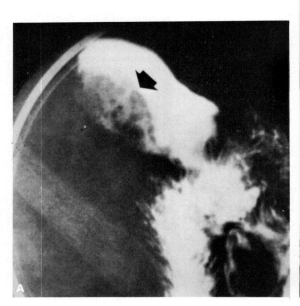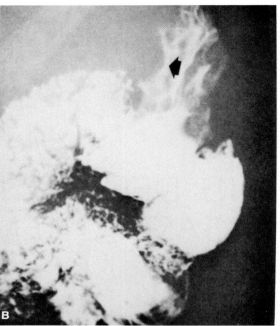

Fig. 19-1. *Surgical deformity (Hofmeister defect). (A) Large defect on the lesser curvature and posterior aspect of the gastric remnant (arrow) several weeks after surgery. (B) Smaller defect (arrow) 4 years later. (Fisher MS: The Hofmeister defect: A normal change in the postoperative stomach. AJR 84:1082–1086, 1960. Copyright 1960. Reproduced with permission)*

This lesion appears as a well-defined, rounded filling defect at the level of the surgical anastomosis. Although asymptomatic and merely an incidental finding, the radiographic appearance can mimic a gastric neoplasm and lead to unnecessary reoperation. Because suture granulomas occur only after gastric surgery with nonabsorbable suture material,

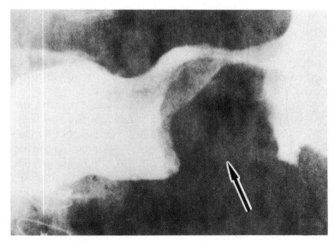

Fig. 19-2. *Suture granuloma. A large mass at the greater curvature side of the antrum (arrow) projects as a smooth tumor into the gastric lumen. (Gueller HA, Shapiro HA, Nelson JA et al: Suture granulomas simulating tumors: A preventable postgastrectomy complication. Dig Dis 21:223–228, 1976)*

the use of completely absorbable sutures should eliminate them as well as other complications related to nonabsorbable sutures, such as suture-line ulcers, abscesses, and adhesions.

BEZOAR

Bezoars in the gastric remnant are a not infrequent complication following partial gastric resection with Billroth-I or -II anastomoses. The chief constituent of postgastrectomy bezoars is the fibrous, pithy component of fruits (especially citrus) and vegetables. These congeal to form masses that entrap varying amounts of stems, seeds, fruit skins, and fat globules. The resulting conglomerate mass of fiber becomes coated by gastric mucus secretions. Masses containing yeast organisms have also been reported in the gastric remnant, but these bezoars usually disappear without any therapy.

Both acid–pepsin secretion and the mixing and agitation of gastric contents are essential for the digestion of fibrous foods, especially oranges. After vagotomy, hydrochloric acid secretion is markedly reduced, if not eliminated. Resection of the pylorus and antral portion of the stomach results in loss of the normal gastric churning action. Inadequate chewing of food related to impaired dentition is also a contributing factor in the development of postgastrectomy bezoars. Stenosis of the anastomosis does

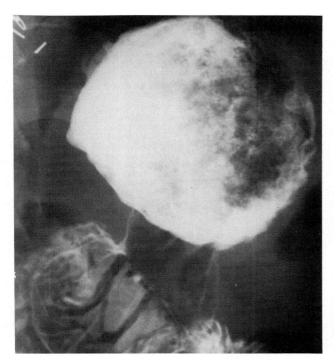

Fig. 19-3. Bezoar in the gastric remnant. A mottled filling defect simulates a mass of retained food particles.

not appear to predispose to bezoar formation in the gastric remnant, since, in most cases, the size of the stoma is adequate for the passage of food of up to 4 cm in diameter.

Bezoars in the gastric remnant vary in size, consistency, and number. They can be large enough to fill and distend the entire gastric remnant or small and easily overlooked. Their consistency varies from rubbery and firm to mushy and soft. Although most bezoars in the gastric remnant are single, several separate masses can be formed.

Many small bezoars in the gastric remnant are entirely asymptomatic. If there is substantial reduction in gastric volume due to encroachment upon the lumen or retardation of gastric emptying by obstruction of the stoma, a sensation of fullness, early satiety, nausea, vomiting, or epigastric or left upper quadrant pain can result. A ball–valve mechanism can cause intermittent symptoms. Although bezoars can erode the gastric mucosa, blood loss (either acute or chronic) is rarely encountered and, if present, should suggest another diagnosis.

A bezoar in the gastric remnant appears radiographically as a mottled filling defect simulating a mass of retained food particles (Fig. 19-3). It conforms to the gastric outline and tends to trap barium in spongelike fashion within its matrix. When the patient is in the upright position, the bezoar tends to float in the barium column like an iceberg, its convex superior border projecting above the level of the barium into the gastric air bubble. Bezoars are usually freely movable with change in the patient's

position, unlike neoplasms, which are fixed to the gastric wall.

In addition to causing gastric outlet obstruction, a bezoar arising in the gastric remnant can pass into and obstruct the small bowel, usually in the relatively narrow terminal ileum.

To prevent the development of bezoars in the gastric remnant, postgastrectomy patients must be counseled with regard to both the foods they can safely eat and how to chew them properly. All fibrous foods, especially citrus fruits, should be avoided or else minced prior to ingestion. It has been suggested that about 90% of all bezoars in the gastric remnant could be prevented by the elimination of oranges from the diets of postgastrectomy patients.

GASTRIC STUMP CARCINOMA

Gastric stump carcinoma refers to a malignancy occurring in the gastric remnant after resection for

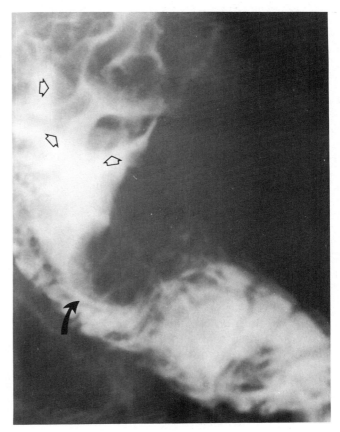

Fig. 19-4. Gastric stump carcinoma. A large, irregular polypoid mass is visible in the proximal portion of the gastric remnant **(open arrows)**. The smooth filling defect at the anastomosis **(curved, solid arrow)** represents a benign leiomyoma.

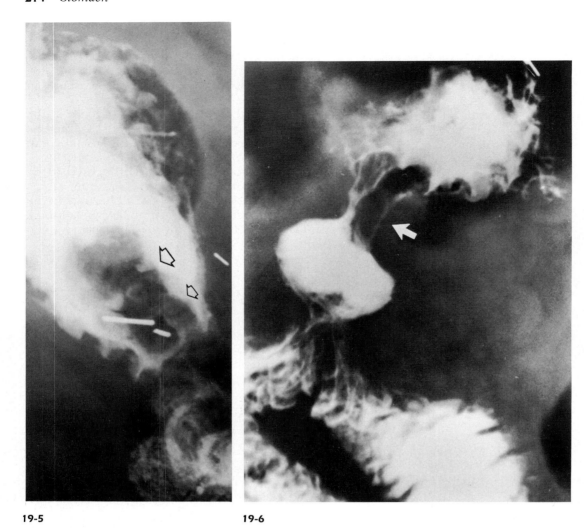

19-5   19-6

Fig. 19-5. Gastric stump carcinoma. A large, irregular polypoid mass **(arrows)** arises near the anastomosis and fills much of the distal gastric remnant.

Fig. 19-6. Gastric stump carcinoma. Tumor infiltration causes narrowing of the lumen **(arrow)**.

peptic ulcer or other benign disease (Fig. 19-4). The development of recurrent symptoms after a long period of relatively good health following partial gastrectomy should suggest the possibility of gastric stump carcinoma. A neoplasm at the anastomotic site can ulcerate and clinically mimic a benign ulcer. However, simple stomal ulceration rarely occurs after many years of freedom from symptoms. For the possibility to be excluded that the carcinoma was undetected at the time of the original resection, most authors stipulate that at least 5 years must have elapsed since the initial gastric surgery.

The incidence of carcinoma in the gastric remnant is two to six times higher than in the intact stomach. This complication is especially high in Europe, where gastric stump carcinoma has been reported to occur in about 15% of patients within 10 years of initial surgery and in about 20% after 20 years. In view of these statistics, some authors advise that gastric resection for benign disease should be avoided whenever possible, especially in young patients. If partial resection of the stomach is performed, an annual endoscopic examination beginning 10 years after the initial surgery is recommended.

The increased incidence of carcinoma in the gastric remnant is probably related to the chronic reflux of bile and pancreatic juice into the gastric remnant after partial gastrectomy. When gastric mucosa is subjected to a constant flow of bile and pancreatic juice, chronic and atrophic gastritis, intestinal metaplasia, adenomatous transformation of gastric mucosa, and submucosal ectopic glandular hyperplasia can occur. These changes may be seen singly or in combination and can vary in degree. The predilection for malignant transformation to occur in the perianastomotic region may well reflect these probably premalignant dysplastic changes in the gastric mucosa. Vagotomy-induced hypochlorhydria may also be a contributing factor in the postoperative development of adenocarcinoma in the stomach.

RADIOGRAPHIC FINDINGS

The rate of detection of gastric stump carcinoma by means of barium swallow has been poor. In most series, a majority of carcinomas have not been demonstrated on upper gastrointestinal series. However, retrospective analysis usually demonstrates signs of stump carcinoma in almost every case, suggesting that meticulous technique aided by a more careful interpretation might allow for earlier detection.

Gastric stump carcinomas usually appear as irregular polypoid masses at the anastomotic margin or in the gastric remnant (Fig. 19-5). Unlike bezoars, they remain fixed in relation to the wall of the stomach with change in patient position. In contrast to benign plication defects found on the lesser curvature proximal to the stoma, gastric stump carci-

noma can cause irregularities on both the greater and the lesser curvatures of the gastric outflow tract.

Gastric stump malignancy can present as a marginal ulceration near the anastomosis. Patients with this carcinoma usually have a long symptom-free period averaging in excess of 20 years. In contrast, the peak incidence of benign mucosal ulcerations is in the first postoperative year, and the majority of the rest occur within the next 2 years. Benign marginal ulcers almost invariably follow surgery for duodenal ulcers; less than 2% develop in patients whose original surgery was for gastric ulcer disease. Benign marginal ulcers usually occur on the jejunal side of the anastomosis. Thus, any ulcer on the gastric side should be considered malignant unless proved otherwise.

Decrease in the size of the gastric remnant can occur secondary to uniform infiltration by carcinoma (Fig. 19-6). This sign of malignancy requires comparison with previous studies and is an excellent reason for obtaining a baseline upper gastrointestinal examination several months after partial gastrectomy (Fig. 19-7). The diagnosis of stump shrinkage cannot be made if there is inadequate distention of the gastric remnant caused by failure to administer enough contrast or by underfilling due to rapid emptying.

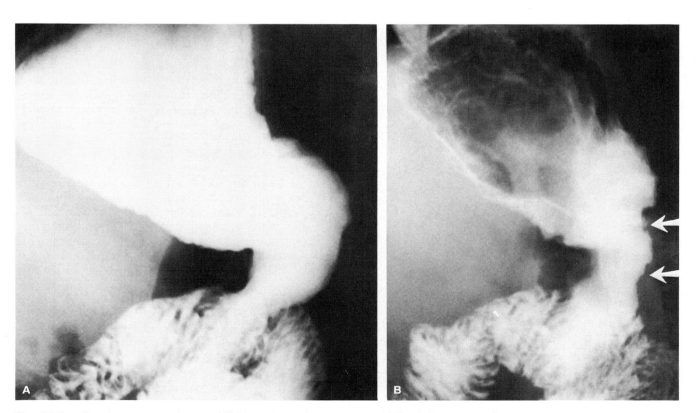

Fig. 19-7. Gastric stump carcinoma. **(A)** Normal gastric remnant and Billroth-II anastomosis following surgery for peptic disease. **(B)** Irregular narrowing of the perianastomotic region **(arrows)** several years later represents a gastric stump carcinoma.

The small bowel appears to be resistant to invasion by carcinoma in the gastric stump. The malignant process tends to terminate abruptly at the anastomotic line, as if stopped by some barrier mechanism. Tumor occasionally infiltrates into deep parts of the jejunal wall, but the mucosa is almost invariably spared. At times, benign rugal hypertrophy causes perianastomotic filling defects that are indistinguishable from malignant tumors. Whenever new radiographic findings develop at the anastomotic site, gastroscopic examination is warranted.

RECURRENT CARCINOMA

Recurrence of previous gastric carcinoma can cause filling defects within the gastric remnant. It is sometimes difficult to distinguish between a recurrent carcinoma and the development of a second primary. Most observers consider a carcinoma in the gastric remnant to represent a second primary if it has occurred 10 years or more since the initial surgical resection for malignant disease. Recurrent carcinoma can appear as a filling defect in the gastric remnant, infiltration of the wall with straightening and loss of normal distensibility, or mucosal destruction with superficial ulceration. The major sign of recurrence at the stoma is symmetric or eccentric narrowing with local mucosal effacement (Fig. 19-8).

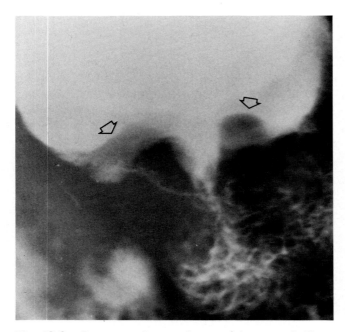

Fig. 19-8. *Recurrent adenocarcinoma of the stomach. There is symmetric narrowing of the stoma with nodular masses* **(arrows)** *on the gastric side of the anastomosis.*

GASTRIC STUMP LYMPHOMA

Malignant gastric lymphoma has been reported to develop 20 or more years following surgery for peptic ulcer disease. The radiographic manifestations are similar to those of lymphoma involving the unoperated stomach and consist of markedly enlarged rugal folds, thickening of the involved portions of the wall, and prominent submucosal nodules (Fig. 19-9A). Despite extensive intramural infiltration by the tumor, the stomach retains its pliability and is fully distensible during the barium examination (Fig. 19-9B). These features differ from those of gastric stump carcinoma, which usually causes a pronounced desmoplastic response leading to significant narrowing of the gastric lumen in addition to mucosal destruction and effacement of the folds.

The underlying mechanism for the development of lymphoma after gastric surgery is unclear. Some studies have shown that the initially resected portion of the stomach, or subsequent endoscopy biopsy specimens of the anastomosis, had histopathologic features of benign lymphoid hyperplasia or pseudolymphoma. This finding has led to speculation that residual inflammatory lymphoid aggregates within the gastric remnant may have the potential for transformation into malignant lymphoma.

HYPERPLASTIC POLYPS/BILE (ALKALINE) REFLUX GASTRITIS

Hyperplastic polyps in the gastric remnant probably represent a reactive response to reflux of bile and pancreatic juices from the jejunum into the stomach. These highly alkaline digestive secretions are normally prevented from entering the stomach by an intact pylorus. When the pyloric mechanism is destroyed or circumvented by partial gastric resection, free reflux can produce severe gastritis and ulceration. Damage to the stomach mucosa is often multifocal or diffuse, resulting in the development of hyperplastic gastric polyps in multiple areas.

Bile reflux gastritis appears radiographically as thickened folds in the gastric remnant (Fig. 19-10). The most severe changes tend to occur near the anastomosis. Extensive swelling of gastric rugae can produce a discrete mass effect. Ulcerations due to bile reflux gastritis occur on the gastric side of the remnant (Fig. 19-11). True stomal ulceration due to the residual action of acid and pepsin on the sensitive intestinal mucosa occurs on the jejunal side of the anastomosis (Fig. 19-12).

Typical symptoms of alkaline reflux gastritis include postprandial pain, bilious vomiting, and weight loss. Gastric analysis demnstrates achlorhydria. If the symptoms of alkaline reflux gastritis cannot be managed effectively by conservative measures (diet, antispasmodics, cholestyramine), a

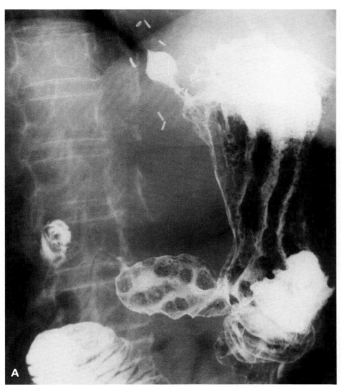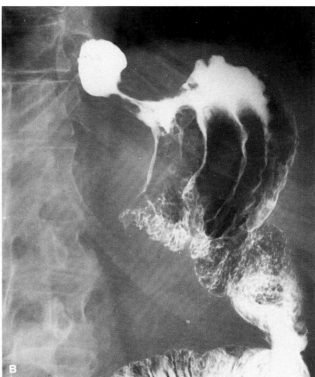

Fig. 19-9. Gastric stump lymphoma. **(A)** Thickened gastric rugal folds associated with multiple submucosal nodules in the antrum that developed 39 years after vagotomy and gastrojejunostomy. **(B)** Giant rugal folds and deformed cardia of an otherwise well-distensible gastric remnant representing extensive lymphoma that developed 20 years after Billroth-II gastrojejunostomy. (Ghahremani GG, Fisher MR: Lymphoma of the stomach following gastric surgery following benign peptic ulcers. Gastrointest Radiol 8:213–217, 1983)

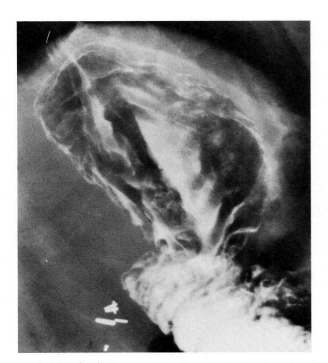

Fig. 19-10. Bile reflux gastritis. There is thickening of rugal folds in the gastric remnant.

surgical procedure is needed to divert bile and other duodenal contents from the gastric remnant.

Discrete polypoid lesions developing in the gastric remnant within a few years of surgery are more likely to be hyperplastic polyps than carcinoma. Nevertheless, endoscopy and biopsy are essential for confirmation of the diagnosis. Most postgastrectomy hyperplastic polyps produce few, if any, symptoms. Progressive increase in the size and number of these polyps, however, can lead to the formation of large conglomerate masses in the gastric remnant immediately proximal to the stoma. Surgical or endoscopic removal of these polyps may be required if they produce symptoms of intermittent gastric outlet obstruction, epigastric pain, vomiting, or gastrointestinal hemorrhage.

JEJUNOGASTRIC INTUSSUSCEPTION

Jejunogastric intussusception is a rare but potentially lethal complication of partial gastrectomy with Billroth-II anastomosis. In this condition, a portion of the full thickness of the jejunum invaginates back into the stomach. The efferent loop alone

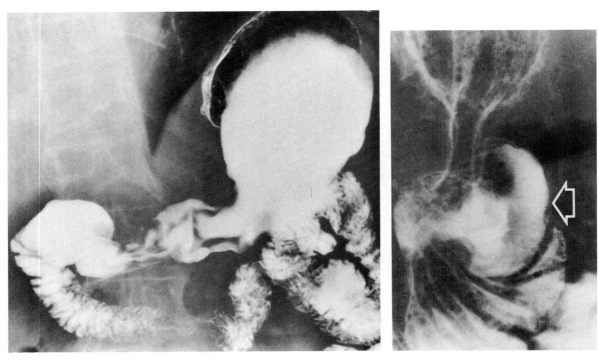

19-11   19-12

Fig. 19-11. Bile reflux gastritis. The patient had undergone gastroenterostomy for previous peptic disease. Because the patient could produce no gastric acid even on stimulation tests, the thickened antral folds and ulceration were attributed to bile reflux gastritis.

Fig. 19-12. Marginal (stomal) ulceration. The large ulcer **(arrow)** has arisen on the jejunal side of the anastomosis.

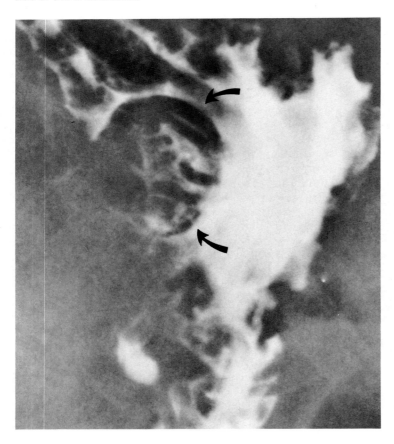

Fig. 19-13. Retrograde jejunogastric intussusception (afferent loop) producing a large, sharply defined filling defect **(arrows)**.

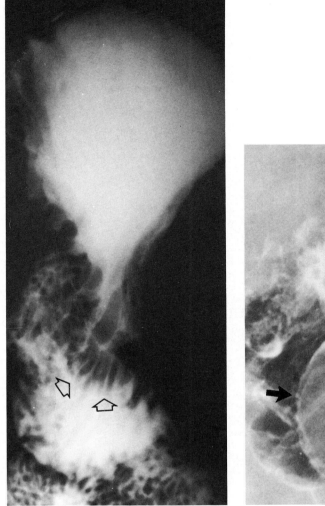

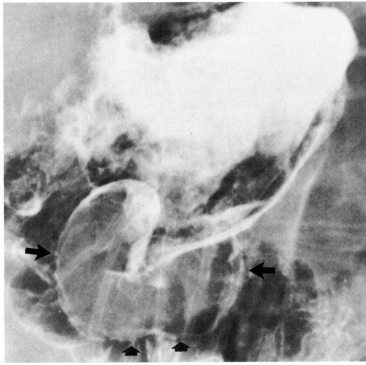

19-14   19-15

Fig. 19-14. Gastrojejunal mucosal prolapse. There is a sharply marginated, smooth mass in the efferent loop **(arrows)**.

Fig. 19-15. Antegrade gastrojejunal mucosal prolapse producing a large, partially obstructing mass in the efferent loop **(arrows)**.

accounts for about 75% of jejunogastric intussusceptions; the afferent loop alone or in combination with the efferent loop constitutes the remaining cases.

The precise etiology of jejunogastric intussusception is unclear. Widely patent gastroenteric anastomoses may favor jejunogastric intussusception by permitting the loose mucosa at the anastomotic site to prolapse into the gastric pouch during normal peristalsis. Hyperperistalsis in the small bowel after gastric surgery, as well as excessive mobility of the jejunum (especially with antecolic anastomoses), are also contributing factors.

Jejunal intussusception can be either acute or chronic recurrent. Acute but delayed jejunogastric intussusception can occur months or years after

gastric surgery. The patient with this condition presents as an acute surgical emergency, with sudden, severe colicky abdominal pain, intractable vomiting, and hematemesis. These symptoms reflect incarceration of the intussusceptum, and mortality rises sharply with delay in surgical decompression of the upper intestinal obstruction.

Chronic jejunogastric intussusception often produces only vague symptoms of recurrent abdominal pain relieved by vomiting. Because chronic recurrent intussusception is intermittent, gastroscopy or laparotomy may fail to demonstrate the lesion.

Retrograde jejunogastric intussusception appears radiographically as a clearly defined spherical or ovoid intraluminal filling defect in the gastric remnant (Fig. 19-13). Contrast material may be seen outlining the jejunal folds and surrounding the intussusceptum. These folds are stretched or enlarged, because of pressure edema, and appear as thin, curvilinear, concentric parallel stripes or striations (coiled-spring appearance).

Recent reports have demonstrated that some jejunogastric intussusceptions can be reduced at fluoroscopy because of the favorable direction of the pressure exerted by the barium. Glucagon-induced hypotonia can also promote reduction of the intussusception.

Antegrade gastrojejunal mucosal prolapse or intussusception occurs more frequently than the retrograde process. It produces a sharply marginated, smooth, occasionally scalloped intraluminal mass in the efferent or afferent loop (Fig. 19-14). External compression or jejunal peristalsis may alter the size and shape of this soft, flexible lesion. A large gastrojejunal mucosal prolapse can cause partial obstruction, especially if the anastomotic stoma is small (Fig. 19-15).

BIBLIOGRAPHY

Bachman AL, Parmer EA: Radiographic diagnosis of recurrence following resection for gastric cancer. Radiology 84:913–924, 1965

Burrell M, Touloukian JS, Curtis AM: Roentgen manifestations of carcinoma in the gastric remnant. Gastrointest Radiol 5:331–341, 1980

Domellof L, Janunger KG: The risk for gastric carcinoma after partial gastrectomy. Am J Surg 134:581–584, 1977

Ghahremani GG, Fisher MR: Lymphoma of the stomach following gastric surgery for benign peptic ulcers. Gastrointest Radiol 8:213–217, 1983

Goldstein HM, Cohen LE, Hagne RO et al: Gastric bezoars: A frequent complication in the postoperative ulcer patient. Radiology 107:341–344, 1973

Gueller R, Shapiro HA, Nelson JA et al: Suture granulomas simulating tumors: A preventable postgastrectomy complication. Am J Dig Dis 21:223–228, 1976

Herrington JL, Sawyers JL, Whitehead WA: Surgical management of reflux gastritis. Ann Surg 180:526–537, 1974

Jay BS, Burrell M: Iatrogenic problems following gastric surgery. Gastrointest Radiol 2:239–257, 1977

Joffe N, Antonioli DA: Atypical appearances of benign hyperplastic gastric polyps. AJR 131:147–152, 1978

Joffe N, Goldman H, Antonioli DA: Recurring hyperplastic gastric polyps following subtotal gastrectomy. AJR 130:301–305, 1978

LeVine M, Boley SJ, Mellins HZ et al: Gastrojejunal mucosal prolapse. Radiology 80:30–38, 1963

Marx WJ: Reduction of jejunogastric intussusception during upper gastrointestinal examination. AJR 131:334–336, 1978

Moskowitz H: Phytobezoars of the small bowel following gastric surgery. Radiology 113:23–26, 1974

Perttala Y, Peltokallio P, Leiviska T et al: Yeast bezoar formation following gastric surgery. AJR 125:365–373, 1975

Poppel MH: Gastric intussusceptions. Radiology 78:602–608, 1968

Rogers LF, Davis EK, Harle TS: Phytobezoar formation and food boli following gastric surgery. AJR 119:280–290, 1973

Sasson L: Tumor-simulating deformities after subtotal gastrectomy JAMA 174:280–283, 1960

Seaman WB: Prolapsed gastric mucosa through a gastrojejunostomy. AJR 110:304–314, 1970

Szemes GC, Amberg JR: Gastric bezoars after partial gastrectomy. Radiology 90:765–768, 1968

Van Heerden JA, Priestly JT, Farrow GM et al: Postoperative alkaline reflux gastritis: Surgical complications. Am J Surg 118:427–433, 1969

Wolf JA Jr, Spjut HJ: Focal lymphoid hyperplasia of the stomach preceding gastric lymphoma: Case report and review of the literature. Cancer 48:2518–2523, 1981

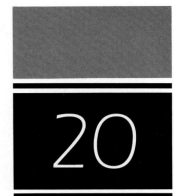

GASTRIC OUTLET OBSTRUCTION

Disease Entities

Peptic ulcer disease
    Duodenal
    Pyloric channel
    Antral
Tumors
    Malignant
        Antral carcinoma
        Carcinoma of the head of the pancreas
        Other malignant tumors causing duodenal
            obstruction
        Lymphoma
        Primary scirrhous carcinoma of the pyloric
            channel
    Benign
Inflammatory disorders
    Crohn's disease
    Pancreatitis
    Cholecystitis
    Corrosive stricture
    Sarcoidosis
    Syphilis
    Tuberculosis
    Amyloidosis
Congenital disorders
    Antral mucosal diaphragm
    Duodenal diaphragm
    Gastric duplication
    Annular pancreas

Miscellaneous disorders
    Gastric volvulus
    Hypertrophic pyloric stenosis
    Gastric bezoar
    Prolapsed antral mucosa

PEPTIC ULCER DISEASE

In adults, peptic ulcer disease is by far the most common cause of gastric outlet obstruction (about 60–65% of cases) (Fig. 20-1). The obstructing lesion in peptic ulcer disease is usually in the duodenum, occasionally in the pyloric channel or prepyloric gastric antrum, and rarely in the body of the stomach. Narrowing of the lumen due to peptic ulcer disease can result from spasm, acute inflammation and edema, muscular hypertrophy, or contraction of scar tissue. In most patients, several of these factors combine to produce gastric outlet obstruction.

    Most patients with peptic disease causing pyloric obstruction have a long history of ulcer symptoms. Indeed, gastric outlet obstruction as the initial manifestation of peptic ulcer disease is very unusual and should raise the suspicion of gastric malignancy. Vomiting is a characteristic clinical symptom. Although the constant presence of large amounts of bile in the retained secretions suggests that the descending duodenum is included in the obstructed segment, bile-stained gastric aspirate is not inconsistent with pyloric stenosis. Vomiting secondary to obstruction is usually delayed for several

281

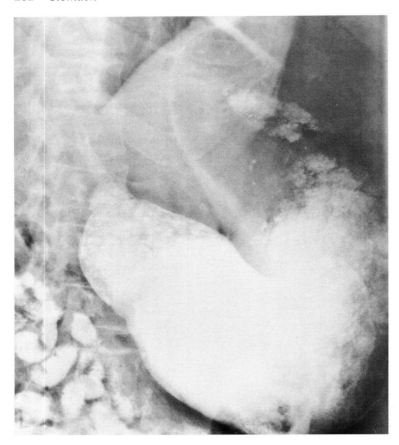

Fig. 20-1. Gastric outlet obstruction caused by peptic ulcer disease.

hours after meals, unlike that which occurs rapidly in response to an irritant in the stomach. In patients with peptic disease who develop gastric outlet obstruction, ulcer pain tends to be constant, and vomiting becomes a major means of pain relief.

RADIOGRAPHIC FINDINGS

Plain abdominal radiographs often demonstrate the shadowy outline of a distended stomach in patients with gastric outlet obstruction. On upright films, there is frequently a fuzzy air-fluid level distinct from the sharp, even air-fluid levels seen elsewhere in the bowel. On barium examination, a mottled density of nonopaque material represents excessive overnight gastric residual (Fig. 20-2A). There is a marked delay in gastric emptying, with barium often retained in the stomach for 24 hr or longer. The stomach may become huge and, with the patient in the upright position, hang down into the lower abdomen or pelvis. The critical differential diagnosis is between a benign (primarily peptic ulcer disease) and malignant cause of gastric outlet obstruction. The presence of a persistent fleck of barium in a narrowed pyloric channel suggests peptic disease. However, a discrete filling defect suggests malignancy, as does nodularity or irregularity of the mucosa proximal to the constricted area. It is essential that every effort be made to ex-

press barium into the duodenal bulb. The finding of distortion and scarring of the bulb with formation of pseudodiverticula makes peptic ulcer disease the most likely etiology (Fig. 20-2B). Conversely, a radiographically normal duodenal bulb increases the likelihood of underlying malignant disease. In many patients, unfortunately, it is impossible to differentiate confidently on barium studies between a benign and a malignant cause of gastric outlet obstruction. In these cases, endoscopy or surgical exploration is required to exclude the possibility of a malignant lesion.

MALIGNANT TUMORS

An annular constricting lesion near the pylorus (Fig. 20-3), representing carcinoma of the antrum, is the second leading cause of gastric outlet obstruction (about 30–35% of cases). Other infiltrative primary malignant tumors or metastatic lesions obliterating the lumen of the distal stomach and proximal duodenum can also produce the radiographic pattern of gastric outlet obstruction.

Unlike patients with gastric outlet obstruction caused by peptic disease, who typically have a long history of ulcer pain, about one-third of patients with obstruction due to malignancy have no pain. A large majority have a history of pain of less than 1

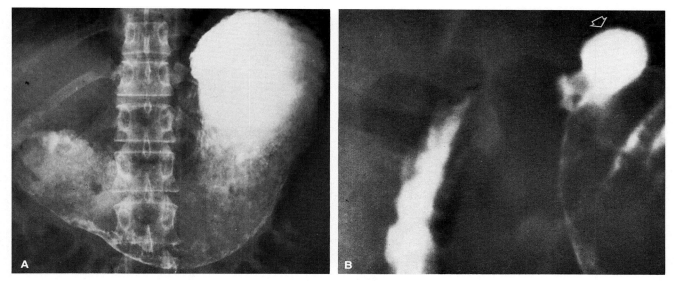

Fig. 20-2.   Gastric outlet obstruction due to a giant duodenal ulcer. **(A)** The mottled density of nonopaque material represents excessive overnight gastric residual. **(B)** A delayed film shows the giant duodenal ulcer **(arrow)**. (Eisenberg RL, Margulis AR, Moss AA: Giant duodenal ulcers. Gastrointest Radiol 2:347–353, 1978)

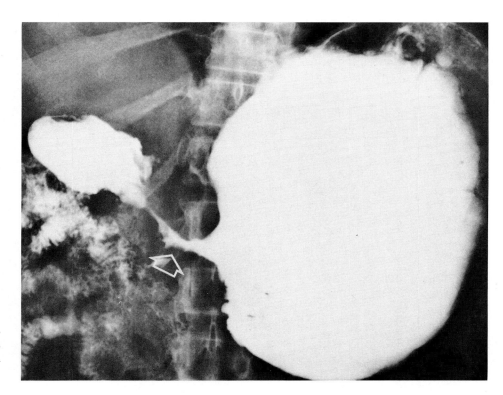

Fig. 20-3.   Gastric outlet obstruction caused by annular constricting carcinoma of the stomach **(arrow)**.

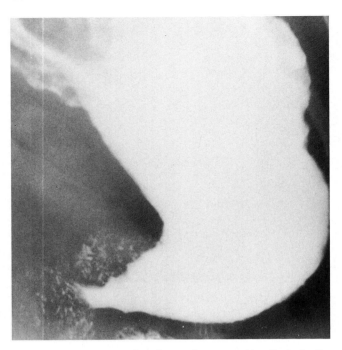

Fig. 20-4. Gastric outlet obstruction caused by Crohn's disease involving the stomach.

year's duration. Vomiting and weight loss are prominent clinical symptoms.

Primary scirrhous carcinoma of the pyloric channel is a cause of gastric outlet obstruction that can be indistinguishable radiographically from benign stricture. The tumor originates in the pyloric channel and grows circumferentially. It has a definite tendency for submucosal, muscular, and serosal invasion with preservation of the mucosal lining. Although the pyloric lesion associated with this tumor appears radiographically to be relatively benign, early development of metastases is the rule. Distal antral involvement can be seen in advanced cases, but the duodenum is usually spared.

The cellular neoplastic and nonspecific inflammatory infiltrate, as well as a secondary desmoplastic reaction, contributes to the formation of a short, concentric stricture without peristalsis. The pylorus is elongated, symmetrically smooth, and rigid, often with gradual tapering of the proximal margin. The major differential point between pyloric narrowing due to primary scirrhous carcinoma and that due to a healed ulcer is the frequent presence of acute ulceration (gastric, antral, pyloric, duodenal) and duodenal deformity in patients with peptic disease.

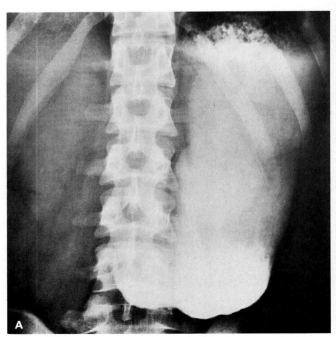

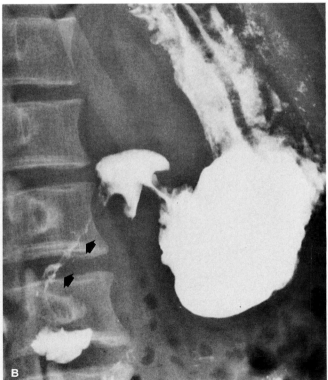

Fig. 20-5. Acute pancreatitis. **(A)** Complete gastric outlet obstruction. **(B)** As the acute inflammatory process subsides, some barium is seen to pass through the severely spastic and narrowed second portion of the duodenum **(arrows)**.

BENIGN TUMORS

Rarely, prolapse of a benign antral polyp into the duodenum produces intermittent gastric outlet obstruction. As the gastric polyp is propelled by peristalsis through the pylorus into the duodenum, it pulls a segment of stomach with it. Radiographically, the prolapsed polyp appears as an intraluminal filling defect in the duodenal bulb (see Fig. 30-42). Shortening of the gastric antrum with convergence of distal gastric folds can sometimes be identified. At fluoroscopy, the defect caused by the polyp can be demonstrated to change position, sometimes being in the pyloric antrum and then prolapsing into the duodenal bulb.

INFLAMMATORY DISORDERS

Inflammatory disease involving the distal stomach and proximal duodenum can cause infiltration or spasm resulting in clinical and radiographic signs of gastric outlet obstruction. Up to two-thirds of patients with Crohn's disease of the stomach develop this complication (Fig. 20-4). Although rare, granulomatous involvement of the stomach in patients with sarcoidosis, syphilis, or tuberculosis can cause sufficient thickening of the gastric wall to produce an obstructive appearance. Severe pancreatitis and cholecystitis can incite inflammatory spasm, which leads to obliteration of the lumen of the proximal duodenum and gastric outlet obstruction (Fig. 20-5). Stricture of the antrum can result from fibrous healing after the ingestion of corrosive substances (Fig. 20-6). On rare occasions, deposition of amyloid in the stomach wall can be so pronounced as to produce severe luminal narrowing and gastric outlet obstruction.

ANTRAL MUCOSAL DIAPHRAGM

Antral mucosal diaphragms are thin membranous septa that are usually situated within 3 cm of the pyloric canal and run perpendicular to the long axis of the stomach. Both congenital and acquired etiologies have been postulated for this entity. The congenital theory is based on the fact that antral webs occur in infants and children, probably resulting from failure of the embryonic foregut to recanalize or from a fetal vascular incident with insult to the bowel. Some antral mucosal diaphragms in adults are also probably congenital. They may become symptomatic in adulthood because of such factors as decreased gastrointestinal motility with increasing age, poor mastication secondary to dental problems, and narrowing of the diaphragmatic lumen from small erosions, gastritis, and mucosal edema. An acquired etiology in the adult has been suggested in view of reports of patients with gastric ulcers that alternatively heal and recur, leading to fibrosis that ultimately forms an antral web. Support for this mechanism of web formation is the large percentage of patients who have peptic ulcer disease when the diagnosis of antral mucosal diaphragm is made. Nevertheless, it should be stressed that an antral mucosal diaphragm histologically is composed of a layer of normal mucosa on either side of a common submucosa and muscularis, usually with no evidence of inflammation or fibrosis.

Clinical symptoms of partial gastric outlet obstruction (upper epigastric pain, fullness, and vomiting, particularly after a heavy meal) correlate with the size of the central aperture of the antral mucosal diaphragm. Symptoms of obstruction do not occur if the diameter of the diaphragm is more than 1 cm. Even with minute central orifices as small as 2 mm, no obstructive symptoms may be produced until adult life. Infrequently, infants with mucosal diaphragms present with projectile vomiting in the neonatal period. In severe obstruction, gastric emptying is greatly delayed, and barium can be seen to pass in a thin stream (jet effect) from the center of the obstruction.

The nonobstructing antral mucosal diaphragm appears radiographically as a persistent, sharply defined, 2-cm- to 3-cm-wide bandlike defect in the barium column that arises at right angles to the gastric wall (Fig. 20-7). Although this appearance can be simulated by a prominent transverse mucosal fold that is often found in the antrum, this fold does not extend across the gastric lumen, nor is it generally perfectly straight. The antral mucosal diaphragm is best seen when the stomach proximal and

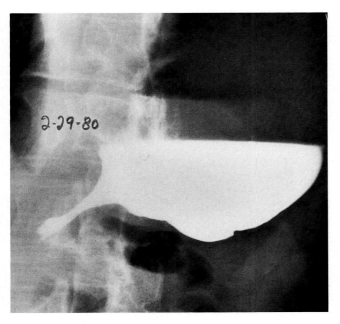

Fig. 20-6. Gastric outlet obstruction. The obstruction was caused by a caustic stricture that developed within 1 month of the ingestion of hydrochloric acid.

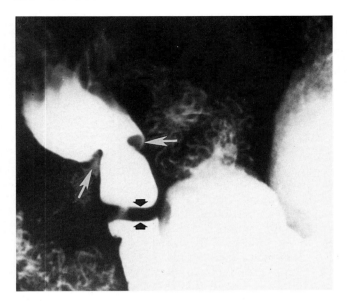

Fig. 20-7. *Antral mucosal diaphragm. The bandlike defect* **(black arrows)** *arises at right angles to the gastric wall. The channel (web aperture) in this patient measures 4 mm; the web is 5 mm thick. The white arrows point to the pyloric canal. (Bjorgvinsson E, Rudzki C, Lewicki AM: Antral web. Am J Gastroenterol 79:663–665, 1984)*

distal to it are distended. The portion of the antrum proximal to the pylorus and distal to the mucosal diaphragm can mimic a second duodenal bulb (Fig. 20-8). The distal antrum can sometimes even be confused with a gastric diverticulum or ulcer, though, on close inspection, it clearly lies within the line of the stomach and changes size and shape during the examination.

Because an antral mucosal diaphragm is readily amenable to surgical correction, it is important that the proper diagnosis be made. The radiologist must suggest the possibility of an antral mucosal diaphragm to the gastroscopist, because the orifice can closely simulate the pylorus on endoscopy and thus be easily overlooked.

GASTRIC DUPLICATION

Gastric duplications infrequently communicate with the stomach. They tend to appear as tumor masses within the gastric lumen, narrowing and deforming the antrum. Although they usually cause only an indentation of the stomach, complete gastric outlet obstruction can occur.

ANNULAR PANCREAS

Annular pancreas most commonly produces an extrinsic impression on the lateral aspect of the descending duodenum. Infrequently, complete luminal obstruction can develop.

GASTRIC VOLVULUS

Gastric volvulus is an uncommon acquired twist of the stomach upon itself that can lead to gastric outlet obstruction (Fig. 20-9). It usually occurs in conjunction with a large esophageal or paraesophageal hernia that permits part or all of the stomach to assume an intrathoracic position. Free upward movement of the stomach is limited by several ligaments that normally anchor the stomach within the abdomen. The most rigid point of attachment is the site at which the second portion of the duodenum assumes a retroperitoneal position and thus becomes fixed to the posterior abdominal wall. The gastrocolic and gastrolienal ligaments also contribute to fixation of the stomach. In paraesophageal hernias, intra-abdominal fixation of the esophagogastric junction also serves to limit free upward movement of the stomach. Because of these anatomic fixation points, torsion of the stomach can occur with significant degrees of gastric herniation. Gastric volvulus can also be secondary to eventration or paralysis of the diaphragm. Cases of idiopathic gastric volvulus without apparent cause have also been reported.

In small herniations, the proximal portion of the stomach enters the hernia sac first. Obstruction or strangulation almost never occurs at this stage. As herniation progresses, the body and a variable portion of the antrum come to lie above the diaphragm, so that the stomach can become an entirely intrathoracic organ and prone to gastric volvulus. Organoaxial volvulus refers to rotation of the stomach upward around its long axis (a line connecting the cardia with the pylorus). In this condition, the

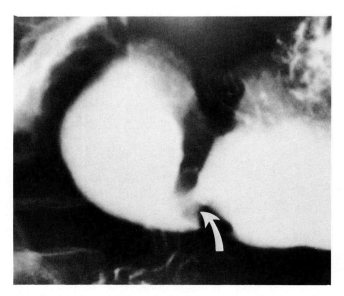

Fig. 20-8. *Antral mucosal diaphragm severely narrowing the lumen* **(arrow)**. *The dilated portion of the antrum distal to the mucosal diaphragm and proximal to the pylorus simulates a second duodenal bulb.*

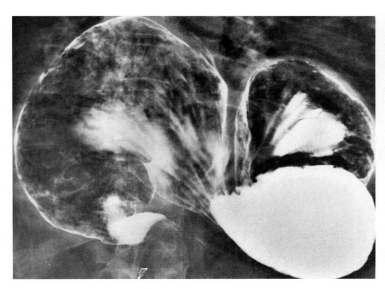

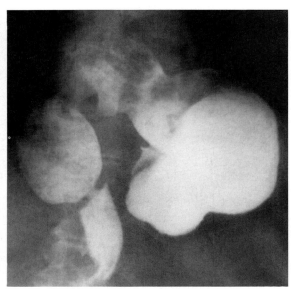

20-9

20-10

Fig. 20-9. Organoaxial volvulus of the stomach with gastric outlet obstruction.

Fig. 20-10. Organoaxial volvulus with gastric outlet obstruction. The greater curvature is above the level of the lesser curvature, and the cardia and pylorus are positioned at about the same level.

antrum moves from an inferior to a superior position. In the mesenteroaxial type of gastric volvulus, the stomach rotates from right to left or left to right about the long axis of the gastrohepatic omentum (a line connecting the middle of the lesser curvature with the middle of the greater curvature).

Gastric volvulus can be asymptomatic if there is no outlet obstruction or vascular compromise. Acute volvulus associated with interference of blood supply is a surgical emergency. The classic clinical triad in this condition consists of violent retching with production of little vomitus, constant, severe epigastric pain, and great difficulty in the advancement of a nasogastric tube past the distal esophagus. Vascular occlusion leads to necrosis, shock, and a mortality rate of about 30%.

The radiographic signs of gastric volvulus are characteristic. They include a double air-fluid level on upright films, inversion of the stomach with the greater curvature above the level of the lesser curvature, positioning of the cardia and pylorus at the same level, and downward pointing of the pylorus and duodenum (Fig. 20-10).

HYPERTROPHIC PYLORIC STENOSIS

The histologic, anatomic, and radiographic abnormalities in adult hypertrophic pyloric stenosis (Fig. 20-11) are indistinguishable from those in the infantile form (Fig. 20-12). Indeed, the disease in adults may be the same entity observed in infants and children but milder and later in clinical appearance.

Most patients with adult hypertrophic pyloric stenosis go unrecognized because they are entirely free of symptoms. Some complain of nausea and vomiting, epigastric pain, weight loss, and anorexia. Unlike children, adults infrequently have high-grade outlet obstruction with hypertrophic pyloric stenosis.

About half of all patients with demonstrable pyloric hypertrophy have concomitant gastric ulceration. This probably reflects the development of an ulcer due to the delayed gastric emptying, which interferes with the passage of semisolid food and results in increased gastrin production and consequent hyperacidity. The possibility of pyloric hypertrophy representing a complication of chronic spasm induced by a proximal gastric ulcer appears to be less likely.

Elongation and narrowing of the pyloric canal are characteristic radiographic findings in adult hypertrophic pyloric stenosis. The pylorus is elongated, measuring 2 cm to 4 cm in length (normal, ≤1 cm in adults). Hypertrophy of the musculature produces a narrowed segment, the contour of which can be smooth or slightly irregular. Invagination of the mucosa into the narrow pyloric canal produces the characteristic "double track" sign. The proximal end of the narrowed pylorus merges gradually with the contiguous stomach, resulting in a smooth, round juncture without the shoulders suggestive of a malignant neoplasm. A classic sign of adult hypertrophic stenosis is a symmetric, concave, crescentic indentation of the base of the duodenal bulb. This mushroom-shaped defect is presumably due to partial invagination of the hypertrophied muscle mass into the bulb. Although generally considered char-

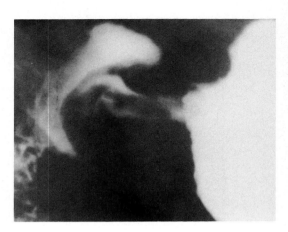

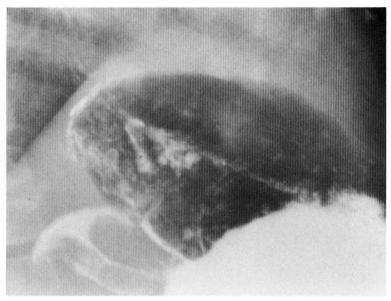

20-11   20-12

Fig. 20-11.   Adult hypertrophic pyloric stenosis. There is narrowing and elongation of the pyloric canal with characteristic concave, crescentic indentation at the base of the duodenal bulb.

Fig. 20-12.   Congenital pyloric stenosis in an infant. There is narrowing and elongation of the pyloric canal with characteristic concave, crescentic indentation at the base of the duodenal bulb.

acteristic of adult hypertrophic pyloric stenosis, the concave impression has also been described in patients with scirrhous carcinoma of the pyloric channel.

A less common and atypical form of muscular hypertrophy has been termed "focal hypertrophy" or "torus hyperplasia." It is the result of a localized muscle hypertrophy on the lesser curvature, at the level where normal muscle fibers usually converge to form a muscular prominence called the "torus." An additional uneven hypertrophy of the muscle fibers along the greater curvature leads to the development of a characteristic radiographic appearance. The distal antrum and pyloric canal are asymmetrically narrowed, the lesser curvature is flattened or concave, and the greater curvature is slightly serrated (Fig. 20-13).

Ultrasound has emerged as a noninvasive alternative to the upper gastrointestinal study and is now the imaging modality of choice for demonstrating pyloric stenosis. The criteria for the sonographic diagnosis of hypertrophic pyloric stenosis include the demonstration of a sonolucent doughnut lesion consisting of a prominent anechoic rim of thickened muscle (measuring 0.3 cm or greater) and an echogenic center of mucosa and submucosa (Fig. 20-14A); the demonstration on longitudinal sections of continuity between the anechoic rim of thickened muscle and the thin muscle of the gastric antrum; evidence of gastric outlet obstruction (lack of

opening of the pyloric canal); and the demonstration of an elongated pyloric canal (1.4 cm or greater) (Fig. 20-14B). If the findings meet the sonographic criteria for hypertrophic pyloric stenosis,

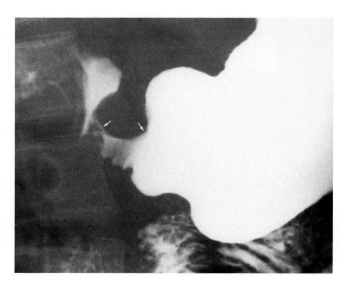

Fig. 20-13.   Focal pyloric hypertrophy or torus hyperplasia. The lesser curvature of the distal antrum has a smooth concave configuration **(arrows)**, whereas the opposite wall on the greater curvature is irregular and serrated. (Balthazar EJ: Hypertrophic pyloric stenosis in adults: Radiographic features. Am J Gastroenterol 78:449–453, 1983)

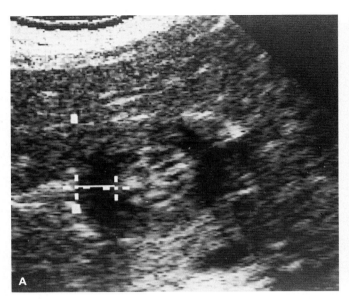
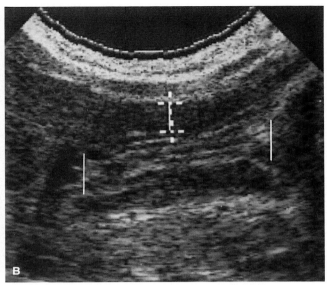

Fig. 20-14. Ultrasound of hypertrophic pyloric stenosis. **(A)** Characteristic doughnut lesion consisting of a prominent anechoic rim of thickened muscle and an echogenic center of mucosa and submucosa. The thickness of the muscle between the cursors measured 6 mm. **(B)** On a longitudinal view, the elongated pyloric canal **(between vertical white lines)** measures 2.5 cm. Note the alternating echolucent and echogenic channels within the pyloric canal, corresponding to the "double-track" mucosa sign on barium studies. The thickness of the pyloric muscle again measures 6 mm **(between cursors)**.

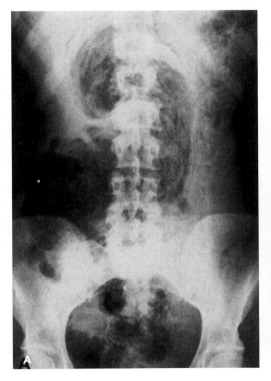
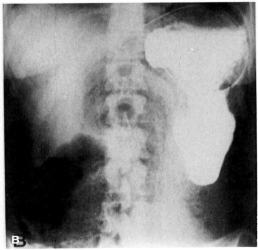

Fig. 20-15. Massive phytobezoar in the right colon causing gastric outlet obstruction. **(A)** Plain radiograph shows the large collection of mottled and curvilinear lucencies assuming a whorled appearance in the epigastrium and extending down to the right iliac fossa. **(B)** Contrast examination shows complete obstruction of the distended stomach due to extrinsic compression of the antrum and pylorus by the bezoar. (Agha FT, Nostrant TT, Fiddian–Green RG: "Giant colonic bezoar": A medication bezoar due to psyllium seed husks. Am J Gastroenterol 79:319–321, 1984)

an upper gastrointestinal contrast study is not needed.

BEZOAR/PROLAPSED ANTRAL MUCOSA

Masses of foreign material in the stomach rarely produce bezoars of sufficient size to cause gastric outlet obstruction. One case has been reported of a massive phytobezoar in the right colon (due to psyllium seed husks) causing complete gastric outlet obstruction by extrinsic compression (Fig. 20-15). Intermittent pyloric obstruction is occasionally caused by prolapse of antral mucosa. The prolapsed mucosa can undergo erosion or ulceration, leading to gastrointestinal bleeding and iron deficiency anemia.

BIBLIOGRAPHY

Agha FP, Nostrant TT, Fiddian–Green RG: "Giant colonic bezoar": A medication bezoar due to psyllium seed husks. Am J Gastroenterol 79:319–321, 1984

Aranha GV, Prinz RA, Greenlee HB et al: Gastric outlet and duodenal obstruction from inflammatory pancreatic disease. Arch Surg 119:833–835, 1984

Balthazar EJ: Hypertrophic pyloric stenosis in adults: Radiographic features. Am J Gastroenterol 78:449–453, 1983

Balthazar EJ, Rosenberg H, Davidian MM: Scirrhous carcinoma of the pyloric channel and distal antrum. AJR 134:669–673, 1980

Bjorgvinsson E, Rudzki C, Lewicki AM: Antral web. Am J Gastroenterol 79:663–665, 1984

Clements JL, Jinkins JR, Torres WE et al: Antral mucosal diaphragms in adults. AJR 133:1105–1111, 1979

Dworkin HJ, Roth HP: Pyloric obstruction associated with peptic ulcer. JAMA 180:1007–1010, 1962

Gerson DE, Lewicki AM: Intrathoracic stomach: When does it obstruct? Radiology 119:257–264, 1976

Goldstein H, Jamin M, Schapiro M et al: Gastric retention associated with gastroduodenal disease. Am J Dig Dis 11:887–897, 1966

Kozoll DD, Meyer KA: Obstructing duodenal ulcer, symptoms and signs. Arch Surg 89:491–498, 1964

Kreel L, Ellis H: Pyloric stenosis in adults: A clinical and radiological study of 100 consecutive patients. Gut 6:253–261, 1965

Scott RL, Felker R, Winer–Muram H et al: The differential retrocardiac air–fluid level: A sign of intrathoracic gastric volvulus. J Can Assoc Radiol 37:119–121, 1986

GASTRIC DILATATION WITHOUT OUTLET OBSTRUCTION

Disease Entities

Postabdominal surgery
Abdominal trauma
    Ruptured spleen
    Fractures
    Retroperitoneal hematoma
    Urinary tract injury
Severe pain
    Renal colic
    Biliary colic
    Migraine headaches
Infection and inflammation
    Peritonitis
    Pancreatitis
    Appendicitis
    Subphrenic abscess
    Septicemia
Immobilization
    Body plaster cast
    Paraplegia
    Postoperative state
Diabetes mellitus
Neurologic abnormalities
    Brain tumor
    Bulbar poliomyelitis
    Vagotomy
    Tabes dorsalis
Muscular abnormalities
    Scleroderma

Polymyositis/dermatomyositis
    Muscular dystrophy
Drug-induced disorders
    Atropine or atropine-like drugs
    Morphine
    Ganglionic blocking agents
Electrolyte/acid-base imbalance
    Diabetic ketoacidosis
    Hypercalcemia
    Hypocalcemia
    Hypokalemia
    Hepatic coma
    Uremia
    Myxedema
Lead poisoning
Porphyria
Emotional distress

Acute or chronic dilatation of the stomach with prolonged retention of food and barium can occur without any organic gastric outlet obstruction. Gastric retention is defined as vomiting of food eaten more than 6 hr earlier or the presence of food in the stomach at the time of an upper gastrointestinal series (assuming that the patient has not eaten for 8–10 hr). It is critical to remember that gastric retention does not necessarily mean gastric outlet obstruction and that "corrective" surgery may be contraindicated.

The appearance of gastric dilatation without obstruction on plain radiographs is indistinguishable from that of organic gastric outlet obstruction. Huge quantities of air and fluid fill a massively enlarged stomach that can extend even to the floor of the pelvis (Fig. 21-1). Administration of barium demonstrates a large amount of solid gastric residue (Fig. 21-2). Persistalsis is irregular, sluggish, and ineffectual. The failure of radiographic studies to demonstrate an organic cause for gastric outlet obstruction in patients with dilation of the stomach does not imply at all that no abnormality exists. In addition, when retained food is seen in the stomach during a barium examination, the various nonobstructive causes of gastric retention must be excluded before the patient can be accused of disregarding instructions and eating just before the examination.

ACUTE GASTRIC DILATATION

Acute gastric dilatation is sudden and excessive distention of the stomach by fluid and gas, usually accompanied by vomiting, dehydration, and peripheral vascular collapse (Fig. 21-3). Within minutes or hours, a normal stomach can expand into a hyperemic, cyanotic, atonic sac that fills the abdomen.

Most cases of acute gastric dilatation occur during the first several days after abdominal surgery. The incidence of this postoperative complication has dramatically decreased with the advent of nasogastric suction, improved anesthetics, close monitoring of acid-base and electrolyte balance, and meticulous care in the handling of tissues at surgery. Acute gastric dilatation can also be a complication of other medical or surgical diseases. Abdominal trauma, especially involving the back, is often followed by acute gastric dilatation (Fig. 21-4). Although the exact etiology is unclear, some reflex paralysis of the gastric motor mechanisms secondary to surgery or trauma most likely permits the stomach to distend abnormally as fluid and air accumulate within it. Patients with severe pain and patients with inflammatory processes in the peritoneal cavity can also develop acute gastric dilatation through a reflex neurologic pathway. Immobilization, primarily in patients with body casts or with paraplegia, causes gastric dilatation by making belching difficult as well as by compressing the transverse portion of the duodenum.

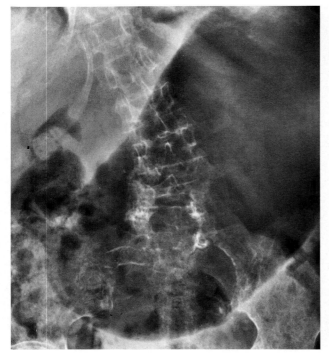

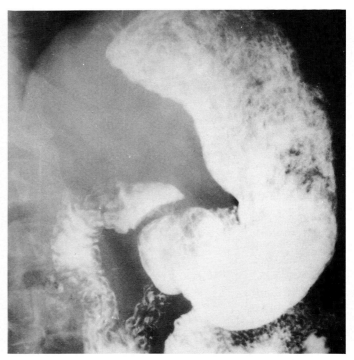

21-1   21-2

Fig. 21-1. Gastric dilatation. A plain abdominal radiograph demonstrates a huge quantity of air and fluid filling a massively enlarged stomach that extends to the lower portion of the pelvis.

Fig. 21-2. Dilated, atonic stomach with a substantial solid gastric residue in a patient with diabetic gastric neuropathy. There is no evidence of gastric outlet obstruction. (Gramm HF, Reuter K, Costello P: The radiologic manifestations of diabetic gastric neuropathy and its differential diagnosis. Gastrointest Radiol 3:151–155, 1978)

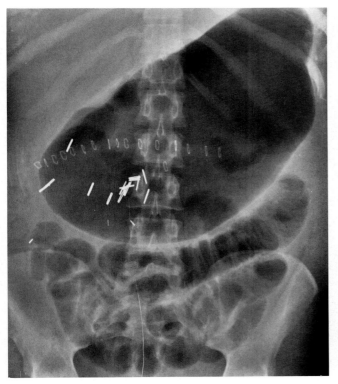

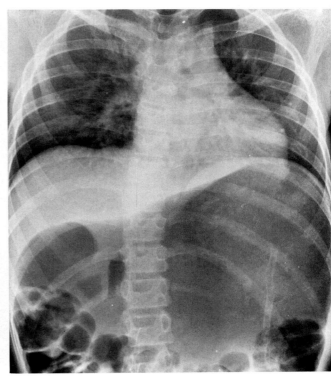

21-3

21-4

Fig. 21-3. Acute gastric dilatation following abdominal surgery.

Fig. 21-4. Acute gastric dilatation following trauma.

The danger of acute gastric dilatation lies in its potential for complications and death if untreated. Prompt response to appropriate therapy can usually be achieved if early signs are appreciated. Unfortunately, pain is seldom severe until gastric dilatation is pronounced. Distention can progress rapidly due to aerophagia or air-sucking. Sudden relaxation of the gastric cardia can lead to copious vomiting, aspiration, asphyxiation, and cardiac arrest. Acute gastric dilatation can cause gastric perforation with peritonitis or result in severe fluid and electrolyte disturbances, dehydration, decreased urinary output, and shock.

CHRONIC GASTRIC DILATATION

The development of gastric dilatation can be indolent and essentially asymptomatic. Gastric motor abnormalities occur in 20% to 30% of diabetics, primarily those who have long-term disease under relatively inadequate control and evidence of peripheral neuropathy or other complications. Diabetics who have delayed gastric emptying may complain of vague abdominal discomfort and, on occasion, protracted vomiting. Chronic gastric dilatation in this disease is probably secondary to an autonomic neuropathy, since an identical appearance can be produced following vagotomy. Radiographically, the stomach is large and distended (Fig. 21-5). It contains substantial amounts of retained fluid and food and demonstrates little, if any, peristalsis. Although gastric emptying is severely prolonged, some barium usually can be manipulated to outline a patent pylorus and proximal duodenum. Many diabetics have gastric mucosal atrophy and diminished secretions, which may explain the reported low incidence of duodenal ulcer disease in these patients. However, complications of peptic ulcer disease tend to be more severe in diabetics than in other patients, since the vascular abnormalities associated with diabetes make bleeding more profuse and difficult to control. In diabetics who are out of medical control, ketoacidosis can lead to acute gastric dilatation and a possibly catastrophic outcome.

Patients with neurologic abnormalities (brain tumor, bulbar poliomyelitis, tabes dorsalis) may develop chronic gastric retention. In these conditions, however, decreased peristalsis and dilatation more commonly involve the esophagus. Surgical or chemical vagotomy (atropine or drugs with an atropine-like action) can also result in gastric dilatation.

Gastric manifestations of scleroderma are uncommon but not rare. Diffuse hypotonia and prolonged emptying time produce nonobstructive gas-

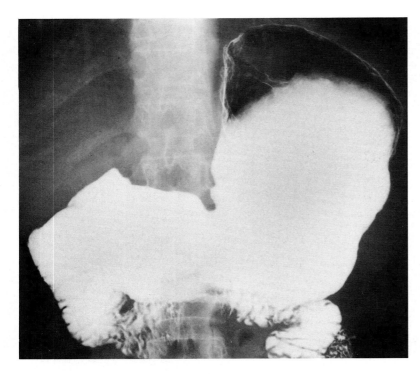

Fig. 21-5. Gastric dilatation due to chronic diabetic neuropathy.

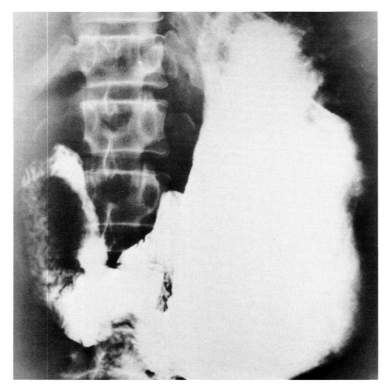

Fig. 21-6. Gastric dilatation without obstruction in a patient with scleroderma.

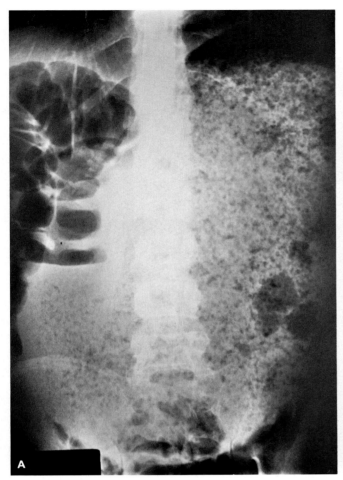
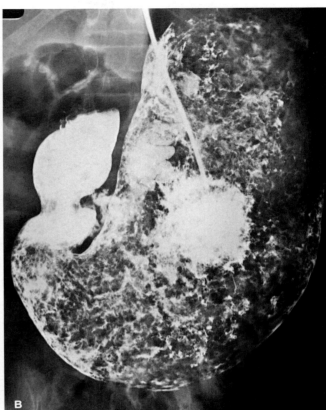

Fig. 21-7. Chronic gastric dilatation due to severe electrolyte and acid–base imbalance in a diabetic patient. **(A)** Plain film and **(B)** contrast study show a tremendous amount of particulate material in the massively distended stomach.

tric dilatation (Fig. 21-6). Effacement of mucosal folds can result in a smooth gastric outline. A similar pattern of chronic gastric dilatation has been reported in patients with polymyositis, dermatomyositis, and myotonic muscular dystrophy.

Electrolyte and acid-base imbalances tend to produce dilatation of abdominal viscera, presumably because of alteration in muscle tone (Fig. 21-7). Although these metabolic disorders are more likely to cause megacolon than dilatation of the stomach, the latter does occur. Alteration in muscle tone is also the probable mechanism for gastric distention secondary to lead poisoning and porphyria. In patients under severe emotional stress, gastric dilatation can be due to a reflex neurologic abnormality or to hyperventilation associated with excessive swallowing of air.

BIBLIOGRAPHY

Berk RN, Coulson DB: The body cast syndrome. Radiology 94:303–305, 1970

Feldman M, Schiller LR: Disorders of gastrointestinal motility associated with diabetes mellitus. Ann Intern Med 98:378–384, 1983

Gramm HF, Reuter K, Costello P: The radiologic manifestations of diabetic gastric neuropathy and its differential diagnosis. Gastrointest Radiol 3:151–155, 1978

Horowitz M, McNeil JD, Maddern GJ et al: Abnormalities of gastric and esophageal emptying in polymyositis and dermatomyositis. Gastroenterology 90:434–439, 1986

Joffe N: Some unusual roentgenologic findings associated with marked gastric dilatation. AJR 119:291–299, 1973

Nowak TV, Ionasescu V, Anuras S: Gastrointestinal manifestations of the muscular dystrophies. Gastroenterology 82:800–810, 1982

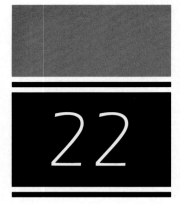

INTRINSIC/EXTRINSIC MASSES OF THE FUNDUS

Disease Entities

Neoplasms
  Primary malignancies of the stomach
    Carcinoma
    Lymphoma
    Leiomyosarcoma
  Extragastric malignancies
    Carcinoma of the body or tail of the pancreas
    Carcinoma of the splenic flexure of the colon
    Tumors of adjacent organs (liver, adrenal, kidney)
    Lymphoma or metastases to adjacent lymph nodes
  Benign tumors of the stomach
    Spindle cell tumor
    Adenoma
Extrinsic pressure by normal or enlarged structures
  Liver
  Spleen
  Splenic flexure
  Kidney
  Aorta
  Heart
  Cardiac aneurysm
Intrinsic benign gastric lesions
  Esophagogastric herniation/reduced hiatal hernia
  Gastric varices

Giant rugal folds
Postoperative deformities (*e.g.,* Nissen fundoplication, splenectomy)
Regenerated splenosis
Subphrenic abscess
Gastric diverticulum
Hematoma

The gastric fundus is that portion of the stomach lying above an imaginary horizontal line drawn from the esophagogastric junction to the greater curvature of the stomach. Most of the superior surface of the fundus is usually in close contact with the left leaf of the diaphragm. The left lobe of the liver is interposed between the diaphragm and the anteromedial aspect of the fundus; the spleen is usually situated between the diaphragm and the posterolateral aspect of the fundus.

    The gastric fundus is a difficult area to examine by a single-contrast barium study. When the stomach is not distended, crowding of prominent folds tends to obscure surface detail. Instillation of larger volumes of barium makes the fundus so opaque that only contour abnormalities can be identified. The overlying rib cage precludes the possibility of effective compression. Therefore, the double-contrast technique with full distention is essential for optimal visualization of the fundus (Fig. 22-1).

NEOPLASMS

Primary carcinoma of the stomach is the most important lesion involving the fundus. Carcinoma of

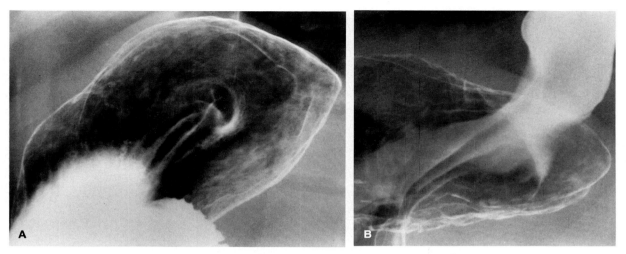

Fig. 22-1. Normal appearance of the fundus with the double-contrast technique. **(A)** Esophageal rosette pattern and **(B)** high transverse fold pattern.

the fundus can produce a discrete filling defect (Fig. 22-2), nodularity (Fig. 22-3), or effacement and nodularity of the esophageal rosette or the fundal mucosal folds (Fig. 22-4). Ulceration is common, and exophytic growth of tumor can cause extrinsic impressions on the fundus. A primary malignant lesion involving the fundus can sometimes be detected by demonstration of a deformed gastric air bubble on upright plain abdominal or chest radiographs (Fig. 22-5). Carcinoma of the fundus frequently extends proximally to involve the distal esophagus as well (Fig. 22-6).

Gastric lymphoma commonly involves the fundus, either alone or in conjunction with disease in the body of the stomach. The radiographic ap-

pearance varies from large, irregular, ulcerated masses (Fig. 22-7) to nodular submucosal infiltration. Although transcardial extension is less common than with carcinoma of the fundus, extension of malignant disease to the distal esophagus has been reported to occur in 2% to 10% of cases of gastric lymphoma.

Leiomyosarcomas are rare gastric tumors that can involve the fundus of the stomach. They tend to be large lesions with central ulcerations, and they often have a large exogastric component (Fig. 22-8).

Malignant tumors developing in adjacent organs can spread to the fundus and produce an appearance mimicking primary intragastric carcinoma. This is most commonly seen in patients with

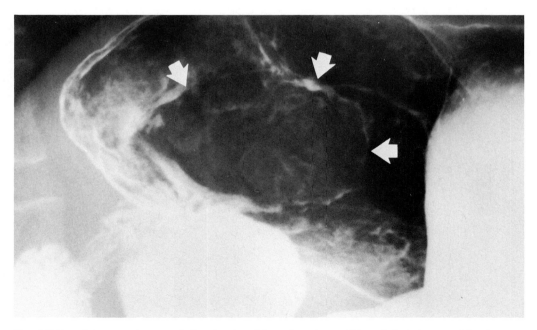

Fig. 22-2. Adenocarcinoma of the fundus. There is a large filling defect **(arrows)** in the region of the esophagogastric junction.

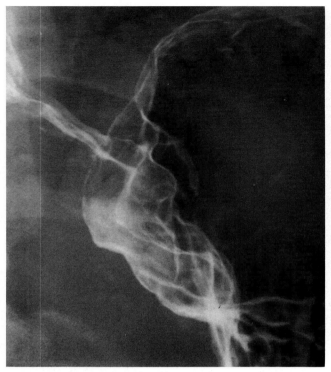

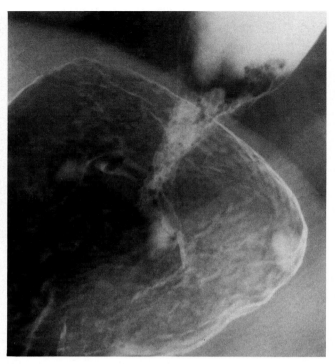

Fig. 22-3. Adenocarcinoma of the fundus. There is nodular irregularity of the medial aspect of the fundus with extension of the tumor into the distal esophagus.

Fig. 22-4. Adenocarcinoma of the fundus. The normal fold pattern at the gastroesophageal junction is absent. Irregular narrowing of the distal esophagus represents proximal spread of the tumor.

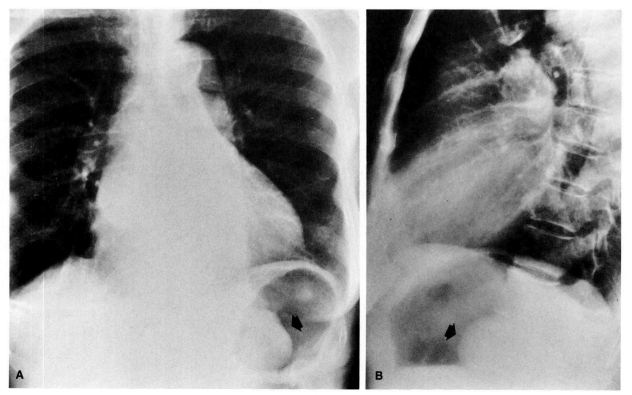

Fig. 22-5. Adenocarcinoma of the fundus. The tumor is seen as a soft-tissue mass **(arrows)** within the gastric air bubble on **(A)** frontal and **(B)** lateral views.

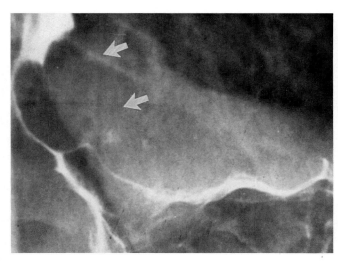

Fig. 22-6. Adenocarcinoma of the fundus. An irregular tumor of the superior aspect of the fundus extends proximally as a large mass **(arrows)**, almost obstructing the distal esophagus.

carcinoma of the pancreas or tumors of the splenic flexure of the colon. Malignant lesions of the liver, adrenal, kidney, and breast (Fig. 22-9) can cause a similar radiographic pattern. Neoplastic enlargement of celiac lymph nodes can produce an extrinsic impression on the medial aspect of the fundus.

Benign neoplasms, such as spindle cell tumors (especially leiomyomas) and adenomas, can present as fundal filling defects that are indistinguishable from malignant tumors (Figs. 22-10, 22-11).

EXTRINSIC PRESSURE BY NORMAL OR ENLARGED STRUCTURES

Many normal variants and extrinsic processes can simulate tumors of the gastric fundus. In one study,

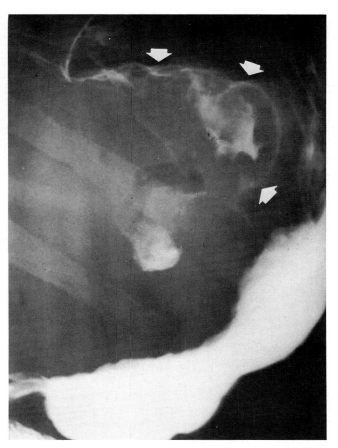

Fig. 22-8. Leiomyosarcoma. The large fundal mass **(arrows)** shows extensive exophytic extension and ulceration.

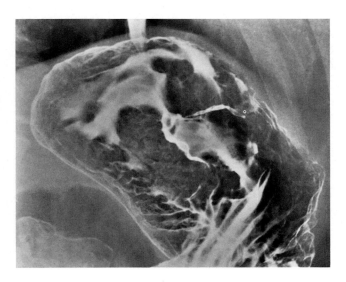

Fig. 22-7. Lymphoma. Large, irregular fundal mass with central ulceration.

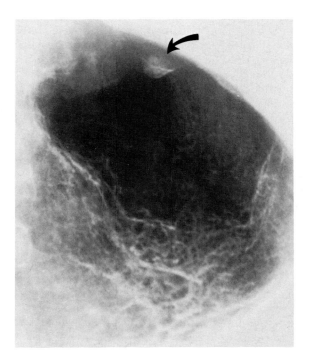

Fig. 22-9. Small, malignant implant in the fundus **(arrow)** representing hematogenous metastasis from carcinoma of the breast.

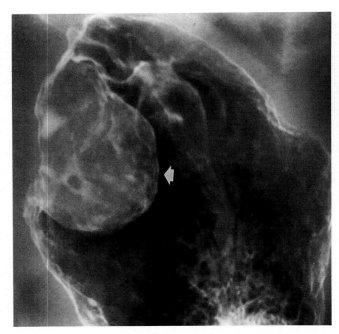

Fig. 22-10. Leiomyoma of the fundus **(arrow)**.

more than 70% of fundal masses proved to be non-neoplastic conditions. About 20% of these patients had pseudotumors, masses that were not seen on subsequent examinations. Therefore, a repeat examination should be performed to confirm the presence of any suspected mass in the fundus.

Both the liver and the spleen can normally flatten the usually rounded contour of the fundus (Fig. 22-12). This flattening is variable and is generally considered to be within normal limits as long as there is no evidence of either splenic or hepatic enlargement. The splenic flexure of the colon can produce a pressure defect simulating a localized lesion, and this condition can readily be diagnosed when the splenic flexure is filled with air or barium. An impression on the posterior aspect of the fundus can sometimes be caused by a normal left kidney. Tortuosity of the aorta can produce an extrinsic impression with no evidence of a mucosal lesion. A normal cardiac silhouette can cause an impression on the fundus (Fig. 22-13*A*), as can a large cardiac aneurysm (Fig. 22-13*B*).

With the patient in the erect position, the soft-tissue space between the diaphragm and the superior margin of the air-distended fundus usually measures 3 mm to 5 mm (a maximum of 15 mm is normal). This represents the combined thickness of the gastric wall and the diaphragm. Although an increase in this space can be due to a true pathologic entity, it can also be the result of incomplete distention of a normal fundus (Fig. 22-14). Infrequently, interposition of the spleen between the fundus and the diaphragm can cause a confusing deformity simulating a malignant process.

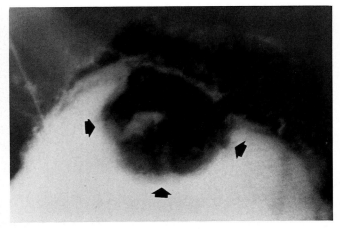

Fig. 22-11. Ulcerated leiomyoma of the fundus **(arrows)**.

Extrinsic pressure on the stomach can be due to an anomalous lobe of the liver or to aberrant positions of the spleen or left kidney. Enlargement of these structures for whatever reason can also produce extrinsic impressions in the fundal region. Radioisotope liver-spleen scanning and excretory urography can differentiate these extrinsic defects from true intragastric lesions.

INTRINSIC BENIGN GASTRIC LESIONS

Invagination or prolapse of the distal esophageal mucosa into the stomach can cause a pseudotumor

Text continues on page 303

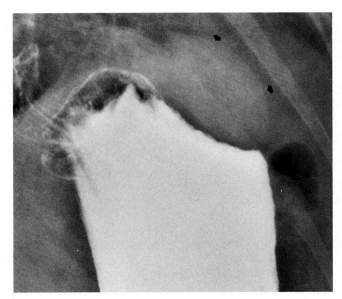

Fig. 22-12. Impression of the normal spleen **(arrows)** on the fundus.

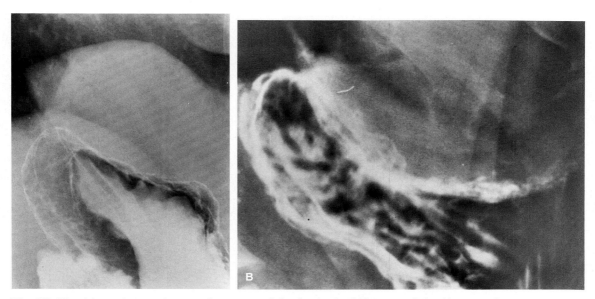

Fig. 22-13. Impression on the superior aspect of the fundus by **(A)** a normal-sized heart and **(B)** a large cardiac aneurysm.

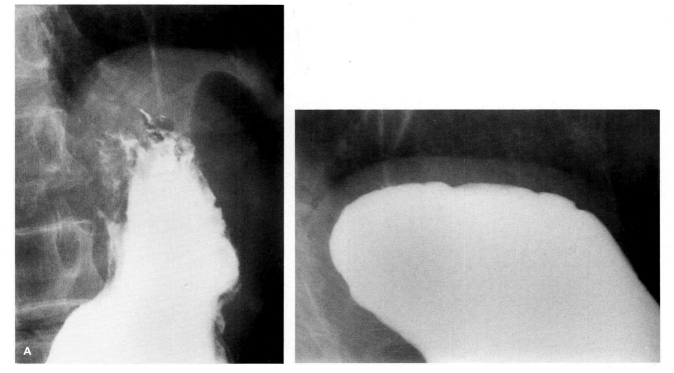

Fig. 22-14. **(A)** Apparently increased soft-tissue space between the hemidiaphragm and the superior margin of the fundus due to incomplete distention of the fundus. **(B)** With full distention of the fundus, the space is shown to be of normal size.

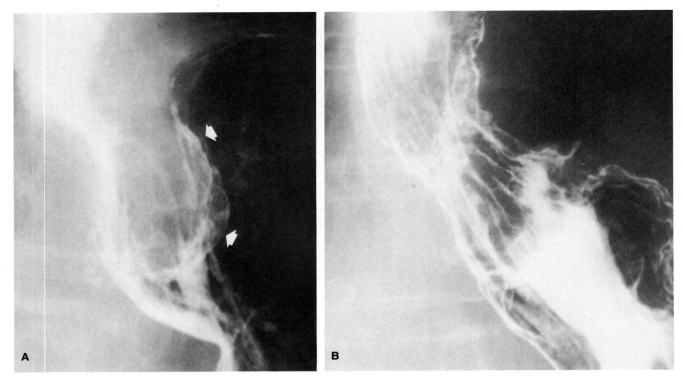

Fig. 22-15. **(A)** Fundal pseudotumor **(arrows)** caused by a reduced hiatal hernia. **(B)** The pseudotumor disappears when the hiatal hernia is fully distended and situated above the diaphragm.

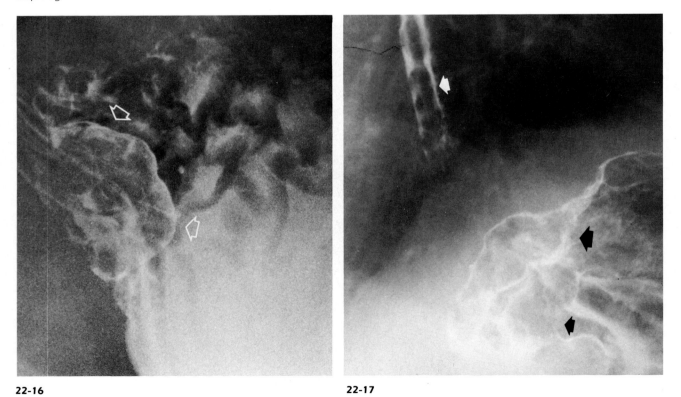

22-16

22-17

Fig. 22-16. Gastric varix. A single fundal mass **(arrows)** in the region of the esophagogastric junction simulates a neoplastic process.

Fig. 22-17. Gastric varices. Irregular filling defects in the fundus **(black arrows)** are associated with serpiginous varices in the esophagus **(white arrow)**.

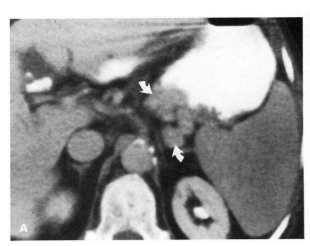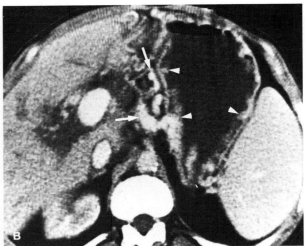

Fig. 22-18. Gastric varices. **(A)** Large enhancing venous channels within the posterior wall of the proximal stomach **(arrows)**. Note the scalloped configuration of the posterior gastric wall. **(B)** In another patient who had chronic pancreatitis and splenic vein thrombosis, a CT scan obtained while the stomach was distended with water shows enhancing venous channels within the lesser omentum **(arrows)** and along the circumference of the proximal stomach **(arrowheads)**. (Balthazar EJ: Miscellaneous disorders of the stomach. In Taveras JM, Ferrucci JT (eds): Radiology: Diagnosis–Imaging–Intervention. Philadelphia, JB Lippincott, 1987)

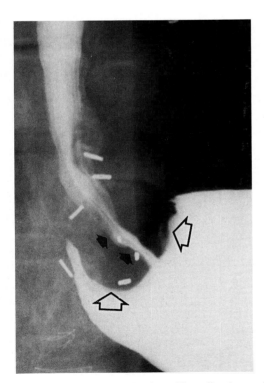

Fig. 22-19. Nissen fundoplication. The distal esophagus **(closed arrows)** passes through the fundal pseudotumor **(open arrows)**. (Skucas J, Mangla JC, Adams JT et al: An evaluation of the Nissen fundoplication. Radiology 118:539–543, 1976)

in the fundus. Erosion of the herniated portion often leads to gastric bleeding. Redundancy of soft tissue associated with a reduced hiatal hernia can produce a discrete mass in the fundus (Fig. 22-15*A*). In some patients, a notchlike defect is seen. This form of fundal pseudotumor disappears when the hiatal hernia is fully distended and is located above the diaphragm (Fig. 22-15*B*).

Gastric varices can be difficult to distinguish from a primary fundal tumor (Fig. 22-16), especially without esophageal varices, splenomegaly, or a history of cirrhosis. The thick, tortuous mucosal folds or lobulated polypoid mass caused by varices frequently demonstrate alteration in size and shape when the patient changes position and phase of respiration (Fig. 22-17). On CT scanning, gastric varices appear as well-defined clusters of rounded or tubular soft-tissue densities within the posterior and posteromedial wall of the proximal stomach (Fig. 22-18). The wall of the stomach is scalloped, and there is no cleavage plane between the gastric lumen and the varicosities. In some patients, CT may show the underlying pathogenesis of gastric varices by identifying such conditions as hepatic cirrhosis, calcific pancreatitis, and pancreatic carcinoma.

Thickened gastric rugae in the fundus may be caused by a true pathologic process or may merely be due to poor distention. When prominent fundal folds reflect a clinically significant entity, there are

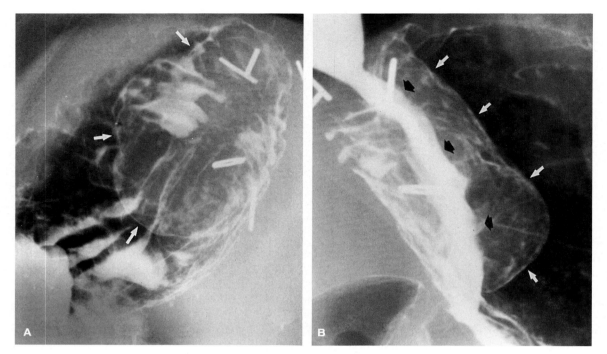

Fig. 22-20. Fundoplication mimicking neoplasm. **(A)** With the distal esophagus emptied of barium, the pseudotumor of the fundoplication **(arrows)** is indistinguishable from a large fundal mass. **(B)** On a later film during the examination, barium in the distal esophagus **(black arrows)** passes through the fundal pseudotumor **(white arrows)**.

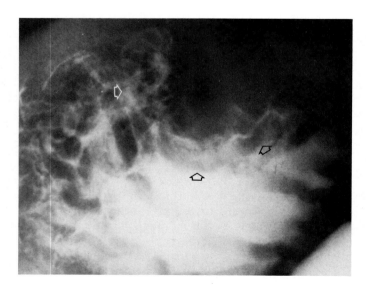

Fig. 22-21. Postsplenectomy gastric deformity. Oblique view from an upper gastrointestinal examination 2 months after splenectomy shows a characteristic masslike indentation on the upper greater curvature of the stomach **(arrows)**. (Ansel HJ, Wasserman NF: Postsplenectomy gastric deformity. AJR 139:99–101, 1982)

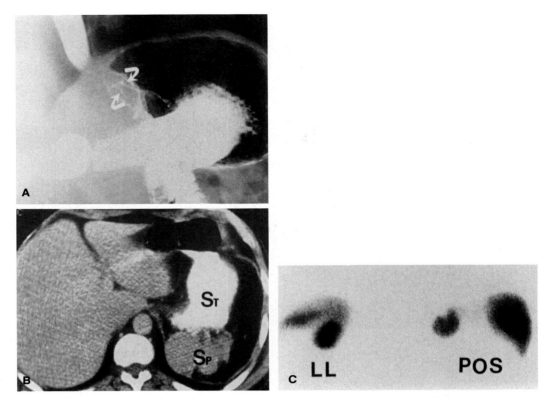

Fig. 22-22. Regenerated splenosis. **(A)** Distortion of the gastric fundus by a mass lesion with overlying linear ulceration **(arrows)**. The sharp margins of the mass suggest an intramural-extramucosal location. **(B)** CT scan at the level of the fundus shows a lobulated homogeneous mass indenting the gastric fundus from behind and medially. Note the absence of the spleen because of a previous splenectomy. **(ST,** stomach; **Sp,** regenerated spleen). **(C)** Radionuclide liver–spleen scan confirms that the mass indenting the gastric fundus indeed represents splenic tissue **(LL,** left lateral; **POS,** posterior). (Agha FP: Regenerated splenosis masquerading as gastric fundic mass. Am J Gastroenterol 79:576–578, 1984)

usually similar changes elsewhere in the stomach that offer a clue to the diagnosis. If thickened mucosal folds are localized to the fundus and cannot be effaced by overdistention of the stomach, gastroscopy is required to exclude the possibility of malignancy.

Postoperative distortion of normal anatomic relationships can cause extrinsic masses in the fundus. A typical example is the pseudotumor secondary to a Nissen fundoplication. This method of hiatal hernia repair involves wrapping the gastric fundus around the lower esophagus to create an intra-abdominal esophageal segment with a natural valve mechanism at the esophagogastric junction. The surgical procedure characteristically results in a prominent filling defect at the esophagogastric junction (Fig. 22-19) that is generally smoothly marginated and symmetric on both sides of the distal esophagus. An irregular outline may be present if part of the stomach is incompletely filled with bar-

ium or air. The distal esophagus appears to pass through the center of the concave mass (pseudotumor), which impresses the superomedial aspect of the fundus. If an adequate clinical history has not been obtained, the pseudotumor may be confused with a neoplasm in this area, especially if radiographs are obtained without the distal esophagus being filled with contrast material (Fig. 22-20). Demonstration of a preserved esophageal lumen and mucosal pattern, as well as good delineation of the gastroesophageal junction, should permit exclusion of the possibility of a neoplastic process.

Mass- or polyplike defects of the gastric fundus may occur following splenectomy. During splenectomy, the short gastric vessels between the spleen and greater curvature of the fundus of the stomach are ligated and cut. Rather than individually ligating these vessels, the surgeon often ligates several together. This may cause an infolding of the gastric wall and account for the defect seen in some post-

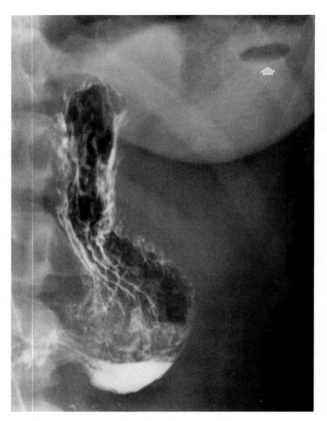

Fig. 22-23. Left subphrenic abscess. The mass narrows the fundus and displaces it from the hemidiaphragm. Note the collection of gas **(arrow)** in the abscess.

splenectomy patients (Fig. 22-21). An anterior or medial impression on the fundus and narrowing of the distal esophagus may represent a postoperative deformity following the placement of a valve conduit from the apex of the left ventricle to the abdominal aorta for relief of left ventricular outlet obstruction in patients in whom conventional aortic valve replacement is not safe or feasible.

Regenerated splenosis may masquerade as a gastric fundal mass (Fig. 22-22A). The spleen develops from the dorsal mesogastrium, and some residual tissue may remain there after full splenic development. After splenectomy, splenules may even grow in the wall of the stomach, producing a contour abnormality simulating an intramural neoplasm. A radionuclide or CT scan can accurately demonstrate that the indentation on the gastric fundus is caused by regenerated splenic tissue and thus preclude the need for angiography and exploratory surgery (Fig. 22-22B, C).

A left subphrenic abscess can displace the fundus of the stomach caudad, abnormally widening the distance between it and the diaphragm (Fig. 22-23). Concomitant findings of splinting of the left hemidiaphragm, irritative phenomena at the base of the left lung, or the presence of gas within the abscess can clarify the diagnosis. This pattern can be simulated by a large infrapulmonary effusion that appears to widen the distance between the left hemidiaphragm and fundus in the absence of a true abdominal process. Abscesses can also extrinsically

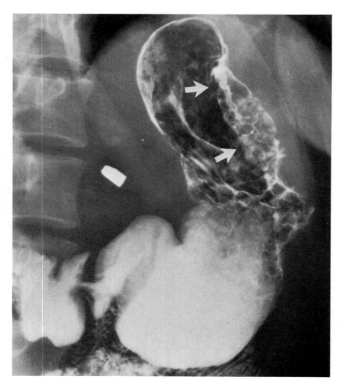

Fig. 22-24. Post-traumatic abscess extrinsically impressing the fundus **(arrows)** without widening the space between the fundus and the left hemidiaphragm. The patient sustained a gunshot wound in which the bullet penetrated the pancreas and left kidney.

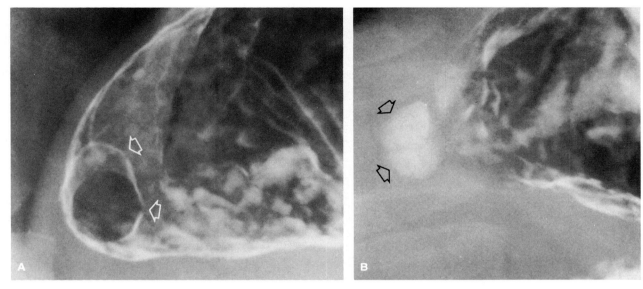

Fig. 22-25. **(A)** Gas-filled gastric diverticulum mimicking a discrete fundal mass **(arrows)**. **(B)** On repeat examination, barium within the diverticulum **(arrows)** is clearly separated from the fundus, revealing the true nature of the process.

impress the fundus without widening the space between it and the left hemidiaphragm (Fig. 22-24).

An apparent filling defect in the posterior portion of the fundus can be due to a large gastric diverticulum that fails to fill with gas or barium and mimics a smooth-bordered, submucosal mass (Fig. 22-25*A*). On repeat examination, barium can usually be demonstrated to enter the diverticulum, thereby establishing the diagnosis (Fig. 22-25*B*). At times, a collection of barium may pool in a gastric diverticulum and mimic an acute ulceration (Fig. 22-26). Inflammatory or neoplastic enlargement of celiac

lymph nodes can cause a pressure defect upon the medial aspect of the fundus that is difficult to distinguish from an impression due to a normal left lobe of the liver. In one instance, a large, irregular polypoid filling defect in the fundus was reported to represent a hematoma secondary to a Mallory-Weiss tear.

BIBLIOGRAPHY

Agha FP: Regenerated splenosis masquerading as gastric fundic mass. Am J Gastroenterol 79:576–578, 1984

Ansel HJ, Wasserman NF: Postsplenectomy gastric deformity. AJR 139:99–101, 1982

Balthazar EJ, Megibow A, Naidich D et al: Computed tomographic recognition of gastric varices. AJR 142:1121–1125, 1984

Bickers GH, Williams SM, Harned RK et al: Gastroesophageal deformities of left ventricular-abdominal aortic conduit. AJR 138:867–869, 1982

Feigen DS, James AE, Stitik FP et al: The radiological appearance of hiatal hernia repairs. Radiology 110:71–77, 1974

Font RG, Sparks RD, Herbert GA: Ectopic spleen mimicking an intrinsic fundal lesion of the stomach. Am J Dig Dis 15:49–56, 1970

Freeny PC: Double-contrast gastrography of the fundus and cardia: Normal landmarks and their pathologic change. AJR 133:481–487, 1979

Freeny PC, Marks WM: Adenocarcinoma of the gastroesophageal junction: Barium and CT examination. AJR 138:1077–1084, 1982

Glick SN, Teplick SK, Levine MS et al: Gastric cardia metastasis in esophageal carcinoma. Radiology 160:627–630, 1986

Herlinger H, Grossman R, Laufer I et al: The gastric cardia in double-contrast study: Its dynamic image. AJR 135:21–29, 1980

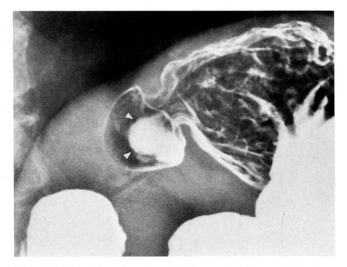

Fig. 22-26. Gastric diverticulum. Pooling of barium **(arrows)** simulates an acute ulceration.

Kaye JJ, Stassa G: Mimicry and decption in the diagnosis of tumors of the gastric cardia. AJR 110:295–303, 1970

Laufer I: A simple method for routine double-contrast study of the upper gastrointestinal tract. Radiology 117:513–518, 1975

Levine MS, Laufer I, Thompson JJ: Carcinoma of the gastric cardia in young people. AJR 140:69–72, 1983

Skucas J, Mangla JC, Adams JT et al: An evaluation of the Nissen fundoplication. Radiology 118:539–543, 1976

Thoeni RF, Moss AA: The radiographic appearance of complications following Nissen fundoplication. Radiology 131:17–21, 1979

Wohl GT, Shore L: Lesions of the cardiac end of the stomach simulating carcinoma. AJR 82:1048–1057, 1959

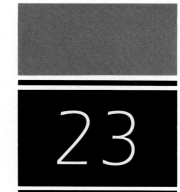

WIDENING OF THE RETROGASTRIC SPACE

Disease Entities

Generalized widening without a discrete mass
  Obesity
  Previous surgery
  Ascites
  Gross hepatomegaly
  Hernias involving the omentum
  Emphysema
Discrete retrogastric masses
  Pancreatic masses
    Carcinoma
    Pseudocysts
    Pancreatitis
    Cystadenoma
  Retroperitoneal masses
    Neoplasms
    Lymph node enlargement
    Abscesses
    Hematoma
  Masses on the posterior wall of the stomach
  Aortic aneurysm
  Choledochal cyst

The midline posterior gastric wall is separated from the anterior vertebral body by two layers of peritoneum that enclose the lesser sac, the prepancreatic (properitoneal) fat layer, the pancreatic neck (about 1–1.5 cm thick in the midline), the aortic lymph nodes, and the aorta. Numerous methods have been suggested for measuring the distance from the stomach to the spine to quantitatively determine enlargement of the retrogastric space. Unfortunately, the wide range of normal variation has made it clear that measurements alone are of little value in the detection of a retrogastric mass. In order for the existence of a true retrogastric mass to be demonstrated on the lateral view of a barium upper gastrointestinal series, an extrinsic impression must be identified. Attempts at measuring the retrogastric space to detect anterior displacement when an impression is lacking have proved unreliable.

At times, the "wrap-around" effect of barium surrounding a mass can camouflage the existence of an enlarged retrogastric space. A mass behind the stomach indents and displaces that portion of the posterior wall of the stomach immediately in contact with it. With overfilling of the stomach by barium, the posterior wall on either side of the mass may not be displaced, resulting in the radiographic appearance of a normal retrogastric space. A well-penetrated lateral radiograph demonstrates the extrinsic impression on that portion of the stomach immediately in contact with the mass and can differentiate this area from the uninvolved remainder of the posterior wall of the stomach.

GENERALIZED WIDENING WITHOUT A DISCRETE MASS

Several conditions can cause the radiographic appearance of generalized widening of the retrogastric space without a discrete mass. In obese patients,

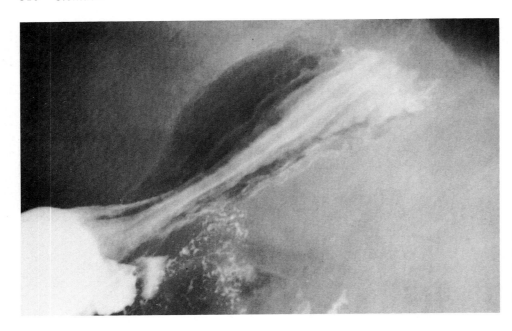

Fig. 23-1. Enlargement of the retrogastric space caused by obesity. Note that there is no evidence of a discrete mass impressing the posterior margin of the stomach.

increased thickness of the retroperitoneal fat can anteriorly displace the stomach (Fig. 23-1). Anterior displacement of the stomach after upper abdominal surgery may be due to disruption of normal anatomic attachments or to postoperative adhesions. Therefore, measurements of an enlarged retrogastric space following surgery have little significance.

Generalized ascites can cause widening of the retrogastric space. A similar radiographic pattern can be produced by gross hepatomegaly (especially of the caudate lobe), though diffuse enlargement of the liver usually displaces the stomach posteriorly. Any abdominal hernia leading to anterior or superior displacement of the omentum (such as ventral

and foramen of Morgagni hernias) causes widening of the retrogastric space. Slight widening of the retrogastric space has also been reported in patients with emphysema in whom the diaphragm is abnormally low after expiration.

PANCREATIC MASSES

Pancreatic masses are the most common causes of discrete lesions producing widening of the retrogastric space. Acute and chronic pancreatitis, pancreatic pseudocysts, and cystadenomas of the pancreas can have similar radiographic appearances

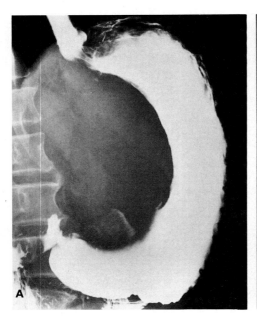
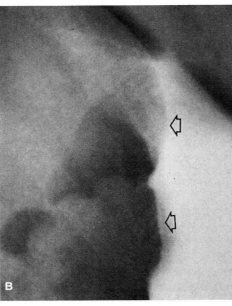

Fig. 23-2. Widening of the retrogastric space due to pancreatic pseudocyst. **(A)** Large smooth impression on the posterior wall of the stomach. **(B)** In another patient, there is a lobulated impression **(arrows)** on the posterior gastric wall.

(Fig. 23-2). Lesions in the head of the pancreas tend to produce extrinsic impressions on the posterior and inferior aspects of the antrum; those in the body and tail of the pancreas generally deform the body and fundus of the stomach, respectively. In addition to a smooth impression and pad effect, splaying of the mucosal folds is often identified. The possibility of invasion of the stomach by pancreatic carcinoma should be strongly considered if there is associated fixation of the gastric wall, mucosal destruction or ulceration, or high-grade gastric outlet obstruction.

Obvious widening of the retrogastric space in a patient with pancreatic carcinoma does not necessarily imply that the tumor itself is large. Much of the anterior displacement of the stomach may be due to pancreatitis accompanying the malignant neoplasm.

RETROPERITONEAL MASSES

In addition to pancreatic masses, a variety of retroperitoneal lesions, both benign and malignant, can result in widening of the retrogastric space. Retroperitoneal neoplasms (sarcomas, renal or adrenal carcinomas) can displace the stomach anteriorly (Fig. 23-3). A similar appearance can be produced by enlargement of retroperitoneal lymph nodes due

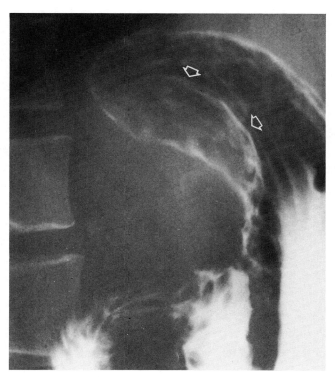

Fig. 23-4. Widening of the retrogastric space with a large impression on the posterior wall of the stomach **(arrows)** due to an adrenal cyst.

to lymphoma or tuberculosis and by retroperitoneal cysts (Fig. 23-4), abscesses, and hematomas.

OTHER CAUSES

Large tumor masses arising from the posterior wall of the stomach itself can widen the retrogastric space. This appearance is most commonly seen with tumors that have large exogastric components, such as leiomyomas and leiomyosarcomas. A similar pattern can be caused by large aortic aneurysms or choledochal cysts.

BIBLIOGRAPHY

Beranbaum SL: Carcinoma of the pancreas: A bidirectional roentgen approach. AJR 96:447–463, 1966

Herbert WW, Margulis AR: Diagnosis of retroperitoneal masses by gastrointestinal roentgenographic measurements: A computer study. Radiology 84:52–57, 1965

Mani JR, Zboralske FF, Margulis AR: Carcinoma of the body and tail of the pancreas. AJR 96:429–446, 1966

Poole GJ: A new roentgenographic method of measuring the retrogastric and retroduodenal spaces: Statistical evaluation of reliability and diagnostic utility. Radiology 97:71–81, 1970

Schultz EH: Measurements of the retrogastric space. Radiology 84:58–65, 1965

Whalen JP, Bader LM, Wolfman R: Evaluation of the retrogastric space: Normal appearance and variation. AJR 121:348–356, 1974

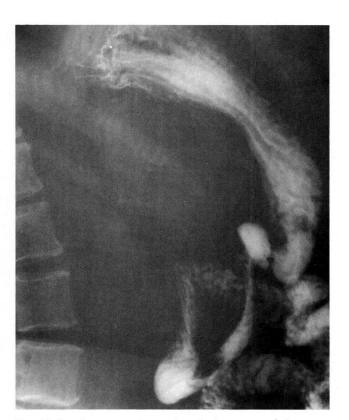

Fig. 23-3. Pronounced anterior displacement of the stomach and duodenum caused by a retroperitoneal sarcoma.

24

GAS IN THE WALL
OF THE STOMACH

Disease Entities

Emphysematous gastritis
Corrosive gastritis
Severe necrotizing gastroenteritis
Ischemia
Recent gastroduodenal surgery
Peptic ulcer with intramural perforation
Gastric outlet obstruction (*e.g.,* malignancy,
    volvulus)
Traumatic emphysema of the stomach
  Gastroscopy
  Esophagoscopy
Gastric pneumatosis
Bullus ruptured into the esophageal wall

The presence of gas in the wall of the stomach is not a distinct pathologic entity but a sign of an underlying abnormality, such as infection, ischemia, increased intraluminal pressure, or severe vomiting. Its clinical importance depends on the severity of the underlying disorder, which can vary from a high-mortality condition, such as phlegmonous gastritis, to a benign, transient sequela of gastroscopy.

Emphysematous gastritis is a severe form of phlegmonous gastritis in which gas in the wall of the stomach is caused by coliform organisms, hemolytic streptococci, or *Clostridia welchii* (Fig. 24-1). One case has been described in which emphysematous gastritis was due to diffuse necrosis of the gastric mucosa caused by the filariform larvae of *Strongyloides stercoralis* in an immunosuppressed

patient rather than by infection of the gastric wall with gas-forming organisms (Fig. 24-2). Emphysematous gastritis has an explosive onset of severe epigastric pain, nausea, and hematemesis that simulates acute perforation of an intra-abdominal viscus. The disease generally progresses rapidly, involving all layers of the stomach and frequently resulting in death (Fig. 24-3). A pathognomonic event that occurs in a large number of patients with emphysematous gastritis is spontaneous separation of the gastric mucosa as a necrotic cast shortly after the onset of the acute episode. If the patient survives the acute illness, cicatricial stenosis almost invariably occurs, resulting in gastric outlet obstruction. Gastric sinus tract formation is another serious complication of the disease.

Any severe inflammatory disease that impairs gastric mucosal integrity can predispose to the development of gas in the wall of the stomach. Peptic ulcer disease with intramural perforation and severe necrotizing gastroenteritis can damage the gastric mucosa and permit intraluminal gas and bacteria to enter the deep portions of the gastric wall. Gas in the wall of the stomach can also occur secondary to the ingestion of corrosives (*e.g.,* concentrated hydrochloric acid) or gastric infarction, or following recent gastroduodenal surgery.

The radiographic appearance of gas in the wall of the stomach in patients with severe inflammatory disease can vary from a mottled gastric shadow to an irregular radiolucent band of innumerable small gas bubbles outlining the stomach wall. These bubbles maintain a constant relationship to each other despite changes of body position. The radiographic

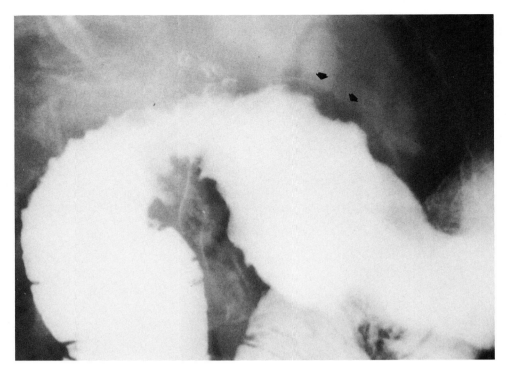

Fig. 24-1. Phlegmonous emphysematous gastritis. There is severe, irregular ulceration of the distal stomach with air in the wall **(arrows)**.

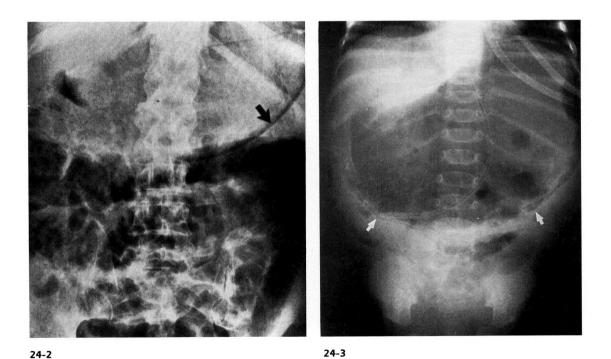

24-2   24-3

Fig. 24-2. Emphysematous gastritis due to strongyloidiasis. Thin lucent rim **(arrow)** outlines the distended stomach. (Williford ME, Forster WL, Halvorsen RA et al: Emphysematous gastritis secondary to disseminated strongyloidiasis. Gastrointest Radiol 7:123–126, 1982)

Fig. 24-3. Emphysematous gastritis. There are submucosal gas collections along the greater curvature of the distended stomach **(arrows)** and within the portal veins of this infant. (Udassin R, Aviad I, Vinograd I et al: Isolated emphysematous gastritis in an infant. Gastrointest Radiol 9:9–12, 1984)

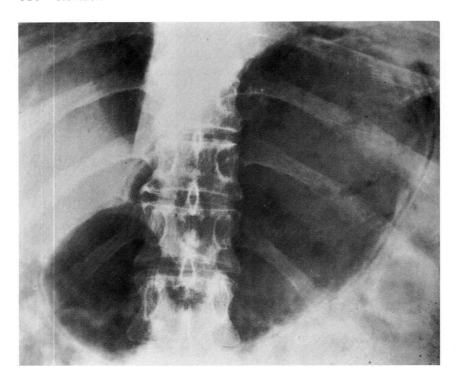

Fig. 24-4. Linear collection of intramural air surrounding the stomach. This represents a complication of endoscopy.

findings faithfully reflect the pathologic features of tiny blebs in the submucosa that cause bulging of the mucosa into the lumen throughout the stomach, giving its surface a cobblestone appearance. Intramucosal penetration of contrast medium and sinus tracts can also be seen.

Gas in the gastric wall can be related to overdistention of the stomach. This can be caused by gastric outlet obstruction (often with focal ischemia) due to stomach malignancy or volvulus or be a complication of gastric or esophageal endoscopy. In such a complication, the gas pattern tends to be finely linear and sharply defined (Fig. 24-4) rather than irregular and mottled; there is no associated thickening of the stomach wall or mucosal destruction.

Unfortunately, the morphologic characteristics of intramural gas in the stomach are not reliable parameters for differential diagnosis. The presence of gas in the gastric wall merely reflects a loss of integrity of the gastric epithelium; all diagnostic possibilities must be considered.

Gas in the wall of the stomach can rarely be demonstrated in the absence of severe inflammation, obstruction, or direct trauma to the esophagus or stomach. Pneumatosis intestinalis can affect the wall of the stomach, though it far more commonly involves the small bowel. Nonbacterial gastric emphysema can also result from spontaneous traumatic rupture of a pulmonary bullus into the areolar tissue around the esophagus. Changes in intrapulmonary pressure force the gas into the upper portion of the esophagus, creating a valvelike mechanism with gradual downward extension of gas into the submucosal or subserosal layers of the gastric wall. When the radiographic appearance of gas in the wall of the stomach is seen in a patient who is not prostrate, gastric pneumatosis intestinalis, traumatic emphysema of the stomach secondary to endoscopic perforation, and rupture of a pulmonary bullus into the esophageal wall are the most likely diagnostic possibilities.

BIBLIOGRAPHY

Lee S, Rutledge JN: Gastric emphysema. Am J Gastroenterol 79:899–904, 1984

Martel W: Radiologic features of esophagogastritis secondary to extremely caustic agents. Radiology 103:31–36, 1972

Meyers HI, Parker JJ: Emphysematous gastritis. Radiology 89:426–431, 1967

Seaman WB, Fleming RJ: Intramural gastric emphysema. AJR 101:431–436, 1967

Smith TJ: Emphysematous gastritis associated with adenocarcinoma of the stomach. Am J Dig Dis 11:341–345, 1966

Udassin R, Aviad I, Vinograd I et al: Isolated emphysematous gastritis in an infant. Gastrointest Radiol 9:9–12, 1984

Williford ME, Foster WL Jr, Halvorsen RA et al: Emphysematous gastritis secondary to disseminated strongyloidiasis. Gastrointest Radiol 7:123–126, 1982

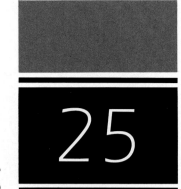

SIMULTANEOUS INVOLVEMENT OF THE GASTRIC ANTRUM AND DUODENAL BULB

Disease Entities

Malignant lesions
    Lymphoma
    Carcinoma
Peptic ulcer disease
Crohn's disease
Tuberculosis
Strongyloidiasis
Eosinophilic gastroenteritis

MALIGNANT LESIONS

The radiographic demonstration of transpyloric extension of a gastric tumor to involve the duodenal bulb has long been considered essentially pathognomonic evidence of lymphoma (Fig. 25-1). Indeed, transpyloric extension of tumor, which can appear radiographically as contour deformities, polypoid filling defects, or ulceration of the duodenal bulb (Fig. 25-2), has been described in up to 33% of patients with this malignant disease (Fig. 25-3). In contrast, adenocarcinoma involving the distal stomach has been said to result almost invariably in gastric outlet obstruction before it can be seen to grossly extend to the duodenal bulb. Recent studies, however, have shown radiographically detectable invasion of the duodenum in 5% of patients with gastric carcinoma (Fig. 25-4); microscopic involvement of the duodenum was demonstrated in 18%. The radiographic abnormalities in the duodenum vary from irregularity of the base of the bulb to narrowing and distortion extending well into the second portion of the duodenum (Fig. 25-5).

Although the incidence of gastric lymphoma is rising while adenocarcinoma of the stomach is becoming less common, carcinoma of the stomach still occurs about 50 times more frequently than gastric lymphoma. Therefore, even though transpyloric extension of tumor is far more frequently associated with lymphoma, the demonstration of duodenal involvement by an antral tumor in an individual patient favors carcinoma as the more likely diagnosis (Fig. 25-6).

PEPTIC ULCER DISEASE

Benign inflammatory processes can also simultaneously affect the antrum and the duodenal bulb. Peptic ulcer disease commonly causes mucosal thickening and/or ulceration of both areas. Fibrotic healing can produce narrowing and deformity involving both sides of the pylorus.

CROHN'S DISEASE

The blending of the antrum, pylorus, and duodenal bulb into a single tubular or funnel-shaped structure is suggestive of Crohn's disease (Fig. 25-7). In this condition, the pylorus and duodenal bulb lose their identity as recognized anatomic landmarks between the antrum and second portion of the duodenum. The somewhat abrupt transition from normal

Text continues on page 318

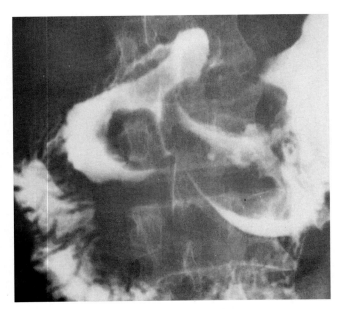

Fig. 25-1. Gastric lymphoma. There are large lymphomatous masses in the distal stomach and duodenal bulb with irregular ulcerations.

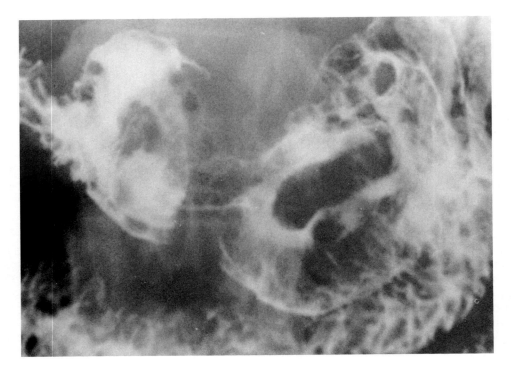

Fig. 25-2. Gastric lymphoma. Polypoid filling defects and thickened folds involve the antrum and duodenal bulb.

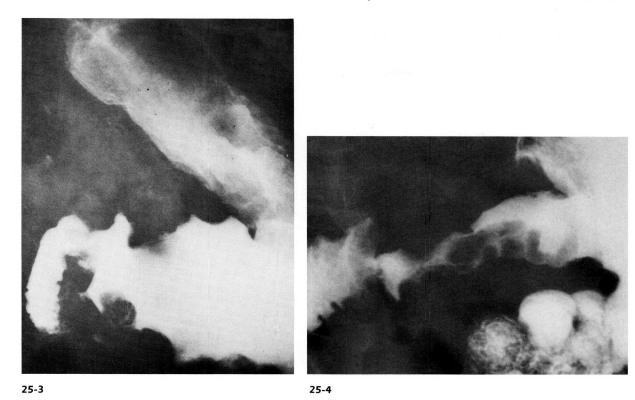

25-3

25-4

Fig. 25-3. Gastric lymphoma. Diffuse thickening of folds involves the distal stomach and duodenal bulb.

Fig. 25-4. Adenocarcinoma of the antrum. Rigid, abnormal folds in the distal stomach extend to involve the base of the duodenal bulb.

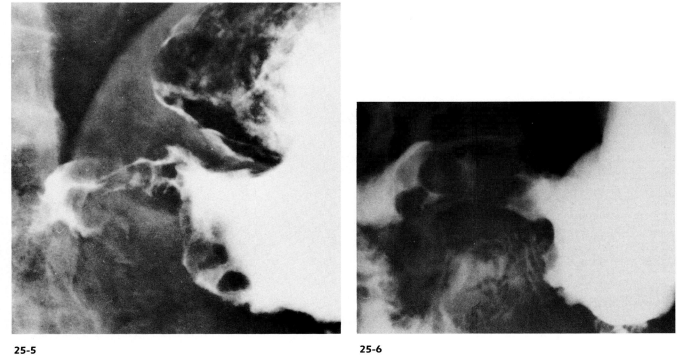

25-5

25-6

Fig. 25-5. Adenocarcinoma of the antrum. Thickened folds and antral narrowing characterize this malignant tumor, which extends across the pylorus to involve the duodenal bulb.

Fig. 25-6. Adenocarcinoma of the antrum. The neoplastic process causes filling defects on both the antral and the duodenal sides of the pylorus.

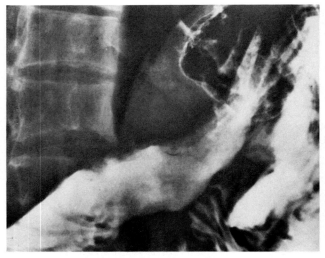

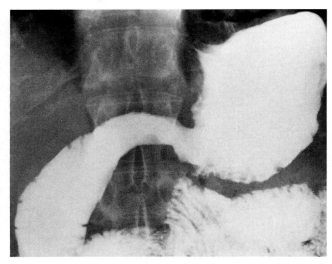

25-7   25-8

Fig. 25-7. Crohn's disease (pseudo-Billroth-I pattern). There are no recognizable anatomic landmarks between the antrum and the second portion of the duodenum.

Fig. 25-8. Radiographic appearance following Billroth-I anastomosis (gastroduodenostomy).

gastric antrum to the diseased, tube-shaped segment that extends into the second portion of the duodenum can closely simulate the radiographic appearance in a patient who has undergone a Billroth-I type of gastroduodenostomy (pseudo-Billroth-I pattern) (Fig. 25-8). The presence of residual pliability, distensibility, and lack of nodularity in the diseased area favors an inflammatory process rather than a neoplastic one. At times, the mucosa can appear shaggy and nodular, resembling the granulomatous changes seen in the ileum and colon.

TUBERCULOSIS

Duodenal involvement has been described in about 10% of patients with gastric tuberculosis; it occurs in more than half of those in whom the pylorus is involved. The pyloroduodenal area demonstrates mural nodularity and ulceration, often with a short area of narrowing. However, tuberculosis of the stomach and duodenum is a rare entity, even in patients with pulmonary or intestinal tuberculosis.

STRONGYLOIDIASIS

In advanced cases of strongyloidiasis, both the stomach and the duodenum can be involved with nodular intramural defects, ulceration of the mucosa, and narrowing of the lumen due to severe inflammatory changes and diffuse fibrosis within the gastric and duodenal walls.

EOSINOPHILIC GASTROENTERITIS

Long, contiguous spread of mural narrowing and mucosal fold thickening is not infrequently demonstrated in patients with eosinophilic gastroenteritis (Fig. 25-9). Transpyloric extension of disease combined with peripheral eosinophilia and specific food allergies should suggest this diagnosis.

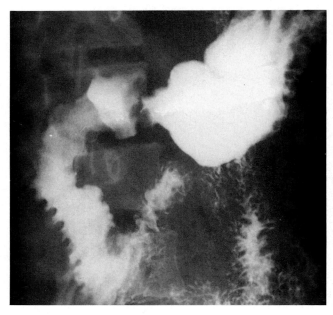

Fig. 25-9. Eosinophilic gastroenteritis. Irregular fold thickening involves the antrum and proximal duodenum.

BIBLIOGRAPHY

Balikian JR, Yenikomshian SM, Jidejian YD: Tuberculosis of the pyloroduodenal area. AJR 101:414–420, 1967

Berkmen YM, Rabinowitz J: Gastrointestinal manifestations of the strongyloidiasis. AJR 115:306–311, 1972

Farman J, Faegenburg D, Dallemand S et al: Crohn's disease of the stomach: The "ram's horn" sign. AJR 123:242–251, 1975

Goldberg HI, O'Kieffe D, Jenis EH et al: Diffuse eosinophilic gastroenteritis. AJR 119:342–351, 1973

Gonzalez G, Kennedy T: Crohn's disease of the stomach. Radiology 113:27–29, 1974

Hricak H, Thoeni RF, Margulis AR et al: Extension of gastric lymphoma into the esophagus and duodenum. Radiology 135:309–312, 1980

Koehler RE, Hanelin LG, Laing FC et al: Invasion of the duodenum by carcinoma of the stomach. AJR 128:201–205, 1977

Meyers MA, Katzen B, Alonso DR: Transpyloric extension to duodenal bulb in gastric lymphoma. Radiology 115:575–580, 1975

Nelson SW: Some interesting and unusual manifestations of Crohn's disease ("regional enteritis") of the stomach, duodenum and small intestine. AJR 107:86–101, 1969

PART FOUR

DUODENUM

POSTBULBAR ULCERATION OF THE DUODENUM

26

Disease Entities

Peptic ulcer disease
Zollinger–Ellison syndrome
Benign tumors
Malignant tumors
  Primary duodenal malignancy
  Metastatic malignancy
    Contiguous invasion (pancreas, right colon, right kidney, gallbladder)
    Invasion from lymph node metastases
    Hematogenous metastases (melanoma)
Crohn's disease
Tuberculosis
Aorticoduodenal fistula
Lesions simulating ulceration
  Ectopic pancreas
  Duodenal diverticulum

PEPTIC ULCER DISEASE

Ulceration in the postbulbar region represents only about 5% of duodenal ulcers secondary to benign peptic disease. Postbulbar ulcerations are often difficult to detect radiographically, though their identification is important because they are so frequently the cause of obstruction, pancreatitis, gastrointestinal bleeding, and atypical abdominal pain. Hyperactive peristalsis, mucosal edema, and poor barium coating can obscure the ulcer niche. Severe spasm of the duodenum in the area of ulceration can narrow and deform the lumen and prevent barium from filling the ulcer crater.

RADIOGRAPHIC FINDINGS

The classic radiographic appearance of a benign postbulbar ulcer is a shallow, flattened niche on the medial aspect (rarely the lateral) of the upper second portion of the duodenum (Fig. 26-1) or just past the apex of the duodenal bulb (Fig. 26-2). The ulcer is usually associated with an incisura, an indentation defect on the opposite duodenal margin at the same level as the ulcer crater. This incisura is produced by spasm secondary to acute ulceration and points toward the ulcer crater, causing eccentric narrowing of the lumen (Fig. 26-3). It can persist if there is chronic ulceration or fibrotic scarring during the healing phase of the postbulbar ulcer.

Chronic postbulbar ulceration can also result in a ring stricture, a discrete circumferential narrowing of the lumen that is almost always situated in the upper descending duodenum (Fig. 26-4). No mucosal pattern is visible in these strictures. They are usually 2 mm to 3 mm wide and show an abrupt transition to a normal duodenal caliber at either end. Even if an ulcer crater is not visible on barium studies, a ring stricture is indicative of peptic ulcer disease. Ring strictures are not quiescent lesions but are chronic and progressive. Patients who have them are frequently severely symptomatic, with intractable pain, recurrent bleeding, and vomiting due to residual or increasing narrowing of the lumen.

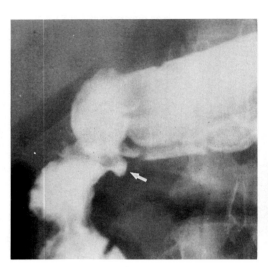

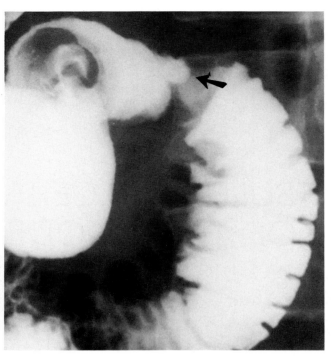

26-1   26-2

Fig. 26-1. Postbulbar ulcer **(arrow)** on the medial aspect of the second portion of the duodenum.

Fig. 26-2. Postbulbar ulcer **(arrow)** situated just distal to the apex of the duodenal bulb.

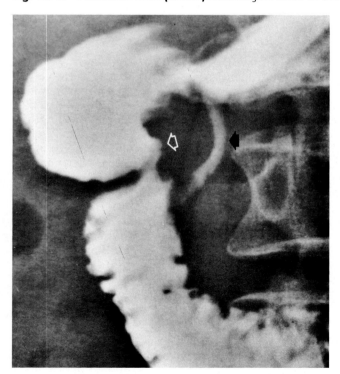

Fig. 26-3. Deep incisura on the lateral margin of the second portion of the duodenum pointing toward a postbulbar ulcer **(open arrow)** on the medial wall. Note the reflux of barium into the common bile duct **(closed arrow)**. This can occasionally be related to postbulbar ulcer disease near the papilla of Vater.

Penetration of a postbulbar ulcer into the pancreas results in a large ulcer niche (Fig. 26-5), medial retraction of the duodenal lumen, flattening of mucosal folds, and nodular defects along the upper duodenal margin (Fig. 26-6). This complication is often associated with an inflammatory mass in the head of the pancreas due to subacute pancreatitis. If an ulcer niche cannot be demonstrated in patients with a postbulbar ulcer and pancreatitis, the combination of effacement of plical folds, rigid narrowing of the lumen, and an extrinsic pressure defect on the medial aspect of the duodenal sweep may simulate the radiographic appearance of a pancreatic neoplasm.

ZOLLINGER–ELLISON SYNDROME

Although most duodenal ulcers in the Zollinger–Ellison syndrome occur in the duodenal bulb and are indistinguishable from those secondary to benign peptic disease, about one-fourth of the ulcers in this condition occur in the postbulbar region, the second and third portions of the duodenum, or the proximal jejunum. The combination of multiple ulcers distal to the duodenal bulb, thickening of gastric and duodenal folds, and evidence of hypersecretion should suggest the presence of an islet cell tumor of the pancreas and the Zollinger–Ellison syndrome (Fig. 26-7). A feature of the ulcers in this condition is their failure to respond to traditional

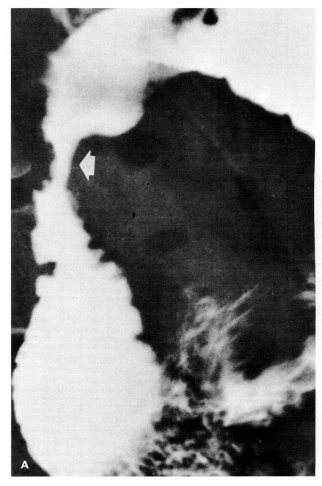

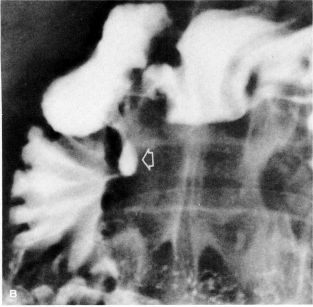

Fig. 26-4. Ring stricture. **(A)** Circumferential narrowing of the lumen of the second portion of the duodenum **(arrow)**. **(B)** Previous postbulbar ulcer in the same patient **(arrow)**. Note the duodenal folds radiating to the edge of the crater.

medical and surgical therapy for benign peptic ulcer disease. A common radiographic pattern is evidence of simultaneous healing of an ulcer in one location and development or extension of an ulcer at another site in a patient already being treated for ulcer disease. Recurrent ulcers are characteristic after surgery in patients with the Zollinger–Ellison syndrome. They tend to occur at the anastomosis or distal to the site of the surgical procedure and may be associated with severe complications such as hemorrhage or perforation.

BENIGN TUMORS

Ulceration in a benign duodenal neoplasm can simulate the radiographic appearance of a mound of edema surrounding a peptic postbulbar ulcer. This finding is most common in patients with spindle cell tumors, especially leiomyomas.

MALIGNANT TUMORS

The most frequent cause of nonpeptic postbulbar ulceration is duodenal malignancy. Tumors of the duodenum can cause narrowing and ulceration at any point along the duodenal sweep. Most primary malignancies of the duodenum are adenocarcinomas, but ulcerating lymphomas and sarcomas also occur.

Malignant tumors arising in the head of the pancreas, colon, right kidney, or gallbladder can invade the duodenum by contiguous spread. Cancer of the right colon, right kidney, or gallbladder tends to involve the duodenal bulb or outer aspects of the duodenal sweep. In contrast, carcinoma of the head of the pancreas usually produces an irregular, ulcerating lesion on the medial aspect of the duodenal sweep at any point from the apex of the bulb to the ligament of Treitz. Metastases to periduodenal lymph nodes or lymphoma arising at this site can

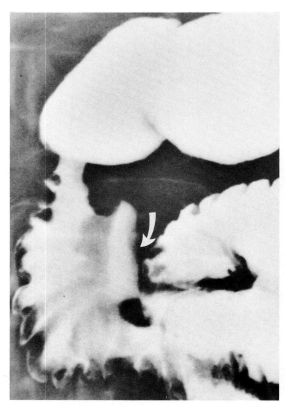
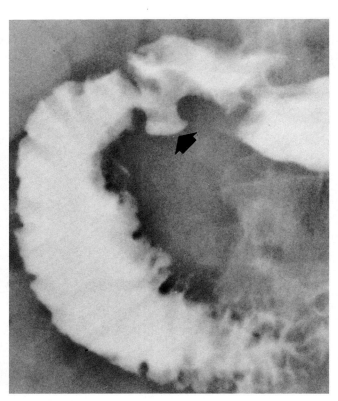

26-5   26-6

Fig. 26-5. Large postbulbar ulcer **(arrow)** on the medial wall of the second portion of the duodenum. The ulcer has penetrated into the head of the pancreas.

Fig. 26-6. Nodular defect along the medial border of the duodenum surrounding a postbulbar ulcer **(arrow)**, which has penetrated into the head of the pancreas.

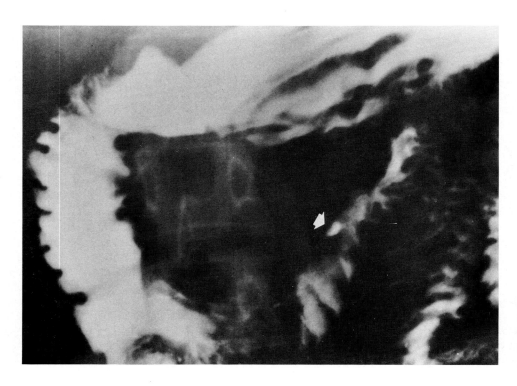

Fig. 26-7. Zollinger-Ellison syndrome. An ulcer **(arrow)** is seen in the fourth portion of the duodenum. Note the thickened gastric and duodenal folds.

also invade the wall of the duodenum and produce an ulcerated mass. Hematogenous metastases to the duodenum (especially melanoma) produce relatively flat filling defects. These often ulcerate centrally and can lead to massive ulcers and fatal hemorrhage.

GRANULOMATOUS DISEASE

Crohn's disease can cause duodenal nodularity and postbulbar ulceration (Fig. 26-8). It can usually be readily differentiated from benign peptic ulcer dis-

ease, since duodenal involvement with Crohn's disease is almost invariably associated with evidence of the same process elsewhere in the gastrointestinal tract. Tuberculosis involving the duodenum can also cause postbulbar ulceration, which is usually associated with severe spasm and mucosal edema (Fig. 26-9).

AORTICODUODENAL FISTULA

In patients who have had abdominal aneurysms or who have undergone reconstructive surgery and

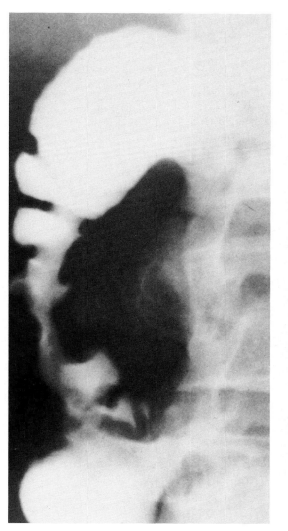

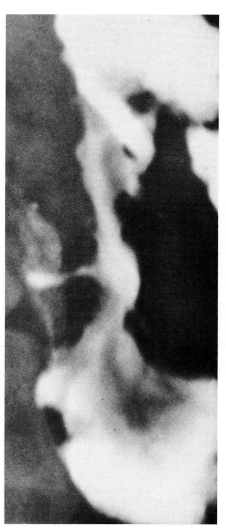

26-8

26-9

Fig. 26-8. Crohn's disease of the duodenum. Deep ulcerations are associated with thickening of mucosal folds and a short stricture.

Fig. 26-9. Tuberculosis of the duodenum. There are multiple ulcers and sinus tracts with marked swelling of the duodenal mucosa. (Tishler JMA: Duodenal tuberculosis. Radiology 130:593–595, 1979)

placement of a prosthetic Dacron graft, rupture into the adjacent duodenum can occur. This aortico-duodenal fistula (which can also be spontaneous) may result in compression or displacement of the third portion of the duodenum by an extrinsic mass, which sometimes contains a central ulceration. On rare occasions, barium may be seen outlining the wall of the abdominal aorta.

LESIONS SIMULATING ULCERATION

An ectopic pancreas with a small fleck of barium filling the rudimentary central duct can simulate a postbulbar ulceration surrounded by a mound of edema. In this condition, however, no characteristic incisura is produced. A small diverticulum of the medial wall of the descending duodenum, especially if partially filled or distorted, may occasionally mimic an ulceration. However, the distinction between diverticulum and ulceration can usually be made without difficulty. Intact mucosal folds are frequently demonstrated running into duodenal diverticula. Diverticula change shape or fill and empty with barium on serial radiographs, unlike ulcer craters, which have a constant, rigid shape.

BIBLIOGRAPHY

Bilbao MK, Frische LH, Rösch J et al: Postbulbar duodenal ulcer and ring-stricture: Cause and effect. Radiology 100:27–35, 1971

Blatt CJ, Bernstein RG, Lopez F: Uncommon roentgenologic manifestation of pancreatic carcinoma. AJR 113:119–124, 1971

Christoforidis AJ, Nelson SW: Radiological manifestations of ulcerogenic tumors of the pancreas. JAMA 198:511–516, 1966

Eaton SB, Ferrucci JT: Radiology of the Pancreas and Duodenum. Philadelphia, WB Saunders, 1973

Kaufman SA, Levene G: Post-bulbar duodenal ulcer. Radiology 69:848–852, 1957

Legge DA, Carlson HC, Judd ES: Roentgenologic features of regional enteritis of the upper gastrointestinal tract. AJR 110:355–360, 1970

McCort JJ: Roentgenographic appearance of metastases to the central lymph nodes of the superior mesenteric artery in carcinoma of the right colon. Radiology 60:641–646, 1953

Paterson DE, Hancock DM: Duodenal stenosis due to postbulbar ulcer. Br J Radiol 31:660–665, 1958

Teplick JG: Duodenal loop changes in posterior penetration of duodenal ulcer. Ann Intern Med 44:958–974, 1956

Treitel H, Meyers MA, Maya V: Changes in the duodenal loop secondary to carcinoma of the hepatic flexure of the colon. Br J Radiol 43:209–213, 1970

Zboralske FF, Amberg JR: Detection of the Zollinger–Ellison syndrome: The radiologist's responsibility. AJR 104:529–543, 1968

THICKENING OF DUODENAL FOLDS

27

Disease Entities

Inflammatory disorders
  Peptic ulcer disease
  Brunner's gland hyperplasia
  Zollinger–Ellison syndrome
  Duodenitis
  Pancreatitis
  Cholecystitis
  Uremia (chronic dialysis)
  Crohn's disease
  Tuberculosis
  Parasitic infestation (giardiasis, strongyloi-
    diasis)
  AIDS-related infections
  Nontropical sprue
Neoplastic disorders
  Lymphoma
  Metastases to peripancreatic lymph nodes
  AIDS-related malignancy
Diffuse infiltrative disorders
  Whipple's disease
  Amyloidosis
  Mastocytosis
  Eosinophilic enteritis
  Intestinal lymphangiectasia
Vascular disorders
  Duodenal varices
  Mesenteric arterial collaterals
  Intramural hemorrhage
  Chronic duodenal congestion
Cystic fibrosis (mucoviscidosis)

The mucosal folds in the duodenal bulb are relatively sparse and usually disappear completely when the bulb is distended. In the remaining portions of the duodenum, even when distended, there is a rich mucosal pattern. These criss-crossing mucosal folds produce a fine serration of the margin of the barium-filled duodenum.

INFLAMMATORY DISORDERS

PEPTIC ULCER DISEASE

Any disease process resulting in inflammatory edema of the mucosal or submucosal layers of the duodenum can result in thickening of duodenal folds. The most common cause of duodenal fold thickening is peptic ulcer disease (Fig. 27-1). It is clinically of little importance whether this fold thickening represents mucosal edema or diffuse hyperplasia of Brunner's glands, which also reflects the response of the duodenal mucosa to an ulcer diathesis. In Brunner's gland hyperplasia, the fold thickening often appears nodular and has a cobblestone appearance (Fig. 27-2). Compression of the bulb can be helpful in distinguishing between coarsened folds secondary to the edema of peptic ulcer disease and thickened folds due to Brunner's gland hyperplasia. In peptic disease, the coarse folds can be obliterated by compression; in Brunner's gland hyperplasia, the filling defects are not obliterated and appear constant on serial films.

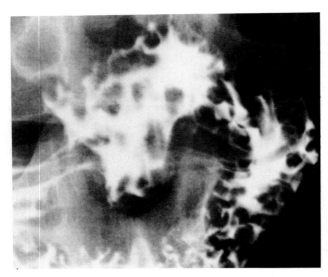

Fig. 27-1. Thickening of folds in the duodenal bulb and proximal sweep secondary to peptic ulcer disease.

ZOLLINGER–ELLISON SYNDROME

The Zollinger–Ellison syndrome can cause diffuse thickening of duodenal mucosal folds (Fig. 27-3). This disease should be suggested whenever thickened duodenal folds are associated with enlarged

gastric rugae and ulcerations in atypical positions (third and fourth duodenum, proximal jejunum) (Fig. 27-4).

DUODENITIS

Nonerosive duodenitis is commonly observed endoscopically, though it may be difficult to diagnose radiographically because the endoscopic spectrum of the condition can range from mere erythema to thickened nodular folds and duodenal erosions. Although the significance of nonspecific duodenitis is controversial, some authors report that it may be a more frequent cause of epigastric pain than duodenal ulcer. Prior to the widespread use of fiberoptic endoscopy, it was unclear whether duodenitis could exist as an entity separate from peptic ulcer disease. However, it is now evident that most cases of duodenitis are not accompanied by peptic ulcer and that the majority of patients do not have gastric hypersecretion. Thickening of duodenal folds ($\geq$5 mm) is the most sensitive but least specific radiographic sign of duodenitis (Fig. 27-5). Many patients with nonspecific duodenal fold thickening are shown to be normal at endoscopy. Nodularity (Fig. 27-6), deformity, and erosions (Fig. 27-7) are other manifestations of this condition, and in some patients the duodenum shows hyperactive peristalsis or irritability. In view of the wide range of normal

Text continues on page 333

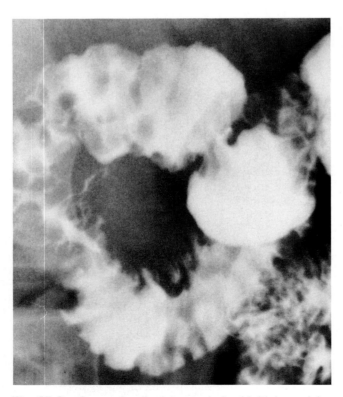

Fig. 27-2. Brunner's gland hyperplasia. Multiple nodules produce a cobblestone appearance involving the duodenal bulb and proximal sweep.

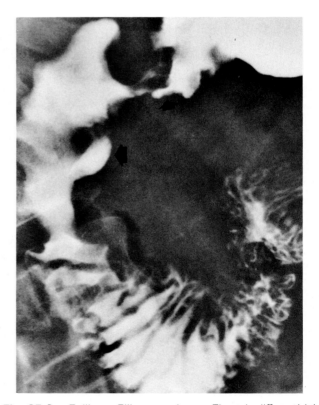

Fig. 27-3. Zollinger-Ellison syndrome. There is diffuse thickening of folds in the proximal duodenal sweep with bulbar and postbulbar ulceration **(arrows)**.

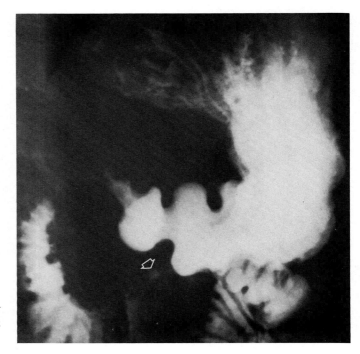

Fig. 27-4. Zollinger-Ellison syndrome. Note the ulcer **(arrow)** in the fourth portion of the duodenum. There is diffuse thickening of folds in the duodenal sweep.

Fig. 27-5. Duodenitis. Thickening of folds in the duodenal bulb and proximal sweep. (Gelfand DW, Dale WJ, Ott DJ et al: Duodenitis: Endoscopic-radiologic correlation in 272 patients. Radiology 157:577–581, 1985)

Fig. 27-6. Duodenitis. Scattered mucosal nodules throughout the second portion of the duodenum. (Gelfand DW, Dale WJ, Ott DJ et al: Duodenitis: Endoscopic-radiologic correlation in 272 patients. Radiology 157:577–581, 1985)

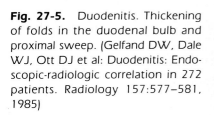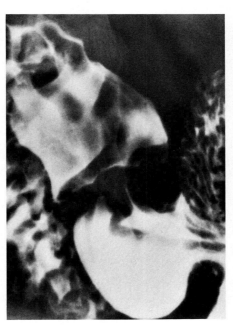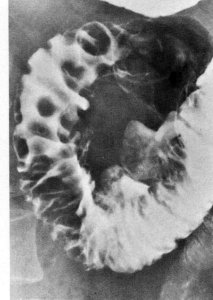

27-5 27-6

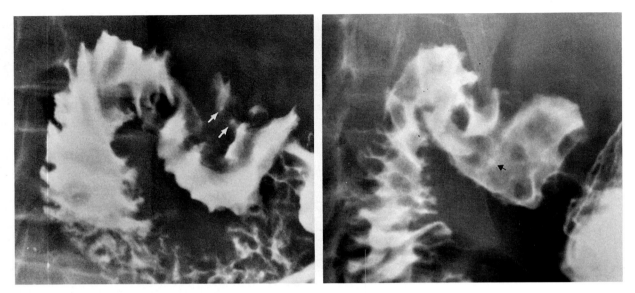

Fig. 27-7. Duodenitis. Two examples of erosions **(arrows)** in the duodenal bulb in patients with duodenitis. (Gelfand DW, Dale WJ, Ott DJ et al: Duodenitis: Endoscopic-radiologic correlation in 272 patients. Radiology 157:577–581, 1985)

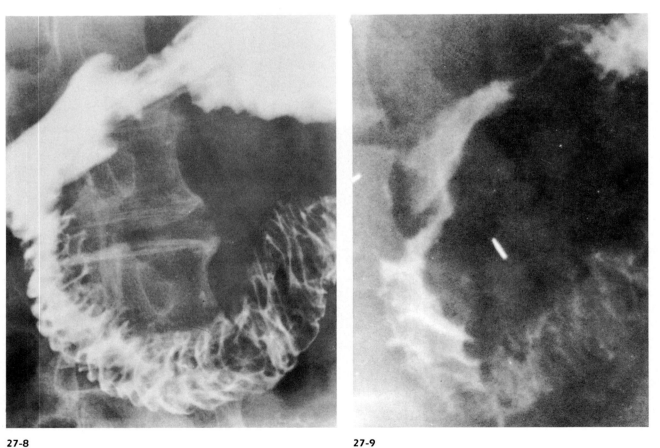

27-8   27-9

Fig. 27-8. Acute pancreatitis causing thickening of duodenal folds. Note the widening of the duodenal sweep, the double-contour effect, and sharp spiculations.

Fig. 27-9. Acute hemorrhagic pancreatitis following pancreatic biopsy. There is diffuse thickening of duodenal folds, although the severe inflammatory spasm makes the duodenal sweep so irritable that it does not completely fill with barium.

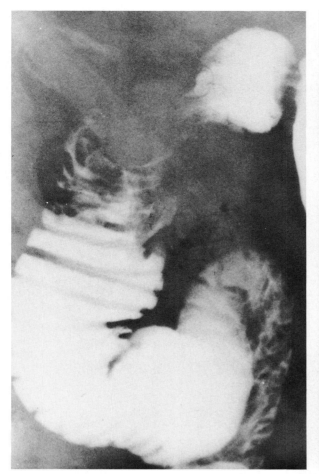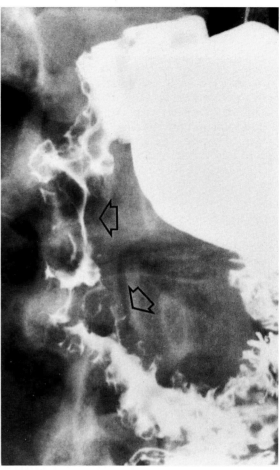

27-10   27-11

Fig. 27-10. Acute cholecystitis. An adjacent inflammatory process produces fold thickening, luminal narrowing, and a mass effect involving the proximal second portion of the duodenum.

Fig. 27-11. Chronic renal failure. Irregular thickening of folds in the duodenal sweep simulates pancreatitis.

folds in the duodenum, the radiographic differentiation of normal thick folds from enlarged folds secondary to duodenitis or peptic ulcer disease may be difficult, and it may be impossible to distinguish between the two pathologic conditions. The nodularity and thickened folds seen radiographically reflect the pathologic finding of patchy inflammatory and fibrous infiltrate distorting the lamina propria and villi.

Duodenitis has an increased occurrence in patients with end-stage renal disease. Because there is also an increased incidence of peptic ulcers in these patients, it has been suggested that duodenitis may be part of the spectrum of acid peptic disease.

PANCREATITIS/CHOLECYSTITIS

Acute pancreatitis is the other major cause of thickening of duodenal folds (Fig. 27-8). Severe inflam-

matory spasm secondary to pancreatitis can make the duodenal sweep so irritable that it does not completely fill with barium (Fig. 27-9). The radiographic appearance of edematous, thickened folds in the periampullary region and proximal second portion of the duodenum, especially if associated with elevation of serum amylase and a mass impression on the duodenum from the swollen head of the pancreas, should suggest the diagnosis of acute pancreatitis. Thickening of duodenal folds, often with narrowing of the lumen, can also be associated with other types of adjacent periduodenal inflammation, such as acute cholecystitis (Fig. 27-10).

UREMIA (CHRONIC DIALYSIS)

Gastrointestinal complaints such as nausea and vomiting are not infrequent long-term complications in uremic patients undergoing chronic dialysis. Prominence of the mucosal pattern can be seen with irregular, swollen, and stiffened folds in the duodenal bulb and second portion of the duodenum (Fig. 27-11). Although an increase in the incidence of peptic ulceration has been reported in patients on chronic dialysis, the nodular thickening of duodenal folds is apparently not related to hyperacidity or peptic ulcer disease. Indeed, the thickening of duodenal folds in patients on chronic dialysis often simulates the appearance of pancreatitis, a disease that frequently complicates prolonged uremia and may be responsible for producing the radiographic pattern.

CROHN'S DISEASE/TUBERCULOSIS

Chronic inflammatory disorders can also cause thickening of duodenal folds. Crohn's disease can affect the duodenum and produce a spectrum of radiographic appearances, including mucosal thickening, ulceration, and stenosis (Fig. 27-12). Al-

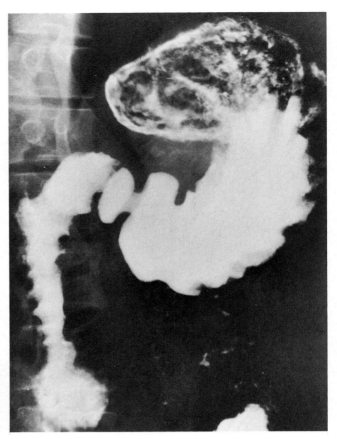

Fig. 27-13.   Tuberculosis of the duodenum. There is diffuse fold thickening, spasm, and ulceration of the proximal duodenum.

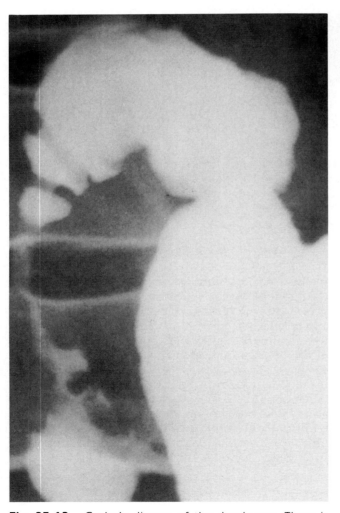

Fig. 27-12.   Crohn's disease of the duodenum. There is thickening of mucosal folds in a narrowed second portion of the duodenum.

though duodenal involvement is occasionally an isolated process in Crohn's disease, concomitant disease in the terminal ileum can usually be detected. Tuberculosis of the duodenum, although rare even in patients with pulmonary or gastrointestinal disease, can produce a pattern of nodular, hyperplastic fold thickening, diffuse ulceration, and luminal narrowing identical to that seen in Crohn's disease (Fig. 27-13). When tuberculosis involves the duodenum, associated antral and pyloric disease is almost always present.

OTHER INFLAMMATORY DISORDERS

Nodular thickening of duodenal folds can be seen with parasitic infestations such as giardiasis and strongyloidiasis (Fig. 27-14). In giardiasis, hyperperistalsis and increased secretions produce a blurred, thickened, edematous mucosal fold pattern involving the duodenum and jejunum. Strongyloides infestation of the duodenum causes diffuse coarse thickening of folds, ulceration, and luminal stenosis that can closely simulate Crohn's disease. In patients with AIDS, thickening of duodenal folds with dilatation of the lumen may be caused by a variety of infectious agents such as *Cryptosporidium*

(Fig. 27-15), cytomegalovirus, and *Mycobacterium avium-intracellulare.* A bizarre pattern of thickened or nodular folds in the bulb and second portion of the duodenum, which may be associated with focal erosions, has been reported as a common finding in patients with nontropical sprue (Fig. 27-16).

NEOPLASTIC DISORDERS

Lymphoma occasionally involves the duodenal bulb and sweep and produces a radiographic pattern of coarse, nodular, irregular folds (Fig. 27-17). Metastases to peripancreatic lymph nodes can result in localized impressions on the duodenum simulating thickened folds (Fig. 27-18). Fold thickening can also be secondary to impaired lymphatic drainage due to malignant replacement of normal lymph node architecture (Fig. 27-19). In patients with AIDS, submucosal infiltration by Kaposi's sarcoma or lymphoma may cause thickening of duodenal folds indistinguishable from that caused by opportunistic infection occurring in these immunocompromised patients.

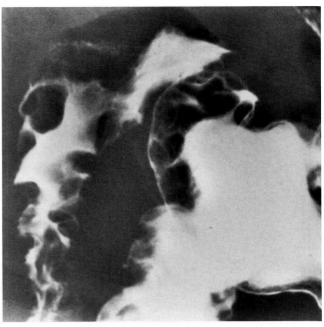

Fig. 27-15. Cryptosporidiosis. Diffuse coarse thickening of duodenal and antral folds.

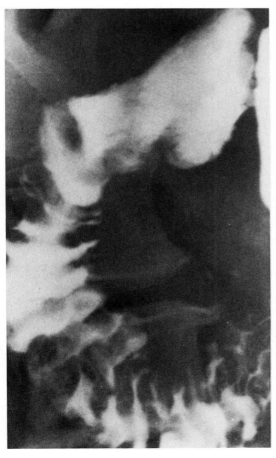

Fig. 27-14. Strongyloidiasis. Irregular, at times nodular, thickening of folds throughout the duodenal sweep.

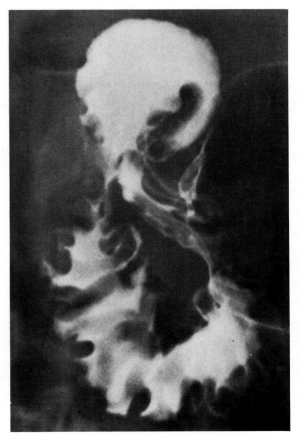

Fig. 27-16. Nontropical sprue. Coarse thickening of folds involving the duodenal sweep. (Marn CS, Gore RM, Ghahremani GG: Duodenal manifestations of nontropical sprue. Gastrointest Radiol 11:30–35, 1986)

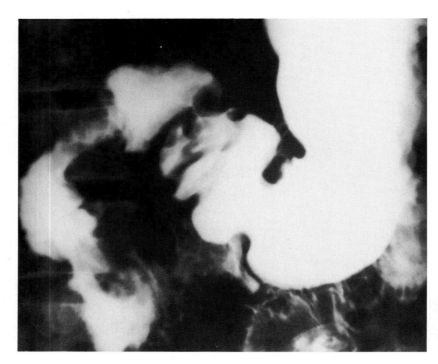

Fig. 27-17. Lymphoma. There is localized luminal narrowing of the proximal second portion of the duodenum with a pattern of coarse, nodular, irregular folds.

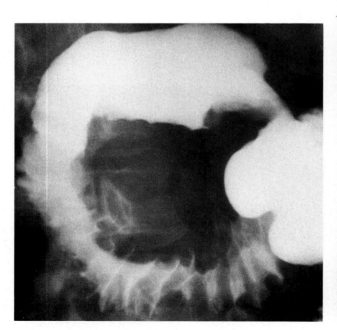

27-18

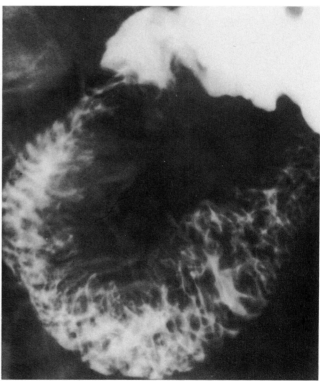

27-19

Fig. 27-18. Metastases to peripancreatic lymph nodes causing localized impressions on the duodenum. The impressions simulate thickened folds.

Fig. 27-19. Metastases to peripancreatic lymph nodes. Impaired lymphatic drainage, which is due to tumor replacement of normal lymph nodes, causes a pattern of diffuse fold thickening in the duodenal sweep.

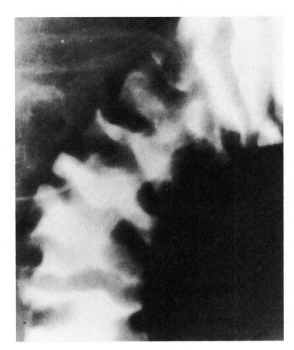

Fig. 27-20. Mastocytosis. The duodenal folds are thickened.

INFILTRATIVE DISORDERS

Diffuse small bowel infiltrative diseases can also affect the duodenum, though duodenal involvement as an isolated finding has not been reported. In Whipple's disease, periodic acid-Schiff (PAS)-positive macrophages can infiltrate the duodenal submucosa and produce diffuse thickening of folds. A similar pattern can be caused by infiltration of the duodenal wall in amyloidosis, mastocytosis (Fig. 27-20), and eosinophilic enteritis. The gross dilatation of lymphatics seen in patients with intestinal lymphangiectasia can also present the radiographic appearance of thickening of duodenal folds.

VASCULAR DISORDERS

DUODENAL VARICES

Duodenal varices are collateral vessels that can result from extrahepatic obstruction of the portal or splenic veins as well as from intrahepatic portal hypertension. Esophageal varices are almost always also present. Duodenal varices have four major radiographic appearances. First, collateral flow in a dilated superior pancreaticoduodenal vein can cause a vertical compression defect on the duodenal bulb about 1 cm distal to the pylorus. Second, small varices produce a diffuse polypoid mucosal pattern in the duodenum that can be difficult to distinguish from inflammatory fold thickening due to Brunner's gland hyperplasia. Third, larger, di-

lated submucosal veins can project into the lumen and cause serpiginous filling defects similar to the typical appearance of esophageal varices (Fig. 27-21). Finally, an isolated duodenal varix occasionally presents as a discrete filling defect on the medial aspect of the descending duodenum. In patients with known portal hypertension, unusual polypoid, mural, or extrinsic defects in the duodenum should suggest the possibility of duodenal varices.

MESENTERIC ARTERIAL COLLATERALS

Arteriosclerotic occlusive disease of the mesenteric vessels primarily involves the origins of the celiac axis and superior mesenteric artery. Occlusion of either of these arterial trunks causes enlargement and tortuosity of the collateral pathways between them. The initial loops of the pancreaticoduodenal arcade lie roughly parallel and in close proximity to the descending duodenum. The gastroduodenal artery also lies adjacent and parallel to the descending duodenum for a variable distance. When these arteries serve as enlarged collaterals, they can appear as serpiginous, nodular filling defects simulating thickened duodenal folds (Fig. 27-22). In addition, enlarged arterial collaterals can produce discrete filling defects on the medial aspect of the duodenum with widening of the sweep. Tortuous enlargement of an aberrant right hepatic artery arising from the

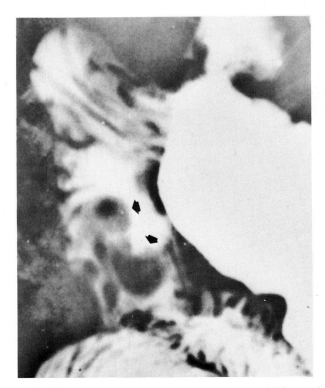

Fig. 27-21. Duodenal varices presenting as multiple serpiginous filling defects **(arrows)**.

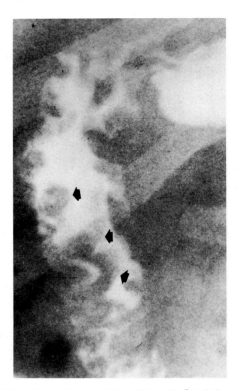

Fig. 27-22. Duodenal arterial collaterals. Serpiginous nodular filling defects **(arrows)** simulate thickened folds in a patient with occlusion of the origin of the celiac axis.

superior mesenteric artery instead of from the celiac axis can cause a sharply marginated extrinsic defect on the superior aspect of the duodenal bulb.

INTRAMURAL HEMORRHAGE/DUODENAL CONGESTION

Hemorrhage into the duodenal wall can produce the radiographic pattern of mucosal fold thickening (stacked-coins appearance). Duodenal intramural hemorrhage can be caused by anticoagulant therapy or a bleeding diathesis or can be a complication of trauma to the upper abdomen. Chronic congestion of the duodenum secondary to portal hypertension (cirrhosis) or congestive heart failure can also give rise to peptic symptoms and thickening of duodenal mucosal folds.

CYSTIC FIBROSIS

A thickened, coarse fold pattern in the duodenum is commonly demonstrated in patients with cystic fibrosis of the pancreas (mucoviscidosis) (Fig. 27-23). Associated findings include nodular indentations along the duodenal wall, smudging or poor definition of the mucosal fold pattern, and redundancy, distortion, and kinking of the duodenal contour. These changes are usually confined to the first and

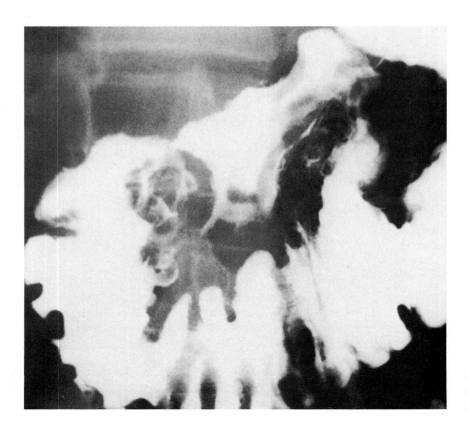

Fig. 27-23. Cystic fibrosis of the pancreas (mucoviscidosis). The duodenal folds have a thick, coarse pattern.

second portions of the duodenum, though the thickened fold pattern occasionally extends into the proximal jejunum. The cause of duodenal fold thickening in cystic fibrosis is obscure. It is postulated that the lack of pancreatic bicarbonate in patients with cystic fibrosis results in inadequate buffering of normal amounts of gastric acid, causing mucosal irritation and muscular contractions that produce the thickened mucosal folds.

BIBLIOGRAPHY

Bateson EM: Duodenal and antral varices. Br J Radiol 42:744–747, 1969

Baum S, Stein GN, Baue A: Extrinsic pressure defects on the duodenal loop in mesenteric occlusive disease. Radiology 85:866–874, 1965

Dallemand S, Waxman M, Farman J: Radiological manifestations of *Strongyloides stercoralis*. Gastrointest Radiol 8:45–51, 1983

Dodds WJ, Spitzer RM, Friedland GW: Gastrointestinal roentgenographic manifestations of hemophilia. AJR 110:413–416, 1970

Eaton SB, Ferrucci JT: Radiology of the Pancreas and Duodenum. Philadelphia, WB Saunders, 1973

Fleming RJ, Seaman WB: Roentgenographic demonstration of unusual extra-esophageal varices. AJR 103:281–290, 1968

Fraser GM, Pitman RG, Lawrie JH et al: The significance of the radiological finding of coarse mucosal folds in the duodenum. Lancet 2:979–982, 1964

Gelfand DW, Dale WF, Ott DJ et al: Duodenitis: Endoscopic-radiologic correlation in 272 patients. Radiology 157:577–581, 1985

Govoni AF: Benign lymphoid hyperplasia of the duodenal bulb. Gastrointest Radiol 1:267–269, 1976

Itzchak Y, Glickman MG: Duodenal varices in extrahepatic portal obstruction. Radiology 124:619–624, 1977

Legge DA, Carlson HC, Judd ES: Roentgenologic features of regional enteritis of the upper gastrointestinal tract. AJR 110:355–360, 1970

Levine MS: Crohn's disease of the upper gastrointestinal tract. Radiol Clin North Am 25:79–91, 1987

Marn CS, Gore RM, Ghahremani GG: Duodenal manifestations of nontropical sprue. Gastrointest Radiol 11:30–35, 1986

Megibow AJ, Balthazar EJ, Hulnick DH: Radiology of nonneoplastic gastrointestinal disorders in acquired immune deficiency syndrome. Semin Roentgenol 22:31–41, 1987

Perez CA, Dorfman RF: Benign lymphoid hyperplasia of the stomach and duodenum. Radiology 87:505–510, 1966

Phelan MS, Fine DR, Zentler–Munro L et al: Radiographic abnormalities of the duodenum in cystic fibrosis. Clin Radiol 34:573–577, 1983

Schulman A: The cobblestone appearance of the duodenal cap, duodenitis and hyperplasia of Brunner's glands. Br J Radiol 43:787–795, 1970

Shimkin PM, Pearson KD: Unusual arterial impressions upon the duodenum. Radiology 103:295–297, 1972

Taussig LM, Saldino RM, di Sant'Agnese PA: Radiographic abnormalities of the duodenum and small bowel in cystic fibrosis of the pancreas (mucoviscidosis). Radiology 106:369–376, 1973

Wiener SN, Vertes V, Shapiro H: The upper gastrointestinal tract in patients undergoing chronic dialysis. Radiology 92:110–114, 1969

Zukerman GR, Mills BA, Koehler RE et al: Nodular duodenitis: Pathologic and clinical characteristics in patients with end-stage renal disease. Dig Dis Sci 28:1018–1024, 1983

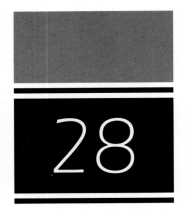

28
WIDENING OF THE DUODENAL SWEEP

Disease Entities

Normal variant
Pancreatic lesions
   Pancreatitis
   Pancreatic pseudocyst
   Pancreatic cancer
   Metastatic replacement of the pancreas
   Cystadenoma/cystadenocarcinoma
Lymph node enlargement
   Metastases
   Lymphoma
   Inflammation
Cystic lymphangioma of the mesentery
Mesenteric arterial collaterals
Retroperitoneal masses (tumors, cysts)
Aortic aneurysm
Choledochal cyst

Widening of the duodenal sweep is often considered evidence suggestive of malignancy or inflammation in the head of the pancreas. However, this finding frequently does not represent pancreatic pathology and thus must be interpreted with great caution. There is great variation in the configuration of the duodenal sweep among normal patients, and slight degrees of enlargement are difficult to recognize with confidence. In heavy patients, the combination of a high transverse stomach and long vertical course of the descending duodenum can create the illusion of a large sweep, which is actually within normal limits. In addition, widening of the sweep can be related to upward pressure on the duodenal bulb or downward pressure on the third portion of the duodenum rather than to an impression by the head of the pancreas on the medial aspect of the second portion of the duodenum.

Enlargement of the duodenal sweep can reflect benign pancreatic disease (pancreatitis or pseudocyst) or pancreatic malignancy. Although there are numerous radiographic criteria for distinguishing between benign and malignant pancreatic disease, a precise diagnosis is often extremely difficult to make.

ACUTE PANCREATITIS

Most patients with acute pancreatitis have a history of alcohol abuse. Abdominal pain is almost universal; radiation of pain to the back occurs in about half of patients. Nausea, vomiting, and a feeling of prostration are common, as are fever and epigastric tenderness.

In acute pancreatitis, the gland may enlarge to three times its normal size. Involvement of the head of the pancreas may produce a smooth mass indenting the inner border of the duodenal sweep (Fig. 28-1). Duodenal paresis and edema of duodenal folds is common, as is edema of the papilla of Vater (Fig. 28-2). Gastric atony and dilatation, as well as edema of folds in the proximal jejunum, can

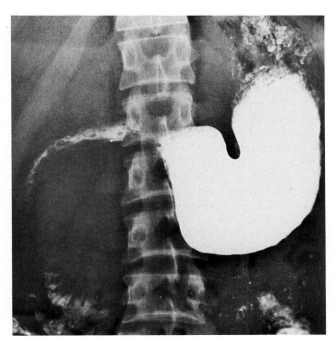

Fig. 28-1. Acute pancreatitis. Severe inflammation causes widening of the sweep and a high-grade duodenal obstruction.

be seen. Swelling of the pancreas can also cause an extrinsic impression on the posterior surface or greater curvature of the stomach.

RADIOGRAPHIC FINDINGS

Abnormalities on chest or plain abdominal radiographs can suggest the diagnosis of acute pancreatitis. Hemidiaphragmatic elevation, platelike subsegmental atelectasis, consolidation (pneumonia or segmental atelectasis), and pleural effusion are frequently seen in patients with acute pancreatitis. Except for pleural effusion, these findings occur with equal frequency on both sides and are commonly bilateral; pleural effusion is much more common on the left side than on the right. Although the precise mechanism is unclear, direct spread of the inflammatory process (chemical and enzymatic irritation) may occur through the diaphragm itself, by way of the hiatal orifices between the chest and abdomen, or through retroperitoneal tissues. The rich transdiaphragmatic lymphatic connections may also play a role in the spread of acute inflammation. Patients with acute pancreatitis sometimes demonstrate a gasless abdomen, a nonspecific finding that can be seen in normal patients and in patients with high intestinal obstruction. The reverse pattern of generalized adynamic ileus also can be noted. Sentinel loops (localized segments of gas-filled, dilated small bowel adjacent to an acute inflammation) can often be demonstrated in the midabdomen.

The "colon cut-off" sign, though infrequently seen, has been considered highly suggestive of acute pancreatitis. Contrary to the initial theory that pancreatitis tends to produce gaseous distention of the ascending colon and hepatic flexure with a sharp cut-off in the proximal transverse colon, gaseous distention of the right and entire transverse colon with an abrupt cut-off of the gas column at the splenic flexure is more commonly seen (Fig. 28-3). The mechanism for this phenomenon probably depends on the anatomic position of the transverse mesocolon, which connects the transverse colon with the anterior surface of the pancreas and permits the inflammatory exudate from acute pancreatitis to spread to involve the transverse colon. Although the colon cut-off sign is suggestive of acute pancreatitis, it is nonspecific. A similar appearance can be seen in colonic obstruction at the splenic flexure, mesenteric vascular thrombosis, or ischemic colitis.

Computed tomography (CT) and ultrasound are the imaging modalities that can most precisely define the degree of pancreatic inflammation and the pathways of its spread throughout the abdomen. They are also of great clinical importance in the early diagnosis of complications of acute pancreatitis, such as abscess, hemorrhage, and pseudocyst formation. In acute pancreatitis, CT demonstrates diffuse or focal enlargement of the gland (Fig. 28-4). In the normal patient, the margins of the pancreas

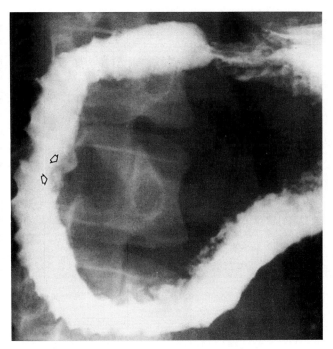

Fig. 28-2. Hemorrhagic pancreatitis with severe inflammatory changes involving the duodenal sweep (thickened folds and mucosal ulcerations) and probably edematous enlargement of the papilla of Vater **(arrows)**.

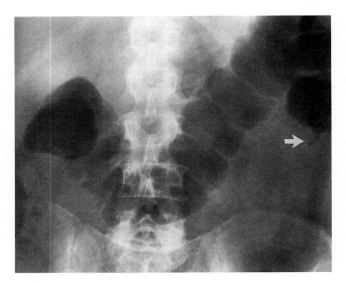

Fig. 28-3. Colon cut-off sign of acute pancreatitis. The colon gas column is abruptly cut off just distal to the splenic flexure **(arrow)**.

Acute pancreatitis may alter both the size and the parenchymal echogenicity of the gland on ultrasound (Fig. 28-6). Although the pancreas usually enlarges symmetrically and retains its initial shape, nonspecific enlargement of the pancreatic head or tail can simulate focal pancreatic carcinoma. The accompanying interstitial inflammatory edema causes the pancreas to appear relatively sonolucent when compared to the adjacent liver. However, in the presence of hemorrhage or necrosis, fat, clotted blood, or peripancreatic debris may produce areas of increased echogenicity. Ultrasound is an excellent method for demonstrating cholelithiasis, an important cause of acute pancreatitis; however, it is less precise than CT in defining fascial compartments and pathways of extraperitoneal spread of inflammation. One limitation of ultrasound in patients with acute pancreatitis is the frequent occurrence of adynamic ileus with excessive intestinal gas, which may prevent adequate visualization of the gland.

CHRONIC PANCREATITIS

are sharply delineated by surrounding peripancreatic fat. Extrapancreatic spread of inflammation and edema (especially into the anterior perirenal space, lesser peritoneal sac, and transverse mesocolon) obscures the peripancreatic soft tissues and often thickens the surrounding fascial planes (Fig. 28-5).

More than half of patients with chronic pancreatitis have a history of alcoholism. Biliary tract disease (usually with gallstones) is seen in about one-third. Almost all patients report one or more episodes of abdominal pain often radiating to the back. Weight loss is nearly universal, though jaundice is rare ex-

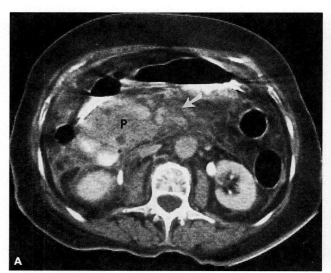
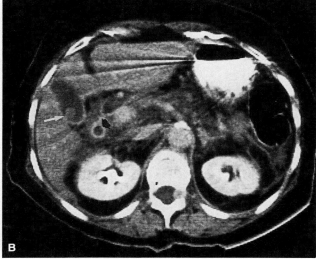

Fig. 28-4. Acute gallstone pancreatitis. **(A)** There is enlargement of the head of the pancreas **(P)** with inflammatory reaction of surrounding peripancreatic fat planes. **(B)** At a higher level, a stone **(white arrow)** is seen in the gallbladder, and the common bile duct is enlarged **(black arrow)**. (Eisenberg RL: Diagnostic Imaging in Surgery. New York, McGraw–Hill, 1987)

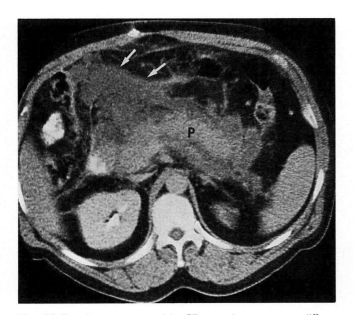

Fig. 28-5. Acute pancreatitis. CT scan demonstrates diffuse enlargement of the pancreas **(P)** with obliteration of peripancreatic fat planes by the inflammatory process. Note the extension of the inflammatory reaction into the transverse mesocolon **(arrows)**. (Jeffrey RB, Federle MD, Laing FC: Computed tomography of mesenteric involvement in fulminant pancreatitis. Radiology 147:185–192, 1983)

cept during acute exacerbations of pancreatitis. Malabsorption and diabetes can also be complications of chronic pancreatitis.

Radiographically visible pancreatic calcification is seen in about 30% of patients with chronic pancreatitis. Progressive displacement of calcium on serial films can provide a clue to the presence of an enlarging tumor or developing pseudocyst. On rare occasions, calcification disappears with the development of pancreatic cancer.

About 5% of patients with chronic pancreatitis have osseous abnormalities such as medullary infarction or aseptic necrosis of the femoral or humeral heads. This is probably related to episodes of necrosis of medullary fat, a process similar to necrosis of intraperitoneal fat, which also occurs during episodes of acute pancreatitis.

RADIOGRAPHIC FINDINGS

The most common and specific radiographic abnormality in patients with chronic pancreatitis is fold effacement (Fig. 28-7). This appears as straightening of the upper inner margin of the descending duodenum and flattening of the normal interfold crevices, usually with a slight reduction in luminal caliber. Fold effacement reflects chronic inflammatory

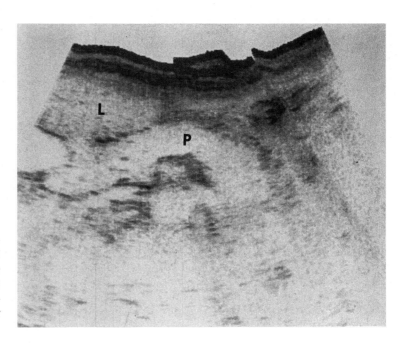

Fig. 28-6. Acute pancreatitis. Transverse sonogram demonstrates diffuse enlargement of the gland with retention of its normal shape. Note the relative sonolucency of the pancreas **(P)** when compared with the echogenicity of the adjacent liver **(L)**. (Eisenberg RL: Diagnostic Imaging in Surgery. New York, McGraw–Hill, 1987)

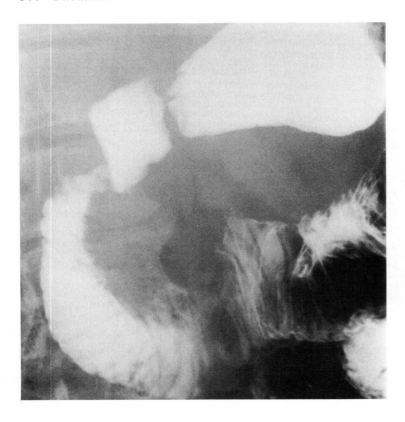

Fig. 28-7. Chronic pancreatitis. Fold effacement is seen as flattening of the medial wall of the duodenum due to the fibrosis of chronic inflammatory disease.

change with fibrosis and rigidity of the duodenal wall. Serrations and spiculation of the mucosa (Fig. 28-8), as well as enlargement of the papilla, can be seen, though identical findings can be demonstrated in patients with pancreatic carcinoma and impacted ampullary gallstones, respectively. Unusual appearances in chronic pancreatitis include thumbprint-like indentations on the duodenal bulb and nodular, bulbar filling defects with central ulceration.

Alteration of the intrinsic echo pattern is a major feature of the ultrasound diagnosis of chronic pancreatitis. This indicates generalized or local increased tissue reflectivity that is particularly obvious in calcific pancreatitis (Fig. 28-9) but can also be due to fibrosis in noncalcific disease. The pancreas often is atrophic in chronic pancreatitis; in subacute disease or with acute recurrence, however, the pancreas can be significantly enlarged, and the echo pattern can become increasingly sonolucent. Dilatation of the pancreatic duct due to gland atrophy and obstruction can be seen (Fig. 28-10), though a similar pattern can be produced by ductal obstruction in pancreatic cancer. Computed tomography can also demonstrate ductal dilatation, calcification, and atrophy of the gland in patients with chronic pancreatitis (Fig. 28-11). However, since similar information can be obtained less expensively and without ionizing radiation by ultrasound, CT is usually reserved for patients with chronic pancreatitis in whom technical factors make ultrasound suboptimal.

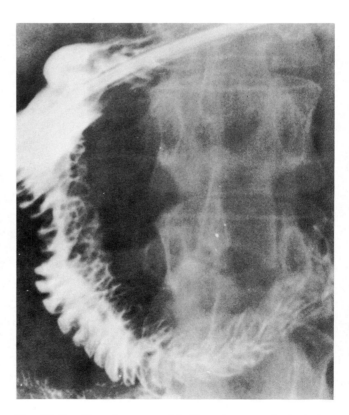

Fig. 28-8. Chronic pancreatitis. There is mucosal spiculation along the inner border of the descending duodenum. Note the mass impression on the duodenal sweep by the markedly enlarged head of the pancreas.

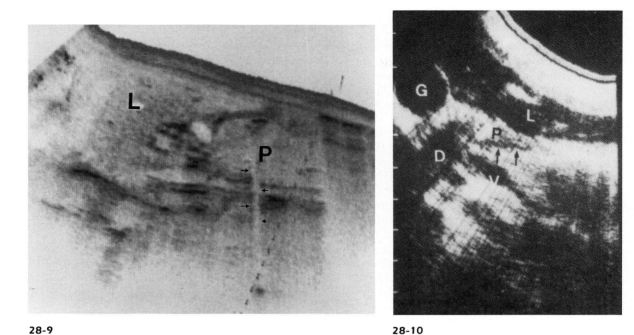

28-9   28-10

Fig. 28-9. Chronic pancreatitis. Transverse sonogram shows a large pancreas **(P)** containing calcification that produces acoustic shadowing **(arrows)**. The intrahepatic bile ducts are not enlarged. **L,** liver. (Eisenberg RL: Diagnostic Imaging in Surgery. New York, McGraw–Hill, 1987)

Fig. 28-10. Chronic pancreatitis. Sonogram performed in the left posterior oblique position (because of gas shadowing) demonstrates dilatation of the pancreatic duct **(arrows)**. The pancreas **(P)** is displayed between the splenic vein **(V)** and the liver **(L)**. **G,** gallbladder; **D,** duodenal shadow. (Weill FS: Ultrasonography of Digestive Diseases. St. Louis, CV Mosby, 1982)

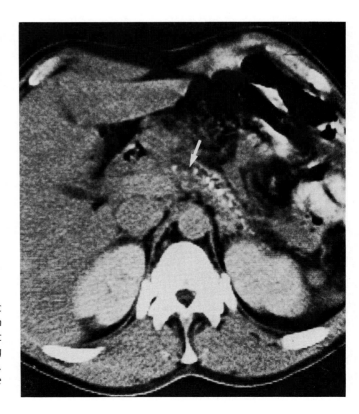

Fig. 28-11. Chronic pancreatitis. CT scan shows pancreatic atrophy along with multiple intraductal calculi and dilatation of the pancreatic duct **(arrow)**. The calcifications were not seen on plain abdominal radiographs. (Federle MP, Goldberg HI: Computed tomography of the pancreas. In Moss AA, Gamsu G, Genant HK (eds): Computed Tomography of the Body. Philadelphia, WB Saunders, 1983)

PANCREATIC PSEUDOCYST

Pancreatic pseudocysts are encapsulated collections of fluid with a high concentration of pancreatic enzymes. They are so named because they do not possess the epithelial lining that is characteristic of true cysts. A pseudocyst can develop following a severe episode of acute pancreatitis (especially if secondary to alcohol abuse) in which pancreatic juices exuding from the surface of the gland or from ductal disruption are walled off by adjacent serosal, mesenteric, and peritoneal surfaces. Because of the high protein content, osmotic pressure draws fluid into the pseudocyst and increases its size. If the fluid within the cyst is not resorbed, the inflamed membranes become a thickened and fibrotic cyst wall. The true incidence of pseudocysts complicating pancreatitis is not known. With the advent of ultrasound, pseudocysts can now be demonstrated in more than half of patients with pancreatitis.

Pseudocysts can develop after injury to the pancreas. Although most commonly the result of blunt abdominal trauma, pseudocysts can also be secondary to iatrogenic damage from previous abdominal surgery. Up to 20% of pseudocysts arise in the absence of any known predisposing pancreatic disorder.

About 70% of pseudocysts arise from the body and tail of the pancreas. Those arising from the head of the gland cause widening and compression of the duodenal sweep. Pancreatic pseudocysts can appear to migrate and have been demonstrated in the mediastinum, chest, and even the neck. The great majority, however, develop between the pancreas and the stomach, though they can become large enough to fill the entire abdomen.

Small pancreatic pseudocysts are often asymptomatic. Like patients with chronic pancreatitis, patients with large pseudocysts complain of abdominal pain frequently radiating to the back. An upper abdominal mass can sometimes be palpated. Although jaundice is uncommon, it can be caused by compression of the bile duct due to a pseudocyst in the head of the pancreas. Jaundice can also be due to underlying hepatocellular disease in the absence of any extrahepatic biliary obstruction.

RADIOGRAPHIC FINDINGS

Plain abdominal radiographs often demonstrate pancreatic calcification consistent with chronic alcoholic pancreatitis. Rarely, calcification occurs in the wall of the pseudocyst itself. On barium examination, pseudocysts tend to produce large mass im-

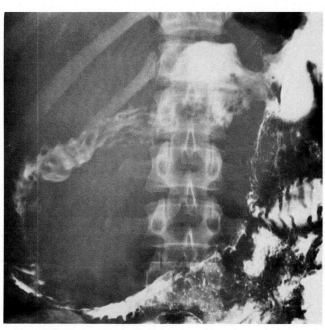

Fig. 28-12. Pancreatic pseudocyst. There is huge enlargement of the duodenal sweep.

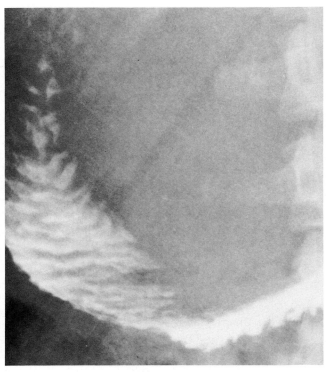

Fig. 28-13. Pancreatic pseudocyst. There is a pad effect (impression without invasion) on the inner aspect of the duodenal sweep.

pressions on the inner border of the second portion of the duodenum or on the inferior or posterior wall of the stomach (Fig. 28-12). These impressions are usually smooth, without any evidence of invasion (pad effect) (Fig. 28-13). At times, however, the adjacent stomach or duodenal wall appears irregular or ragged (Fig. 28-14), implying invasion of the pseudocyst into adjacent viscera due to enzymatic action, pressure necrosis, or intense inflammation. In these instances, it can be extremely difficult to differentiate radiographically between a pseudocyst and a pancreatic malignancy.

On ultrasound, a pseudocyst typically appears as an echo-free cystic structure with a sharp posterior wall (Fig. 28-15). Hemorrhage into the pseudocyst produces a complex fluid collection containing septations or echogenic areas (Fig. 28-16). Computed tomography demonstrates pseudocysts as sharply marginated, fluid-filled collections that are often best delineated after intravenous contrast material is given (Fig. 28-17). Because of its ability to image the entire body, CT may demonstrate pseudocysts that have dissected superiorly into the mediastinum or to other ectopic locations (Fig. 28-18), such as the lumbar or inguinal regions or within the liver, spleen, or kidney.

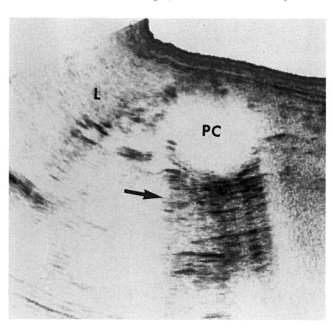

Fig. 28-15. Pancreatic pseudocyst. Longitudinal sonogram of the right upper quadrant demonstrates an irregularly marginated pseudocyst **(PC)** with acoustic shadowing **(arrow)**. **L**, liver. (Eisenberg RL: Diagnostic Imaging in Surgery. New York, McGraw–Hill, 1987)

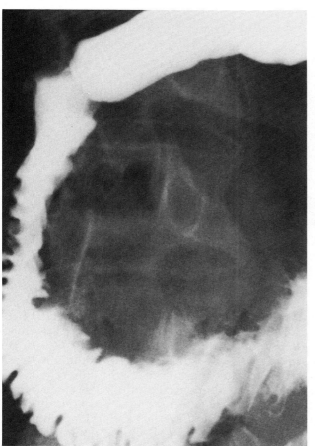

Fig. 28-14. Pancreatic pseudocyst. The irregular, ragged appearance of the inner margin of the duodenal sweep reflects intense adjacent inflammation.

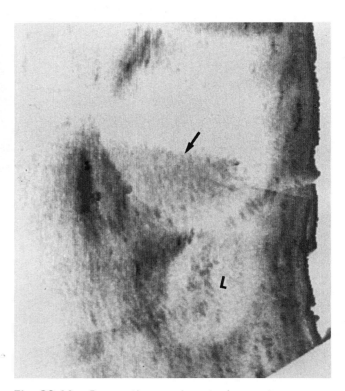

Fig. 28-16. Pancreatic pseudocyst. An erect sonogram demonstrates a fluid–debris level **(arrow)** in the pseudocyst. **L**, left kidney. (Eisenberg RL: Diagnostic Imaging in Surgery. New York, McGraw–Hill, 1987)

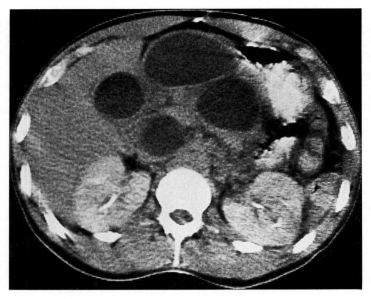

28-17

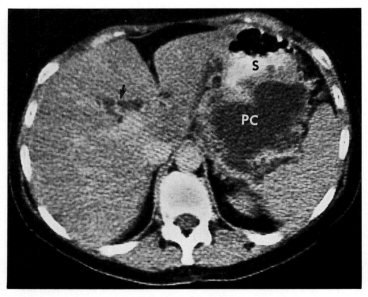

28-18

Fig. 28-17. Multiple pancreatic pseudocysts. CT scan following the intravenous administration of contrast material demonstrates four sharply marginated, fluid-filled collections. (Eisenberg RL: Diagnostic Imaging in Surgery. New York, McGraw–Hill, 1987)

Fig. 28-18. Ectopic pancreatic pseudocyst. CT scan shows the pseudocyst **(PC)** in the superior recess of the lesser sac posterior to the stomach **(S)**. Note the dilated intrahepatic bile ducts **(arrow)**. (Eisenberg RL: Diagnostic Imaging in Surgery. New York, McGraw–Hill, 1987)

COMPLICATIONS

Infection, rupture, and hemorrhage can complicate pancreatic pseudocysts. Infection by organisms from the adjacent stomach and bowel produces a high fever, chills, and leukocytosis. Sudden perforation of a pseudocyst into the peritoneal cavity results in a severe chemical peritonitis with boardlike abdominal rigidity, intense pain, and an often fatal outcome. Hemorrhage from a pancreatic pseudocyst can be caused by enzymatic digestion of small vessels lining the cyst wall, erosion into nearby major vessels (*e.g.*, gastroduodenal, spnic), or perforation into an adjacent viscus. Like cyst rupture, hemorrhage from a pancreatic pseudocyst is associated with a high mortality rate.

CARCINOMA OF THE PANCREAS

In patients with a malignancy in the head of the pancreas, significant widening of the duodenal sweep generally indicates advanced disease. Because diffuse widening of the duodenal sweep is such a late sign of carcinoma of the pancreas, subtle changes in the duodenum produced by enlargement of the head of the pancreas must be carefully evaluated. These include flattening and indentation of the medial wall, formation of double contours, deformity and displacement of diverticula, and alteration of the height, width, and direction of mucosal folds on the medial aspect of the duodenum. The extent of radiographic abnormalities does not necessarily

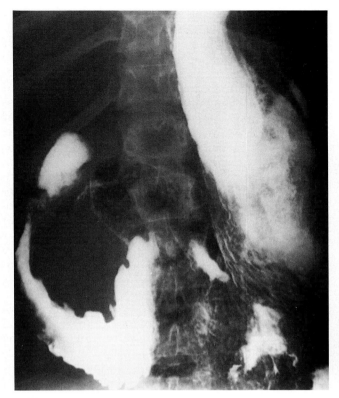

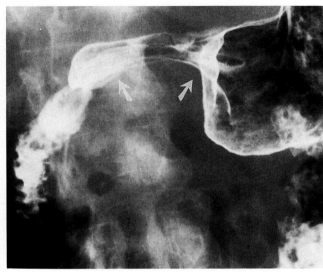

28-19   28-20

Fig. 28-19. Gastrin-secreting islet cell carcinoma of the pancreas causing widening of the duodenal sweep. Pronounced irregularity of the duodenal margin indicates neoplastic invasion.

Fig. 28-20. Antral pad sign **(arrow)** caused by carcinoma of the pancreas.

reflect the size of the pancreatic lesion. Small, strategically located tumors close to the duodenum or stomach produce radiographic abnormalities at a much earlier stage than large lesions arising at points relatively removed from these organs.

RADIOGRAPHIC FINDINGS

Masses in the head of the pancreas typically cause impressions on either the stomach or the duodenal sweep (Fig. 28-19). Indentation on the greater curvature of the antrum results in the "antral pad" sign (Fig. 28-20). More commonly, mass impressions on the inner aspect of the duodenum create a double-contour effect (Fig. 28-21). This appearance results from differential filling of the duodenum, with the interfold spaces along the inner aspect of the sweep containing less barium than the corresponding spaces along the outer aspect. Localized impressions on the sweep can cause nodular indentations. Malignant disease infiltrating the wall of the duodenum can produce an "inverted-3" (Frostberg) sign (Fig. 28-22), though this nonspecific sign, which is seen in fewer than 10% of patients with pancreatic carcinoma, is probably more common in inflamma-

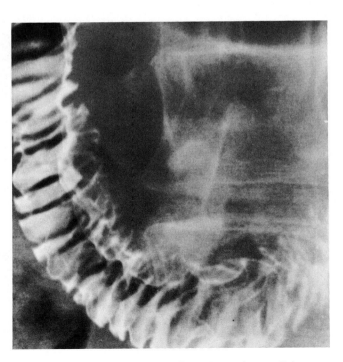

Fig. 28-21. Double-contour effect along the medial aspect of the duodenal sweep caused by carcinoma of the pancreas.

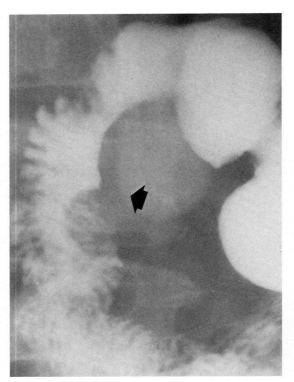

Fig. 28-22. Frostberg's inverted-3 sign **(arrow)** in a patient with carcinoma of the head of the pancreas.

tory disorders such as acute pancreatitis (Fig. 28-23) and postbulbar ulcer disease (Fig. 28-24). An identical appearance may be produced by enlargement of pancreaticoduodenal lymph nodes (Fig. 28-25). The central limb of the "3" represents the point of fixation of the duodenal wall where the pancreatic and common bile ducts insert into the papilla. The impressions above and below this point reflect either tumor mass, edema of the minor and major papillae, or smooth muscle spasm and edema in the duodenal wall.

Distortion of a duodenal diverticulum is an infrequent but highly suggestive indication of an enlarging mass in the pancreas (Fig. 28-26). This finding is not pathognomonic but merely indicates an expanding process in the head of the pancreas or peripancreatic area. Flattening, indentation, or any other contour distortion of a duodenal diverticulum is more suggestive of malignancy than is mere displacement.

Fine or coarse sharpening and elongation of barium-filled crevices between duodenal plical folds (spiculation) is secondary to mucosal edema and neuromuscular irritation. This appearance can be seen in patients with pancreatitis (Fig. 28-27) or pancreatic carcinoma (Fig. 28-28). Displacement or frank splaying of the spikes suggests tumor infiltra-

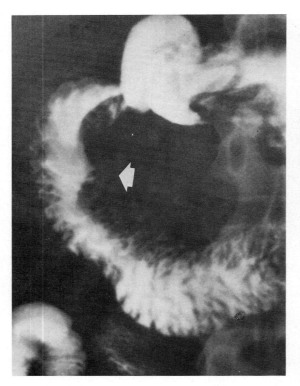

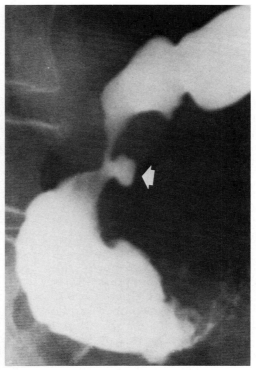

28-23

28-24

Fig. 28-23. Frostberg's inverted-3 sign **(arrow)** in a patient with acute pancreatitis and no evidence of malignancy.

Fig. 28-24. Frostberg's inverted-3 sign in a patient with a large postbulbar ulcer **(arrow)** and no evidence of malignancy.

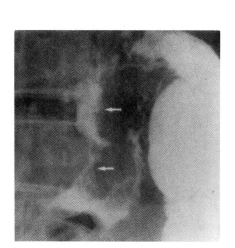

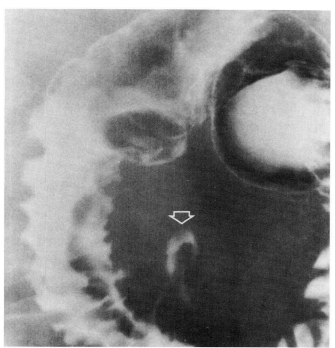

28-25   28-26

Fig. 28-25. Pancreaticoduodenal lymphadenopathy. Invasion of the duodenal sweep in a jaundiced patient with non-Hodgkin lymphoma produces a reverse-3 configuration. (Zeman RK, Schiebler M, Clark LR et al: The clinical and imaging spectrum of pancreaticoduodenal lymph node enlargement. AJR 144:1223–1227, 1985. Copyright 1985. Reproduced with permission)

Fig. 28-26. Distorted duodenal diverticulum **(arrow)** in a patient with carcinoma of the pancreas. Note the double contour (mass effect) and spiculations.

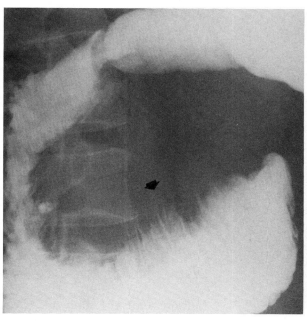

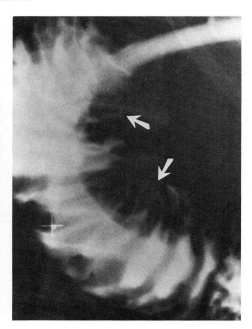

28-27   28-28

Fig. 28-27. Spiculation of duodenal folds in acute pancreatitis **(arrow)**.

Fig. 28-28. Spiculation of duodenal folds in carcinoma of the pancreas **(arrows)**. Note the mass effect on the medial wall of the descending duodenum.

tion of the wall causing traction and fixation of folds.

Irregular nodularity along the medial aspect of the second portion of the duodenum is more suggestive of malignancy than inflammation. This finding is of importance primarily in the duodenum distal to the papilla, since postbulbar peptic disease can also produce nodular filling defects in the proximal duodenum.

Although mucosal flattening with fold effacement and a slight reduction in luminal caliber can be seen in patients with pancreatic carcinoma, this appearance is more consistent with chronic pancreatitis. Severe tumor involvement can cause ulceration and frank duodenal obstruction.

Ultrasound and CT are the procedures of choice for detecting and evaluating the extent of carcinoma of the pancreas. Ultrasound can demonstrate most tumors over 2 cm in diameter that lie in the head of the pancreas; lesions in the body and tail of the gland are more difficult to detect by this modality. Pancreatic carcinoma typically causes the gland to have an irregular contour and a semisolid pattern of intrinsic echoes (Fig. 28-29). Associated signs can include compression of the inferior vena cava and superior mesenteric vein, dilatation of the biliary tract, and demonstration of hepatic metastases.

Computed tomography is the most effective modality for detecting a pancreatic cancer in any portion of the gland and for defining its extent. It can demonstrate the mass of the tumor as well as ductal dilatation and invasion of neighboring structures. Following the administration of intravenous contrast material, the relatively avascular tumor appears as an area of decreased attenuation when compared with the normal pancreas (Fig. 28-30). Computed tomography is a valuable noninvasive tool for the staging of pancreatic carcinoma and may prevent needless surgery in patients with nonresectable lesions. This technique may permit detection of hepatic metastases or involvement of regional vessels and adjacent retroperitoneal lymph nodes. The subtle finding of encasement of superior mesenteric, splenic, or hepatic arteries strongly suggests unresectable carcinoma with extrapancreatic extension (Fig. 28-31).

Cytologic examination of tissue obtained by percutaneous fine-needle aspiration under ultrasound or CT guidance can often provide the precise histologic diagnosis of a neoplastic mass, thus obviating surgical intervention.

METASTATIC LESIONS

Widening of the duodenal sweep can be caused by metastatic replacement of the head of the pancreas. Secondary malignant involvement of the pancreas is usually due to direct extension of a cancer arising in an adjacent organ (stomach, colon, kidney). True hematogenous metastases to the pancreas are rare.

CYSTADENOMA/CYSTADENOCARCINOMA

Although most cystadenomas and cystadenocarcinomas occur in the body or tail of the pancreas, tumors arising in the head of the pancreas can widen the duodenal sweep (Fig. 28-32). These uncommon lesions have certain clinical features that can permit their differentiation from solid neoplasms. They occur in younger persons than pancreatic carcinoma and have a heavy predominance in women. Symptoms are infrequent; the presenting complaint is usually a poorly defined upper abdominal mass that is not tender. The incidence of concomitant metabolic and endocrine abnormalities (diabetes, obesity, sterility, infertility, thyroid dysfunction, hypertension) is high. Cystadenocarcinomas of the pancreas have a much better prognosis than solid adenocarcinomas. Many of the tumors are surgically resectable, and complete excision is associated with a high cure rate.

LYMPH NODE ENLARGEMENT

Enlargement of lymph nodes near the head of the pancreas can widen the duodenal sweep. The subpyloric lymph nodes lie below the flexure that forms the junction between the first and second portions of the duodenum. The pancreaticoduodenal nodes lie medial to the head of the pancreas in the groove between it and the duodenum. Any enlargement of

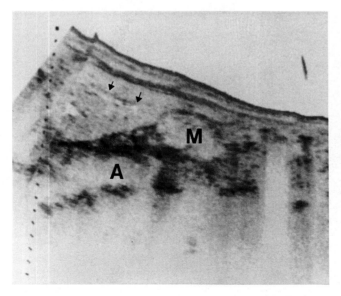

Fig. 28-29. *Carcinoma of the pancreas. Longitudinal sonogram demonstrates an irregular mass* **(M)** *with a semisolid pattern of intrinsic echoes. There is associated dilatation of the intrahepatic bile ducts* **(arrows)**. **A**, *aorta. (Eisenberg RL: Diagnostic Imaging in Surgery. New York, McGraw–Hill, 1987)*

Text continues on page 356

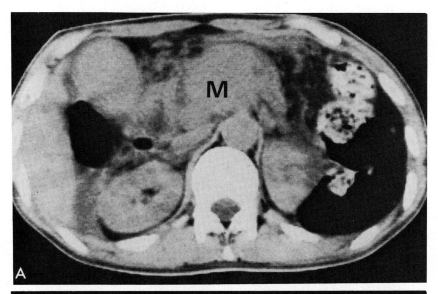

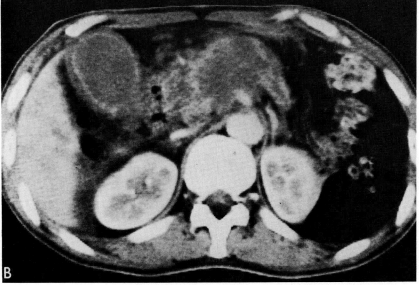

Fig. 28-30. Carcinoma of the pancreas. **(A)** Noncontrast CT scan demonstrates a homogeneous mass **(M)** in the body of the pancreas. **(B)** After the administration of an intravenous bolus of contrast material, a CT scan at the time of maximum aortic contrast shows enhancement of the surrounding vascular structures and normal pancreatic parenchyma while the pancreatic carcinoma remains unchanged and thus appears as a low-density mass. (Federle MP, Goldberg HI: Computed tomography of the pancreas. In Moss AA, Gamsu G, Genant HK (eds): Computed Tomography of the Body. Philadelphia, WB Saunders, 1983)

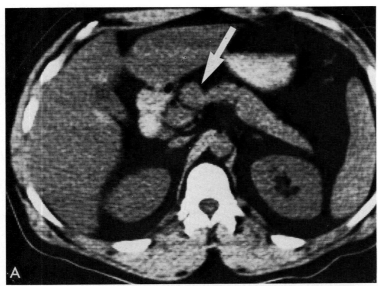

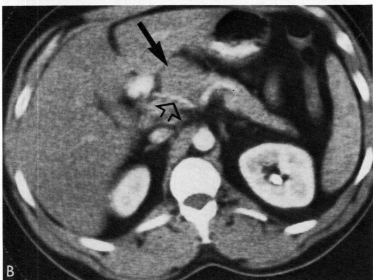

Fig. 28-31. Rapid growth and arterial encasement of pancreatic carcinoma. **(A)** CT scan demonstrates a focal change in the shape of the ventral contour of the pancreas at the junction of the body and head **(arrow)**. No enlargement of the pancreatic tissue is present. This was initially interpreted as representing an anatomic variant. **(B)** Three months later, a repeat CT scan shows a focal tumor mass **(closed arrow)** in the location of the focal contour abnormality seen in **A**. A dynamic CT scan after the intravenous bolus injection of contrast material demonstrates the splenic and hepatic arteries at the base of the tumor. Note that the hepatic artery **(open arrow)** has an irregular contour. Arteriography showed encasement by this unresectable tumor. (Federle MP, Goldberg HI: Computed tomography of the pancreas. In Moss AA, Gamsu G, Genant HK (eds): Computed Tomography of the Body. Philadelphia, WB Saunders, 1983)

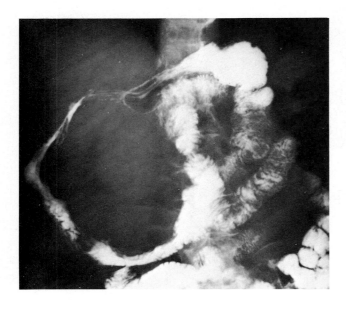

Fig. 28-32. Cystadenoma. Widening of the duodenal sweep with striking lateral displacement of the descending duodenum and inferior displacement of the horizontal portion. It would be unlikely for a typical pancreatic carcinoma to grow this large. (Ferrucci JT: The postbulbar duodenum. In Taveras JM, Ferrucci JT (eds): Radiology: Diagnosis–Imaging–Intervention. Philadelphia, JB Lippincott, 1987)

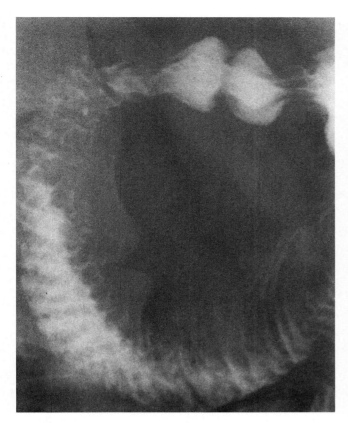

Fig. 28-33. Lymphoma involving the peripancreatic lymph nodes and causing widening of the duodenal sweep. Note the spiculations and double-contour effect simulating primary pancreatic carcinoma.

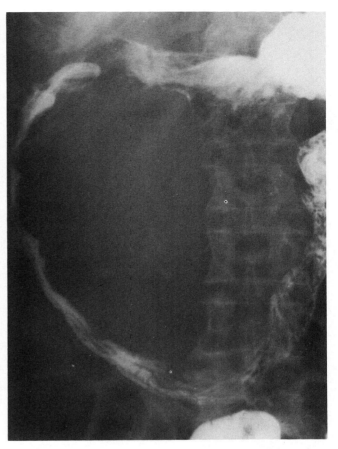

Fig. 28-34. Cystic lymphangioma of the mesentery. Note the scattered clumps of calcification in the lesion.

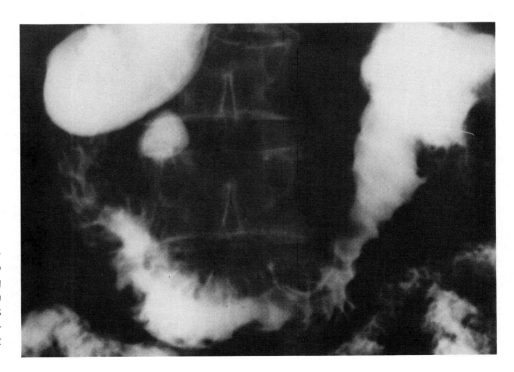

Fig. 28-35. Squamous carcinoma of the lung metastatic to the retroperitoneum. Widening of the duodenal sweep with multiple nodular indentations and spiculation simulates the appearance of primary pancreatic carcinoma.

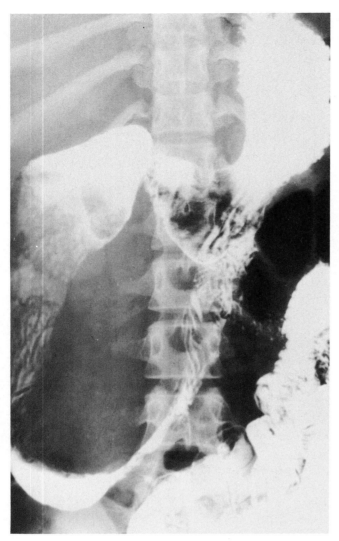

Fig. 28-36. Huge choledochal cyst causing generalized widening of the duodenal sweep.

these peripancreatic lymph nodes (due to lymphoma, metastases to lymph nodes, or inflammatory disease) can produce the radiographic pattern of widening of the duodenal sweep (Fig. 28-33).

OTHER CAUSES

Cystic lymphangiomas of the mesentery can also widen the duodenal sweep (Fig. 28-34). These benign, unilocular or multilocular cystic structures contain serous or chylous fluid. They can be the result of congenital or developmental misplacement and obliteration of draining lymphatics or be secondary to acquired lymphatic obstruction (*e.g.,*

trauma). Similar to the findings in lymphangiectasia, associated protein-losing enteropathy and hypoproteinemic edema have been reported in cystic lymphangiomas.

Dilated pancreaticoduodenal collateral vessels in patients with occlusion of the celiac axis or superior mesenteric artery infrequently produce a smooth, concave impression on the medial aspect of the descending duodenum. This double-contour effect can simulate a mass in the head of the pancreas.

Retroperitoneal masses (primary or metastatic neoplasms, cysts) can widen the duodenal sweep (Fig. 28-35). Downward displacement of the third portion of the duodenum by an aortic aneurysm can produce a similar radiographic appearance. Choledochal cysts (localized dilatations of the common bile duct) occurring near the ampulla of Vater can result in generalized widening of the duodenal sweep (Fig. 28-36) or a localized impression near the papilla.

BIBLIOGRAPHY

Bellon EM, George CR, Schreiber H: Pancreatic pseudocysts of the duodenum. AJR 133:827–831, 1979

Beranbaum SL: Carcinoma of the pancreas: A bidirectional roentgen approach. AJR 96:447–467, 1966

Eaton SB, Ferrucci JT: Radiology of the Pancreas and Duodenum. Philadelphia, WB Saunders, 1973

Eaton SB, Ferrucci JT, Margulis AR et al: Unusual roentgen findings in pancreatic disease. AJR 116:396–405, 1972

Ferrucci JT, Wittenberg J, Black EB et al: Computed body tomography in chronic pancreatitis. Radiology 130:175–182, 1979

Frostberg N: Characteristic duodenal deformity in cases of different kinds of perivaterial enlargement of the pancreas. Acta Radiol 19:164–173, 1938

Lee JKT, Stanley RJ, Melson GL et al: Pancreatic imaging by ultrasound and computed tomography. Radiol Clin North Am 16:105–117, 1979

Leonidas JC, Kopel FB, Danese CA: Mesenteric cyst associated with protein loss in the gastrointestinal tract. AJR 112:150–154, 1971

Renert WA, Hecht HL: Lymphangiographic demonstration of impression upon the duodenum by retroperitoneal lymph nodes. Br J Radiol 44:189–194, 1971

Renert WA, Pitt MJ, Capp MP: Acute pancreatitis. Semin Roentgenol 8:405–414, 1973

Sarti DA, King W: The ultrasonic findings in inflammatory pancreatic diseases. Semin Ultrasound 1:178–191, 1980

Silverstein W, Isikoff MB, Hill MC et al: Diagnostic imaging of acute pancreatitis: Perspective study using CT and sonography. AJR 157:497–502, 1981

Weyman PJ, Stanley RJ, Levitt RG: Computed tomography in the evaluation of the pancreas. Semin Roentgenol 16:301–311, 1981

Zeman RK, Schiebler M, Clark LR et al: The clinical and imaging spectrum of pancreaticoduodenal lymph node enlargement. AJR 144:1223–1227, 1985

EXTRINSIC PRESSURE ON THE DUODENUM

Disease Entities

Bile ducts
  Normal impression
  Enlargement
  Choledochal cyst
Gallbladder
  Normal impression
  Enlargement
    Hydrops
    Courvoisier phenomenon
  Carcinoma
  Pericholecystic abscess
Liver
  Generalized hepatomegaly (especially
      enlargement of the caudate lobe)
  Cyst
  Tumor
  Lymphadenopathy in the periportal region
Right kidney
  Enlargement due to bifid collecting system/
      hydronephrosis
  Multiple cysts/polycystic disease
  Hypernephroma
    Mass effect
    Direct invasion of duodenum
Right adrenal
  Enlargement (Addison's disease)
  Carcinoma
Pancreas
  Annular pancreas
  Carcinoma (wrapped around the duodenum)

Postbulbar ulcer (lateral incisura
      appearance)
Colon
  Duodenocolic apposition
  Carcinoma of the hepatic flexure
Vascular structures
  Duodenal varices
  Mesenteric arterial collaterals
  Aortic aneurysm
  Intramural or mesenteric hematoma

The duodenal bulb and sweep are intimately related anatomically to other structures in the right upper quadrant. The liver and gallbladder are in immediate contact with the anterior-superior aspect of the first portion of the duodenum. The transverse colon normally crosses the second portion of the duodenum anteriorly. A mesenteric bridge attaches the hepatic flexure of the colon to the lower portion of the descending duodenum. Posteriorly, the duodenum is extraperitoneal and has a variable relationship to the medial portion of the anterior aspect of the right kidney in the neighborhood of the hilus. As the superior mesenteric artery and vein emerge from the root of the mesentery, they cross the transverse portion of the duodenum near the midline. Thus, any disease state involving an organ within the right upper quadrant can cause displacement of or extrinsic pressure on the duodenal bulb and sweep.

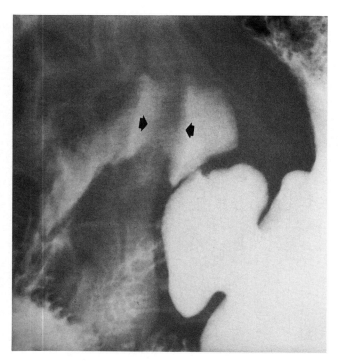

Fig. 29-1. Dilated common bile duct producing a tubular impression **(arrows)** on the duodenum near the apex of the bulb.

BILE DUCTS

Even when normal, the common bile duct can produce a linear or small, rounded impression on the duodenal bulb. A dilated common bile duct tends to cause a large tubular impression on the duodenal bulb or the postbulbar area (Fig. 29-1). This broad radiolucent defect arises superiorly and to the right of the barium-filled duodenum.

A choledochal cyst is a segmental dilatation of the common bile duct that can also involve the adjacent cystic and common hepatic ducts. Much more common in females than in males, about 60% occur in children under the age of 10. The classic clinical triad of jaundice, right upper quadrant abdominal mass, and abdominal pain is found in less than 40% of cases. Depending on the size of the cyst and the portion of the bile duct involved, various patterns of impression and displacement of the duodenal bulb and sweep can be seen. A choledochal cyst can become so large that it widens and stretches the duodenal loop; it can even displace the stomach upward.

GALLBLADDER

The normal gallbladder can cause an impression on the upper outer margin of the duodenal bulb and proximal sweep (Fig. 29-2). This is especially prone to occur in patients with hepatomegaly or a low-lying diaphragm. Hydrops of the gallbladder is usually a complication of acute cholecystitis that develops when the cystic duct remains obstructed even after the acute inflammation has subsided. This leads to distention of the gallbladder lumen with clear mucoid fluid. On plain radiographs, the enlarged gallbladder can appear as a soft-tissue mass often impressing or displacing the duodenal bulb and sweep. Acute hydrops of the gallbladder without obvious inflammation or obstruction (idiopathic) can occur in children from early infancy to adolescence.

Enlargement of the gallbladder in patients with jaundice usually indicates a malignant cause for ex-

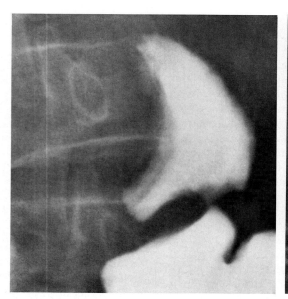
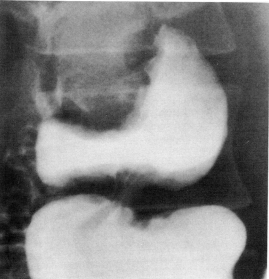

Fig. 29-2. Two examples of normal gallbladders causing impressions on the duodenal bulb.

trahepatic biliary obstruction (Courvoisier phenomenon). The gallbladder is capable of enlarging into a palpable, nontender right upper quadrant mass only if it has not been scarred or lost its pliability because of previous inflammatory disease. In the patient with jaundice secondary to an obstructing common bile duct stone, the gallbladder is not distensible because it has been the site of chronic cholecystitis for many years.

Carcinoma of the gallbladder is an unusual tumor that occasionally produces a right upper quadrant mass displacing and impressing the duodenal bulb or sweep. Carcinoma of the gallbladder primarily affects the elderly and, like cholecystitis, occurs at a far higher incidence in women than in men. Many patients with this neoplasm have coexisting gallstones; a relationship has been suggested between the presence of gallstones and subsequent malignant degeneration in the gallbladder. Therefore, carcinoma of the gallbladder should be considered as a possible etiology whenever an elderly patient with acute or chronic cholecystitis presents with a palpable right upper quadrant mass.

Carcinoma frequently arises in a gallbladder that has calcification within its wall (porcelain gallbladder). Most carcinomatous gallbladders are not visible on oral cholecystography; in well-visualized gallbladders, malignant lesions occasionally appear as irregular filling defects. On an upper gastrointestinal series, carcinoma of the gallbladder can cause a large mass impression that indents the duodenal bulb and sweep and displaces them inferiorly and medially. If ulceration into the duodenum occurs, gas can be seen in the biliary ductal system.

Abscess formation around the gallbladder secondary to acute cholecystitis can cause an irregular mass impression on the lateral aspect of the duodenal sweep. Additional radiographic findings include such inflammatory changes as fold thickening and spiculation.

LIVER

Hepatomegaly or anomalous lobes of the liver can cause marked leftward displacement of the duodenal bulb and sweep. This is especially prominent when there is hypertrophy of the caudate lobe. A similar pattern can be produced by an anomalous lobe of normal hepatic tissue that is attached by a wide pedicle to the left lobe of the liver. Hepatic cysts and tumors, as well as metastatic lymphadenopathy in the periportal region, can also cause an extrinsic impression on the duodenal bulb and sweep.

RIGHT KIDNEY/ADRENAL

Although the descending duodenum is usually thought to be related to the midportion of the right kidney, its position is somewhat variable (Fig. 29-3). Masses in any portion of the right kidney or adrenal can impress the posterolateral aspect of the duodenal sweep. Generalized renal enlargement (secondary to a bifid collecting system or hydronephrosis), multiple cysts, polycystic disease, or hypernephroma can also impress and displace the duodenum (Fig. 29-4). In addition, direct invasion by a malignant renal tumor may result in irregular mass impressions, ulcerations, or frank intraluminal polypoid filling defects. Anterior displacement of the duodenum can be caused by enlargement of the right adrenal gland in patients with Addison's disease (Fig. 29-5) or adrenal carcinoma.

PANCREAS/POSTBULBAR ULCER

A discrete single nodular defect on the lateral aspect of the second portion of the duodenum can be due to annular pancreas, carcinoma of the head of the pancreas, or a postbulbar peptic ulcer. In annular pancreas, a portion of the constricting ring of pancreatic tissue is responsible for the localized mass effect (Fig. 29-6). Tumor infiltration in patients with carcinoma of the pancreas can lead to a fixed lateral defect (wrap-around effect) (Fig. 29-7). In postbulbar peptic ulcer disease, acute inflammatory spasm characteristically produces an indentation (incisura) on the lateral wall of the descending duodenum. As fibrotic healing progresses, this may become a fixed defect.

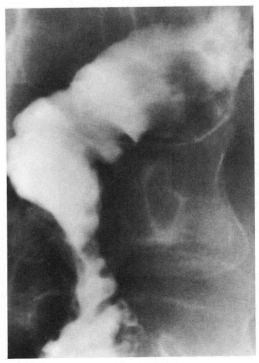

Fig. 29-3. Impression on the posterior aspect of the duodenal sweep caused by a normal right kidney.

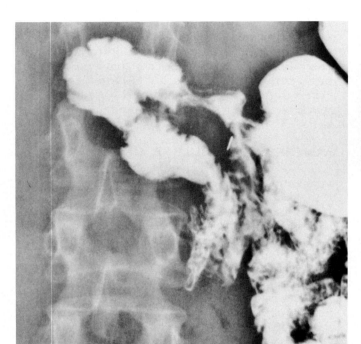

29-4

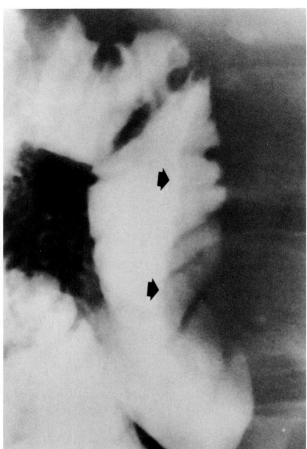

29-5

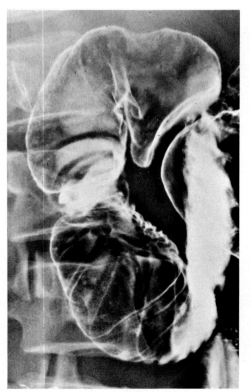

29-6

Fig. 29-4. Marked displacement of the duodenum to the left of the spine due to an enormous polycystic right kidney. The surgical clip represents the site of a previous left nephrectomy for polycystic disease.

Fig. 29-5. Posterior impression with a double-contour effect **(arrows)** on the duodenal sweep in a patient with Addison's disease and enlargement of the right adrenal gland.

Fig. 29-6. Annular pancreas. Eccentric lateral defect in the descending portion of the duodenum. (Margulis AR, Burhenne HJ (eds): Alimentary Tract Radiology, St. Louis, CV Mosby, 1983)

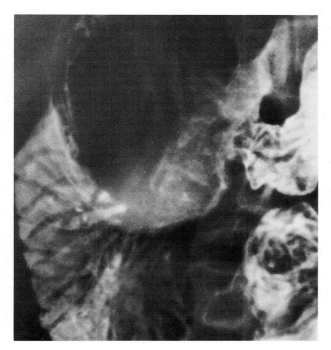

Fig. 29-7. Leiomyosarcoma of the pancreas. The huge retroperitoneal neoplastic mass causes a large extrinsic impression on the duodenal bulb and proximal sweep.

COLON

The midportion of the descending duodenum is crossed anteriorly by the transverse colon. In some patients (up to 3%), there is a closer than normal positional relationship between these two structures resulting in some degree of mutual indentation. This duodenocolic apposition appears to be related to anomalies of peritoneal fixation, with persistence of a fold of the embryologic anterior mesogastrium extending from the liver or gallbladder across the ventral surface of the duodenum to the transverse mesocolon. The resulting convex impression on the lateral border of the duodenum caused by the gas-filled colon has no clinical significance.

Carcinoma of the right side of the colon, especially of the hepatic flexure, can result in an extrinsic pressure defect on the outer border of the descending duodenum. This can be caused by lymph node enlargement from metastatic spread or be due to direct extension of the neoplastic process across the short fascial plane of the lateral reflection of the transverse mesocolon, which attaches the hepatic flexure of the colon to the lower portion of the descending duodenum. Large mass impressions distort the mucosal folds. Irregular ulcerations and duodenal-colic fistulas can develop.

VASCULAR STRUCTURES

Dilated vessels can produce single or multiple impressions on the outer wall of the duodenal bulb and sweep. Duodenal varices usually develop in conjunction with esophageal varices and are secondary to portal hypertension. Dilated arterial collateral pathways can result from occlusion of the celiac axis or superior mesenteric artery. Extension of aortic aneurysms can cause posterior impression and anterior displacement of the transverse duodenum. Bleeding into the duodenal wall (because of trauma, anticoagulant therapy, or bleeding diathesis) can simulate an extrinsic impression on the second or third portion of the duodenum and produce a high-grade stenosis.

BIBLIOGRAPHY

Bateson EM: Duodenal and antral varices. Br J Radiol 42:744–747, 1969

Bluth I, Vitale P: Right renal enlargement causing alterations in the descending duodenum: A radiographic demonstration. Radiology 76:777–784, 1961

Chon H, Arger PH, Miller WT: Displacement of duodenum by an enlarged liver. AJR 119:85–88, 1973

Eaton SB, Ferrucci JT: Radiology of the Pancreas and Duodenum. Philadelphia, WB Saunders, 1973

Eaton SB, Ferrucci JT, Margulis AR et al: Unfamiliar roentgen findings in pancreatic disease. AJR 116:396–405, 1972

Fleming RJ, Seaman WB: Roentgenographic demonstration of unusual extraesophageal varices. AJR 103:281–290, 1968

Kattan KR, Moskowitz M: Position of the duodenal bulb and liver size. AJR 119:78–84, 1973

Khilnani MT, Wolf BS, Finkel M: Roengen features of carcinoma of the gallbladder on barium-meal examination. Radiology 79:264–273, 1962

McConnell F: Malignant neoplasm of the gallbladder: Roentgenological diagnosis. Radiology 69:720–725, 1957

Meyers HI, Jacobson G: Displacements of stomach and duodenum by anomalous lobes of the liver. AJR 79:789–793, 1958

Poppel MH: Duodenocolic apposition. AJR 83:851–856, 1960

Shimkin PM, Pearson KD: Unusual arterial impressions upon the duodenum. Radiology 103:295–297, 1972

Treitel H, Meyers MA, Maza V: Changes in the duodenal loop secondary to carcinoma of the hepatic flexure of the colon. Br J Radiol 43:209–213, 1970

30

DUODENAL FILLING DEFECTS

Disease Entities

Pseudotumors
    Gallbladder impression
    Acute ulcer mound
    Blood clot
    Foreign body (fruit pit, gallstone)
    Stitch abscess
    Gas-filled duodenal diverticulum
    Flexure defect
Nonneoplastic masses
    Brunner's gland hyperplasia
    Benign lymphoid hyperplasia
    Heterotopic gastric mucosa
    Nonerosive duodenitis
    Sprue
    Ectopic pancreas
    Prolapsed antral mucosa
    Enlarged papilla
    Choledochocele
    Duplication cyst
    Pancreatic pseudocyst
    Duodenal varices/mesenteric arterial
        collaterals
    Anomalous vessel
    Intramural hematoma
    Adjacent abscess
Benign tumors
    Adenomatous polyp
    Leiomyoma
    Lipoma

    Hamartoma (Peutz–Jeghers syndrome)
    Neurogenic tumors
    Cavernous lymphangioma
    Prolapsed/intussuscepted antral polyp
    Brunner's gland adenoma
Tumors with variable malignant potential
    Villous adenoma
    Carcinoid-islet cell tumor
Malignant tumors
    Adenocarcinoma
    Ampullary carcinoma
    Sarcoma
    Lymphoma
    Metastases
    Kaposi's sarcoma

PSEUDOTUMORS

Several types of pseudotumors can present radiographically as duodenal filling defects. A prominent gallbladder can impress the bulb and simulate an intrinsic duodenal lesion (Fig. 30-1). Severe edema surrounding a small ulcer crater can mimic a mass lesion. A retained blood clot can appear as a duodenal filling defect (Fig. 30-2); if there is a collection of barium on its surface, the clot may simulate an ulcerating tumor (Fig. 30-3). Ingested material, especially fruit pits, can lodge in the duodenal bulb. This is especially common in patients with chronic scarring in the apical or postbulbar region secondary to peptic ulcer disease. Erosion of a gallstone

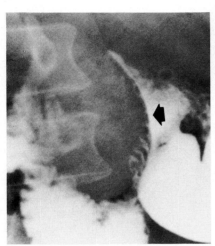
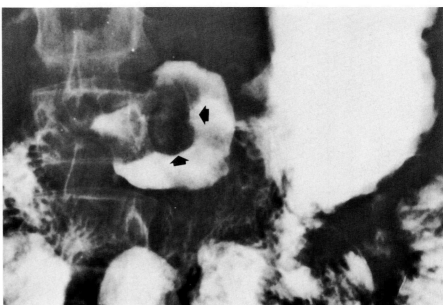

30-1   30-2

Fig. 30-1. *Gallbladder impression* **(arrow)** *on the duodenal bulb simulating an intrinsic mass.*

Fig. 30-2. *Large blood clot* **(arrows)** *in a giant ulcer of the duodenal bulb.*

into the duodenum can present as an obstructing mass (Fig. 30-4). In this instance, the appearance of barium in the biliary tree should suggest an intraluminal gallstone as the likely diagnosis. A feeding gastrostomy tube sometimes prolapses into the bulb and mimics a discrete duodenal mass (Fig. 30-5). Following surgery, an apparent duodenal filling defect can represent a stitch abscess (Fig. 30-6). A gas-filled duodenal diverticulum can simulate an intraluminal or intramural lesion (Fig. 30-7A), but filling of the diverticulum with barium clearly indicates the true nature of the mass (Fig. 30-7B). The pylorus seen on end occasionally mimics a mass in the duodenal bulb (Fig. 30-8).

The flexure defect is a pseudotumor that often occurs in normal persons on the inner (inferior) margin of the junction between the first and second portions of the duodenum (Fig. 30-9A). The acute change in the axis of the duodenum at this point causes the heaping up of redundant loose mucosa, and this creates an apparent filling defect (Fig. 30-9B). A circular or swirled configuration of plical folds is typically produced. When the duodenal folds are edematous and thickened, small amounts of barium trapped between them can mimic an ulcer crater or bull's-eye lesion. The flexure defect can usually be distinguished from a true lesion by virtue of its typical location and variable appearance on different projections.

NONNEOPLASTIC MASSES

NORMAL MUCOSAL SURFACE PATTERN OF THE DUODENAL BULB

Most technically satisfactory double-contrast examinations of the normal duodenum demonstrate a smooth, featureless surface. In about 5% to 10% of cases, a fine, lacy reticular pattern is seen (Fig. 30-10A), occasionally extending into the descending duodenum. Visualization of this pattern requires adequate distention and fold effacement as well as the absence of mucus, which otherwise fills the sulci to produce the more common featureless surface. When the mucosal surface can be demonstrated, it may contain small, rounded lucent areas of uniform size representing the villi. Occasionally, discrete punctate (Fig. 30-10B) or even larger collections of barium (Fig. 30-10C) are seen in the duodenal bulb (Fig. 30-10D). These collections are usually numerous, uniformly distributed, and often extend to the apex of the bulb or to the descending duodenum. When seen in profile, they appear as triangular barium spiculations of uniform size and shape (Fig. 30-11). Such spiculations and barium collections must be distinguished from duodenal erosions and barium precipitates. Erosions are neither as uniformly distributed nor as numerous; they tend to be more punctate and focal, are usually located in the

Text continues on page 367

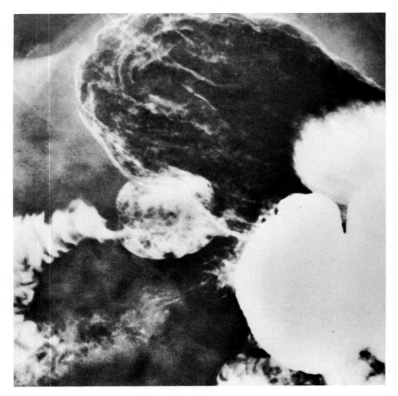

30-3

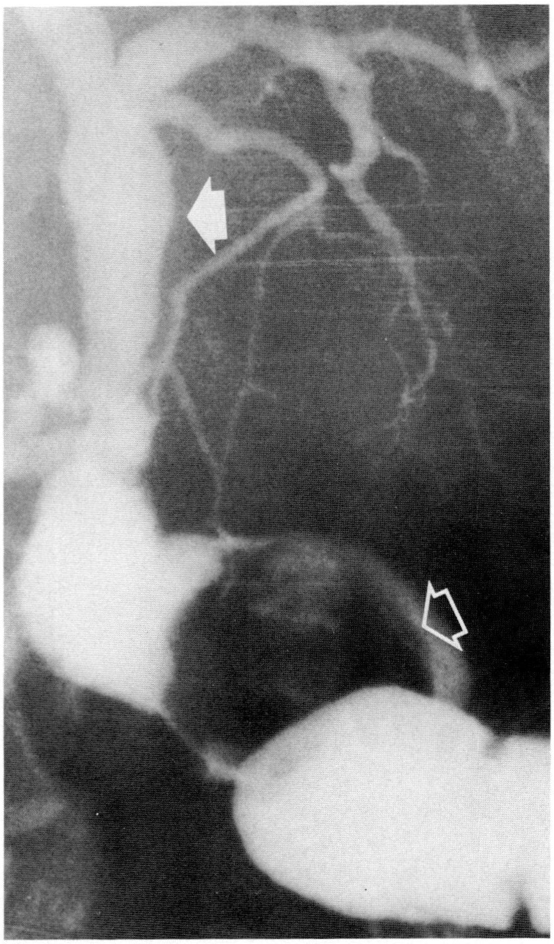

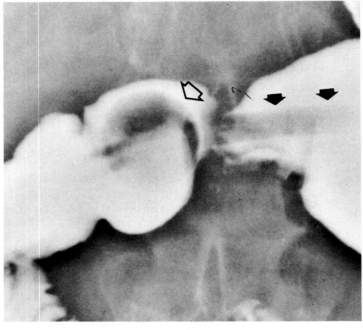

30-5

Fig. 30-3. Blood clot bezoar in the duodenal bulb. The collection of barium on the surface of the clot produces an appearance simulating that of an ulcerating tumor.

Fig. 30-4. Gallstone **(open arrow)** lodged within the duodenal bulb. The appearance of barium within the biliary tree **(solid arrow)** should suggest the proper diagnosis.

Fig. 30-5. Feeding gastrostomy tube **(open arrow)** prolapsed into the duodenal bulb. The tube could be mistaken for a polyp on a long stalk **(solid arrows)**.

30-4

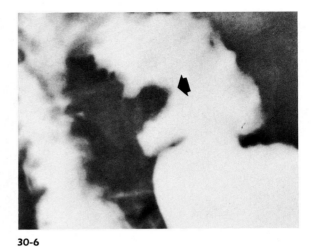

Fig. 30-6. Stitch abscess **(arrow)** in the duodenal bulb.

Fig. 30-7. Duodenal diverticulum simulating a discrete filling defect. **(A)** The gas-filled duodenal diverticulum **(arrows)** simulates a mass in the second portion of the duodenum. **(B)** Filling of the diverticulum with barium **(arrow)** clearly indicates the true nature of this pseudolesion.

30-6

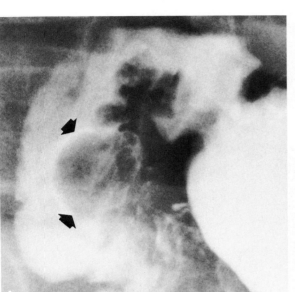

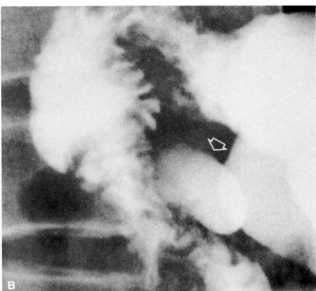

30-7

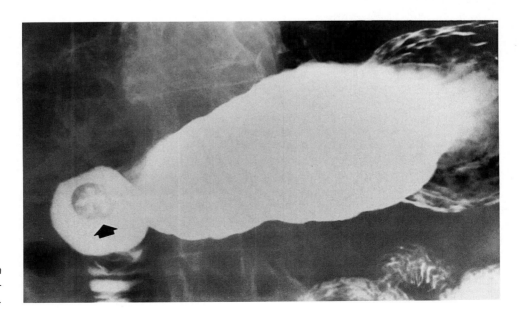

Fig. 30-8. Pylorus, seen on end **(arrow)**, simulating a discrete mass in the duodenal bulb.

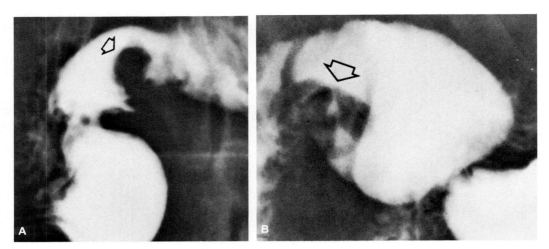

Fig. 30-9. Two examples of flexure defects producing duodenal pseudotumors **(arrows)** at the junction between the first and second portions of the duodenum.

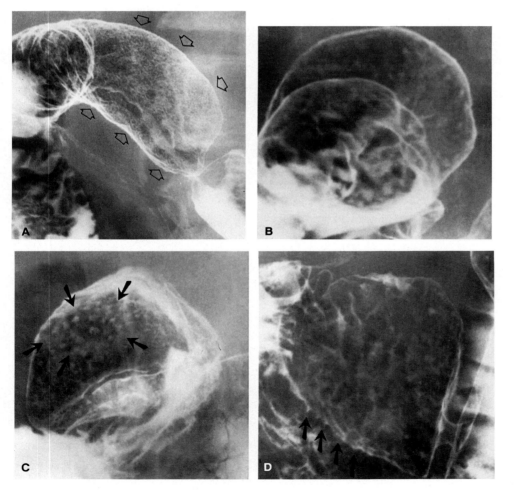

Fig. 30-10. Normal surface patterns in the duodenal bulb range from a fine reticular mosaic **(arrowheads) (A)** to a varying speckled *en face* appearance **(B, C, arrows)**. In profile, uniform, equally spaced spiculations are seen **(arrows) (D)**. All of these patients had normal-appearing duodenal mucosa on endoscopy. (Glick SN, Gohel VK, Laufer I: Mucosal surface patterns of the duodenal bulb: Subject review. Radiology 150:317–322, 1984)

proximal duodenal bulb, do not usually project tangentially, and are often surrounded by a faint radiolucent halo representing edema. These erosions are usually related to peptic disease but may also be present in Crohn's disease. Barium precipitates appear more discrete and dense, may also be seen as barium clumps on the mucosal surface when viewed tangentially, and may disappear during the course of the study.

In addition to duodenal erosions, several other pathologic conditions discussed below may alter or replace the normal surface pattern of the duodenum. These include Brunner's gland hyperplasia, benign lymphoid hyperplasia, heterotopic gastric mucosa, and nonerosive duodenitis.

BRUNNER'S GLAND HYPERPLASIA

Brunner's gland hyperplasia can produce multiple nodular filling defects in the duodenum (Fig. 30-12). Brunner's glands are elaborately branched acinar glands containing both mucus and serous secretory cells. They are arranged in 0.5-mm to 1-mm lobules and fill much of the submucosal space of the duodenal bulb and proximal half of the second portion of the duodenum. Brunner's glands are also found in the distal antrum and distal duodenum; isolated islets can extend into the jejunum. The alkaline secretions from Brunner's glands are rich in mucus

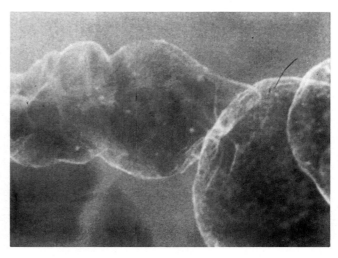

Fig. 30-11. Normal surface pattern in the duodenal bulb. The distal stomach and duodenal bulb exhibit multiple small, punctate, dense barium collections caused by clumps of improperly mixed powder, which should not be mistaken for erosions. Distinguishing features are the lack of an inflammatory halo surrounding the particles, their universal distribution, and their tendency to change position during the course of the examination. In profile, barium precipitates cling to the inner aspect of the bowel wall and do not project beyond the mucosal outline. (Glick SN, Gohel VK, Laufer I: Mucosal surface patterns of the duodenal bulb: Subject review. Radiology 150:317–322, 1984)

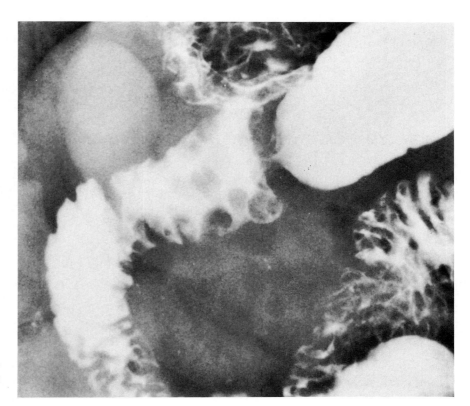

Fig. 30-12. Brunner's gland hyperplasia. Note the multiple filling defects within the duodenal bulb.

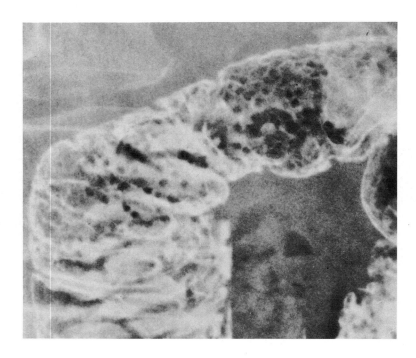

Fig. 30-13. *Benign lymphoid hyperplasia. Multiple round elevations are evenly spread over the duodenal surface. (Langkamper R, Hoek AC, Dekker W et al: Elevated lesions in the duodenal bulb caused by heterotopic gastric mucosa. Radiology 137:621–624, 1980)*

and bicarbonate, which protects the sensitive duodenal mucosa from erosion by stomach acid. Brunner's gland hyperplasia probably represents a response of the duodenal mucosa to peptic ulcer disease. The diffuse form appears as generalized nodular thickening of folds usually limited to the first portion of the duodenum. Scattered, discrete, well-defined filling defects may be seen in the nodular type of Brunner's gland hyperplasia. Occasionally, these lesions have a central depression and may be difficult to distinguish from erosions, though in Brunner's gland hyperplasia the filling defects tend to be more discrete and sharply defined.

BENIGN LYMPHOID HYPERPLASIA

Benign lymphoid hyperplasia in the gastrointestinal tract is characterized by proliferation of lymphoid aggregates without any infiltrative or inflammatory changes. The duodenum is usually incidentally affected by the reactive type of benign lymphoid hyperplasia rather than by the nodular form, which is generally associated with hypogammaglobulinemia. Benign lymphoid hyperplasia most commonly presents as innumerable tiny nodular defects evenly scattered throughout the duodenum (Fig. 30-13). Occasionally, larger, umbilicated masses simulating thickened folds occur. Unlike those seen in peptic disease, the nodular defects or thickened folds found in benign lymphoid hyperplasia are associated with normal distensibility of the duodenal bulb and an unchanging appearance with compression and on serial films.

HETEROTOPIC GASTRIC MUCOSA

Heterotopic gastric mucosa in the duodenal bulb can present as multiple elevated lesions. These abruptly marginated, angular filling defects range from 1 mm to 6 mm in diameter and are scattered over the surface of the bulb in one or more clusters, predominantly in the juxtapyloric region (Fig. 30-14). They are best visualized on double-contrast

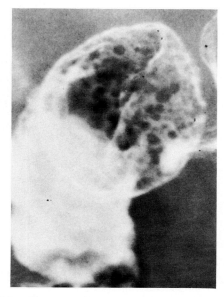

Fig. 30-14. *Heterotopic gastric mucosa in the duodenal bulb producing a diffuse, finely nodular pattern.*

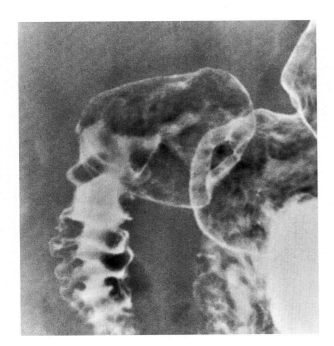

Fig. 30-15. Duodenitis. Thickening of folds involving the second portion of the duodenum. (Gelfand DW, Dale WJ, Ott DJ et al: Duodenitis: Endoscopic-radiologic correlation in 272 patients. Radiology 157:577–581, 1985)

views of an optimally distended bulb. The irregular clusters of elevated lesions caused by heterotopic gastric mucosa must be differentiated from other causes of multiple filling defects in the bulb. In benign lymphoid hyperplasia, the smoothly demarcated, round elevations are similar in size and are evenly scattered on the duodenal surface rather than being restricted to the bulb. In Brunner's gland hyperplasia, the elevations tend to be larger and more uniform in size, rather round, and often less numerous.

NONEROSIVE DUODENITIS

Nonerosive duodenitis produces a subtle coarsening in the surface pattern of the duodenum (Fig. 30-15). The normal fine velvety pattern is replaced by larger lucent areas of variable size, which are surrounded by barium-filled grooves and resemble the areae gastricae. A more nodular form of duodenitis with patchy, inflammatory, and fibrous infiltrate distorting the lamina propria and villi has been reported to be a common finding in patients with end-stage renal disease. Although this pattern may be radiographically impossible to separate from the peptic ulcer disease that often occurs in patients with uremia, most cases of nonerosive duodenitis are not accompanied by peptic ulcer, and the majority of patients with this appearance do not have gastric hypersecretion.

SPRUE

Small (1–4 mm) hexagonal filling defects in the duodenal bulb have been reported in patients with unresponsive (atypical) sprue (Fig. 30-16). The nodules are similar in size and shape to those described with heterotopic gastric mucosa, but produce an unusual mosaic pattern ("bubbly bulb"). This radiographic appearance most likely results from a combination of Brunner's gland hyperplasia due to peptic duodenitis and the inherent changes of sprue. Flattening of the villi and the abnormal motility due to sprue may allow these nodular submucosal and mucosal aggregations of Brunner's glands to become visible as bumps on the otherwise smooth mucosal surface. The demonstration of duodenal bulb nodularity in patients with sprue may help to delineate a subgroup who are relatively resistant to gluten withdrawal and in whom the addition of an antipeptic regimen may result in clinical improvement.

ECTOPIC PANCREAS

Ectopic pancreas is a nonneoplastic embryologic anomaly that can present as a discrete filling defect in the proximal second portion of the duodenum (Fig. 30-17A). Pancreatic rests are usually single and occur most frequently in the distal stomach (especially along the greater curvature of the antrum).

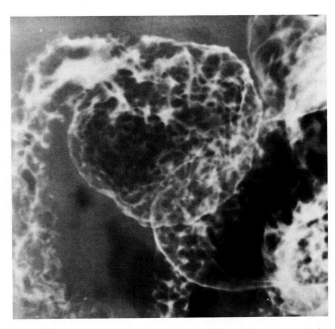

Fig. 30-16. Bubbly bulb in sprue. Multiple hexagonal defects associated with nodularity and fold thickening in the descending duodenum. (Jones W, Bayless TM, Hamilton SR et al: "Bubbly" duodenal bulb in celiac disease: Radiologic-pathologic correlation. AJR 142:119–122, 1984. Copyright 1984. Reproduced with permission)

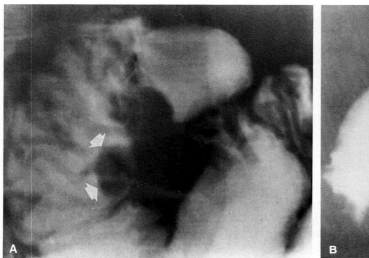
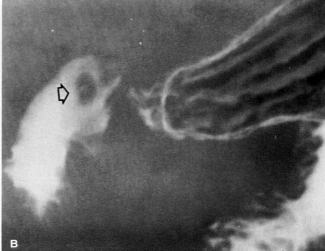

Fig. 30-17. Two examples of ectopic pancreas. **(A)** Discrete filling defect **(arrows)** in the proximal second portion of the duodenum. **(B)** Filling defect in the duodenal bulb **(arrow)**. The central collection of barium within the mass represents the filling of miniature duct-like structures within the nodule of aberrant pancreatic tissue.

Whether in the stomach or duodenum, ectopic pancreas is usually asymptomatic and is detected as an incidental finding. The discovery of a round or oval, smooth, well-demarcated filling defect in the duodenum suggests the presence of a benign tumor. A characteristic radiographic sign of ectopic pancreas is a central collection of barium (dimple) within the mass representing filling of miniature duct-like structures present in the nodule of pancreatic tissue (Fig. 30-17*B*). Although this appearance can simulate an ulcerated mass, the ulceration in a benign tumor is more likely to be eccentrically placed.

PROLAPSED ANTRAL MUCOSA

Redundant mucosa of the gastric antrum can prolapse through the pylorus under the influence of active peristalsis, resulting in single or lobulated filling defects at the base of the duodenal bulb (Fig. 30-18). Mucosal folds in the prepyloric area of the stomach can usually be traced through the pylorus to the base of the bulb, where they become continuous with the characteristic mushroom, umbrella, or cauliflower-shaped prolapsed mass. When the prolapse is extensive, the antral folds may fill a major

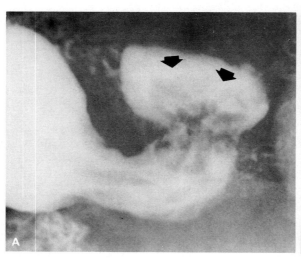
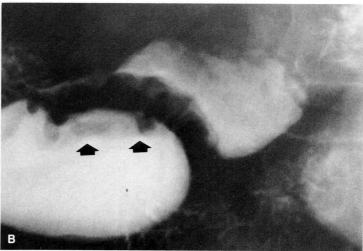

Fig. 30-18. Prolapse of gastric antral folds through the pylorus. **(A)** Appearance of a mass **(arrows)** in the duodenal bulb. **(B)** With reduction of the prolapse, the mass in the base of the bulb disappears and the redundant antral folds become evident **(arrows)**.

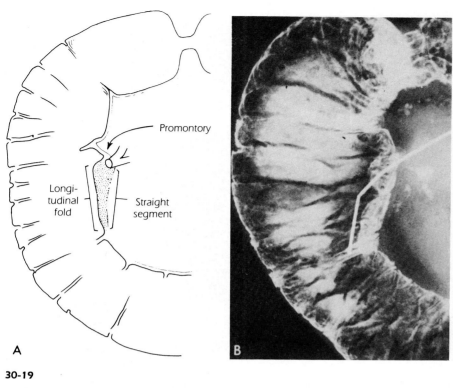

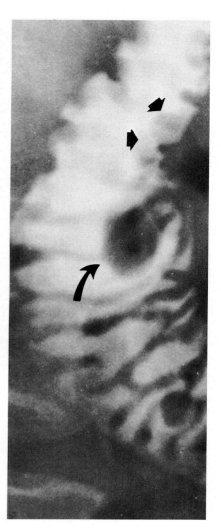

30-19

30-20

Fig. 30-19. Normal duodenal anatomy on hypotonic study. **(A)** Schematic representation of the descending duodenum showing the typical arrangement of the promontory, papilla, straight segment, and longitudinal fold. **(B)** Radiograph of a specimen demonstrating the characteristic appearance of the inner duodenal profile. Note the relationship of the papilla to the promontory and the position of the longitudinal fold along the straight segment. (Eaton SB, Ferrucci JT: Radiology of the Pancreas and Duodenum. Philadelphia, WB Saunders, 1973)

Fig. 30-20. Benign polyp in the duodenal sweep. The large polyp **(curved arrow)** is clearly separate from the duodenal papilla **(straight arrows)**.

portion of the bulb. Under fluoroscopy, mucosal prolapse can be detected as a gastric peristaltic wave passes through the antrum. As the wave relaxes, the mucosal folds tend to return into the antrum, and the defect in the base of the bulb diminishes or completely disappears.

The significance of prolapsed antral mucosa is controversial. Slight degrees of mucosal prolapse are observed frequently during gastrointestinal examinations. Although some investigators have believed antral prolapse to be a frequent cause of ulceration and bleeding, most authors agree that this finding is of little clinical significance.

PAPILLA OF VATER

In patients with filling defects in the second portion of the duodenum, it is essential that it be determined whether the mass represents the duodenal papilla, an elevated mound of tissue projecting into the duodenal lumen. The duodenal papilla can usually be precisely localized on hypotonic studies by identification of the promontory, straight segment, and longitudinal fold (Fig. 30-19). The papilla generally sits on or immediately below the promontory, a localized bulging along the medial contour of the mid-descending duodenum that results in slight widening of the lumen. The straight segment is the flat, smooth portion of the medial wall of the duodenum that extends 2 cm to 3 cm inferior to the promontory. Contrary to the appearance on the lateral wall at this level, regular interfold indentations are not visible within the straight segment. The longitudinal fold is a vertically oriented ridge of mucosa and submucosa that arises as a mucosal hood above the papilla and extends distally for 2 cm to 3 cm parallel to the straight segment. This fold runs perpendicular to the typical transverse plical folds of the duodenum. Any filling defects situated within the triangle bordered by these three structures is most likely related to the papilla. Lesions outside this area should suggest another pathologic process (Fig. 30-20).

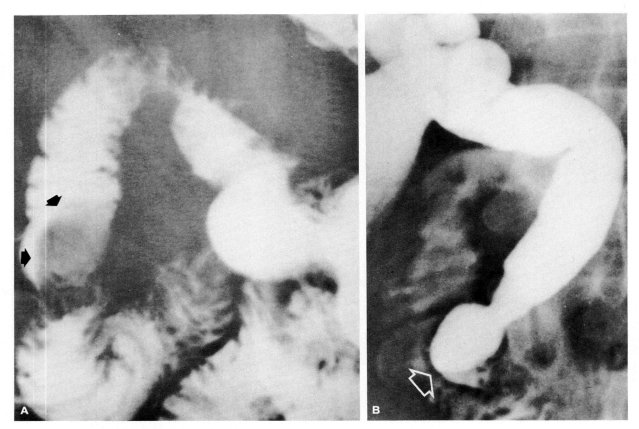

Fig. 30-21. Choledochocele. **(A)** On barium study, the lesion appears as a smooth filling defect **(arrows)** projecting into the lumen on the medial wall of the descending duodenum. **(B)** At cholangiography, the bulbous terminal portion of the common bile duct is evident **(arrow)**

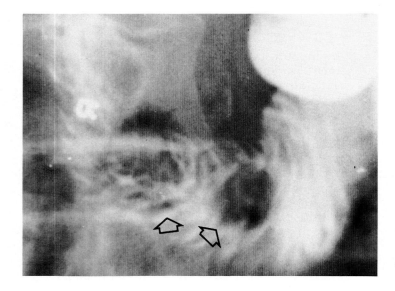

Fig. 30-22. Duodenal duplication cyst. A lobulated filling defect **(arrows)** may be seen in the region of the junction of the second and third portions of the duodenum.

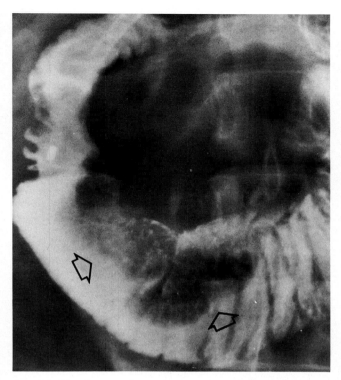

Fig. 30-23. Pancreatic pseudocyst extending into the wall of the duodenum and producing a large intramural filling defect **(arrows)**.

Enlargement of the papilla (greater than 1.5 cm in length) can be due to papillary edema or neoplasm of the ampulla of Vater (the slightly dilated segment of bile duct within the papilla). Differential diagnosis of enlargement of the papilla is discussed in Chapter 64.

CHOLEDOCHOCELE

A choledochocele is a cystic dilatation of the intraduodenal portion of the common bile duct in the region of the ampulla of Vater. On barium studies of the upper gastrointestinal tract, a choledochocele causes a well-defined, smooth filling defect projecting into the lumen on the medial wall of the descending duodenum (Fig. 30-21*A*). At cholangiography, the bulbous terminal portion of the common bile duct is evident (Fig. 30-21*B*).

DUPLICATION CYST

Duodenal duplication cysts can appear as intramural filling defects and are usually detected early in life (Fig. 30-22). Communication with the duodenal lumen has been reported to occur in about 10% to 20% of these rare congenital lesions. Duodenal duplication cysts most commonly present as abdominal masses, often with nausea and vomiting. They

Fig. 30-24. Duodenal bulb varix presenting as a solitary filling defect **(arrows)**.

Fig. 30-25. Duodenal varices. Diffuse, serpiginous thickening of mucosal folds **(arrows)**.

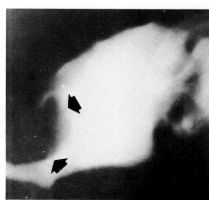

30-24

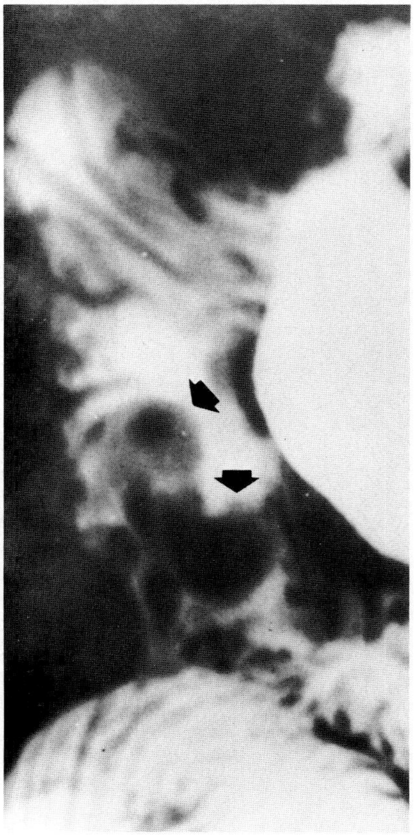

30-25

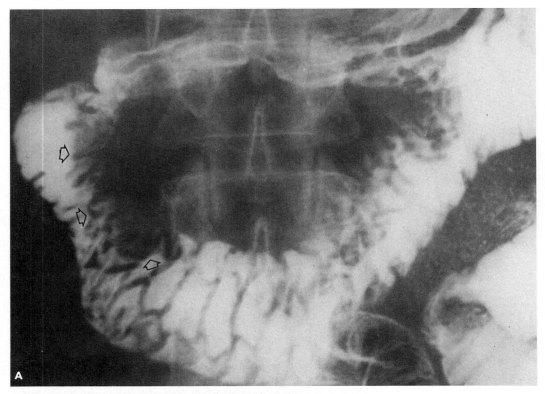

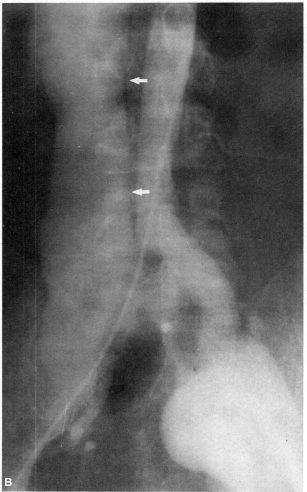

Fig. 30-26. Iliac arteriovenous fistula. **(A)** Smooth medial indentation of the second portion of the duodenum **(arrows)**. **(B)** Abdominal aortogram shows a fistula between the left iliac artery and vein with marked dilatation of the inferior vena cava **(arrows)**. (Liu CI, Cho SR, Shaw CI et al: Medial indentation of the duodenal sweep by a dilated inferior vena cava. AJR 141:1287–1288, 1983. Copyright 1983. Reproduced with permission)

are occasionally so large as to cause duodenal obstruction.

Two radiographic patterns of duodenal duplication cysts have been described. The first is a well-defined oval filling defect. The second and more characteristic pattern is a sharply defined intramural defect, usually situated in the concavity of the first and second portions of the duodenum. Because the cysts are filled with fluid, they often change shape with compression and on serial films.

PANCREATIC PSEUDOCYST

Rarely, pancreatic pseudocysts extend into the wall of the duodenum and produce an intramural filling defect (Fig. 30-23). If a pseudocyst is tensely distended, the bulging mucosa or muscularis can compromise the lumen and cause varying degrees of duodenal obstruction.

VASCULAR STRUCTURES

An isolated duodenal varix can present as a solitary filling defect (Fig. 30-24). More commonly, duodenal varices produce diffuse, serpiginous thickening of mucosal folds (Fig. 30-25). They occur secondary to portal obstruction at any level but are most frequent with subhepatic portal vein occlusion. Duodenal varices are almost always associated with esophageal varices and can be complicated by gastrointestinal bleeding. Enlarged mesenteric arterial collaterals in patients with occlusion of the celiac trunk or superior mesenteric artery can cause smooth filling defects on the inner aspect of the second portion of the duodenum. In one case, an extrinsic filling defect along the medial wall of the second portion of the duodenum was caused by dilatation of the inferior vena cava due to an iliac arteriovenous fistula (Fig. 30-26).

Anomalous vessels traversing the duodenum can cause sharply defined marginal filling defects similar to those seen when anomalous vessels cross the esophagus or ureter. Although rarely responsible for symptoms, they can mimic intramural tumors and occasionally require surgical confirmation.

INTRAMURAL HEMATOMA

Intramural duodenal hematoma is a recognized complication of blunt trauma to the abdomen. More than 80% of reported cases have occurred in children or young adults, and child abuse is a major cause in infants and young children. It is believed that the hematoma results from the bowel being crushed between the anterior abdominal wall and the vertebral column. Because the retroperitoneal second and third portions of the duodenum are relatively fixed, these areas are prone to such injury if enough force is applied to the anterior abdominal wall. Once the mucosa is separated from the loose submucosa, bleeding leads to dissection along the submucosal compartments. Duodenal intramural hematomas can also occur in patients with congenital bleeding diatheses, in persons receiving anticoagulants, or as an unusual complication of endoscopic biopsy.

Intramural duodenal hematomas can present as circumscribed intramural masses with well-de-

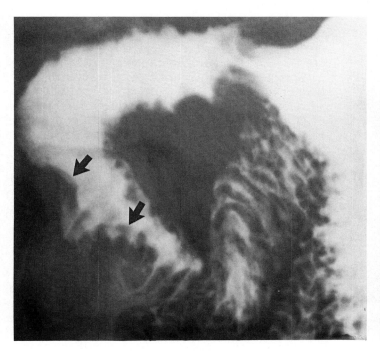
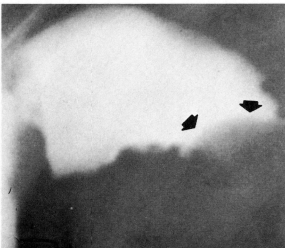

30-27 **30-28**

Fig. 30-27. *Intramural duodenal hematoma. Two well-defined mural defects* **(arrows)** *arising from the greater curvature aspect of the duodenum. There is associated mucosal fold thickening. (Kleinman PK, Brill PW, Winchester P: Resolving duodenal–jejunal hematoma in abused children. Radiology 160:747–750, 1986)*

Fig. 30-28. *Intramural duodenal hematoma. A sharply defined intramural mass* **(arrows)** *obstructs the lumen in the immediate postbulbar area. The patient complained of abdominal pain and vomiting following an automobile accident.*

fined margins (Fig. 30-27). Some degree of stenosis and occasionally complete obstruction are usually present (Fig. 30-28). The right psoas margin can be obliterated because of associated retroperitoneal bleeding. A "coiled-spring" appearance has been described, and late rupture into the peritoneal or retroperitoneal space may occur (Fig. 30-29).

ADJACENT ABSCESS

A localized inflammatory mass, such as an abscess arising from rupture of the gallbladder following acute cholecystitis, occasionally simulates an intramural duodenal lesion (Fig. 30-30).

BENIGN TUMORS

Almost 90% of duodenal bulb tumors are benign. In the second and third portions of the duodenum, benign and malignant tumors occur with approximately equal frequency. In the fourth portion of the

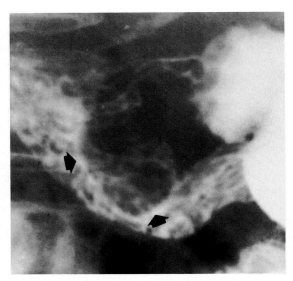

Fig. 30-30. Periduodenal abscess. The mass **(arrows)**, which appears to be intramural, developed after the patient's gallbladder ruptured during an acute attack of cholecystitis.

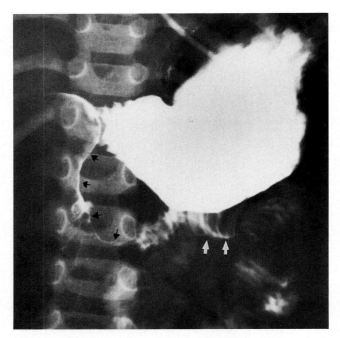

Fig. 30-29. Acute duodenal hematoma. In this 2-year-old abused child, an extensive duodenal hematoma arises from the lateral aspect of the descending duodenum and the inferior aspect of the third portion of the duodenum. A small amount of barium is trapped between the mass and the medial and superior margins of the second and third portions of the duodenum, respectively **(black arrows)**. Fold thickening is present in the fourth portion of the duodenum, and a coiled-spring pattern is noted in the proximal jejunum **(white arrows)**. (Kleinman PK, Brill PW, Winchester P: Resolving duodenal–jejunal hematoma in abused children. Radiology 160:747–750, 1986)

duodenum, there is a heavy predominance of malignant lesions.

Benign duodenal neoplasms are often asymptomatic and incidental findings on upper gastrointestinal series. However, benign tumors can ulcerate and cause acute or chronic gastrointestinal hemorrhage and abdominal pain. In contrast, malignant tumors are frequently associated with constitutional symptoms such as weight loss and anorexia. Those arising near the papilla or metastasizing to regional lymph nodes in the porta hepatis can produce obstructive jaundice.

Adenomas, leiomyomas, and lipomas are the most common benign tumors of the duodenum. Although they are usually solitary, multiple lesions do occur. A pedunculated tumor can serve as the leading edge of an intussusception.

ADENOMA

Adenomas are usually small (1 cm), smooth or lobulated intraluminal polyps that produce sharply circumscribed, rounded filling defects in the barium column (Fig. 30-31*A*). Many are pedunculated and move over some distance under the effect of peristalsis. The point of attachment of the lucent stalk can cause an inward tenting of the wall as the pedicle is placed under tension by a peristaltic wave (Fig. 30-31*B*). Foreign bodies or air bubbles sometimes simulate adenomatous polyps (Fig. 30-32). These artifacts can be excluded by demonstration of the attachment of the polyp to the wall on profile views or by demonstration that the lesion is in the same position on a repeat examination after fasting.

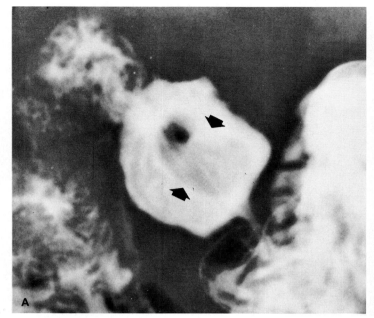

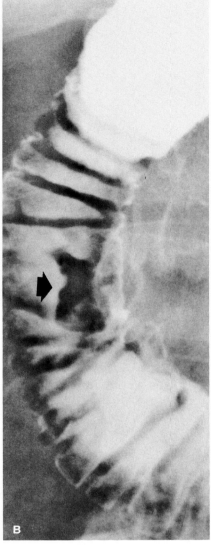

Fig. 30-31. **(A)** Adenomatous polyp of the duodenal bulb **(arrows)**. **(B)** Adenomatous polyp of the duodenal sweep **(arrow)**. Note the inward tenting of the base of the polyp.

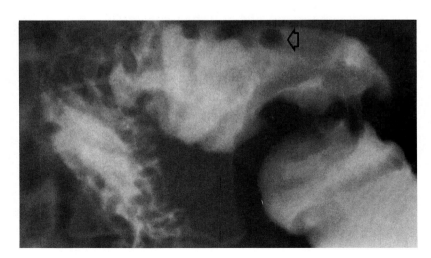

Fig. 30-32. Gas bubble **(arrow)** in the duodenal bulb mimicking a true polyp.

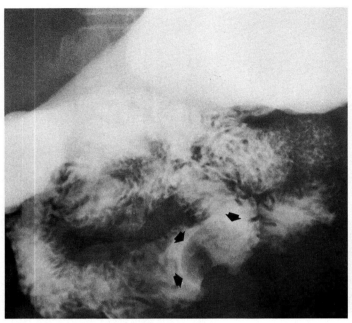

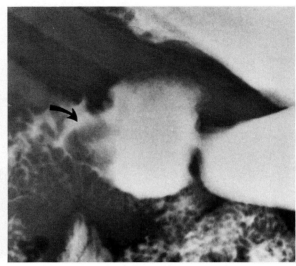

30-33   30-34

Fig. 30-33. Leiomyoma of the third portion of the duodenum **(arrows)**. The submucosal tumor forms a characteristic smooth, convex bulge into the lumen.

Fig. 30-34. Leiomyoma at the apex of the duodenal bulb **(arrow)**. The mass is well defined, with smooth margins and central ulceration.

LEIOMYOMA

A leiomyoma is an intramural tumor arising in the submucosa. The tumor characteristically forms a smooth, convex bulge into the duodenal lumen, producing a fairly sharp angle at the junction of the defect and the normal duodenal wall (Fig. 30-33). Stretched but intact mucosal folds are visualized over its surface. A spectrum of radiographic findings can be produced if a leiomyoma preferentially develops in an intraluminal or extrinsic location. As with leiomyomas elsewhere in the bowel, central, punched-out ulcerations are common and can lead to severe gastrointestinal bleeding (Fig. 30-34). Unfortunately, because smooth-surfaced adenomas and leiomyomas can be histologically malignant, the radiographic appearance of these tumors is not a reliable criterion for distinguishing between benign and malignant lesions.

LIPOMA

Lipomas are submucosal tumors that often develop pedicles and present as intraluminal masses. The soft consistency of these smooth lesions allows

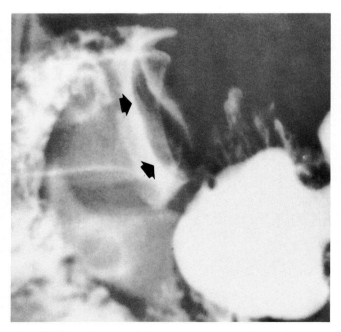

Fig. 30-35. Lipoma of the duodenal bulb. The soft consistency of the tumor allows it to conform its shape to the lumen of the bulb **(arrows)**.

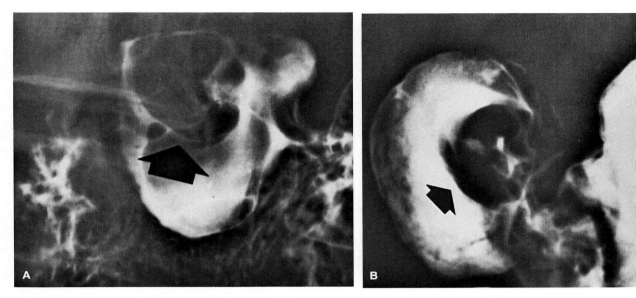

Fig. 30-36. Lipoma of the duodenal bulb **(arrows)**. Note the difference in the contour of the tumor between the two films.

Fig. 30-37. Duodenal lipoma. Low-density mass **(arrow)** with an attenuation value of −86 HU in the second portion of the duodenum. (Farah MC, Jafri SZH, Schwab RE et al: Duodenal neoplasms: Role of CT. Radiology 162:839–843, 1987)

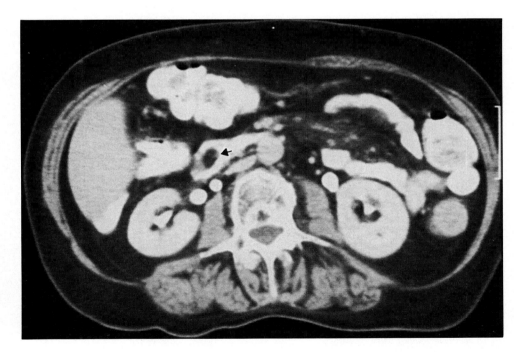

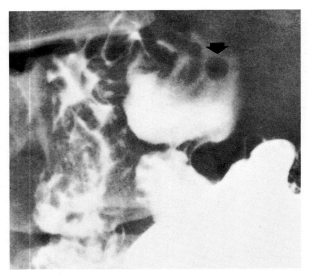

Fig. 30-38. *Peutz-Jeghers syndrome. A hamartomatous polyp* **(arrow)** *mimics a smooth gas bubble in the duodenal bulb.*

them to have an elliptical appearance that conforms to the lumen of the bowel (Fig. 30-35). Like lipomas elsewhere in the bowel, these tumors can change shape under the influence of peristalsis and demonstrate an altered contour on serial films (Fig. 30-36); however, this finding is nonspecific, since a similar appearance has been reported with rare duodenal duplication cysts and cavernous lymphangiomas. CT scans can document the characteristic low attenuation of these fatty neoplasms (Fig. 30-37).

HAMARTOMA

Small hamartomatous polyps can cause single or multiple filling defects in the duodenum in patients with the Peutz–Jeghers syndrome (Fig. 30-38).

NEUROGENIC TUMORS

Solitary or multiple neurogenic tumors in the duodenum distal to the bulb have been reported in pa-

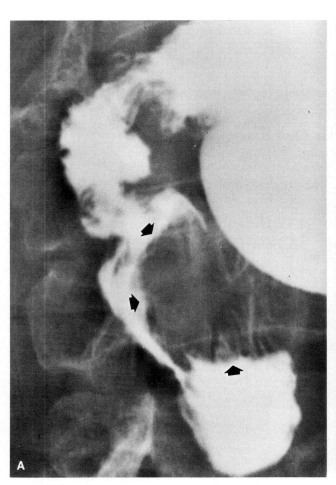
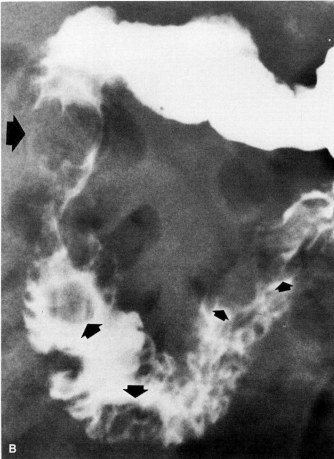

Fig. 30-39. *Neurofibromatosis.* **(A)** *Large submucosal mass in the descending duodenum* **(arrows)**. **(B)** *Numerous submucosal masses in the second and third portions of the duodenum. Twelve distinct neurofibromas were identified on the resected duodenal specimen. (Tishler JM, Han SY, Colcher H et al: Neurogenic tumor of the duodenum in patients with neurofibromatosis. Radiology 149:51–53, 1983)*

tients with neurofibromatosis (Fig. 30-39). The tumors usually arise from the subserosal nerves, Auerbach plexus, or, less often, from the submucosal plexus. Neurogenic duodenal tumors may cause ulceration of the overlying mucosa and bleeding, duodenal obstruction secondary to tumor bulk or intussusception, or jaundice due to tumor obstruction of the common bile duct. The lesions are generally benign and have a very low potential for malignant degeneration. Gangliocytic paraganglioma is a rare neurogenic tumor that is exclusively a solid tumor of the second portion of the duodenum (Fig. 30-40).

CAVERNOUS LYMPHANGIOMA

Cavernous lymphangiomas are composed of numerous irregularly dilated lymphatic channels lined with benign-appearing endothelial cells. They rarely affect the intestinal tract and are usually discovered incidentally in asymptomatic persons. Occasionally, the lesions are large enough to cause obstruction or intussusception, but in most instances complaints,

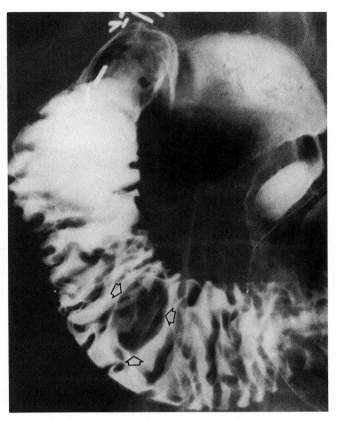

Fig. 30-41. Cavernous lymphangioma. Smooth oblong mass **(arrows)** at the junction of the second and third portions of the duodenum. (Davis M, Fenoglio–Preiser C, Haque AK: Cavernous lymphangioma of the duodenum: Case report and review of the literature. Gastrointest Radiol 12:10–12, 1987)

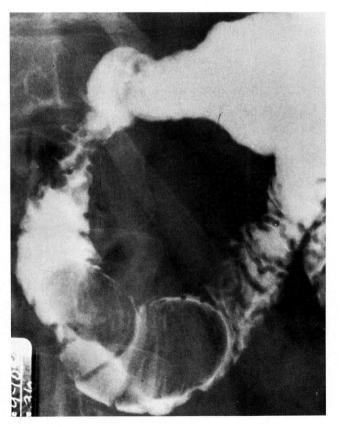

Fig. 30-40. Gangliocytic paraganglioma. Large tumor mass at the junction of the second and third portions of the duodenum. (Olmsted WW, Ros PR, Hjermstead BM et al: Tumors of the small intestine with little or no malignant predisposition: A review of the literature and report of 56 cases. Gastrointest Radiol 12:231–239, 1987)

if present, are those of intermittent abdominal pain and spasm. Radiographically, cavernous lymphangiomas are very difficult to differentiate from other intramural masses (Fig. 30-41). Like lipomas, the lesions are pliable and at fluoroscopy can be seen to change shape with compression.

PROLAPSED ANTRAL POLYP

Pedunculated polyps of the antrum can prolapse through the pylorus and present as solitary or multiple filling defects in the base of the duodenal bulb (Fig. 30-42*A*). These benign tumors are typically round or oval and have either a smooth or a slightly lobulated surface. Patients with prolapsed polyps are often anemic; abdominal pain is not infrequent. Most prolapsing antral polyps are adenomas. Ulceration within the lesion should suggest the diagnosis of leiomyoma. Like prolapsed antral mucosal folds, prolapsed antral tumors change location or completely reduce on serial films (Fig. 30-42*B*).

Any polypoid gastric tumor can pull a segment of stomach with it as it is pushed by peristalsis through the pylorus. In the resulting intussuscep-

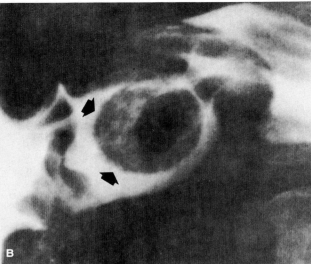

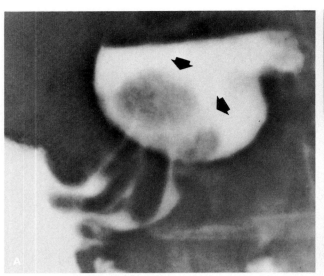

Fig. 30-42. Prolapsing antral polyp. **(A)** Prolapsed polyp presenting as a solitary filling defect **(arrows)** in the base of the duodenal bulb. **(B)** With reduction of the prolapse, the true origin of the polyp within the antrum becomes evident **(arrows)**.

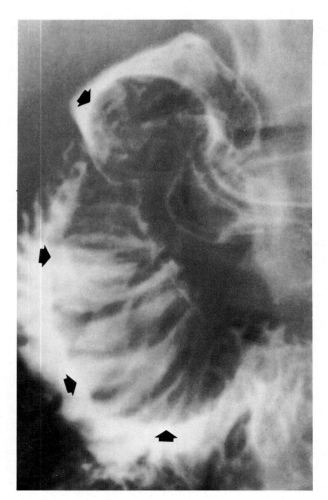

Fig. 30-43. Brunner's gland adenoma. A large filling defect **(arrows)** involves the duodenal bulb and sweep.

tion, the entire gastric wall is invaginated into the duodenum, not just the mucosa, as with prolapse of antral folds. Symptoms of gastric intussusception into the duodenum vary from acute obstruction and incarceration to more chronic gastrointestinal complaints. In addition to the radiographic appearance of an intraluminal duodenal mass, there can be shortening of the antrum, complete or incomplete gastric outlet obstruction, converging of distal gastric rugae, and compression of pyloric and duodenal folds.

BRUNNER'S GLAND ADENOMA

A Brunner's gland adenoma can present as a discrete filling defect in the bulb or second portion of the duodenum (Fig. 30-43). The "adenoma" probably represents a localized area of hypertrophy and hyperplasia rather than a true neoplasm.

TUMORS OF VARIABLE MALIGNANT POTENTIAL

VILLOUS ADENOMA

Villous adenomas and carcinoid-islet cell tumors of the duodenum have a variable malignant potential; about half have histologic evidence of malignancy. Villous adenomas of the duodenum are unusual lesions that have a radiographic appearance similar to tumors of the same cell type in the colon (Fig. 30-44). Because the ampullary region is the most frequent location for duodenal villous adenomas, obstructive jaundice is the most common clinical

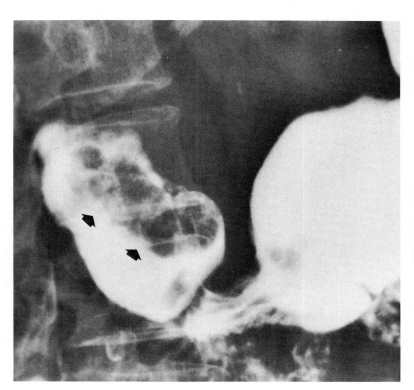

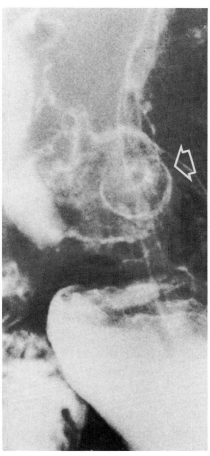

30-44   30-45

Fig. 30-44. Villous adenoma of the duodenal bulb. A bulky mass with irregular margins and barium may be seen entering the interstices in the tumor **(arrows)**. Note the radiolucent defect in the antrum, which represents a benign gastric polyp.

Fig. 30-45. Carcinoid-islet cell tumor in the duodenal bulb **(arrow)**.

presentation. Jaundice can be secondary to infiltrative growth into the ampulla or to exophytic growth physically blocking the common bile duct. Because the appearance of jaundice depends on the size of the villous adenoma and its relationship to the papilla, this physical finding can occur in benign lesions. The diffuse mucorrhea and potassium loss that is frequently associated with villous adenoma of the colon and rectum is not seen with these duodenal lesions.

Villous adenomas of the duodenum appear radiographically as lobulated filling defects covered by fine networks of barium coating the interstices between the fine, frond-like projections of the tumor. Because of their soft consistency, villous adenomas can change contour on serial films. As with tumors of this cell type in the colon, there are no definite radiographic criteria with which to differ-

entiate benign villous adenomas of the duodenum from lesions with early carcinomatous transformation.

CARCINOID-ISLET CELL TUMOR

Carcinoid-islet cell tumors of the duodenum have morphologic and functional features of both carcinoid and islet cell tumors of the pancreas (Fig. 30-45). Both carcinoid and islet cell tumors appear to arise from a common neuroectodermal precursor that is related to the argentaffin cell. Clinically, progressive and intractable peptic ulceration or severe diarrhea is present in most patients. The patient frequently has a history of one or more operative procedures for ulcer disease. Carcinoid-islet cell tumors have remarkable endocrine activity; serotonin, insulin, and gastrin-like substances have

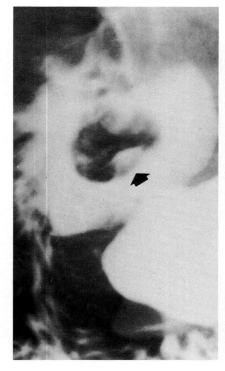

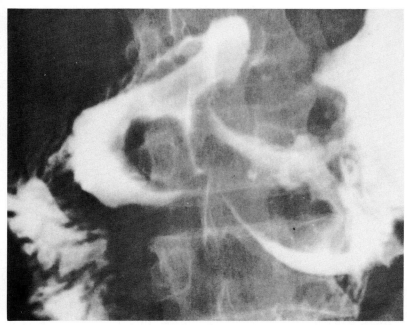

30-46

30-47

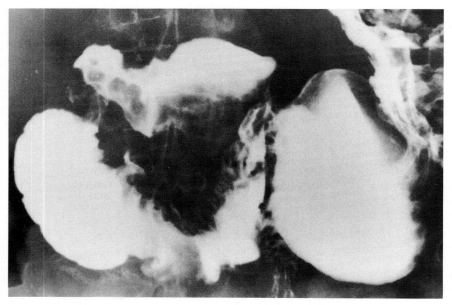

30-48

Fig. 30-46. Polypoid carcinoma of the duodenal bulb **(arrow)**.

Fig. 30-47. Nodular filling defects in the duodenal bulb caused by transpyloric extension of lymphoma arising in the gastric antrum.

Fig. 30-48. Pancreatic carcinoma. There is an annular constriction of the proximal second portion of the duodenum. A large mass effect with spiculations involves most of the duodenal sweep.

been extracted from tumor tissue. Patients with these tumors may have multiple endocrine adenomatosis (parathyroid, pancreatic, and duodenal tumors) or evidence of neural ectodermal dysplasia.

Carcinoid-islet cell tumors are most commonly found in a submucosal location on the anterior or medial wall of the first or second portion of the duodenum proximal to the papilla. Although they are usually solitary, multiple tumors are occasionally present. Malignant tumors of this cell type often produce lymph node metastases in the region of the head of the pancreas.

MALIGNANT TUMORS

Primary duodenal malignancies are rare. Of all duodenal cancers, 80% to 90% are adenocarcinomas; most occur at or distal to the papilla. In addition to polypoid intraluminal masses (Fig. 30-46), adenocarcinomas can appear as annular constricting lesions with mucosal destruction and ulceration. Clinical symptoms vary according to the location of the lesion; they include obstructive jaundice, bowel obstruction, and hemorrhage. Carcinomas of the ampulla of Vater occur on the medial aspect of the second portion of the duodenum; they will be discussed in subsequent sections.

Sarcomas, primarily leiomyosarcomas, are rare duodenal lesions that generally present as lobulated intramural filling defects, often with central ulceration. Sinus tracts often extend into the necrotic central portion of the mass, which may be large, bulky, and primarily extramural in location.

Primary lymphoma of the duodenum is rare. It can present as a polypoid mass or as multiple small nodules that produce a cobblestone appearance simulating thickened mucosal folds.

Metastases can involve the duodenum by direct invasion from adjacent structures or by hematogenous spread. Gastric carcinoma or lymphoma can extend across the pylorus and produce contour deformities and filling defects in the duodenal bulb (Fig. 30-47). Carcinoma of the pancreas can cause ulcerating and constricting lesions that are indistinguishable from primary duodenal carcinoma (Fig. 30-48). Direct extension of primary malignancies of the gallbladder, colon, or kidney can produce a similar radiographic appearance. Rarely, retroperitoneal node involvement from distal tumors distorts or invades the duodenum. Duodenal filling defects with central necrosis and ulceration (bull's-eye lesions) suggest hematogenous metastases, most of which are due to melanoma (Fig. 30-49). Occasionally, metastases present as multiple filling defects simulating thickened mucosal folds (Fig. 30-50).

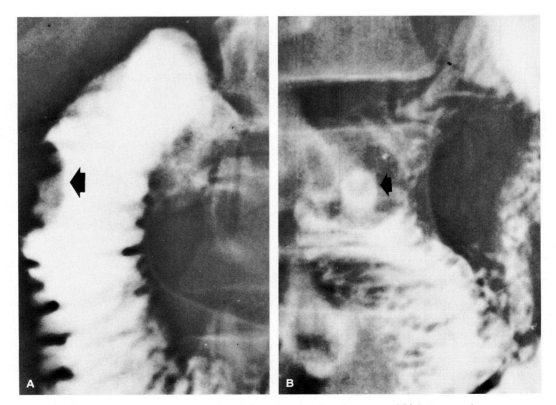

Fig. 30-49. Metastatic melanoma involving the duodenal sweep. **(A)** Intramural mass **(arrow)** on the lateral border of the descending duodenum. **(B)** Central ulceration **(arrow)** in the intramural mass suggests a hematogenous metastasis.

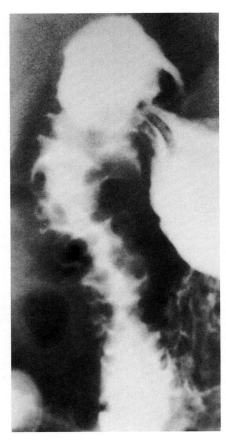

Fig. 30-50. *Carcinoma of the lung metastatic to the duodenal sweep. Multiple filling defects simulate diffuse thickening of mucosal folds.*

KAPOSI'S SARCOMA

In patients with AIDS, Kaposi's sarcoma may produce duodenal filling defects ranging from minimally elevated submucosal plaques, some with central ulceration, to discrete submucosal nodules.

BIBLIOGRAPHY

Basemann EF, Auerbach SH, Wolfe WW: The importance of roentgenologic diagnosis of aberrant pancreatic tissue in the gastrointestinal tract. AJR 107:71–76, 1969

Bateson EM: Duodenal and antral varices. Br J Radiol 42:744–747, 1969

Burrell M, Toffler R: Flexural pseudotumors of the duodenum. Radiology 120:313–315, 1976

Clements JL, Roche RR: Carcinoid of the duodenum: A report of six cases. Gastrointest Radiol 9:17–21, 1984

Davis M, Fenoglio–Preiser C, Haque AK: Cavernous lymphangioma of the duodenum: Case report and review of the literature. Gastrointest Radiol 12:10–12, 1987

Delpy JC, Bruneton JN, Drouillard J et al: Non-Vaterian duodenal adenomas: Report of 24 cases and review of the literature. Gastrointest Radiol 8:135–141, 1983

Eaton SB, Ferrucci JT: Radiology of the Pancreas and Duodenum. Philadelphia, WB Saunders, 1973

Faegenburg D, Bosniak M: Duodenal anomalies in the adult. AJR 88:642–657, 1962

Farah MC, Jafri SZH, Schwab RE et al: Duodenal neoplasms: Role of CT. Radiology 162:839–843, 1987

Gelfand DW, Dale WJ, Ott DJ et al: Duodenitis: Endoscopic-radiologic correlation in 272 patients. Radiology 157:577–581, 1985

Ghishan FK, Werner M, Vieira et al: Intramural duodenal hematoma: An unusual complication of endoscopic small bowel biopsy. Am J Gastroenterol 82:368–370, 1987

Glick SN, Gohel VK, Laufer I: Mucosal surface patterns of the duodenal bulb. Radiology 150:317–322, 1984

Halasz NA: Gallstone obstruction of the duodenal bulb (Boeveret's syndrome). Am J Dig Dis 9:856–861, 1964

Jacobson HG, Shapiro JH, Pisano D et al: The Vaterian and peri-Vaterian segments in peptic ulcer. AJR 79:793–798, 1958

Jones B, Bayless TM, Hamilton SR et al: "Bubbly" duodenal bulb in celiac disease: Radiologic-pathologic correlation. AJR 142:119–122, 1984

Kleinman PK, Brill PW, Winchester P: Resolving duodenal–jejunal hematoma in abused children. Radiology 160:747–750, 1986

Kundrotas LW, Camara DS, Meenaghan MA et al: Heterotopic gastric mucosa: A case report. Am J Gastroenterol 80:253–256, 1985

Langkemper R, Hoek AC, Dekker W et al: Elevated lesions in the duodenal bulb caused by heterotopic gastric mucosa. Radiology 137:621–624, 1980

Liu CI, Cho SR, Shaw CI et al: Medial indentation of the duodenal sweep by a dilated inferior vena cava. AJR 141:1287–1288, 1983

McWay P, Dodds WJ, Slota T et al: Radiographic features of heterotopic gastric mucosa. AJR 139:380–382, 1982

Miller JH, Gisvold JJ, Weiland LH: Upper gastrointestinal tract: Villous tumors. AJR 134:933–936, 1980

Nelson JA, Sheft DJ, Minagi H et al: Duodenal pseudopolyp–The flexure fallacy. AJR 123:262–267, 1975

Olmsted WW, Ros PR, Hjermstad BM et al: Tumors of the small intestine with little or no malignant predisposition: A review of the literature and report of 56 cases. Gastrointest Radiol 12:231–239, 1987

Peison B, Benisch B: Brunner's gland adenoma of the duodenal bulb. Am J Gastroenterol 77:276–278, 1982

Ring EJ, Ferrucci JT, Eaton SB et al: Villous adenomas of the duodenum. Radiology 104:45–48, 1972

Rose HS, Balthazar EJ, Megibow AJ et al: Alimentary tract involvement in Kaposi sarcoma: Radiographic and endoscopic findings in 25 homosexual men. AJR 139:661–666, 1982

Shimkin PM, Pearson KD: Unusual arterial impressions upon the duodenum. Radiology 103:295–297, 1972

Short WF, Young BR: Roentgen demonstration of prolapse of benign polypoid gastric tumors into the duodenum, including a dumbbell-shaped leiomyoma. AJR 103:317–320, 1968

Stassa G, Klingensmith WC: Primary tumors of the duodenal bulb. AJR 107:105–110, 1969

Tishler JM, Han SY, Colcher H et al: Neurogenic tumors of the duodenum in patients with neurofibromatosis. Radiology 149:51–53, 1983

Weichert RF, Roth LM, Krementz ET et al: Carcinoid–islet cell tumors of the duodenum: Report of twenty-one cases. Am J Surg 121:195–205, 1971

Weinberg PE, Levin B: Hyperplasia of Brunner's glands. Radiology 84:259–262, 1965

Zukerman GR, Mills BA, Koehler RE et al: Nodular duodenitis: Pathologic and clinical characteristics in patients with end-stage renal disease. Dig Dis Sci 28:1018–1024, 1983

DUODENAL NARROWING/ OBSTRUCTION

Disease Entities

Congenital obstruction
    Duodenal atresia
    Annular pancreas
    Duodenal diaphragm (web)
    Intraluminal diverticulum
    Midgut volvulus
    Extrinsic bands (Ladd's)
    Duodenal duplication cyst
Inflammatory disorders of the duodenum
    Postbulbar ulcer
    Crohn's disease
    Tuberculosis
    Strongyloidiasis
    Nontropical sprue
Inflammatory disorders of the pancreas
    Acute pancreatitis
    Chronic pancreatitis
    Pseudocyst of the pancreas
Malignancies
    Primary pancreatic lesions
    Primary duodenal lesions
    Metastatic lesions
Intramural duodenal hematoma
Intraluminal duodenal diverticulum
Aorticoduodenal fistula
Radiation injury
Preduodenal portal vein
Superior mesenteric artery syndrome

A variety of congenital abnormalities can result in partial or complete obstruction of the gastrointestinal tract at the level of the duodenum. Except for annular pancreas, these congenital lesions are usually recognized during infancy. If the degree of stenosis is not severe, however, symptoms may not be manifest for weeks or months. In some instances, the physical characteristics of the anomaly are such that the first symptoms do not occur until adulthood.

CONGENITAL OBSTRUCTION

DUODENAL ATRESIA

Duodenal atresia is *complete* obliteration of the intestinal lumen at the level of the duodenum (Fig. 31-1). The obstruction usually occurs distal to the ampulla of Vater, though the proximal duodenum is affected in 20% of cases. Duodenal atresia results from failure of the duodenum to recanalize between the 6th and 11th weeks of fetal life. The duodenum proximal to the atretic segment thus has a long time during which it can become dilated before birth. This is in contrast to other types of congenital obstruction that develop at a later stage in intrauterine life or are incomplete and therefore result in a lesser degree of proximal duodenal dilatation.

Duodenal atresia is the most common cause of congenital obstruction of the duodenum. In this condition, vomiting (usually containing bile) begins

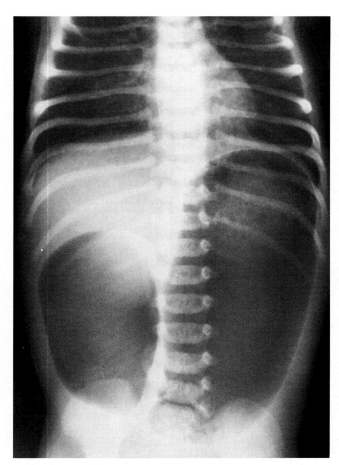

Fig. 31-1. Duodenal atresia. There is complete obstruction of the intestinal lumen at the level of the duodenum.

within a few hours of birth or following the first feeding. Because the obstruction is so high in the gastrointestinal tract, the frequent vomiting and consequent loss of fluids and electrolytes can cause rapid clinical deterioration unless a surgical diverting procedure is promptly performed. There is a higher than normal incidence of duodenal atresia in infants with Down's syndrome. Vertebral and rib anomalies, intestinal malrotation, imperforate anus, and various urinary tract anomalies can be associated with duodenal atresia. However, since such anomalies can also occur in patients with annular pancreas, the presence of one or more of them in conjunction with congenital duodenal obstruction is of little help in differentiating between these two conditions.

The classic radiographic appearance of duodenal atresia is the "double bubble" sign (Fig. 31-2). Large amounts of gas are present in both a markedly dilated stomach (left bubble) and that portion of the duodenum that is proximal to the obstruction (right bubble). In duodenal atresia, there is a total absence of gas in the small and large bowel distal to the level of the complete obstruction. In high-grade but incomplete congenital stenosis of the duodenum, there is some gas in the bowel distal to the obstruction (Fig. 31-3).

ANNULAR PANCREAS

Annular pancreas is an anomalous ring of pancreatic tissue encircling the duodenal lumen usually at

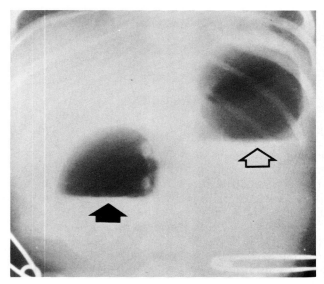

31-2 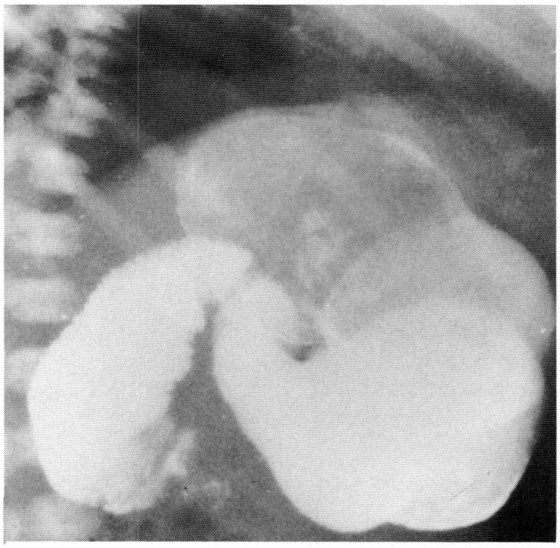   31-3

Fig. 31-2. Duodenal atresia with double bubble sign. The left bubble **(open arrow)** represents air in the stomach; the right bubble **(solid arrow)** reflects duodenal gas. There is no gas in the small or large bowel distal to the level of the complete obstruction.

Fig. 31-3. Congenital duodenal stenosis. The presence of small amounts of gas distal to the obstruction indicates that the stenosis is incomplete.

or above the level of the ampulla of Vater. The pancreas develops from two entirely distinct entodermal outgrowths (dorsal and ventral pancreas) that fuse to form a single organ. The ventral pancreatic bud is bilobed. The left bud usually degenerates, though it can persist and develop its own pancreatic lobe, which then grows around the left side of the duodenum to join the other two parts of the pancreas in the dorsal mesentery. Severe congenital anomalies of the gastrointestinal tract (*e.g.*, duodenal atresia, malrotation with bands, duodenal diaphragm) frequently coexist with annular pancreas; Down's syndrome is seen in about 30% of patients. Annular pancreas may be asymptomatic or produce symptoms consistent with varying degrees of duodenal obstruction.

Infants with symptomatic annular pancreas have the radiographic appearance of a double bubble sign (Fig. 31-4). Unlike duodenal atresia, annular pancreas almost always results in an *incomplete* obstruction. A small but recognizable amount of gas can be demonstrated within the bowel distal to the level of the high-grade duodenal stenosis. These tiny collections of gas distal to a partially obstructing annular pancreas can be easily missed. However, they must be carefully sought, since their presence excludes the possibility of duodenal atresia.

When symptoms arising from an annular pancreas are delayed until adulthood, some complicating condition must be suspected. Inflammatory edema of an annular pancreas can result in suffi-

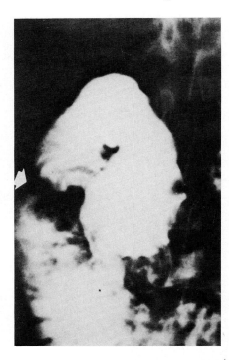

Fig. 31-5. Annular pancreas (adult). Extrinsic narrowing of the second portion of the duodenum **(arrow)** causes partial obstruction (large duodenal bulb). (Glazer GM, Margulis AR: Annular pancreas: Etiology and diagnosis using endoscopic retrograde cholangiopancreatography. Radiology 133:303–306, 1979)

cient luminal narrowing to cause duodenal obstruction. Duodenal ulceration often accompanies symptomatic annular pancreas in adults, though it is unclear whether the ulcer precedes the duodenal obstruction or is a consequence of it.

The radiographic appearance of annular pancreas in adults is a notchlike defect on the lateral duodenal wall causing an eccentric narrowing of the lumen (Fig. 31-5). This appearance must be differentiated from a postbulbar ulcer (with deep incisura) or a malignant tumor, both of which can produce a similar deformity. Unlike the pattern seen with postbulbar disease, the duodenal mucosal folds in annular pancreas are intact, and no discrete ulcer crater can be identified. With malignant disease, the constriction is usually more irregular and involves a longer segment of the duodenum, and the mucosal pattern is destroyed through the area of constriction. Very rarely, pancreatic cancer develops in an annular pancreas and is indistinguishable from an intrinsic duodenal malignancy.

DUODENAL DIAPHRAGM

Congenital duodenal diaphragms are web-like projections of the mucous membrane that occlude the lumen of the duodenum to varying degrees (Fig. 31-6). The majority of reported cases have occurred

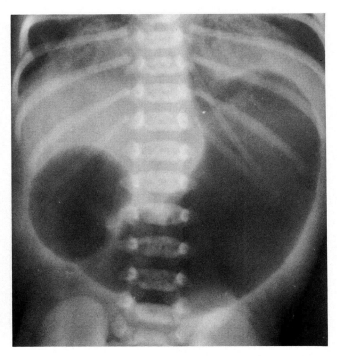

Fig. 31-4. Annular pancreas (infant). In this patient, there was complete duodenal obstruction and no evidence of distal gas.

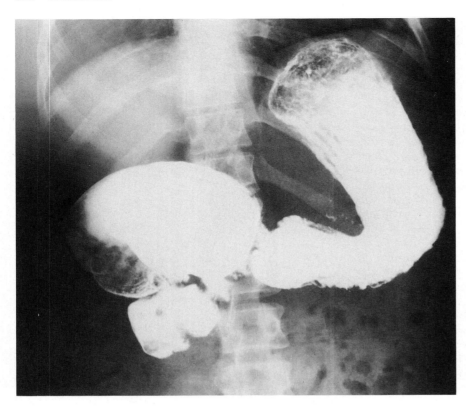

Fig. 31-6. Duodenal diaphragm. There is high-grade stenosis of the second portion of the duodenum. The presence of gas in the bowel distal to the diaphragm indicates that the obstruction is not complete.

in the second part of the duodenum near the ampulla of Vater. Radiographically, the congenital duodenal diaphragm presents as a thin, radiolucent line extending across the lumen, often with proximal duodenal dilatation. Because the duodenal obstruction is incomplete, small amounts of gas are scattered through the more distal portions of the bowel. On rare occasions, the thin diaphragm balloons out distally, producing a rounded barium-filled, comma-shaped sac (intraluminal diverticulum).

MIDGUT VOLVULUS

Midgut volvulus is an infrequent complication that occurs in patients with incomplete rotation of the bowel (Fig. 31-7). Normal rotation of the gut results in a broad mesenteric attachment of the small bowel that effectively precludes the development of a midgut volvulus. Incomplete rotation, however, leads to a narrow mesenteric attachment of the small bowel that can permit rotation around the axis of the superior mesenteric artery and result in a midgut volvulus. Although often an isolated finding, incomplete rotation coexists in about 20% of patients with congenital duodenal obstruction from

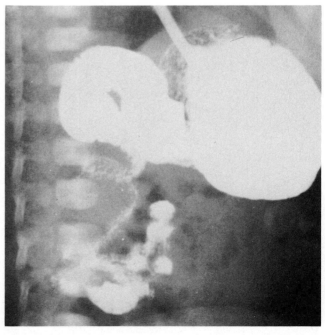

Fig. 31-7. Midgut volvulus. There is duodenal obstruction and spiraling of the small bowel. (Swischuk LE: Emergency Radiology of the Acutely Ill or Injured Child. Baltimore, Williams & Wilkins, 1979)

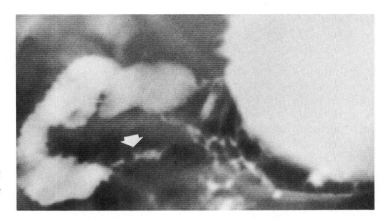

Fig. 31-8.   Ladd's bands. Obstruction of the third portion of the duodenum in this newborn infant is due to dense fibrous bands.

duodenal atresia, annular pancreas, or duodenal diaphragm. Therefore, it is probably prudent to perform a barium enema in any newborn infant with congenital obstruction of the duodenum so as to demonstrate the position of the cecum and exclude the possibility of incomplete rotation of the gut being a potential complicating factor. If the cecum is shown to be in an abnormal position in the mid-abdomen or on the left side, an upper gastrointestinal series is indicated to determine whether a midgut volvulus is the cause of the partial duodenal obstruction. The combination of a duodenojejunal junction (ligament of Treitz) located inferiorly and to the right of its expected position and a spiral course of bowel loops on the right side of the abdomen is diagnostic of midgut volvulus.

CONGENITAL PERITONEAL BANDS

Congenital peritoneal bands (Ladd's bands) can produce extrinsic duodenal obstruction in newborn infants (Fig. 31-8). These dense, fibrous bands extend from an abnormally placed, malrotated cecum or hepatic flexure over the anterior surface of the second or third portion of the duodenum to the right gutter and inferior surface of the liver. Obstructing Ladd's bands can be an isolated process or be found in conjunction with malrotation, annular pancreas, preduodenal portal vein, or duplication of the duodenum. They cause episodes of acute obstruction or, more commonly, intermittent partial obstruction, which can be aggravated by food intake or change in position. Standing can result in tightening of the bands and increased symptoms; lying down often relaxes them.

DUPLICATION CYST

A duodenal duplication cyst is an uncommon spherical or tubular structure filled with serous fluid, mucus, or even bile (if the bile duct empties into the

cyst). A duplication cyst is usually situated within the muscular layer of the duodenum but occasionally lies in a submucosal, subserosal, or even intramesenteric location. The cyst can encroach on the lumen of the duodenum and present as an intramural or extrinsic mass. Most duodenal duplications are asymptomatic and are found only incidentally at laparotomy during surgery for an unrelated problem. Extremely rarely, a duplication cyst causes high-grade stenosis or complete obstruction of the duodenum (Fig. 31-9).

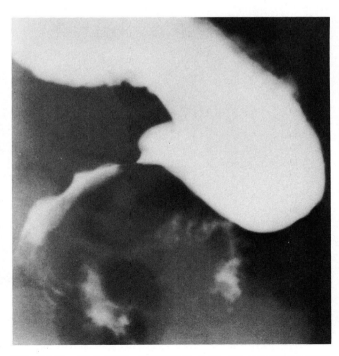

Fig. 31-9.   Duodenal duplication cyst. An intramural mass causes high-grade stenosis of the duodenal sweep.

INFLAMMATORY DISORDERS

POSTBULBAR ULCER

Postbulbar ulcers account for only a small percentage of all duodenal ulcers. Although they can be difficult to diagnose clinically or radiographically, it is important that they be recognized, because they may be the source of obstruction, pancreatitis, gastrointestinal hemorrhage, and atypical pain. The classic appearance of a postbulbar ulcer crater is a shallow, flat niche on the medial aspect of the second portion of the duodenum. The ulcer is usually accompanied by an incisura, an indrawing of the lateral wall of the duodenum caused by muscular spasm. In chronic ulceration or after healing of a postbulbar ulcer, the incisura may become a fixed and permanent stricture, producing a ring-like narrowing of the duodenum (Fig. 31-10). Although this pattern closely resembles the appearance in annular pancreas, the effaced, granular-appearing mucosa in the narrowed segment suggests healed ulceration.

CROHN'S DISEASE

Crohn's disease can cause narrowing and partial obstruction of the duodenum (Fig. 31-11). Although isolated duodenal involvement by this granulomatous process can occur, the disease is usually present elsewhere in the small bowel. The radiographic spectrum of Crohn's disease in the duodenum is similar to that in the ileum. In some patients, there are spiculated ulcers, linear ulcers, and a cobblestone appearance, usually associated with some nar-

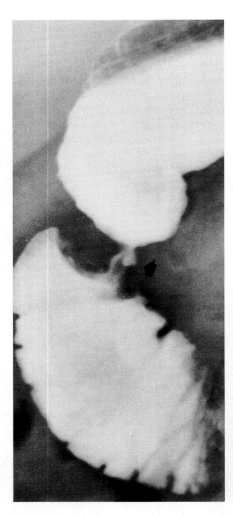

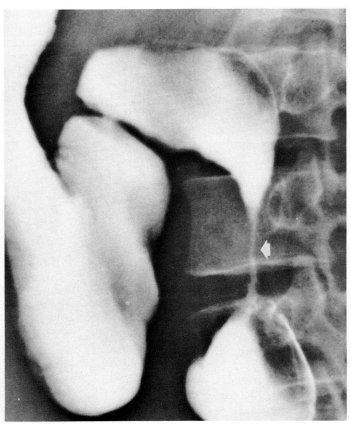

31-10   **31-11**

Fig. 31-10. Deep incisura, associated with a medial-wall postbulbar ulcer **(arrow)**, causing severe narrowing of the second portion of the duodenum.

Fig. 31-11. Crohn's disease. There is a tight stricture of the midportion of the descending duodenum **(arrow)**.

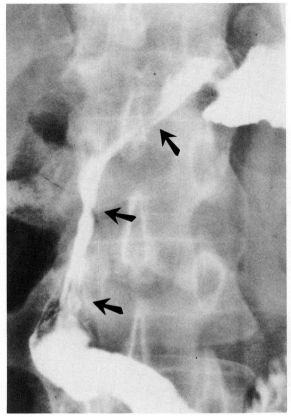

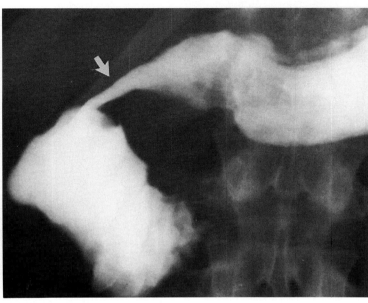

31-12

31-13

Fig. 31-12. Crohn's disease. A long stenosis **(arrows)** involves the first and second portions of the duodenum with effacement of the normal mucosal pattern.

Fig. 31-13. Crohn's disease. There is fusiform, concentric narrowing of the apical and post-bulbar areas **(arrow)**.

rowing. In others, there are long stenotic areas with effacement of the normal mucosal pattern (Fig. 31-12). These areas of narrowing tend to be fusiform and concentric (Fig. 31-13), unlike the puckering or "clover-leaf" type of deformity that is associated with duodenal ulcer disease (Fig. 31-14). In most cases of Crohn's disease of the duodenum, the stomach is also involved, resulting in a characteristic tubular or funnel-shaped narrowing of the antrum, pylorus, and proximal duodenum.

TUBERCULOSIS

Tuberculosis of the duodenum is extremely rare, even in patients with pulmonary or gastrointestinal disease. Isolated duodenal involvement has been reported, though tuberculosis of the duodenum is almost always associated with antral and pyloric disease. The radiographic pattern of nodular hyperplastic thickening of folds, diffuse ulceration, and luminal narrowing caused by a constricting inflammatory mass may be indistinguishable from Crohn's

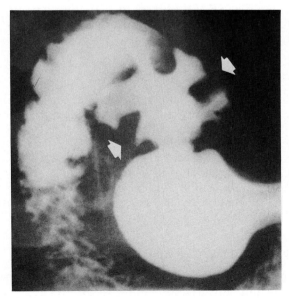

Fig. 31-14. Duodenal ulcer disease. A typical "clover-leaf" deformity is visible **(arrows)**.

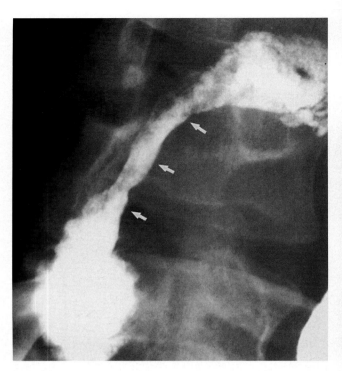

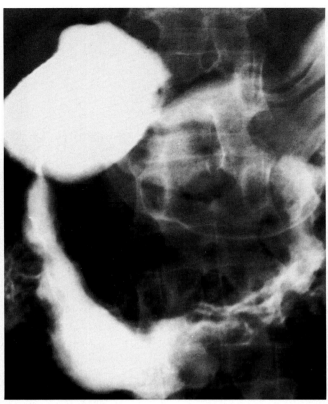

31-15   31-16

Fig. 31-15. Tuberculosis. There is narrowing of the second portion of the duodenum **(arrows)** with ulceration and diffuse mucosal irregularity.

Fig. 31-16. Strongyloidiasis. There is diffuse mucosal inflammation and ulceration with luminal narrowing.

disease (Fig. 31-15). Caseation with abscess formation can lead to fistulas and the development of sinus tracts.

STRONGYLOIDIASIS/SPRUE

Strongyloidiasis involving the duodenum can also simulate Crohn's disease. Diffuse ulceration, mucosal inflammation, and abnormal peristalsis result in severe atony and duodenal dilatation. Fibrotic healing can lead to stenotic narrowing of the lumen (Fig. 31-16). Duodenal or jejunal ulceration in longstanding cases of nontropical sprue can cause multiple areas of stenosis and postobstructive dilatation of the duodenum.

PANCREATITIS/CHOLECYSTITIS

Severe acute inflammation of the pancreas can result in sufficient irritability and spasm to cause narrowing of the duodenal lumen. In addition, retroperitoneal inflammation due to acute pancreatitis can thicken the bowel wall and root of the mesentery in the space between the aorta and the superior mesenteric artery (aorticomesenteric angle), producing high-grade obstruction of the third portion of the duodenum. The postinflammatory fibrosis of chronic pancreatitis can cause narrowing and deformity of the second portion of the duodenum, with tapering stenosis, mucosal thickening, and spiculation (Fig. 31-17). A similar appearance involving the postbulbar area can be due to acute cholecystitis (Fig. 31-18).

PANCREATIC PSEUDOCYST

Pseudocysts arising in the head of the pancreas can compress the duodenal sweep and produce partial or complete duodenal obstruction (Fig. 31-19). The mass effect of a pseudocyst causes the mucosal folds of the duodenum to be thickened, splayed, and distorted. The duodenal mucosa is not destroyed in patients with large pseudocysts, unlike that in patients with pancreatic cancer.

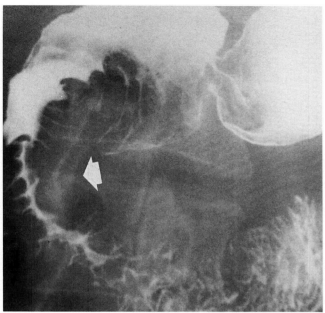

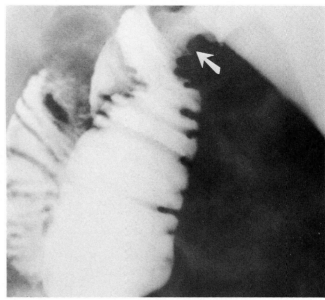

31-17

31-18

Fig. 31-17. Chronic pancreatitis with acute exacerbation. The inflammatory mass narrows the second portion of the duodenum and causes marked mucosal edema and spiculation **(arrow)**.

Fig. 31-18. Acute cholecystitis causing intense inflammation and narrowing of the adjacent portion of the duodenal sweep **(arrow)**. The appearance simulates a malignant process.

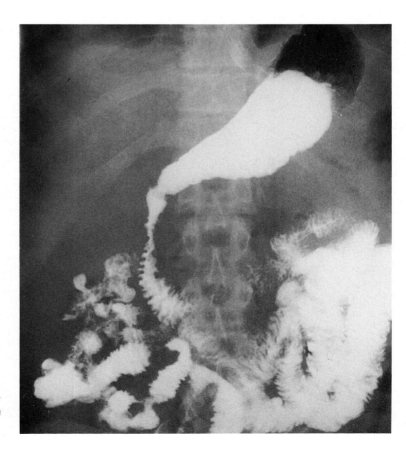

Fig. 31-19. Pancreatic pseudocyst. There is narrowing of the second portion of the duodenum with widening of the duodenal sweep.

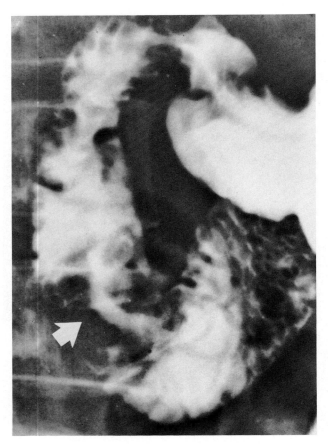

Fig. 31-20. Adenocarcinoma of the pancreas presenting as an annular constricting lesion of the duodenum **(arrow)**. The radiographic appearance is indistinguishable from that of primary duodenal carcinoma.

MALIGNANCIES

CARCINOMA OF THE PANCREAS

Pancreatic cancer can invade and narrow the duodenum at any level and produce duodenal obstruction with proximal dilatation (Fig. 31-20). About 70% of pancreatic carcinomas arise in the head of the gland and tend to compress the second portion of the duodenum. Carcinomas arising in the body (20%) and tail (10%) of the pancreas have a tendency to narrow the third and fourth portions of the duodenum, respectively (Fig. 31-21). The most common symptom in pancreatic cancer is jaundice, which occurs in 60% to 95% of patients. Painless jaundice has long been considered characteristic of cancer of the head of the pancreas, but most patients suffer from dull, steady, and often intense epigastric pain. Weight loss with anorexia is very frequent; pruritus is seen in a substantial minority of patients.

An enlarging pancreatic cancer can exert extrinsic pressure at any point along the duodenal sweep, resulting in a mass impression and "double-contour" effect. As the disease progresses, ulceration, stricture formation, and obstruction can occur. Pancreatic cancers can also involve the stomach, producing a typical indentation defect on the greater curvature of the gastric antrum (antral pad sign).

Differentiation of pancreatic cancer from pancreatitis can be difficult on barium examination. The presence of duodenal mucosal destruction suggests malignancy. However, pancreatic tumors can

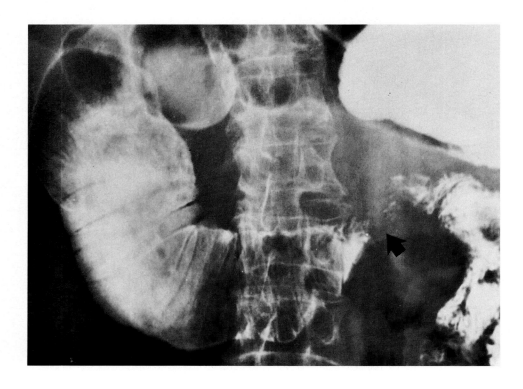

Fig. 31-21. Adenocarcinoma of the body of the pancreas causing a high-grade obstruction of the distal duodenum **(arrow)**.

infiltrate the submucosa and produce stenosis without mucosal destruction (especially in the third portion of the duodenum). In patients with cancer of the head of the pancreas, a combination of tumor infiltration and neuromuscular irritation (wraparound effect) can produce a fixed, partially obstructing lateral defect in the second portion of the duodenum.

OTHER MALIGNANCIES

Primary neoplasms of the duodenum, as well as metastases, can cause obstructive lesions of the duodenum and proximal duodenal dilatation. Adenocarcinomas, which constitute 80% to 90% of all duodenal malignancies, most commonly arise at or distal to the ampulla of Vater. Tumors in a periampullary location produce extrahepatic jaundice; those arising proximally or distally tend to cause bleeding, ulceration, or obstruction. The radiographic appearance of adenocarcinomas of the duodenum is similar to that associated with tumors of the same cell type arising at any level in the gastrointestinal tract. They most commonly present as annular constricting lesions with overhanging edges, nodular mucosal destruction, and frank ulceration (Fig. 31-22). Primary duodenal sarcomas, often with ulceration, also occur (Fig. 31-23). It is frequently impossible to differentiate primary duodenal malignancy from secondary neoplastic invasion of the duodenum by the extension of tumors arising in the pancreas, gallbladder, or colon.

Much of the duodenum is surrounded by groups of lymph nodes. The descending duodenum is encircled by peripancreatic lymph nodes; celiac and para-aortic nodes lie along the third portion of the duodenum. Metastatic enlargement of these nodes can produce a mass effect on the duodenal lumen with ulceration or obstructive narrowing. In the patient with a stenotic lesion of the third portion of the duodenum and a history of previous abdominal malignancy, the possibility of metastases to lymph nodes must be considered.

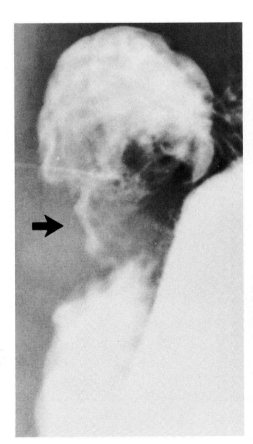

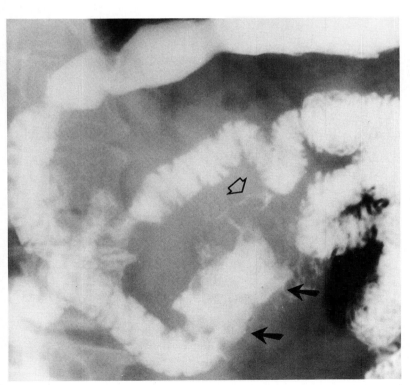

31-22   **31-23**

Fig. 31-22. Primary adenocarcinoma of the duodenum. Note the "apple-core" lesion **(arrow)**, which is similar to primary carcinoma at other levels of the gastrointestinal tract.

Fig. 31-23. Ulcerated fibrosarcoma of the third portion of the duodenum **(solid arrows)** causing luminal narrowing **(open arrow)**.

INTRAMURAL HEMATOMA

More than 80% of the reported cases of intramural duodenal hematoma have occurred in children or young adults, and child abuse is a major cause in infants and young children. Intramural duodenal hematomas can also be secondary to anticoagulant therapy or to an abnormal bleeding diathesis or be a rare complication of endoscopic biopsy. Hemorrhage into the duodenal wall produces a tumorlike intramural mass that can become so large that it obstructs the lumen and results in proximal duodenal dilatation (Fig. 31-24).

INTRALUMINAL DUODENAL DIVERTICULUM

Intraluminal duodenal diverticulum is a rare congenital anomaly that primarily involves the second portion of the duodenum and may cause duodenal obstruction. When filled with barium, the intraluminal diverticulum typically appears as a fingerlike sac separated from contrast in the duodenal lumen by a radiolucent band representing the wall of the diverticulum ("halo sign") (see Fig. 44-13).

AORTICODUODENAL FISTULA

Aorticoduodenal fistula can occur primarily as a complication of abdominal aortic aneurysm or be secondary to placement of a prosthetic Dacron graft. Pressure necrosis of the third portion of the duodenum, which is fixed and apposed to the anterior wall of an aortic aneurysm, can lead to digestion of that wall by enteric secretions and a primary aorticoduodenal fistula. Secondary fistulas result from pseudoaneurysm formation with erosion into the adherent duodenum or dehiscence of the suture line due to infection caused by the leak of intestinal contents through the duodenum, the blood supply of which has been compromised at surgery. Aorticoduodenal fistula is an often fatal condition that presents clinically with abdominal pain, gastrointestinal bleeding, and a palpable, pulsatile mass.

Aorticoduodenal fistulas cause compression or displacement of the third portion of the duodenum by an extrinsic mass (Fig. 31-25). Central ulceration can also occur. On rare occasions, extraluminal contrast tracking along the graft into the paraprosthetic space outlines the wall of the abdominal aorta.

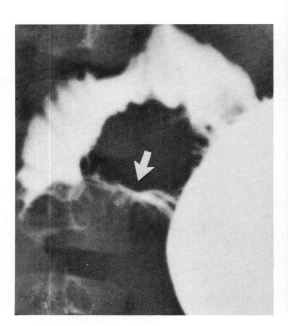

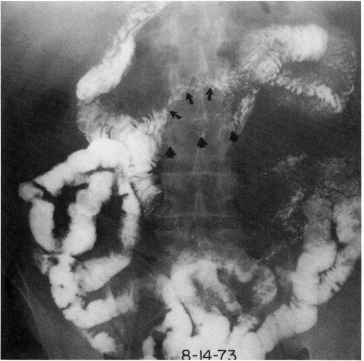

31-24

31-25

Fig. 31-24. Intramural duodenal hematoma. This high-grade stenotic lesion **(arrow)** was seen in a young child who had been kicked in the abdomen by his father.

Fig. 31-25. Aorticoduodenal fistula causing extrinsic pressure on the third portion of the duodenum **(large arrows)**. A jejunal loop is also slightly displaced **(small arrows)**. (Wyatt GM, Rauchway MI, Spitz HB: Roentgen findings in aortoenteric fistulae. AJR 126:714–722, 1976. Copyright 1976. Reproduced with permission)

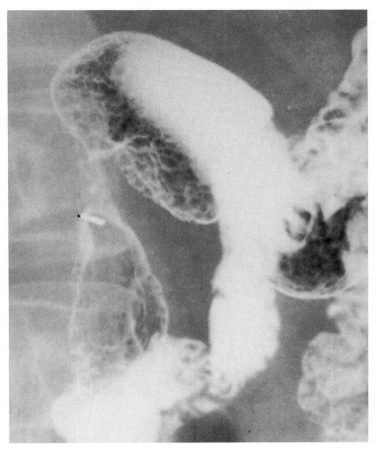

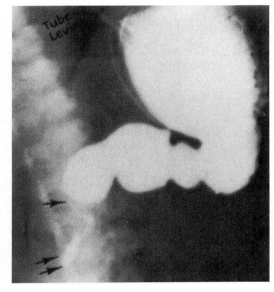

31-26

31-27

Fig. 31-26. Radiation injury. This postbulbar duodenal stricture with irregular mucosa appeared 13 months after irradiation for an angiosarcoma of the right kidney. (Rogers LF, Goldstein HM: Roentgen manifestations of radiation injury to the gastrointestinal tract. Gastrointest Radiol 2:281–291, 1977).

Fig. 31-27. Preduodenal portal vein. Dilatation of the first and second portions of the duodenum with a small amount of barium trickling along the third and fourth portions **(arrows)**. (Braun P, Collin PP, Ducharme JC: Preduodenal portal vein: A significant entity? Report of two cases and a review of the literature. Can J Surg 17:316–322, 1974)

RADIATION INJURY

Duodenal changes can develop following radiation therapy to the upper abdomen. These primarily involve the second portion and vary from ulcerations to smooth strictures (Fig. 31-26).

PREDUODENAL PORTAL VEIN

Preduodenal portal vein refers to the rare situation in which the portal vein crosses in front of, rather than behind, the duodenum. It has been reported that the anterior position of the preduodenal portal vein can cause duodenal obstruction (Fig. 31-27), though it is difficult to understand how the low venous pressure within a thin-walled vessel can cause intestinal blockage. Preduodenal portal vein is associated with a very high incidence of malformations (*e.g.*, duodenal bands, annular pancreas, and malrotation) which most likely cause the clinical picture of duodenal obstruction and lead to the incidental discovery of the abnormal position of the vessel. The main surgical implication of the preduodenal portal vein is that the anomaly must be recognized to avoid injury to the vessel during operations on the biliary tract and duodenum.

SUPERIOR MESENTERIC ARTERY SYNDROME

The broad spectrum of conditions producing the superior mesenteric artery syndrome, which is characterized by obstruction of the third portion of the duodenum and proximal dilatation, is discussed in the next section.

BIBLIOGRAPHY

Alberti–Flor JJ, Johnson AC, Dunn GD: Intraluminal duodenal diverticulum. Am J Gastroenterol 80:500–502, 1985

Aranha GV, Prinz RA, Greenlee HB et al: Gastric outlet and duodenal obstruction from inflammatory pancreatic disease. Arch Surg 119:833–835, 1984

Beranbaum SL: Carcinoma of the pancreas: A bidirectional roentgen approach. AJR 96:447–467, 1966

Berdon WE, Baker DH, Bull S et al: Midgut malrotation and volvulus: Which films are most helpful? Radiology 96:375–383, 1970

Braun P, Collin PP, Ducharme JC: Preduodenal portal vein: A significant entity? Can J Surg 17:316–322, 1974

Eaton SB, Ferrucci JT: Radiology of the Pancreas and Duodenum. Philadelphia, WB Saunders, 1973

Faegenburg D, Bosniak M: Duodenal anomalies in the adult. AJR 88:642–657, 1962

Fonkalsrud EW, DeLorimier AA, Hays DM: Congenital atresia and stenosis of the duodenum: A review compiled from the members of the surgical section of the American Academy of Pediatrics. Pediatrics 43:79–83, 1969

Free EA, Gerald B: Duodenal obstruction in the newborn due to annular pancreas. AJR 103:321–329, 1968

Ghishan FK, Werner M, Vieira P et al: Intramural duodenal hematoma: An unusual complication of endoscopic small bowel biopsy. Am J Gastroenterol 82:368–370, 1987

Glazer GM, Margulis AR: Annular pancreas: Etiology and diagnosis using endoscopic retrograde cholangiopancreatography. Radiology 133:303–306, 1979

Lautin EM, Friedman AC: A complicated case of aortoduodenal fistula. Gastrointest Radiol 4:401–404, 1979

Levine MS: Crohn's disease of the upper gastrointestinal tract. Radiol Clin North Am 25:79–90, 1987

Louisy CL, Barton CJ: The radiological diagnosis of *Strongyloides stercoralis* enteritis. Radiology 98:535–541, 1971

Pratt AD: Current concepts of the obstructing duodenal diaphragm. Radiology 100:637–643, 1971

Simon M, Lerner MA: Duodenal compression by the mesenteric root in acute pancreatitis and inflammatory conditions of the bowel. Radiology 79:75–81, 1962

Thompson WM, Cockrill H, Rice RP: Regional enteritis of the duodenum. AJR 123:252–261, 1975

Wyatt GM, Rauchway MI, Spitz HB: Roentgen findings in aortoenteric fistulae. AJR 126:714–722, 1976

DUODENAL DILATATION (SUPERIOR MESENTERIC ARTERY SYNDROME)

Disease Entities

Normal variant
Congenital small vascular angle or childhood growth spurt
Prolonged bed rest in supine position
  Body cast syndrome
  Whole-body burns
  Surgery
Loss of retroperitoneal fat
Multiple pregnancies with loss of muscle tone
Decreased duodenal peristalsis
  Smooth muscle or neuromuscular junction dysfunction
    Scleroderma
    Dermatomyositis/systemic lupus erythematosus
    Aganglionosis
    Chagas' disease
  Vagus or splanchnic nerve dysfunction
    Surgical or chemical vagotomy
    Neuropathy (diabetes, porphyria, thiamine deficiency)
  Inflammatory disorders
    Pancreatitis
    Cholecystitis
    Peptic ulcer disease
  Trauma
  Altered emotional states
Thickening of the bowel wall or root of the mesentery

Crohn's disease
Tuberculous enteritis
Pancreatitis
Peptic ulcer disease
Strongyloidiasis
Metastatic lesions
Exaggerated lumbar lordosis
Abdominal aortic aneurysm
Aorticoduodenal fistula
Chronic idiopathic intestinal pseudo-obstruction

The transverse portion of the duodenum lies in a fixed position in a retroperitoneal location. It is situated in a closed compartment bounded anteriorly by the root of the mesentery, which carries the superior mesenteric vessel sheath (artery, vein, nerve), and posteriorly by the aorta and lumbar spine (at the L2-L3 level, where lumbar lordosis is most pronounced). Any factor that compresses or fills this compartment can favor the development of narrowing of the transverse duodenum with proximal duodenal dilatation and stasis (superior mesenteric artery syndrome). Regardless of the underlying cause, the radiographic pattern is similar.

    Even in normal persons, there is often a transient delay of barium at the point at which the transverse duodenum crosses the spine (Fig. 32-1). This can be associated with mild, inconstant proximal duodenal dilatation (Fig. 32-2). Casts of the duodenum from cadavers with normal gastrointestinal

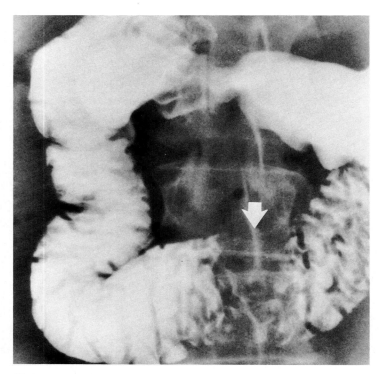

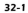

32-1

Fig. 32-1. Normal patient. There is a transient delay of barium at the point at which the transverse duodenum crosses the spine **(arrow)**.

Fig. 32-2. Normal patient. **(A)** A frontal projection shows apparent obstruction of the third portion of the duodenum **(arrow)**, suggesting the superior mesenteric artery syndrome. **(B)** A right anterior oblique view obtained slightly later shows the duodenal sweep to be entirely normal, without any evidence of organic obstruction.

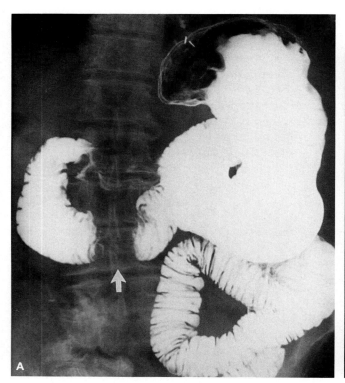

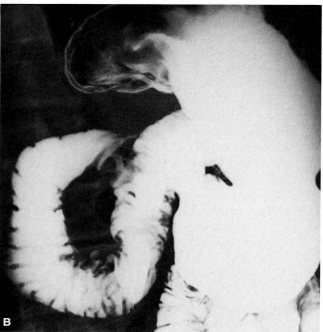

32-2

tracts sometimes demonstrate grooves on the anterior and posterior duodenal walls, most likely secondary to impression by the superior mesenteric artery and aorta, respectively.

NARROWING OF AORTICOMESENTERIC ANGLE

Any process that tends to close the nutcracker-like jaws of the aorticomesenteric angle results in some degree of compression of the transverse portion of the duodenum. It is most common in asthenic persons, especially those who have lost substantial weight. This condition can be detected in children who have a congenitally small vascular angle or in children who are growing rapidly without a corresponding gain in weight. Prolonged bed rest or immobilization in the supine position (patients with body casts or whole-body burns or patients who are fixed in a position of hyperextension after spinal injury or surgery) causes the superior mesenteric artery to fall back and anteriorly compress the transverse duodenum, resulting in relative duodenal obstruction (Fig. 32-3). In patients who lose weight and retroperitoneal fat because of a debilitating illness, the increased dragging effect of the mesenteric root narrows the aorticomesenteric compartment. Similarly, conditions leading to relaxation of abdominal wall musculature (*e.g.*, multiple pregnancies) can obstruct the transverse duodenum.

REDUCED DUODENAL PERISTALSIS

In patients with diseases causing reduced duodenal peristaltic activity, especially when they are placed in a supine position, the combination of lumbar spine, aorta, and superior mesenteric artery can constitute enough of a barrier to cause significant obstruction of the transverse duodenum. Muscular atrophy and intramural fibrosis in patients with scleroderma produce atony and dilatation of the duodenum as part of a diffuse process involving all of the small bowel (Fig. 32-4). Other collagen diseases, such as dermatomyositis and systemic lupus erythematosus, can cause the same radiographic pattern (Fig. 32-5). Aganglionosis, the absence of cells in Auerbach's plexus, is associated with a similar histologic finding in the distal esophagus and rectum and can result in pronounced proximal duodenal dilatation. In Chagas' disease, inflammatory destruction of intramural autonomic plexuses due to trypanosomes can lead to generalized gastrointestinal aperistalsis and dilatation. This most frequently involves the esophagus and colon but can also affect the duodenum.

As in other portions of the bowel, dysfunction of the vagus or splanchnic nerves can result in dilatation of the duodenum and the radiographic appearance of the superior mesenteric artery syndrome. This can occur after surgical vagotomy for peptic disease or following chemical vagotomy due to ingestion of such drugs as atropine, morphine, or Lomotil (diphenoxylate). Disordered duodenal motil-

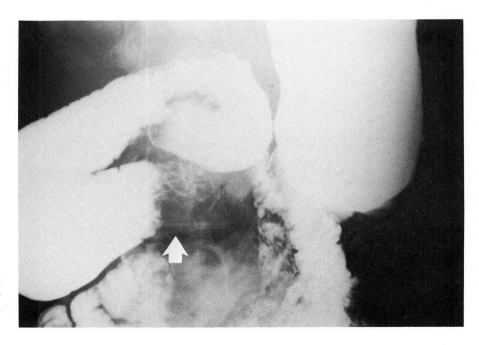

Fig. 32-3. Relative duodenal obstruction **(arrow)** in a bedridden patient who sustained a severe burn several weeks earlier.

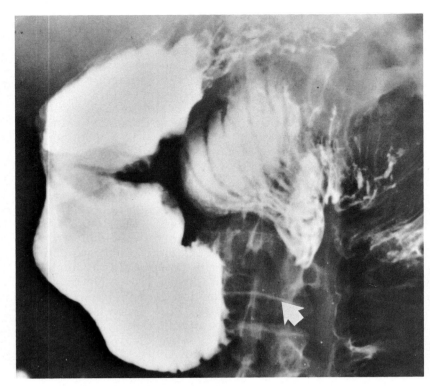

32-4

Fig. 32-4. Scleroderma. There is severe atony and dilatation of the duodenum proximal to the aorticomesenteric angle (arrow).

Fig. 32-5. Systemic lupus erythematosus. Atony and dilatation of the proximal duodenum are indistinguishable from the pattern in scleroderma.

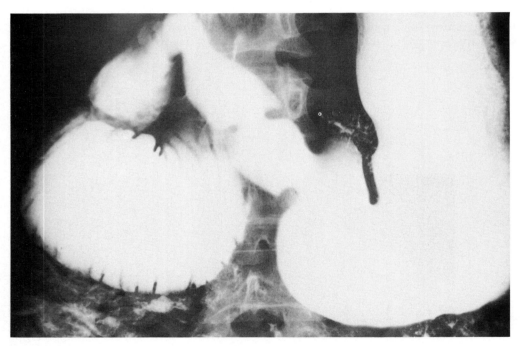

32-5

ity with dilatation can also be seen in patients with neuropathies secondary to diabetes, porphyria, and thiamine deficiency.

Adynamic ileus caused by any acute upper abdominal inflammatory process can affect the duodenum and cause pronounced dilatation proximal to the midline barrier of normal structures (spine, aorta, superior mesenteric artery). This duodenal atony is seen in patients with acute pancreatitis, cholecystitis, and peptic ulcer disease. Adynamic ileus of the duodenum (as well as of the stomach) can occur in patients who have sustained severe trauma or acute burns. A controversial concept is the possible relationship of duodenal ileus to hysterical syndromes or other abnormal emotional states.

OTHER CAUSES

Any space-occupying process within the aorticomesenteric angle can also compress the transverse duodenum. Inflammatory thickening of the bowel wall or mesenteric root (*e.g.*, pancreatitis [Fig. 32-6], Crohn's disease, tuberculous enteritis, peptic ulcer disease, strongyloidiasis) or metastases to the mesentery or mesenteric nodes can lead to relative duodenal obstruction.

Increased lumbar lordosis diminishes the size of the compartment occupied by the transverse duodenum. This forces the duodenum to lie on a slightly convex surface, leading to a greater risk of mesenteric compression. A similar mechanism can occur when the transverse duodenum lies in a low position over the 4th lumbar vertebra.

A rare cause of relative obstruction of the transverse duodenum is an abdominal aortic aneurysm (Fig. 32-7). This etiology should be suspected whenever duodenal stasis first occurs in an elderly patient with arteriosclerosis, especially if plain radiographs demonstrate calcification of a dilated aorta in this region. After reconstructive arterial surgery, aorticoduodenal fistulas can cause partial obstruction of the third portion of the duodenum.

Severe dilatation of the duodenum mimicking the superior mesenteric artery syndrome has been described as the first manifestation of chronic idiopathic intestinal pseudo-obstruction (Fig. 32-8). As this disease of unknown etiology progresses, more segments of the small bowel become dilated; dilatation can eventually involve the colon and stomach.

Symptoms attributed to the superior mesenteric artery syndrome include epigastric or periumbilical pain, which typically occurs several hours after eating and is relieved by a prone or knee–chest position. Bilious vomiting is also a common complaint. High-grade obstruction of the transverse du-

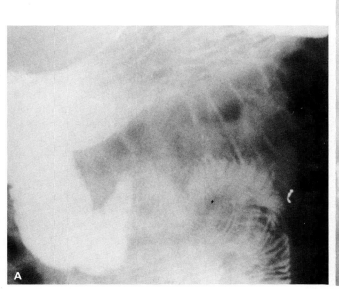
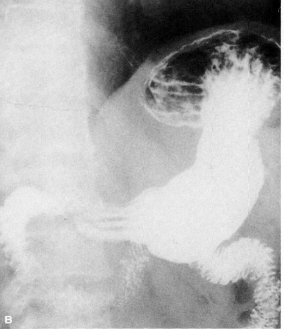

Fig. 32-6. Acute pancreatitis. **(A)** Distention of the proximal duodenum is unrelieved by the knee-chest crouch position. **(B)** Fourteen days later, following clinical recovery, the duodenal distention is no longer present. (Simon M, Lerner MA: Duodenal compression by the mesenteric root in acute pancreatitis and inflammatory conditions of the bowel. Radiology 79:75–81, 1962)

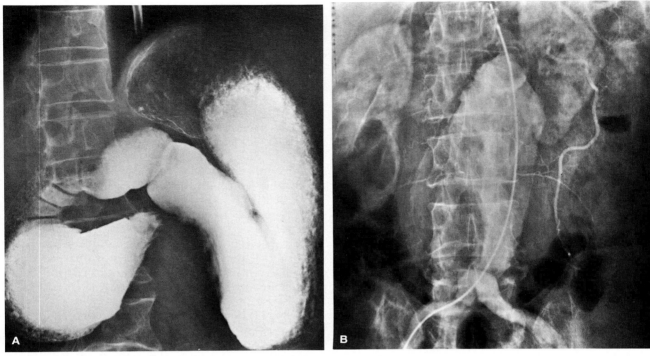

Fig. 32-7. Abdominal aortic aneurysm. **(A)** Obstruction of the third portion of the duodenum with proximal dilatation. **(B)** Arteriogram demonstrates the large aneurysm, which is causing the obstruction.

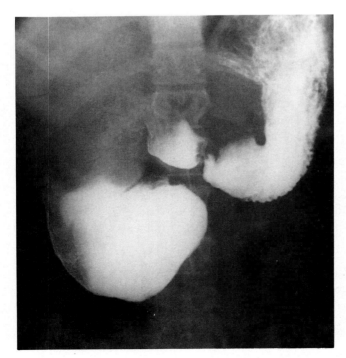

Fig. 32-8. Chronic idiopathic intestinal pseudo-obstruction. Severe dilatation of the duodenum mimicking the superior mesenteric artery syndrome was the first manifestation of the disease in this patient.

odenum can lead to emaciation and nutritional deficiency, with such striking loss of weight that a provisional diagnosis of malignancy is made.

RADIOGRAPHIC FINDINGS

Regardless of the underlying pathologic mechanism, the radiographic appearance is almost identical in all patients with the superior mesenteric artery syndrome. Pronounced dilatation of the first and second portions of the duodenum (and frequently the stomach) is associated with a vertical, linear extrinsic pressure defect in the transverse portion of the duodenum overlying the spine. The duodenal mucosal folds are intact but compressed. For the superior mesenteric artery syndrome to be differentiated from an organic obstruction, the patient should be turned to a prone, left decubitus, or knee–chest position. With the traction drag by the mesentery on the transverse duodenum thus decreased (through widening of the aorticomesenteric angle), barium can usually be seen to promptly pass the "obstruction," confirming the diagnosis of superior mesenteric artery syndrome. Because the aorticomesenteric angle is not reduced in patients with thickening of the bowel wall or root of the mesentery, postural change provides much less relief of duodenal compression. In these conditions, relative duodenal obstruction is primarily related to the clinical activity of the inflammatory process. If there is no emptying of the duodenum with change in position or evidence of intra-abdominal inflammation, the possibility of an organic duodenal obstruction (*e.g.*, metastases to the mesentery, direct spread of carcinoma of the body of the pancreas) must be excluded.

BIBLIOGRAPHY

Berk RN, Coulson DB: The body cast syndrome. Radiology 94:303–305, 1970

Bitner WP: Arteriomesenteric occlusion of duodenum. AJR 79:807–814, 1958

Christoforidis AJ, Nelson SW: Radiographic manifestations of ulcerogenic tumors of the pancreas. JAMA 198:511–516, 1966

Eaton SB, Ferrucci JT: Radiology of the Pancreas and Duodenum. Philadelphia, WB Saunders, 1973

Edwards KC, Katzen BT: Superior mesenteric artery syndrome due to large dissecting abdominal aortic aneurysm. Am J Gastroenterol 79:72–74, 1984

Evarts CM, Winters RB, Hall JE: Vascular compression of duodenum associated with treatment of scoliosis. J Bone Joint Surg (Am) 53:431–444, 1971

Fischer HW: The big duodenum. AJR 83:861–875, 1960

Gondos B: Duodenal compression defect and the "superior mesenteric artery syndrome." Radiology 123:575–580, 1977

Lee CS, Mangla JC: Superior mesenteric artery compression syndrome. Am J Gastroenterol 70:141–150, 1978

Mindell HJ, Holm JL: Acute superior mesenteric artery syndrome. Radiology 94:299–302, 1970

Nugent FW, Braasch JW, Epstein H: Diagnosis and surgical treatment of arteriomesenteric obstruction of the duodenum. JAMA 196:1091–1093, 1966

Simon M, Lerner MA: Duodenal compression by the mesenteric root in acute pancreatitis and in inflammatory conditions of the bowel. Radiology 79:75–81, 1962

Wallace RG, Howard WB: Acute superior mesenteric artery syndrome in the severely burned patient. Radiology 94:307–310, 1970

PART FIVE

SMALL BOWEL

Introduction to Diseases of the Small Bowel

At first glance, the multitude of diseases that involve the small bowel produce a bewildering array of radiographic findings. On closer reflection, however, it is seen that this extensive list can be subdivided into manageable categories of differential diagnosis by analysis of the following:

Caliber of the small bowel
Thickness and regularity of folds
Ulceration
Nodules
Concomitant gastric involvement
Filling defects
Mesenteric impressions
Desmoplastic response
Distribution of lesions

Through a combination of these various factors, rational lists of differential diagnoses can be established and provide a practical radiographic approach to small bowel disease.

BIBLIOGRAPHY

Goldberg HI, Sheft DJ: Abnormalities in small intestine contour and caliber: A working classification. Radiol Clin North Am 14:461–475, 1976
Osborn AG, Friedland GW: A radiological approach to the diagnosis of small bowel disease. Clin Radiol 24:281–301, 1973
Tully TE, Feinberg SB: A roentgenographic classification of diffuse diseases of the small intestine presenting with malabsorption. AJR 121:283–290, 1974

SMALL BOWEL OBSTRUCTION

Mechanical small bowel obstruction occurs whenever there is an intrinsic or extrinsic blockage of the normal flow of bowel contents. Without medical therapy, complete small bowel obstruction has about a 60% mortality rate. Prompt diagnosis and institution of optimal treatment, as well as recognition of the importance of replacing fluid and electrolytes and maintaining an adequate circulating blood volume, can reduce the mortality rate to less than 5%. The classic symptoms of small bowel obstruction include crampy abdominal pain, bloating, nausea, vomiting, and decreased stool output. Diffuse abdominal tenderness and peritoneal signs are common. An abdominal examination usually reveals distention and increased, high-pitched bowel sounds with rushes and tinkles. However, it is extremely important to remember that the typical clinical signs and symptoms can be absent, even in a high-grade small bowel obstruction. In patients with fluid-filled loops containing little or no gas, there can be little abdominal distention; bowel sounds can be normal or diminished because there are no gas bubbles to gurgle. Absence of bowel sounds late in the course of obstruction can be due to the inability of the fatigued bowel to contract effectively or to associated peritonitis.

RADIOGRAPHIC FINDINGS

Distended loops of small bowel containing gas and fluid can usually be recognized within 3 hr to 5 hr of the onset of complete obstruction. Almost all gas proximal to a small bowel obstruction represents swallowed air. In the upright or lateral decubitus view, the interface between gas and fluid forms a straight horizontal margin (Fig. 33-1). Gas–fluid levels are occasionally present normally. However, more than two gas–fluid levels in the small bowel is generally considered to be abnormal. The presence of gas–fluid levels at different heights in the same loop has traditionally been considered excellent evidence for mechanical obstruction (Fig. 33-2). Unfortunately, this pattern can also be demonstrated in some patients with adynamic ileus rather than mechanical obstruction (Fig. 33-3).

Abdominal radiographs in patients with mechanical obstruction usually demonstrate large quantities of gas within distended loops of bowel (Fig. 33-4). The small bowel is capable of huge distention and can become so enlarged as to be almost indistinguishable from colon. To make the critical differentiation between small and large bowel obstruction, it is essential to determine which loops of bowel contain abnormally large amounts of gas. Small bowel loops generally occupy the more central portion of the abdomen, whereas colonic loops are positioned laterally around the periphery of the abdomen or inferiorly in the pelvis (Fig. 33-5). Gas within the lumen of the small bowel outlines the valvulae conniventes, which completely encircle the bowel (Fig. 33-6). In contrast, colonic haustral markings occupy only a portion of the transverse diameter of the bowel. Valvulae conniventes are finer and closer together than colonic haustra. In

Text continues on page 415

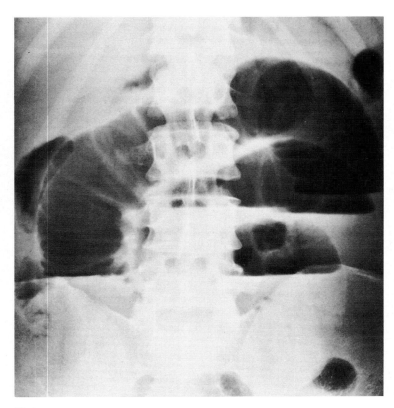

33-1

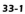

Fig. 33-1. Small bowel obstruction. The interfaces between gas and fluid form straight horizontal margins within small bowel loops proximal to the obstruction.

Fig. 33-2. Small bowel obstruction. Gas-fluid levels are at different heights within the same loop **(arrows)**.

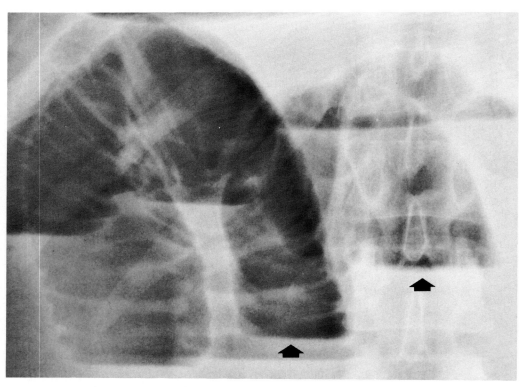

33-2

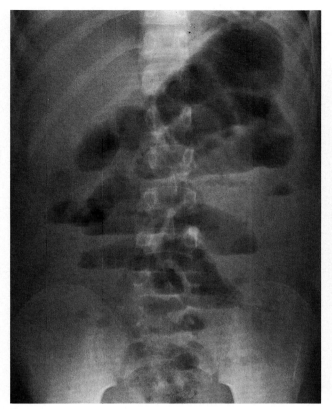

33-3

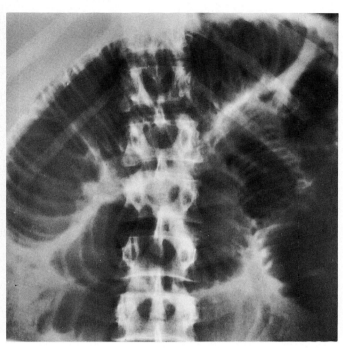

33-4

Fig. 33-3. Adynamic ileus in a patient with acute appendicitis. Although mechanical obstruction was suggested by gas-fluid levels at different heights in the same loop, no evidence of obstruction was found at surgery.

Fig. 33-4. Small bowel obstruction. Gas-filled loops of small bowel are greatly distended.

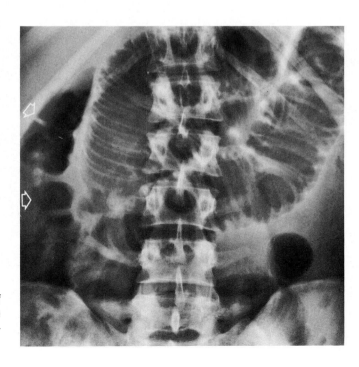

Fig. 33-5. Small bowel obstruction. The dilated loops of small bowel occupy the central portion of the abdomen, with the nondilated cecum and ascending colon positioned laterally around the periphery of the abdomen **(arrows)**.

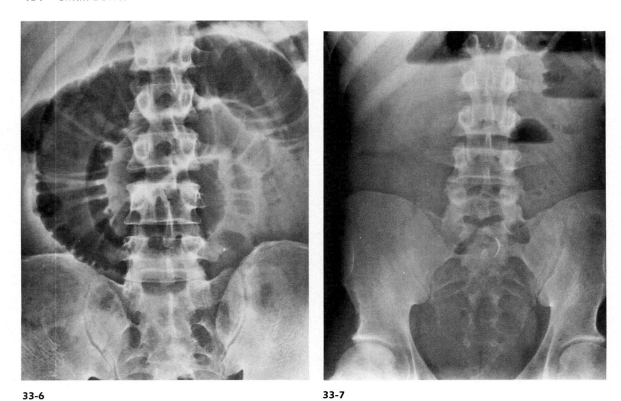

33-6   33-7

Fig. 33-6. Small bowel obstruction. Gas within the lumen of the bowel outlines the valvulae conniventes, which completely encircle the bowel.

Fig. 33-7. Jejunal obstruction. The few dilated loops of small bowel are located in the left upper abdomen.

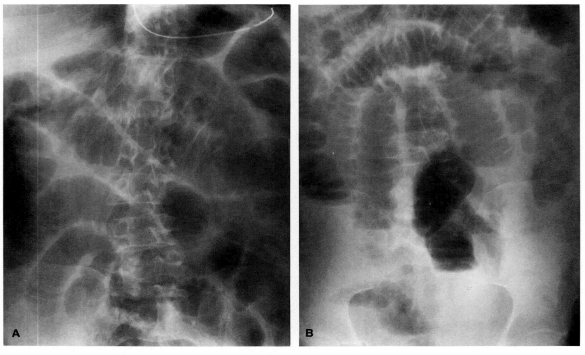

Fig. 33-8. Low small bowel obstruction. The involvement of multiple small bowel loops extends to the right lower quadrant. **(A)** Supine and **(B)** upright views.

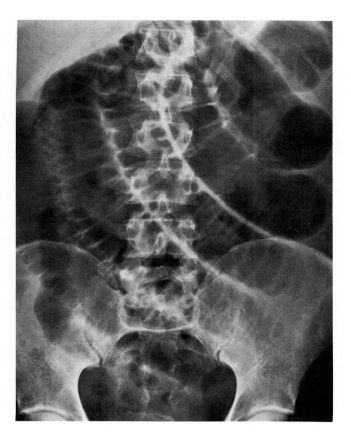

Fig. 33-9. Low small bowel obstruction. The dilated loops of gas-filled bowel appear to be placed one above the other, upward and to the left, producing a characteristic stepladder appearance.

the jejunum, simple distention, no matter how severe, will not completely efface these mucosal folds.

The site of obstruction can usually be predicted with considerable accuracy if the number and position of dilated bowel loops are analyzed. The presence of a few dilated loops of small bowel located high in the abdomen (in the center or slightly to the left) indicates an obstruction in the distal duodenum or jejunum (Fig. 33-7). Involvement of more small bowel loops suggests a lower obstruction (Fig. 33-8). As additional loops are affected, they appear to be placed one above the other, upward and to the left, producing a characteristic ''stepladder'' appearance (Fig. 33-9). This inclined direction is due to fixation of the mesentery, which extends from the right iliac fossa to the upper pole of the left kidney. The point of obstruction is always distal to the lowest loop of dilated bowel.

In patients with complete mechanical small bowel obstruction, little or no gas is found in the colon (Fig. 33-10). This is a valuable differential point between mechanical obstruction and adynamic ileus, in which gas is seen within distended loops throughout the bowel. Small amounts of gas or fecal accumulations may be present in the colon if an examination is performed within the first few hours of the onset of symptoms. The presence of gas in the colon in the late stages of a complete small bowel obstruction can be the result of putrefaction or represent air introduced during administration of an enema. In patients with an incomplete small bowel obstruction, some gas can pass into the colon, though the caliber of the distended small

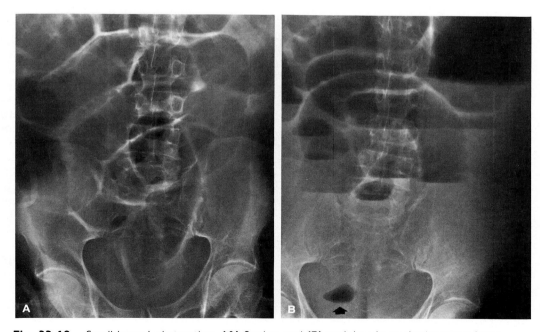

Fig. 33-10. Small bowel obstruction. **(A)** Supine and **(B)** upright views demonstrate large amounts of gas in dilated loops of small bowel but only a single, small collection of gas **(arrow)** in the colon.

bowel will be far larger than the normal or decreased width of the colon. The presence of large amounts of gas in the colon effectively eliminates the diagnosis of small bowel obstruction.

An analysis of the position and amount of abdominal gas can be difficult to make on a single examination; serial observations are often extremely valuable. If gas-filled loops are the result of obstruction, the amount of intraluminal gas and the degree of bowel distention will increase rapidly over several hours.

Small amounts of gas in obstructed loops of bowel can produce the characteristic "string-of-beads" appearance of small gas bubbles in an oblique line (Fig. 33-11). This sign apparently depends on a combination of fluid-filled bowel and peristaltic hyperactivity. Although often considered diagnostic of mechanical obstruction, the string-of-beads sign occasionally appears in adynamic ileus secondary to inflammatory disease.

The bowel proximal to an obstruction can contain no gas but be completely filled with fluid (Fig. 33-12). This pattern is seen in patients who swallow little air or have it removed by effective gastric suction. Large quantities of fluid produce sausage-shaped water-density shadows that can be difficult to diagnose. This pseudotumor, consisting of a large soft-tissue density combined with gaseous distention of the intestine proximal to it, is very likely to represent a strangulation obstruction.

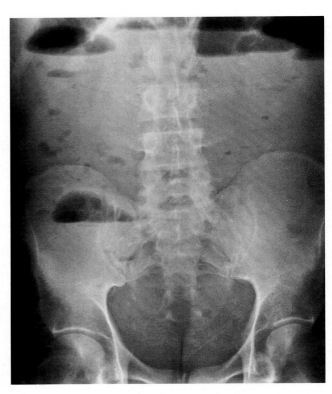

Fig. 33-12. Distal small bowel obstruction. Most of the loops of small bowel proximal to the point of obstruction are filled with fluid and contain only a very small amount of gas.

CONTRAST EXAMINATION

Plain abdominal radiographs are occasionally not sufficient for a distinction to be made between small and large bowel obstruction. In these instances, a contrast examination is required. A carefully performed barium enema will document or eliminate the possibility of large bowel obstruction. If it is necessary to determine the precise site of small bowel obstruction, barium can be administered in either a retrograde or an antegrade manner. A retrograde examination of the small bowel can be successfully performed in about 90% of patients. Radiographs of the small bowel can be obtained once the colon is emptied. Oral barium, *not* water-soluble agents, is the most effective contrast for demonstrating the site of small bowel obstruction. The large amount of fluid proximal to a small bowel obstruction keeps the mixture fluid, so that the trapped barium does not harden or increase the degree of obstruction. Barium is far superior to water-soluble agents in evaluating a small bowel obstruction. The density of barium permits visualization far into the intestine (Fig. 33-13), unlike aqueous agents, which are lost to sight because of dilution and absorption. In addition, the problem of electrolyte imbalance due to the hyperosmolality of water-soluble contrast agents may be significant. However, it is important to remember that oral barium should not be used unless the colon has been excluded as the site of mechanical obstruction; the piling up of hardened barium proximal to a distal colonic obstruction en-

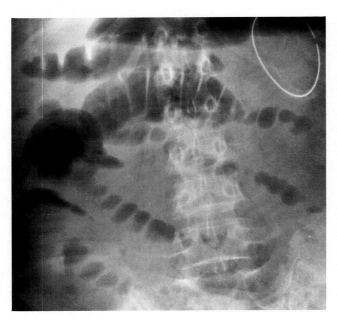

Fig. 33-11. Small bowel obstruction. "String-of-beads" appearance.

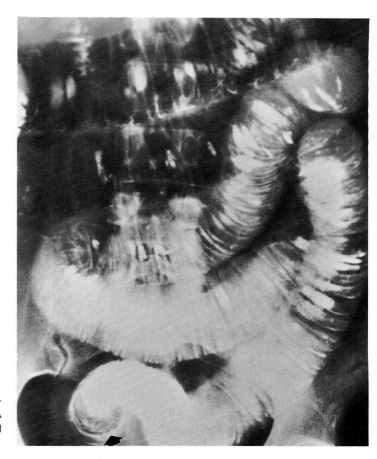

Fig. 33-13. Antegrade administration of barium demonstrating the precise site of a small bowel obstruction. A radiolucent gallstone **(arrow)** is causing the distal ileal obstruction.

tails some risk. Obviously, if plain radiographs clearly demonstrate a mechanical small bowel obstruction, any contrast examination is superfluous.

STRANGULATED OBSTRUCTION

Strangulation of bowel refers to interference with the blood supply associated with an obstruction that is not necessarily complete. In a closed-loop obstruction, both the afferent and the efferent limbs of a loop of bowel become obstructed. Examples of this type of obstruction include volvulus, incarcerated hernia, and loops of small bowel trapped by an adhesive band or passing through an abnormal loop in the mesentery. This is a clinically dangerous form of obstruction, since the continuous outpouring of fluid into the enclosed space can raise the intraluminal pressure and rapidly lead to occlusion of the blood supply to that segment of bowel. Because venous pressure is normally lower than arterial pressure, blockage of venous outflow from the strangulated segment occurs before obstruction of the mesenteric arterial supply. Ischemia can rapidly cause necrosis of the bowel with sepsis, peritonitis, and a potentially fatal outcome.

Strangulation of the bowel can lead to other serious complications. High-grade small bowel obstruction results in an enormous increase in the bacterial population in the stagnant, obstructed segment. Because there is no absorption from this distended bowel, the bacteria-laden fluid within the obstructed segment is of little danger to the patient. If strangulation leads to frank hemorrhagic infarction and gangrenous bowel, intestinal contents can pass into the peritoneal cavity even if no gross perforation is evident. Bacteria can then become absorbed into the systemic circulation and cause severe toxicity and a fatal outcome. Severe hemorrhage into the lumen of the bowel, bowel wall, and peritoneal cavity can be fatal depending on the length of the strangulated segment.

Strangulation of an obstructed loop of small bowel is often difficult to diagnose radiographically. Several signs, though not pathognomonic of strangulated obstruction, are found often enough with strangulation to be an indication for immediate therapy.

An obstructed closed loop bent on itself assumes the shape of a coffee bean, the doubled width of the apposed bowel walls resembling the cleft of the bean. The points of fixation and the length of the involved segment determine whether the loop will bend on itself. Additional evidence of strangulation is a bowel wall that is smooth and featureless because of flattening of the valvulae by edema or hemorrhage. A similar appearance can be seen in the twisted portion of the colon in sigmoid volvulus.

The involved segment of bowel in a closed-loop obstruction is usually filled with fluid and presents radiographically as a tumor-like mass of water density (Fig. 33-14). The outline of this pseudotumor is easier to detect if there is gas distention of bowel above the obstruction than if there are no gas-distended loops. The pseudotumor sign must be differentiated from the fluid-filled loops that are seen in simple mechanical obstruction. In closed-loop obstruction, the pseudotumor sign reflects a loop that is fixed and remains in the same position on multiple projections. This is probably due to the combination of fixation of the bowel loop at both ends and vascular compromise, which prevents the normal tendency of bowel to change configuration and position. When an abdominal mass is apparent radio-graphically but cannot be palpated, the radiologist must be alerted to the possibility of a strangulated loop of bowel.

The absence of gas proximal to a strangulating obstruction sometimes results in a normal-appearing abdomen on plain radiographs. In the patient with clinical signs of obstruction, a film of the abdomen showing no abnormality should alert the radiologist to search very closely for subtle signs of strangulation.

Complications of strangulation obstruction can be detected radiographically. Exudate and free fluid in the peritoneal cavity can cause separation of adjacent loops of bowel and shifting fluid density in the abdomen and pelvis. Frank perforation produces free gas, which can be demonstrated on upright or lateral decubitus views. If necrosis develops, gas can be found in the wall of the involved loop of bowel or in the portal venous system.

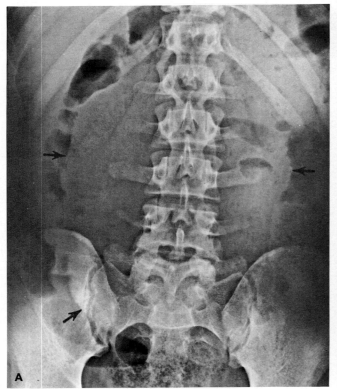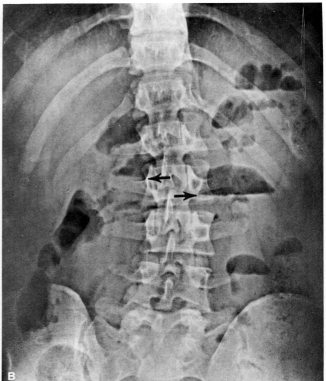

Fig. 33-14. Pseudotumor. **(A)** Supine film showing fluid-filled loops as a tumor-like density in the midabdomen with a polycyclic outline indenting adjacent gas-containing loops **(arrows)**. **(B)** Upright film showing fluid levels in the pseudotumor **(arrows)**. (Bryk D: Strangulating obstruction of the bowel: A reevaluation of radiographic criteria. AJR 130:835–843, 1978. Copyright 1978. Reproduced with permission)

CAUSES OF SMALL BOWEL OBSTRUCTION

Extrinsic bowel lesions
  Adhesions
    Previous surgery
    Previous peritonitis
  Hernias
    External
    Internal
  Extrinsic masses
    Neoplasm
    Abscess
  Volvulus
  Congenital bands
Luminal occlusion
  Tumor
  Gallstone
  Enterolith
  Foreign body
  Bezoar
  Intestinal tube balloon
  Intussusception
  Meconium ileus
Intrinsic lesions of the bowel wall
  Strictures
    Neoplastic
    Inflammatory
    Chemical
    Anastomotic
    Radiation-induced
    Amyloid
  Vascular insufficiency
    Arterial occlusion
    Venous occlusion
  Congenital atresia or stenosis
    Jejunal
    Ileal
    Segmental dilatation of the ileum

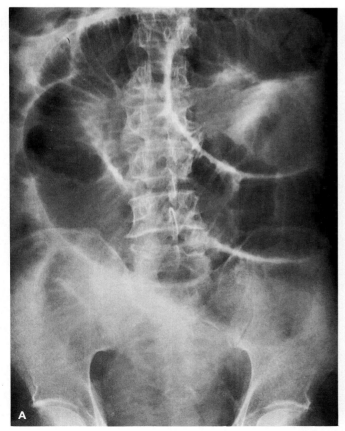 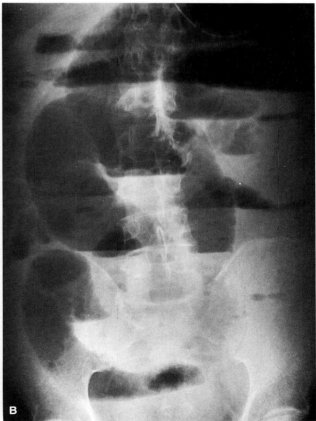

Fig. 33-15.   Small bowel obstruction due to adhesions from previous surgery. **(A)** Supine and **(B)** upright views.

EXTRINSIC BOWEL LESIONS

Fibrous adhesions caused by previous surgery or peritonitis account for almost 75% of all small bowel obstructions (Fig. 33-15). Because the right lower quadrant and pelvis are the site of most abdominal inflammatory processes and a majority of operative procedures, small bowel obstructions due to adhesions most frequently occur in the ileum. In patients with mechanical obstruction, the abdomen should be examined for evidence of surgical scars. Adhesions can produce obstruction by kinking or angulating bowel loops or by forming bands of tissue that compress the bowel.

External hernias (inguinal, femoral, umbilical, incisional) are the second most frequent cause of mechanical small bowel obstruction (Fig. 33-16). Indeed, the risk of intestinal obstruction is a major reason for the decision to electively repair external hernias. The inguinal and obturator foramen areas should always be closely evaluated on abdominal radiographs of patients with mechanical small bowel obstruction. Greater soft-tissue density on one side than the other or tapering of a bowel loop toward the groin should suggest an inguinal or femoral hernia as the underlying cause.

Internal hernias result from congenital abnormalities or surgical defects within the mesentery. If a loop of small bowel is trapped within the mesenteric defect, obstruction can result. More than half of all internal abdominal hernias are paraduodenal, mostly on the left. In this condition, small bowel loops are packed together and displaced under the transverse colon to the left of the midline. In the much less common herniation of small bowel through the foramen of Winslow, abnormal loops are seen along the lesser curvature medial and posterior to the stomach.

Neoplasms (Fig. 33-17) or inflammatory disease (Fig. 33-18) involving the bowel wall or mesentery can cause extrinsic compression and small bowel obstruction. In small intestinal volvulus, anomalies of the mesentery with defective fixation of bowel permit abnormal rotation. Twisting of the bowel about itself results in kinking and mechanical obstruction, frequently with occlusion of the blood supply to that intestinal segment. Another type of volvulus occurs when a segment of the intestine is fixed by adhesions and thus acts as a pivot for other portions of the small bowel to rotate about. In children, congenital fibrous bands are a not uncommon cause of extrinsic mechanical small bowel obstruction.

LUMINAL OCCLUSION

Large polypoid tumors, either benign or malignant, can occlude the bowel lumen and produce small bowel obstruction. Gallstones, enteroliths, foreign

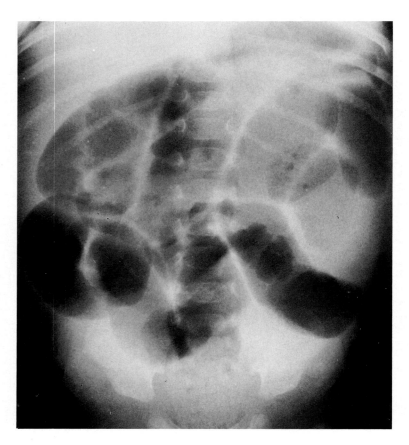

Fig. 33-16. *Small bowel obstruction caused by an inguinal hernia in a child.*

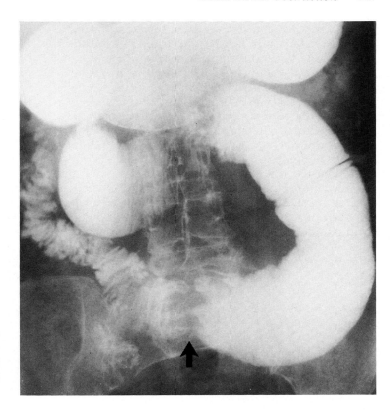

Fig. 33-17. Small bowel obstruction due to carcinoma of the jejunum. Antegrade administration of barium shows pronounced dilatation of the duodenum and proximal jejunum to the level of the annular constricting tumor **(arrow)**.

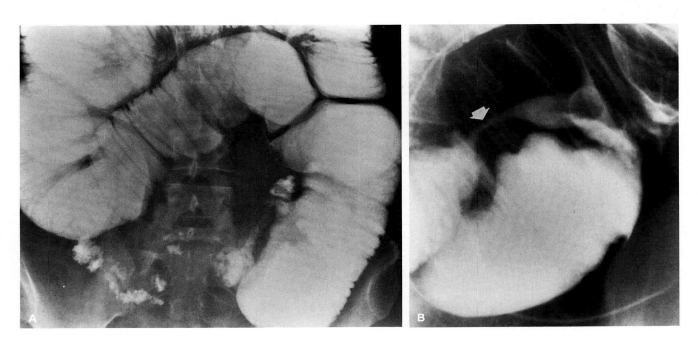

Fig. 33-18. Small bowel obstruction due to Crohn's disease involving the jejunum. **(A)** Antegrade barium study demonstrates markedly dilated proximal small bowel. **(B)** An inflammatory stricture **(arrow)** is seen to be the cause of the small bowel obstruction.

bodies, and bezoars can obstruct the small bowel if they are sufficiently large to be trapped and block the lumen. The combination of small bowel obstruction and gas in the biliary tree from a cholecystoenteric fistula makes gallstone ileus the most likely diagnosis (Fig. 33-19). The offending gallstone can often be found at the site of obstruction (Fig. 33-20). Bezoars causing small bowel obstruction are most commonly seen in patients who are mentally retarded or edentulous or who have undergone a partial gastric resection (Fig. 33-21). Intestinal tubes used for the relief of intestinal obstruction can, although rarely, lead to obstruction themselves when the mercury balloon becomes distended with gas or fluid. Radiographically, there is lack of advancement of the tube tip and persistent small bowel distention. An oval or sausage-shaped lucency is present around the tube tip when the balloon is filled with gas (Fig. 33-22A). If the balloon is filled with fluid, oral contrast is necessary to permit its visualization (Fig. 33-22B). Percutaneous needle balloon puncture is often necessary to relieve gaseous distention of the balloon of a single-lumen intestinal tube; aspiration of the balloon port is usually successful with the double-lumen type.

Intussusception

Intussusception is a major cause of small bowel obstruction in children; it is much less common in adults. Intussusception is the invagination of one part of the intestinal tract into another due to peristalsis, which forces the proximal segment of bowel to move distally within the ensheathing outer portion. Once such a lead point has been established, it gradually progresses forward and causes increased

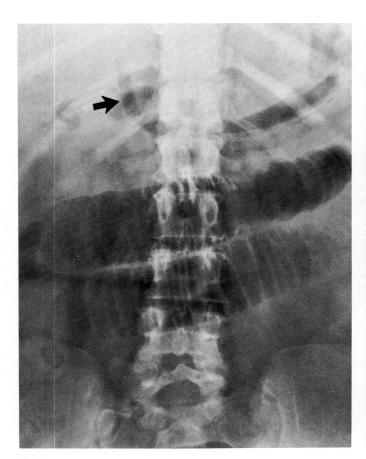

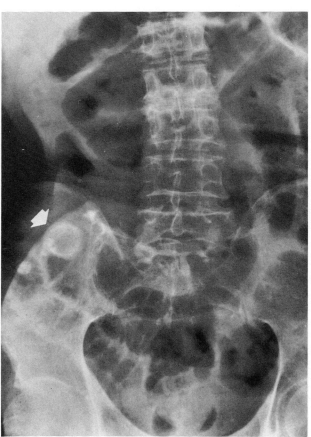

33-19

33-20

Fig. 33-19.   Gallstone ileus. Dilated, gas-filled loops of obstructed small bowel are combined with gas in the biliary tree **(arrow)**.

Fig. 33-20.   Gallstone ileus. There is dilatation of gas-filled loops of small bowel that extend to the level of an obstructing gallstone in the ileum **(arrow)**.

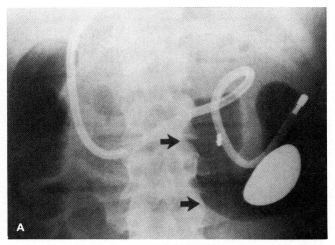

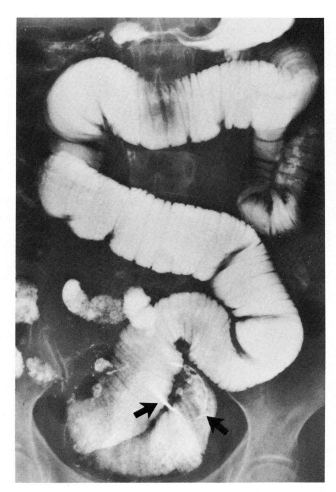

Fig. 33-21. Small bowel obstruction due to an impacted bezoar **(arrows)**.

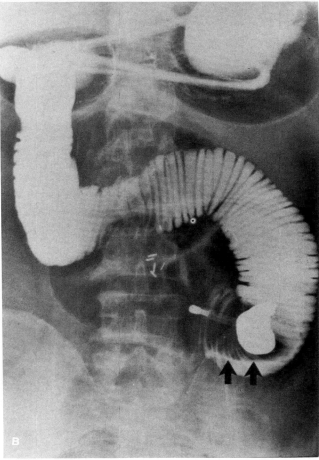

Fig. 33-22. Small bowel obstruction caused by long intestinal tube. **(A)** Plain abdominal radiograph shows the distended mercury balloon filled with gas **(arrows)** and situated in the proximal jejunum. **(B)** In another patient, a barium examination shows dilated small bowel proximal to an occluding fluid-filled mercury balloon **(arrows)**. (Shapir J, Braver J: Distention of intestinal tube balloons causing small bowel obstruction. J Can Assoc Radiol 37:203–205, 1986)

obstruction. This can compromise the vascular supply and produce ischemic necrosis of the intussuscepted bowel. In children, intussusception is most common in the region of the ileocecal valve. The clinical onset tends to be abrupt, with severe abdominal pain, blood in the stools ("currant jelly"), and often a palpable right-sided mass. If the diagnosis is made early and therapy instituted promptly, the mortality rate of intussusception in children is less than 1%. However, if treatment is delayed more than 48 hr after the onset of symptoms, the mortality rate increases dramatically. In adults, intussusception is often chronic or subacute and is characterized by irregular, recurrent episodes of colicky pain, nausea, and vomiting. The leading edge of an intussusception in the adult is usually a pedunculated polypoid tumor, often a lipoma. Other causes include malignant tumors, Meckel's diverticulum

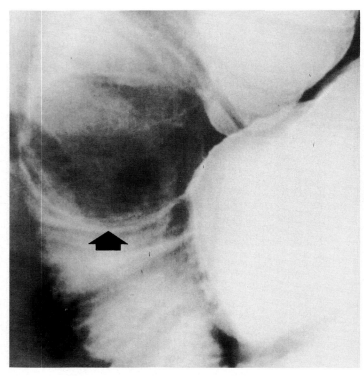

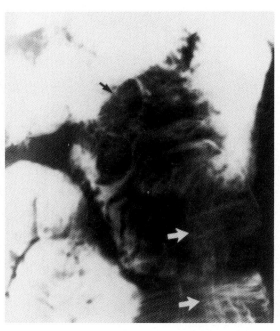

33-23   33-24

Fig. 33-23. Intermittent small bowel obstruction caused by an inverting Meckel's diverticulum. The Meckel's diverticulum presents as a large filling defect in the distal ileum **(arrow).**

Fig. 33-24. Heterotopic gastric mucosa causing jejunal intussusception. The polypoid lesion **(black arrow)** acts as the lead point of the intussusception. The central lumen of the intussusception is outlined by **white arrows**. (McWey P, Dodds WJ, Slota T et al: Radiographic features of heterotopic gastric mucosa. AJR 139:380–382, 1982. Copyright 1982. Reproduced with permission.)

(Fig. 33-23), chronic ulcers, adhesions and bands, aberrant pancreas, a polypoid mass of heterotopic gastric mucosa (Fig. 33-24), and foreign bodies. No cause for the intussusception can be demonstrated in about 10% to 20% of adults; in contrast, intussusceptions in infants and children almost always occur without any apparent anatomic etiology.

The classic radiographic sign of an intussusception is the coiled-spring appearance of barium trapped between the intussusceptum and surrounding portions of bowel (Fig. 33-25). Other findings include a narrow channel of barium representing the compressed lumen of the intussusceptum, a soft-tissue mass on either side of this channel due to hypertrophy and edema of the walls of the intussusceptum and intussuscipiens, and a mass lesion at the distal end of the narrow channel. Computed tomography often can demonstrate an intussusception by identifying the individual layers of bowel wall, contrast material, and mesenteric fat (Fig. 33-26). If mesenteric fat is seen, three individual layers of bowel wall can be identified; in portions of the intussusception where mesenteric fat is not present, only two layers are visible. Because of the asymmetric location of the invaginated mesenteric

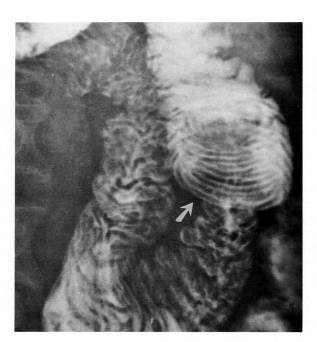

Fig. 33-25. Small bowel obstruction caused by a jejunojejunal intussusception. Note the characteristic coiled-spring appearance **(arrow).**

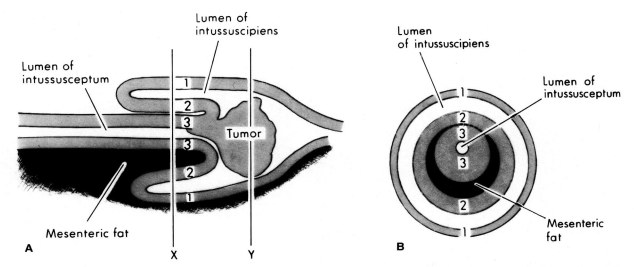

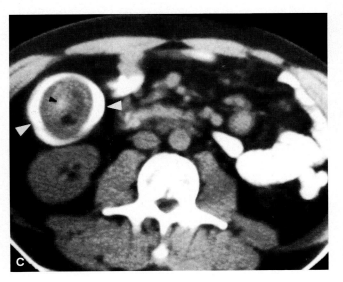

Fig. 33-26.   Computed tomography of intussusception. **(A)** A diagram of a longitudinal section through an intussusception. **1,** wall of intussuscipiens; **2, 3,** folded layers of bowel wall that constitute the intussusceptum. Note how invaginated mesenteric fat is attached to one side of the intussusceptum and separates the wall of the intussusceptum into two individual layers. **(B)** A diagram of the cross section of the intussusception at level X in **A.** Note the eccentric lumen of the intussusceptum. Where mesenteric fat is present, three distinct layers **(1, 2, 3)** can be seen. Only two layers are visible where there is no mesenteric fat, because layers 2 and 3 cannot be distinguished. **(C)** In this patient with an ileocolic intussusception, a cross-sectional view shows contrast material in the ascending colon **(white arrowheads)** surrounding the intussuscepted ileum and associated mesenteric fat. A tiny amount of contrast material was seen in the ileal lumen **(black arrowhead).** Lymphoma of the ileum formed the leading mass. (From Mauro MA, Koehler RE: Alimentary tract. In Lee JKT, Sagel SS, Stanley RJ et al (eds): Computed Body Tomography. New York, Raven, 1983)

fat, the lumen of the intussusceptum often is eccentrically positioned.

Although an intussusception in infants and children after abdominal operations is a well-known cause of bowel obstruction in about 15% of cases, its counterpart in adults is rarely considered among causes of postoperative bowel obstruction (Fig. 33-27). The most frequent postoperative intussusceptions are retrograde jejunogastric intussusception after Billroth-II partial gastrectomy with gastrojejunostomy and intussusception of the excluded intestinal segment after jejunoileal bypass operation for morbid obesity. Postoperative intussusception in adults may be related to a variety of predisposing factors, including suture lines, ostomy closure sites, adhesions, long intestinal tubes, bypassed intestinal segments, submucosal edema, abnormal bowel motility, electrolyte imbalance, and chronic dilatation of the bowel. Unfortunately, the classic clinical signs of intussusception are rarely present and the abdominal pain in these postoperative patients is generally attributed to the surgical wound. Therefore, a high index of suspicion is necessary for the diagnosis of postoperative intussusception.

Meconium Ileus

Meconium ileus is a cause of distal small bowel obstruction in infants, in whom the thick and sticky meconium cannot be readily propelled through the bowel (Fig. 33-28). The excessive viscidity of the meconium is due to the absence of normal pancreatic and intestinal gland secretions during fetal life. Meconium ileus is frequently associated with cystic fibrosis of the pancreas (mucoviscidosis). The unusually viscid intestinal contents in infants with meconium ileus present radiographically as a bubbly or frothy pattern superimposed on numerous dilated loops of small bowel. On barium enema examination, the colon is seen to have a very small caliber (microcolon), since it has not been used during fetal life.

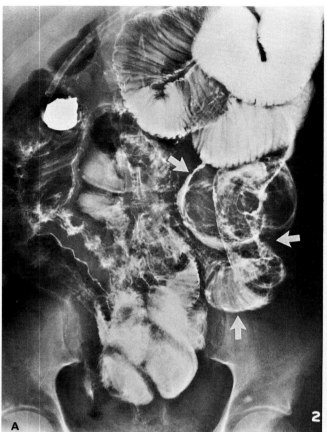

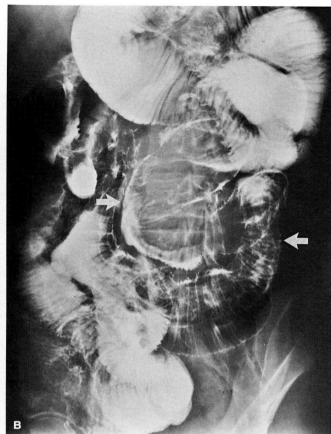

33-27

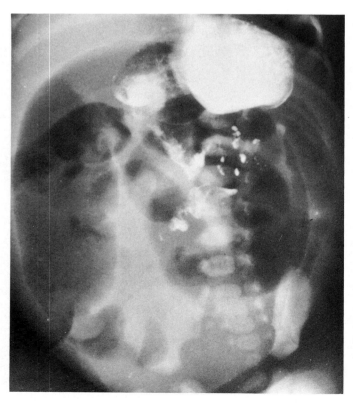

33-28

Fig. 33-27. Adult postoperative intussusception. **(A)** Supine and **(B)** oblique views from a small bowel series in a patient with a Cantor tube in the duodenum demonstrate jejunal dilatation proximal to a long segment of tremendously widened jejunum. This segment contains the large intussusceptum that, in many areas, effaces the typical coiled-spring fold pattern **(arrows)**. (Hertz I, Train J, Keller R et al: Adult postoperative enteroenteric intussusception in Crohn's disease. Gastrointest Radiol 7:131–134, 1982)

Fig. 33-28. Meconium ileus causing small bowel obstruction.

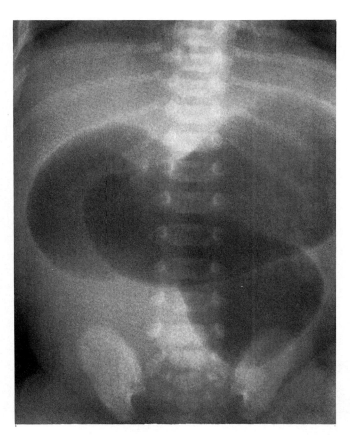

Fig. 33-29. *Jejunal atresia. Dilatation of only proximal small bowel loops indicates a jejunal lesion.*

INTRINSIC LESIONS OF THE BOWEL WALL

Strictures due to intrinsic abnormalities of the bowel wall can produce small bowel obstruction. Such strictures can be caused by constricting primary or metastatic neoplasms, or by inflammatory processes, such as Crohn's disease, tuberculous enteritis, and parasitic infections. Unusual causes include chemical irritation, such as from enteric-coated potassium chloride tablets, which produce ulceration and subsequent fibrosis; postoperative strictures at the level of previous small bowel anastomosis; complications of radiation therapy; and massive deposition of amyloid.

Intestinal ischemia, whether arterial or venous, can heal with intense fibrosis, which may lead to stenosis and small bowel obstruction. Intramural hematomas, due to either abdominal trauma or complications of anticoagulant therapy, can be large enough to occlude the intestinal lumen.

Congenital Atresia or Stenosis

Congenital jejunal (Fig. 33-29) or ileal (Fig. 33-30) atresia or stenosis is a major cause of mechanical small bowel obstruction in infants and young children. In children with obstruction of the jejunum or proximal ileum, distention of the proximal small bowel makes the diagnosis readily apparent on plain radiographs. In jejunal atresia, the characteristic "triple bubble" sign (stomach, duodenum,

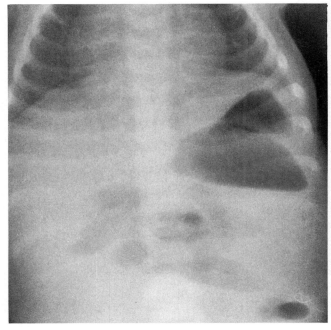

33-30

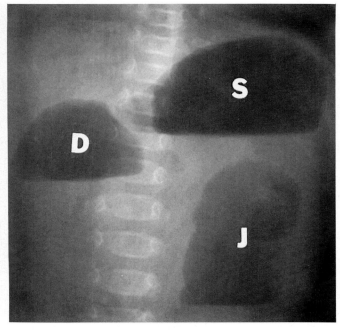

33-31

Fig. 33-30. *Ileal atresia. Dilated loops of gas- and fluid-filled small bowel extend to the left lower quadrant.*

Fig. 33-31. *Jejunal atresia. Note the characteristic triple bubble sign (stomach, duodenum, proximal jejunum).*

proximal jejunum) can often be demonstrated (Fig. 33-31). With lower ileal obstruction, on the other hand, it may be difficult to determine whether the dilated intestinal loops seen on plain radiographs represent large or small bowel. A barium enema may be necessary for this differentiation to be made.

In ileal atresia, little or no small bowel contents reach the colon during fetal life, and the colon therefore remains thin and ribbon-like (Fig. 33-32). This microcolon appearance is most pronounced in infants with complete low small bowel obstructions. It is progressively less marked in babies with higher obstructions, in whom some intestinal secretions have reached the colon. Infants with duodenal atresia often have colons of normal caliber.

Meconium peritonitis is a complication of small bowel atresia. This condition develops *in utero* and is presumed to be the result of a proximal perforation that permits meconium to pass into the peritoneal cavity and incite an inflammatory reaction. Meconium peritonitis frequently causes calcifications, which are usually evident at birth. These calcifications can appear as small flecks scattered throughout the abdomen, curvilinear densities on the serosa of the bowel wall, or larger conglomerates of calcium along the inferior surface of the liver or concentrated in the flanks.

A rare cause of intestinal obstruction in the neonatal period is segmental dilatation of the ileum. The characteristic radiographic appearance is localized dilatation of a single, well-defined segment of intestine with more or less abrupt transition to normal bowel proximally and distally (Fig. 33-33). Possible etiologies include temporary obstruction of a loop of intestine early in development or heterotopic tissue within the bowel that may reflect an early insult to the developing gut or represent a primary dysplasia. The presence of the heterotopic tissue in the bowel wall may interfere with the functional continuity of the normally innervated bowel musculature and lead to dilatation. The definitive treatment is resection of the dilated segment with

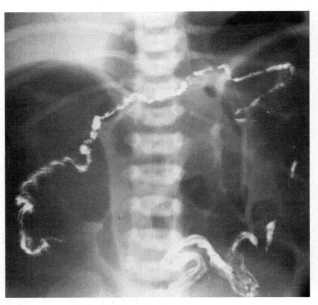

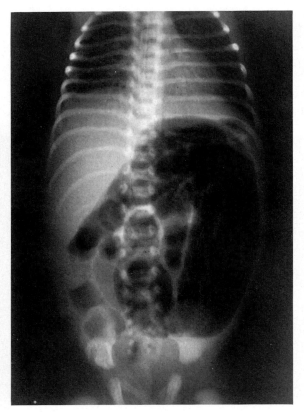

33-32   **33-33**

Fig. 33-32.   Ileal atresia with microcolon. Barium enema examination shows the colon to be thin and ribbon-like. Note the markedly distended loops of small bowel extending to the point of obstruction in the lower ileum.

Fig. 33-33.   Segmental dilatation of the ileum. There is a solitary distended loop of bowel in the left abdomen, but air is present throughout the bowel. A fluid level is present in the loop but there is none proximally. There is no mechanical small bowel obstruction. (Brown A, Carty H: Segmental dilatation of the ileum. Br J Radiol 57:371–374, 1984)

end-to-end anastomosis, which restores functional continuity to the bowel.

BIBLIOGRAPHY

Agha FP: Intussusception in adults: AJR 146:527–531, 1986

Beal SL, Walton CB, Bodai BI: Enterolith ileus resulting from small bowel diverticulosis. Am J Gastroenterol 82:162–164, 1987

Berdon WE, Baker DH, Santulli TV et al: Microcolon in newborn infants with intestinal obstruction. Radiology 90:878–885, 1968

Brown A, Carty H: Segmental dilatation of the ileum. Br J Radiol 57:371–374, 1984

Bryk D: Functional evaluation of small bowel obstruction by successive abdominal roentgenograms. AJR 116:262–275, 1972

Bryk D: Strangulating obstruction of the bowel. A re-evaluation of radiographic criteria. AJR 130:835–843, 1978

Caroline DF, Herlinger H, Laufer I et al: Small-bowel enema in the diagnosis of adhesive obstruction. AJR 142:1133–1139, 1984

Daneman A, Reilly BJ, de Silva M et al: Intussusception on small bowel examinations in children. AJR 139:299–304, 1982

Hertz I, Train J, Keller R et al: Adult postoperative enteroenteric intussusception in Crohn's disease. Gastrointest Radiol 7:131–134, 1982

Levin B: Mechanical small bowel obstruction. Semin Roengenol 8:281–297, 1973

Leonidas J, Berdon WE, Baker DH et al: Meconium ileus and its complications. AJR 108:598–609, 1970

Louw JH: Jejunoileal atresia and stenosis. J Pediatr Surg 1:8–23, 1966

Mauro MA, Koehler RE: Alimentary tract. In Lee JKT, Sagel SS, Stanley RS et al (eds): Computed Body Tomography. New York, Raven, 1983

McWey P, Dodds WJ, Slota T et al: Radiographic features of heterotopic gastric mucosa. AJR 139:380–382, 1982

Miller RE: The technical approach to the acute abdomen. Semin Roentgenol 13:267–275, 1973

Miller RE, Brahme F: Large amounts of orally administered barium for obstruction of the small intestine. Surg Gynecol Obstet 129:1185–1188, 1969

Nelson SW, Christoforidis AJ: The use of barium sulfate suspension in the diagnosis of acute diseases of the small intestine. AJR 104:505–521, 1968

Rigler LG, Pogue WL: Roentgen signs of intestinal necrosis. AJR 94:402–409, 1965

Schwartz SS: The differential diagnosis of intestinal obstruction. Semin Roentgenol 8:323–338, 1973

Shapir J, Braver J: Distention of intestinal tube balloons causing small bowel obstruction. J Can Assoc Radiol 37:203–205, 1986

Shauffer IA, Ferris EJ: The mass sign in primary volvulus of the small intestine in adults. Radiology 84:374–378, 1965

Strauss S, Rubinstein ZJ, Shapira Z et al: Food as a cause of small intestinal obstruction: A report of five cases without previous gastric surgery. Gastrointest Radiol 2:17–20, 1977

Tomchik FS, Wittenberg J, Ottinger LW: The roentgenographic spectrum of bowel infarction. Radiology 96:249–260, 1970

Williams JL: Fluid-filled loops in intestinal obstruction. AJR 88:677–686, 1962

Williams JL: Obstruction of the small intestine. Radiol Clin North Am 2:21–31, 1964

34 ADYNAMIC ILEUS

Adynamic ileus is a common disorder of intestinal motor activity in which fluid and gas do not progress normally through a nonobstructed small and large bowel. A variety of neural, humoral, and metabolic factors can precipitate reflexes that inhibit intestinal motility. The clinical appearance of patients with adynamic ileus varies from minimal symptoms to generalized abdominal distention with a marked decrease in the frequency and intensity of bowel sounds. The radiographic hallmark of adynamic ileus is retention of large amounts of gas and fluid in a dilated small and large bowel (Fig. 34-1). Unlike the appearance in mechanical small bowel obstruction (Fig. 34-2), the entire small and large bowel in adynamic ileus appear almost uniformly dilated with no demonstrable point of obstruction. Concomitant distention of the gas-filled stomach, an infrequent occurrence with mechanical small bowel obstruction, is often seen in patients with adynamic ileus (especially if it is secondary to peritonitis).

CAUSES

Surgical procedure
Peritonitis
Medication
Electrolyte imbalance
Metabolic disorder
Abdominal trauma
Retroperitoneal hemorrhage
Gram-negative sepsis/shock

Renal or ureteral calculus
Acute chest disease (pneumonia, myocardial infarction, congestive heart failure)
Mesenteric vascular occlusion
Myotonic muscular dystrophy

SURGICAL PROCEDURE

Adynamic ileus occurs to some extent in almost every patient who undergoes abdominal surgery (Fig. 34-3). Although the precise etiology is unclear, postoperative ileus may be related to drying of the bowel while it is outside the peritoneal cavity, excessive traction on the bowel or its mesentery, or even mere handling of the bowel during operation. Gas-fluid levels may not be seen in postoperative ileus, even though the bowel loops are markedly dilated. Postoperative adynamic ileus usually resolves spontaneously or clears with the aid of intubation and suction. However, if the ileus progresses and bowel loops become greatly distended, intestinal rupture and pneumoperitoneum can result.

PERITONITIS

Dilated loops of large and small bowel with multiple gas-fluid levels is a common appearance in patients with peritonitis (Fig. 34-4). As the motor activity of the intestine decreases, the gas-fluid levels in each loop tend to stand at the same height, in contrast to mechanical obstruction, in which the gas-fluid levels in the same loop are often seen at different

Text continues on page 433

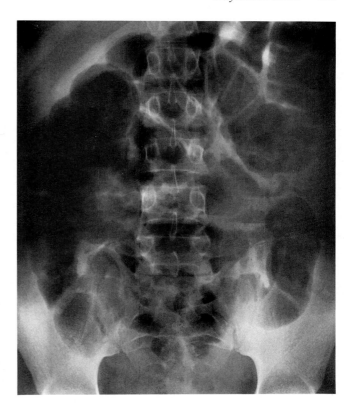

Fig. 34-1. Adynamic ileus. Large amounts of gas and fluid are retained in loops of dilated small and large bowel. The entire small and large bowel appear almost uniformly dilated with no demonstrable point of obstruction.

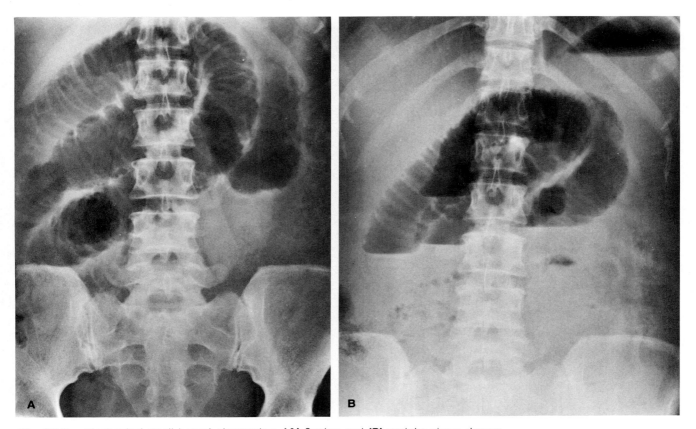

Fig. 34-2. Mechanical small bowel obstruction. **(A)** Supine and **(B)** upright views demonstrate only a few dilated, gas-filled loops of small bowel proximal to the point of obstruction. This is unlike the general dilatation of the entire small and large bowel seen in adynamic ileus.

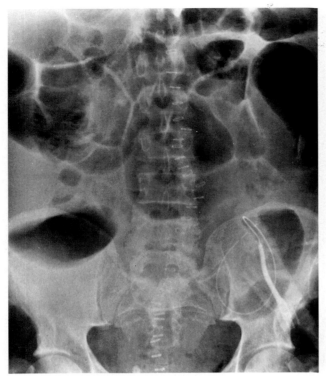

34-3

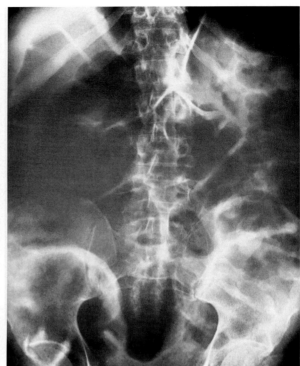

34-4

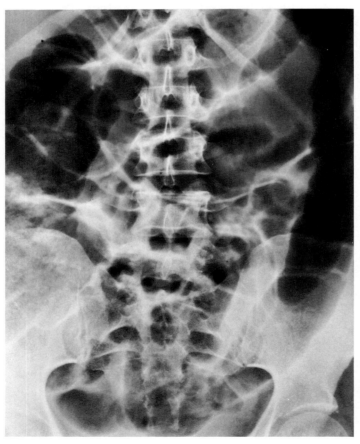

34-5

Fig. 34-3. Adynamic ileus following abdominal surgery.

Fig. 34-4. Adynamic ileus in a patient with peritonitis.

Fig. 34-5. Adynamic ileus in a patient with severe gastroenteritis but without peritonitis.

heights. Peritonitis is a likely cause of adynamic ileus whenever there is associated blurring of the mucosal pattern and intestinal edema, evidence of free peritoneal fluid, restricted diaphragmatic movement, or pleural effusion. Even without peritonitis, gastroenteritis or enterocolitis can present as generalized adynamic ileus (Fig. 34-5).

Some intra-abdominal inflammatory processes can cause both a mechanical block and adynamic ileus. Both conditions may be present at the same time and produce a confusing appearance. For example, an acute periappendiceal abscess can cause true mechanical obstruction in addition to the characteristic adynamic ileus seen in patients with appendicitis. Clinical correlation, serial radiographs, and even a barium enema examination may be necessary to establish the diagnosis.

MEDICATION

Many drugs with muscarinic (atropine-like) effects can produce a radiographic pattern of adynamic ileus (Fig. 34-6). In addition to atropine, this appearance can be caused by morphine, Lomotil (diphenoxylate), L-dopa, barbiturates, and other sympathomimetic agents.

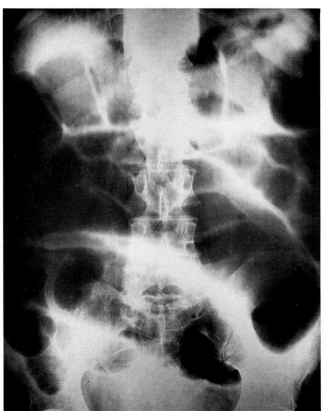

Fig. 34-7. Adynamic ileus in a patient with severe hypokalemia.

ELECTROLYTE IMBALANCE

Electrolyte imbalances can lead to adynamic ileus by interfering with normal ionic movements during contractions of the smooth muscle of the large and small bowel. Hypokalemia (Fig. 34-7) is the most common electrolyte imbalance to cause this pattern, but adynamic ileus can also be seen in patients with hypochloremia and in persons with calcium or magnesium abnormalities. Hormonal deficits, such as hypothyroidism and hypoparathyroidism, can present a similar radiographic appearance.

OTHER CAUSES

Abdominal trauma, retroperitoneal hemorrhage, and spinal or pelvic fractures can also result in adynamic ileus. Generalized gram-negative sepsis, shock, and hypoxia are often associated with decreased intestinal motility, as is the colicky pain due to the passage of renal or ureteral stones. Generalized dilatation of the small and large bowel can be seen in patients with acute chest diseases such as pneumonia, myocardial infarction, and congestive heart failure. Vascular occlusion resulting in mesenteric ischemia and infarction often causes segmental or generalized adynamic ileus. Chronic dila-

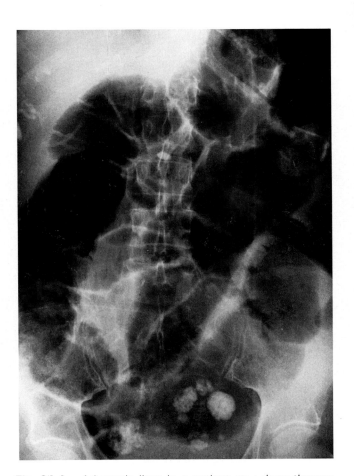

Fig. 34-6. Adynamic ileus in a patient on L-dopa therapy (atropine-like effect).

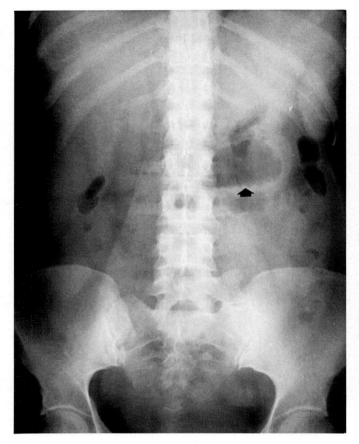

34-8

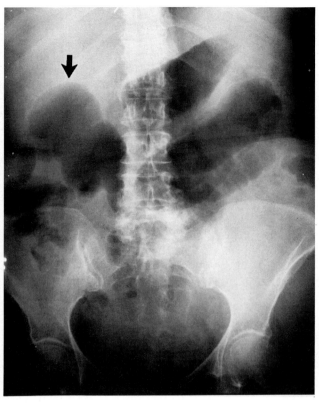

34-9

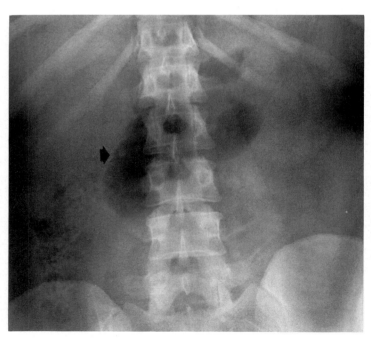

34-10

Fig. 34-8. Localized ileus **(arrow)** in a patient with acute pancreatitis.

Fig. 34-9. Localized ileus **(arrow)** in a patient with acute cholecystitis.

Fig. 34-10. Localized ileus in a patient with acute ureteral colic. The **arrow** points to the impacted ureteral stone.

tation of small intestinal loops and delayed transit of barium can be caused by dystrophy and fatty infiltration of smooth muscle in patients with myotonic muscular dystrophy.

VARIANTS

LOCALIZED ILEUS

An isolated distended loop of small or large bowel reflecting a localized adynamic ileus (sentinel loop) is often associated with an adjacent acute inflammatory process. The portion of the bowel involved can offer a clue to the underlying disease. Localized segments of the jejunum or transverse colon are frequently dilated in patients with acute pancreatitis (Fig. 34-8). Similarly, the hepatic flexure of the colon can be distended in acute cholecystitis (Fig. 34-9), the terminal ileum can be dilated in acute appendicitis, the descending colon can be distended in acute diverticulitis, and dilated loops can be seen along the course of the ureter in acute ureteral colic (Fig. 34-10).

COLONIC ILEUS

Some patients demonstrate selective or disproportionate gaseous distention of the large bowel without an organic obstruction (colonic ileus) (Fig. 34-11). Massive distention of the cecum, which is often horizontally oriented, characteristically dominates the radiographic appearance. There is often much more gas in the right and transverse colon than in the rectum, sigmoid, and descending colon.

Although the pathogenesis of colonic ileus is not known, it is probably related to an imbalance between sympathetic and parasympathetic innervation to the large bowel. Colonic ileus usually accompanies or follows an acute abdominal inflammatory process or abdominal surgery, but it can also occur with any of the etiologic factors associated with adynamic ileus (Figs. 34-12, 34-13). Indeed, acute colonic ileus must be suspected in any hospitalized patient who develops abdominal distention. The clinical importance of this disorder is the need to differentiate it from mechanical obstruction and the risk of colonic ischemia and perforation secondary to dilatation.

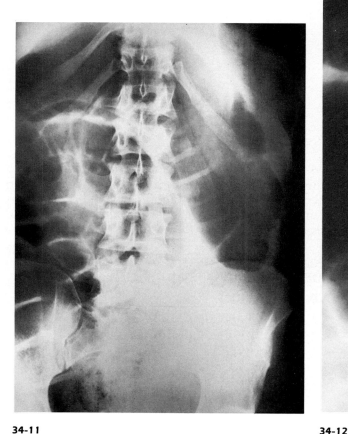

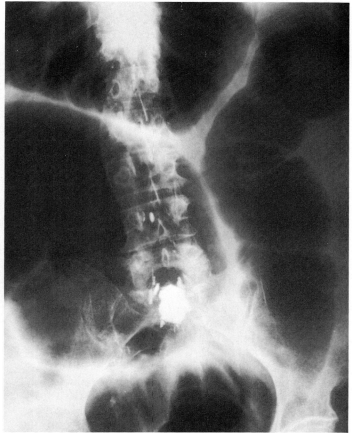

34-11

34-12

Fig. 34-11. Colonic ileus related to an overdose of Thorazine (chlorpromazine)

Fig. 34-12 Colonic ileus in a patient with severe diabetes and hypokalemia.

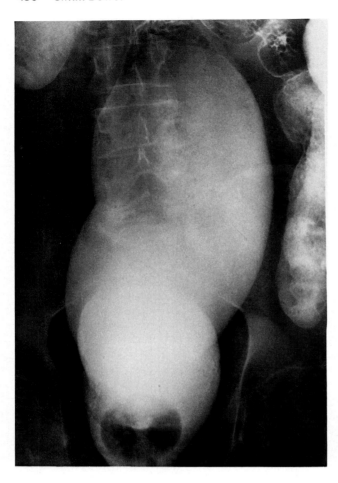

Fig. 34-13 Colonic ileus in a patient on Cogentin (benztropine) therapy. Barium enema examination reveals a massively dilated colon without any point of obstruction.

The clinical presentation of colonic ileus simulates that of mechanical obstruction of the colon. Because colonic ileus usually represents acute dilatation of a previously normal colon, it tends to appear radiographically as pronounced dilatation of part or all of the large bowel with preserved haustrations, thin, well-defined septae, and smooth inner colonic contours. In colonic obstruction, in contrast, mucosal edema, adherent fecal matter, and secretions result in an accentuation of haustrations with numerous, closely packed septations; loss or shallowness of haustrations; large amounts of fecal retention; thickened, ill-defined, irregular septae; and a ragged inner colonic contour. Nevertheless, it can often be difficult to distinguish between colonic ileus and obstruction on plain abdominal radiographs. A barium enema examination is usually necessary to exclude the possibility of an obstructing lesion.

Sequential abdominal radiographs should be obtained to evaluate the size of the cecum. Perforation is likely to occur when the cecal diameter is larger than 9 to 12 cm, and this complication leads to cecal peritonitis and a mortality rate exceeding 40%. Traditionally, tube cecostomy has been performed to decompress the massively distended cecum. More recently, colonoscopy and even percutaneous cecostomy have been used as alternatives to a surgical procedure.

ADYNAMIC ILEUS SIMULATING MECHANICAL OBSTRUCTION

Disease Entities

Chronic idiopathic intestinal
       pseudo-obstruction
Pelvic surgery
Urinary retention
Pancreatitis
Acute intermittent porphyria
Ceroidosis
Neonatal adynamic ileus
   Systemic
   Chemical/hormonal
   Abdominal

CHRONIC IDIOPATHIC INTESTINAL PSEUDO-OBSTRUCTION

Chronic idiopathic intestinal pseudo-obstruction is a rare condition in which there is pronounced distention of the bowel (especially the small intestine) mimicking intestinal obstruction without a demonstrable obstructive lesion (Fig. 34-14). A disease of unknown etiology, chronic idiopathic intestinal pseudo-obstruction may be related to an intrinsic smooth muscle lesion or an abnormality involving the intramural nerve plexuses. Recognition of the true nature of this nonobstructive condition is essential if the patient is to be prevented from undergoing an unnecessary laparotomy.

PELVIC SURGERY

An unusual type of adynamic ileus simulating reversible small bowel obstruction can develop after transabdominal hysterectomy or other pelvic surgery, especially when the procedure involves manipulation of the small bowel. Typically, the patient becomes distended and begins vomiting between the second and fifth postoperative days. Bowel sounds are hyperactive, and plain abdominal radiographs demonstrate the classic appearance of small bowel obstruction. This phenomenon is probably related to impeded peristalsis due to local paralysis of the small bowel secondary to inflammation or

manipulation. Although the radiographic picture is typical of high-grade mechanical small bowel obstruction, surgery is seldom required. If the patient can be kept comfortable by intestinal intubation for a few days, the signs and symptoms of obstruction invariably disappear.

URINARY RETENTION AND PANCREATITIS

Adynamic ileus simulating bowel obstruction can be secondary to urinary retention. Emptying of the distended bladder can result in complete disappearance of symptoms. Adynamic ileus mimicking bowel obstruction can also be seen in patients with acute pancreatitis (Fig. 34-15).

ACUTE INTERMITTENT PORPHYRIA

Acute intermittent porphyria is a familial metabolic disease characterized by attacks of severe, colicky, abdominal pain in association with obstipation. Clinical and radiographic symptoms and signs often lead to the erroneous diagnosis of bowel obstruction (Fig. 34-16). Although many patients are operated upon for this reason, no organic obstruction is found. The diagnosis is usually made from the chance observation that the urine becomes dark on exposure to light or on the basis of the development of characteristic neurologic symptoms, which lead

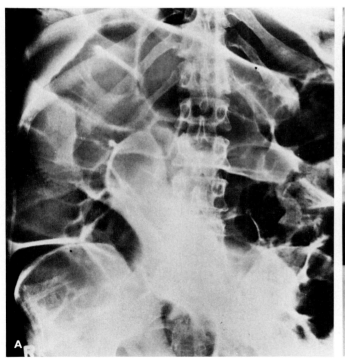
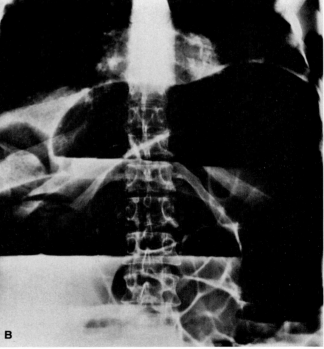

Fig. 34-14 *Idiopathic intestinal pseudo-obstruction.* **(A)** *Supine and* **(B)** *upright views show a massively dilated stomach and small and large bowel with nondifferential gas-fluid levels in all three portions of the gastrointestinal tract. (Teixidor HS, Heneghan MA: Idiopathic intestinal pseudo-obstruction in a family. Gastrointest Radiol 3:91–95. 1978)*

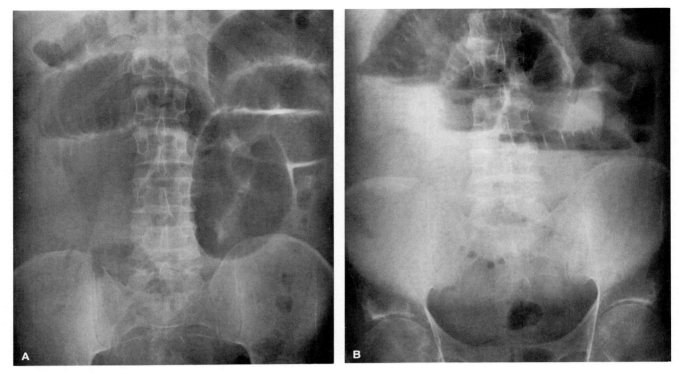

Fig. 34-15. Adynamic ileus mimicking mechanical obstruction in a patient with pancreatitis. **(A)** Supine and **(B)** upright views.

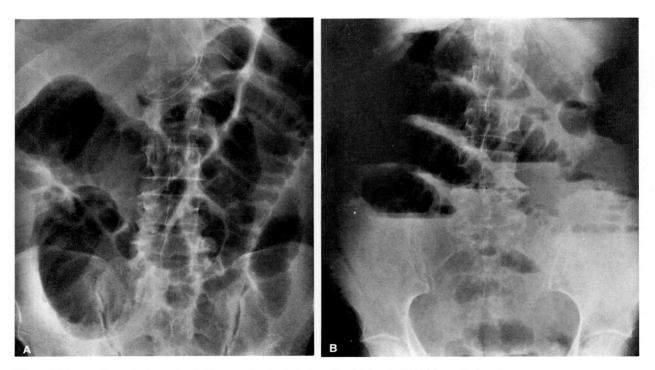

Fig. 34-16. Adynamic ileus simulating mechanical obstruction in a patient with acute intermittent porphyria. **(A)** Supine and **(B)** upright views.

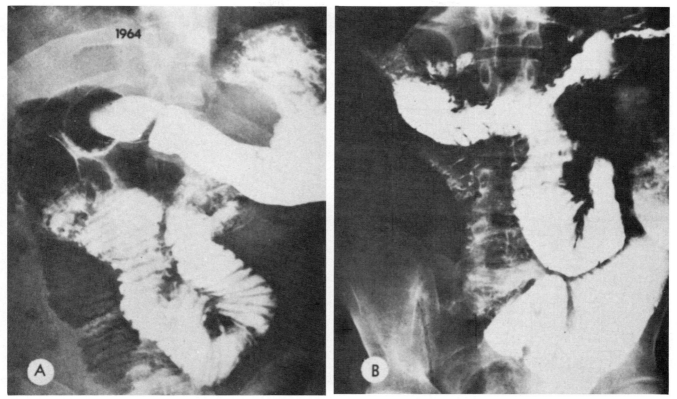

Fig. 34-17. Ceroidosis. **(A)** Barium study showing dilatation of the stomach, duodenum, and proximal jejunum with thickening of valvulae conniventes. **(B)** Follow-up 8½ hr later showing barium still in the diffusely dilated jejunum and proximal ileum. Thickening of valvulae conniventes is again apparent (Boller M, Fiocchi C, Brown CH: Pseudo-obstruction in ceroidosis. AJR 127:277–279. 1976. Copyright 1976. Reproduced with permission)

to a search for the presence of abnormal porphyrins in the urine and feces.

CEROIDOSIS

Ceroidosis is the diffuse accumulation of a brown lipofuscin pigment in the muscularis propria of the gastrointestinal tract (brown bowel syndrome). It is not a primary disease but rather an irreversible consequence of long-standing malabsorption and prolonged depletion of vitamin E. The progressive dilatation and hypomotility of the entire gastrointestinal tract demonstrated by radiographic studies (Fig. 34-17) is probably related to infiltration of ceroid pigment in the smooth muscle cells with resulting functional impairment. As with chronic idiopathic pseudo-obstruction, the correct diagnosis of

ceroidosis is essential to prevent unnecessary bowel resection for a nonexistent obstruction.

NEONATAL ADYNAMIC ILEUS

In neonates and young children, adynamic ileus can predominantly affect the small bowel, producing a radiographic appearance resembling mechanical intestinal obstruction (Fig. 34-18). In most cases, adynamic ileus results from nongastrointestinal ailments such as septicemia, hormonal or chemical deficits, hypoxia-induced vasculitis, or the respiratory distress syndrome. Intestinal infection, peritonitis, mesenteric thrombosis, and infusion of fluid into an umbilical venous line can produce a similar radiographic appearance.

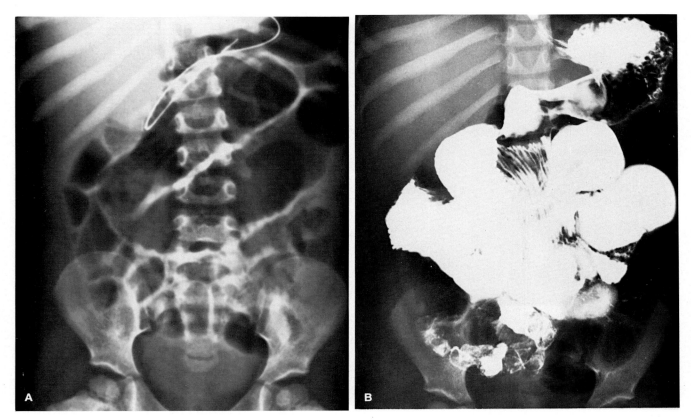

Fig. 34-18 *Adynamic ileus resembling mechanical intestinal obstruction in a child. Vasculitis with localized paralysis of the jejunum is seen in a 3-year-old girl with mucocutaneous lymph node syndrome.* **(A)** *The plain film shows that the proximal jejunum is dilated disproportionately with respect to the remainder of the bowel.* **(B)** *An antegrade barium study confirmed the jejunal dilatation, but contrast passed slowly into a normal-caliber bowel without an abrupt transition of caliber. (Franken EA, Smith WL, Smith JA: Paralysis of the small bowel resembling mechanical intestinal obstruction. Gastrointest Radiol 5:161–167. 1980)*

BIBLIOGRAPHY

Adler YT, Draths KG, Markey WS: Pseudo-obstruction in the geriatric population. RadioGraphics 6:995–1005, 1986

Anuras S, Shirazi SS: Colonic pseudo-obstruction. Am J Gastroenterol 79:525–532, 1984

Boller M, Fiocchi C, Brown CH: Pseudo-obstruction in ceroidosis. AJR 127:277–279, 1976

Casola G, Withers C, vanSonnenberg E et al: Percutaneous cecostomy for decompression of the massively distended cecum. Radiology 158:793–794, 1986

Franken EA, Smith WL, Smith JA: Paralysis of the small bowel resembling mechanical intestinal obstruction. Gastrointest Radiol 5:161–167, 1980

Hohl RD, Nixon RK: Myxedema ileus. Arch Intern Med 115:145–150, 1965

Johnson CD, Rice RP, Kelvin FM et al: The radiologic evaluation of gross cecal distention: Emphasis on cecal ileus. AJR 145:1211–1217, 1985

Legge DA, Wollaeger EE, Carlson HC: Intestinal pseudo-obstruction in systemic amyloidosis. Gut 11:764–767, 1970

Meyers MA: Colonic ileus. Gastrointest Radiol 2:37–40, 1977

Moss AA, Golberg HI, Brotman M: Idiopathic intestinal pseudo-obstruction. AJR 115:312–317, 1972

Nowak TV, Ionasescu V, Anuras S: Gastrointestinal manifestations of the muscular dystrophies. Gastroenterology 82:800–810, 1982

Rohrmann CA, Ricci MT, Krishnamurthy S et al: Radiologic and histologic differentiation of neuromuscular disorders of the gastrointestinal tract: Visceral myopathy, visceral neuropathy, and progressive systemic sclerosis. AJR 143:933–941, 1981

Shirazi KK, Agha FP, Strodel WE et al: Non-obstructive colonic dilatation: Radiologic findings in 50 patients following colonoscopic treatment. J Can Assoc Radiol 35:116–119, 1984

Treacy WL, Bunting WL, Gambill EE et al: Scleroderma presenting as an obstruction of the small bowel. Mayo Clin Proc 37:607–616, 1962

Vanek VW, Al-Salti M: Acute pseudo-obstruction of the colon (Ogilvie's syndrome). Dis Colon Rectum 29:203–210, 1986

DILATATION WITH NORMAL FOLDS

Disease Entities

Mechanical obstruction
Adynamic ileus
Vagotomy (surgical or chemical)
Sprue
Lymphoma
Connective tissue disease
    Scleroderma
    Dermatomyositis
Diabetes with hypokalemia
Lactase deficiency
Vascular insufficiency
    Mesenteric ischemia
    Systemic lupus erythematosus
    Amyloidosis
Chronic idiopathic intestinal pseudo-
        obstruction
Chagas' disease

The normal small bowel measures up to 3 cm in width (up to 4 cm in the proximal small bowel with the enteroclysis technique). Generalized small bowel dilatation is usually easy to recognize. An isolated loop of small bowel that appears to be dilated must be approached with caution until it is certain that it does not merely represent a segment undergoing an active peristaltic rush. Mucosal folds in the small bowel normally measure 2 mm to 3 mm in width and are regular in appearance.

MECHANICAL OBSTRUCTION/ ADYNAMIC ILEUS

The radiographic pattern of dilated small bowel with normal folds is most commonly seen in patients with mechanical small bowel obstruction (Figs. 35-1, 35-2) or adynamic ileus. In mechanical obstruction, there is a distinct difference in caliber between loops proximal and loops distal to the point of obstruction (Fig. 35-2). The muscular activity of the small bowel is usually increased, resulting in active peristalsis that corresponds to the clinical finding of hyperactive, high-pitched bowel sounds. There is generally a paucity of colonic gas.

Adynamic ileus can usually be readily distinguished from mechanical obstruction. Gas is seen throughout the small bowel and colon; there is no point at which the caliber of the bowel dramatically changes. Unlike mechanical obstruction, adynamic ileus is associated with decreased muscular activity and the clinical finding of hypoactive bowel sounds.

VAGOTOMY

Sectioning of the major anterior and posterior vagal trunks during surgical treatment for peptic ulcer disease interrupts the parasympathetic nerve supply to the gastrointestinal tract. This results in prolonged transit time and dilatation of the small bowel with normal folds (Fig. 35-3). A history of previous ulcer surgery is usually easy to elicit. Even if this

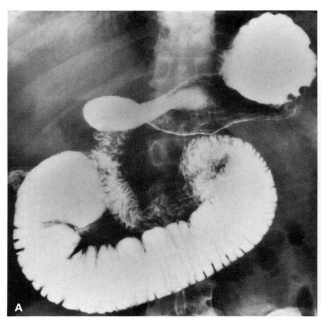
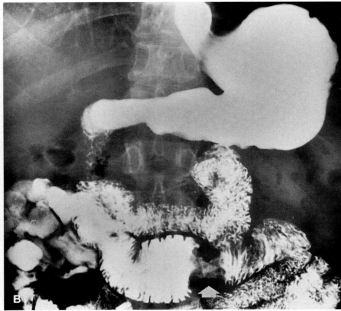

Fig. 35-1. Mechanical small bowel obstruction caused by small bowel metastases from carcinoma of the lung. **(A)** Markedly dilated small bowel with normal folds. **(B)** An annular constricting lesion **(arrow)** is demonstrated as the cause of the partial obstruction. Note the dramatic decrease in the caliber of the small bowel distal to the obstruction.

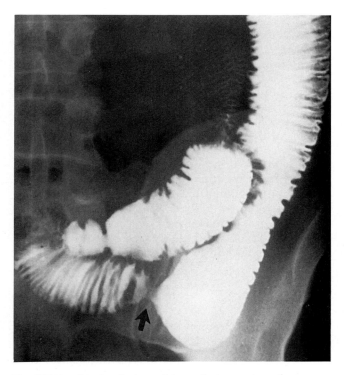

Fig. 35-2. Mechanical small bowel obstruction due to stenosing lymphoma of the jejunum **(arrow)**. Note the dramatic decrease in the caliber of the small bowel immediately distal to the point of partial obstruction.

information is lacking, vagotomy clips are generally apparent on chest or abdominal radiographs.

In contrast, evidence of chemical vagotomy is often difficult to obtain. Medications containing atropine or atropine-like substances are frequently prescribed for a variety of abdominal complaints. In addition, numerous other drugs (*e.g.,* morphine, L-dopa, Lomotil [diphenoxylate], barbiturates) also have atropine-like effects that mimic vagotomy and result in decreased smooth muscle activity, prolonged transit time, and a dilated small bowel with normal folds.

Many of the other conditions that produce the radiographic pattern of dilated small bowel with normal folds present with the clinical syndrome of malabsorption. This all-inclusive term applies to a diverse group of diseases that have in common the defective absorption of nutrients from the small intestine. These disorders generally result in steatorrhea (the passage of bulky, fatty, and foul-smelling stools) and, frequently, in vitamin and mineral deficiencies (folic acid, vitamin-B complex, vitamin B_{12}, vitamin K, calcium, iron, and magnesium).

SPRUE

The classic disease of malabsorption is sprue. This term is used to refer to any of three diseases, all of

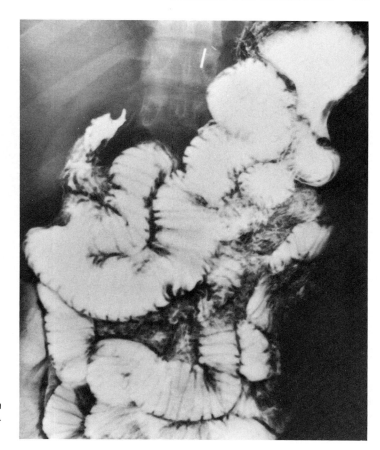

Fig. 35-3. Small bowel dilatation with normal folds in a patient who has undergone vagotomy, partial gastrectomy, and Billroth-II anastomosis.

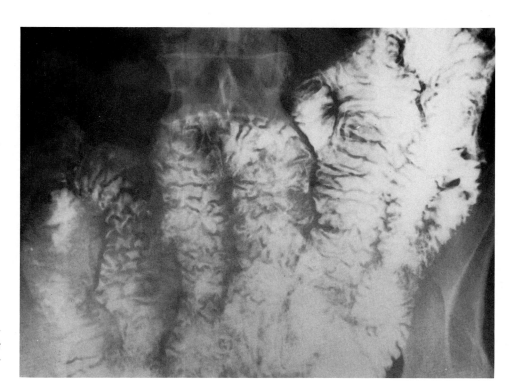

Fig. 35-4. Idiopathic (nontropical) sprue. There is diffuse small bowel dilatation with hypersecretion.

which are similar clinically: idiopathic (nontropical) sprue (Fig. 35-4); tropical sprue (Fig. 35-5); and celiac disease of children. The small bowel dilatation in sprue is usually best visualized in the mid and distal jejunum, though diffuse dilatation of the entire small bowel and colon can occur (Fig. 35-6). The degree of dilatation is generally related to the severity of the disease and is most pronounced in advanced cases. Although the long and tortuous loops sometimes superficially resemble the appearance of mechanical obstruction, the dilated loops in sprue are flaccid and contract poorly. Segmentation and flocculation of barium have traditionally been considered indicative of sprue or other malabsorption disorders. In recent years, however, the use of nondispersible barium with suspending agents has all but eliminated these radiographic signs.

An excessive amount of fluid in the bowel lumen (hypersecretion) is a constant phenomenon in patients with sprue. This fluid may represent either excessive movement of water into the lumen or deficient absorption of water by the deranged mucosa. As a result of hypersecretion, gas–fluid levels are occasionally seen on upright films. The barium in the small bowel has a coarse, granular appearance (Fig. 35-7), unlike barium in the normal intestine, which has a homogeneous quality.

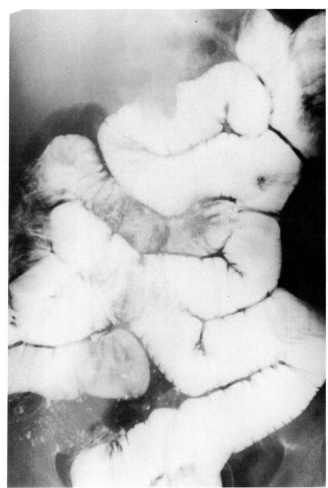

Fig. 35-6. Idiopathic (nontropical) sprue. There is diffuse dilatation of the entire small bowel with pronounced hypersecretion.

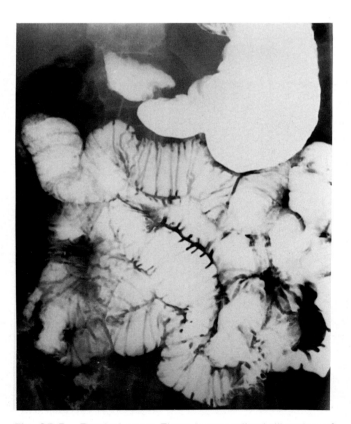

Fig. 35-5. Tropical sprue. There is generalized dilatation of the small bowel with normal fold thickness.

The *"moulage"* sign describes a radiographic appearance of the jejunum in sprue. The French term means "moulding" or "casting" and refers to the smooth contour and unindented margins of barium-filled small bowel loops (Fig. 35-8). This tubular appearance in sprue is probably due to atrophy and effacement of the jejunal mucosal folds.

Reversal of the jejunoileal fold pattern (increase in the ileal fold pattern with concomitant decrease in the jejunal fold pattern) has been reported as a radiographic appearance distinctive for nontropical sprue (Fig. 35-9). This pattern indicates long-standing disease, with chronic inflammation and atrophy of the jejunum and compensatory hypertrophy (adaptation) of the ileum.

Intussusception is a not uncommon finding in patients with sprue (Fig. 35-10). The diagnosis is based on the typical findings of a localized filling defect with stretched and thin valvulae conniventes overlying it (coiled-spring appearance). Because the

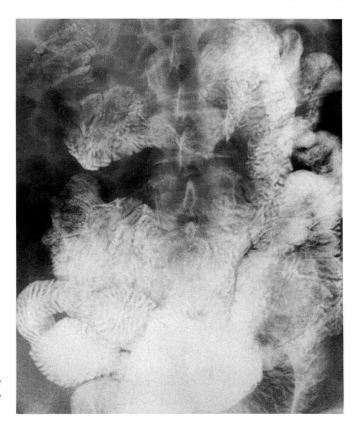

Fig. 35-7. Idiopathic (nontropical) sprue. The barium in the dilated loops of small bowel has a coarse, granular appearance due to hypersecretion.

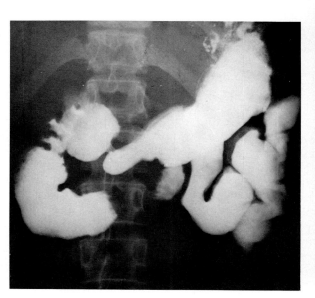

35-8

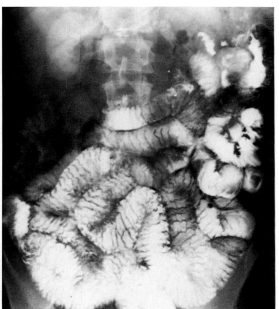

35-9

Fig. 35-8. *Moulage* sign in sprue. The duodenum and jejunum are completely featureless, a characteristic appearance of advanced disease. (Feczko P, Halpert R, Gedgaudas–McClees RK: Radiology of the small bowel. In Gegaudas–McClees RK (ed): Gastrointestinal Imaging, New York, Churchill Livingstone, 1987)

Fig. 35-9. Reversal of jejunoileal fold pattern in sprue. Note the dilatation and the markedly increased number of folds in the ileum. The jejunum is smooth and atrophic, and there is dilution of the barium due to increased secretions. (Bova JG, Friedman AC, Weser E et al: Adaptation of the ileum in nontropical sprue: Reversal of the jejunoileal fold pattern. AJR 144: 299–302, 1985)

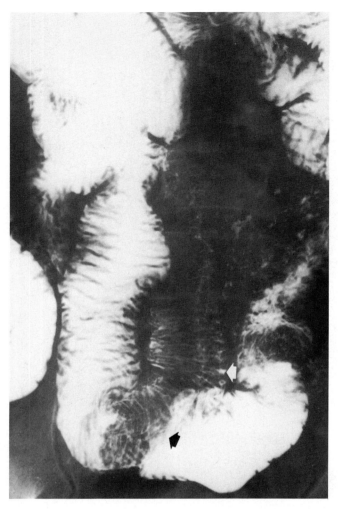

Fig. 35-10. Intussusception **(arrows)** in idiopathic (nontropical) sprue. Note the characteristic coiled-spring appearance.

considered whenever a patient with sprue shows a sudden refractoriness to treatment or develops fever, bowel perforation, or hemorrhage. It should also be considered when a patient with sprue has severe constitutional symptoms and malabsorption at the time of initial presentation. Not only is there the risk of developing lymphoma in sprue, but the prognosis of such a lymphoma is extremely poor (average survival of only 9 months as compared with an almost 50% 5-year survival rate for primary intestinal lymphoma). Primary diffuse intestinal lymphoma is rare in the Western world but relatively frequent in adolescents and young adults in populations native to Middle Eastern countries. Symptoms and signs of intestinal malabsorption are a prominent feature, and the radiographic findings may be indistinguishable from sprue. More commonly, lymphoma produces thickening of the bowel wall, displacement of intestinal loops, and extraluminal masses, any of which can be superimposed on the classic sprue pattern. There is also a significantly increased incidence of small bowel and esophageal carcinoma in those patients (especially males) with long-established sprue who have not adhered strictly to a gluten-free diet.

CONNECTIVE TISSUE DISEASE

The connective tissue diseases, particularly scleroderma, can also cause the malabsorption syndrome and the radiographic pattern of dilated small bowel with normal folds (Fig. 35-11). The small bowel can be affected at any time during the course of scleroderma; however, skin changes, joint symptoms, or the appearance of Raynaud's phenomenon usually precede changes in the small bowel. In scleroderma, smooth muscle atrophy and deposition of connective tissue in the submucosal, muscular, and serosal layers result in hypomotility of the small bowel and an extremely prolonged transit time. Although dilatation is often most marked in the duodenum proximal to the site at which the transverse portion passes between the aorta and superior mesenteric artery, the entire small bowel can be diffusely involved (Fig. 35-12). In scleroderma, there is frequently a relative decrease in the distance between the valvulae conniventes for any given degree of small bowel dilatation. This "hidebound" sign of folds that are abnormally packed together despite bowel dilatation (Fig. 35-13) is in sharp contrast to the typical wide longitudinal separation of valvulae seen with bowel dilatation in sprue and small bowel obstruction. Pseudosacculations, large broad-necked outpouchings simulating small bowel diverticula, are also characteristic of scleroderma. Dermatomyositis, another systemic connective tissue disorder, can produce a radiographic pattern identical to that of scleroderma.

intussusceptions in sprue are transient and nonobstructing, they are often missed on a single examination.

The diagnosis of sprue is made by jejunal biopsy, which demonstrates flattening, broadening, coalescence, and sometimes complete atrophy of intestinal villi. A characteristic finding of idiopathic sprue and celiac disease of children is dramatic clinical and histologic improvement after the patient has been placed on a diet free from gluten (the water-insoluble protein fraction of cereal grains). The radiographic and jejunal biopsy findings in tropical sprue are identical to those seen in idiopathic sprue. However, clinical improvement in tropical sprue follows folic acid or antibiotic therapy rather than gluten withdrawal.

LYMPHOMA

Diffuse intestinal lymphoma may complicate longstanding sprue, and this complication should be

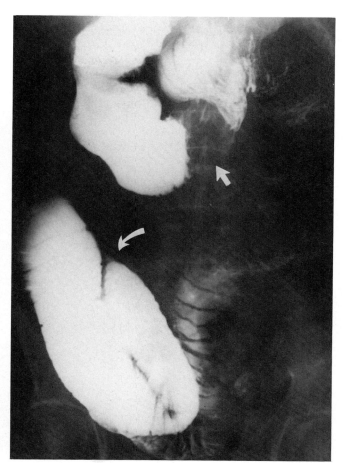

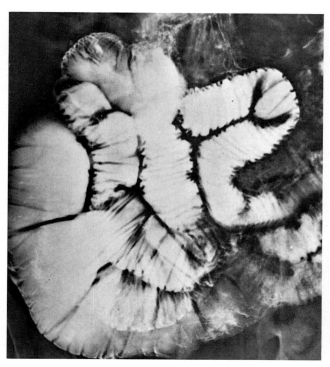

35-11

35-12

Fig. 35-11. Scleroderma causing the malabsorption syndrome and the radiographic pattern of dilated small bowel with normal folds.

Fig. 35-12. Scleroderma. There is diffuse dilatation of distal small bowel loops **(curved arrow)** in addition to severe dilatation of the duodenum proximal to the site at which the transverse portion passes between the aorta and superior mesenteric artery **(straight arrow)**.

Fig. 35-13. Scleroderma. For the degree of dilatation, the small bowel folds are packed strikingly close together ("hidebound" pattern).

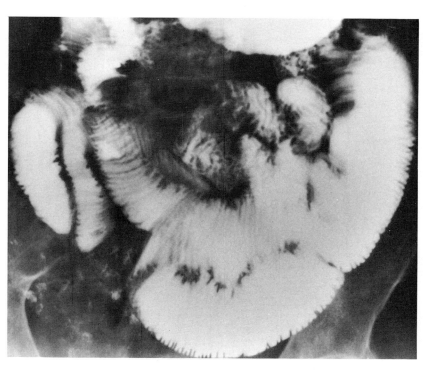

35-13

Scleroderma and sprue can usually be readily distinguished from one another on the basis of radiographic findings. In contrast to the appearance in scleroderma, the small bowel in patients with sprue has relatively normal motility, is most often dilated in the mid and distal jejunum, and generally demonstrates increased secretions.

DIABETES WITH HYPOKALEMIA

Although the small bowel examination in patients with diabetes mellitus is usually normal, dilatation of the small bowel with normal folds has been described when this disease is complicated by hypokalemia. The underlying pathologic mechanism, which occasionally results in severe diarrhea and malabsorption, is probably a visceral neuropathy.

LACTASE DEFICIENCY

Lactase deficiency, the most common of the disaccharidase-deficiency syndromes, is an isolated enzyme defect in which the patient is unable to hydrolyze and absorb lactose properly. In some

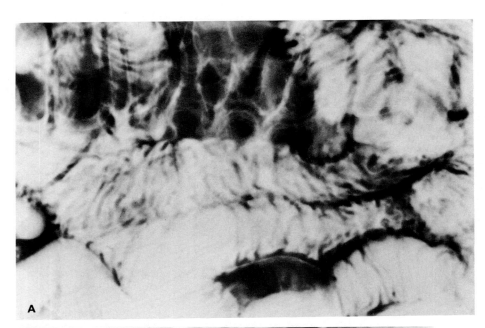

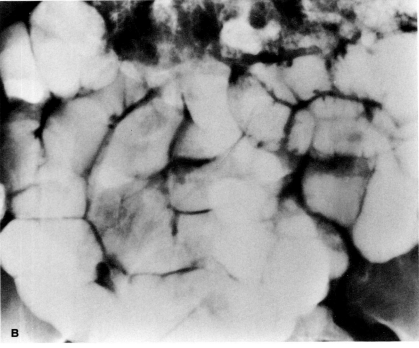

Fig. 35-14. Lactase deficiency. **(A)** Normal conventional small bowel examination. **(B)** After the addition of 50 g of lactose to the barium mixture, there is marked dilatation of the small bowel with dilution of barium, rapid transit, and reproduction of symptoms.

population groups, such as North American blacks, Mexicans, and Chinese, more than 75% of all adults have lactase deficiency. Even among whites in North America and Northern Europe, groups that are the least affected, this enzyme defect can be demonstrated in 3% to 20% of adults. The diagnosis of lactase deficiency should be suggested whenever a patient experiences abdominal discomfort, cramps, and watery diarrhea within 30 minutes to several hours of ingesting milk or milk products. Although conventional small bowel examinations are normal in patients with lactase deficiency (Fig. 35-14*A*), the addition of 25 g to 100 g of lactose to the barium mixture results in marked dilatation of the small bowel with dilution of barium, rapid transit, and reproduction of symptoms (Fig. 35-14*B*).

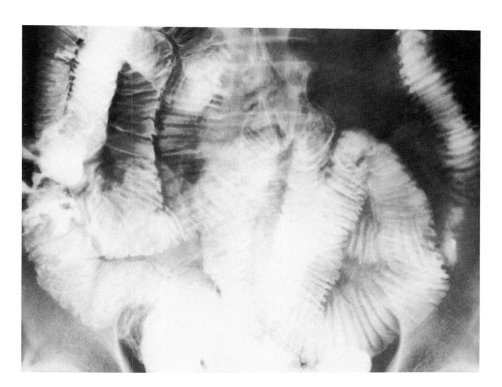

Fig. 35-15. Systemic lupus erythematosus. The small bowel is dilated with normal folds.

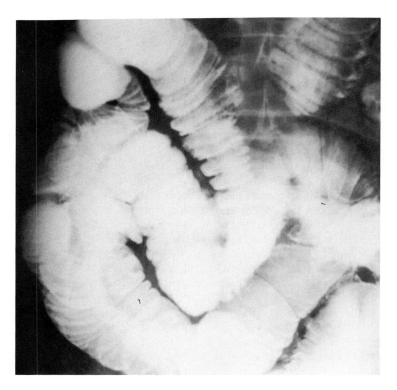

Fig. 35-16. Amyloidosis. The small bowel is dilated with normal folds.

VASCULAR INSUFFICIENCY

Vascular insufficiency of the muscular layer of the small bowel can produce ischemic alteration of motility, which causes delayed intestinal transit and bowel dilatation. Although regular thickening of mucosal folds is characteristic of mesenteric ischemia with hemorrhage, a normal fold pattern is occasionally seen if the disturbance of intestinal motility, rather than intramural bleeding, is the major abnormality. Increased intraluminal fluid dilutes the barium column.

Mesenteric ischemia secondary to atherosclerosis in patients over the age of 50 is the major vascular cause of malabsorption and the radiographic pattern of dilated small bowel with normal folds. A similar appearance can be demonstrated in patients with vasculitis due to systemic lupus erythematosus (Fig. 35-15) and in patients with massive deposition of amyloid in perivascular and muscular tissues of the small bowel (Fig. 35-16).

CHRONIC IDIOPATHIC INTESTINAL PSEUDO-OBSTRUCTION

Chronic idiopathic intestinal pseudo-obstruction is a rare condition characterized by repeated bouts of signs and symptoms of mechanical obstruction without an organic lesion (Fig. 35-17). Although the etiology is unclear, chronic idiopathic intestinal pseudo-obstruction is probably related to various abnormalities of smooth muscle and the intramural nerve plexuses. Exclusion of the possibility of a true mechanical obstruction is important to prevent the patient from undergoing an unnecessary and unrevealing laparotomy. A similar pattern of small bowel dilatation with normal folds can be seen in Chagas' disease, in which trypanosomes extensively invade the smooth muscle and destroy intrinsic neurons and ganglion cells in the bowel wall.

SMALL BOWEL BIOPSY

If radiographic and clinical findings are not sufficient to distinguish among the diseases producing the pattern of dilated small bowel with normal folds, a small bowel biopsy may be required. A normal small bowel pattern suggests surgical or chemical vagotomy, chronic idiopathic intestinal pseudo-obstruction, or diabetes, although degeneration of the myenteric plexus can occasionally be demonstrated in severe diabetics. In sprue, the small bowel biopsy shows villous atrophy and submucosal plasma cell infiltration. In diffuse intestinal lymphoma, there is lymphomatous infiltration into the submucosa. Small bowel biopsy in scleroderma and dermatomyositis demonstrates normal villi but collagenous replacement of the muscularis and varying degrees of vasculitis. Patients with Chagas' disease have sig-

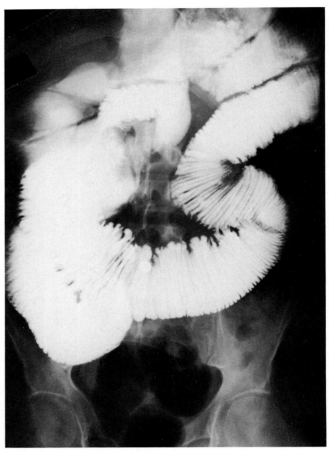

Fig. 35-17. Chronic idiopathic intestinal pseudo-obstruction. There is diffuse small bowel dilatation with normal folds. (Maldonado JE, Gregg JA, Green PA et al: Chronic idiopathic intestinal pseudo-obstruction. Am J Med 49:203–212, 1970)

nificant destruction of the submucosal and myenteric autonomic plexuses in the small bowel; an intermediate form of the causative organism can be found in the blood, bone marrow, spleen, or enlarged lymph nodes.

BIBLIOGRAPHY

Bova JG, Friedman AC, Weser E et al: Adaptation of the ileum in nontropical sprue: Reversal of the jejunoileal fold pattern. AJR 144:299–302, 1985

Burrows FGO, Toye DKM: Barium studies (in coeliac disease). Clin Gastroenterol 3:91–107, 1974

Cooper BT, Holmes GKT, Ferguson R et al: Celiac disease and malignancy. Medicine (Baltimore) 59:249–261, 1980

Couris GD, Block MA, Rupe CE: Gastrointestinal complications of collagen diseases. Arch Surg 89:695–700, 1964

Feldman F, Marshak RH: Dermatomyositis with significant involvement of the gastrointestinal tract. AJR 90:746–752, 1963

Horowitz AL, Meyers MA: The "hide-bound" small bowel of

scleroderma: Characteristic mucosal fold pattern. AJR 119:332–334, 1973

Isbell RG, Carlson HC, Hoffman HN: Roentgenologic pathologic correlation in malabsorption syndromes. AJR 107:158–169, 1969

Jones B, Bayless TM, Fishman EK et al: Lymphadenopathy in celiac disease: Computed tomographic observations. AJR 142:1127–1132, 1984

Legge DA, Wollaeger EE, Carlson HC: Intestinal pseudo-obstruction in systemic amyloidosis. Gut 11:764–767, 1970

Lewicki AM, Kleinhaus U, Brooks JR et al: The small bowel following pyloroplasty and vagotomy. Radiology 109:539–544, 1973

Maldonado JE, Gregg JA, Green PA et al: Chronic idiopathic pseudo-obstruction. Am J Med 49:203–212, 1970

Meyers MA, Kaplowitz N, Bloom AA: Malabsorption secondary to mesenteric ischemia. AJR 119:352–358, 1973

Morrison WJ, Christopher NL, Bayless TM et al: Low lactase levels: Evaluation of the radiologic diagnosis. Radiology 111:513–518, 1974

Moss AA, Goldberg HI, Brotman M: Idiopathic intestinal pseudo-obstruction. AJR 115:312–317, 1972

Poirier T, Rankin G: Gastrointestinal manifestations of progressive systemic sclerosis, based on a review of 364 cases. Am J Gastroenterol 58:30–44, 1972

Preger L, Amberg JR: Sweet diarrhea: Roentgen diagnosis of disaccharidase deficiency. AJR 101:287–295, 1967

Rohrmann CA Jr, Ricci MT, Krishnamurthy S et al: Radiologic and histologic differentiation of neuromuscular disorders of the gastrointestinal tract: Visceral myopathy, visceral neuropathy, and progressive systemic sclerosis. AJR 143:933–941, 1981

Teixidor HS, Heneghan MA: Idiopathic intestinal pseudo-obstruction in a family. Gastrointest Radiol 3:91–95, 1978

Wruble LD, Kalser MH: Diabetic steatorrhea: A distinct entity. Am J Med 37:118–129, 1964

36

DILATATION WITH THICKENED MUCOSAL FOLDS

Disease Entities

Zollinger-Ellison syndrome
Vascular insufficiency states
Diseases affecting the bowel wall and
    mesentery
  Metastases
  Crohn's disease
  Tuberculosis
  Radiation enteritis
Infectious enteritis
Amyloidosis
Lymphoma
Abetalipoproteinemia
Hypoalbuminemia

ZOLLINGER–ELLISON SYNDROME

The Zollinger–Ellison syndrome is caused by a non-beta islet cell tumor of the pancreas that continually secretes gastrin (Fig. 36-1). The persistently high blood level of this hormone results in a strong stimulus to the gastric parietal cells and the development of large gastric rugal folds. Voluminous gastric hypersecretion and hyperacidity produce a clinical picture of severe, often intractable, peptic ulcer disease. Although most ulcers in patients with the Zollinger–Ellison syndrome occur in the stomach or duodenal bulb, up to 25% may be in an atypical location in more distal portions of the duodenum and in the jejunum. Giant duodenal ulcers,

though not pathognomonic, should suggest the possibility of the Zollinger–Ellison syndrome.

The unusual location of the peptic ulcers seen distal to the duodenal bulb is due to the excessively large volume of highly acid gastric fluid that bathes the duodenum and proximal jejunum and overwhelms the alkaline biliary and pancreatic secretions. The resultant chemical enteritis produces severe ulceration and inflammatory fold thickening in the vulnerable distal duodenum and proximal jejunum, which are not normally exposed to such an acid environment. Because the normal succus entericus in the more distal portions of the small bowel dilutes the acid gastric contents and raises the pH, the mucosal pattern of the distal jejunum and the ileum is usually normal.

Massive gastric hypersecretion in the Zollinger–Ellison syndrome leads to large amounts of fluid entering the small intestine from the stomach and, consequently, to small bowel dilatation. This phenomenon also results in considerable dilution of the barium, which appears to have a gray, watery appearance.

Although most gastrin-secreting tumors of the pancreas are very small, about 50% are malignant. Metastases (usually to regional lymph nodes or the liver) continue to secrete gastrin and stimulate the gastric parietal cell mass even after the primary tumor of the pancreas has been removed or a total pancreatectomy has been performed. In about 10% of cases, the tumor lies in an ectopic location (stomach, duodenum, splenic hilum). Therefore, the proper treatment is removal of the entire target

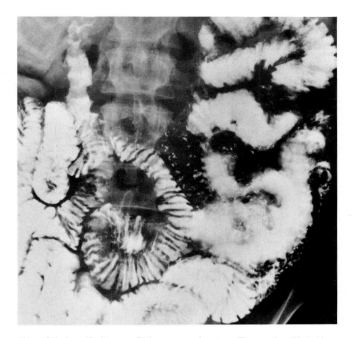

Fig. 36-1. *Zollinger-Ellison syndrome. There is dilatation with fold thickening involving proximal small bowel loops. Characteristic findings of the Zollinger-Ellison syndrome demonstrated on this radiograph include thickening of gastric rugae, markedly edematous folds in the second portion of the duodenum, and a gray, watery appearance of the barium in the proximal small bowel. The latter finding reflects dilution by a large amount of intestinal fluid.*

organ (*i.e.*, the parietal cell mass of the stomach) by total gastrectomy. If the proper diagnosis of Zollinger–Ellison syndrome is not made, death is usually caused by complications of fulminant peptic ulcer disease, which can rapidly recur following repeated ordinary peptic ulcer operations.

The Zollinger–Ellison syndrome frequently coexists with multiple endocrine adenomatosis. In addition to the pancreas, the most commonly involved endocrine glands are the adrenals, parathyroids, and pituitary.

VASCULAR INSUFFICIENCY

In vascular insufficiency states, the radiographic pattern of small bowel dilatation and thickened mucosal folds is produced by a combination of adynamic ileus and submucosal hemorrhage and edema. This condition can be secondary to venous obstruction, embolic arterial occlusion, or hypoperfusion due to atherosclerotic disease or low cardiac output.

DISEASES AFFECTING THE BOWEL WALL AND MESENTERY

Diseases affecting both the bowel wall and the mesentery can produce small bowel dilatation with

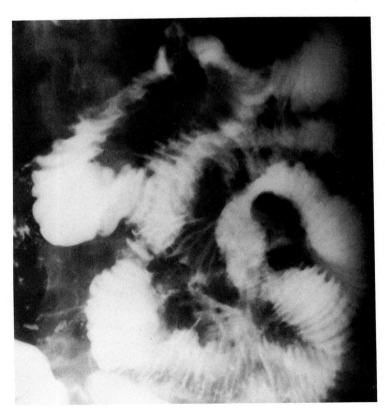

Fig. 36-2. *Tuberculosis. Small bowel dilatation with fold thickening is due to inflammatory disease involving both the small bowel and the mesentery.*

thickening of mucosal folds. The major disorders in this group are metastases, Crohn's disease, tuberculosis (Fig. 36-2), and radiation enteritis. In all three conditions, there is initial thickening of mucosal folds resulting from infiltration of the bowel wall (metastatic, inflammatory, or granulomatous) often combined with edema (secondary to lymphatic or venous blockage by the infiltrating process). If the mesentery is also thickened by infiltration or fibrotic response, kinking and twisting of bowel around the mesentery can lead to bowel obstruction and subsequent proximal dilatation.

INFECTIOUS ENTERITIS

Thickened folds and dilatation involving the jejunum and ileum appear to be nonspecific responses to infectious enteritis, especially in patients with compromised immune systems. This pattern has been reported in patients with enteritis due to *Salmonella, Strongyloides stercoralis, Candida,* cy-

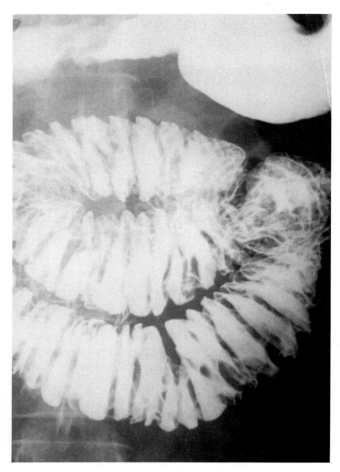

Fig. 36-4. Hypoalbuminemia. Marked dilatation of the jejunum with regular thickening of folds is seen in this patient with cirrhosis, portal hypertension, and hypoalbuminemia (serum albumin of 1.5 g/dl). (Farthing MJG, McLean AM, Bartram CI et al: Radiologic features of the jejunum in hypoalbuminemia. AJR 136:883–886, 1981. Copyright 1981. Reproduced with permission)

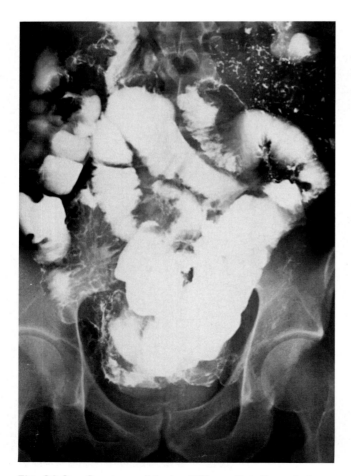

Fig. 36-3. Cryptosporidiosis. Diffuse dilatation of the small bowel with irregular fold thickening in a patient with AIDS. (Berk RN, Wall SD, McCardle CB et al: Cryptosporidiosis of the stomach and small intestine in patients with AIDS. AJR 143:549–554, 1984. Copyright 1984. Reproduced with permission)

tomegalovirus, cryptosporidiosis (Fig. 36-3), and *Mycobacterium avium-intracellulare* (see Fig. 38-25).

OTHER CAUSES

Unusual causes of small bowel dilatation with associated thickening of mucosal folds include amyloidosis, lymphoma, and abetalipoproteinemia. These are primarily infiltrative processes. Lymphoma predominantly involves the submucosa, in contrast to amyloidosis, in which amyloid is deposited around small blood vessels in the submucosa and between fibers in the muscular layer. In abetalipoproteinemia, there are excessive numbers of fat droplets in mucosal cells. Small bowel dilatation is unusual in these diseases and occurs only at a late stage, when the infiltrating material has caused destruction or dysfunction of the bowel musculature or, in the case of lymphoma, when the tumor mass has obstructed the lumen.

Dilatation of the jejunum has been reported to accompany the characteristic regular thickening of folds in patients with hypoalbuminemia due to cirrhosis or the nephrotic syndrome (Fig. 36-4). The degree of jejunal dilatation was shown to be closely related to the level of serum albumin; no dilatation was noted unless the serum albumin was 2.7 g/dl or less (albumin threshold).

BIBLIOGRAPHY

Berk RN, Wall SD, McArdle CB et al: Cryptosporidiosis of the stomach and small intestine in patients with AIDS. AJR 143:549–554, 1984

Christoforidis AJ, Nelson SW: Radiological manifestations of ulcerogenic tumors of the pancreas: The Zollinger–Ellison syndrome. JAMA 198:511–516, 1966

Dallemand S, Waxman M, Farman J: Radiological manifestations of *Strongyloides stercoralis*. Gastrointest Radiol 8:45–51, 1983

Dent DM, Duys PJ, Bird AR et al: Cytomegalovirus infection of bowel in adults. S Afr Med J 49:669–672, 1975

Farthing MJG, McLean AM, Bartram CI: Radiologic features of the jejunum in hypoalbuminemia. AJR 136:883–886, 1981

Legge DA, Carlson HC, Wollaeger EE: Roentgenologic appearance of systemic amyloidosis involving the gastrointestinal tract. AJR 110:406–412, 1970

Radin DR, Fong TL, Halls JM et al: Monilial enteritis in acquired immune deficiency syndrome. AJR 141:1289–1290, 1983

Rubin P, Casarett GW: Clinical Radiation Pathology, Vol 1, pp 193–240. Philadelphia, WB Saunders, 1968

Weinstein MA, Pearson KD, Agus SG: Abetalipoproteinemia. Radiology 108:269–273, 1973

Wiot JF: Intramural small intestinal hemorrhage—A differential diagnosis. Semin Roentgenol 1:219–233, 1966

Zboralske FF, Amberg JR: Detection of the Zollinger–Ellison syndrome: The radiologist's responsibility. AJR 104:529–543, 1968

37 REGULAR THICKENING OF SMALL BOWEL FOLDS

Disease Entities

Hemorrhage into the bowel wall
  Anticoagulant therapy
  Ischemic bowel disease or infarction
  Vasculitis
    Connective tissue diseases
    Thromboangiitis obliterans (Buerger's
      disease)
    Henoch–Schönlein syndrome
  Hemophilia
  Idiopathic thrombocytopenic purpura
  Trauma
  Coagulation defects secondary to other
     diseases
    Hypoprothrombinemia
    Leukemia
    Multiple myeloma
    Lymphoma
    Metastatic carcinoma
    Hypofibrinogenemia/circulating anticoag-
      ulants/fibrinolytic system activation
Intestinal edema
  Hypoproteinemia
    Cirrhosis
    Nephrotic syndrome
    Protein-losing enteropathy
  Lymphatic blockage
    Tumor infiltration
    Lymphangiitis secondary to irradiation
      damage

  Fibrosis of the mesentery
  Angioneurotic edema
  Intestinal lymphangiectasia
    Primary
    Secondary
  Abetalipoproteinemia
  Eosinophilic enteritis
  Amyloid vasculitis
  Xanthomatosis
  Pneumatosis intestinalis

Thickening of small bowel mucosal folds (>3 mm) can be caused by any process that increases the volume of fluid or cells in the submucosal or mucosal region. The thickened folds associated with hemorrhage or edema (as well as with the other entities discussed in this section) are usually regular in appearance, widest at the base and progressively narrower toward the tip. They are perpendicular to the bowel lumen and parallel to neighboring folds. In contrast, the extensive group of diseases that infiltrate the bowel wall with deposition of cells or other amorphous material produce thickened folds that may be distorted and irregular, not perpendicular to the lumen, and angled with respect to neighboring folds.

HEMORRHAGE INTO THE BOWEL WALL

Any cause of bleeding into the bowel wall can lead to uniform, regular thickening of small bowel folds

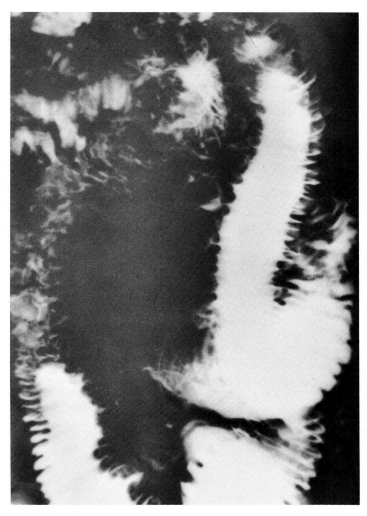

Fig. 37-1. Hemorrhage into the wall of the small bowel. The symmetric, spike-like configuration mimics a stack of coins.

Fig. 37-2. Intramural hemorrhage in a patient receiving Coumadin (warfarin) therapy. **(A)** Eccentric mass with shouldering and partial obstruction **(arrow)**, suggesting a neoplastic process. **(B)** Complete resolution following withdrawal of the drug and conservative treatment. The **arrow** points to the previously involved loop.

37-1

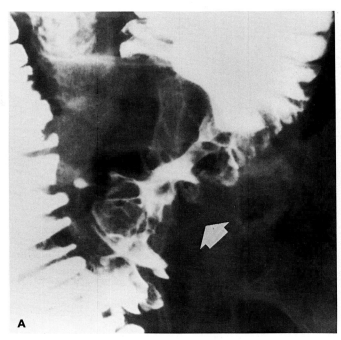

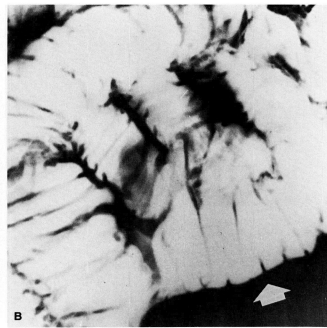

37-2

with sharply delineated margins. The parallel arrangement produces a symmetric, spike-like configuration simulating a stack of coins or picket fence (Fig. 37-1). This appearance is more striking in the jejunum than distally because of the better development and normally greater prominence of jejunal folds. With some causes of intestinal hemorrhage, increased secretions and edema blur the sharpness and symmetry of the folds. Localized hemorrhage produces scalloping and thumbprinting. Concomitant bleeding into the mesentery (especially in hemophiliacs and in patients receiving anticoagulant therapy) often results in an intramural or extrinsic mass (Fig. 37-2), flattening of folds on the mesenteric side of the bowel, and separation and uncoiling of bowel loops (Fig. 37-3).

ISCHEMIC BOWEL DISEASE

Ischemic bowel disease is relatively common among elderly patients with cardiac failure and arteriosclerosis. It can also be caused by thrombosis or embolic occlusion of a major mesenteric artery or vein or its peripheral branches. Ischemic disease can be a complication of the use of hormonal contraceptive pills by young women. Trauma, surgery on the abdominal aorta, and the endarteritis with vascular occlusion that may follow radiation therapy (>5000 rad) to the small bowel can also result in ischemic bowel disease. The presenting symptom is usually colicky periumbilical pain, which may be-

come more diffuse and continuous. Vomiting, abdominal distention, and bloody diarrhea also commonly occur.

The broad spectrum of radiographic appearances in patients with mesenteric vascular insufficiency depends on the rapidity of onset, the length of intestine involved, and the extent of collateral circulation. Rapid occlusion of the major mesenteric vessels results in massive bowel necrosis and death from peritonitis and shock. However, if segmental rather than major vessels are involved, and if the occlusion is slow enough to allow collateral blood flow to develop, total intestinal infarction will not occur. In these cases, the relative degrees of damage and healing give rise to a variety of radiographic findings (Fig. 37-4).

Bleeding into the bowel wall secondary to ischemic mesenteric vascular disease classically produces the radiographic pattern of regular thickening of small bowel folds. Other manifestations of bowel ischemia include ulceration, thumbprinting, sacculation, and stricture formation.

VASCULITIS

Vasculitis can compromise the blood supply to a segment of the small bowel and cause ischemic or hemorrhagic changes in the bowel wall. In systemic connective tissue diseases (rheumatoid arthritis, polyarteritis nodosa, systemic lupus erythematosus, dermatomyositis), a necrotizing vasculitis can in-

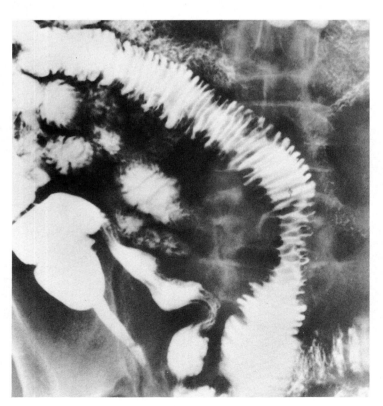

Fig. 37-3. Bleeding into the bowel wall and mesentery due to an overdose of Coumadin (warfarin). In addition to regular thickening of folds, note the separation and uncoiling of bowel loops.

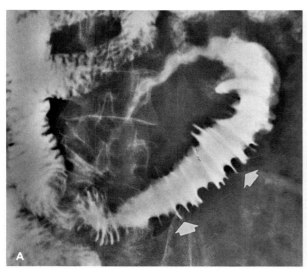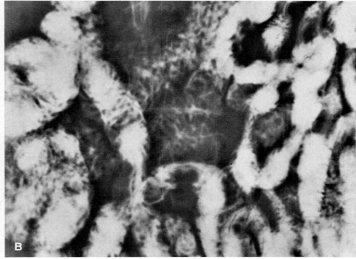

Fig. 37-4. *Small bowel ischemia.* **(A)** *Segmental ischemia in a picket-fence pattern of regular thickening of small bowel folds* **(arrows)**. **(B)** *Complete resolution of the ischemic process following conservative therapy.*

volve small arteries, arterioles, and veins in the bowel wall (Fig. 37-5). In severe cases, massive bleeding, multiple infarctions, and perforation may also occur.

Thromboangiitis obliterans, which is usually found in relatively young men who are heavy smokers, is generally considered to be a peripheral vascular disease. However, this condition can also affect the gastrointestinal tract and produce inflammation of the mesenteric vessels, resulting in ischemic changes in the bowel wall and regular thickening of small bowel folds.

The Henoch–Schönlein syndrome is an acute arteritis characterized by purpura, nephritis, abdominal pain, and joint pain. The disease tends to be self-limited and frequently develops several weeks after a streptococcal infection. Like other causes of vasculitis, Henoch–Schönlein purpura causes a radiographic pattern of regular thickening of small bowel folds (Fig. 37-6). Large amounts of edema and hemorrhage can lead to scalloping, thumbprinting, and dilution of contrast. Henoch–Schönlein purpura can also affect the colon, causing circumferential submucosal lesions with marked luminal narrowing simulating carcinoma.

HEMOPHILIA

Hemophilia is an inherited (sex-linked recessive) anomaly of blood coagulation that appears clinically only in males. Patients with this disease have a decreased or absent serum concentration of antihe-

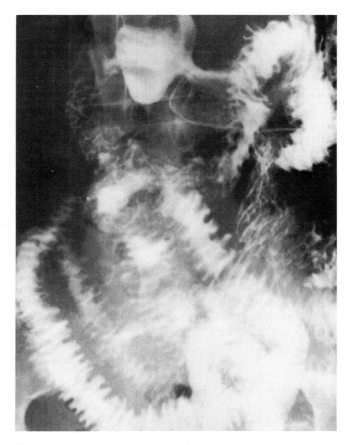

Fig. 37-5. *Systemic lupus erythematosus causing ischemic and hemorrhagic changes in the bowel wall and the radiographic pattern of regular thickening of small bowel folds.*

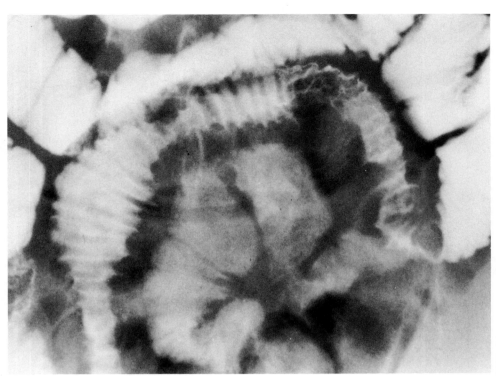

Fig. 37-6. Henoch-Schönlein purpura causing regular thickening of small bowel folds.

mophilic globulin and suffer a life-long tendency for spontaneous hemorrhage. Bleeding into the intestinal wall is more frequently found in the small bowel than in the colon. The extent of bleeding is variable, and either a short or a long segment of small bowel can display the radiographic appearance of regular thickening of folds.

IDIOPATHIC THROMBOCYTOPENIC PURPURA

Acute idiopathic thrombocytopenic purpura typically presents with the sudden onset of severe purpura 1 to 2 weeks after a sore throat or upper respiratory infection in an otherwise healthy child. The manifestations of acute idiopathic thrombocytopenic purpura include extensive petechial hemorrhages and gingival, gastrointestinal, and genitourinary bleeding. In more than 80% of patients, this disorder is self-limited and clears spontaneously within 2 weeks.

Unlike the acute form, chronic idiopathic thrombocytopenic purpura occurs primarily in young female adults. The disease usually has an insidious onset, with a relatively long history of easy bruising and menorrhagia. Because most patients with this condition have a circulating platelet autoantibody that develops without underlying disease or significant exposure to drugs, chronic idiopathic thrombocytopenic purpura is generally considered to be an autoimmune disorder. Although steroid therapy leads to complete recovery in some patients, splenectomy is required in most cases. This can result in long-term and even permanent remission, presumably due to removal of a major site of platelet destruction as well as elimination of a major source of synthesis of platelet antibodies.

Hemorrhage into the small bowel caused by either acute or chronic idiopathic thrombocytopenic purpura produces characteristic uniform, regular thickening of mucosal folds in the affected intestinal segment (Fig. 37-7).

TRAUMA

Intramural hemorrhage secondary to trauma can present as localized, regular thickening of small bowel folds. In children, intramural hemorrhage is most commonly seen in boys who suffer abdominal injuries in athletics. In adults, small bowel contusion may occur after automobile accidents, especially in persons wearing seat belts. In addition to regular thickening of folds, traumatic small bowel hemorrhage can result in the formation of an intramural hematoma, a mass lesion that can narrow and even obstruct the lumen.

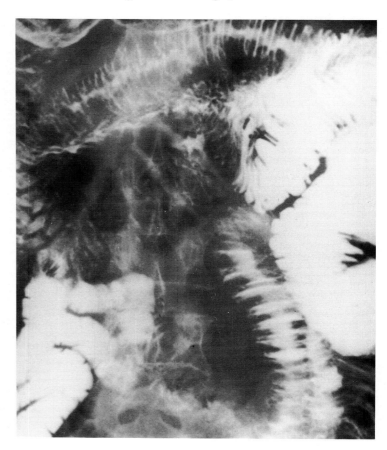

Fig. 37-7. Chronic idiopathic thrombocytopenic purpura. Hemorrhage into the wall of the small bowel causes regular thickening of mucosal folds.

COAGULATION DEFECTS

Any disease associated with defects in coagulation can cause intramural intestinal bleeding and the radiographic appearance of regular thickening of small bowel folds. In severe hepatic disease, the inability of the liver to properly synthesize clotting factors results in a bleeding diathesis. Coagulation defects are also frequently seen as complications of malignant conditions such as leukemia, multiple myeloma, lymphoma, and metastatic carcinoma. This may be due in part to replacement of bone marrow and deposition of large quantities of abnormal cells in reticuloendothelial organs (liver, spleen), leading to a decreased number of platelets and resultant intramural bleeding. Hypofibrinogenemia, circulating anticoagulants, and activation of the fibrinolytic system can also lead to intramural bleeding.

INTESTINAL EDEMA

HYPOPROTEINEMIA

Hypoproteinemia is the most common cause of intestinal edema. When the serum albumin level is 2 g/dl or lower, cell-free infiltrate accumulates in the bowel wall and causes regular, uniform thickening of small bowel folds (Fig. 37-8). Hypoalbuminemia can result from liver disease (cirrhosis) (Fig. 37-9), kidney disease (nephrotic syndrome), or protein loss from the gastrointestinal tract (due to protein-losing enteropathies such as Menetrier's disease, Crohn's disease, Whipple's disease, lymphoma, carcinoma, ulcerative colitis, and intestinal lymphangiectasia). Protein loss from the gastrointestinal tract can also complicate such apparently unrelated conditions as congestive heart failure, constrictive pericarditis, exudative skin lesions, burns, and allergic reactions. A similar pattern can be produced by edema of the wall of the bowel due to metastases in the liver or porta hepatis and obstruction of portal blood flow (Fig. 37-10).

LYMPHATIC BLOCKAGE

Obstruction of lymphatic channels draining the small bowel can result in intestinal edema and regular thickening of small bowel folds. Lymphatic blockage can be due to bowel wall or mesenteric infiltration by tumor, lymphangiitis secondary to ra-

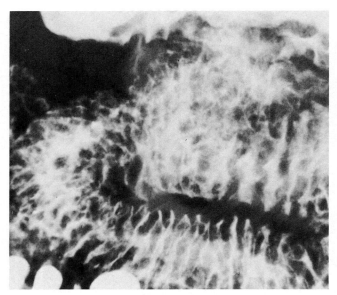

Fig. 37-8. Hypoproteinemia causing regular thickening of small bowel folds in a patient with cirrhosis.

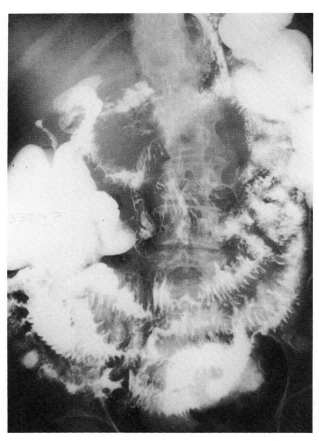

Fig. 37-10. Regular thickening of small bowel folds in a patient with edema of the bowel wall due to diffuse liver metastases and obstruction of portal blood flow.

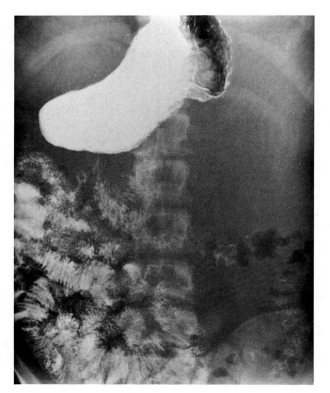

Fig. 37-9. Cirrhosis. There is regular thickening of small bowel folds. Note the marked splenomegaly.

diation damage, or fibrosis of the mesentery caused by inflammatory bowel disease or the desmoplastic response accompanying certain small bowel and mesenteric neoplasms.

ANGIONEUROTIC EDEMA

Angioneurotic edema is characterized by edematous, frequently localized, swellings of the skin, mucous membranes, or viscera. In this inherited disorder (dominant trait with irregular penetrance), visceral manifestations may be the first or the only presenting symptoms, and the patient may be initially thought to have an acute surgical abdomen. Clinical attacks are periodic and occur at irregular intervals. The most serious complication of angioneurotic edema is laryngeal edema, which is associated with a significant mortality rate.

The regular thickening of small bowel folds in angioneurotic edema tends to be more localized than the generalized intestinal edema seen in patients with hypoproteinemia (Fig. 37-11A). Adjacent loops of small bowel are often separated due to mural and mesenteric thickening. The radiographic

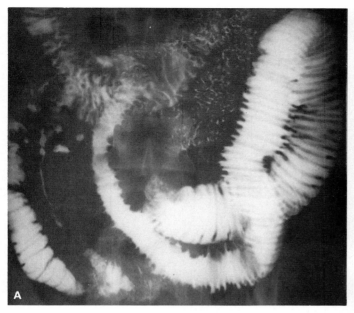

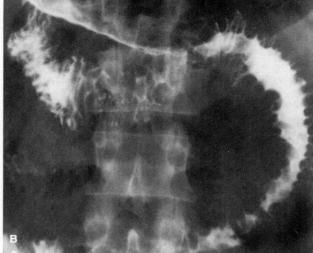

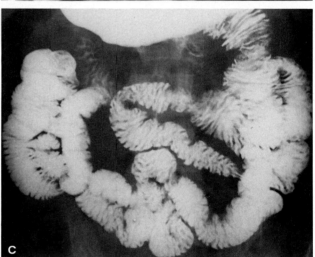

Fig. 37-11. Angioneurotic edema. **(A)** Regular thickening of folds in a portion of the distal jejunum during an acute attack. Areas of thumbprinting are also seen. **(B)** Regular thickening of proximal jejunal folds with thumbprinting during a previous acute attack in the same patient. **(C)** A repeat small bowel barium examination 36 hr after **(B)** demonstrates a dramatic return to a normal bowel pattern. (Pearson KD, Buchignani JS, Shimkin PM et al: Hereditary angioneurotic edema of the gastrointestinal tract. AJR 116:256–261, 1972. Copyright 1972. Reproduced with permission)

findings in angioneurotic edema are present only when the patient is in visceral crisis (Fig. 37-11*B*); they rapidly revert to normal as the attack subsides (Fig. 37-11*C*). This complete reversibility, combined with the characteristic family history and evidence of previous angioneurotic reaction, should allow differentiation of angioneurotic edema from other causes of regular thickening of small bowel folds.

INTESTINAL LYMPHANGIECTASIA

The hallmark of intestinal lymphangiectasia is gross dilatation of the lymphatics in the small bowel mucosa and submucosa. The primary form probably represents a congenital mechanical block to lymphatic outflow; secondary intestinal lymphangiectasia is a complication of inflammatory or neoplastic lymphadenopathy. The intestinal mucosa is filled with abundant foamy macrophages containing large, dense lipid droplets.

Regular thickening of small bowel mucosal folds is caused by a combination of intestinal edema and lymphatic dilatation (Fig. 37-12). Intestinal edema in patients with lymphangiectasia can be due to either lymphatic obstruction or severe loss of protein into the gastrointestinal tract. Diffuse intestinal edema in a patient (especially a child or young adult) with no evidence of liver, kidney, or heart disease should suggest the diagnosis of intestinal lymphangiectasia.

ABETALIPOPROTEINEMIA

Abetalipoproteinemia is a rare, recessively inherited disease manifested clinically by malabsorption of fat, progressive neurologic deterioration, and ret-

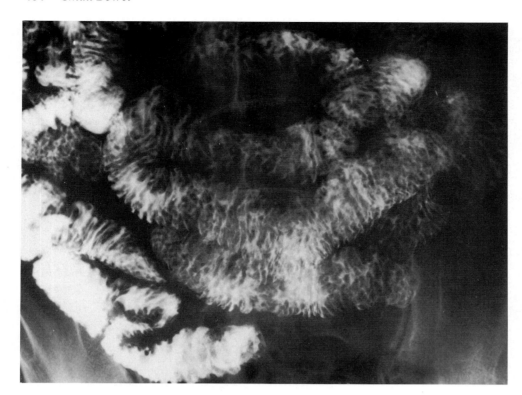

Fig. 37-12. Secondary lymphangiectasia. Lymphatic obstruction due to infiltration of the bowel wall and mesentery by metastatic carcinoma.

initis pigmentosa. An inability to produce the apoprotein moiety of the beta-lipoprotein leads to failure to transport lipid material out of the intestinal epithelial cell. This results in fat malabsorption, with no plasma beta-lipoproteins and markedly reduced serum levels of cholesterol, phospholipids, carotenoids, and vitamin A. Acanthocytosis, a thorny appearance of the red blood cells, is a characteristic finding. Jejunal biopsy reveals accumulation of foamy lipid material in the cytoplasm of intestinal epithelial cells, a pathognomonic lesion.

Abetalipoproteinemia presents radiographically as small bowel dilatation with mild to moderate thickening of mucosal folds (Fig. 37-13). Although most marked in the duodenum and jejunum, fold thickening is present throughout the small bowel. The folds may be uniformly thickened, demonstrate an irregular, more disorganized appearance, or even have a nodular pattern.

OTHER CAUSES

Regular thickening of small bowel mucosal folds can occur in the early phase of eosinophilic enter-

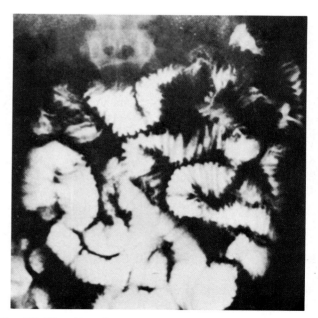

Fig. 37-13. Abetalipoproteinemia. There is regular thickening of folds in the jejunum with less marked changes in the ileum. Dilution and mild dilatation are also present. (Weinstein MA, Pearson KD, Agus SG: Abetalipoproteinemia. Radiology 108:269–273, 1973)

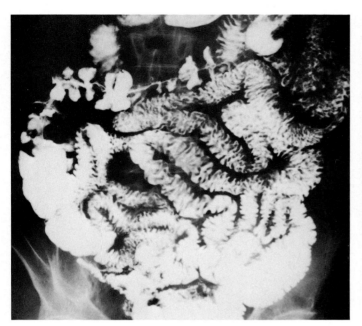

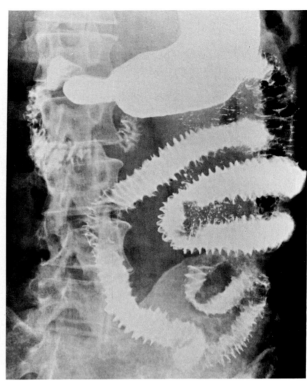

37-14   **37-15**

Fig. 37-14. Amyloidosis. There is relatively regular thickening of small bowel folds in this patient with clinical malabsorption. (Legge DA, Carlson HC, Wallaeger EE: Roentgenologic appearance of systemic amyloidosis involving gastrointestinal tract. AJR 110:406–412, 1970. Copyright 1970. Reproduced with permission)

Fig. 37-15. Xanthomatosis. Minimal dilatation of the jejunum with regular thickening of mucosal folds. (Pope TL, Shaffer H: Small bowel xanthomatosis: Radiologic-pathologic correlation. AJR 144:1215–1216, 1985. Copyright 1985. Reproduced with permission)

itis, when the considerable edema that accompanies the eosinophilic infiltrate has not yet extended through the bowel wall. As the disease progresses and infiltration becomes more extensive, the more characteristic distorted, irregular thickening of small bowel folds is seen. Amyloid involvement of the small bowel can cause symmetric thickening of folds due to vasculitis, infiltration, and edema (Fig. 37-14). In xanthomatosis, which is primarily a cutaneous disorder, multicentric proliferation of lipid-laden cells within the bowel wall can cause regular thickening of small bowel folds (Fig. 37-15). Narrowing of the stomach and colon have also been described in this condition. In patients with pneumatosis intestinalis involving the small bowel, the technical impossibility of demonstrating the outer walls of the radiolucent gas cysts can produce an appearance simulating regular thickening of small bowel folds.

BIBLIOGRAPHY

Dodds WJ, Spitzer RM, Friedland GW: Gastrointestinal roentgenographic manifestations of hemophilia. AJR 110:413–416, 1970

Ellis K, McConnell DJ: Hereditary angioneurotic edema involving the small intestine. Radiology 92:518–519, 1969

Ghahremani GG, Meyers MA, Farman J et al: Ischemic disease of the small bowel and colon associated with oral contraceptives. Gastrointest Radiol 2:221–228, 1977

Khilnani MT, Marshak RH, Eliasoph J et al: Intramural intestinal hemorrhage. AJR 92:1061–1071, 1964

Kumpe DA, Jaffe RB, Waldman TA et al: Constrictive pericarditis and protein-losing enteropathy: An imitator of intestinal lymphangiectasia. AJR 124:365–373, 1975

MacPherson RI: The radiologic manifestations of Henoch–Schoenlein purpura. J Can Assoc Radiol 25:275–281, 1974

Marshak RH, Khilnani MT, Eliasoph J et al: Intestinal edema. AJR 101:379–387, 1967

Marshak RH, Lindner AE, Maklansky D: Ischemia of the small intestine. Am J Gastroenterol 66:309–400, 1976

Marshak RH, Wolf BS, Cohen N et al: Protein-losing disorders of the gastrointestinal tract: Roentgen features. Radiology 77:893–906, 1961

Mueller CF, Morehead R, Alter AJ et al: Pneumatosis intestinalis in collagen disorders. AJR 115:300–305, 1972

Olmsted WW, Madewell JE: Lymphangiectasia of the small intestine: Description and pathophysiology of the roentgenographic signs. Gastrointest Radiol 1:241–243, 1976

Pearson KD, Buchignani JS, Shimkin PM et al: Hereditary angioneurotic edema of the gastrointestinal tract. AJR 116:256–261, 1972

Pope TL, Shaffer H: Small bowel xanthomatosis: Radiologic-pathologic correlation. AJR 144:1215–1216, 1985

Schwartz S, Boley S, Schultz L et al: A survey of vascular diseases of the small intestine. Semin Roentgenol 1:178–218, 1966

Shimkin PM, Waldmann TA, Krugman RL: Intestinal lymphangiectasia. AJR 110:827–841, 1970

Weinstein MA, Pearson KD, Agus SG: Abetalipoproteinemia. Radiology 108:269–273, 1973

Wiot JF: Intramural small intestinal hemorrhage—A differential diagnosis. Semin Roentgenol 1:219–233, 1966

GENERALIZED, IRREGULAR, DISTORTED SMALL BOWEL FOLDS

Disease Entities

Whipple's disease
Giardiasis
Lymphoma
Amyloidosis
Eosinophilic enteritis
Lymphangiectasia
Crohn's disease
Tuberculosis
Histoplasmosis
Mastocytosis
Strongyloidiasis
Yersinia enterocolitica
Typhoid fever
Other infections
   Campylobacter jejuni
   Shigella
   Escherichia coli
   Anisakiasis
   Cryptosporidium
   Mycobacterium avium-intracellulare
Alpha chain disease
Abetalipoproteinemia

Generalized, irregular, distorted mucosal folds without dilatation is the radiographic appearance of a wide variety of diseases that infiltrate the wall of the small bowel. Whether the infiltration is due to an infectious process, a nonspecific inflammation, or a malignancy, the disruption of normal architecture produces irregular thickening of the valvulae conniventes. To distinguish among the many diseases causing this pattern, the physician must carefully consider the site of the lesions, associated radiographic findings, and the patient's clinical history. In Whipple's disease, the lamina propria is extensively infiltrated by large macrophages filled with multiple glycoprotein granules that react positively to the periodic acid-Schiff (PAS) stain (Fig. 38-1). In patients with active disease, numerous small, gram-positive, rod-shaped bacilli also invade the involved tissues and produce a distinctive, usually diagnostic, histologic pattern. Most patients with Whipple's disease present with a generalized malabsorption syndrome; diarrhea is a prominent complaint. Extraintestinal symptoms (arthritis, fever, lymphadenopathy) are common and may precede gastrointestinal complaints by many years. The extensive thickening and distortion of the small bowel folds is most frequently seen in the duodenum and proximal jejunum; in severe cases, the distal jejunum and ileum may also be abnormal. The intestinal villi can swell to such an extent that they become bulbous structures visible to the naked eye. The lumen of the bowel can be normal or slightly dilated. Following successful treatment of Whipple's disease with antibiotic therapy, the irregular thickening of small bowel folds becomes less apparent, and the radiographic appearance may even revert to normal.

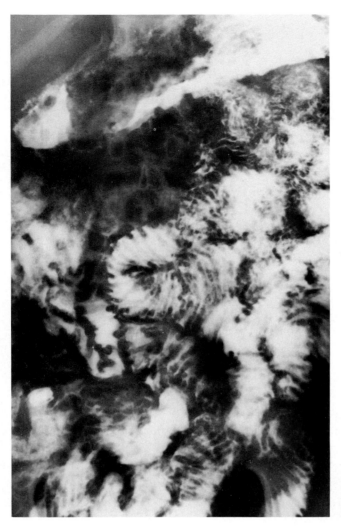

Fig. 38-1. Whipple's disease. Note the diffuse, irregular thickening of small bowel folds.

GIARDIASIS

Giardia lamblia is a protozoan parasite harbored by millions of asymptomatic individuals throughout the world. Clinically significant infestations occur predominantly in children, postgastrectomy patients, and travelers to endemic areas (*e.g.*, Leningrad, India, and the Rocky Mountains of Colorado). The infection is apparently acquired through drinking water. Clinical symptoms range from a mild gastroenteritis to a severe, protracted illness with profuse diarrhea, cramping, malabsorption, and weight loss. In children, the disease can cause a chronic malabsorption syndrome that appears identical to celiac sprue. A striking association has been noted between giardiasis and the gastrointestinal immunodeficiency syndromes.

The irregular, distorted, thickened small bowel mucosal folds in giardiasis are most apparent in the duodenum and jejunum (Fig. 38-2). Diffuse mucosal

inflammation, along with proliferative changes in the mucosal glands, edema of the lamina propria, and widespread infiltration by inflammatory cells, results in irregularly tortuous folds that present a distinctly nodular appearance when seen on end. Hypersecretion and hypermotility (rapid transit time) are also frequently noted. The lumen of the bowel is often narrowed because of spasm. When giardiasis complicates an immunodeficiency state, the irregularly thickened folds can be superimposed on a pattern of multiple tiny filling defects characteristic of nodular lymphoid hyperplasia.

An unequivocal diagnosis of *Giardia lamblia* infestation can be made through identification of the characteristic cysts in the stool. However, these cysts may be absent from the stool even in patients with severe disease. In such patients, the organism may be found only in smears of the jejunal mucus or by careful examination of the intervillous spaces on stained sections of a small bowel biopsy. Irradication of the parasite after treatment with Atabrine (quinacrine) or Flagyl (metronidazole) results in a return of the small bowel pattern to normal.

LYMPHOMA

Intestinal lymphoma can either originate in the small bowel (primary) or be a manifestation of a

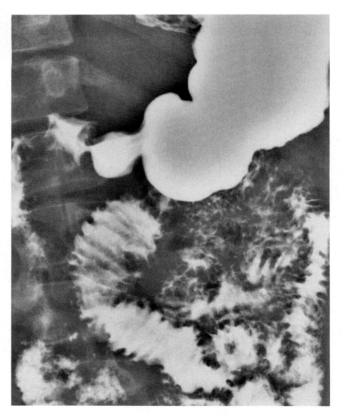

Fig. 38-2. Giardiasis. Irregular fold thickening is most prominent in the proximal small bowel.

disseminated lymphomatous process that affects many organs (secondary). In either case, the disease can be localized to a single intestinal segment, be multifocal, or diffusely involve most of the small bowel (Fig. 38-3). In primary lymphoma, the neoplasm arises in the lamina propria or lymph follicles and is localized to one segment in about 75% of patients. The disease is most frequent in the ileum, where the greatest amount of lymphoid tissue is present. Tumor destruction of the overlying epithelium causes ulceration. Isolated or multifocal polypoid tumor masses can develop and, if large enough or acting as the leading edge of an intussusception, can even obstruct the intestinal lumen. At times, the bowel wall becomes circumferentially infiltrated, resulting in a constricting napkin-ring lesion (Fig. 38-4). Neoplastic involvement of the adjacent mesentery and lymph nodes is common.

Approximately 25% of patients with disseminated lymphoma are found at autopsy to have small bowel involvement. A majority have multifocal intestinal lesions. Unlike the situation in primary intestinal lymphoma, the small bowel involvement in most patients with disseminated lymphoma is merely incidental; specific gastrointestinal symptoms are frequently absent.

A classic radiographic appearance of primary intestinal lymphoma is infiltration of the bowel wall with thickening or obliteration of mucosal folds (Fig. 38-5). Segmental constriction of the bowel is less commonly noted. If lymphoma produces large masses in the bowel that necrose and cavitate, the central core may slough into the bowel lumen and produce aneurysmal dilatation of the bowel (Fig. 38-6).

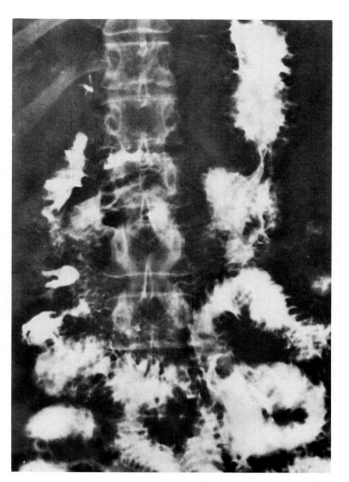

Fig. 38-3. Lymphoma. There is diffuse, irregular thickening of small bowel folds with mesenteric involvement and separation of bowel loops.

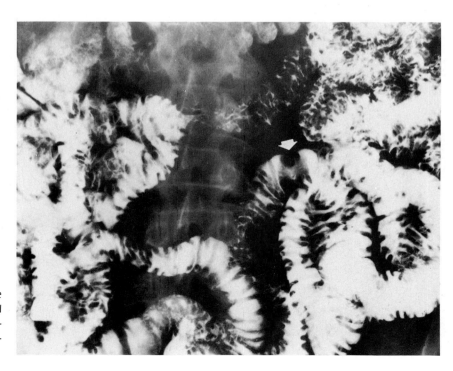

Fig. 38-4. Lymphoma. In addition to the generalized, irregular thickening of small bowel folds, there is segmental circumferential infiltration by tumor causing a constricting napkin-ring lesion **(arrow)**.

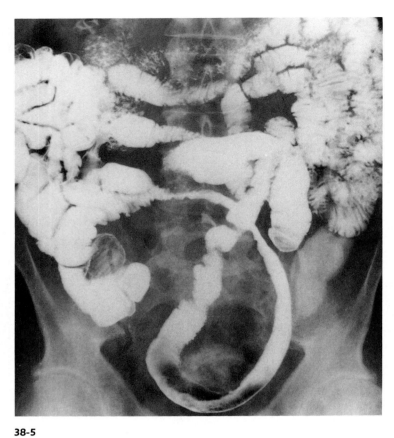

38-5

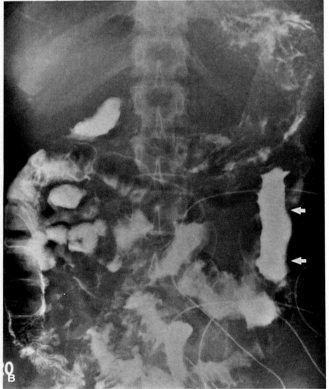

Fig. 38-5. Primary intestinal lymphoma. There is smooth narrowing of a segment of ileum with obliteration of mucosal folds. The elongated bowel loop is displaced around a large suprapubic mass.

Fig. 38-6. Aneurysmal lymphoma. Localized dilatation of a segment of small bowel **(arrows)** on two separate examinations is due to sloughing of the necrotic central core of the neoplastic mass.

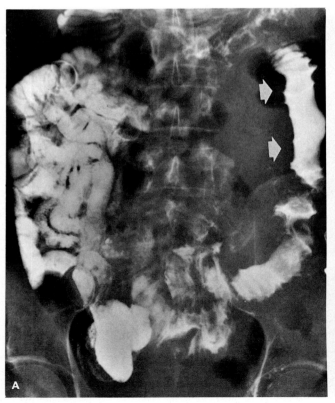

38-6

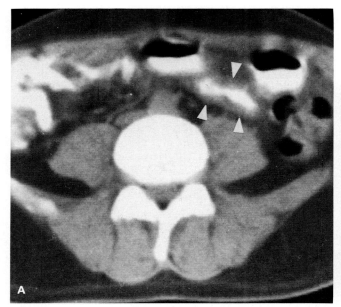

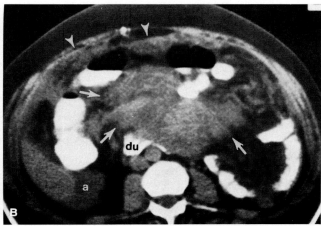

Fig. 38-7. CT of intestinal lymphoma. **(A)** Uniform thickening of the wall **(arrowheads)** in the affected segment of ileum. **(B)** In another patient with abdominal lymphoma, there is infiltration of the mesentery **(arrows)** and omentum **(arrowheads)**, compression of the third portion of the duodenum **(du)**, and ascites **(a)** within the hepatorenal space. (**[A]** Mauro MA, Koehler RE: Alimentary tract. In Lee JKT, Sagel SS, Stanley RJ (eds): Computed Body Tomography, New York, Raven 1983; **[B]** from Levitt RG: Abdominal wall and peritoneal cavity. In Lee JKT, Sagel SS, Stanley RJ (eds): Computed Body Tomography. New York, Raven, 1983)

Computed tomography (CT) in the patient with intestinal lymphoma can demonstrate localized thickening of the bowel wall as well as exophytic and mesenteric tumor masses (Fig. 38-7A). The major value of this modality is to detect disease in other areas of the abdomen, especially enlargement of the mesenteric and retroperitoneal lymph nodes (Fig. 38-7B) and spread of tumor to the liver, spleen, kidneys, and adrenals.

AMYLOIDOSIS

Small intestinal involvement occurs in at least 70% of cases of generalized amyloidosis. Amorphous, eosinophilic amyloid is deposited in and around the walls of small blood vessels and between muscle fibers of the muscularis mucosa and major muscular layers. As deposition of amyloid increases, the entire bowel wall can become involved and appear as a rigid tube. Occlusion of small blood vessels can cause ischemic enteritis with ulceration, intestinal infarction, and hemorrhage. The deposition of amyloid in the muscular layers produces impairment of peristaltic activity. Symptoms include dysphagia, gastric retention, constipation or diarrhea, and intestinal obstruction. Muscular deposition combined with ischemia can cause mucosal atrophy leading to erosion and ulceration. As the bowel wall thickens, the lumen becomes increasingly narrow; even complete obstruction can occur. Generalized deposition of amyloid can also result in a protein-losing enteropathy and malabsorption.

Amyloidosis can be primary and occur without any antecedent disease. More commonly, amyloidosis is secondary to some chronic inflammatory or necrotizing process (*e.g.,* tuberculosis, osteomyelitis, ulcerative colitis, rheumatoid arthritis, malignant neoplasm), multiple myeloma, or hereditary diseases such as familial Mediterranean fever.

The diagnosis of amyloidosis requires demonstration of the characteristic eosinophilic material in affected intestinal tissues. Rectal biopsy has long been considered the most convenient diagnostic procedure in patients with generalized amyloidosis. More recently, peroral jejunal biopsy has proved to be a safe procedure with an equivalently high accuracy rate. Radiographically, amyloidosis is characterized by sharply demarcated thickening of folds throughout the small bowel (Fig. 38-8). The folds can be symmetric and present a uniform appearance or be irregular, with nodularity and tumorlike defects. The appearance of prominent ileal folds resembling valvulae conniventes of the jejunum (jejunization) should suggest amyloidosis as the underlying disorder.

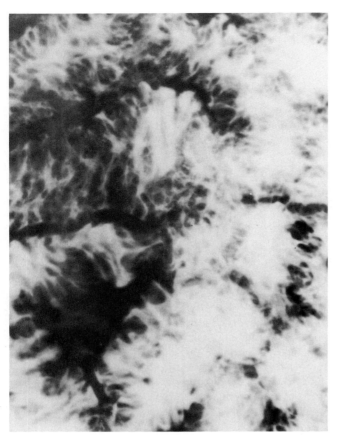

Fig. 38-8. *Amyloidosis. There is irregular thickening of small bowel folds.*

EOSINOPHILIC ENTERITIS

Diffuse infiltration of the small bowel by eosinophilic leukocytes produces the thickened folds seen in eosinophilic enteritis (Fig. 38-9). The jejunum is most prominently involved, though the entire small bowel is sometimes affected. Concomitant eosinophilic infiltration of the stomach is common. Involvement of the mucosa and lamina propria initially results in regular thickening of small bowel folds. More extensive, transmural involvement causes irregular fold thickening, angulation, and a saw-toothed contour of the small bowel. This can be associated with rigidity of the bowel and hyperplastic mesenteric nodes that simulate Crohn's disease. However, peripheral eosinophilia and the typical history of gastrointestinal symptoms related to the ingestion of specific foods usually permit differentiation between these two entities.

CROHN'S DISEASE

Although Crohn's disease most often involves the terminal ileum, it can affect any part of the alimentary canal. The process is frequently discontinuous, with diseased segments of bowel separated by apparently healthy portions. In Crohn's disease, there is diffuse transmural inflammation with edema and infiltration of lymphocytes and plasma cells in all layers of the gut wall. Ulceration is common, and intramural tracking within the submucosal and

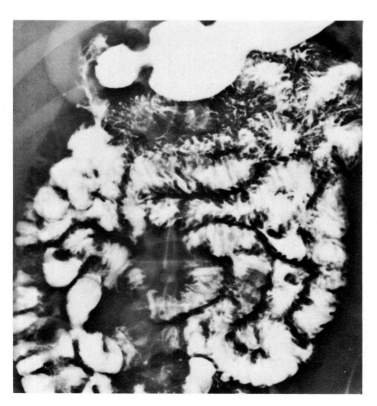

Fig. 38-9. *Eosinophilic enteritis. Irregular thickening of folds primarily involves the jejunum. No concomitant involvement of the stomach is identified.*

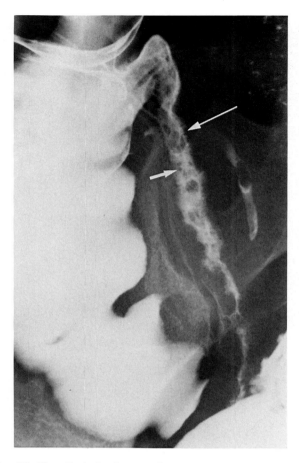

Fig. 38-10. Crohn's disease. Compression view of the stenotic terminal ileum shows a diffuse granular mucosal pattern both *en face* **(arrow)** and tangentially **(arrowhead)**. (Glick SN, Teplick FK: Crohn disease of the small intestine: Diffuse mucosal granularity. Radiology 154:313–317, 1954)

luria. Almost one-third of all patients hospitalized for Crohn's disease eventually develop a small bowel obstruction. Fistula formation is seen in at least half of patients with chronic Crohn's disease, and chronic indurated rectal fissures and fistulas with associated perirectal abscesses occur in about one-third. After surgical resection of an involved segment of small bowel, there is a high incidence of Crohn's disease recurring adjacent to the anastomosis.

RADIOGRAPHIC FINDINGS

The earliest small bowel change in Crohn's disease is a diffuse granular mucosal pattern of the involved bowel (Fig. 38-10). This is produced by a reticular network of radiolucent foci 0.5 to 1 mm in diameter and may be the only evidence of small bowel involvement. Pathologically, this pattern represents widening and blunting of villi with lymphocytic infiltration. As the disease progresses, there is the development of characteristic irregular thickening and distortion of the valvulae conniventes due to submucosal inflammation and edema (Fig. 38-11). Transverse and longitudinal ulcerations can separate islands of thickened mucosa and submucosa, leading to a characteristic rough cobblestone appearance (Fig. 38-12). Rigid thickening of the entire

muscular layers is not infrequent. Fistulas are created when deep ulcerations burrow through the serosa into adjacent loops of bowel. They can extend to the colon, bladder, and even the skin or can end blindly in intraperitoneal or retroperitoneal abscess cavities or in the mesentery.

The clinical spectrum of Crohn's disease is broad, ranging from an indolent course with unpredictable exacerbations and remissions to severe diarrhea and an acute abdomen. Extraintestinal complications (large joint migratory polyarthritis, ankylosing spondylitis, sclerosing cholangitis) occur with a higher frequency than normal in patients with Crohn's disease. In the genitourinary system, infections can result from enterovesical fistulas, hydronephrosis can develop from ureteral obstruction due to involvement of the ureter in the granulomatous inflammatory process, and renal oxalate stones can be caused by increased absorption of dietary oxalate and consequent hyperoxa-

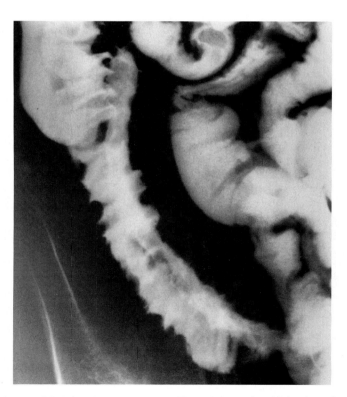

Fig. 38-11. Crohn's disease. There is irregular thickening of the valvulae conniventes in the terminal ileum.

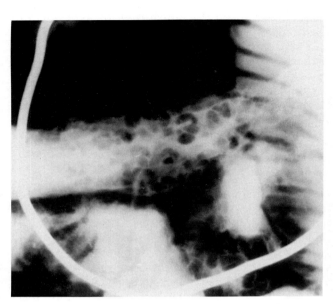

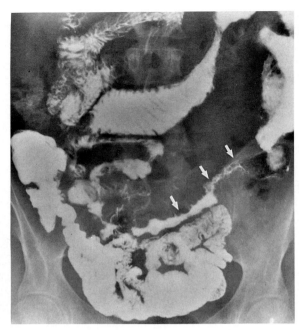

38-12

38-13

Fig. 38-12. Crohn's disease. A cobblestone appearance is produced by transverse and longitudinal ulcerations separating islands of thickened mucosa and submucosa.

Fig. 38-13. Crohn's disease. There is severe segmental narrowing in the jejunum **(arrows)**. The jejunum shows pronounced involvement, although there is no clear evidence of terminal ileal disease.

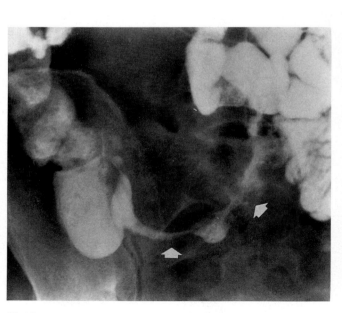

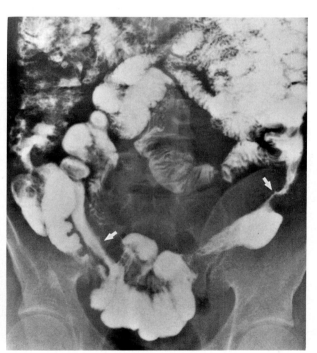

38-14

38-15

Fig. 38-14. String sign in Crohn's disease. The mucosal pattern is lost in a severely narrowed, rigid segment of the terminal ileum **(arrows)**.

Fig. 38-15. Skip lesions in Crohn's disease of the small bowel. The **arrows** point to widely separated areas of disease.

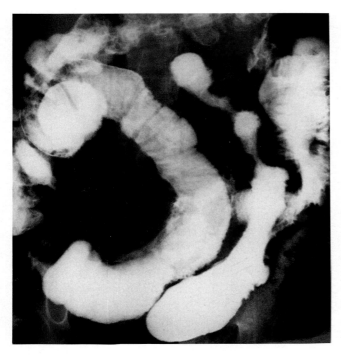

Fig. 38-16. Crohn's disease. Marked separation of bowel loops is due to thickening of the bowel wall and mesenteric involvement.

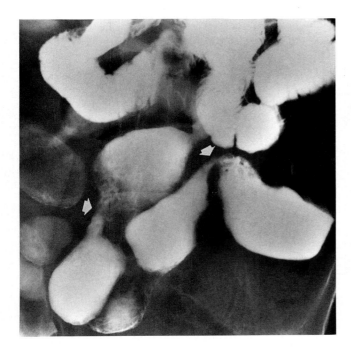

Fig. 38-17. Crohn's disease. Irregular strictures **(arrows)** alternate with areas of dilated small bowel.

bowel wall produces pipe-like narrowing (Fig. 38-13). Continued inflammation and fibrosis can result in a severely narrowed, rigid segment of small bowel in which the mucosal pattern is lost ("string" sign) (Fig. 38-14). When several areas of small bowel are diseased, involved segments of varying length are often sharply separated from radiographically normal segments ("skip" lesions) (Fig. 38-15).

Loops of small bowel involved with Crohn's disease often appear to be separated from one another due to thickening of the bowel wall (Fig. 38-16). Mass effects on involved loops can be produced by adjacent abscesses, thickened indurated mesentery, or enlarged and matted lymph nodes. Irregular strictures are not uncommon (Fig. 38-17). Localized perforations and fistulas from the small bowel to other visceral organs can sometimes be demonstrated.

Computed tomography is valuable for demonstrating mural, serosal, and mesenteric abnormalities in Crohn's disease and for defining the nature of mass effects, separation, or displacement of small bowel segments seen on barium studies. A CT scan can show thickening of the bowel wall, fibrofatty proliferation of mesenteric fat, mesenteric abscesses, inflammatory reactions of the mesentery, and mesenteric lymphadenopathy (Fig. 38-18).

TUBERCULOSIS

Tuberculous involvement of the small bowel can produce a radiographic pattern indistinguishable from Crohn's disease (Fig. 38-19). Tuberculosis tends to be more localized than Crohn's disease and predominantly affects the ileocecal region.

HISTOPLASMOSIS

Although histoplasmosis is primarily a benign, self-limited pulmonary disease caused by the fungus *Histoplasma capsulatum*, it can rarely cause a systemic or disseminated disease that affects the gastrointestinal tract. Symptoms include nausea, vomiting, diarrhea, abdominal colic, anorexia, and weight loss. A protein-losing enteropathy has been described with this disease; generalized lymphadenopathy may mimic malignancy. Infiltration of enormous numbers of *Histoplasma*-laden macrophages into the lamina propria, accompanied by intense villous edema, produces irregularly thickened and distorted small bowel folds (Fig. 38-20). When seen on end, the folds appear as innumerable filling defects varying in size from sand-like pinpoints to nodules greater than 2 mm in diameter. Focal stenotic lesions may closely resemble neoplastic disease.

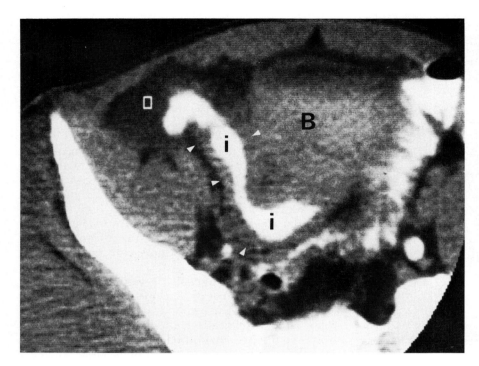

Fig. 38-18. CT of Crohn's disease. There is thickening of the wall **(arrowheads)** of a long abnormal segment of contrast-filled ileum **(i)**. Note the mass of water density **(box)**, which proved to be a mesenteric abscess. **B**, bladder. (Moss AA, Thoeni RF: Computed tomography of the gastrointestinal tract. In Moss AA, Gamsu G, Genant HK (eds): Computed Tomography of the Body.) Philadelphia, WB Saunders, 1983)

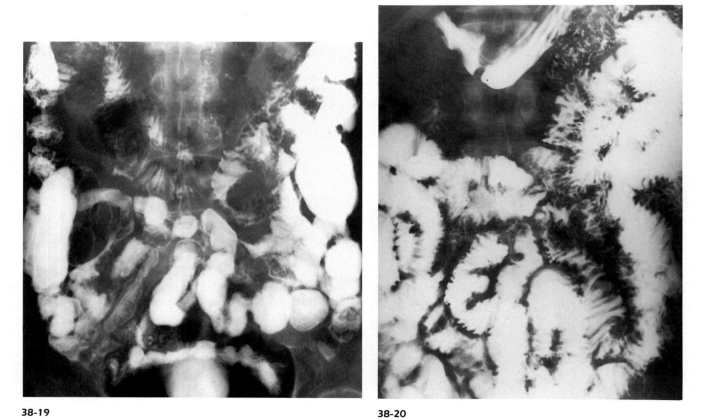

38-19

38-20

Fig. 38-19. Tuberculosis. Irregular thickening of folds, segmental narrowing, and separation of bowel loops produce a pattern indistinguishable from Crohn's disease.

Fig. 38-20. Histoplasmosis. There is irregular thickening and distortion of folds throughout the small bowel.

MASTOCYTOSIS

Systemic mastocytosis is characterized by mast cell proliferation in the reticuloendothelial system and skin (urticaria pigmentosa). Because the lamina propria of the intestinal mucosa is an important component of the reticuloendothelial system, involvement of the small bowel by mastocytosis is not uncommon. Infiltration of lymph nodes and hepatosplenomegaly are frequent; sclerotic bone lesions can also occur. The episodic release of histamine from mast cells causes such symptoms as pruritus, flushing, tachycardia, asthma, and headaches. Nausea, vomiting, abdominal pain, and diarrhea are common gastrointestinal complaints. The incidence of peptic ulcers is high (presumably because of histamine-mediated acid secretion), and malabsorption occurs not infrequently.

Mast cell infiltration into the lamina propria produces the radiographic appearance of generalized irregular, distorted, thickened folds (Fig. 38-21). At times, a diffuse pattern of sand-like nodules is seen. Urticaria-like lesions of the gastric and intestinal mucosa have also been described.

STRONGYLOIDIASIS

Strongyloides stercoralis is a round worm that exists in warm, moist climates in areas in which there is frequent fecal contamination of the soil. When parasitic females of the species are swallowed, they invade the mucosa and produce an infection that predominantly involves the proximal small bowel but can affect any part of the gastrointestinal tract from the stomach to the anus. Mild intestinal disease is

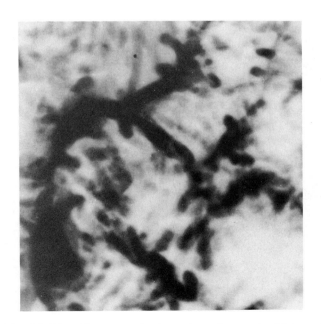

Fig. 38-21. Mastocytosis. Irregular, distorted, thickened folds are visible.

often asymptomatic, but severe symptoms of abdominal pain, nausea, vomiting, weight loss, and fever can occur. Severe diarrhea and steatorrhea can mimic acute tropical sprue.

Radiographically, strongyloidiasis produces irritability and irregular thickening of the mucosal folds of the duodenum and proximal jejunum. Severe infestation can involve the entire small and large bowel and be associated with spasm, ulceration, and stricture. Small bowel dilatation is significant, and in overwhelming infestation toxic dilatation with paresis results. A definitive diagnosis requires detection of the worms or larvae in duodenal secretions.

YERSINIA ENTEROCOLITICA

Yersinia enterocolitica is a gram-negative rod resembling *Escherichia coli*. In children, *Yersinia* infections most frequently cause acute enteritis with fever and diarrhea; in adolescents and adults, acute terminal ileitis or mesenteric adenitis simulating appendicitis more commonly occurs. *Yersinia* usually causes a focal disease involving short segments of the terminal ileum, though it can also affect the colon and rectum.

Coarse, irregular thickening of small bowel mucosal folds is the most common radiographic pattern with *Yersinia* infection (Fig. 38-22A). Nodular filling defects and ulceration are also seen (Fig. 38-22B). Densely packed nodules surrounded by deep ulcerations can produce a pattern resembling the cobblestone appearance of Crohn's disease. Pathologically, acute and chronic nonspecific inflammatory changes are seen in the mucosa. During the healing phases of the disease, the mucosal thickening decreases and tiny filling defects appear (follicular ileitis). These can persist for months following an acute *Yersinia* infection.

TYPHOID FEVER

Irregular thickening and nodularity of the mucosal folds is effectively limited to the terminal ileum in patients with typhoid fever (Fig. 38-23A). This acute, often severe illness, caused by *Salmonella typhosa*, is transmitted by bacterial contamination of food and water by human feces. Once in the gastrointestinal tract, the organisms are phagocytized by lymphoid tissue, particularly in the Peyer's patches of the terminal ileum. The organisms multiply there and produce raised plaques, which appear as thickened mucosal folds. Necrosis of the overlying mucosa causes ulceration. After treatment, the small bowel usually returns to normal (Fig. 38-23B), though healing with fibrosis and stricture can occur.

Typhoid fever must be distinguished radiographically from Crohn's disease of the terminal

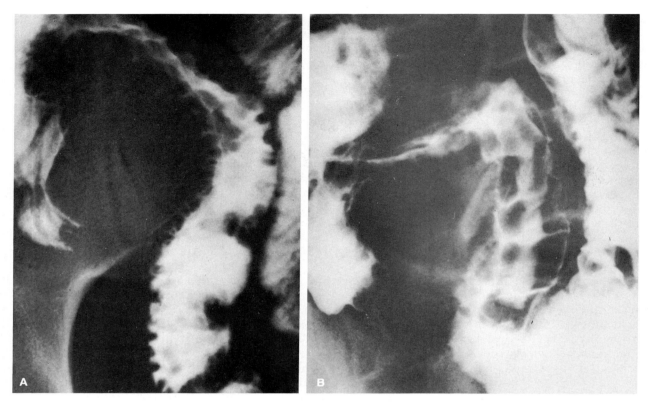

Fig. 38-22. *Yersinia* enterocolitis. **(A)** Numerous small nodules, marked edema, and moderate narrowing of the lumen combine to give the terminal ileum an appearance of irregularly thickened folds. **(B)** Nodular pattern. (Ekberg O, Sjostrom B, Brahme F: Radiological findings in *Yersinia* ileitis. Radiology 123:15–19, 1977)

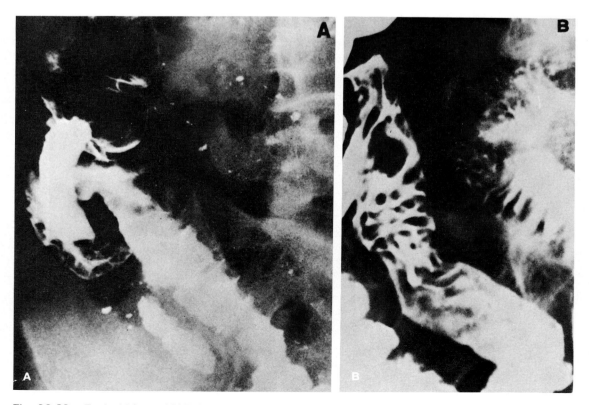

Fig. 38-23. Typhoid fever. **(A)** Thickened, coarse mucosal folds and marginal irregularity of the terminal ileum. **(B)** After therapy, the ileum returns to normal. (Francis RS, Berk RN: Typhoid fever. Radiology 112:583–585, 1974)

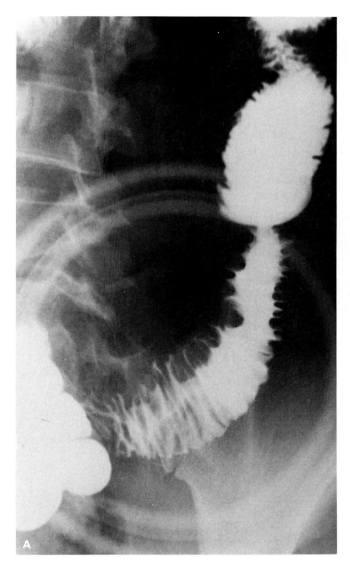

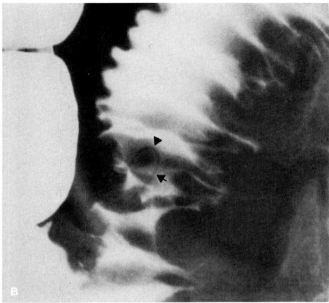

Fig. 38-24. Anisakiasis. **(A)** Compression radiograph shows irregular thickening of mucosal folds. **(B)** Close-up view shows a thread-like filling defect **(arrows)** representing the worm. (Matsui T, Iida M, Murakami M et al: Intestinal anisakiasis: Clinical and radiologic features. Radiology 157:299–302, 1985)

ileum. Ileal involvement in typhoid fever is symmetric; skip areas and fistulas do not occur. In addition, most patients with typhoid fever have clinical and radiographic evidence of splenomegaly.

OTHER INFECTIONS

Many infectious agents can cause inflammation of the small bowel due to either direct invasion or the elaboration of an enterotoxin. *Campylobacter jejuni*, a small, curved, gram-negative rod resembling *Vibrio*, causes hemorrhagic or congested lesions producing irregular mucosal thickening of the small bowel. Birds and domestic animals serve as reservoirs for this organism and transmission occurs by contaminated water, raw milk, and improperly cooked food. *Shigella* and *Escherichia coli* may produce a similar radiographic pattern. Anisa-

kiasis can cause irregular thickening of mucosal folds that most commonly involves the ileocecal region but can affect any portion of the small bowel (Fig. 38-24A). A worm can occasionally be visualized radiographically as a thread-like defect in the barium column (Fig. 38-24B). Irregular thickening of small bowel folds, often associated with substantial dilatation, is a manifestation of various types of opportunistic infection in patients with AIDS and other immunocompromised patients. Infestation by the parasitic protozoan *Cryptosporidium* produces a cholera-like diarrhea (see Fig. 36-3), as can candidal enteritis. A similar pattern may be due to *Mycobacterium avium-intracellulare* (MAC), a slow-growing, ubiquitous bacillus that rarely produces disease even in immunocompromised patients (Fig. 38-25). Because the clinical and histologic patterns in this condition are similar to those seen in Whipple's disease, small-bowel infection with MAC has been

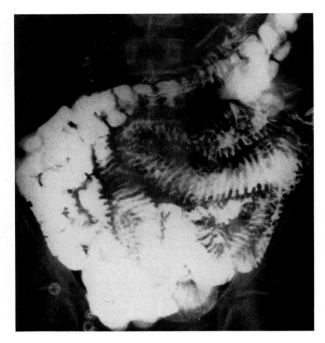

Fig. 38-25. *Mycobacterium avium-intracellulare* enteritis. Moderately irregular thickening of mucosal folds throughout the small bowel. The folds in this condition may vary from regularly thickened to wild and redundant. (Vincent ME, Robbins AH: *Mycobacterium avium-intracellulare* complex enteritis: Pseudo-Whipple's disease in AIDS. AJR 144:921–922, 1985. Copyright 1985. Reproduced with permission)

termed pseudo-Whipple's disease. The significant distinguishing characteristic between these two conditions is the reaction to acid-fast stain: MAC is positive; Whipple's bacilli are negative.

ALPHA CHAIN DISEASE

Alpha chain disease is a disorder of immunoglobulin peptide synthesis and assembly of IgA. Major gastrointestinal symptoms, which include diarrhea and malabsorption, are possibly related to the inability of a defective secretory IgA system to prevent bacteria from penetrating the intestinal epithelial cells. The lamina propria is infiltrated by mononuclear cells (predominantly plasma cells), causing distorted villous architecture and a radiographic pattern of coarsely thickened, irregular mucosal folds. A diffuse pattern of small nodules is occasionally seen. There is often associated mesenteric lymphadenopathy that may cause extrinsic compression and displacement of the bowel and the appearance of strictures.

ABETALIPOPROTEINEMIA

Abetalipoproteinemia is a rare, recessively inherited disease characterized by malabsorption of fat, progressive neurologic deterioration, and retinitis

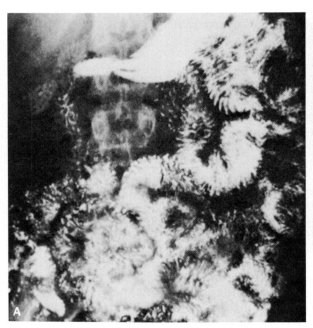

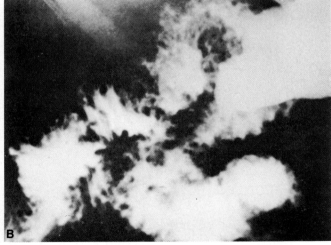

Fig. 38-26. Abetalipoproteinemia. **(A)** Moderately disorganized fold pattern. **(B)** Nodular or cobblestone pattern of folds in the duodenum and jejunum. (Weinstein MA, Pearson KD, Agus SG: Abetalipoproteinemia. Radiology 108:269–273, 1973)

pigmentosa. In addition to producing regular thickening of small bowel folds, abetalipoproteinemia can also cause moderate disorganization of the mucosal fold pattern (Fig. 38-26*A*) or a nodular or cobblestone pattern of folds (Fig. 38-26*B*).

BIBLIOGRAPHY

Balikian JP, Nassar NT, Shamma'A NH et al: Primary lymphomas of the small intestine including the duodenum: A roentgen analysis of 29 cases. AJR 107:131–141, 1969

Bank S, Trey C, Gans I et al: Histoplasmosis of the small bowel with "giant" intestinal villi and secondary protein-losing enteropathy. Am J Med 39:492–501, 1965

Berk RN, Wall SD, McArdle CB et al: Cryptosporidosis of the stomach and small intestine in patients with AIDS. AJR 143:549–554, 1984

Carlson HC, Breen JF: Amyloidosis and plasma cell dyscrasias: Gastrointestinal involvement. Semin Roentgenol 21:128–138, 1986

Clemett AR, Fishbone G, Levine RJ et al: Gastrointestinal lesions in mastocytosis. AJR 103:405–412, 1968

Clemett AR, Marshak RH: Whipple's disease: Roentgen features and differential diagnosis. Radiol Clin North Am 7:105–111, 1969

Dallemand S, Waxman M, Farman J: Radiological manifestations of *Strongyloides stercoralis*. Gastrointest Radiol 8:45–51, 1983

Fisher CH, Oh KS, Bayless TM et al: Current perspectives on giardiasis. AJR 125:207–217, 1975

Fishman EK, Wolf EJ, Jones B et al: CT evaluation of Crohn's disease: Effect on patient management. AJR 148:537–540, 1987

Francis RS, Berk RN: Typhoid fever. Radiology 112:583–585, 1974

Gardiner R, Smith C: Infective enterocolitides. Radiol Clin North Am 25:67–78, 1987

Goldberg HI, Gore RM, Margulis AR et al: Computed tomography in the evaluation of Crohn's disease. AJR 140:277–282, 1983

Goldberg HI, O'Kieffe D, Jenis EH et al: Diffuse eosinophilic enteritis. AJR 119:342–351, 1973

Kelvin FM, Gedgaudas RK: Radiologic diagnoses of Crohn's disease (with emphasis on its early manifestations). CRC Crit Rev Diagn Imaging 16:43–62, 1981

Lee JKT, Sagel SS, Stanley RJ: Computed Body Tomography. New York, Raven, 1983

Legge DA, Carlson HC, Wollaeger EE: Roentgenologic appearance of systemic amyloidosis involving the gastrointestinal tract. AJR 110:406–412, 1970

Marshak RH, Lindner AE: Radiology of the Small Intestine. Philadelphia, WB Saunders, 1976

Marshak RH, Ruoff M, Lindner AE: Roentgen manifestations of giardiasis. AJR 104:557–560, 1968

Matsui T, Iida M, Murakami M et al: Intestinal anisakiasis: Clinical and radiologic features. Radiology 157:299–302, 1987

Moss AA, Thoeni RF: Computed tomography of the gastrointestinal tract. In Moss AA, Gamsu G, Genant HK (eds): Computed Tomography of the Body. Philadelphia, WB Saunders, 1983

Olmsted WW, Reagin DE: Pathophysiology of enlargement of the small bowel fold. AJR 127:423–428, 1976

Philips RL, Carlson HC: The roentgenographic and clinical findings in Whipple's disease. AJR 123:268–273, 1975

Radin DR, Fong GL, Halls JM et al: Monilial enteritis in acquired immunodeficiency syndrome. AJR 141:1289–1290, 1983

Reeder MM, Hamilton LC: Radiologic diagnosis of tropical diseases of the gastrointestinal tract. Radiol Clin North Am 7:57–81, 1969

Robbins AH, Schimmel EM, Rao KC: Gastrointestinal mastocytosis: Radiologic alterations after ethanol ingestion. AJR 115:297–299, 1972

Schulman A, Morton PCG, Dietrich BE: Eosinophilic gastroenteritis. Clin Radiol 31:101–105, 1980

Shimkin PM, Waldmann TA, Krugman RL: Intestinal lymphangiectasia. AJR 110:827–841, 1970

Vantrappen G, Agg HO, Ponette E et al: *Yersinia* enteritis and enterocolitis: Gastroenterological aspects. Gastroenterology 72:220–227, 1977

Vessal K, Dutz W, Kohout E et al: Immunoproliferative small intestinal disease with duodenojejunal lymphoma: Radiologic changes. AJR 135:491–497, 1980

Vincent ME, Robbins AH: *Mycobacterium avium-intracellulare* complex enteritis: Pseudo-Whipple's disease in AIDS. AJR 144:921–922, 1985

SOLITARY FILLING DEFECTS IN THE JEJUNUM AND ILEUM

Disease Entities

Benign neoplasms
    Leiomyoma
    Adenoma
    Lipoma
    Hemangioma
    Neurofibroma
    Peutz–Jeghers hamartoma
    Fibroma/lymphangioma/teratoma
Malignant neoplasms
    Adenocarcinoma
    Lymphoma
    Leiomyosarcoma
    Metastases
Neoplasms with variable malignant potential
    Carcinoid tumor
Gallstone ileus
Inflammatory fibroid polyp
Endometrioma
Pseudotumors
    Parasitic (ascariasis, strongyloidiasis)
    Inflammatory
Duplication cyst
Heterotopic gastric mucosa
Small bowel varix
Inverted Meckel's diverticulum
Blood clot
Foreign body/bezoar/pill

Most solitary filling defects in the jejunum and ileum represent neoplasms. Many of these small bowel neoplasms are asymptomatic and are either incidentally discovered or undetected during the patient's life. Most asymptomatic tumors are benign; a majority of all symptomatic tumors prove to be malignant. The most common symptoms are pain, bleeding, obstruction, a palpable mass, and weight loss.

A small bowel tumor can produce one of five major radiographic appearances, depending on the relationship of the neoplasm to the lumen and wall of the intestine (Fig. 39-1). First, a *pedunculated* intraluminal tumor appears as a filling defect completely surrounded by contrast medium with the exception of its attachment to the bowel wall by a stalk (which is often invisible). Although its appearance remains constant, the filling defect can be moved up and down the lumen for a distance approximately double the length of the pedicle. Second, intraluminal tumors that are *sessile* are seen to project within the lumen when viewed in profile but do not demonstrate a stalk. Unlike pedunculated masses, these lesions cannot be moved up and down the lumen. Third, neoplasms that are mostly *intramural* appear when viewed in profile as curved filling defects projecting into the lumen. This type of tumor has a base that is wider than its projection into the lumen. Because it arises outside the mucosa, a normal mucosal pattern is often seen overlying the mass. As the tumor grows, the mucosa is

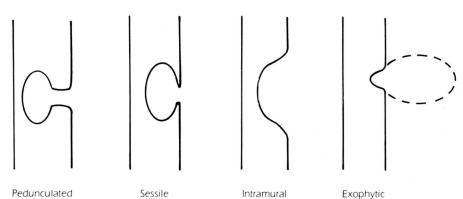

Fig. 39-1. Major radiographic appearances of small bowel tumors.

Pedunculated   Sessile   Intramural   Exophytic

stretched and eventually can become effaced and ulcerated. Fourth, *exophytic* small bowel neoplasms arise in the subserosal region and predominantly project into the peritoneal cavity. In this instance, the barium column is not deformed until the mass grows to a huge size and the tumor displaces adjacent opacified loops. Fifth, the development of gross lobulations, especially in neoplasms of smooth muscle origin, can produce a complex radiographic appearance. For example, if one lobule is sessile and intraluminal while another primarily extends into the peritoneal cavity, the resultant "dumbbell tumor" is seen radiographically both as an intraluminal filling defect and as a mass displacing nearby bowel loops.

BENIGN NEOPLASMS

LEIOMYOMA

Leiomyomas are the most common benign neoplasms of the small bowel (Fig. 39-2). They are usually single (in about 97% of cases) and, although found at all levels of the small bowel, are most frequent in the jejunum. Leiomyomas arise as subserosal or submucosal lesions but can extend intraluminally and become pedunculated. Although the surface of a leiomyoma exhibits a rich blood supply, the central portion of the tumor is often virtually avascular and tends to undergo central necrosis and ulceration causing gastrointestinal hemorrhage. A leiomyoma with a large intraluminal component can be the leading point of an intussusception.

Many leiomyomas project from the serosal surface and are detectable radiographically only when they are large enough to displace adjacent barium-filled loops of small bowel. An intramural leiomyoma is seen in profile as a characteristic broad filling defect, its base wider than its projection into the lumen. Intraluminal tumors often lead to intussusception if they are located in the jejunum or ileum but almost never do so when they are situated in the duodenum. Retention of barium in a superficial mucosal ulceration that communicates with a

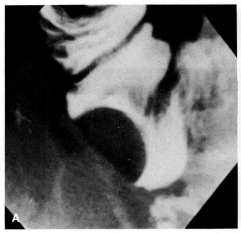 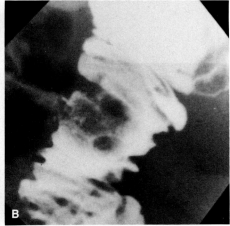

Fig. 39-2. Leiomyoma of the ileum. **(A)** Classic smoothly marginated submucosal defect on a profile view. **(B)** On an *en face* view, the features are less typical. (Maglinte DDT: The small bowel: Neoplasms. In Taveras JM, Ferrucci JT (eds): Radiology: Diagnosis–Imaging–Intervention. Philadelphia, JB Lippincott, 1987)

relatively deep pit in the tumor is a finding that is characteristic of leiomyoma.

ADENOMA

Adenomas are the second most common benign small bowel neoplasms (Fig. 39-3). They can be found throughout the small bowel but are most frequent in the ileum. Most adenomas are single, well-circumscribed polyps, though multiple lesions do occur. These polyps are usually intraluminal and

pedunculated and are therefore prone to act as the leading point of an intussusception.

LIPOMA

Lipomas are the third most frequent benign tumors of the small bowel (Fig. 39-4). Although most are found in the distal ileum and ileocecal valve area, they can occur anywhere in the small bowel. Lipomas arise in the submucosa but tend to protrude into the lumen. On barium studies, lipomas charac-

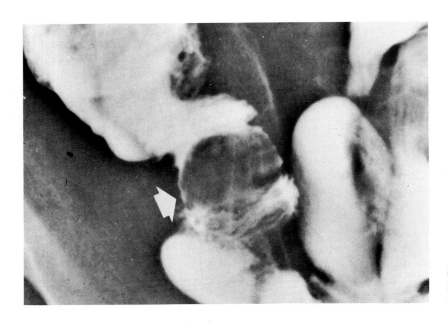

Fig. 39-3. Adenoma. A smooth polypoid mass **(arrow)** fills most of the lumen of the terminal ileum.

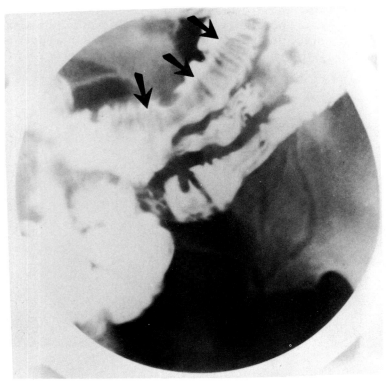

Fig. 39-4. Lipoma. A long pedunculated tumor produces an intraluminal filling defect. (Good CA: Tumors of the small intestine. AJR 89:685–705, 1963. Copyright 1963. Reproduced with permission)

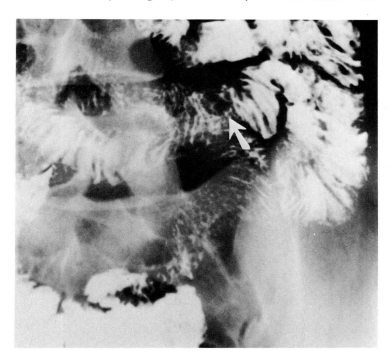

Fig. 39-5. Hemangioma. A filling defect **(arrows)** may be seen in the jejunum. (Good CA: Tumors of the small intestine. AJR 89:685–705, 1963. Copyright 1963. Reproduced with permission)

teristically appear as intraluminal filling defects with a smooth surface and a broad base of attachment indicating their intramural origin. The fatty consistency of these tumors permits them to be easily deformed by palpation. Pedunculated lipomas can be associated with intussusception.

HEMANGIOMA

Hemangiomas are tumors composed of endothelium-lined, blood-containing spaces (Fig. 39-5). Though far less common than other benign small bowel tumors, hemangiomas are clinically important because of their propensity for bleeding. Less than 25% of hemangiomas are solitary tumors. Most are relatively sessile lesions that are frequently missed on barium studies because of their small size and easy compressibility. The uncommon demonstration of phleboliths in the wall of an involved segment is a pathognomonic sign of hemangioma. Some authors do not distinguish between hemangiomas (true tumors) and telangiectasias (dilatation of existing vascular structures). Telangiectasias can be associated with several abnormalities, the best known of which is the Osler-Weber-Rendu syndrome, in which there is a familial history of repeated hemorrhage from the nasopharynx and gastrointestinal tract and multiple telangiectatic lesions involving the nasopharyngeal, buccal, and gastrointestinal mucosa.

NEUROFIBROMA

Neurofibromas are unusual tumors of the small bowel that most frequently occur in the ileum. Most

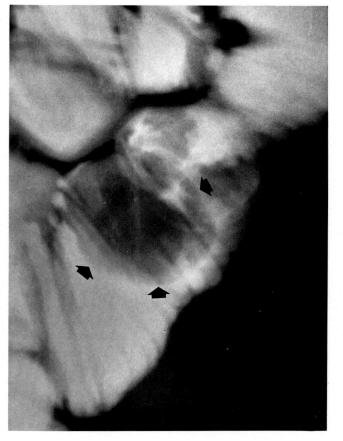

Fig. 39-6. Peutz–Jeghers hamartoma. Lobulated mass **(arrows)** in the jejunum. (Olmsted WW, Ros PR, Hjermstad BM et al: Tumors of the small intestine with little or no malignant predisposition: A review of the literature and report of 56 cases. Gastrointest Radiol 12:231–239, 1987)

arise in the subserosal layer (presumably from Auerbach's plexus) and present as pedunculated masses growing in an extraluminal direction along the antimesenteric border. Neurofibromas originating in the muscularis or submucosa tend to grow toward the lumen and cause well-demarcated polypoid filling defects. Neurofibromas can ulcerate, and, if the crater is large or irregular, malignancy is likely. The presence of multiple lesions suggests underlying neurofibromatosis (see Fig. 40-8).

PEUTZ–JEGHERS HAMARTOMA

The Peutz–Jeghers hamartoma is composed of a core of branching smooth muscle folded into fronds and lined by normal intestinal epithelial cells. It may be solitary or multiple (Peutz–Jeghers syndrome) and typically measures less than 5 cm. These hamartomas may affect any portion of the gastrointestinal tract, but are most often found in the jejunum and ileum (Fig. 39-6). Radiographically, solitary or multiple polyps, which may be lobular, are usually noted in the distal small intestine.

MALIGNANT NEOPLASMS

Primary small bowel malignancies can present as solitary filling defects. Although a given type of primary tumor can be found anywhere in the small bowel, carcinomas tend to cluster around the ligament of Treitz, whereas sarcomas occur more frequently in the ileum. Like benign tumors, a malignant lesion with a large intraluminal component can be the leading point of an intussusception.

CARCINOMA

Adenocarcinomas are the most common malignant tumors of the small bowel. They tend to be aggressively invasive and extend rapidly around the circumference of the bowel, inciting a fibrotic reaction and luminal narrowing that soon cause obstruction (Fig. 39-7). Occasionally, adenocarcinomas of the small bowel appear as broad-based intraluminal masses; extremely rarely, they present as pedunculated polyps.

LYMPHOMA

One of the many appearances of small bowel lymphoma is a discrete polypoid mass that is often large and bulky and has irregular ulcerations (Fig. 39-8). If there is no substantial intramural extension, the intraluminal mass can be drawn forward by peristalsis to form a pseudopedicle and even become the lead point of an intussusception. Displacement of adjacent loops of bowel is common, as are mesenteric impressions and a diffuse desmoplastic response.

SARCOMA

Leiomyosarcomas are most often large, bulky, irregular lesions usually more than 5 cm in diameter (Fig. 39-9). Like benign leiomyomas, leiomyosarcomas have a tendency for central necrosis and ulceration leading to massive gastrointestinal hemorrhage and the radiographic appearance of an umbilicated lesion. Because more than two-thirds of leiomyosarcomas primarily project into the peri-

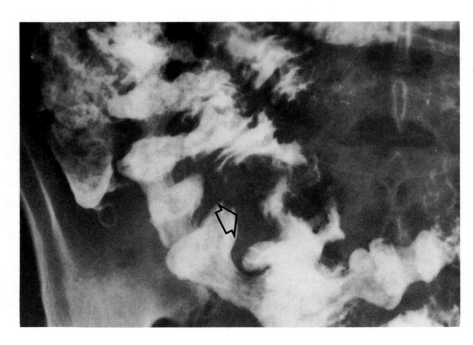

Fig. 39-7.   *Primary adenocarcinoma of the ileum* **(arrow)** *appearing as an annular constricting lesion.*

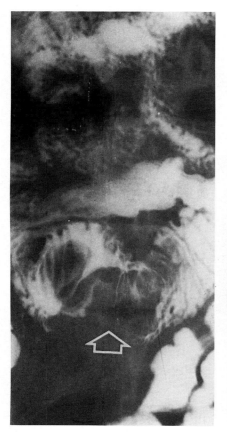

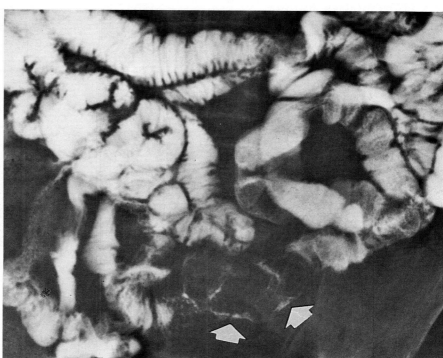

39-8   **39-9**

Fig. 39-8.   Lymphoma. Note the large, bulky, irregular lesion **(arrow)**.

Fig. 39-9.   Leiomyosarcoma. Note the large, bulky, irregular lesion **(arrows)**.

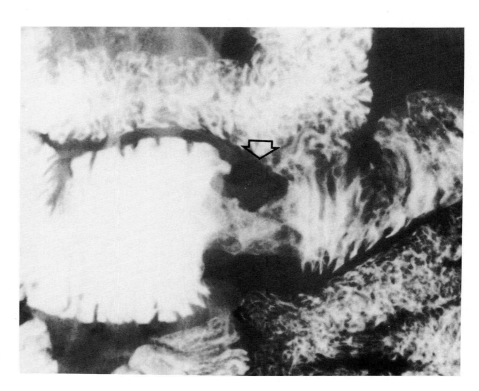

Fig. 39-10.   Adenocarcinoma of the lung metastatic to the jejunum **(arrow)**.

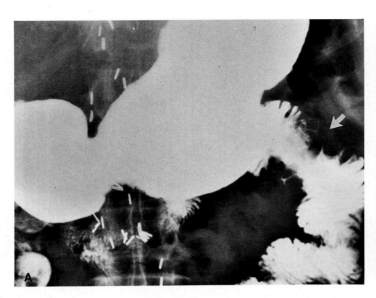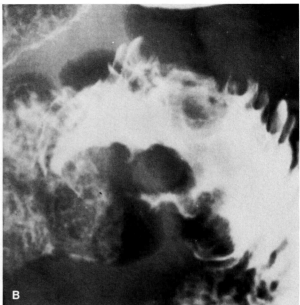

Fig. 39-11. Hypernephroma metastatic to the jejunum. **(A)** Full and **(B)** coned views show the multilobulated nodular mass **(arrow)** in the proximal jejunum.

toneal cavity, the major manifestation of this type of tumor is displacement of adjacent, uninvolved, barium-filled loops of small bowel.

METASTASES

Metastases to the small intestine (especially from such primaries as melanoma, lung, kidney, and breast) can appear as single intraluminal or intramural small bowel masses, which may have an annular configuration with mucosal destruction and shelflike margins mimicking primary adenocarcinoma (Figs. 39-10, 39-11). However, most metastases to the small bowel are multiple. Single metastatic lesions that present as huge cavitary lesions with irregular, amorphous ulcerations can simulate leiomyosarcoma or lymphoma. Metastases are often masked by the spread of tumor to the adjoining mesentery or by a reactive desmoplastic response.

CARCINOID TUMOR

Carcinoid tumors are the most common primary neoplasms of the small bowel (Fig. 39-12). The "rule of one-third" has been applied to small bowel carcinoids: they account for one-third of gastrointestinal carcinoid tumors, one-third of them show metastases, one-third present with a second malignancy, and about one-third are multiple. Although carcinoids of the small bowel can occur at any site, they are most frequently seen in the ileum.

The characteristic carcinoid syndrome consists of skin flushing and diarrhea as well as cyanosis, asthmatic attacks, and lesions of the tricuspid and pulmonic valves. The clinical symptoms are due to circulating serotonin produced by the carcinoid tumor. Because serotonin released into the portal venous system is inactivated in the liver, the carcinoid syndrome is seen almost exclusively in patients with liver metastases (Fig. 39-13), in whom serotonin is released directly into the systemic circulation without being inactivated. The primary tumor site in almost all patients with carcinoid syndrome is the small intestine; however, only a minority of small bowel lesions present with this endocrine syndrome.

Small carcinoids present as sharply defined, small submucosal lesions. At this stage of development, they are usually asymptomatic and are rarely detected on routine small bowel examination. Most carcinoids tend to grow extraluminally, infiltrating the bowel wall, lymphatic channels, and eventually the regional lymph nodes and mesentery. Local release of serotonin leads to hypertrophic muscular thickening and intense desmoplastic response, which results in the characteristic radiographic appearance of separation, fixation, and angulation of intestinal loops and diffuse luminal narrowing (Fig. 39-14).

The presence of metastases from carcinoid tumors is directly related to the size of the primary lesion. Metastases are rare in primary tumors of under 1 cm; they are seen in half of tumors between 1 cm and 2 cm in size and in about 90% of primary lesions larger than 2 cm.

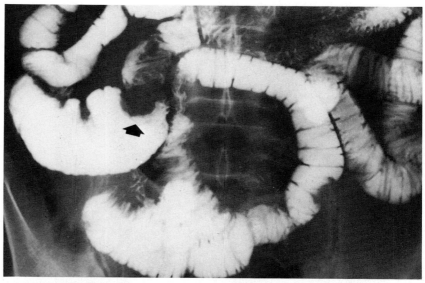

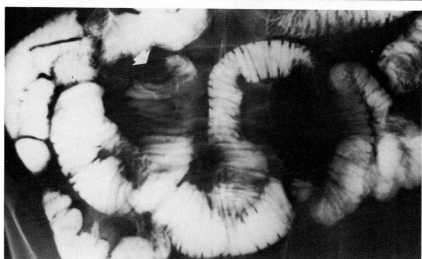

Fig. 39-12. Carcinoid tumor. Two views show the polypoid filling defect **(arrows)**.

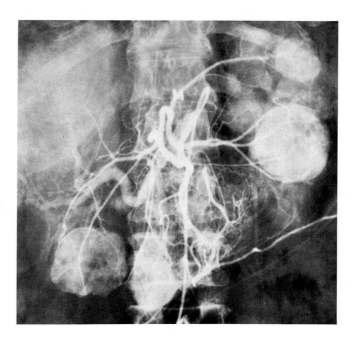

Fig. 39-13. Carcinoid syndrome. There are multiple large, extremely vascular metastases from a carcinoid tumor of the small bowel.

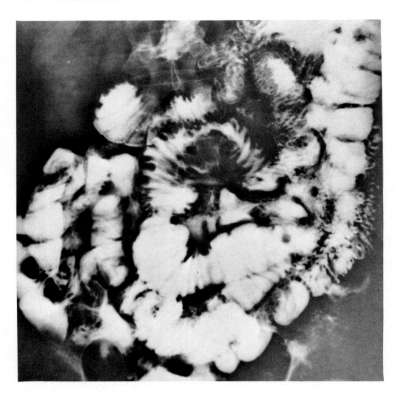

Fig. 39-14. Carcinoid tumor. Separation, fixation, and angulation of intestinal loops and diffuse luminal narrowing are caused by the intense desmoplastic response incited by the tumor.

GALLSTONE ILEUS

The combination of a filling defect in the ileum or jejunum, mechanical small bowel obstruction, and gas or barium in the biliary tree is virtually pathognomonic of gallstone ileus (Fig. 39-15). In this condition, which primarily occurs in elderly women, a large gallstone enters the small bowel by way of a fistula from the gallbladder or common bile duct to the duodenum. As the stone temporarily lodges at various levels in the small bowel, intermittent symptoms of abdominal cramps, nausea, and vomiting can simulate a recurrent partial obstruction. Complete obstruction develops when the gallstone finally reaches a portion of bowel too narrow to allow further progression. This usually occurs in the ileum, which is the narrowest segment of the small bowel. Far less commonly, a gallstone enters the colon (either by traversing the entire small bowel or by passing directly through a cholecystocolonic fistula). However, gallstone obstruction of the colon is unusual because of the large size of the lumen. When it does occur, the obstructing stone usually lodges in a segment that has been narrowed by another disease process (*e.g.*, chronic sigmoid diverticulitis).

On plain abdominal radiographs, the demonstration of an opaque gallstone in the small bowel associated with typical findings of small bowel obstruction and gas in the biliary tree is sufficient for the diagnosis of gallstone ileus to be made. If a barium examination is performed, the obstructing gallstone may appear as a lucent filling defect, and contrast material is often seen in the biliary ductal system.

INFLAMMATORY FIBROID POLYP

An inflammatory fibroid polyp is composed of loose connective tissue containing fibroblasts, vascular tissue, and eosinophils. Although often termed "eosinophilic granuloma," it is unrelated to histiocytosis X and has none of the clinical symptoms of eosinophilic gastroenteritis. Inflammatory fibroid polyps of the small bowel are rare lesions seen in the sixth and seventh decades of life. They are usually solitary and almost exclusively located in the ileum (Fig. 39-16). Although the etiology is unclear, an inflammatory fibroid polyp most likely represents a benign process reflecting a nonspecific inflammatory infiltrate in response to an unknown injury. Large inflammatory fibroid polyps can serve as the leading point of an intussusception.

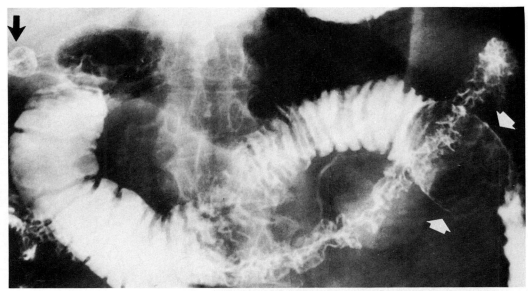

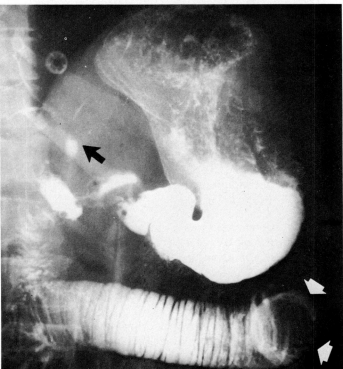

Fig. 39-15. Two patients with gallstone ileus. Obstructing stones **(white arrows)** are present, and there is evidence of barium in the biliary tree **(black arrows)**.

OTHER CAUSES

Several unusual conditions can produce solitary filling defects in the small bowel that are indistinguishable from primary neoplasms. In premenopausal women with pelvic endometriosis, a polypoid lesion in the small bowel can represent an endometrioma. In patients from endemic areas or nonnatives who have spent time in the tropics, a filling defect in the region of the ileocecal valve can represent a pseu-dotumor caused by invasion of the gut wall by roundworms (*Ascaris* or *Strongyloides*) or a bolus of ascaris worms in the intestinal lumen. A duplication cyst can appear radiographically as a solitary intra-mural filling defect. Duplication cysts tend to change in contour with external pressure and can be associated with vertebral abnormalities. They occasionally communicate with the small bowel lumen and fill with contrast. Heterotopic gastric mucosa in the small bowel can produce a polypoid

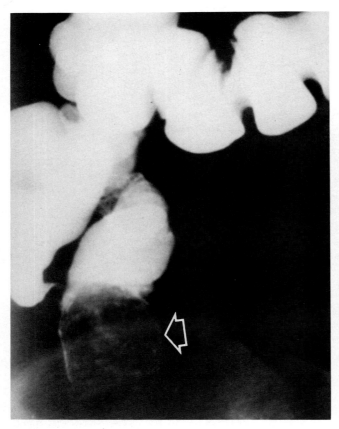

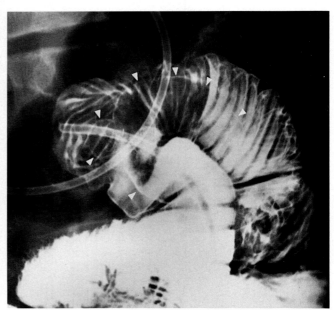

39-16   39-17

Fig. 39-16.   Inflammatory fibroid polyp. Large, smooth-surfaced filling defect in the ileum **(arrow)**. (Olmsted WW, Ros PR, Hjermstad BM et al: Tumors of the small intestine with little or no malignant predisposition: A review of the literature and report of 56 cases. Gastrointest Radiol 12:231–239, 1987)

Fig. 39-17.   Heterotopic gastric mucosa. Lobulated mass **(arrows)** projecting into the proximal jejunum. (Lodge JPA, Brennan TG, Chapman AH: Heterotopic gastric mucosa presenting as small-bowel obstruction. Br J Radiol 60:710–712, 1987)

lesion (Fig. 39-17) that may serve as the lead point for an intussusception (see Fig. 33-24). Small bowel varices, which occur almost exclusively in patients with portal hypertension, may appear as serpiginous or nodular filling defects on barium studies (Fig. 39-18). Patients with this rare lesion typically present with recurrent, often massive, gastrointestinal hemorrhage and usually have a history of chronic liver disease. A traumatic neuroma is a rare cause of a filling defect at the site of an intestinal anastomosis (Fig. 39-19). This nonneoplastic proliferative mass of Schwann cells may develop at the proximal end of a severed or injured nerve. Although it most commonly occurs in an extremity following amputation, traumatic neuromas occasionally develop in the nerves innervating the digestive tract following intestinal surgery. Rarely, an inverted Meckel's diverticulum appears as a characteristic oblong filling defect in the distal ileum (Fig. 39-20). Its margins are smooth, and palpation usually demonstrates a soft, pliable lesion with a

dimple at the site of invagination. In a patient who is actively bleeding from a gastric or duodenal ulcer or neoplasm, a single filling defect in the jejunum or ileum can represent a blood clot.

Foreign bodies, food particles, bezoars, and pills can present as solitary masses in the small bowel. Fruit pits (*e.g.*, prune, apricot) can become trapped in areas of narrowed bowel, such as in patients with Crohn's disease, or be found in areas of stasis, such as a Meckel's diverticulum or a blind loop. The pit can become calcified and radiopaque. The resulting enterolith can lead to ulceration and stenosis or be a cause of small bowel obstruction (see Fig. 33-21). Although bezoars in the small bowel are uncommon, they can be seen in patients who have had gastric resections or are edentulous. Barium entering the interstices of the bezoar produces a characteristic mottled appearance. Ingested enteric-coated pills that are not completely broken down in the stomach can also be a cause of single or multiple filling defects in the small bowel.

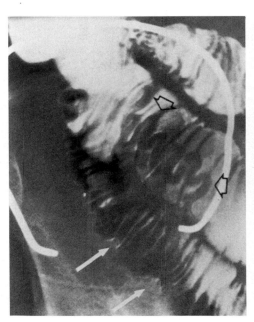

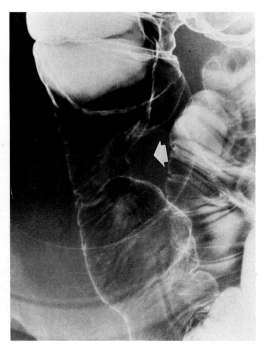

39-18

39-19

Fig. 39-18. Small bowel varix. Long serpiginous filling defect **(arrowheads)** represents a varix in the ileum. Note evidence of serosal metastases **(arrows)** in an adjacent segment of ileum. (Radin DR, Siskind BN, Alpert S et al: Small bowel varices due to mesenteric metastasis. Gastrointest Radiol 11:183–184, 1986)

Fig. 39-19. Traumatic neuroma. Extramucosal mass on the medial side of the ascending colon **(arrow)** at the site of an ileocolic anastomosis. (Chandrasoma P, Wheeler D, Radin DR: Traumatic neuroma of the intestine. Gastrointest Radiol 10:161–162, 1985)

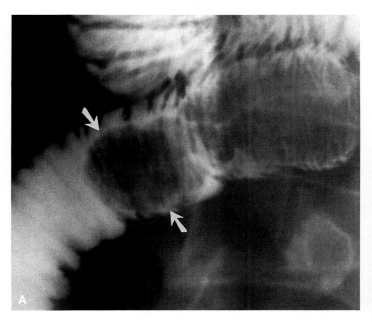

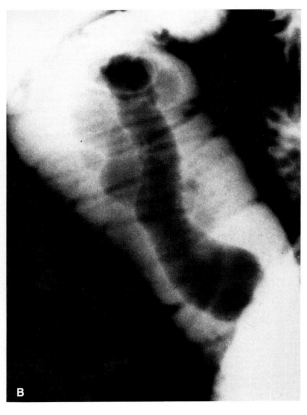

Fig. 39-20. Inverted Meckel's diverticulum and intussuscepted jejunal polyp. **(A)** Initial examination of the small bowel demonstrates an intussuscepted polypoid mass in the distal jejunum **(arrows)**. **(B)** An inverted Meckel's diverticulum was identified in the terminal ileum. (Freeny PC, Walker JH: Inverted diverticula of the gastrointestinal tract. Gastrointest Radiol 4:57–59, 1979)

BIBLIOGRAPHY

Agarwal D, Scholz FJ: Small-bowel varices demonstrated by enteroclysis. Radiology 140:350, 1981

Balthazar EJ: Carcinoid tumors of the alimentary tract: Radiographic diagnosis. Gastrointest Radiol 3:47–56, 1978

Campbell WL, Green WM, Seaman WB: Inflammatory pseudotumor of the small intestine. AJR 121:305–311, 1974

Chavez CM, Timmis HH: Duplication cysts of the gastrointestinal tract. Am J Surg 110:960–963, 1965

Eisenman JI, Finck EJ, O'Loughlin BJ: Gallstone ileus: A review of the roentgenographic findings and report of a new roentgen sign. AJR 101:361–366, 1967

Freeny PC, Walker JH: Inverted diverticula of the gastrointestinal tract. Gastrointest Radiol 4:57–59, 1979

Ginsburg LD: Eccentric polyposis of the small bowel: A possible radiographic sign of plexiform neurofibromatosis of the small bowel and its mesentery. Radiology 116:561–562, 1975

Good CA: Tumors of the small intestine. AJR 89:685–705, 1963

Jeffree MA, Barter SJ, Hemingway AP et al: Primary carcinoid tumors of the ileum: The radiological appearances. Clin Radiol 35:451–455, 1984

Levine MS, Drooz AT, Herlinger H: Annular malignancies of the small bowel. Gastrointest Radiol 12:53–58, 1987

LiVolsi VA, Perzin KH: Inflammatory pseudotumors (inflammatory fibrous polyps) of the small intestine. A clinicopathologic study. Am J Dig Dis 20:325–336, 1975

Marshak RH, Freund S, Maklansky D: Neurofibromatosis of the small bowel. Am J Dig Dis 8:478–483, 1963

Marshak RH, Lindner AE: Radiology of the Small Intestine. Philadelphia, WB Saunders, 1976

McWey P, Dodds WJ, Slota T et al: Radiographic features of heterotopic gastric mucosa. AJR 139:380–382, 1982

Meyers MA, McSweeney J: Secondary neoplasms of the bowel. Radiology 105:1–11, 1972

Olmsted WW, Ros PR, Hjermstad BM et al: Tumors of the small intestine with little or no malignant predisposition: A review of the literature and report of 56 cases. Gastrointest Radiol 12:231–239, 1987

Radin DR, Siskind BN, Alpert S et al: Small-bowel varices due to mesenteric metastasis. Gastrointest Radiol 11:183–184, 1986

Zornoza J, Goldstein HM: Cavitating metastases of the small intestine. AJR 129:613–615, 1977

MULTIPLE FILLING DEFECTS IN THE SMALL BOWEL

Disease Entities

Multiple polyps
  Peutz-Jeghers syndrome
  Gardner's syndrome
  Disseminated gastrointestinal polyposis
  Generalized gastrointestinal juvenile
    polyposis
  Cronkhite–Canada syndrome
  Ruvalcaba–Myhre–Smith syndrome
  Simple adenomatous polyps
Hemangiomas
Leiomyomas
Lipomas
Carcinoid tumors
Neurofibromas
Metastases (especially melanoma, breast
    carcinoma, lung carcinoma)
Lymphoma
Crohn's disease
Nodular lymphoid hyperplasia
Food particles, seeds, foreign bodies, pills
Parasites
  Ascaris lumbricoides
  Strongyloides stercoralis
  Ancylostoma duodenale (hookworm)
  Taenia solis (tapeworm)
Gallstones
Blood clots
Varices
Behcet's syndrome

MULTIPLE POLYPS

PEUTZ-JEGHERS SYNDROME

Several inherited multiple polyposis syndromes of the gastrointestinal tract affect the small bowel. The most common is Peutz-Jeghers syndrome, in which multiple gastrointestinal polyps are associated with mucocutaneous pigmentation (Fig. 40-1). Excessive melanin deposits can be found about the mouth, nostrils, palms, fingers, dorsum of the hands, soles of the feet, and perianal regions, though hyperpigmentation involving the buccal mucosa is characteristic and virtually diagnostic of the disease. The polyps in Peutz-Jeghers syndrome are hamartomas consisting of an arborizing fibromuscular stroma that appears to originate from a central smooth muscle mass in the muscularis layer of the bowel wall. The polyps are most prominent in the small bowel but can occur in the stomach, colon, and rectum. Severe, recurrent colicky abdominal pain is frequent, as is rectal bleeding. Intussusception and bowel obstruction may occur when the polyps increase in size. The hamartomatous polyps in Peutz-Jeghers syndrome are benign and apparently do not undergo malignant transformation. Nevertheless, 2% to 3% of patients with this syndrome develop adenocarcinomas of the intestinal tract (most commonly in the duodenum and proximal small bowel), and 5% of women with the disease have ovarian cysts and tumors.

495

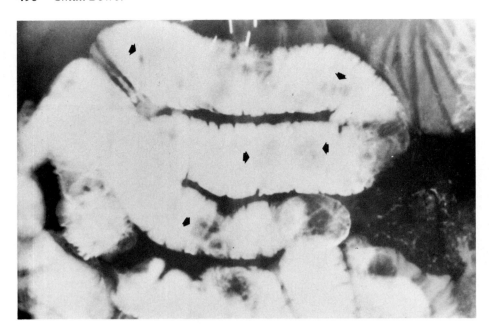

Fig. 40-1. Peutz-Jeghers syndrome. Multiple small bowel hamartomas are present in a patient with mucocutaneous pigmentation. The **arrows** point to a few of the many filling defects in the barium column.

GARDNER'S SYNDROME

In Gardner's syndrome, diffuse colonic polyposis is associated with osteomas and soft-tissue tumors. The adenomatous polyps in this condition predominantly involve the colon, though they can sometimes be found in the ileum or proximal small bowel (Fig. 40-2). Essentially all patients with Gardner's syndrome develop colorectal carcinoma. In addition, these patients have an increased risk of developing small bowel carcinoma, especially in the pancreaticoduodenal region.

OTHER CAUSES

If multiple adenomatous polyps (similar to those in familial polyposis) involve the stomach or small bowel as well as the colon, yet do not have the extraintestinal stigmata of the Peutz-Jeghers or Gardner's syndrome, the term disseminated gastrointestinal polyposis is applied. Patients with this extremely rare condition have a very high risk of developing carcinoma somewhere in their gastrointestinal tracts.

Generalized gastrointestinal juvenile polyposis refers to the presence of juvenile polyps in the stomach, small bowel, and colon without any extraintestinal manifestations. The juvenile polyps in this condition are hamartomas and are not premalignant; nevertheless, several instances of gastrointes-

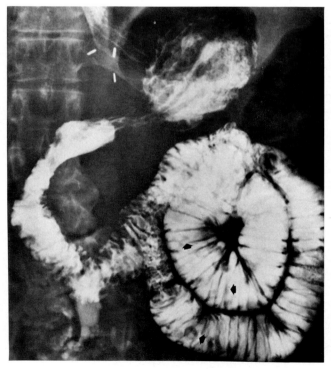

Fig. 40-2. Gardner's syndrome. Diffuse polyposis involves the proximal small bowel in a patient with extensive colonic polyposis. The **arrows** point to a few of the many filling defects in the barium column.

tinal carcinoma have been described in patients with generalized juvenile polyposis.

The association of diffuse juvenile polyps with alopecia, onychodystrophy, hyperpigmentation, and malabsorption is termed the Cronkhite-Canada syndrome. The juvenile polyps in this rare condition are hamartomas without malignant potential that are scattered throughout the stomach, small bowel, and colon.

In the Ruvalcaba–Myhre–Smith syndrome, hamartomatous polyps that diffusely involve the gastrointestinal tract are associated with macrocephaly and pigmented genital lesions (Fig. 40-3). No malignancies have been reported in patients with this extremely rare condition.

Although adenomatous polyps in the small bowel are usually single, multiple polyps can occur as an isolated event and not as part of an inherited disorder.

OTHER TUMORS

Hemangiomas of the small bowel are generally multiple but tend to be so small that they are frequently missed on barium studies. The combination of phleboliths and multiple filling defects in the small bowel is pathognomonic of multiple hemangiomas (Fig. 40-4).

Leiomyomas, though the most common benign tumors of the small bowel, are very rarely multiple. A few cases have been reported of extensive involvement of the small bowel by multiple lipomas causing large intramural and mesenteric masses and separation of bowel loops (Fig. 40-5). These fatty lesions produce characteristic low attenuation on CT (Fig. 40-6), which can also distinguish intestinal lipomatosis from liposarcoma by the homogeneity of the lesions and the absence of areas of increased density.

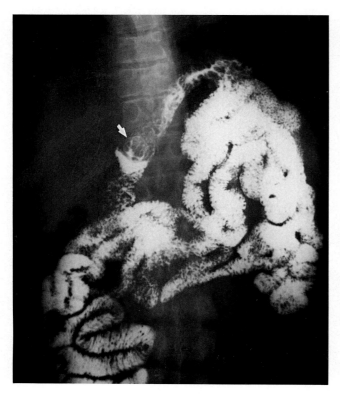

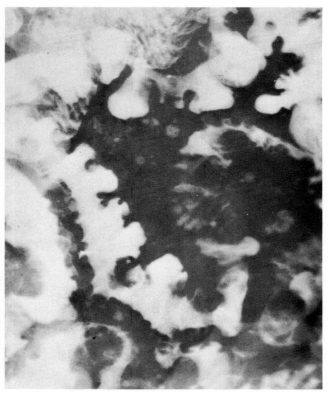

40-3   40-4

Fig. 40-3. Ruvalcaba–Myhre–Smith syndrome. Multiple discrete polypoid filling defects in the ileum. Note the large gastric antral polyp **(arrow)**. (Foster MA, Kilcoyne RF: Ruvalcaba–Myhre–Smith syndrome: New consideration in the differential diagnosis of intestinal polyposis. Gastrointest Radiol 11:349–350, 1986)

Fig. 40-4. Hemangiomatosis of the small bowel and mesentery. Characteristic phleboliths are associated with multiple filling defects in the small bowel.

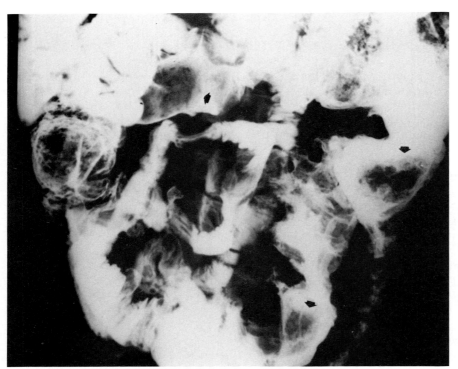

Fig. 40-5. Polypoid lipomatosis of the small bowel. Multiple loops of the distal small bowel display segmental, irregular dilatation with pronounced distortion of the bowel lumen and mucosal pattern. The bowel loops appear separated and impressed extrinsically by multiple mesenteric masses **(arrows)**. (Margolin FR, Lagios MD: Polypoid lipomatosis of the small bowel. Gastrointest Radiol 5:59–60. 1980)

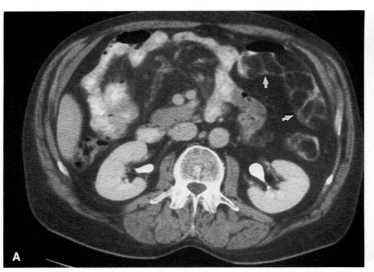

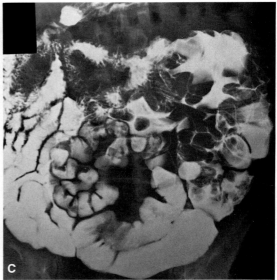

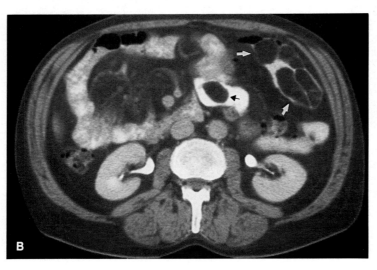

Fig. 40-6. Polypoid lipomatosis of the small bowel. **(A)** and **(B)** CT scans show multiple radiolucent ovoid masses **(arrows)** outlined by contrast material in the intestinal lumen. The lesions are of the same radiolucency as normal abdominal fat. **(C)** Barium study shows multiple smooth-walled radiolucent masses projecting into the lumen of the jejunum and upper ileum. (Ormson MJ, Stephens DH, Carlson HC: CT recognition of intestinal lipomatosis. AJR 144:313–314, 1985. Copyright 1985. Reproduced with permission)

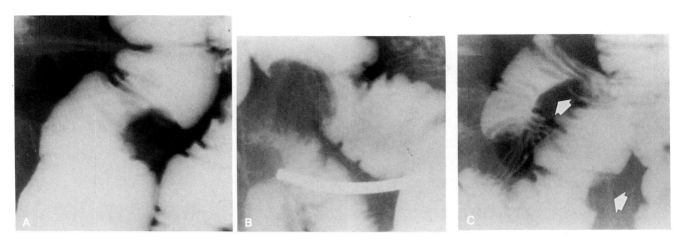

Fig. 40-7. Multiple carcinoid tumors. (Jeffree MA, Nolan DJ: Multiple ileal carcinoid tumours. Br J Radiol 60:402–403, 1987)

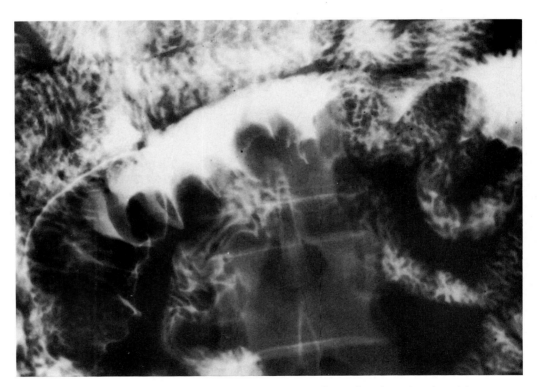

Fig. 40-8. Neurofibromatosis. The polyps are both sessile and pedunculated and have a characteristic eccentric location. (Ginsburg LD: Eccentric polyposis of the small bowel. Radiology 116:561–562, 1975)

Carcinoid tumors are multiple in about one-third of cases (Fig. 40-7). They can show central ulceration or umbilication. However, the tumors are usually small, and multiple lesions are rarely demonstrated radiographically.

In patients with von Reklinghausen's disease, neurofibromas occasionally produce multiple small bowel filling defects. Unlike the intestinal polyposis syndromes, multiple small bowel neurofibromas have an eccentric distribution (Fig. 40-8).

Multiple intraluminal or intramural filling defects are a common presentation of metastatic disease to the small bowel, especially in patients with melanoma and primary carcinomas of the breast

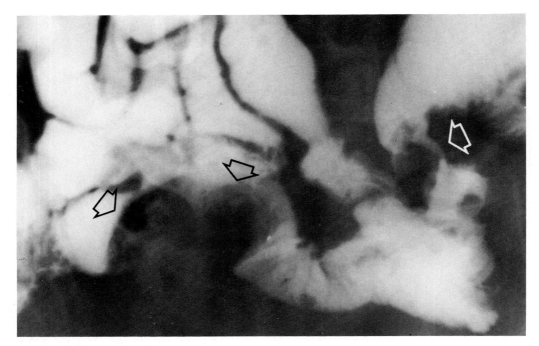

Fig. 40-9. Carcinoma of the breast metastatic to the small bowel and mesentery producing large mass impressions **(black arrows)** and an annular constricting lesion **(white arrow)**.

and lung (Fig. 40-9). Other less frequent sites of primary neoplasms include ovary, pancreas, kidney, stomach, and uterus, and Kaposi's sarcoma. Primary or secondary lymphoma can cause a similar pattern (Fig. 40-10). In small bowel metastases, central ulceration is extremely common as the lesion outgrows its blood supply. This produces a characteristic target or bull's-eye appearance.

As in the colon, hyperplastic, inflamed mucosa that remains between areas of ulceration in Crohn's disease can produce pseudopolyps and a cobblestone appearance of the small bowel (see Fig. 38-12). In a case report, filiform pseudopolyps in a patient with Crohn's disease produced elongated, thin, and fingerlike filling defects in the small bowel (Fig. 40-11).

NODULAR LYMPHOID HYPERPLASIA

Although most commonly presenting as small, regular filling defects diffusely scattered throughout the small bowel (Fig. 40-12), nodular lymphoid hyperplasia can appear as larger filling defects suggesting multiple polypoid masses (Fig. 40-13).

INGESTED MATERIAL

Ingested material can present as multiple filling defects within the small bowel. Fruit pits, especially those from prunes, can be trapped in areas of chronic obstruction (Crohn's disease) or in areas of stasis (Meckel's diverticulum or blind loop). These enteroliths are frequently calcified and can cause ulceration, stenosis, or small bowel obstruction. Food particles, seeds, and pills can present radiographically as filling defects in the small bowel. In patients with previous gastric resection who are edentulous, multiple bezoars can form in the small bowel lumen.

PARASITES

Multiple linear intraluminal defects in the small bowel are usually related to parasitic infection. *Ascaris lumbricoides* is the most common small bowel parasite. After the ingestion of contaminated vegetables, water, or soil, larvae of the worm hatch in the small bowel. Following a complicated migration through the bowel wall, lung, and tracheo-

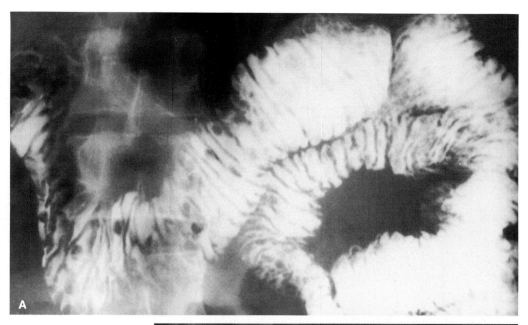

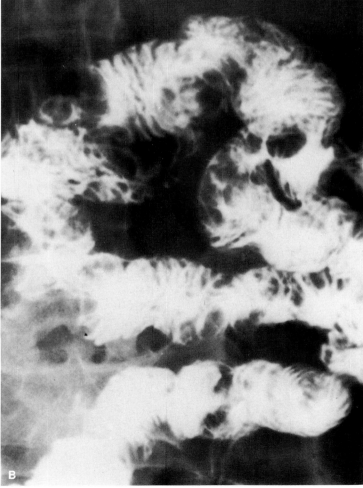

Fig. 40-10. Two patients with lymphoma of the small bowel demonstrating **(A)** small and **(B)** large nodular patterns.

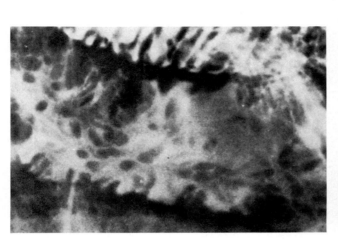

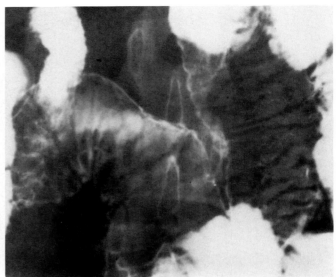

40-11

40-12

Fig. 40-11. Crohn's disease. Close-up view of a segment of small bowel demonstrates numerous filiform polyps. (Bray JF: Filiform polyposis of the small bowel in Crohn's disease. Gastrointest Radiol 8:155–156, 1983)

Fig. 40-12. Nodular lymphoid hyperplasia. Innumerable small, regular filling defects are diffusely scattered throughout the small bowel.

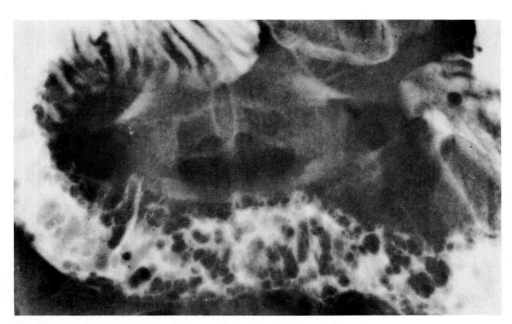

Fig. 40-13. Nodular lymphoid hyperplasia. Large filling defects suggest multiple polypoid masses.

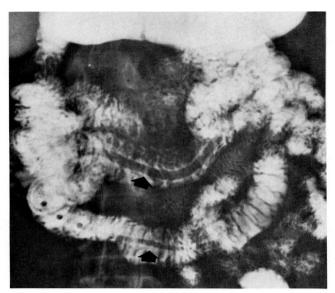

Fig. 40-14. *Ascaris lumbricoides.* On barium studies, the worms appear as elongated, radiolucent filling defects **(arrows)**.

bronchial tree, the larvae again enter the alimentary tract and reach the small bowel, where they mature into adult worms. If they are not in large numbers, the mere presence of adult worms in the small bowel is usually asymptomatic or associated with vague and nonspecific abdominal complaints. Complications of ascariasis include intestinal obstruction, peritonitis (if the worms penetrate the bowel), biliary colic (if the worms enter the bile duct), and hemoptysis (as the worms pass through the lungs en route to the bowel).

On barium studies, the worms appear as elongated radiolucent filling defects (Fig. 40-14). If the patient has been fasting for 12 hr or longer, an ascaris often ingests barium, and the gastrointestinal tract of the worm then appears as a thin longitudinal opaque density bisecting the length of the lucent filling defect (Fig. 40-15). At times, masses of coiled worms clump together and produce one or more rounded intraluminal filling defects in the small bowel. In endemic areas, a similar radiographic appearance can occur with parasitic infes-

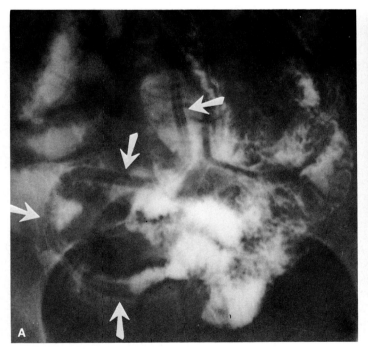

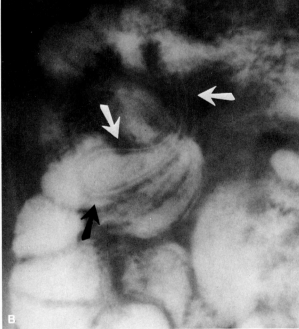

Fig. 40-15. *Ascaris lymbricoides.* Barium can be seen in the intestinal tract of the worm **(arrows)**. (Weissberg DL, Berk RN: Ascariasis of the gastrointestinal tract. Gastrointest Radiol 3:415–418, 1978)

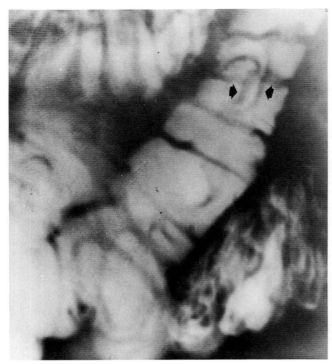

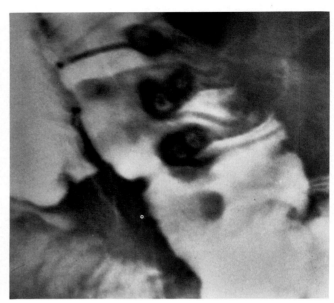

40-16   40-17

Fig. 40-16. *Taenia solis* (tapeworm). Multiple small filling defects **(arrows)** are visible in this segment of small bowel.

Fig. 40-17. Behcet's syndrome. Multiple large, discrete nodular lesions with central ringlike barium collections. (McLean AM, Simms DM, Homer MJ: Ileal ring ulcers in Behcet syndrome. AJR 140:947–948, 1983. Copyright 1983. Reproduced with permission)

tations of the small bowel caused by *Strongyloides stercoralis*, *Ancylostoma duodenale* (hookworm), or *Taenia solis* (tapeworm) (Fig. 40-16).

OTHER CAUSES

Gallstones in the small bowel are usually single. Infrequently, several gallstones enter the bowel through fistulas from the biliary tree to adjacent duodenum, colon, or stomach. Gallstones characteristically progress through the small bowel until they become impacted in the relatively narrow terminal ileum, where they produce distal small bowel obstruction. The majority of patients with gallstone ileus are elderly women, most of whom have a history compatible with chronic gallbladder disease. When multiple filling defects in the small bowel are associated with mechanical obstruction and gas within the biliary tree, gallstone ileus should be considered the most likely diagnosis.

In patients who are actively bleeding from an upper gastrointestinal tract ulcer or tumor, multiple filling defects in the jejunum or ileum can be due to blood clots.

Jejunal and ileal varices are extremely rare. They can appear radiographically as multiple polypoid or serpiginous filling defects throughout the small bowel (see Fig. 39-18). Dilatation of jejunal veins can occur as part of a syndrome (multiple phlebectasia involving the jejunum, oral mucosa, tongue, and scrotum) and should be suspected as a possible cause of upper gastrointestinal hemorrhage if mucocutaneous manifestations are present.

One patient with Behcet's syndrome has been reported with multiple large nodular small bowel lesions containing central ringlike collections of barium (Fig. 40-17).

BIBLIOGRAPHY

Bancks NH, Goldstein HM, Dodd GD: The roentgenologic spectrum of small intestinal carcinoid tumors. AJR 123:274–280, 1975

Bartholomew LG, Dahlin DC, Waugh JM: Intestinal polyposis associated with mucocutaneous melanin pigmentation (Peutz–Jeghers syndrome). Gastroenterology 32:434–451, 1957

Bray JF: Filiform polyposis of the small bowel in Crohn's disease. Gastrointest Radiol 8:155–156, 1983

Cavanaugh RC, Buchignani JS, Rulon DB: Metastatic melanoma of the small intestine. RPC of the month from the AFIP. Radiology 101:195–200, 1971

Cronkhite LW, Canada WJ: Generalized gastrointestinal polyposis: An unusual syndrome of pigmentation, alopecia, and onychotrophia. N Engl J Med 252:1011–1015, 1955

Dodds WJ: Clinical and roentgen features of the intestinal polyposis syndromes. Gastrointest Radiol 1:127–142, 1976

Dodds WJ, Schulte WJ, Hensley GT et al: Peutz–Jeghers syndrome and gastrointestinal malignancy. AJR 115:374–377, 1972

Fleming RJ, Seaman WB: Roentgenographic demonstration of unusual extraesophageal varices. AJR 103:281–290, 1968

Foster MA, Kilcoyne RF: Ruvalcava–Myhre–Smith syndrome: A new consideration in the differential diagnosis of intestinal polyposis. Gastrointest Radiol 11:349–350, 1986

Ginsburg LD: Eccentric polyposis of the small bowel: A possible radiologic sign of plexiform neurofibromatosis of the small bowel and its mesentery. Radiology 116:561–562, 1975

Jeffree MA, Nolan DJ: Multiple ileal carcinoid tumors. Br J Radiol 60:402–403, 1987

Jeghers H, McKusick VA, Katz KH: Generalized intestinal polyposis and melanin spots of the oral mucosa, lips and digits: A syndrome of diagnostic significance. N Eng J Med 241:933–1005, 1031–1036, 1949

Johnson GK, Soergel KH, Hensley GT et al: Cronkhite–Canada syndrome: Gastrointestinal pathophysiology and morphology. Gastroenterology 63:140–152, 1972

Macdonald JM, Davis WC, Crago HR et al: Gardner's syndrome and periampullary malignancy. Am J Surg 113:425–430, 1967

Margolin FR, Lagios MD: Polypoid lipomatosis of the small bowel. Gastrointest Radiol 5:59–60, 1980

Marshak RH, Freund S, Maklansky D: Neurofibromatosis of the small bowel. Am J Dig Dis 8:478–483, 1963

McLean AM, Simms DM, Homer MJ: Ileal ring ulcers in Behcet syndrome. AJR 140:947–948, 1983

Meyers MA, McSweeney J: Secondary neoplasms of the bowel. Radiology 105:1–11, 1972

Ormson MJ, Stephens DH, Carlson HC: CT recognition of intestinal lipomatosis. AJR 144:313–314, 1985

Smith SJ, Carlson HC, Gisvold JJ: Secondary neoplasms of the small bowel. Radiology 125:29–33, 1977

Weissberg DL, Berk RN: Ascariasis of the gastrointestinal tract. Gastrointest Radiol 3:415–418, 1978

Zboralske FF, Bessolo RJ: Metastatic carcinoma to the mesentery and gut. Radiology 88:302–310, 1967

41 SANDLIKE LUCENCIES

Disease Entities

Macroglobulinemia
Mastocytosis
Histoplasmosis
Lymphoid hyperplasia
Intestinal lymphangiectasia
Whipple's disease
Crohn's disease
Yersinia enterocolitis
Eosinophilic enteritis
Cronkhite–Canada syndrome
Amyloidosis
Food particles/gas bubbles
Radiation enteritis
Pancreatic glucagonoma
Protein-losing enteropathy
Small bowel ischemia

Massive enlargement of small bowel villi can produce multiple fine, punctate lucencies in the barium column that appear sandlike and granular. In most instances, these innumerable tiny, nodular lucencies are superimposed on a diffusely thickened fold pattern.

MACROGLOBULINEMIA

Primary macroglobulinemia (Waldenstrom's syndrome) is a plasma cell dyscrasia involving those cells that synthesize macroglobulins (IgM) (Fig. 41-1). Large amounts of IgM are found in the sera of patients with the disorder. It has an insidious onset in late adult life and is characterized clinically by anemia, bleeding, lymphadenopathy, and hepatosplenomegaly. Although gastrointestinal symptoms are unusual, malabsorption can occur. In Waldenstrom's syndrome, the lacteals and lamina propria of the small bowel villi are filled with a macroglobulin proteinaceous material. As the villi become greatly extended and even visible to the naked eye, a sandlike radiographic pattern is produced. Tiny barium droplets adhering to the surface tips of the enlarged villi may produce a stippled punctate pattern.

MASTOCYTOSIS

In mastocytosis, diffuse infiltration of the lamina propria by a cellular infiltrate containing a large number of tissue mast cells causes enlargement of the small bowel villi and the radiographic appearance of punctate filling defects (Fig. 41-2). This pattern is superimposed on a generally irregular, thickened fold pattern produced by edema and urticaria-like lesions of the intestinal mucosa.

HISTOPLASMOSIS

Although histoplasmosis is primarily a benign, self-limited pulmonary disease, disseminated infection

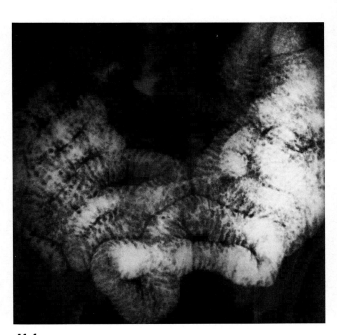

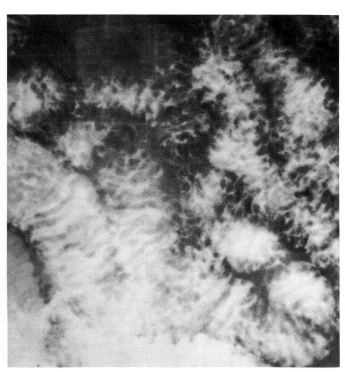

41-1   **41-2**

Fig. 41-1. Waldenstrom's macroglobulinemia.

Fig. 41-2. Mastocytosis. Nodular filling defects are superimposed on a pattern of irregular thickened folds.

can affect the gastrointestinal tract. In this condition, the lamina propria is infiltrated by enormous numbers of histoplasma-laden macrophages. When seen on end, they can appear in a pattern of innumerable filling defects that seem to diffusely blanket the small bowel with a sandlike covering superimposed on irregular, distorted folds (Fig. 41-3).

NODULAR LYMPHOID HYPERPLASIA

Nodular lymphoid hyperplasia primarily involves the jejunum but can occur throughout the entire small bowel. Lymphoid hyperplasia is often seen in children without any immunodeficiency problems. In adults, however, it is almost invariably associated with late-onset immunoglobulin deficiency. The chronically reduced concentration of serum globulins results in an increased susceptibility to respiratory and other infections. Diarrhea and malabsorption are frequent complaints; *Giardia lamblia* infection can be demonstrated in up to 90% of patients with this condition. There is a relatively high incidence of carcinoma of the stomach and benign thymoma (Good's syndrome) in young persons with nodular lymphoid hyperplasia.

The hyperplastic lymph follicles in the lamina propria cause effacement of the villous pattern,

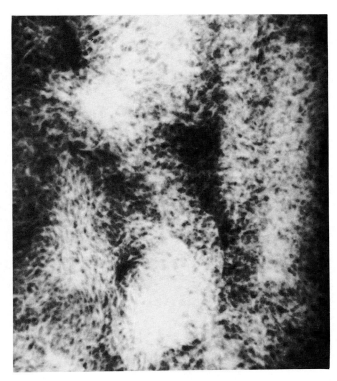

Fig. 41-3. Histoplasmosis. Innumerable filling defects diffusely blanket the small bowel with a sandlike covering superimposed on irregular distorted folds.

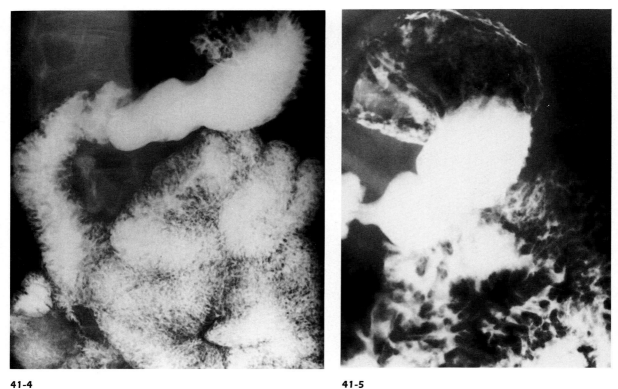

41-4   41-5

Fig. 41-4. Nodular lymphoid hyperplasia. Innumerable tiny polypoid masses are uniformly distributed throughout the involved segments of small bowel. The underlying small bowel fold pattern is normal in this patient, who had no evidence of associated disease.

Fig. 41-5. Nodular lymphoid hyperplasia in a patient with an immunodeficiency and *Giardia lamblia* infestation. The relatively larger nodules are superimposed on an irregularly thickened and grossly distorted underlying fold pattern.

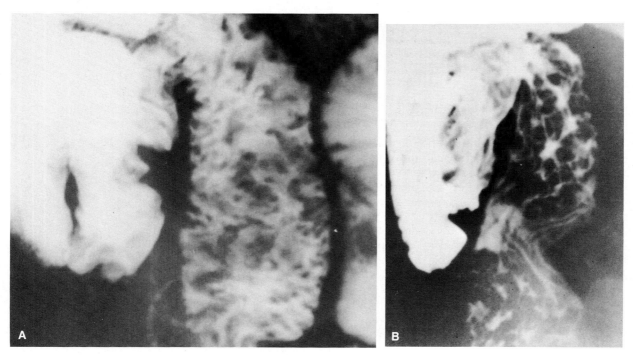

Fig. 41-6. Normal terminal ileum in two adolescents. **(A)** Multiple small nodules in the terminal ileum representing normal prominence of lymphoid follicles. **(B)** Larger nodules of lymphoid follicles.

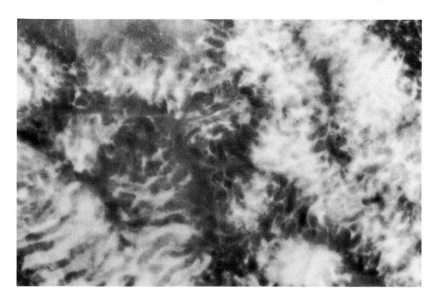

Fig. 41-7. *Intestinal lymphangiectasia. Note the diffuse nodularity and irregular folds.*

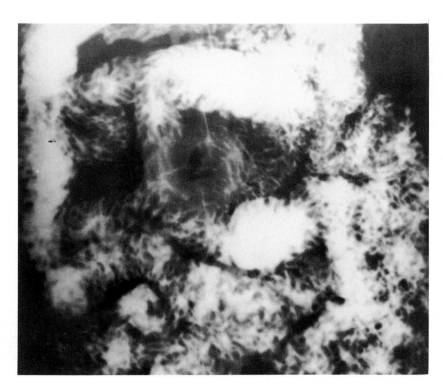

Fig. 41-8. *Whipple's disease. Multiple nodules are superimposed on a grossly distorted small bowel fold pattern.*

making the bowel appear to be studded with innumerable tiny polypoid masses uniformly distributed throughout the involved segment of intestine (Fig. 41-4). The filling defects are round and regular in outline and have no recognizable ulceration. If there is no associated disease, the sandlike nodules of lymphoid hyperplasia are superimposed on a background of normal small bowel folds. When *Giardia* infection is also present, however, the underlying fold pattern is irregularly thickened and grossly distorted (Fig. 41-5). In children and young adults, the presence of multiple small, symmetric nodules of lymphoid hyperplasia in the terminal ileum is a normal finding (Fig. 41-6).

INTESTINAL LYMPHANGIECTASIA

Intestinal lymphangiectasia is characterized by the early onset of massive edema, hypoproteinemia, and lymphocytopenia. The dilated, telangiectatic

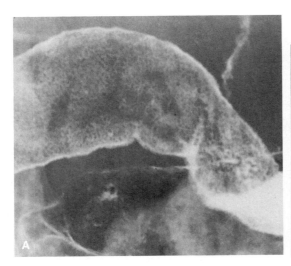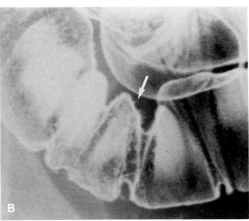

Fig. 41-9. Crohn's disease. **(A)** Diffuse, uniform pattern of tiny, round filling defects along with fine scalloping of the inferior contour in an otherwise normal segment of the small bowel. **(B)** In another patient, diffuse granularity in an otherwise normal segment of the small bowel is seen both en face and tangentially as fine spicules **(arrow)** representing barium located between filling defects. (Glick SN, Teplick SK: Crohn disease of the small intestine: Diffuse mucosal granularity. Radiology 154:313–317, 1985)

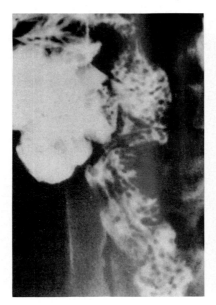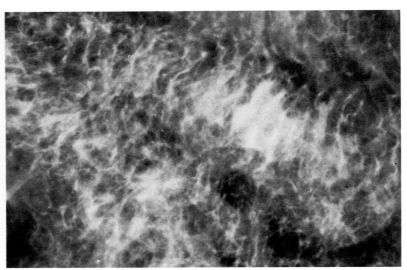

41-10   41-11

Fig. 41-10. *Yersinia* enterocolitis. Multiple small filling defects in the terminal ileum during the healing stage of the disease.

Fig. 41-11. Amyloidosis. Magnified view of the small bowel shows multiple fine filling defects, many containing tiny flecks of barium, superimposed on generalized thickening of mucosal folds. (Smith TR, Cho KC: Small intestine amyloidosis producing a stippled punctate mucosal pattern: Radiological–pathological correlation. Am J Gastroenterol 81:477–479, 1986)

lymphatic vessels in the small bowel cause marked enlargement of the villi, which produces diffuse nodularity and a sandlike pattern (Fig. 41-7) as well as radiographic evidence of hypersecretion.

WHIPPLE'S DISEASE

In Whipple's disease, extensive infiltration of the lamina propria with large periodic acid-Schiff (PAS)-positive macrophages causes marked swelling of the intestinal villi and thickened, irregular mucosal folds (primarily in the duodenum and proximal jejunum). When these bulbous structures become large enough to be macroscopically visible, they may appear as innumerable small filling defects superimposed on the irregularly thickened fold pattern (Fig. 41-8).

CROHN'S DISEASE

Diffuse mucosal granularity has been reported as the earliest radiographic abnormality in Crohn's disease involving the small bowel (Fig. 41-9). This appearance is produced by a reticular network of tiny radiolucent foci that pathologically represents widening and blunting of villi with lymphocytic infiltration. At times, the granular mucosal pattern may be the only evidence of Crohn's disease. A similar appearance may also be seen following extensive small bowel resection in patients with Crohn's disease, possibly due to villous enlargement resulting from intestinal adaptation. This refers to a compensatory acceleration of epithelial cell turnover in the small bowel villi and crypts with an increase in villous height and crypt depth due to villous hyperpla-

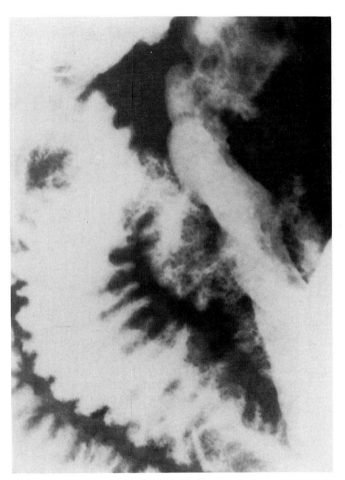

Fig. 41-12. Radiation jejunitis. Diffuse granularity and minimal fold thickening involving several loops of proximal jejunum. (Jones B, Hamilton SR, Rubesin SE et al: Granular small bowel mucosa: A reflection of villous abnormality. Gastrointest Radiol 12:219–225, 1987)

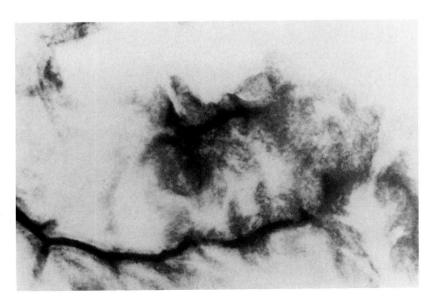

Fig. 41-13. Pancreatic glucagonoma. Coned view of the jejunum demonstrates granularity consisting of a coalescence of innumerable tiny filling defects representing the elongated villi. (Jones B, Hamilton SR, Rubesin SE et al: Granular small bowel mucosa: A reflection of villous abnormality. Gastrointest Radiol 12:219–225, 1987)

sia, the magnitude of which appears to be directly proportional to the amount of resected intestine.

YERSINIA ENTEROCOLITIS

Yersinia enterocolitis characteristically causes a radiographic pattern of coarse, irregularly thickened mucosal folds predominantly affecting the terminal ileum. During the healing stages of this disease, tiny filling defects of 1 mm to 2 mm in diameter appear, producing a granular pattern (follicular ileitis) that can persist for many months (Fig. 41-10).

OTHER CAUSES

Innumerable tiny nodules in the small bowel presenting a sandlike pattern have been described in eosinophilic enteritis (often with gastric involvement), the Cronkhite–Canada syndrome (associated with colonic polyposis), and mucoviscidosis. Diffuse deposition of amyloid in the lamina propria can produce a similar pattern, which may appear stippled due to tiny adherent droplets of barium (Fig. 41-11). Food particles and gas bubbles are inconstant nodular defects that can be moved by manipulation at fluoroscopy. Diffuse mucosal granularity simulating the appearance in early Crohn's disease has been recently reported in patients with radiation enteritis (Fig. 41-12), pancreatic glucagonoma (Fig. 41-13), protein-losing enteropathy, and small bowel ischemia. The unifying feature of these entities on microscopic examination is a change in the morphology of the small bowel villi, which may be due to edema, hyperplasia, clubbing, or fusion.

BIBLIOGRAPHY

Ajdukiewicz AB, Youngs GR, Bouchier IAD: Nodular lymphoid hyperplasia with hypogammaglobulinemia. Gut 13:589–595, 1972

Ament ME, Rubin CE: Relation of giardiasis to abnormal intestinal structure and function in gastrointestinal immunodeficiency syndromes. Gastroenterology 62:216–226, 1972

Bank S, Trey C, Gans I et al: Histoplasmosis of the small bowel with "giant" intestinal villi and secondary protein-losing enteropathy. Am J Med 39:492–501, 1965

Bedine MS, Yardley JH, Elliott HL et al: Intestinal involvement in Waldenstrom's macroglobulinemia. Gastroenterology 65:308–315, 1973

Clemett AR, Fishbone G, Levine RJ et al: Gastrointestinal lesions in mastocytosis. AJR 103:405–412, 1968

Clemett AR, Marshak RH: Whipple's disease: Roentgen features and differential diagnosis. Radiol Clin North Am 7:105–111, 1969

Hodgson JR, Hoffman HN, Huivenga KA: Roentgenologic features of lymphoid hyperplasia of the small intestines associated with dysgammaglobulinemia. Radiology 88:883–888, 1967

Khilnani MT, Keller RJ, Cuttner J: Macroglobulinemia and steatorrhea: Roentgen and pathologic findings in the intestinal tract. Radiol Clin North Am 7:43–55, 1969

Shimkin PM, Waldmann TA, Krugman RL: Intestinal lymphangiectasia. AJR 110:827–841, 1970

Smith TR, Cho KC: Small intestinal amyloidosis producing a stippled punctate mucosal pattern: Radiological–pathological correlation. Am J Gastroenterol 81:477–479, 1986

Vantrappen G, Agg HO, Ponette E et al: *Yersinia* enteritis and enterocolitis: Gastroenterological aspects. Gastroenterology 72:220–227, 1977

THICKENED SMALL BOWEL FOLDS WITH CONCOMITANT INVOLVEMENT OF THE STOMACH

Disease Entities

Lymphoma
Crohn's disease
Eosinophilic gastroenteritis
Zollinger-Ellison syndrome
Menetrier's disease
Gastric varices with hypoproteinemia
Amyloidosis
Whipple's disease

LYMPHOMA

Involvement of both the stomach and the small bowel is one of the many manifestations of gastrointestinal lymphoma (Fig. 42-1). In the stomach, lymphoma can present as large gastric folds, a discrete intraluminal mass, a nodular lesion, or a large malignant ulceration. Irregular thickening of mucosal folds is one appearance of small bowel lymphoma. Lymphoma of the small bowel can also manifest itself as a polypoid filling defect or ulcerated intramural lesion. Extrinsic impressions and separation of small bowel loops can be due to extension into the mesentery and enlargement of mesenteric nodes.

CROHN'S DISEASE

Although the ileum, especially its terminal portion, is the most common site of Crohn's disease, this condition can affect any portion of the gastrointestinal tract and produce concomitant small bowel and gastric lesions. Crohn's disease causes a broad spectrum of small bowel abnormalities, ranging from ulceration, fold thickening, and "cobblestoning" to strictures, fistulas, and sinus tracts. Granulomatous inflammatory infiltration of the antrum results in deformity, tubular narrowing, limited distensibility, and poor peristalsis, which can mimic an infiltrating gastric carcinoma. Crohn's disease involving both sides of the pyloric channel leads to a characteristic funnel-shaped pseudo-Billroth-I deformity (see Fig. 25-7).

EOSINOPHILIC GASTROENTERITIS

Combined gastric and small bowel involvement is a typical finding in eosinophilic gastroenteritis (Fig. 42-2). This disease, which is of allergic or immunologic etiology, is characterized by peripheral eosinophilia and infiltration of the bowel wall by eosinophilic leukocytes. Clinically, gastrointestinal symptoms and signs follow the ingestion of specific foods.

Eosinophilic gastroenteritis most commonly presents radiographically as coarsening and nodularity of folds in the distal stomach and small bowel, particularly the jejunum. The folds can be distorted and irregularly angulated, producing a sawtooth contour of the bowel (often appearing rigid at fluoroscopy) with separation of bowel loops. When eosinophilic gastroenteritis primarily involves the muscular layer, marked thickening and rigidity of

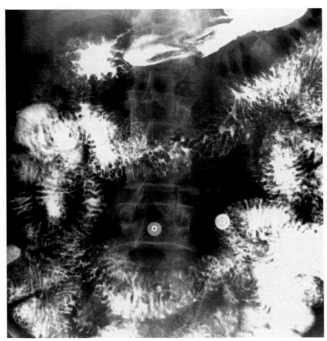

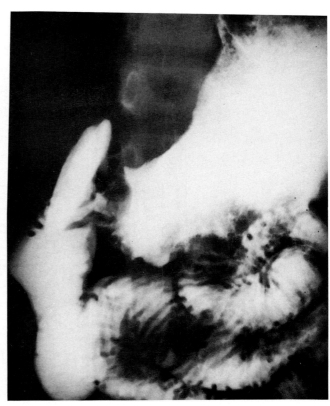

42-1   42-2

Fig. 42-1. Lymphoma. Fold thickening and nodularity diffusely involve the stomach and small bowel.

Fig. 42-2. Eosinophilic gastroenteritis. Fold thickening involves both the stomach and the proximal small bowel.

the antrum and pylorus can simulate an infiltrating carcinoma, peptic disease, or Crohn's disease affecting the stomach. Extensive mural thickening and rigidity of the duodenum and small bowel are also frequently seen. Symptoms of gastric outlet obstruction or incomplete small bowel obstruction are not uncommon. The radiographic differentiation between eosinophilic gastroenteritis and Crohn's disease can be difficult. A characteristic clinical distinction is the self-limited nature of eosinophilic gastroenteritis and the return of the small bowel pattern to normal in response to steroid therapy.

ZOLLINGER-ELLISON SYNDROME

The gastric rugal folds in patients with the Zollinger-Ellison syndrome are extremely prominent, reflecting an abnormal hypersecretory state in response to a gastrin-secreting islet cell tumor of the pancreas (Fig. 42-3). The stomach can contain large

amounts of fluid without any demonstrable gastric outlet obstruction. The excessive volume of hyperacidic gastric secretions floods the small bowel and produces a chemical enteritis manifested by dilatation and thickening of small bowel folds. Ulcerations are often demonstrated in unusual locations in the distal duodenum or jejunum.

MENETRIER'S DISEASE

The radiographic hallmark of Menetrier's disease is giant hypertrophy of gastric rugal folds. Once thought to involve only the body of the stomach, Menetrier's disease is now known to potentially affect the entire organ. Menetrier's disease is one of the "protein-losing enteropathies" in which large amounts of protein (especially albumin and gamma-globulin) are lost into the lumen of the stomach. The precise mechanism involved is unclear, but it may be related to impaired metabolism of surface epithelial cells or to mucosal disease

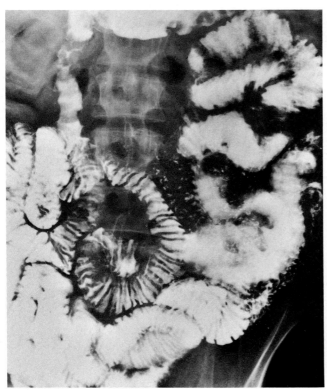

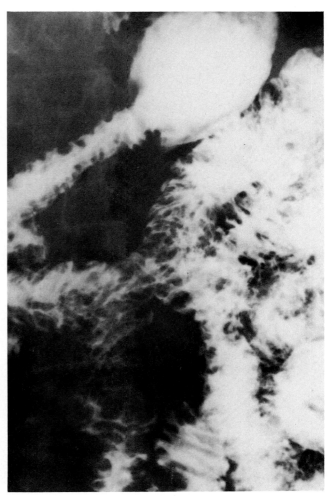

42-3   42-4

Fig. 42-3. Zollinger-Ellison syndrome. There is prominent thickening of gastric and duodenal folds and dilatation and fold thickening in the small bowel. Excessive secretions in the small bowel cause the barium to have a granular, indistinct quality.

Fig. 42-4. Amyloidosis. Diffuse thickening of mucosal folds involves the stomach, duodenum, and visualized small bowel.

without ulceration, either of which may lead to altered mucosal permeability to protein or an increase in cell desquamation. The resulting systemic hypoproteinemia can cause regular thickening of small bowel folds, which is indistinguishable from the thickening caused by hypoproteinemia related to severe liver disease.

GASTRIC VARICES WITH HYPOPROTEINEMIA

The combination of gastric varices and hypoproteinemia in patients with severe liver disease can result in prominent gastric rugae or nodular fundal masses in association with regular thickening of small bowel folds. Although esophageal varices are usually also present, gastric varices can exist independently and mimic the radiographic findings of Menetrier's disease or malignant neoplasm of the stomach.

AMYLOIDOSIS/WHIPPLE'S DISEASE

Amyloidosis (Fig. 42-4) and Whipple's disease are unusual causes of large gastric rugae in combination with diffusely thickened small bowel folds. Both conditions can also infiltrate the wall of the distal stomach and narrow the antrum.

BIBLIOGRAPHY

Burhenne JH: Eosinophilic (allergic) gastroenteritis. AJR 96:332–338, 1966

Christoforidis AJ, Nelson SW: Radiological manifestations of ulcerogenic tumors of the pancreas: The Zollinger-Ellison syndrome. JAMA 198:511–516, 1966

Clemett AR, Marshak RH: Whipple's disease: Roentgen features and differential diagnosis. Radiol Clin North Am 7:105–111, 1969

Cohen WN: Gastric involvement in Crohn's disease. AJR 101:425–430, 1967

Dodds WJ, Geenen JE, Stewart ET: Eosinophilic enteritis. Am J Gastroenterol 61:308–312, 1974

Farman J, Faegenburg D, Dallemand S et al: Crohn's disease of the stomach: The "ram's horn" sign. AJR 123:242–251, 1975

Goldberg HI, O'Kieffe D, Jenis EH et al: Diffuse eosinophilic gastroenteritis. AJR 119:342–351, 1973

Legge DA, Carlson HC, Wollaeger EE: Roentgenologic appearance of systemic amyloidosis involving the gastrointestinal tract. AJR 110:406–412, 1970

Muhletaler CA, Gerlock AJ, Goncharenko V et al: Gastric varices secondary to splenic vein occlusion: Radiographic diagnosis and clinical significance. Radiology 132:593–598, 1979

Reese DF, Hodgson JR, Dockerty MB: Giant hypertrophy of the gastric mucosa (Menetrier's disease): A correlation of the roentgenographic, pathologic and clinical findings. AJR 88:619–626, 1962

SEPARATION OF SMALL BOWEL LOOPS

Disease Entities

Processes that thicken or infiltrate the bowel
    wall or mesentery
    Crohn's disease
    Tuberculosis
    Intestinal hemorrhage or mesenteric
        vascular occlusion
    Whipple's disease
    Amyloidosis
    Lymphoma
    Primary carcinoma of the small bowel
    Radiation-induced enteritis
    Carcinoid tumor
    Neurofibromatosis of the small bowel
Ascites
    Hepatic cirrhosis
    Peritonitis
    Congestive failure/constrictive pericarditis
    Peritoneal carcinomatosis
    Primary or metastatic disease of the
        lymphatic system
Neoplasms
    Primary tumors of the peritoneum
    Primary tumors of the mesentery
    Metastases (peritoneal carcinomatosis)
Intraperitoneal abscess
Retractile mesenteritis
Retroperitoneal hernia
Graft-versus-host disease (GVHD)

THICKENING OR INFILTRATION OF THE BOWEL WALL OR MESENTERY

Any process that infiltrates or thickens the bowel wall or mesentery can produce the radiographic appearance of separation of small bowel loops. A classic example of this mechanism is Crohn's disease of the small bowel (Fig. 43-1). In this condition, transmural inflammation results in thickening of all layers of the small bowel wall. The mesentery is markedly thickened, fatty, and edematous; mesenteric nodes are enlarged, firm, and often matted together to form an irregular mass (Fig. 43-2). Narrowing of the bowel lumen further enhances the radiographic appearance of separation of small bowel loops (Fig. 43-3). A similar appearance of irregular narrowing and separation of loops can be due to tuberculosis involving the small bowel (Fig. 43-4) or to cytomegalovirus infection in patients with AIDS (Fig. 43-5).

In patients with intestinal hemorrhage or mesenteric vascular occlusion, bleeding into the bowel wall or mesentery causes separation of bowel loops (Fig. 43-6). Thickening of the mesentery, infiltration of the bowel wall, and enlargement of mesenteric lymph nodes cause separation of small bowel loops in patients with Whipple's disease (Fig. 43-7) and amyloidosis. In primary lymphoma of the small bowel, diffuse submucosal infiltration combined with mesenteric involvement produce the appearance of separated bowel loops (Fig. 43-8). Primary carcinoma of the small bowel (Fig. 43-9) infrequently presents a similar pattern.

517

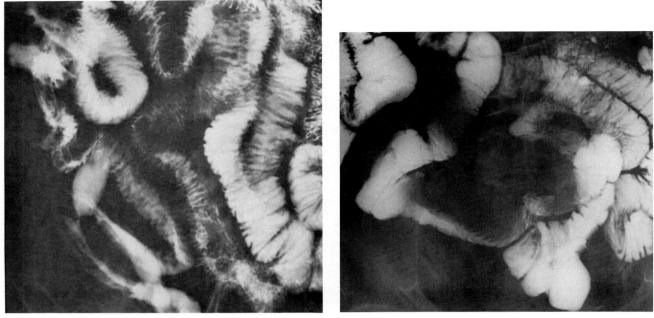

43-1   43-2

Fig. 43-1. Crohn's disease. There is diffuse mesenteric involvement with separation of small bowel loops.

Fig. 43-2. Crohn's disease. Marked thickening of the mesentery and mesenteric nodes produces a lobulated mass widely separating small bowel loops.

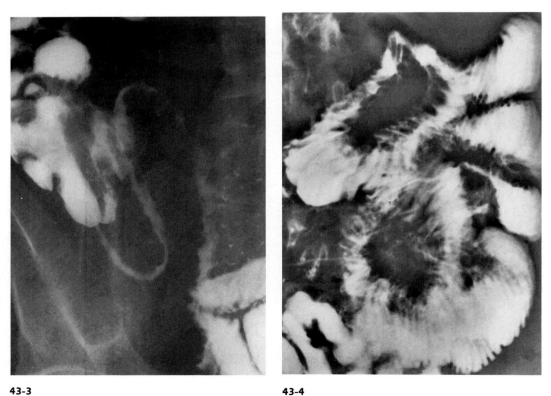

43-3   43-4

Fig. 43-3. Crohn's disease. Severe narrowing of the lumen enhances the radiographic appearance of separation of bowel loops.

Fig. 43-4. Tuberculous enteritis and peritonitis. There is separation of bowel loops, irregular narrowing, fold thickening, and angulation.

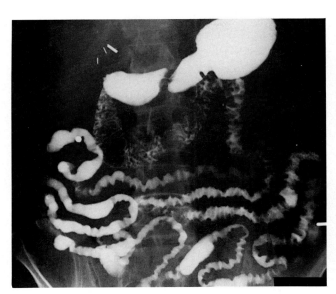

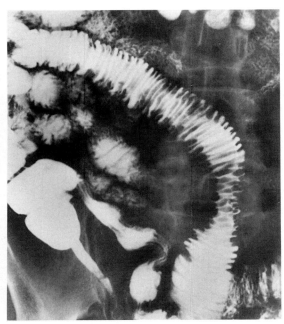

43-5   **43-6**

Fig. 43-5. Cytomegalovirus enteritis. In addition to separation of bowel loops, there is blunting and thickening of mucosal folds, luminal narrowing, and some small ulcers. At autopsy, 90 cm of proximal small bowel showed diffusely congested mucosa with small ulcerations. (Teixidor HS, Honig CL, Norsoph E et al: Cytomegalovirus infection of the alimentary canal: Radiologic findings with pathologic correlation. Radiology 163:317–323, 1987)

Fig. 43-6. Intestinal hemorrhage. This patient, who was on Coumadin (warfarin) therapy, shows radiographic evidence of bleeding into the bowel wall and mesentery.

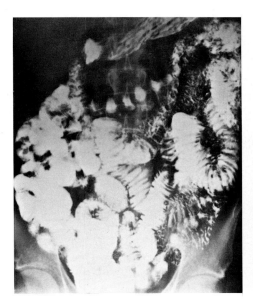

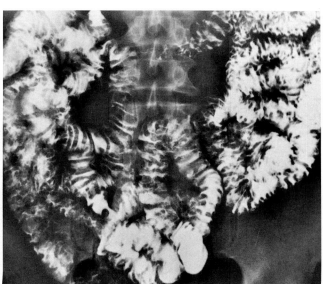

43-7   **43-8**

Fig. 43-7. Whipple's disease. Separation of bowel loops containing grossly distorted, irregular folds. (Phillips RL, Carlson HC: The roentgenographic and clinical findings in Whipple's disease. AJR 123:268–273, 1975. Copyright 1975. Reproduced with permission)

Fig. 43-8. Lymphoma. Submucosal infiltration and mesenteric involvement produce a pattern of generalized irregular fold thickening and separation of bowel loops.

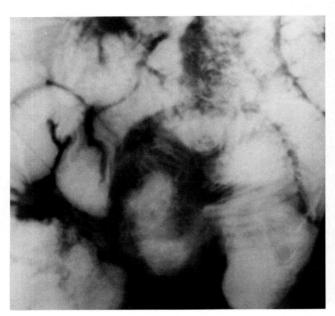

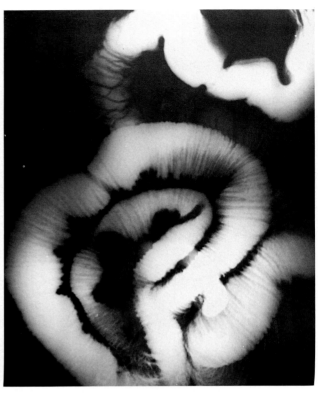

43-9   43-10

Fig. 43-9. Primary adenocarcinoma of the jejunum. Separation of bowel loops is visible in the region of the tumor mass.

Fig. 43-10. Radiation enteritis and mesenteritis. Thickening of the bowel wall and multiple nodular masses cause separation of small bowel loops. The patient had received 7000 rad for treatment of metastatic carcinoma of the cervix.

RADIATION INJURY

Clinically significant radiation damage to the gastro-intestinal tract can occur following radiotherapy to the abdomen (Fig. 43-10). This radiation injury is thought to be secondary to an endarteritis with vascular occlusion and bowel ischemia. Radiographic manifestations include shallow ulceration of the mucosa, submucosal thickening with straightening of folds, and nodular filling defects. Thickening of the bowel wall due to submucosal edema and fibrosis is an almost universal finding in radiation enteritis and leads to separation of adjacent small bowel loops.

CARCINOID TUMOR

Carcinoid tumors initially appear as sharply defined, small submucosal lesions. As they develop, most carcinoids tend to grow extraluminally, infiltrating the bowel wall, lymphatic channels, and eventually regional lymph nodes and the mesentery. Local release of serotonin causes hypertrophic muscular thickening and severe fibroblastic proliferation, which lead to diffuse luminal narrowing and

separation of intestinal loops with external compression and localized abrupt angulation (Fig. 43-11). The presence of one or several intramural nodules coexisting with severe intestinal kinking and a bizarre pattern of small bowel loops is characteristic of carcinoid tumors (Fig. 43-12).

NEUROFIBROMATOSIS

Plexiform neurofibromatosis, a manifestation of von Recklinghausen's disease, consists of the enlargement of many nerve trunks in a given area. When the disease involves the small bowel, multiple polypoid filling defects and thickening of the mesentery cause separation of loops. A characteristic finding in this disorder is eccentric polyposis of the small bowel, the defects being seen entirely on the mesenteric side (Fig. 43-13).

ASCITES

The accumulation of ascitic fluid in the peritoneal cavity can be caused by abnormalities in venous

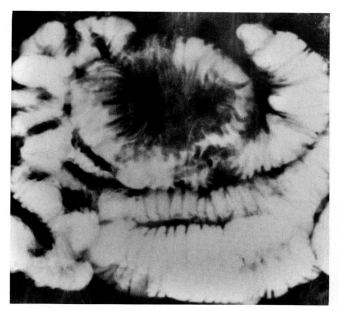

Fig. 43-11. Carcinoid tumor. Separation of bowel loops, luminal narrowing, and fibrotic tethering of mucosal folds are evident.

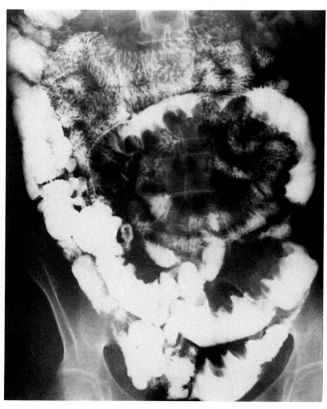

Fig. 43-13. Neurofibromatosis (von Recklinghausen's disease). The mesentery is thickened, and there is separation of small bowel loops. Multiple polypoid filling defects are present along the mesenteric side of the small bowel. (Ginsburg LD: Eccentric polyposis of the small bowel. Radiology 116:561–562, 1975)

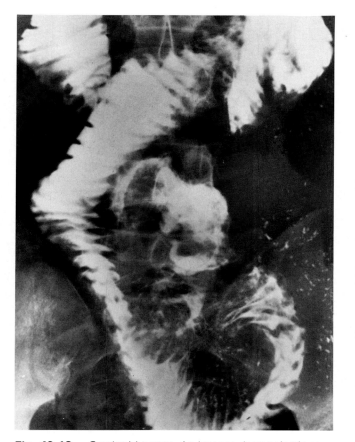

Fig. 43-12. Carcinoid tumor. An intense desmoplastic reaction incited by the tumor causes kinking and angulation of the bowel and separation of small bowel loops in the midabdomen.

pressure, plasma colloid osmotic pressure, hepatic lymph formation, splanchnic lymphatic drainage, renal sodium and water excretion, or subperitoneal capillary permeability. In almost 75% of patients with ascites, the underlying disease is hepatic cirrhosis, in which there is elevated portal venous pressure and a decreased serum albumin level. Extrahepatic portal venous obstruction can also produce ascites, though it rarely does so in the absence of liver disease or hypoalbuminemia. The permeability of subperitoneal capillaries is increased in a broad spectrum of inflammatory and neoplastic diseases. Large amounts of intraperitoneal fluid are seen in patients with peritonitis secondary to infectious processes such as bacterial infection, tuberculosis, typhoid fever, and various fungal and parasitic infestations. Altered capillary permeability is most likely responsible for the development of ascites in patients with peritoneal carcinomatosis, as well as in patients with myxedema, ovarian disease, and allergic vasculitis. Primary or metastatic diseases of the lymphatic system can obstruct lymphatic vessels

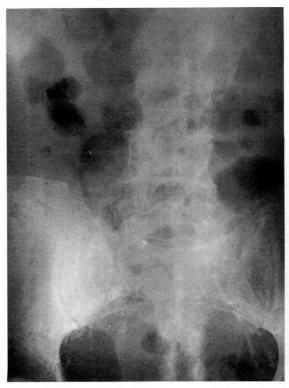

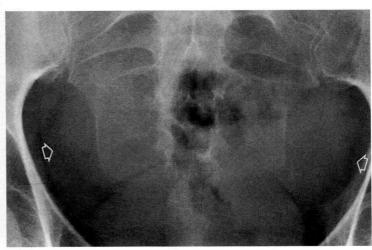

43-14   **43-15**

Fig. 43-14.   Ascites. Note the general abdominal haziness ("ground-glass" appearance).

Fig. 43-15.   Ascites. Supine abdominal radiograph demonstrates a large amount of ascitic fluid within the pelvic peritoneal reflections **(arrows)**.

or the thoracic duct and produce ascites by blocking the normal splanchnic lymphatic drainage.

Large amounts of ascitic fluid are easily detectable on plain abdominal radiographs as a general abdominal haziness ("ground-glass" appearance) (Fig. 43-14). There may be elevation of the diaphragm due to the increased volume of abdominal contents. With the patient in a supine position, the peritoneal fluid continues to gravitate to dependent portions of the pelvis and accumulate within the pelvic peritoneal reflections, thus filling the recesses on both sides of the bladder and producing a symmetric density resembling dog's ears (Fig. 43-15). Smaller amounts of fluid (800–1000 ml) may widen the flank stripe, obliterate the right lateral inferior margin of the liver (hepatic angle), or produce a pencil-thin vertical fat line projecting over the iliac crest representing the properitoneal fat interface accentuated by a small amount of fluid between the visceral and parietal peritoneum. On barium examination, ascitic fluid causes separation of adjacent loops of small bowel.

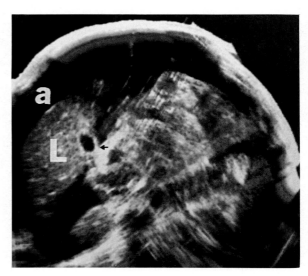

Fig. 43-16.   Ultrasound of ascites. A large amount of sonolucent ascitic fluid **(a)** separates the liver **(L)** and other soft-tissue structures from the anterior abdominal wall. Note the relative thickness of the gallbladder wall **(arrow)**.

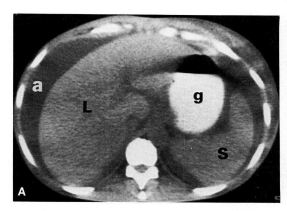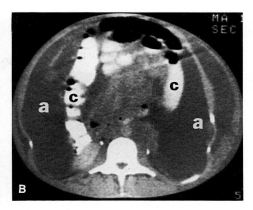

Fig. 43-17. CT of ascites. **(A)** CT scan through the upper abdomen shows the low-density ascitic fluid **(a)** lateral to the liver **(L)** and spleen **(S)** and separating these structures from the abdominal wall; **g**, barium in the stomach. **(B)** CT scan through the lower abdomen shows a huge amount of low-density ascitic fluid **(a)** with medial displacement of the ascending and descending colon **(c)**.

Ultrasound demonstrates ascites as mobile, echo-free fluid regions shaped by adjacent structures (Fig. 43-16). The smallest volumes of fluid in the supine patient appear first around the inferior tip of the right lobe of the liver, the superior right flank, and in the cul-de-sac of the pelvis. Fluid then collects in the pericolic gutters, as well as lateral and anterior to the liver. The distribution of fluid is not determined solely by gravity but is influenced by volume, the boundaries of peritoneal compartments, the fluid density, and intraperitoneal pressures, as well as the origin of the fluid.

Computed tomography shows ascites as an extravisceral collection of fluid with an attenuation value less than that of adjacent soft-tissue organs (Fig. 43-17). This modality is of special value in patients with noncirrhotic ascites, in whom it may detect the underlying lesion producing the excessive amounts of intra-abdominal fluid.

NEOPLASMS

PERITONEAL TUMORS

Primary neoplasms of the peritoneum (mesotheliomas) are extremely rare. They are usually seen in middle-aged to elderly persons, predominantly men. Like tumors of the same cell type involving the pleura, peritoneal mesotheliomas appear to be closely related to exposure to asbestos. In addition

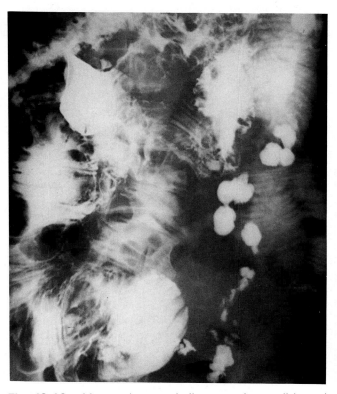

Fig. 43-18. Metastatic mesothelioma to the small bowel from a lung primary. Separation of bowel loops is evident, with multiple intrinsic and extrinsic nodular masses and areas of annular constriction and ulceration.

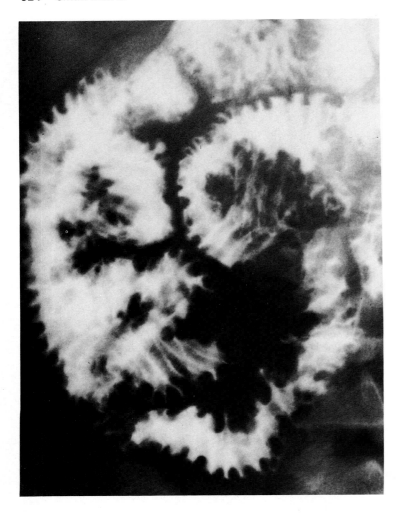

Fig. 43-19. Primary lymphangioma of the small bowel and mesentery. Diffuse mesenteric infiltration causes prominent nodularity and separation of bowel loops.

to having a large bulk, peritoneal mesotheliomas are associated with severe ascites, which contributes to the separation of small bowel loops. Metastatic mesothelioma from a lung primary can produce a similar radiographic appearance (Fig. 43-18).

MESENTERIC TUMORS

Primary tumors of the mesentery are also rare. Almost two-thirds of mesenteric tumors are benign, primarily fibromas or lipomas. Many are discovered incidentally during operations for other diseases. Most primary malignant tumors of the mesentery are fibrosarcomas or leiomyosarcomas arising from the smooth muscle of mesenteric blood vessels. They can grow to an extremely large size before producing symptoms or metastasizing. Malignant lymphoid tumors of the mesentery are rare lesions that can be locally infiltrative and cause separation of bowel loops (Fig. 43-19). Mesenteric lymphoid tumors can also be benign and present with systemic manifestations such as fever, leukocytosis,

hyperglobulinemia, and anemia. Rather than true lymphoid neoplasms, these benign lesions probably represent giant lymph node hyperplasia secondary to an inflammatory or infectious process.

METASTASES

Intraperitoneal seeding occurs as a result of tumor cells floating freely in ascitic fluid and implanting themselves on peritoneal surfaces. Metastatic tumors to the peritoneum commonly occur in the terminal stages of cancer of the intraperitoneal organs (Fig. 43-20), most being due to adenocarcinoma (Fig. 43-21). Neoplasms of the ovary and stomach are especially prone to widespread seeding of the peritoneal surfaces. However, a variety of mesenchymal tumors (Fig. 43-22), lymphoma, and leukemia can also infiltrate the peritoneum. Major areas of intraperitoneal seeding include the pouch of Douglas at the rectosigmoid junction; the right lower quadrant at the lower end of the small bowel mesentery; the left lower quadrant along the superior border of the sigmoid mesocolon and colon;

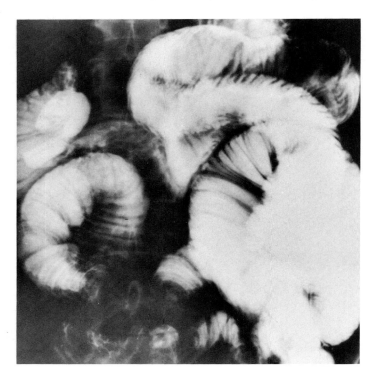

Fig. 43-20. Abdominal carcinomatosis (sigmoid primary).

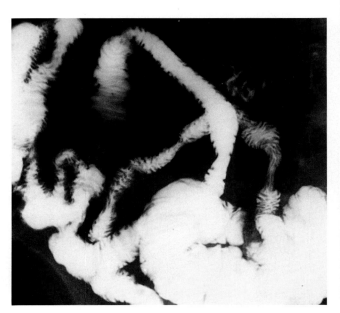

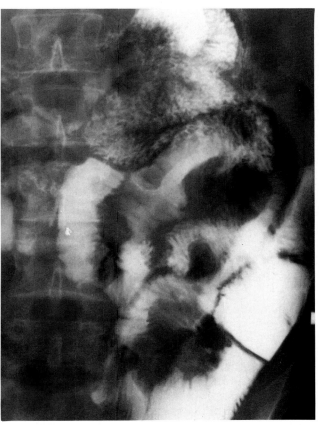

43-21   43-22

Fig. 43-21. Metastatic carcinoma (lung primary) to the mesentery and peritoneal cavity causing wide separation of small bowel loops.

Fig. 43-22. Leiomyosarcoma of the ileum metastatic to the small bowel and mesentery. Multiple nodular masses cause separation of small bowel loops.

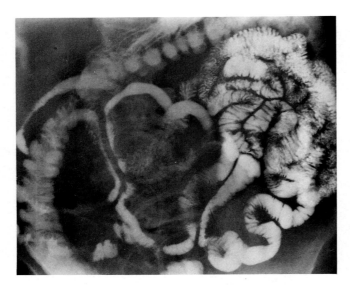

Fig. 43-23. *Retractile mesenteritis. Separation of small bowel folds remained constant on successive studies. (Clemett AR, Tracht DG: The roentgen diagnosis of retractile mesenteritis. AJR 107:787, 1969. Copyright 1969. Reproduced with permission)*

and the right pericolic gutter lateral to the cecum and ascending colon. Metastases to the peritoneum usually produce large volumes of ascites, and the diagnosis of intraperitoneal carcinomatosis can often be made by cytologic examination of aspirated ascitic fluid. In addition to separation of intestinal loops by ascites, peritoneal carcinomatosis can cause mesenteric masses, nodular impressions, or angulated segments of small bowel. Stretching and fixation of mucosal folds transverse to the longitudinal axis of the bowel lumen (transverse stretch) is reported to be highly indicative of secondary neoplastic involvement of the small bowel.

INTRAPERITONEAL ABSCESS

Intraperitoneal abscesses are localized collections of pus that can follow either generalized peritonitis or a more localized intra-abdominal disease process or injury. The location of intraperitoneal abscesses depends on the site of the primary underlying disease. For example, appendicitis leads to abscesses in the right pericolic gutter and pelvis, and sigmoid diverticulitis produces abscesses in the left pericolic gutter and pelvis. Pancreatitis and perforated gastric or duodenal ulcers lead to abscesses in the lesser sac, whereas Crohn's disease generally results in abscesses in the center of the peritoneal cavity. Radiographically, intraperitoneal abscesses appear as soft-tissue masses displacing and separating small bowel loops. A critical radiographic sign of an intra-

peritoneal abscess is the presence of extraluminal bowel gas, which can appear as discrete, round lucencies, multiple small lucencies ("soap bubbles"), or linear radiolucent shadows that follow fascial planes. Localized ileus (sentinel loop) is often seen adjacent to an intraperitoneal abscess, though this is a nonspecific finding.

RETRACTILE MESENTERITIS

Retractile mesenteritis is a disease characterized by fibro-fatty thickening and sclerosis of the mesentery. A poorly understood condition, it probably represents a slowly progressive mesenteric inflammatory process. Three major pathologic features are usually present to some extent: fibrosis, inflammation, and fatty infiltration. When fibrosis is the dominant feature, the disease is known as retractile mesenteritis. When fatty infiltration is the most prominent feature, the condition is called lipomatosis or isolated lipodystrophy of the mesentery. Mesenteric panniculitis is the term used whenever chronic inflammation is the major pathologic feature. For all practical purposes, these three different terms describe the same process, or perhaps different stages of a single disease.

The small bowel mesentery is the usual site of origin of retractile mesenteritis, though the sigmoid

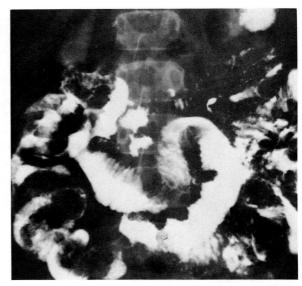

Fig. 43-24. *Retractile mesenteritis. Marked separation of bowel loops with segmental dilatation and abrupt angulation of the mid-small bowel associated with indentations on the concave border. The more severely involved bowel was arranged distally in a spiral pattern of continuous curves smoothly narrowed on the inside of the loop. (Aach RD, Kahn LJ, Frech RS: Obstruction of the small intestine due to retractile mesenteritis. Gastroenterology 54:594–598, 1968)*

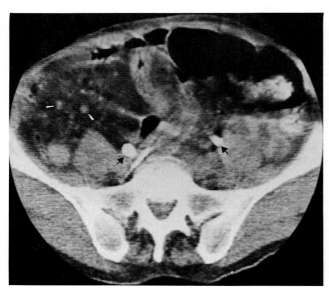

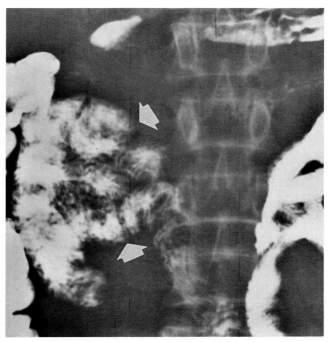

43-25

43-26

Fig. 43-25. CT of retractile mesenteritis. There is a poorly defined but fairly localized fat-density mass within the right lower quadrant. Multiple small areas of increased density within the mass **(white arrowheads)** represent enhanced neurovascular bundles due to the administration of contrast material during the performance of the CT scan. Both ureters are well opacified **(black arrows)**. (Seigel RS, Kuhns LR, Borlaza GS et al: Computed tomography and angiography in ileal carcinoid tumor and retractile mesenteritis. Radiology 134:437–440, 1980)

Fig. 43-26. Right paraduodenal hernia. The loops of bowel crowded together in the hernia sac are widely separated from other segments of small bowel that remain free in the peritoneal cavity.

mesentery can also be affected. The radiographic appearance is that of a diffuse mesenteric mass that separates and displaces small bowel loops (Fig. 43-23). When prominent fibrosis causes adhesions and retractions, the bowel tends to be drawn into a central mass with kinking, angulation, and conglomeration of adherent loops (Fig. 43-24).

Computed tomography demonstrates retractile mesenteritis as a localized fat-density mass containing areas of increased density representing fibrosis (Fig. 43-25).

RETROPERITONEAL HERNIA

Retroperitoneal hernias occur in fossae formed by peritoneal folds and are generally found in paraduodenal, paracecal, or intersigmoidal locations. The herniated portion of intestine is almost always a part of the small bowel. Although the loops of bowel within the hernia sac appear to be crowded closely together in a small, confined space, they are widely separated from those segments of small bowel that remain free in the peritoneal cavity (Fig. 43-26).

GRAFT-VERSUS-HOST DISEASE (GVHD)

Graft-versus-host disease (GVHD), a life-threatening complication of allogeneic bone marrow transplantation, is probably due to an immunologic reaction mounted by engrafted lymphocytes against the host. Necrosis of crypt epithelium leading to glandular depopulation is most marked in the ileum and colon and generally produces abdominal cramps and diarrhea. Mural thickening due to edema or fibrosis leads to an increased distance between barium-filled small bowel loops (Fig. 43-27). Concomitant loss of mucosal folds and luminal narrowing causes the bowel to have a ribbonlike appearance.

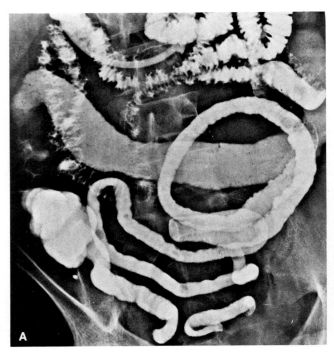
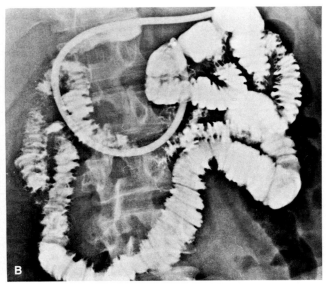

Fig. 43-27. Graft-versus-host disease. **(A)** Separation of ribbonlike ileal loops with loss of mucosal markings. **(B)** Edematous pattern of jejunal folds. (Schimmelpenninck M, Zwaan F: Radiographic features of small intestinal injury in human graft-versus-host disease. Gastrointest Radiol 7:29–33, 1982)

It should be noted that after bone marrow transplantation, patients are also at risk for developing overwhelming gastrointestinal infection with opportunistic organisms, such as cytomegalovirus, which can also result in profuse diarrhea and an indistinguishable radiographic appearance.

BIBLIOGRAPHY

Aach RD, Kahn LI, Frech RS: Obstruction of the small intestine due to retractile mesenteritis. Gastroenterology 54:594–598, 1968

Balikian JP, Nassar NT, Shamma'A NH et al: Primary lymphomas of the small intestine including the duodenum: A roentgen analysis of 29 cases. AJR 107:131–141, 1969

Balthazar EJ: Carcinoid tumors of the alimentary tract: Radiographic diagnosis. Gastrointest Radiol 3:47–56, 1978

Banner MP, Gohel VK: Peritoneal mesothelioma. Radiology 129:637–640, 1978

Bundrick TJ, Cho SR, Brewer WH et al: Ascites: Comparison of plain film radiographs with ultrasonograms. Radiology 152:503–506, 1984

Clemett AR, Marshak RH: Whipple's disease: Roentgen features and differential diagnosis. Radiol Clin North Am 7:105–111, 1969

Clemett AR, Tracht DG: The roentgen diagnosis of retractile mesenteritis. AJR 107:787, 1969

Gefter WB, Arger PH, Edell SL: Sonographic patterns of ascites. Semin Ultrasound 2:226–232, 1981

Jolles H, Coulam CM: CT of ascites. AJR 135:315–322, 1980

Jones B, Fishman EK, Kramer SS et al: Computed tomography of gastrointestinal inflammation after bone marrow transplantation. AJR 146:691–695, 1986

Khilnani MT, Marshak RH, Eliasoph J et al: Intramural intestinal hemorrhage. AJR 92:1061–1071, 1964

Legge DA, Carlson HC, Wollaeger EE: Roentgenologic appearance of systemic amyloidosis involving the gastrointestinal tract. AJR 110:406–412, 1970

Marshak RH, Lindner AE, Maklansky DM: Lymphoreticular disorders of the gastrointestinal tract: Roentgenographic features. Gastrointest Radiol 4:103–120, 1979

Rogers LF, Goldstein HM: Roentgen manifestations of radiation injury to the gastrointestinal tract. Gastrointest Radiol 2:281–291, 1977

Schimmelpennick M, Zwaan F: Radiographic features of small intestinal injury in human graft-versus-host disease. Gastrointest Radiol 7:29–33, 1982

Seigel RS, Kuhns LR, Borlaza GS et al: Computed tomography and angiography in ileal carcinoid tumor and retractile mesenteritis. Radiology 134:437–440, 1980

Smith SJ, Carlson HC, Gisvold JJ: Secondary neoplasms of the small bowel. Radiology 125:29–33, 1977

Tedeschi CG, Botta GC: Retractile mesenteritis. N Engl J Med 266:1035–1040, 1962

Teixidor HS, Honig CL, Norsoph E et al: Cytomegalovirus infection of the alimentary canal: Radiologic findings with pathologic correlation. Radiology 163:317–323, 1987

SMALL BOWEL DIVERTICULA AND PSEUDODIVERTICULA

Disease Entities

True diverticula
   Duodenal
   Jejunal
   Meckel's
   Ileal
Pseudodiverticula
   Giant duodenal ulcer
   Peptic disease
   Intraluminal diverticula
   Scleroderma
   Crohn's disease
   Lymphoma
   Communicating ileal duplication

DUODENAL DIVERTICULA

Diverticula of the duodenum are incidental findings in 1% to 5% of barium examinations of the upper gastrointestinal tract. They are acquired lesions consisting of a sac of mucosal and submucosal layers herniated through a muscular defect, and they fill and empty by gravity as a result of pressures generated by duodenal peristalsis. Although most commonly found along the medial border of the descending duodenum in the periampullary region (Fig. 44-1), diverticula frequently arise in the third (Fig. 44-2) and fourth portions of the duodenum (30%–40%) and can even occur on the lateral border of the descending duodenum (Fig. 44-3).

On barium examinations, duodenal diverticula typically have a smooth rounded shape, are often multiple, and generally change configuration during the course of the study. The lack of inflammatory reaction (spasm, distortion of mucosal folds) permits a duodenal diverticulum to be differentiated from a postbulbar ulcer. Bizarre multilobulated diverticula (racemose) occasionally occur (Fig. 44-4). Filling defects representing inspissated food particles, blood clots, or gas can be identified in a duodenal diverticulum (Fig. 44-5); these are inconstant and may change in appearance or disappear during observation.

Although the overwhelming majority of duodenal diverticula are asymptomatic, serious complications can develop. Duodenal diverticulitis mimics numerous abdominal diseases (cholecystitis, peptic ulcer disease, pancreatitis) and is a diagnosis of exclusion. Complications of inflammation of duodenal diverticula include hemorrhage, perforation, abscesses, and fistulas. Because duodenal diverticula are retroperitoneal structures, perforation occurs without signs of peritonitis and with no free intraperitoneal gas. The most common radiographic finding of a perforated duodenal diverticulum is retroperitoneal gas localized to the area surrounding the duodenum and the upper pole of the right kidney. A very large diverticulum occasionally causes symptoms of partial upper gastrointestinal obstruction.

Anomalous insertion of the common bile duct and pancreatic duct into a duodenal diverticulum can be demonstrated in about 3% of carefully per-

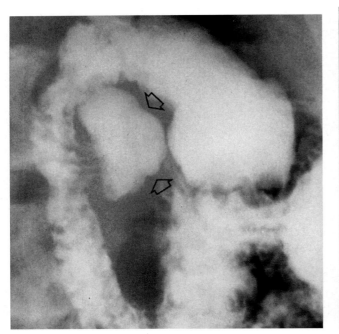

44-1

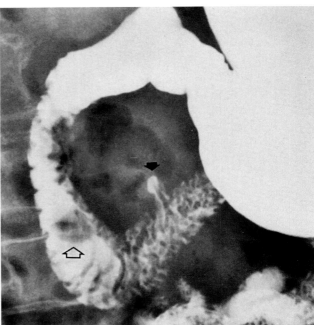

44-2

Fig. 44-1. Diverticulum **(arrows)** arising from the second portion of the duodenum.

Fig. 44-2. Diverticulum arising from the third portion of the duodenum **(solid arrow)**. Of incidental note is an adenomatous polyp **(open arrow)** in the second portion of the duodenum.

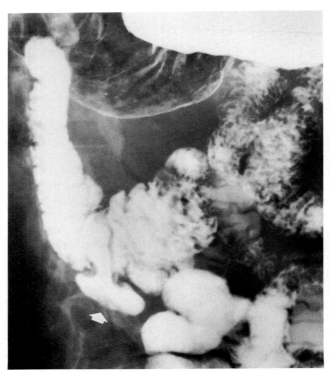

44-3

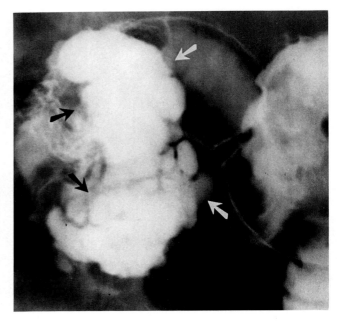

44-4

Fig. 44-3. Diverticulum arising on the lateral aspect of the duodenum at the junction of the second and third portions **(arrow)**.

Fig. 44-4. Bizarre multilobulated diverticulum (racemose).

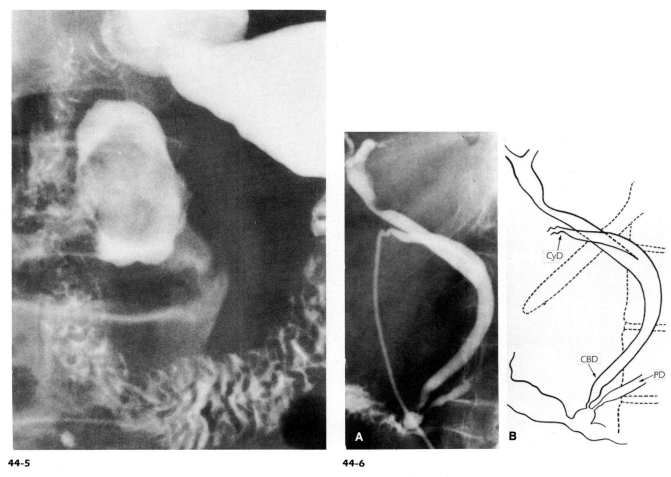

44-5

44-6

Fig. 44-5. Irregular filling defect representing a blood clot within a duodenal diverticulum in a patient with severe upper gastrointestinal bleeding.

Fig. 44-6. **(A)** Operative cholangiogram and **(B)** corresponding line drawing. These illustrations clearly demonstrate the insertion of the common bile duct and pancreatic duct into the dome of a small duodenal diverticulum. (Nelson JA, Burhenne HJ: Anomalous biliary and pancreatic duct insertion into duodenal diverticula. Radiology 120:49–52, 1976)

formed T-tube cholangiograms (Fig. 44-6). This anatomic arrangement appears to interfere with the normal emptying mechanism of the ductal systems and predisposes to obstructive biliary and pancreatic disease. The absence of an ampullary sphincter mechanism permits spontaneous reflux of barium from the diverticulum into the common bile duct, and this can be a cause of ascending infection.

Duodenal diverticula occasionally become very large and present on plain abdominal radiographs as confusing collections of gas. Because diverticula on the medial wall are usually limited in size by surrounding pancreatic tissue, these "giant" diverticula tend to arise laterally (Fig. 44-7). A gas-filled giant duodenal diverticulum may be incorrectly interpreted as an abscess, dilated cecum, colonic diverticulum, or pseudocyst of the pancreas.

GIANT DUODENAL ULCER

Giant duodenal ulcers occasionally mimic diverticula arising from the first portion of the duodenum. In contrast to the vast majority of ulcers, which are small and involve only a small portion of the duodenal bulb, giant duodenal ulcers range from 2 cm to 6 cm in size and often completely replace the bulb (Fig. 44-8). Unlike the normal duodenal bulb or a duodenal diverticulum, a giant duodenal ulcer is a rigid-walled cavity that remains constant in size and shape throughout the gastrointestinal examination and lacks a normal mucosal pattern (Fig. 44-9). Narrowing of the pylorus proximally and of the duodenum distal to the giant ulcer can be severe enough to produce gastric outlet obstruction. In some cases, nodular filling defects in the floor of the

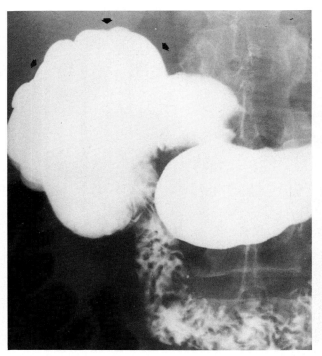

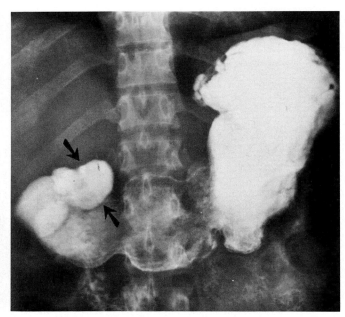

44-7   44-8

Fig. 44-7.   Giant diverticulum **(arrows)** arising laterally from the junction of the first and second portions of the duodenum.

Fig. 44-8.   Giant duodenal ulcer **(arrows)** completely replacing the duodenal bulb. (Eisenberg RL, Margulis AR, Moss AA: Giant duodenal ulcers. Gastrointest Radiol 2:347–353, 1978)

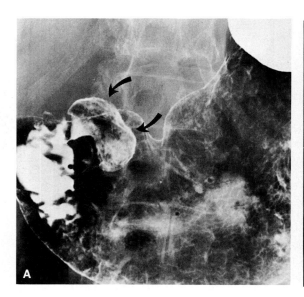

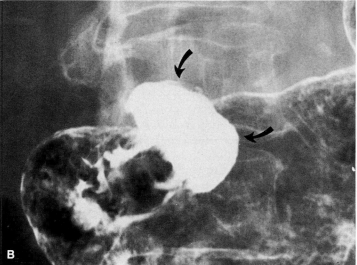

Fig. 44-9.   Giant duodenal ulcer. There is little change in the appearance of the rigid-walled cavity **(arrows)** in air-contrast and barium-filled views. (Eisenberg RL, Margulis AR, Moss AA: Giant duodenal ulcers. Gastrointest Radiol 2:347–353, 1978)

ulcer or prominence of a surrounding edematous mass may simulate an ulcerated neoplasm (Fig. 44-10). A not uncommon finding is the "ulcer within an ulcer" appearance, which represents a small area of deeper ulceration within the giant duodenal ulcer (Fig. 44-11).

Most patients with giant duodenal ulcers have moderate to severe abdominal pain, often radiating to the back, and a long history of prior ulcer disease. Because giant duodenal ulcers have been reported to have a great propensity for perforation and massive hemorrhage and to be associated with mortality rates of up to 40%, prompt correct diagnosis and the institution of appropriate therapy are essential.

PSEUDODIVERTICULA OF THE DUODENUM

Pseudodiverticula are exaggerated outpouchings of the inferior and superior recesses which are located at the base of the bulb and are related to duodenal ulcer disease (Fig. 44-12). In addition to inflammation of the area containing the ulcer, the deformity results from spasm of the circular muscles opposite the ulcer, a mechanism similar to that of an incisura opposite a gastric or postbulbar ulcer. The degree of deformity is not directly related to ulcer size; small

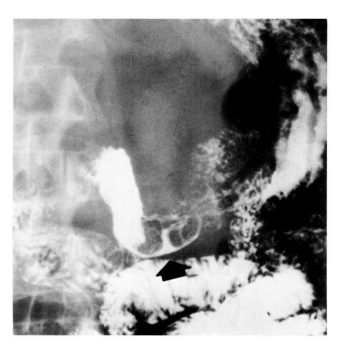

Fig. 44-10. Giant duodenal ulcer. The markedly enlarged fold at the base of the ulcer **(arrow)** simulates a neoplastic process. (Eisenberg RL, Margulis AR, Moss AA: Giant duodenal ulcers. Gastrointest Radiol 2:347–353, 1978)

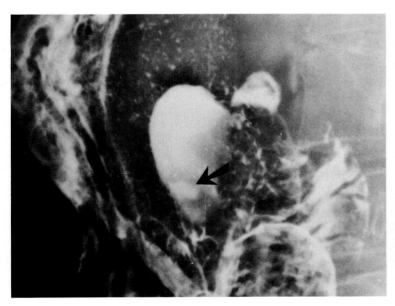

44-11

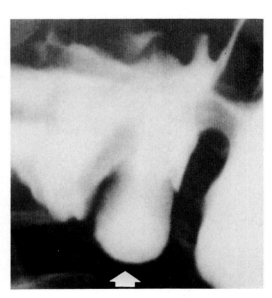

44-12

Fig. 44-11. Giant duodenal ulcer. Note the "ulcer within an ulcer" appearance **(arrow)**. (Eisenberg RL, Margulis AR, Moss AA: Giant duodenal ulcers. Gastrointest Radiol 2:347–353, 1978)

Fig. 44-12. Pseudodiverticulum of the duodenal bulb. Exaggerated outpouching **(arrow)** of the inferior recess, which is located at the base of the bulb and is related to duodenal ulcer disease.

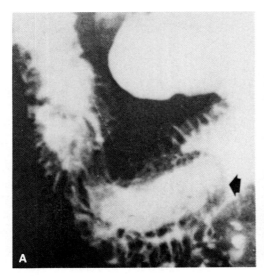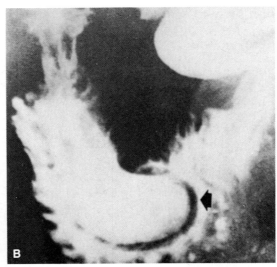

Fig. 44-13. Intraluminal duodenal diverticulum. "Halo" sign **(arrow)** seen with the diverticulum **(A)** partially and **(B)** completely filled. (Laudan JCH, Norton GI: Intraluminal duodenal diverticulum. AJR 90:756–760, 1963. Copyright 1963. Reproduced with permission)

ulcers may produce large deformities, and huge ulcers may produce little alteration in bulb contour.

INTRALUMINAL DIVERTICULA

An intraluminal duodenal diverticulum is a sac of duodenal mucosa originating in the second portion of the duodenum near the papilla of Vater (Fig. 44-13). Formation of the diverticulum in adults from a congenital duodenal web or diaphragm appears to be due to purely mechanical factors, such as forward pressure by food and strong peristaltic activity. When filled with barium, the intraluminal duodenal diverticulum appears as a fingerlike sac separated from contrast in the duodenal lumen by a radiolucent band representing the wall of the diverticulum ("halo sign"). When empty of barium, it can simulate a pedunculated polyp. Complications of intraluminal duodenal diverticula include retention of food and foreign bodies and partial duodenal obstruction. Increased intraluminal pressure can cause reflux of duodenal contents into the pancreatic duct and an acute attack of pancreatitis.

Intraluminal duodenal diverticulum and its predecessor, the congenital duodenal diaphragm, frequently occur in association with other anomalies, including annular pancreas, midgut volvulus, situs inversus, choledochocele, congenital heart disease, Down's syndrome, imperforate anus, Hirschsprung's disease, omphalocele, hypoplastic kidneys, and exstrophy of the bladder.

JEJUNAL DIVERTICULA

Jejunal diverticula are herniations of mucosa and submucosa through muscular defects at points of entrance of blood vessels on the mesenteric side of the small bowel (Fig. 44-14). These thin-walled outpouchings lack muscular components and are atonic; they are filled and emptied by the activity of adjacent bowel. Jejunal diverticula are found twice as frequently in men than in women and occur almost exclusively in persons over the age of 40. Associated diverticula are frequently found in the colon and duodenum of the same patient.

The most common complication of jejunal diverticulosis is the blind loop syndrome, in which the population of bacteria within the stagnant diverticula becomes so large as to cause steatorrhea with increased numbers of bowel movements, malabsorption, anemia, and weight loss. Most symptomatic patients have multiple diverticula; however, the development of complications of bacterial overgrowth has been reported in a few patients with a single large jejunal diverticulum.

Jejunal diverticulitis is a rare complication. The larger size and wider necks of jejunal as opposed to colonic diverticula may mitigate against the inspissation of bowel contents and obstruction of the diverticular opening, thereby decreasing the incidence of inflammatory disease. Radiographically, jejunal diverticulitis can present as incomplete jejunal obstruction, an omental mass displacing jejunal loops, leakage of barium into an adjacent mes-

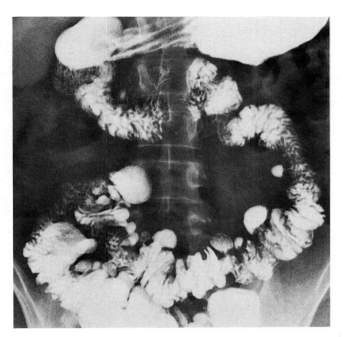

Fig. 44-14. *Jejunal diverticulosis.*

enteric abscess, or extrinsic serosal changes involving the transverse colon.

Jejunal diverticulosis is one of the leading gastrointestinal causes of pneumoperitoneum without peritonitis or surgery. It is postulated that gas passes through small perforations in the wall of the diver-

ticula during periods of hyperperistalsis. Although the perforations are so small that gas can pass through them, the intestinal contents are filtered free of fecal matter, so peritonitis does not develop. Other rare complications of jejunal diverticulosis include bleeding (usually chronic), enterolith formation, and impaction of a foreign body, which can ultimately result in perforation with peritonitis.

PSEUDODIVERTICULA OF THE JEJUNUM OR ILEUM

Sacculation of the small bowel in scleroderma can simulate jejunal diverticulosis (Fig. 44-15). These pseudodiverticula are the result of smooth muscle atrophy and fibrosis accompanied by vascular occlusion. They involve only one wall of the bowel and have an appearance similar to the characteristic sacculation in the colon in patients with scleroderma.

Radiographically, pseudodiverticula due to scleroderma are large sacs with squared, broad bases that resemble colonic haustra. Sacculations are readily differentiated from true diverticula of the small bowel, which have narrow necks and are usually smaller.

Pseudodiverticula can also be demonstrated in Crohn's disease (Fig. 44-16) and lymphoma. In the former, the pseudodiverticula are associated with strictures and characteristic mucosal changes; in the latter, the aneurysmal dilatation is fusiform and not restricted to one wall.

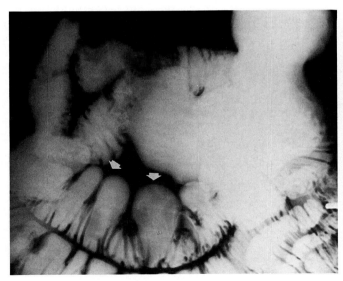

44-15

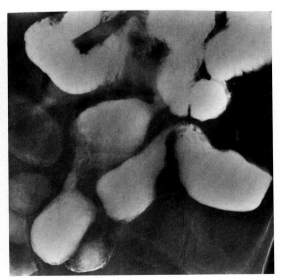

44-16

Fig. 44-15. Sacculations of the small bowel **(arrows)** in scleroderma simulating jejunal diverticulosis (pseudodiverticula).

Fig. 44-16. Sacculations of the small bowel in Crohn's disease simulating intestinal diverticulosis.

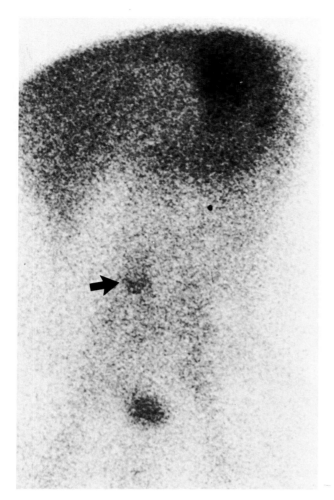

Fig. 44-17. Ectopic gastric mucosa in a Meckel's diverticulum. Pertechnetate scintigraphy shows a "hot spot" **(arrow)** in the lower abdomen. (Maglinte DDT: The small bowel: Miscellaneous considerations. In Taveras JM, Ferrucci JT (eds): Radiology: Diagnosis—Imaging—Intervention. Philadelphia, JB Lippincott, 1987)

MECKEL'S DIVERTICULA

Meckel's diverticulum is the most frequent congenital anomaly of the intestinal tract, having an incidence of 1% to 4% in autopsy reports. The diverticula are blind outpouchings representing the rudimentary omphalomesenteric duct (embryonic communication between the gut and yolk sac), which is normally obliterated between the fifth and seventh weeks of gestation. Meckel's diverticulum usually arises within 100 cm of the ileocecal valve (average, 80–85 cm). It opens into the antimesenteric side of the ileum, unlike other diverticula, which arise on the mesenteric side of the small bowel.

In most patients, Meckel's diverticulum remains asymptomatic throughout life. Of persons presenting with complications, a majority are under 2 years of age, and more than one-third are less than 1 year. In children, the most common symptom of Meckel's diverticulum is bleeding. Usually copious and painless, the bleeding is almost invariably the result of ulceration of ileal mucosa adjacent to heterotopic gastric mucosa in the diverticulum. Because this ectopic gastric mucosa has an affinity for pertechnetate, radionuclide imaging can be helpful in demonstrating the lesion (Fig. 44-17). In adults, the most common symptom is intestinal obstruction, which can be due to invagination and intussusception of the diverticulum (Fig. 44-18), volvulus, inflammation, or adhesions.

Inflammation in a Meckel's diverticulum can produce a clinical picture indistinguishable from acute appendicitis. Resultant stenosis of the neck of the diverticulum or a valvelike flap of mucosa arising from the margin can prevent adequate drainage from the diverticulum. Stasis can precipitate changes in the acid-base balance, causing the development of faceted calculi. Neoplasms in Meckel's

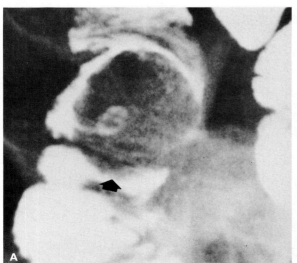
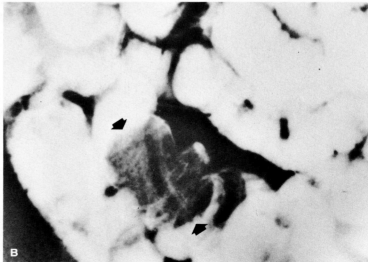

Fig. 44-18. (A) *En face* and **(B)** profile views of an ulcerated lipoma arising from a Meckel's diverticulum and causing an intussusception **(arrows)**.

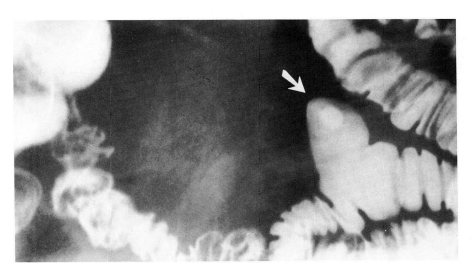

44-19

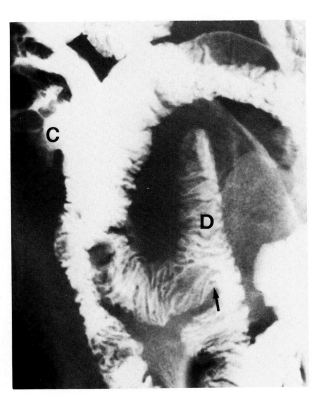

44-20

Fig. 44-19. Meckel's diverticulum **(arrow)** with a small diverticulum (area of increased density) arising from it. Note the mouth of the diverticular sac, the width of which is approximately equal to the width of the intestinal lumen.

Fig. 44-20. Mucosal triangular plateau in Meckel's diverticulum. Characteristic junctional fold pattern **(arrow)**, which is produced by no other small bowel anomaly. **D**, Meckel's diverticulum; **C**, cecum. (Maglinte DDT: The small bowel: Miscellaneous considerations. In Taveras JM, Ferrucci JT (eds): Radiology: Diagnosis—Imaging—Intervention. Philadelphia, JB Lippincott, 1987)

diverticula have been reported; free perforation with peritonitis is rare.

Despite the relative frequency of Meckel's diverticula, preoperative radiographic demonstration is unusual. If a diverticulum is not large, it can be difficult to distinguish from normal loops of small bowel unless careful compression films are obtained. Failure to demonstrate a diverticulum on routine small bowel examination can be due to stenosis of the opening, filling of the diverticulum with intestinal contents or feces, muscular contractions, or rapid emptying and small size of the diverticu-

lum. The use of enteroclysis (antegrade small bowel enema) has been reported to greatly improve the detection rate.

A Meckel's diverticulum appears radiographically as an outpouching arising from the antimesenteric side of the distal ileum. The mouth of the sac is wide, often equal to the width of the intestinal lumen itself (Fig. 44-19). The identification of the meckelian nature of the sac depends on demonstration of the junctional fold pattern, which is the site of exit of the omphalomesenteric duct. A "mucosal triangular plateau" (Fig. 44-20) is the junction iden-

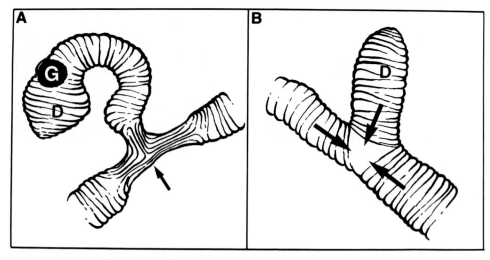

Fig. 44-21. *Schematic drawings of Meckel's junctional fold patterns.* **(A)** *A triradiate fold pattern* **(arrow)** *results when the loops are collapsed.* **(B)** *The mucosal triangular plateau is the junction identified* **(arrows)** *when the loops are distended.* **D**, *Meckel's diverticulum;* **G**, *heterotopic gastric mucosa. (Maglinte DDT: The small bowel: Miscellaneous considerations. In Taveras JM, Ferrucci JT (eds): Radiology: Diagnosis—Imaging—Intervention. Philadelphia, JB Lippincott, 1987)*

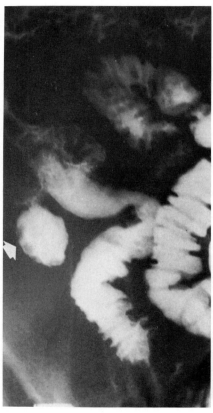

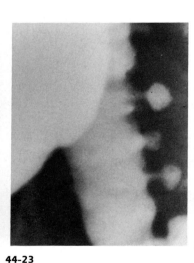

Fig. 44-22. *Ectopic gastric mucosa appearing as multiple filling defects* **(arrow)** *in a Meckel's diverticulum.*

Fig. 44-23. *Ileal diverticula. Note that these diverticula are near the ileocecal valve, unlike Meckel's diverticula, which are situated more proximally.*

44-22   **44-23**

tified when the loops are distended; a "triradiate" fold pattern (Fig. 44-21) results when the loops are collapsed. Filling defects in the diverticulum, irregularity, or distortion of a segment strongly suggests the presence of ectopic gastric mucosa in the diverticulum (Fig. 44-22).

ILEAL DIVERTICULA

Diverticula are less common in the ileum than in the proximal segments of the small bowel. They are generally small and can be multiple. Most ileal diverticula lie in the terminal portion near the ileocecal valve (Fig. 44-23), unlike Meckel's diverticula, which are more proximally situated and generally much larger.

Although diverticula in the terminal ileum resemble those in the sigmoid colon, complications of these distal small bowel diverticula are rare. Acute ileal diverticulitis probably results from irritation or occlusion of the diverticulum by food particles or a foreign body. The clinical symptoms are usually indistinguishable from those of acute appendicitis. Localized abscess formation or generalized peritonitis can result, and postinflammatory fibrosis can cause partial small bowel obstruction.

COMMUNICATING ILEAL DUPLICATION

A communicating ileal duplication can be confused with a Meckel's diverticulum. This rare tubular lesion has an axis parallel to that of the bowel loop. Like ileal diverticula, communicating duplications are differentiated from Meckel's diverticula in that they lie on the mesenteric border and do not demonstrate a junctional fold pattern.

BIBLIOGRAPHY

Bothen NF, Ekloff O: Diverticula and duplications (enterogenous cysts) of stomach and duodenum. AJR 96:375–381, 1966

Dalinka MK, Wunder JF: Meckel's diverticulum and its complications with emphasis on roentgenologic demonstration. Radiology 106:295–298, 1973

Dunn V, Nelson JA: Jejunal diverticulosis and chronic pneumonperitoneum. Gastrointest Radiol 4:165–168, 1979

Eaton SB, Berke RA, White AF: Preoperative diagnosis of common bile duct entering a duodenal diverticulum. AJR 107:43–46, 1969

Eisenberg RL, Margulis AR, Moss AA: Giant duodenal ulcers. Gastrointest Radiol 2:347–353, 1978

Faulkner JW, Dockerty MB: Lymphosarcoma of the small intestine. Surg Gynecol Obstet 95:76–84, 1952

Fisher JK, Fortin D: Partial small bowel obstruction secondary to ileal diverticulitis. Radiology 122:321–322, 1977

Giustra PE, Killoran PJ, Root JA et al: Jejunal diverticulitis. Radiology 125:609–611, 1977

Karoll MP, Ghahremani GG, Port RB et al: Diagnosis and management of intraluminal duodenal diverticulum. Dig Dis Sci 28:411–415, 1983

Loudan JCH, Norton GI: Intraluminal duodenal diverticulum. AJR 90:756–760, 1963

Maglinte DDT, Chernish SM, DeWeese R et al: Acquired jejunoileal diverticular disease: Subject review. Radiology 158:577–580, 1986

Maglinte DDT, Elmore MF, Isenberg M et al: Meckel diverticulum: Radiologic demonstration by enteroclysis. AJR 134:925–932, 1980

Millard JR, Ziter FMH, Slover WP: Giant duodenal diverticula. AJR 121:334–337, 1974

Miller KB, Naimark A, O'Connor JF et al: Unusual roentgenologic manifestations of Meckel's diverticulum. Gastrointest Radiol 6:209–215, 1981

Nelson JA, Burhenne HJ: Anomalous biliary and pancreatic duct insertion into duodenal diverticula. Radiology 120:49–52, 1976

Ohba S, Fakuda A, Kohno S et al: Ileal duplication and multiple intraluminal diverticula: Scintigraphy and barium meal. AJR 136:992–994, 1981

Oueloz JM, Woloshin HJ: Sacculation of the small intestine in scleroderma. Radiology 105:513–515, 1972

Salomonowitz G, Wittich G, Hajek P et al: Detection of intestinal diverticula by double-contrast small bowel enema. Gastrointest Radiol 8:271–278, 1983

White AF, Oh KS, Weber AL et al: Radiologic manifestations of Meckel's diverticulum. AJR 118:86–94, 1973

Wolfe RD, Pearl MJ: Acute perforation of duodenal diverticulum with roentgenographic demonstration of localized retroperitoneal emphysema. Radiology 104:301–302, 1972

PART SIX

ILEOCECAL VALVE AND CECUM

ABNORMALITIES OF THE ILEOCECAL VALVE

The ileocecal valve is a clearly defined radiologic landmark that represents the junction between the terminal ileum and the colon. It is almost always situated at the level of the first complete haustral segment above the tip of the cecum, and it separates the cecum below from the ascending colon above. The valve is composed of an upper and a lower lip which, at their corners of fusion, taper to form transverse folds that are part of the cecal wall. The lips of the ileocecal valve consist of muscular, submucosal, and mucosal layers. The muscularis is derived primarily from the ileum; the mucosa, however, is of the colonic type on the outer (colonic) surface and of the ileal type on the inner surface, the transition being at the free margin of the valve.

The ileocecal valve functions as a true sphincter by preventing the passage of ileal contents into the colon before completion of the digestive process. Further evidence for the role of the ileocecal valve as a sphincter is the protracted diarrhea, suggesting defective motor control, that often follows an ileo-ascending colostomy bypassing the valve. The ileocecal valve also functions as a partial barrier to retrograde flow, preventing contamination of the small intestine by coliform bacterial flora. Nevertheless, in about 90% of patients, reflux of contrast into the terminal ileum can be achieved during barium enema examination.

The ileocecal valve usually appears as a round or oval protuberance arising from the medial or posteromedial wall of the colon at the junction between the cecum and the ascending colon (Fig. 45-1). Infrequently, the valve is located in a poster-

olateral position (Fig. 45-2). The two lips of the valve project into the filled cecum and, when viewed in profile, may be seen to cause elliptical filling defects one above the other. The lips are separated by a small extension of barium that can be continuous with the barium-filled lumen of the distal small bowel if ileal reflux has occurred. The terminal ileum is directed horizontally and slightly downward as it forms a slotlike orifice in the cecum. When filled with barium, it has the configuration of a bird's neck, head, and beak.

On *en face* views, the ileocecal valve can mimic a discrete mass (Fig. 45-3). Its true nature can be determined by the demonstration of radiating mucosal folds converging on a central ostium (stellate or rosette pattern), which represents the orifice of the terminal ileum.

Disease Entities

Lipomatosis (fatty infiltration)
Neoplasms
  Benign tumors
    Lipoma
    Adenomatous polyp
    Villous adenoma
  Tumors of intermediate potential
    Carcinoid tumor
  Malignant tumors
    Adenocarcinoma
    Lymphoma

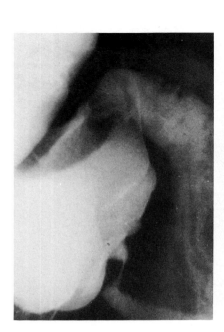

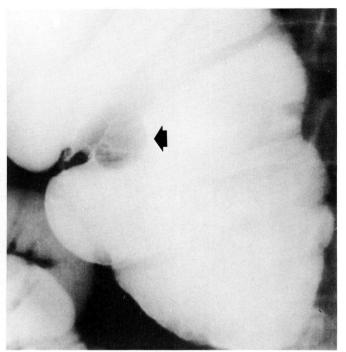

45-1   45-2

Fig. 45-1. Normal ileocecal valve.

Fig. 45-2. Posterolateral position of the ileocecal valve.

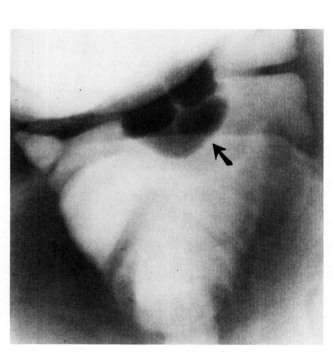

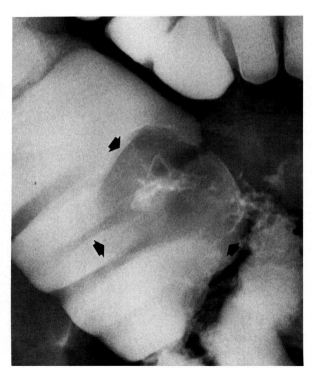

45-3   45-4

Fig. 45-3. *En face* view of a normal ileocecal valve. Note the characteristic appearance of radiating mucosal folds converging on a central ostium (rosette pattern).

Fig. 45-4. Lipomatosis of the ileocecal valve **(arrows)**.

Inflammatory disorders
   Crohn's disease
   Ulcerative colitis
   Tuberculosis
   Amebiasis
   Typhoid fever
   Yersinia enterocolitis
   Anisakiasis
   Actinomycosis
   Cathartic abuse
Prolapse
   Antegrade
   Retrograde
Intussusception
Lymphoid hyperplasia

Because of variations in the size of the ileocecal valve due to magnification, compression, and degree of cecal distention, it is difficult to determine a strict upper limit of normal for measurements of the valve. It is generally considered that the upper and lower lips of the valve should each be no more than 1.5 cm thick. The vertical diameter of the valve is usually 3 cm or less; some authors have considered 4 cm to be the upper limit of normal.

LIPOMATOSIS

Lipomatosis of the ileocecal valve is characterized by enlargement of the valve due to benign submucosal fatty infiltration (Fig. 45-4). It is found predominantly in women and is uncommon in persons under 40 years of age. Many patients are asymptomatic, and prominence of the valve is usually an incidental finding at barium enema examination. Symptoms include vague abdominal distress, cramping, rightsided abdominal pain, and even nausea and vomiting. These complaints may be due to the enlarged valve causing intermittent episodes of chronic intussusception and bowel obstruction.

Lipomatosis of the ileocecal valve appears radiographically as a smooth, masslike enlargement that is sharply demarcated from the surrounding bowel mucosa (Fig. 45-5). The valve can be lobulated and slightly irregular due to contraction of the muscularis, but the surface remains smooth (Fig. 45-6), and the valve is changeable in size and shape. If barium can be refluxed back into the terminal ileum, demonstration of the characteristic stellate appearance of the ileal mucosa on the *en face* view reveals that the process is benign. The stellate pattern indicates that the muscularis is intact and not

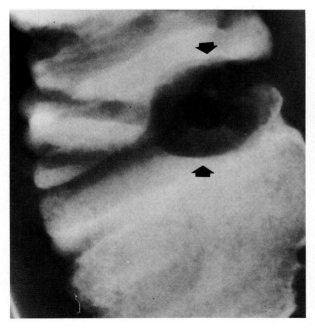

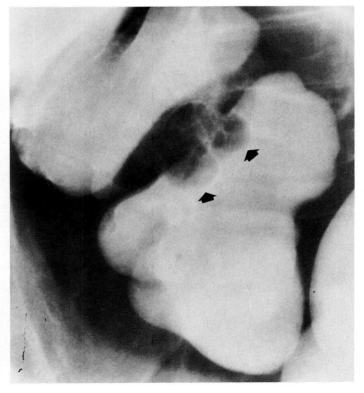

45-5   **45-6**

Fig. 45-5. Lipomatosis of the ileocecal valve presenting as a smooth, masslike enlargement **(arrows)**.

Fig. 45-6. Lipomatosis of the ileocecal valve. Although the valve is lobulated, the surface remains completely smooth **(arrows)**.

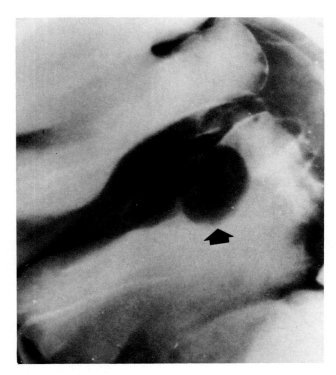

Fig. 45-7. Lipoma of the ileocecal valve. A sharply circumscribed, smooth, rounded mass arises from the lower lip of the valve **(arrow)**.

infiltrated with tumor, since it is contraction of this tissue that presumably causes the wrinkling of the overlying mucosa.

BENIGN TUMORS

LIPOMA

The most common benign neoplasm of the ileocecal valve is a lipoma, which presents as a sharply circumscribed, smooth, rounded mass arising from either lip of the valve (Fig. 45-7). In contrast to lipomatous infiltration, lipomas of the ileocecal valve have a true capsule and are confined to only one portion of the valve. Their appearance, like that of tumors of this cell type elsewhere in the bowel, may change on serial films, reflecting their soft consistency (Fig. 45-8). Lipomas of the ileocecal valve are rarely of clinical significance unless they become so large as to cause substantial bleeding or episodes of intussusception.

ADENOMA/VILLOUS ADENOMA

Adenomatous polyps and villous adenomas (Fig. 45-9) are rare benign tumors arising from the ileocecal valve. The surface of these tumors is usually

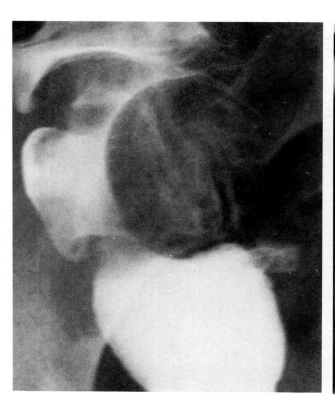
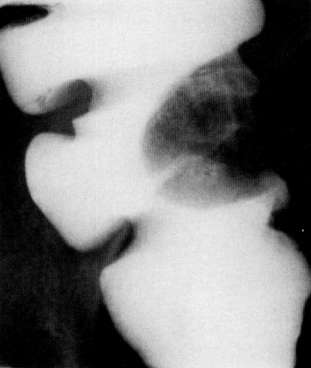

Fig. 45-8. Lipoma of the ileocecal valve. Note the change in appearance on serial views.

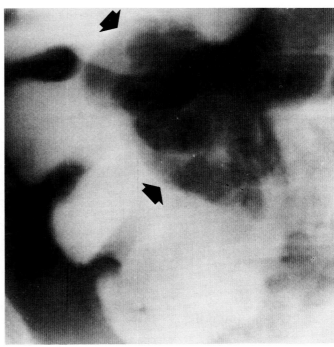

Fig. 45-9. Villous adenoma of the ileocecal valve. This large benign tumor has a moderately irregular surface **(arrows)**.

Fig. 45-10. Carcinoid tumor of the ileocecal valve **(arrows)**. The tumor, which measured 5 cm in diameter, is contained within the lumen of the valve. A few small nodules on the colonic surface of the valve are not visible in this radiograph. Because a carcinoid tumor may cause smooth, symmetric enlargement of the valve, it is important that the terminal ileum be visualized whenever a prominent, nonpliable valve is encountered. (Short WF, Smith BD, Hoy RJ: Roentgenologic evaluation of the prominent or the unusual ileocecal valve. Med Radiogr Photogr 52:2–26, 1976)

Fig. 45-11. Adenocarcinoma of the ileocecal valve. Note the prominent dilatation of the small bowel proximal to this partially obstructing lesion.

45-9

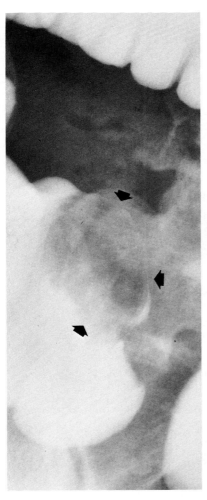

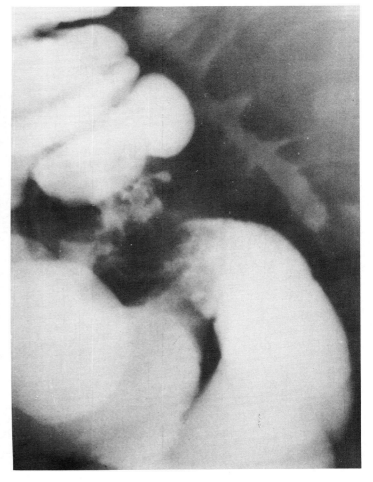

45-10

45-11

shaggy and irregular, in contrast to the invariably smooth, though often lobulated, contours of lipomas and fatty infiltration of the ileocecal valve.

CARCINOID TUMOR

Carcinoid tumors of the ileocecal valve often arise centrally within the lumen of the valve (*i.e.,* within the terminal ileum itself) rather than from either the upper or the lower lip (Fig. 45-10). One characteristic feature of these tumors is the corrugated appearance of the adjacent cecal wall, which most likely reflects edema and spasm of the wall due to plugging of lymphatics by the tumor cells. However, this feature is not specific for carcinoid tumors; it can also be produced by inflammatory lesions in the cecum.

MALIGNANT TUMORS

ADENOCARCINOMA

About 2% of adenocarcinomas of the colon arise from the ileocecal valve (Fig. 45-11). Pronounced lobulation, asymmetry, rigidity, or eccentricity of the ileocecal valve is highly indicative of a malignant tumor (Fig. 45-12). Although they are usually broad-based, irregular polypoid masses, carcinomas of the ileocecal valve can be surprisingly smooth and well-demarcated and indistinguishable from benign lesions. Villous adenocarcinomas frequently present as large, irregular masses with the

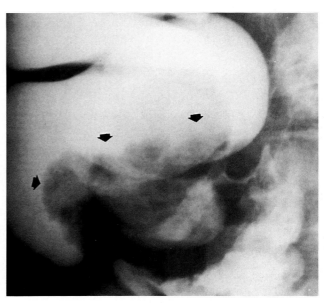

Fig. 45-13. Villous adenocarcinoma of the ileocecal valve. This large, irregular mass **(arrows)** with a typical frondlike shaggy surface is characteristic of this type of tumor elsewhere in the bowel.

typical frondlike shaggy surface that is characteristic of these tumors elsewhere in the bowel (Fig. 45-13). Because of the fluid consistency of the ileal contents, obstruction caused by carcinoma of the ileocecal valve usually appears late. Nevertheless, obstruction is a frequent complication that can be the result of occlusion of the intestinal lumen either by growth of the tumor or by intussusception of the malignant mass.

LYMPHOMA

Lymphoma can present as a polypoid mass arising from the region of the ileocecal valve (Fig. 45-14). It can have a diffusely nodular appearance or be seen as a bulky, ulcerating lesion. Unlike carcinoma, lymphoma often involves the terminal ileum. Because lymphoma typically causes little desmoplastic reaction, the tumor can reach a large size before causing obstructive narrowing of the intestinal lumen.

INFLAMMATORY DISORDERS

Inflammatory diseases involving the terminal ileum and cecum, especially Crohn's disease and ulcerative colitis, can affect the ileocecal valve. In Crohn's disease, extensive panenteric lymphedema frequently produces valvular enlargement, which can be in the form of direct inflammatory enlargement, lipomatous infiltration, or solitary or multiple well-encapsulated lipomas (Fig. 45-15). Small sinus

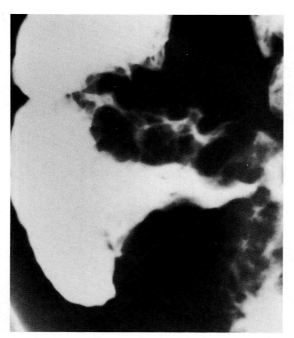

Fig. 45-12. Adenocarcinoma of the ileocecal valve. Note that the mass is rigid and irregular.

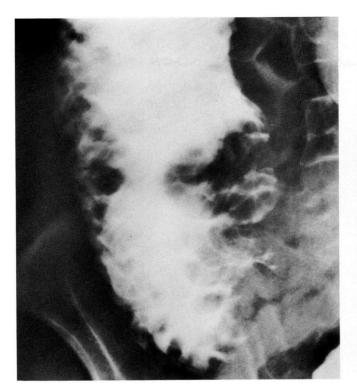
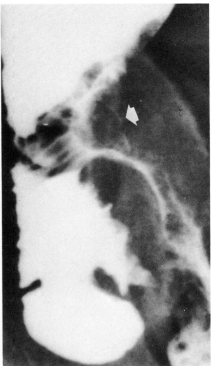

45-14 **45-15**

Fig. 45-14. Lymphoma involving the ileocecal valve, ascending colon, cecum, and terminal ileum. The irregular nodularity and diffuse involvement seen in this radiograph are common features of lymphoma. (Short WF, Smith BD, Hoy, RJ: Roentgenologic evaluation of the prominent or the unusual ileocecal valve. Med Radiogr Photogr 52:2–26, 1976)

Fig. 45-15. Crohn's disease involving the ileocecal valve. Note the fistula **(arrow)** traversing the thickened upper lip of the ileocecal valve. (Short WF, Smith BD, Hoy RJ: Roentgenologic evaluation of the prominent or the unusual ileocecal valve. Med Radiogr Photogr 52:2–26, 1976)

tracts traversing the valve strongly suggest Crohn's disease. In ulcerative colitis (backwash ileitis), the ileocecal valve is often rigid and irregular but usually not enlarged. Indeed, it tends to be thin, patulous, and fixed in an open position (Fig. 45-16). A similar wide-open appearance of the ileocecal valve can be seen in patients with prolonged cathartic abuse.

Thickening of the ileocecal valve is not uncommon in patients with tuberculosis and amebiasis. In tuberculosis, concomitant ileal changes (mucosal ulceration and nodularity, mural rigidity, luminal narrowing, fistulas) are often seen (Fig. 45-17). In amebiasis, in contrast, the terminal ileum is not involved (Fig. 45-18). Typhoid fever, *Yersinia* enterocolitis, anisakiasis (Fig. 45-19), schistosomiasis, and actinomycosis can also alter the appearance of the

ileocecal valve. These inflammatory processes sometimes produce radiographic patterns that are difficult to distinguish from more common conditions, such as Crohn's disease or ulcerative colitis.

PROLAPSE

Prolapse of ileal mucosa through the lips of the ileocecal valve is an unusual cause of apparent valve enlargement and an intracecal mass (Fig. 45-20A). This phenomenon, which is similar to the extension of gastric mucosa across the pylorus into the base of the duodenal bulb, is an asymptomatic condition probably related to lipomatous infiltration of the valve. The prolapsed tissue produces smooth enlargement of the ileocecal valve, causing an appear-

(Text continues on page 552)

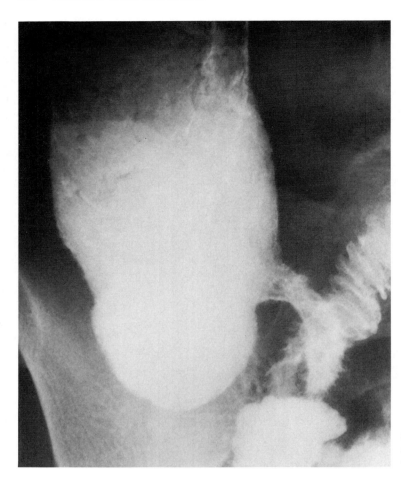

Fig. 45-16. Ulcerative colitis. The ileocecal valve is gaping, and there are inflammatory changes in the terminal ileum (backwash ileitis).

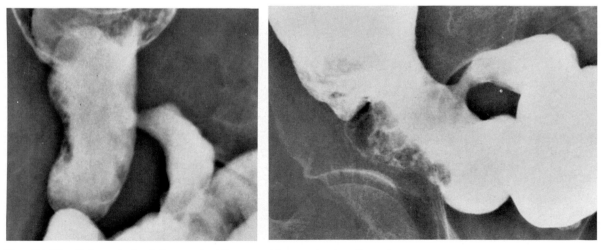

Fig. 45-17. Tuberculosis of the terminal ileum and ileocecal valve. Two views demonstrate a coned cecum, thickening of the ileocecal valve, and mucosal irregularity of the terminal ileum.

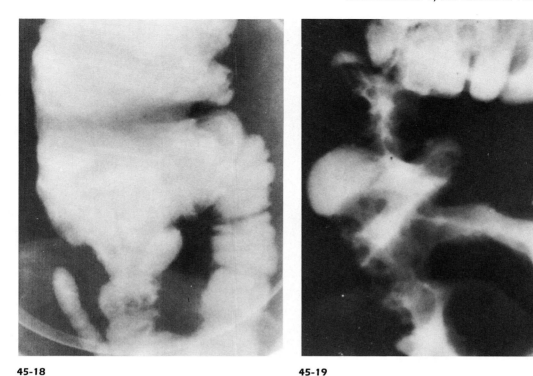

45-18   45-19

Fig. 45-18. Amebiasis of the ileocecal valve and cecum. Note that the terminal ileum is not involved.

Fig. 45-19. Anisakiasis of the ileocecal region. There is irregular thickening of the ileocecal valve with mucosal edema and luminal narrowing in the cecum.

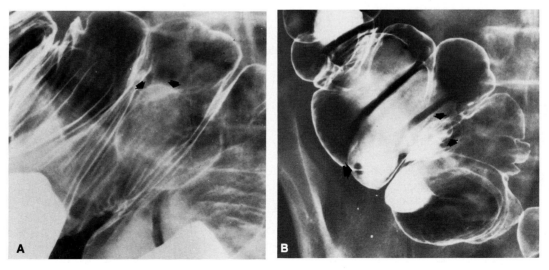

Fig. 45-20. Prolapse of the ileocecal valve. **(A)** Spot film showing a large papillary-shaped valve. Note the smooth, polypoid lobulation of the upper lip **(arrows)**. **(B)** Radiograph made a few minutes later. The valve is much smaller and has a classic spindle shape. Marked change in the volume of a valve that is not attributable to differences in compression or distention of the large intestine is probably the best evidence of prolapse. Note that the smooth, polypoid lobulation of the upper lip **(bottom arrow)** is localized but changeable. An appearance such as this should suggest the possibility of a tumor, particularly a lipoma. Note also the small polyp **(top arrow)** of the ascending colon. Follow-up studies over the next 2 years showed no change in the ileocecal valve. (Short WF, Smith BD, Hoy RJ: Roentgenologic evaluation of the prominent or the unusual ileocecal valve. Med Radiogr Photogr 52:2–26, 1976)

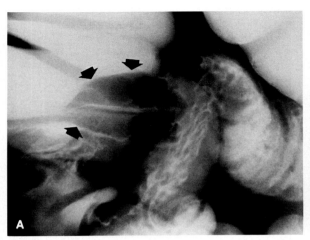
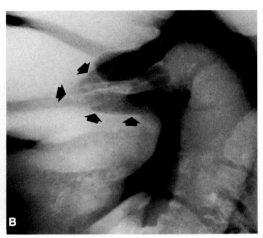
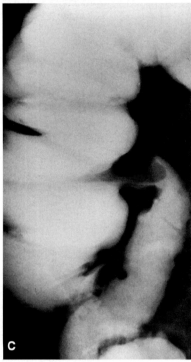

Fig. 45-21. Retrograde prolapse of the ileocecal valve on serial films from a barium enema examination. **(A)** Nondistended colon. Note the filling defect within the cecum **(arrows)**. **(B)** and **(C)** Distention of the cecum by the barium column. **(B)** The ileocecal valve **(arrows)** prolapses in a retrograde manner and **(C)** finally produces an entirely extracecal defect of the terminal ileum. (Hatten HP, Mostowycz L, Higihara PF: Retrograde prolapse of the ileocecal valve. AJR 128:755–757, 1977. Copyright 1977. Reproduced with permission)

ance that is indistinguishable from lipomatosis. Extensive prolapse can simulate a benign or malignant tumor arising from the valve. The correct diagnosis of ileal prolapse can be made if it is shown by appropriate compression that the mass arises between the lips of the ileocecal valve and that there is barium in the center of the mass representing the ileal lumen. If there is substantial change in the volume of a valve on serial films and if this change is clearly not attributable to differences in compression or distention of the cecum, ileal prolapse is probably the cause of the apparent enlargement of the ileocecal valve (Fig. 45-20*B*).

Prolapsing neoplasms of the terminal ileum are rare causes of prominence of the ileocecal valve. Like prolapsing normal ileal mucosa, a prolapsing ileal neoplasm presents in the region of the ileocecal valve as a mass that changes size and shape during barium enema examination. The pressure of the barium column may force the tumor back across the valve, demonstrating the true origin of the lesion to be in the terminal ileum.

Retrograde prolapse of the ileocecal valve results when redundant mucosa produces prominence of the lips of the valve, which is seen as a filling defect within the cecum (Fig. 45-21*A*). With manual palpation or the hydrostatic pressure of the barium column, this prominent ileocecal valve prolapses in a retrograde fashion to produce a tapered defect of the terminal ileum (Fig. 45-21*B, C*). The pliability and changeability of the defect indicates that it represents a benign condition.

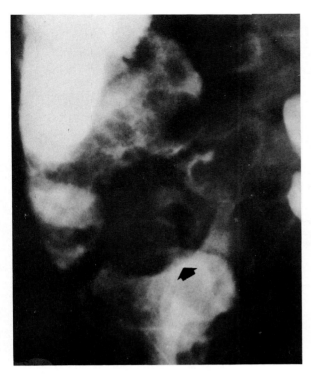

Fig. 45-22. Massive enlargement of the ileocecal valve due to lymphoid hyperplasia. Barium enema reveals a persistent smooth mass (4 cm) in the area of the ileocecal valve. (Selke AC, Jona JZ, Belin RP: Massive enlargement of the ileocecal valve due to lymphoid hyperplasia. AJR 127:518–520, 1976. Copyright 1976. Reproduced with permission)

INTUSSUSCEPTION

Intussusception of the distal ileum into the cecum can present as a discrete mass arising from the region of the ileocecal valve. The distensibility of the colon can permit intussusception of numerous ileal loops, producing the characteristic "coiled-spring" appearance on barium enema examination. With relatively fixed intussusceptions, orally administered barium may only demonstrate the long, very narrow central channel of the intussuscepted small bowel. This appearance suggests some degree of vascular insufficiency and a possible surgical emergency. After reduction of an ileocolic intussuscep-

tion, there may be temporary generalized thickening of the ileocecal valve due to edema from mechanical trauma sustained during the intussusception.

LYMPHOID HYPERPLASIA

Although most cases of benign lymphoid hyperplasia of the small bowel and colon present as multiple small papillary lesions, massive enlargement of the ileocecal valve has also been reported in this condition (Fig. 45-22). Lymphoid hyperplasia occurs primarily in children and is presumed to be a response to nonspecific inflammation.

BIBLIOGRAPHY

Berk RN, Davis GB, Cholhaffy EB: Lipomatosis of the ileocecal valve. AJR 119:323–328, 1973

Boquist L, Bergdahl L, Andersson A: Lipomatosis of the ileocecal valve. Cancer 29:136–140, 1972

Calenoff L: Rare ileocecal lesions. AJR 110:343–351, 1970

Carlson HC: Small intestinal intussusception. An easily misunderstood sign. AJR 110:338–339, 1970

Fleischner FG, Bernstein C: Roentgen—anatomical studies of the normal ileocecal valve. Radiology 54:43–58, 1950

Hatten HP, Mostowycz L, Hagihara PF: Retrograde prolapse of the ileocecal valve. AJR 128:755–757, 1977

Hinkel CL: Roentgenological examination and evaluation of the ileocecal valve. AJR 68:171–182, 1952

Kabakian HA, Nassar NT, Nasrallah SM: Roentgenographic findings in typhoid fever. AJR 125:198–206, 1975

Lasser EC, Rigler LG: Observations on the structure and function of the ileocecal valve. Radiology 63:176–183, 1954

Lasser EC, Rigler LG: Ileocecal valve syndrome. Gastroenterology 28:1–16, 1955

Richman RH, Lewicki AM: Right ileocolitis secondary to anisakiasis. AJR 119:329–331, 1973

Rubin S, Dann DS, Ezekial C et al: Retrograde prolapse of the ileocecal valve. AJR 87:706–708, 1962

Schnur MJ, Seaman WB: Prolapsing neoplasms of the terminal ileum simulating enlarged ileocecal valves. AJR 134:1133–1136, 1980

Selke AC, Jona JZ, Belin RP: Massive enlargement of the ileocecal valve due to lymphoid hyperplasia. AJR 127:518–520, 1976

Short WF, Smith BD, Hoy RJ: Roentgenologic evaluation of the prominent or unusual ileocecal valve. Med Radiogr Photogr 52:2–26, 1976

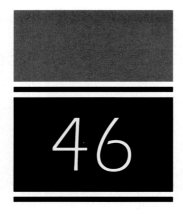

FILLING DEFECTS IN THE CECUM

Disease Entities

Abnormalities of the appendix
    Acute appendicitis
    Abscess
    Crohn's disease
    Inverted appendiceal stump
    Mucocele
    Myxoglobulosis
    Intussusception
    Benign neoplasms (carcinoid tumor; spindle
       cell tumor)
    Malignant neoplasms (adenocarcinoma)
Metastases (pancreas, ovary, colon, stomach)
General causes of colonic filling defects
    Inflammatory diseases
    Benign and malignant primary neoplasms
    Ileocolic intussusception
Unusual abnormalities of the cecum
    Diverticulitis of the ileocecal area
    Solitary benign ulcer of the cecum
    Adherent fecalith (cystic fibrosis)
    Endometriosis
    Intussusception of distal ileum lesion
    Burkitt's lymphoma
    Cecal diaphragm

ABNORMALITIES OF THE APPENDIX

Various abnormalities of the appendix can cause extramucosal filling defects at the base of the cecum. The appendix, which arises from the posteromedial aspect of the cecum at the junction of the three tenia coli, is a narrow and hollow organ with an average length of 5 cm to 10 cm. The origin of the appendix from the cecum has a constant relationship with the ileocecal valve. It is found only between the cecal apex and the ileocecal valve and is always on the same side as the valve. About three-quarters of appendices lie anterior to the cecum or in line with it. Of these, about half are found caudad toward the pelvis, and a similar number lie medial to the cecum; about 5% of appendices are situated lateral to the cecum.

Twenty-five percent of appendices lie in a retrocecal position (Fig. 46-1). The organ is infrequently located in the right upper quadrant and, rarely, can even be found in the left upper or left lower quadrant in patients with appendices of excessive length, malrotations of the colon, unusual cecal mobility, or hernias.

APPENDICITIS/APPENDICEAL ABSCESS

Acute appendicitis is the most common inflammatory disease of the right lower quadrant. Occlusion of the neck of the appendix by a fecalith or postinflammatory scarring creates a closed-loop obstruction within the organ. Because of inadequate drainage, fluid accumulates in the obstructed portion and serves as a breeding ground for bacteria. The wall of the appendix distal to the obstruction is thinned by distention, and the mucosa becomes ulcerated. As the inflammatory process progresses, thrombosis and infarction can develop. Free perforation can

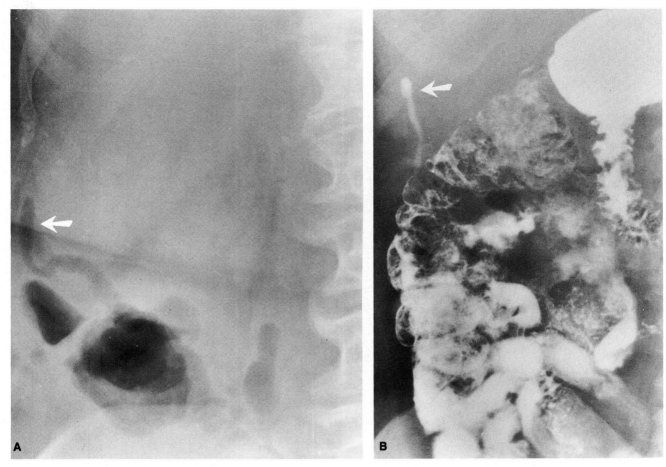

Fig. 46-1. Retrocecal appendix **(arrows). (A)** Plain abdominal radiograph. **(B)** Barium enema examination.

eventually occur and lead to a localized abscess or generalized peritonitis.

The clinical symptoms of acute appendicitis are usually so characteristic that there is no difficulty in making the correct diagnosis. The presence of severe right lower quadrant pain, rebound tenderness, low-grade fever, and slight leukocytosis, especially in males under the age of 40, is presumptive evidence of appendicitis. However, in some patients, especially in elderly persons, the clinical findings may be obscure or minimal. In these instances, a barium enema examination may be necessary for prompt diagnosis and surgical intervention before perforation occurs.

When performing an emergency or semiemergency barium enema in a patient suspected of having appendicitis, it is not necessary to prepare the colon with cleansing enemas or laxatives. Indeed, laxatives may actually be contraindicated. Once the barium reaches the cecum, it is important to evaluate the cecum in various degrees of obliquity to determine if an extrinsic mass is present. Sequentially lowering and raising the enema bag and using intravenous glucagon and postevacuation films are tech-

niques that may help to obtain maximal filling of the appendix. It is impossible to be certain that the appendix is entirely filled unless a globular tip is seen.

Acute appendicitis and appendiceal abscesses can produce characteristic appearances on barium enema examinations. An irregular impression at the base of the cecum due to inflammatory edema, in association with failure of barium to enter the appendix, has been considered virtually pathognomonic of acute appendicitis or appendiceal abscess (Fig. 46-2). Nevertheless, failure of barium to fill the appendix alone is not a reliable sign of appendicitis, since the appendix does not fill in about 20% of normal patients. Sometimes there is partial filling of the appendix with distortion in its shape or caliber (Fig. 46-3). This appearance strongly suggests acute appendicitis, especially if there is a cecal impression. In contrast, a patent appendiceal lumen effectively excludes the diagnosis of acute appendicitis, especially when barium extends to fill the rounded appendiceal tip.

Although highly suggestive of acute appendicitis, especially if there are appropriate clinical symptoms, a mass impression on the cecum with

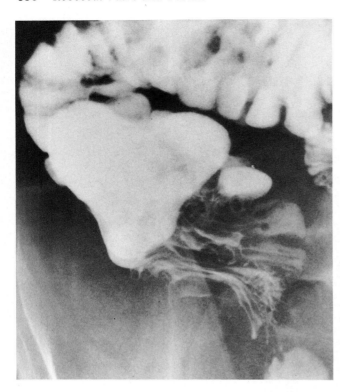

Fig. 46-2. Periappendiceal abscess. There is fixation and a mass effect at the base of the cecum with no filling of the appendix.

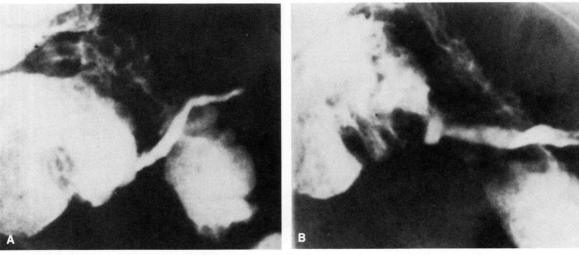

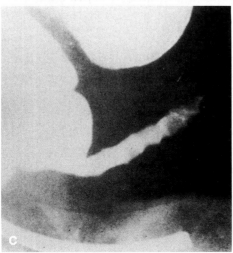

Fig. 46-3. Acute appendicitis. Spot radiographs from the barium enema examinations of three different patients with appendicitis show incomplete filling of the appendix. (Rice RP, Thompson WM, Fedyshin PJ et al: The barium enema in appendicitis: Spectrum of appearances and pitfalls. RadioGraphics 4:393–409, 1984)

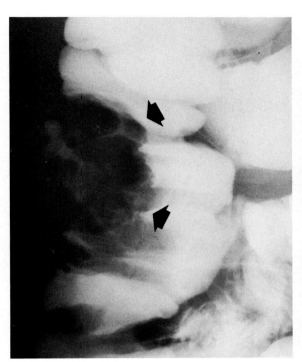

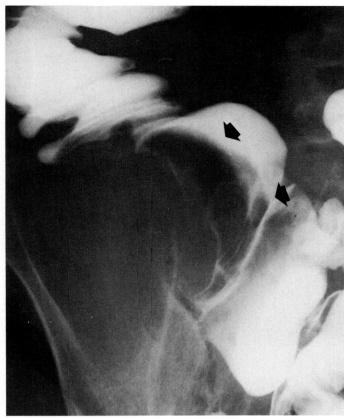

46-4   46-5

Fig. 46-4. Periappendiceal abscess. Severe inflammatory mucosal changes and a mass effect on the lateral aspect of the ascending colon **(arrows)** were seen in a patient with a ruptured retrocecal appendix.

Fig. 46-5. Periappendiceal abscess. This large extrinsic mass involving the lateral aspect of the ascending colon **(arrows)** was seen in a patient with a ruptured retrocecal appendix.

nonfilling of the appendix can be caused by other pathologic entities. Endometriosis, ovarian cyst, and tubo-ovarian abscess can produce an identical radiographic appearance. *Yersinia* enterocolitis is notorious for mimicking appendicitis clinically and, on occasion, may be associated with an inflammatory process suggesting an appendiceal abscess. Crohn's disease is a well-known cause of right lower quadrant inflammatory processes and occasionally may produce a pattern indistinguishable from appendicitis. Patients with distal small bowel obstruction may have dilated, fluid-filled loops of ileum causing extrinsic compression of the cecum that may mimic a pericecal inflammatory mass.

In the proper clinical context, the vast majority of patients with nonfilling of the appendix and a large extrinsic compression of the base of the cecum will have an appendiceal abscess. The contour defect in the cecum adjacent to an appendiceal abscess is accompanied by increased irritability and inflammatory edema of the mucosa with local oblit-

eration of cecal haustration (Fig. 46-4). Depending on the size and extent of the inflammatory process, the contour deformity may involve the cecum, ascending colon, bladder, ileum, ureter, adnexa, uterus, or sigmoid. In rare instances, barium enters the abscess cavity itself, implying that the appendiceal lumen has remained partially patent. Supine plain abdominal radiographs occasionally demonstrate a mottled gas pattern in an appendiceal abscess, and a gas–fluid level can sometimes be noted on upright or decubitus views.

In some patients, a large appendiceal inflammatory process may not involve the tip of the cecum. When the appendix is in a retrocecal position and the inflammatory process is limited to the tip of the appendix, there may be a more proximal mass on the posterolateral aspect of the cecum but sparing of the cecal tip (Fig. 46-5). In some patients an appendiceal abscess may be entirely pelvic in location with an extrinsic process involving the rectum or sigmoid but with no detectable pericecal

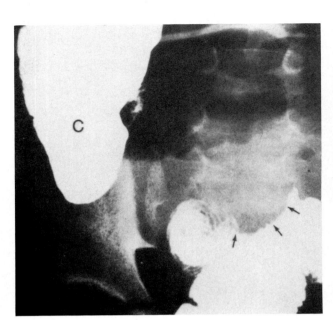

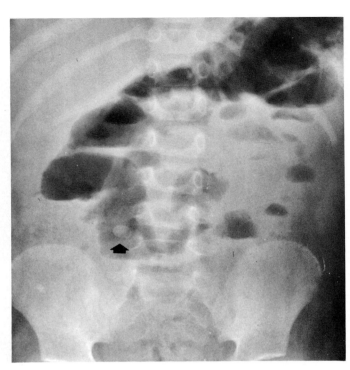

46-6   **46-7**

Fig. 46-6.   Appendiceal abscess. Mass effect with tethering of the sigmoid **(arrows)** in a 4-year-old boy with a 3-day history of abdominal pain. The cecum **(C)** is normal.

Fig. 46-7.   Appendicolith **(arrow)** in a patient with acute appendicitis.

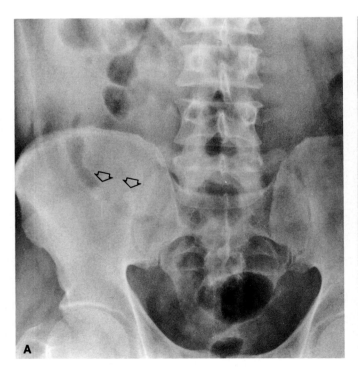

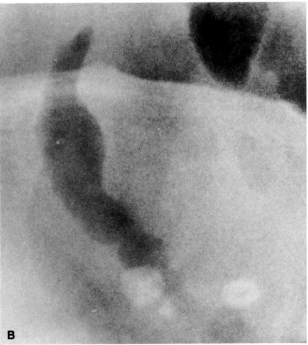

Fig. 46-8.   Appendicoliths in a patient with acute appendicitis and a periappendiceal abscess. **(A)** Full and **(B)** coned views show that the appendicoliths **(arrows)** lie in an abscess outside of the gas-filled appendix.

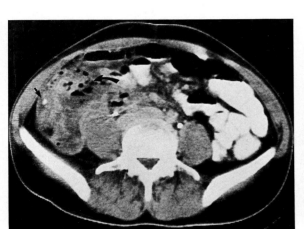

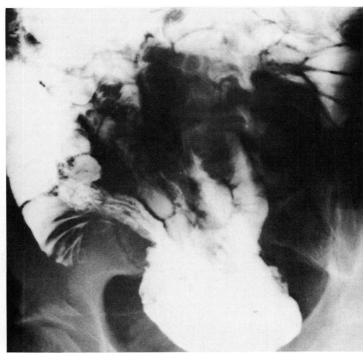

46-9   46-10

Fig. 46-9. Ruptured appendix with periappendiceal abscess. CT scan demonstrates a large soft-tissue mass with ectopic gas **(curved arrow)** and a high-density appendicolith **(arrow)**.

Fig. 46-10. Crohn's disease of the appendix. Pressure film from a barium enema examination reveals a large extrinsic mass impinging upon the cecal tip and medial cecal wall. Note the normal mucosa and the distensibility of the terminal ileum. (Threatt B, Appelman H: Crohn's disease of the appendix presenting as acute appendicitis. Radiology 110:313–317, 1974)

component (Fig. 46-6). In such cases, it may be impossible radiographically to exclude the possibility of an abscess arising from diverticulitis, pelvic inflammatory disease, or some other source. Appendiceal abscesses may be in locations remote from the right lower quadrant because of positional anomalies of the cecum and appendix or as a result of spread of the inflammatory process. Extension of the inflammatory process superiorly from the pelvis into the right or left paracolic gutter may result in a subdiaphragmatic or subhepatic abscess.

Whenever the diagnosis of acute appendicitis is being considered, it is essential that the right lower quadrant be examined for evidence of an appendicolith (Fig. 46-7). If typical clinical signs and symptoms are also present, these round or ovoid, often laminated calcifications are virtually diagnostic of acute appendicitis (Fig. 46-8). In addition, patients with acute appendicitis who have radiographically demonstrable appendicoliths have a much higher incidence than usual of complications, especially perforation and abscess formation.

Computed tomography (CT) may be a valuable adjunct to a conventional contrast enema in assessing the patient with appendicitis, especially in se-

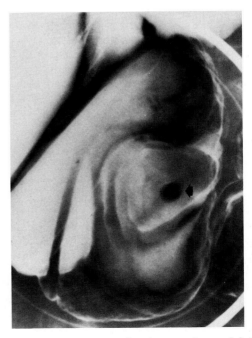

Fig. 46-11. Inverted appendiceal stump **(arrow)** following appendectomy.

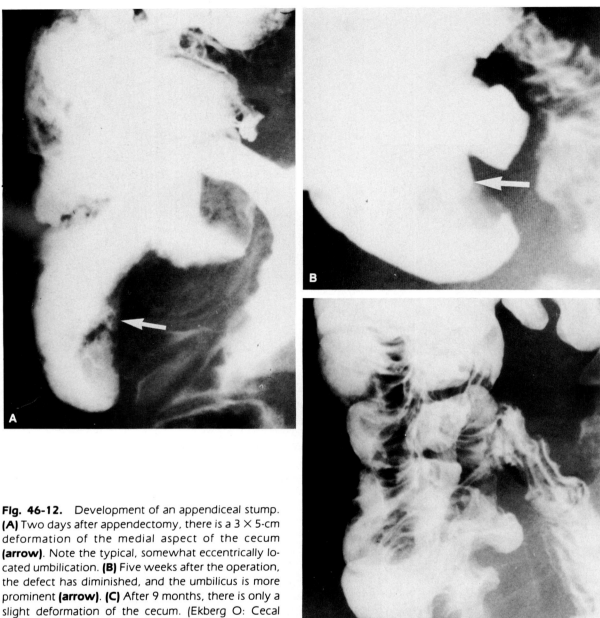

Fig. 46-12. Development of an appendiceal stump. **(A)** Two days after appendectomy, there is a 3 × 5-cm deformation of the medial aspect of the cecum **(arrow)**. Note the typical, somewhat eccentrically located umbilication. **(B)** Five weeks after the operation, the defect has diminished, and the umbilicus is more prominent **(arrow)**. **(C)** After 9 months, there is only a slight deformation of the cecum. (Ekberg O: Cecal changes following appendectomy. Gastrointest Radiol 2:57–60, 1977)

vere disease associated with phlegmons or periappendiceal abscesses. An appendiceal abscess appears as an oval or round mass of soft-tissue density that may contain gas and occasionally a calcified appendicolith (Fig. 46-9). CT provides a more precise evaluation of the nature, extent, and location of the pathologic process than does barium enema examination. In addition, CT can detect intra-abdominal disease unrelated to appendicitis that may explain the patient's clinical presentation. A normal CT scan does not exclude appendicitis, because mild forms without periappendiceal disease may escape detection and abscesses can be missed if terminal ileal loops and the cecum are not adequately visualized.

CROHN'S DISEASE

Rarely, Crohn's disease is limited to the appendix and shows no evidence of terminal ileal involvement. This condition usually occurs in young adults with no previous gastrointestinal problems who present with acute onset of abdominal pain and a palpable right lower quadrant mass simulating acute appendicitis. Barium enema examination generally demonstrates a large extrinsic mass im-

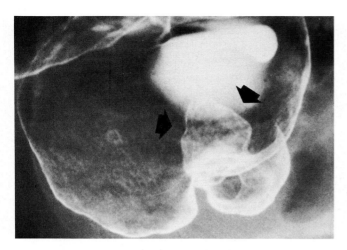

Fig. 46-13. *Inverted appendiceal stump. In this patient, the mass (arrow) is large and irregular, simulating a neoplasm at the base of the cecum.*

pinging upon the cecal tip and medial cecal wall (Fig. 46-10). Crohn's disease can be expected if the appendix is partially patent with an irregular lumen or if there is any evidence of coexistent inflammation and aphthous ulcers in the adjacent cecum, terminal ileum, or both.

INVERTED APPENDICEAL STUMP

An inverted appendiceal stump following appendectomy produces a filling defect in the tip of the cecum at the base of the appendix that may be seen on barium studies (Fig. 46-11). The mass is usually small and localized but can be very prominent for several weeks after surgery until postoperative edema and inflammation subside (Fig. 46-12). The surface of an inverted stump deformity is generally smooth but can be lobulated or irregular. Although an inverted appendiceal stump is essentially asymptomatic, recognition of the entity is essential, because the radiographic appearance can be indistinguishable from a neoplasm at the base of the cecum (Fig. 46-13). A smooth cecal defect in the expected site of the appendix in a patient with a history of previous appendectomy is presumptive evidence for the diagnosis of an inverted appendiceal stump. A negative history of appendectomy, however, does not exclude the diagnosis of appendiceal stump, since many patients have had appendectomies incidental to other surgery without being aware of it. If the cecal defect is large or irregular, colonoscopy or surgical intervention is necessary to exclude the possibility of a neoplastic process.

MUCOCELE

Mucocele of the appendix is an uncommon benign condition in which there is cystic dilatation of the appendix. Most mucoceles are believed to result from proximal luminal obstruction (caused by a fecalith, foreign body, tumor, adhesions, or volvulus), which leads to accumulation of mucus distally in the distended appendix. A few authors suggest that the lesion represents a mucinous cystadenoma arising within the appendix.

Most mucoceles of the appendix are found incidentally during abdominal radiography, at laparotomy, or on portmortem examination. Some patients with mucoceles complain of recurrent vague lower abdominal discomfort; physical examination may reveal a right lower quadrant mass. Significant symptoms are infrequent and reflect complications such as secondary infection or intussusception of the lesion.

Plain radiographs of the abdomen may demonstrate a mottled or rimlike calcification around the periphery of an appendiceal mucocele (see Fig. 73-55). This calcification occurs infrequently but is helpful in establishing the diagnosis. On barium enema examination, a mucocele presents as a sharply outlined smooth-walled, broad-based filling defect indenting the lower part of the cecum, usually on its medial side (Fig. 46-14). There is typically nonfilling of the appendix, though a few cases have been reported in which barium has entered the mucocele through what was probably a recanalized lumen.

Computed tomography and ultrasound have been reported to be of value in diagnosing mucocele of the appendix (Fig. 46-15). In a patient who has not had an appendectomy, the combined findings of a low-density, right lower quadrant mass on CT and a through-transmitting mass with echogenic

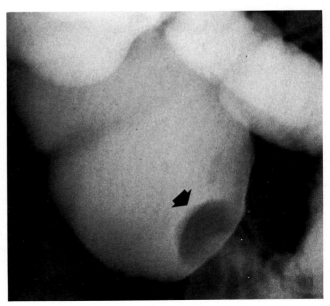

Fig. 46-14. *Mucocele of the appendix. A smooth, broad-based filling defect (arrow) indents the lower part of the cecum. There is no filling of the appendix with barium.*

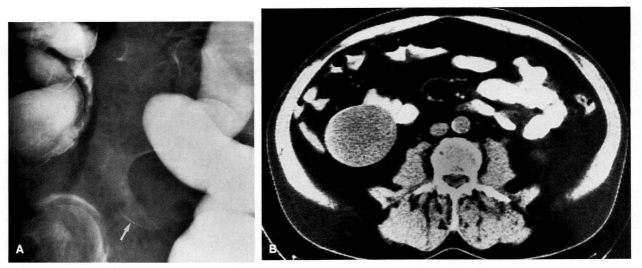

Fig. 46-15. Mucocele of the appendix. **(A)** Barium enema demonstrates curvilinear calcification in the wall of the mucocele **(arrow)**. Note that the mucocele is distant from the cecum and does not impress it. **(B)** CT scan demonstrates the low-attenuation mass with rim calcification in its lateral aspect **(arrow)** and adherence to an adjacent loop of bowel. (Dachman AH, Lichtenstein JE, Friedman AC: Mucocele of the appendix and pseudomyxoma peritonei. AJR 144:923–929, 1985. Copyright 1985. Reproduced with permission)

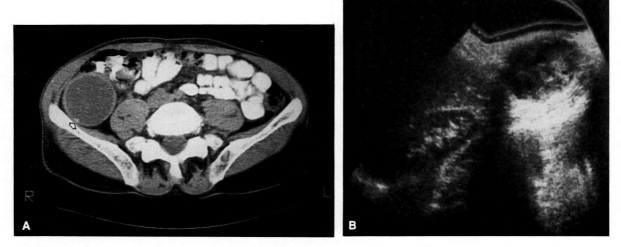

Fig. 46-16. Mucocele of the appendix. **(A)** CT scan shows a low-attenuation (26 HU) mass in the right lower quadrant with anteromedial displacement of the adjacent cecum. Note the high-attenuation area **(arrow)** within the wall posterolaterally, representing a fleck of calcification. **(B)** Right parasagittal sonogram shows a complex lesion with enhanced through transmission. (Horgan JG, Chow PP, Richter JO et al: CT and sonography in the recognition of mucocele of the appendix. AJR 143:959–962, 1984. Copyright 1984. Reproduced with permission)

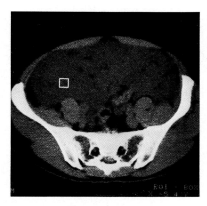

Fig. 46-17. *Pseudomyxoma peritonei. CT scan of the abdomen following rupture of a mucocele of the appendix demonstrates the characteristic appearance of multiple cystic masses throughout the abdomen. (Berk RN: Radiology of the appendix. In Taveras JN, Ferrucci JT (eds): Radiology: Diagnosis— Imaging—Intervention. Philadelphia, JB Lippincott, 1987)*

foci (representing mucus) at sonography are typical of a mucocele (Fig. 46-16). A purely cystic mass on CT and ultrasound is consistent with a fluid-filled mucocele, though the differential diagnosis is broad.

Rupture of a mucocele of the appendix (or ovary) can lead to the development of pseudomyxoma peritonei, a condition characterized by epithelial implants on the peritoneal surface with massive accumulation of gelatinous ascites (Fig. 46-17). Acute, sharp abdominal pain can occur at the time of rupture of the mucocele; this event is often asso-

ciated with straining. Radiographic demonstration of a sudden decrease in the size of a mucocele may indicate that rupture has occurred. Rarely, a mucocele causes ureteral or ileal obstruction, becomes inflamed, twists on itself, or intussuscepts.

MYXOGLOBULOSIS

Myxoglobulosis is a rare type of mucocele of the appendix that is composed of many round or oval translucent globules mixed with mucus. The globules vary from 0.1 cm to 1.0 cm in size and are said to resemble tapioca or fish eggs. Like simple mucoceles of the appendix, myxoglobulosis is usually asymptomatic. Radiographically, myxoglobulosis can present as a smooth extramucosal mass impressing on the cecum and associated with nonfilling of the appendix, a pattern indistinguishable from simple mucocele (Fig. 46-18*A*). The most characteristic features of myxoglobulosis are calcified rims about the periphery of the individual globules. Unlike appendiceal calculi, the calcified spherules in myxoglobulosis usually are annular and nonlaminated, shift within the mucocele, and can layer in the upright position. In contrast to simple mucoceles, in which calcification involves only the wall, in myxoglobulosis the individual globules within the lumen are calcified (Fig. 46-18*B*).

INTUSSUSCEPTION

Primary appendiceal intussusception is an infrequent occurrence in which the appendix invaginates into the cecum and simulates a cecal tumor

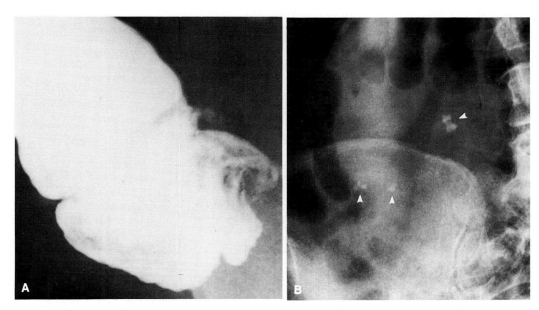

Fig. 46-18. *Myxoglobulosis of the appendix.* **(A)** *A mass effect on the medial wall of the cecum with distortion but no destruction of cecal folds is seen on barium enema examination.* **(B)** *Typical calcifications of myxoglobulosis* **(arrowheads)**. *(Felson B, Wiot JF: Some interesting right lower quadrant entities. Radiol Clin North Am 7:83–95, 1969)*

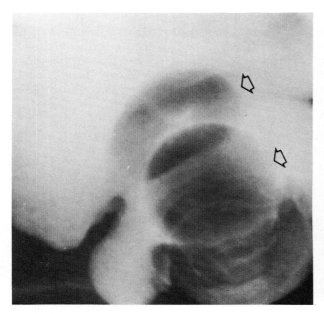
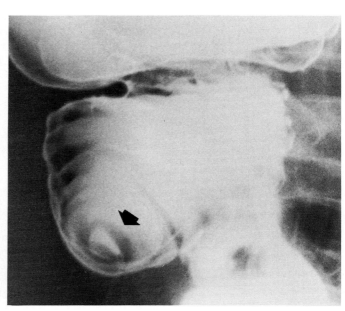

46-19   46-20

Fig. 46-19.   Primary appendiceal intussusception. Lobulated, fingerlike filling defect **(arrows)** projects into the cecum and simulates a cecal tumor.

Fig. 46-20.   Primary appendiceal intussusception **(arrow)**. Following reduction, the cecum and appendix appeared normal on a subsequent barium enema examination.

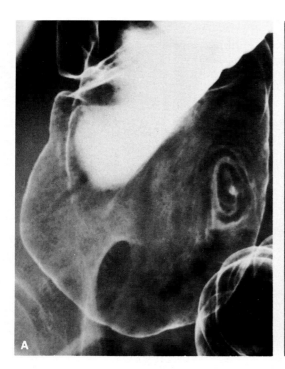
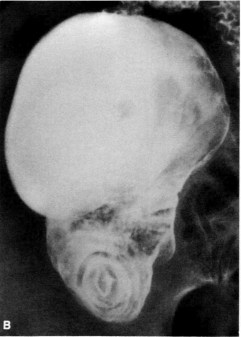

Fig. 46-21.   Coiled-spring cecum in appendicitis. **(A)** Compression spot film shows ring shadows arranged concentrically around a central barium collection in a patient with acute appendicitis without perforation. **(B)** In this patient with acute appendicitis and pericecal abscess, the postevacuation radiograph was the only film to show the coiled-spring appearance and shallow contour defect of the medial cecal wall. (Demos TC, Flisak ME: Coiled-spring sign of the cecum in acute appendicitis. AJR 146:45–48, 1986. Copyright 1986. Reproduced with permission)

(Fig. 46-19). It can present as an acute surgical emergency or as a subacute recurring condition. Intussusception of the appendix can also be asymptomatic and may be noted only during a barium enema examination (Fig. 46-20).

Intussusception is probably caused by increased and abnormal peristalsis of the appendix. This may be related either to an attempt of the organ to extrude an intraluminal abnormality (foreign body, fecalith, polyp, parasite) or to intramural disease (mucocele, tumor, endometriosis, lymphoid follicles).

On barium enema examination, intussusception of the appendix produces an oval, round, or fingerlike filling defect projecting from the medial wall of the cecum. The appendix is not visible. A coiled-spring appearance in the cecum associated with nonfilling of the appendix has been suggested as characteristic of appendiceal intussusception. However, a recent study showed that although the coiled-spring sign was most often caused by acute appendicitis (Fig. 46-21), an identical appearance could also be seen in patients with mucocele, carcinoma, or endometriosis of the appendix.

An intussusception of the appendix demonstrated by barium enema can reduce itself completely during the course of a single examination or be reduced on a subsequent study. After reduction occurs, the cecum and appendix appear radiographically to be entirely normal. Patients with this condition are asymptomatic, and the cause of reducible partial intussusception of a normal appendix is unknown.

BENIGN NEOPLASMS

Although tumors of the appendix can be demonstrated in about 6% of surgical and autopsy specimens, these lesions are rarely diagnosed radiographically because of their small size or the frequent complication of appendicitis. The most common appendiceal neoplasm is the carcinoid tumor, which arises from the argentaffin cells of the crypts of Lieberkuhn. Of all carcinoids, 90% arise in the distal ileum or appendix; of all tumors of the appendix, 90% are carcinoids. These lesions are almost always benign and rarely metastasize or cause the carcinoid syndrome. Most carcinoids are dis-

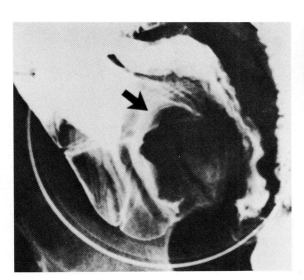

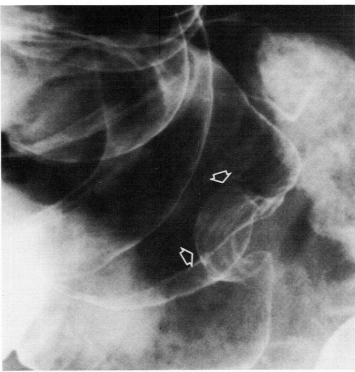

46-22   46-23

Fig. 46-22. Adenocarcinoma arising from the base of the appendix and projecting into the cecal lumen **(arrow)**. Note the sharply defined lobulated contour and acute angle, characteristic of an intrinsic lesion, that are formed by the mass and the adjacent wall of the cecum. (Stiehm WD, Seaman WB: Radiographic aspects of primary carcinoma of the appendix. Radiology 108:275–278, 1973)

Fig. 46-23. Adenocarcinoma of the appendix. The extensive tumor produces a large mass **(arrows)** that mimics an intraluminal cecal neoplasm.

covered in appendices removed incidentally at surgery for another procedure or because of acute appendicitis. Appendiceal carcinoids tend to obstruct the lumen and cause acute appendicitis. This permits such a tumor to be diagnosed relatively early, thereby greatly decreasing the incidence of metastases. Other benign tumors of the appendix include leiomyomas, neuromas, and lipomas. Like carcinoids, these small tumors are generally incidental findings in surgical specimens and are rarely diagnosed by barium studies.

MALIGNANT NEOPLASMS

Adenocarcinoma of the appendix usually arises in the distal third of the appendix, where it frequently results in luminal obstruction and secondary acute appendicitis. The preoperative diagnosis of adenocarcinoma of the appendix is rarely made. In half of the reported cases, patients were initially thought to have acute appendicitis.

Radiographic demonstration of appendiceal carcinoma is unusual. When visualized, these tumors generally present as extrinsic masses deforming and displacing the cecum. If the tumor is extensive enough, the acute angle formed between the mass and the adjacent cecal wall can mimic an intramural (Fig. 46-22) or even an intraluminal (Fig. 46-23) cecal mass. Calcification is occasionally detected in the tumor on plain abdominal radiographs.

METASTASES

A localized defect on the medial aspect of the cecum below the ileocecal valve can represent a metastatic lesion (Fig. 46-24). Metastases in the right lower quadrant producing such defects are most commonly secondary to a primary neoplasm in the ovary, colon, stomach, or pancreas. The relatively common association of primary pancreatic carcinoma with a prominent right lower quadrant metastatic mass is due to the typical routes of spread of this malignancy. The origin of the mesentery near the inferior margin of the pancreas and its insertion in the region of the ileocecal valve provide a pathway for the spread of pancreatic carcinoma to the right lower quadrant of the abdomen. This is analogous to the pattern seen in acute pancreatitis, in which extravasated enzymes dissecting between the leaves of the mesentery cause abscess formation in the ileocecal area. These secondary abscesses can produce a medial cecal deformity identical to that seen in patients with metastatic pancreatic carcinoma. Metastatic spread by intraperitoneal seeding often demonstrates preferential flow along the root of the small bowel mesentery toward the right lower quadrant and then upward in the right pericolic gutter; this can cause extrinsic impressions in the region of the ileocecal junction or the lateral and posterior aspects of the cecum, respectively. In middle-aged or elderly patients with nonspecific abdominal complaints and no clinical evidence of in-

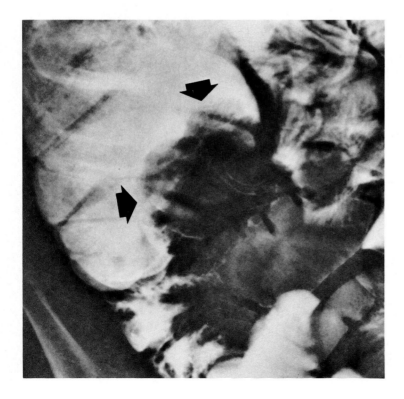

Fig. 46-24. Carcinoma of the pancreas metastatic to the cecum. There is a localized extrinsic pressure defect **(arrows)** on the medial and inferior aspects of the cecum and no filling of the appendix.

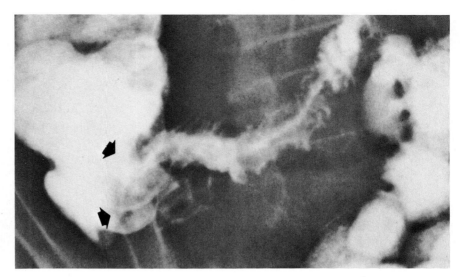

Fig. 46-25. Crohn's disease. This irregular mass on the medial aspect of the cecum **(arrows)** was seen in a patient with extensive disease of the terminal ileum.

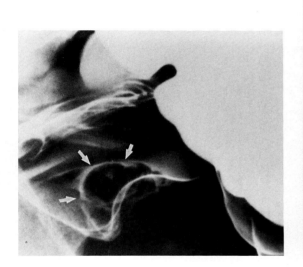

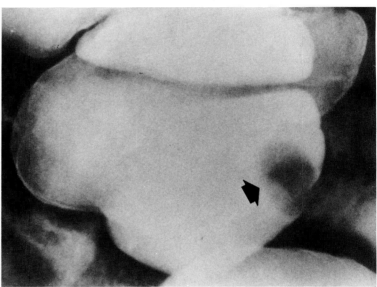

46-26   46-27

Fig. 46-26. Tuberculosis. Filling defect at the base of the cecum **(arrows)** in a young man from Thailand with a 6-week history of right lower quadrant pain.

Fig. 46-27. Benign adenomatous polyp **(arrow)** in the cecum.

flammatory disease in the right lower quadrant, the presence of a localized defect on the medial aspect of the cecum should raise the possibility of metastatic carcinoma.

GENERAL COLONIC LESIONS

Numerous conditions described in detail in other sections can produce filling defects in the barium-filled cecum. These include inflammatory masses (Fig. 46-25, 46-26), especially ameboma, benign (Fig. 46-27) and malignant (Fig. 46-28, 46-29) primary cecal neoplasms, and ileocolic intussusception (Fig. 46-30). Several unusual entities, however, can cause masses or contour deformities that either primarily involve the cecum or have a specific radiographic appearance when the cecum is affected.

ILEOCECAL DIVERTICULITIS

Diverticulitis of the ileocecal area can result in a localized mural abscess in the wall of the colon that

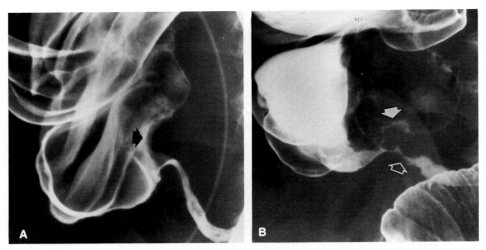

Fig. 46-28. Development of a cecal carcinoma. **(A)** Small, smooth impression on the medial wall of the cecum **(arrow)** that was noted only in retrospect. **(B)** One year later, the malignant mass is irregular **(solid arrow)**, and the tumor has spread to irregularly narrow the appendix **(open arrow)**.

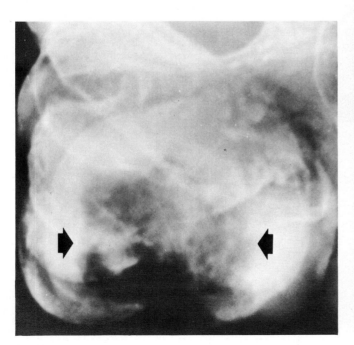

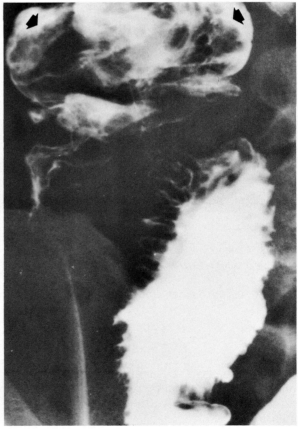

46-29   46-30

Fig. 46-29. Villous adenocarcinoma of the cecum. A huge irregular mass **(arrows)** is visible. Barium fills the interstices of the frondlike tumor.

Fig. 46-30. Ileocolic intussusception due to pseudolymphoma of the distal ileum. A large mass **(arrows)** is visible at the base of the cecum. There are inflammatory (pseudoneoplastic) changes in the distal ileum.

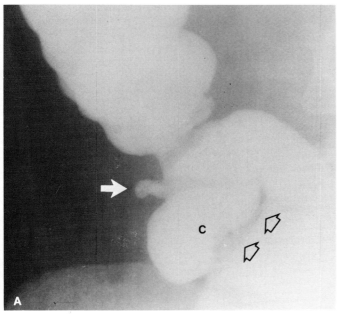

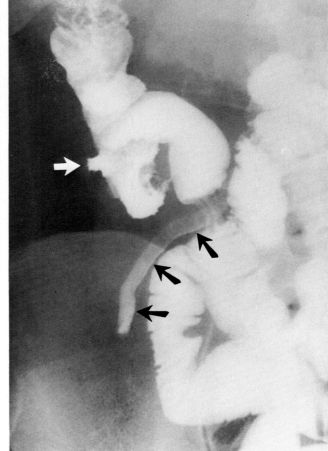

Fig. 46-31. Cecal diverticulitis in a 24-year-old man. **(A)** Solitary cecal diverticulum **(white arrow)** surrounded by an intramural mass. The mucosa over the mass is intact and not ulcerated. The terminal ileum **(black arrows)** is not displaced from the cecum (C). **(B)** Postevacuation spot film demonstrates the cecal diverticulum **(white arrow)** and normal filling of the appendix **(black arrows)**. (Norfray JF, Givens JD, Sparberg MS et al: Cecal diverticulitis in young patients. Gastrointest Radiol 5:379–382, 1980)

presents radiographically as a smooth, eccentric mass that is sharply demarcated from the adjacent colonic wall (Fig. 46-31). Extraluminal barium is occasionally seen as a small fleck in a fistula or in an abscess cavity. Both cecal and ileal diverticula are uncommon. Because the major symptom of acute diverticulitis in the ileocecal area is generalized abdominal pain that eventually localizes to the right lower quadrant, the preoperative diagnosis is almost always acute appendicitis. A major reason for these errors in diagnosis is that cecal diverticulitis often occurs in young patients (up to 50% of cases develop in persons under the age of 30) who are generally not considered to suffer from complications of diverticular disease. A barium enema in patients with diverticulitis of the ileocecal area sometimes demonstrates complete filling of the appendix, excluding the presence of acute appendicitis. A correct preoperative diagnosis of cecal diverticulitis is of great importance, since it may permit medical treatment rather than immediate surgical intervention.

SOLITARY BENIGN ULCER OF THE CECUM

A smooth mass in the base of the cecum can be due to granulation tissue caused by the healing of a solitary benign ulcer of the cecum. In this rare disease, which is of uncertain etiology, the ulcer itself is infrequently visible on barium enema examination. The adjacent inflammatory reaction can be so intense that it simulates a discrete tumor mass. Localized irritability, hypermotility, spasm, and stricture can also be present. Because of the danger of perforation, surgical resection of the cecum is usually performed.

ADHERENT FECALITH

The sticky fecal material that is found in patients with cystic fibrosis can form a persistent tumorlike mass in the colon, particularly in the cecum (Fig.

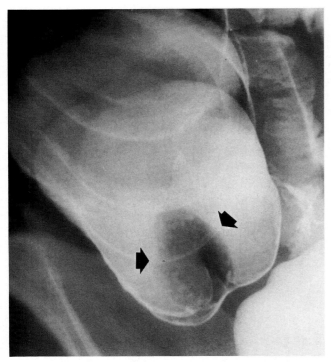

Fig. 46-32.   Adherent fecalith. A tumorlike mass **(arrows)** is visible in the cecum of a patient with cystic fibrosis.

46-32). This can produce a filling defect on barium enema examination that often persists on repeat studies over an interval of several weeks. Palpable adherent fecaliths in cystic fibrosis can simulate colonic neoplasms; associated tenderness can suggest acute appendicitis. Occasionally, an adherent fecalith can be the leading point of an intussusception.

ENDOMETRIOSIS

Endometriosis can present as an intramural, extramucosal lesion of the cecum with a smooth surface and sharp margins (Fig. 46-33). The mucosa overlying the lesion usually remains intact. Cecal endometriosis rarely causes the fibrotic compression and kinking of the colon that are characteristic of the disease in the sigmoid region.

BURKITT'S LYMPHOMA

Burkitt's lymphoma is a distinct childhood tumor of the reticuloendothelial system. The disease predominantly affects African children and is characterized by swelling and bony lesions of the mandible and maxilla. A tumor histologically indistinguishable from the African variety is being increasingly reported in North American children. Most of these

children, unlike their African counterparts, have demonstrated some involvement of the gastrointestinal tract, predominantly masses in the ileocecal area (Fig. 46-34), which often cause intussusception or obstruction.

CECAL DIAPHRAGM

Cecal diaphragm (web) is a rare anomaly that is probably part of the colonic atresia spectrum due to either failure of recanalization or a fetal vascular insult. On single-contrast enema examination, a cecal diaphragm appears as a characteristic band-like stricture at the level of the ileocecal valve. There is usually one or more large filling defects (fecal material) in the cecum proximal to the transverse lucency of the web. Air inflation after evacua-

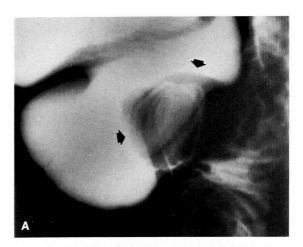

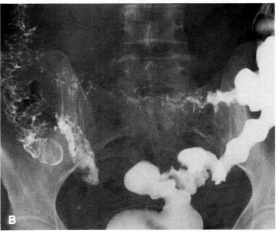

Fig. 46-33.   Endometriosis of the cecum. Note the intramural extramucosal lesion **(arrows)**. The mucosa over the mass is stretched but preserved. (Felson B, Wiot JF: Some interesting right lower quadrant entities. Radiol Clin North Am 7:83–95, 1969)

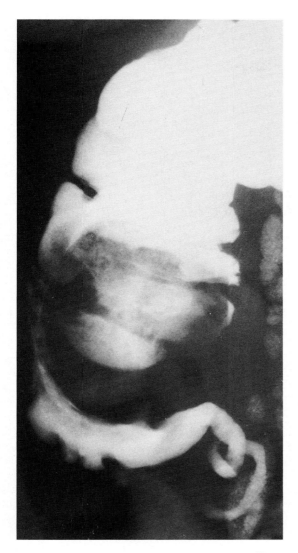

Fig. 46-34. Burkitt's lymphoma. A huge mass fills essentially the entire cecum.

tion will distend the barium-coated cecum and outline the regular, smooth opening of the membrane and the weblike, convergent mucosal folds.

A plain radiograph may reveal retained feces, old barium, or a laminated calcification (fecalith). If the patient has had a previous upper gastrointestinal series, a preliminary radiograph may show a very well-prepared bowel but with retained barium in the cecal area.

BIBLIOGRAPHY

Agha FP, Ghahremani GG, Panella JS et al: Appendicitis as the initial manifestation of Crohn's disease: Radiologic features and prognosis. AJR 149:515–518, 1987

Alcalay J, Alkalay L, Lorent T: Myxoglobulosis of the appendix. Br J Radiol 58:183–184, 1985

Alford BA, Coccia PF, L'Heureux PR: Roentgenographic features of American Burkitt's lymphoma. Radiology 124:763–770, 1977

Bachman AL, Clemett AR: Roentgen aspects of primary appendiceal intussusception. Radiology 101:531–538, 1971

Balthazar EJ, Megibow AJ, Hulnick D et al: CT of appendicitis. AJR 147:705–710, 1986

Beneventano TC, Schein CJ, Jacobson HG: The roentgen aspects of some appendiceal abnormalities. AJR 96:344–360, 1966

Benninger GW, Honig LJ, Fein HD: Nonspecific ulceration of the cecum. Am J Gastroenterol 55:594–601, 1971

Berk RN, Lee FA: The late gastrointestinal manifestations of cystic fibrosis of the pancreas. Radiology 106:377–381, 1973

Collins DC: Seventy-one thousand human appendix specimens. A final report summarizing 40 years' study. Am J Proctol 14:365–381, 1963

Dachman AH, Lichtenstein JE, Friedman AC: Mucocele of the appendix and pseudomyxoma peritonei. AJR 144:923–929, 1985

Demos TC, Flisak ME: Coiled-spring sign of the cecum in acute appendicitis. AJR 146:45–48, 1986

Douglas NJ, Cameron SJ, Nixon MV et al: Intussusception of mucocele of the appendix. Gastrointest Radiol 3:97–100, 1978

Felson B, Wiot JF: Some interesting right lower quadrant entities. Myxoglobulosis of the appendix, ileal prolapse, diverticulitis, lymphoma, endometriosis. Radiol Clin North Am 7:83–95, 1969

Freedman E, Radwin MH, Linsman JF: Roentgen simulation of polypoid neoplasms by invaginated appendiceal stumps. AJR 75:380–385, 1956

Gibbs NM: Mucinous cystadenocarcinoma of vermiform appendix with particular reference to mucocele and pseudomyxoma peritonei. J Clin Pathol 26:413–421, 1973

Gorske K: Intussusception of the proximal appendix into the colon. Radiology 91:791, 1968

Govoni AF: Radiology of para and pericecal lesions. Rev Interam Radiol 9:181–185, 1984

Howard RJ, Ellis CM, Delaney JP: Intussusception of the appendix simulating carcinoma of the cecum. Arch Surg 101:520–522, 1970

Joffe N: Medial cecal defect associated with metastatic pancreatic carcinoma. Radiology 111:297–300, 1974

Levine MS, Trenkner SW, Herlinger H et al: Coiled-spring sign of appendiceal intussusception. Radiology 155:41–44, 1985

Marshak RH, Gerson A: Mucocele of the appendix. Am J Dig Dis 5:49–54, 1960

Norfray JF, Givens JD, Sparberg MS et al: Cecal diverticulitis in young patients. Gastrointest Radiol 5:379–382, 1980

Otto RE, Ghislandi EV, Lorenzo GA et al: Primary appendiceal adenocarcinoma. Am J Surg 120:704–707, 1970

Ponka JL: Carcinoid tumors of the appendix. Report of 35 cases. Am J Surg 126:77–83, 1973

Raymond J, Belliveau P, Arseneau J: The cecal diaphragm. Radiology 147:79–80, 1983

Rice RP, Thompson WM, Fedyshin PJ et al: The barium enema in appendicitis: Spectrum of appearances and pitfalls. RadioGraphics 4:393–409, 1984

Soter CS: The contribution of the radiologist to the diagnosis of acute appendicitis. Semin Roentgenol 8:375–388, 1973

Stiehm WD, Seaman WB: Roentgenographic aspects of primary carcinoma of the appendix. Radiology 108:275–278, 1973

Threatt B, Appelman H: Crohn's disease of the appendix presenting as acute appendicitis. Radiology 110:313–317, 1974

CONED CECUM

Disease Entities

Crohn's disease
Tuberculosis
Amebiasis
Ulcerative colitis
Appendicitis
Carcinoma of the cecum
Perforated cecal diverticulum
Actinomycosis
South American blastomycosis
Anisakiasis
Typhoid fever
Yersinia enterocolitis
Cytomegalovirus
Typhlitis

CROHN'S DISEASE

Once thought to be virtually pathognomonic of amebic infection, concentric narrowing of the normal saclike cecum (coned cecum; Fig. 47-1) can be found in a broad spectrum of inflammatory diseases affecting the right lower quadrant. Deformities of the cecum and ascending colon are frequently associated with terminal ileum involvement in Crohn's disease (Fig. 47-2). A mild concavity on the medial aspect of the cecum can be caused by pressure on the colon by the thickened terminal ileum with its inflamed mesentery. Severe disease can lead to narrowing and rigidity of the cecum and ascending colon (Fig. 47-3), often associated with a thin,

linear collection of barium in the region of the terminal ileum. This barium collection, which resembles a frayed cotton string ("string sign"; Fig. 47-4), represents incomplete filling of the terminal ileum due to the irritability and spasm accompanying severe ulceration and is considered a pathognomonic radiographic manifestation of Crohn's disease.

TUBERCULOSIS

The coned cecum is a characteristic finding of intestinal tuberculosis. Healing of acute tuberculous inflammation of the terminal ileum and cecum results in shortening and narrowing of the purse-shaped cecum. This is most marked opposite the ileocecal valve, where there can be a broad, deep indentation. Further progression of this process causes straightening and rigidity of the ileocecal valve. The terminal ileum can appear to empty directly into the stenotic ascending colon with nonopacification of the fibrotic, contracted cecum (Stierlin's sign; Fig. 47-5). In contrast to those in Crohn's disease, the lesions in tuberculosis tend to have more irregular contours and coarser mucosal markings, and involvement of the colon is usually more prominent than that of the terminal ileum (Fig. 47-6). The majority of patients in the western hemisphere who have gastrointestinal tuberculosis also have pulmonary tuberculous disease, with typical symptoms of cough, fever, night sweats, hemoptysis, anorexia, and weight loss. Without concomitant pulmonary involvement, however, differ-

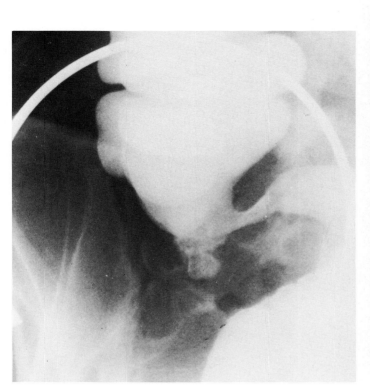

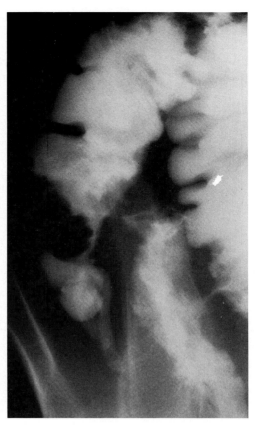

47-1

47-2

Fig. 47-1. Classic coned cecum in a patient with amebiasis. Note that the terminal ileum is not involved.

Fig. 47-2. Crohn's disease. There is severe irregular narrowing of the cecum. Note also the inflammatory involvement of the terminal ileum and ascending colon.

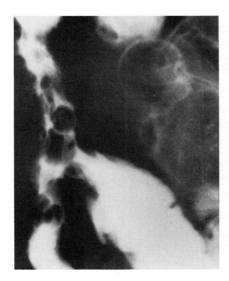

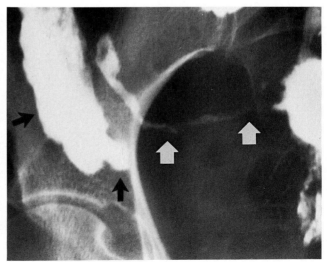

47-3

47-4

Fig. 47-3. Crohn's disease. There is narrowing and rigidity of the cecum and ascending colon.

Fig. 47-4. Crohn's disease. There is incomplete filling of the terminal ileum ("string sign", **right arrows**) in a patient with rigid narrowing of the cecum **(left arrows)**.

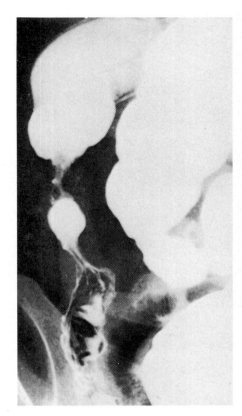

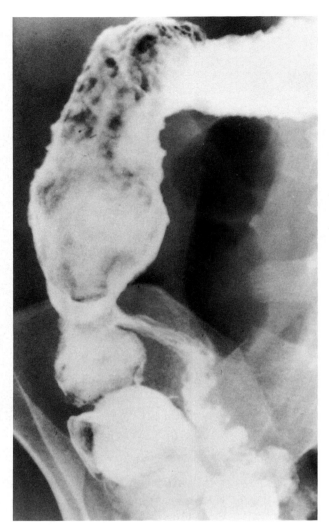

47-5   47-6

Fig. 47-5. Stierlin's sign in tuberculosis. The terminal ileum appears to empty directly into the stenotic ascending colon with nonopacification of the fibrotic, contracted cecum. (Carrera GF, Young S, Lewicki AM: Intestinal tuberculosis. Gastrointest Radiol 1:147–155, 1976)

Fig. 47-6. Tuberculosis. Note that the ulcerative process primarily involves the ascending and transverse colon and essentially spares the terminal ileum, unlike the usual appearance in Crohn's disease.

entiation between tuberculosis and Crohn's disease can be extremely difficult.

AMEBIASIS

The cecum is involved in about 90% of cases of chronic amebiasis. In the early stages of the disease, small, shallow ulcers produce an irregular bowel margin and finely granular mucosa (Fig. 47-7). With continued inflammation and fibrosis, the lumen of the cecum concentrically narrows until it has as-

sumed a cone-shaped configuration (Fig. 47-8). The ileocecal valve often appears to move downward, sometimes lying close to the cecal tip. In contrast to Crohn's disease and tuberculosis, in which terminal ileum involvement is the rule, the terminal ileum in amebic colitis is usually normal. In amebiasis, the ileocecal valve is almost invariably thickened, rigid, and fixed in an open position, permitting free reflux into the terminal ileum; this is in contrast to tuberculosis, in which reflux is infrequent because of intense ileocecal spasm. The combination of a coned cecum, an intact terminal ileum, and skip lesions in

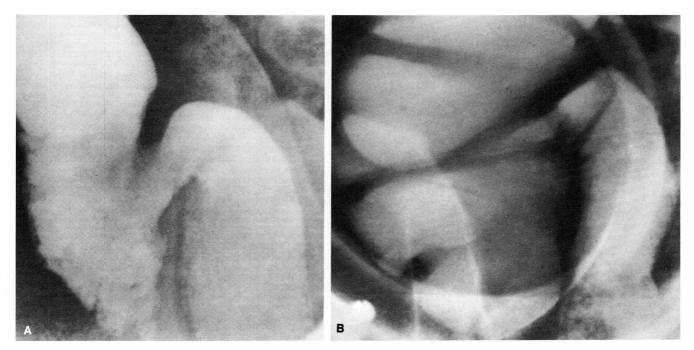

Fig. 47-7. Amebiasis. **(A)** The small, shallow ulcers produce an irregular bowel margin and finely granular mucosa. **(B)** After a course of antiamebic therapy, the cecum and ileocecal valve appear normal.

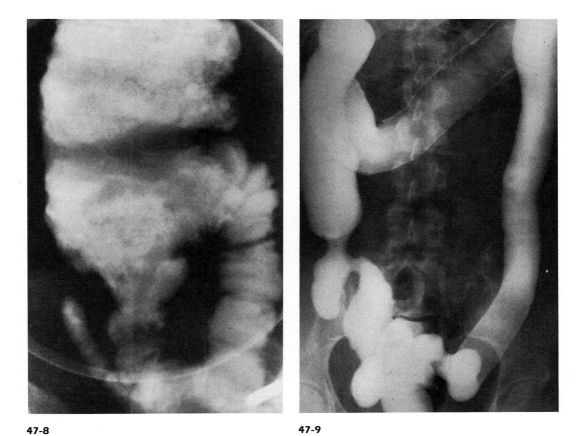

47-8   47-9

Fig. 47-8. Amebiasis. Continued inflammation and fibrosis cause concentric narrowing of the lumen of the cecum until it has assumed a cone-shaped configuration.

Fig. 47-9. Ulcerative colitis. There is concentric narrowing of the cecum. Note the gaping ileocecal valve.

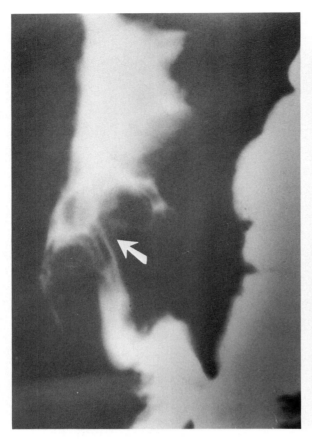

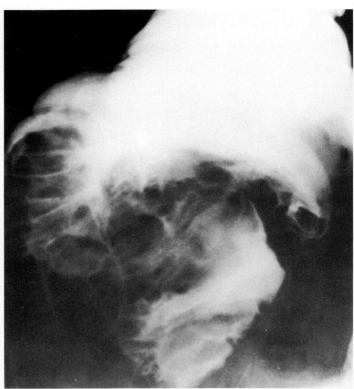

47-10   47-11

Fig. 47-10. Tuberculosis. The ileocecal valve **(arrow)** has an inverted umbrella-like appearance as a result of spasm. Note the severe narrowing and almost complete obliteration of the cecum.

Fig. 47-11. Carcinoma of the cecum with perforation. The patient presented with acute abdominal pain mimicking appendicitis.

the colon is highly suggestive of amebic infection. The diagnosis is made by demonstration of *Entamoeba histolytica* in the stool or rectal biopsy. However, a negative stool examination or rectal biopsy does not rule out amebiasis; similarly, the presence of amebas in the stool does not exclude the possibility of other ulcerative diseases of the colon. Laparotomy as a means for diagnosis or for resection of the lesion is dangerous and is contraindicated in untreated patients. One differential point is the dramatic change in radiographic appearance seen within 2 weeks of the institution of antiamebic therapy (Fig. 47-7*B*).

ULCERATIVE COLITIS/APPENDICITIS

Although ulcerative colitis tends to involve the left colon more than the right, the inflammatory pro-

cess can affect the cecum and result in severe narrowing (Fig. 47-9). Involvement of the terminal ileum in ulcerative colitis (backwash ileitis) occurs in about 10% of patients with generalized colonic disease. Although the appearance can resemble Crohn's disease (thickening of mucosal folds, spasm, irritability), the changes are limited to a short segment, and the degree of narrowing is not pronounced. As in amebiasis, the ileocecal valve is usually gaping in ulcerative colitis. In contrast, the valve is thickened and criss-crossed by ileocecal fistulas in Crohn's disease and appears inverted and umbrella-like (Fig. 47-10) because of spasm of the valve in tuberculosis.

Perforation of an inflamed appendix can lead to the formation of an abscess that causes an eccentric defect at the base of the cecum, most commonly on the medial aspect. Depending on the position of the appendix and the degree of spread of inflammatory

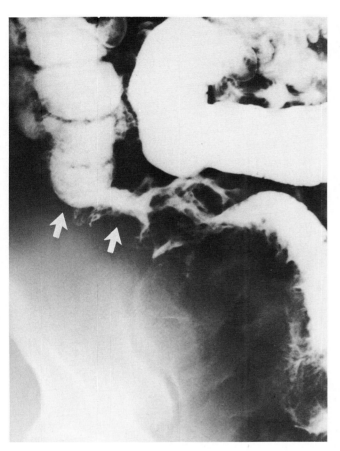

Fig. 47-12. Carcinoma of the cecum with extension to involve the terminal ileum. Severe narrowing and rigidity **(arrows)** give the radiographic appearance of a coned cecum.

These diverticula are relatively uncommon and frequently solitary and are usually situated within 2 cm of the ileocecal valve. Perforation of a cecal diverticulum leads to a walled-off pericecal abscess that can mimic acute appendicitis and produce inflammatory pressure defects on the barium-filled colon.

ACTINOMYCOSIS

Actinomycosis of the bowel is an uncommon infection that tends to involve the cecum and the appendix. Acute disease can simulate appendicitis and be associated with fever, abdominal pain, cachexia, vomiting, and diarrhea. Palpable abdominal masses and draining fistulas often occur. Although exploratory laparotomy is frequently necessary to establish the diagnosis of gastrointestinal actinomycosis, the combination of a palpable abdominal mass and indolent sinus tracts draining through the abdominal wall is highly suggestive of this condition.

SOUTH AMERICAN BLASTOMYCOSIS

Severe narrowing and rigidity of the cecum and terminal ileum can be seen in patients with South

contents, any portion of the cecum can be involved, and a cone-shaped appearance can result.

CARCINOMA OF THE CECUM

Acute abdominal pain mimicking appendicitis can be due to necrosis and perforation of carcinoma of the cecum (Fig. 47-11). The resulting inflammatory reaction can cause stiffness and rigidity of the cecal wall and the radiographic appearance of a coned cecum (Fig. 47-12). A similar pattern can be produced by carcinoma of the cecum without perforation. The cecum narrowed by malignancy is not distensible, unlike the coned cecum due to an inflammatory etiology, which can often be distended with pressure.

PERFORATED CECAL DIVERTICULUM

A rare cause of narrowing and rigidity of the cecum is perforation of a cecal diverticulum (Fig. 47-13).

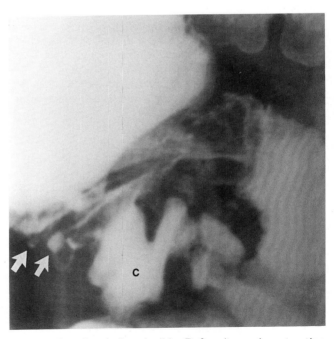

Fig. 47-13. Cecal diverticulitis. Deformity and contraction of the cecum is seen on a barium enema examination performed about 3 weeks following the onset of symptoms in a 27-year-old man. Several diverticula **(arrows)** are seen along the lateral wall of the cecum (C). (Norfray JF, Givens JD, Sparberg MS et al: Cecal diverticulitis in young patients. Gastrointest Radiol 5:379–382, 1980)

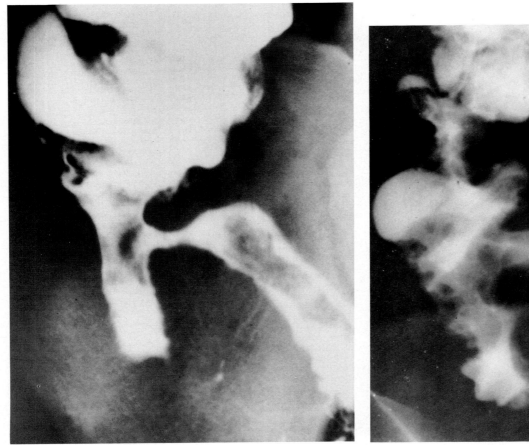
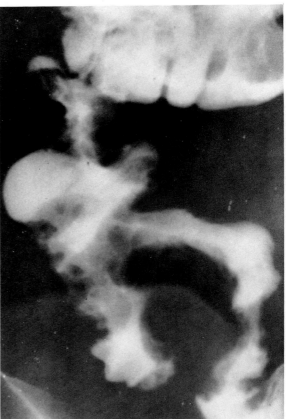

47-14   **47-15**

Fig. 47-14. South American blastomycosis. There is severe narrowing and rigidity of the cecum and terminal ileum. (Avritchir Y, Perroni AA: Radiological manifestations of small intestinal South American blastomycosis. Radiology 127:607–609, 1978)

Fig. 47-15. Anisakiasis. Severe inflammatory changes were seen in the cecum, ascending colon, and ileocecal valve in a patient who developed severe abdominal pain after eating raw fish.

American blastomycosis (Fig. 47-14). This granulomatous disease is caused by *Paracoccidioides brasiliensis*, a round fungus with a double wall that is common in Brazil and occasionally occurs elsewhere in South and Central America. Although the disorder most commonly involves the skin and such visceral organs as the lungs, lymph nodes, liver, spleen and bone, the diagnosis of South American blastomycosis should be considered whenever a patient in an endemic area develops fixed narrowing and mucosal irregularity of the distal small bowel and ileocecal region simulating Crohn's disease.

ANISAKIASIS

Thickening of the bowel wall of the ascending colon or terminal ileum in a patient (especially one from Japan, Holland, or Scandinavia) who is in the habit of eating raw fish should suggest the diagnosis of anisakiasis (Fig. 47-15). This ascaris-like nematode has a marine mammal (whale, dolphin) as its final host; humans are only incidentally affected when they ingest raw, slightly salted, or vinegar-pickled fish containing the intermediate larval stage of the parasite.

TYPHOID / *YERSINIA*

Narrowing and irregularity of the cecum, usually associated with more severe inflammatory changes in the terminal ileum, can develop in patients with typhoid fever (Fig. 47-16) or *Yersinia enterocolitica* infection (Fig. 47-17).

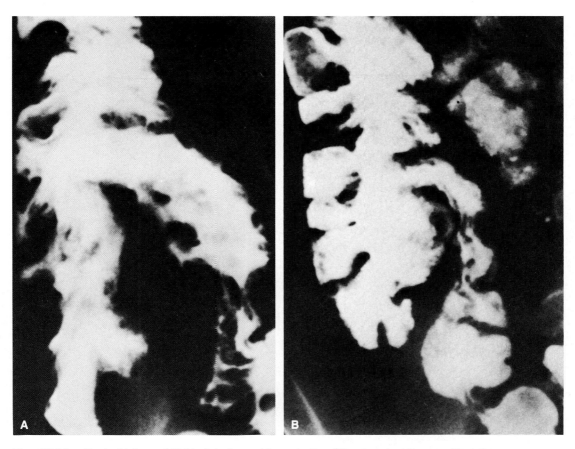

Fig. 47-16. Typhoid fever. **(A)** Nodularity and irregularity of the terminal ileum with deformity of the cecum. **(B)** After therapy, the ileum and cecum returned to normal. (Francis RS, Berk RN: Typhoid fever. Radiology 112:583–585, 1974)

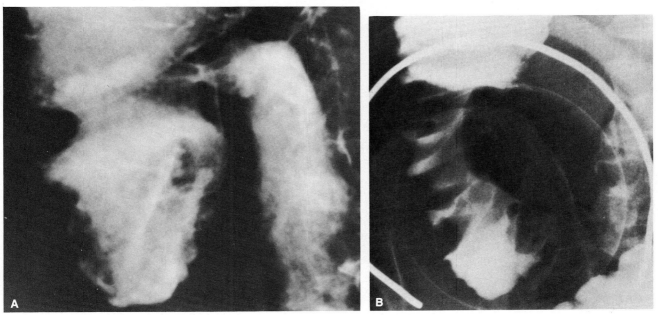

Fig. 47-17. *Yersinia enterocolitica.* **(A)** Conical narrowing and irregular margins of the cecum are present with mild inflammatory changes in the terminal ileum. **(B)** Narrowing and inflammatory fold thickening of the cecum in a young man with acute right lower quadrant pain, fever, and leukocytosis mimicking appendicitis. (**[B]** from Rice RP, Thompson WM, Fedyshin PJ et al: The barium enema in appendicitis: Spectrum of appearances and pitfalls. RadioGraphics 3:393–409, 1984)

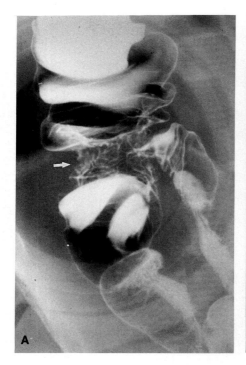

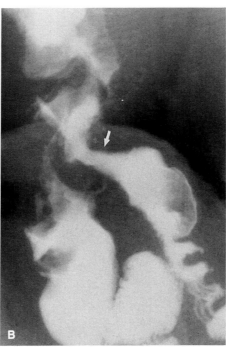

Fig. 47-18. Cytomegalovirus in AIDS. **(A)** Thickened irregular folds in the cecum, mainly at the level of the ileocecal valve. **(B)** The terminal ileum is narrowed **(arrow)** and the cecum is spastic with thick mucosal folds. (Balthazar EJ, Megibow AJ, Fazzini E et al: Cytomegalovirus colitis in AIDS: Radiographic findings in 11 patients. Radiology 155:585–589, 1985)

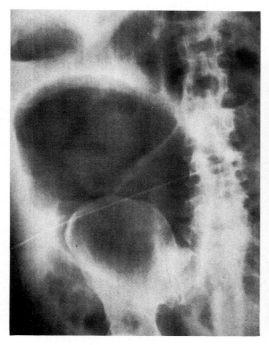

47-19

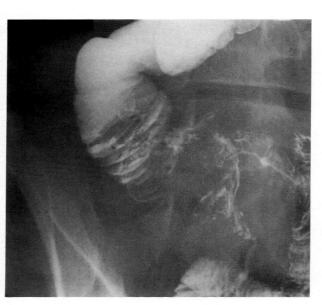

47-20

Fig. 47-19. Typhlitis. Distended, dilated cecum (toxic cecitis). (Cronin TG, Calandra JD, Del Fava RL: Typhlitis presenting as toxic cecitis. Radiology 138:29–30, 1981)

Fig. 47-20. Typhlitis. Coned view of the right lower quadrant shows a distorted irritable cecum with effacement and edema of cecal mucosa. The terminal ileum is displaced smoothly away from the cecum in curvilinear fashion. The appendix appears normal. (Del Fava RL, Cronin TG: Typhlitis complicating leukemia in an adult: Barium enema findings. AJR 129:347–348, 1977. Copyright 1977. Reproduced with permission)

CYTOMEGALOVIRUS

Cytomegalovirus is an opportunistic infection that may involve the cecum in patients with AIDS and other disorders that compromise the immune system. Spasticity and thickening of mucosal folds may be limited to the cecum or diffusely involve the distal ileum and other portions of the colon (Fig. 47-18).

TYPHLITIS

Typhlitis is a necrotizing process of multifactorial origin that predominantly involves the right colon though it may extend to other areas of the intestine. Although most commonly found in children with leukemia, typhlitis may also occur in adults with hematologic malignancy or, less commonly, aplastic anemia or lymphoma. Multiple factors such as intestinal ischemia, neoplastic infiltrate, mucosal hemorrhage, and fecal ulceration may contribute to the pathogenesis. Pathologically, typhlitis is characterized by bowel wall thickening, mucosal ulceration, intramural hemorrhage, and necrosis. Secondary colonization of mucosal ulcers by colonic flora commonly leads to septicemia and pyrexia. The clinical symptoms of typhlitis typically begin 1 to 2 weeks following the initial course of chemotherapy and consist of a variable complex of fever, nausea, vomiting, and abdominal pain.

Plain abdominal radiographs show progressive dilatation of an atonic cecum and right colon, accompanied by prominent haustrations and a thickened bowel wall (Fig. 47-19). If the diagnosis of typhlitis is not made after correlation of clinical and plain film findings, further evaluation is necessary and a contrast enema may be obtained. If the patient has abdominal rebound tenderness or substantial dilatation of the right colon, barium should not be used and the enema should either be deferred or carried out using water-soluble contrast material since colonic perforation is a well-recognized risk in patients with typhlitis. On contrast enemas, rigidity, narrowing, and distortion may be limited to the cecum (Fig. 47-20), or the entire right colon may have a rigid, tubular appearance with loss of haustral markings. Submucosal edema or hemorrhage may produce thumbprinting mimicking ischemic colitis; mucosal disruption with bacterial entry into the bowel wall may lead to the development of intramural air.

BIBLIOGRAPHY

Avritchir Y, Perroni AA: Radiological manifestations of small intestinal South American blastomycosis. Radiology 127:607–609, 1978

Balikian JR, Uthman SM, Khorui NF: Intestinal amebiasis. AJR 122:245–256, 1974

Balthazar EJ, Megibow AJ, Fazzini E et al: Cytomegalovirus colitis in AIDS: Radiographic findings in 11 patients. Radiology 155:585–589, 1985

Berk RN, Lasser EC: Radiology of the Ileocecal Area. Philadelphia, WB Saunders, 1975

Carrera CF, Young S, Lewicki AM: Intestinal tuberculosis. Gastrointest Radiol 1:147–155, 1976

Del Fava RL, Cronin TG: Typhlitis complicating leukemia in an adult: Barium enema findings. AJR 129:347–348, 1977

Ekberg O: Cecal changes following appendectomy. Gastrointest Radiol 2:57–60, 1977

Gardiner R, Smith C: Infective enterocolitides. Radiol Clin North Am 25:67–78, 1987

Kolawole PM, Lewis EA: Radiologic observations on intestinal amebiasis. AJR 122:257–265, 1974

Lockhart–Mummery HE, Morson BC: Crohn's disease of the large intestine. Gut 5:493–509, 1964

Moss JD, Knauer CM: Tuberculous enteritis. Gastroenterology 65:959–966, 1973

Taylor AJ, Dodds WJ, Gonyo JE et al: Typhlitis in adults. Gastrointest Radiol 10:363–369, 1985

Werbeloff L, Novis BH, Bank S et al: The radiology of tuberculosis of the gastrointestinal tract. Br J Radiol 46:329–336, 1973

PART SEVEN

COLON

ULCERATIVE LESIONS OF THE COLON

Disease Entities

Ulcerative colitis
Crohn's colitis
Ischemic colitis
Specific infections
  Protozoan
    Amebiasis
    Schistosomiasis
  Bacterial
    Shigellosis
    Salmonellosis
    Tuberculous colitis
    Gonorrheal proctitis
    Staphylococcal colitis
    Yersinia colitis
    Campylobacter fetus colitis
    Lymphogranuloma venereum
  Fungal
    Histoplasmosis
    Mucormycosis
    Actinomycosis
    Candidiasis
  Viral
    Herpes simplex
    Herpes zoster
    Cytomegalovirus
    Rotavirus
  Helminthic
    Strongyloidiasis

Pseudomembranous colitis
  Postantibiotic colitis
  Postoperative colitis
  Uremia
  Large bowel obstruction
  Hypoxia
Radiation injury
Caustic colitis
Pancreatitis
Malignancy
  Primary carcinoma
  Metastases
  Leukemic infiltration
Amyloidosis
Inorganic mercury poisoning
Behcet's syndrome
Diverticulosis/diverticulitis
Solitary rectal ulcer syndrome
Nonspecific benign ulceration of the colon
Drug-induced colitis
Diversion colitis
Post-rectal biopsy

Ulcerative inflammation of the colon or rectum is a nonspecific response to a host of harmful agents and processes. In many cases, an ulcerating colitis can be attributed to a specific infectious disease, systemic disorder, or toxic agent. However, in a large group of patients, a precise cause cannot be determined. Most of these "nonspecific" inflammatory diseases of the colon are generally placed into one of two categories: ulcerative colitis or Crohn's disease. Although radiographic and pathologic criteria have been established for distinguishing between these two processes, there is a substantial overlap in practice. In at least 10% of colectomy specimens for ulcerating colitis, it is impossible to distinguish between ulcerative colitis and Crohn's disease even with careful gross inspection and multiple microscopic sections. Features of ulcerative colitis and Crohn's disease often coexist, making a precise histologic diagnosis difficult. Such cases can be termed "unclassified colitis" or "colitis, type unknown."

ULCERATIVE COLITIS

Ulcerative colitis is primarily a disease of young adults, the peak incidence being in persons between 20 and 40 years of age. The disease may be first diagnosed at an older age; a second peak incidence has been reported in persons in their sixth and seventh decades. These patients are reputed to have a higher mortality rate than younger persons and often require surgical therapy. It has been suggested, however, that many cases of "ulcerative" colitis in elderly patients actually represent an ischemic process secondary to occlusive vascular disease. This hypothesis is based on the clinical onset and posttreatment course of the disease, which often closely simulate ischemic colitis, and the difficulty in separating the various forms of ulcerating colitis on radiographic or pathologic grounds.

Although the etiology of ulcerative colitis is unknown, current theory points to a hypersensitivity and autoimmune mechanism as the most likely cause of the disease. Evidence for this theory includes the relatively frequent association of ulcerative colitis with connective tissue diseases (rheumatoid arthritis, rheumatic fever, systemic lupus erythematosus), increased serum gamma-globulin in some cases, the response of the disease to steroid and immunosuppressive drugs, and the demonstration of circulating antibodies to colon extract in some patients with ulcerative colitis. Other suggested causes of ulcerative colitis include infection, destructive enzymes and surface irritants, exogenous antigens (food allergies), and psychosomatic or emotional factors.

Ulcerative colitis is not a distinct histopathologic entity. Most of the features of the disease can be seen in other inflammations of the colon of known cause. Therefore, the diagnosis of ulcerative colitis requires a combination of clinical, radiographic, and pathologic criteria. These include the course of the disease, extent and distribution of the anatomic lesions, and exclusion of other forms of ulcerating colitis caused by specific infectious or toxic agents, or associated with systemic diseases.

Except in rare instances, ulcerative colitis is an inflammatory disease confined to the mucosa and, to a lesser extent, to the adjacent submucosa. The deeper muscular layers and serosa of the colon are usually not involved; the process does not extend to regional lymph nodes (except perhaps as a nonspecific reactive hyperplasia). A characteristic microscopic finding in ulcerative colitis is the crypt abscess, which reflects necrosis of the crypt epithelium with extension of polymorphonuclear infiltrate into the crypt. It is associated with a more chronic inflammatory infiltrate and vascular engorgement in the adjacent submucosa. Although often considered pathognomonic of ulcerative colitis, crypt abscess formation can be seen in any infectious colitis and in ischemic disease.

CLINICAL SYMPTOMS AND COURSE

Ulcerative colitis is highly variable in severity, clinical course, and ultimate prognosis. The onset of the disease, as well as subsequent exacerbations, can be insidious or abrupt. Symptoms range from small amounts of rectal bleeding (simulating hemorrhoids) to prominent diarrhea with colonic hemorrhage and prostration. A characteristic feature of ulcerative colitis is alternating periods of remission and exacerbation. Most patients (up to 75%) have intermittent episodes of symptoms with complete remission between attacks. Of the remainder, about half have one attack and no subsequent symptoms and the same number have continuous symptoms without any remission.

A majority of patients have mild ulcerative colitis that is often segmental in distribution and usually involves just the distal colon. In less than 10% of patients, ulcerative colitis presents as an acute fulminating process. Patients with this form of the disease have severe diarrhea, fever, systemic toxicity, and electrolyte depletion or hemorrhage. They also have a far higher incidence than usual of severe complications, such as toxic megacolon and free perforation into the peritoneal cavity.

EXTRACOLONIC MANIFESTATIONS

Extracolonic manifestations of ulcerative colitis are relatively common and include spondylitis, peripheral arthritis, iritis, skin disorders (erythema nodosum, pyoderma gangrenosum), and various liver abnormalities. It is unclear whether these concomitant conditions represent the host's systemic response to the agent causing the colonic disease, a complication of the colonic lesion, or a general abnormality of the autoimmune mechanism. The extracolonic manifestations of ulcerative colitis appear to have little relation to the severity, extent, or duration of bowel disease.

Up to 25% of patients with ulcerative colitis have some form of arthritis: sacroiliitis, spondylitis,

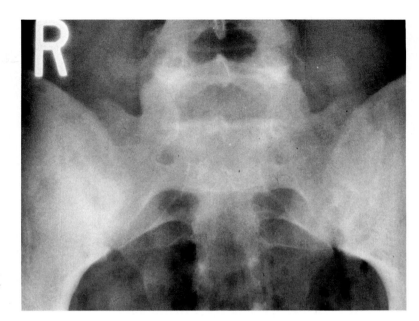

Fig. 48-1. Spondylitis in a patient with ulcerative colitis. Note the symmetric involvement of the sacroiliac joints.

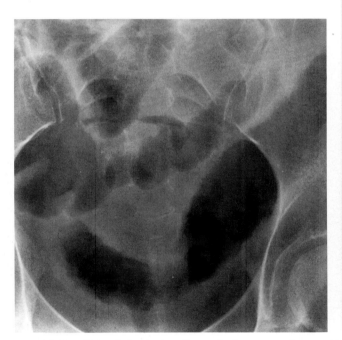

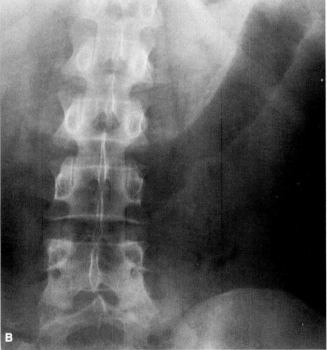

Fig. 48-2. Plain abdominal radiographs in two patients with ulcerative colitis. **(A)** Nodular protrusions of hyperplastic mucosa and the loss of haustral markings involve essentially the entire sigmoid colon. **(B)** Featureless transverse colon with complete loss of normal haustration.

or peripheral arthritis. The sacroiliac joints show symmetric narrowing, erosions, and sclerosis (Fig. 48-1). Spinal involvement is characterized by squaring of the vertebral bodies and syndesmophyte formation. The peripheral arthritis almost always occurs at the same time or after the onset of the colitis. When the arthritis antedates the onset of colitis, it usually flares up again during subsequent

exacerbations of colonic disease. The peripheral arthritis associated with ulcerative colitis tends to be migratory and to involve large joints. Because joint cartilage and bony apposition are generally unaffected, there often is no residual damage.

The most characteristic liver disorder associated with ulcerative colitis is pericholangitis. The term is used to describe inflammation not only about the bile ducts but also involving the connective tissue around the hepatic artery and portal vein (portal triad). Fatty infiltration of the liver, chronic active hepatitis, and primary sclerosing cholangitis are not infrequently seen.

Patients with ulcerative colitis also appear to have a relatively high incidence of thrombotic complications. Although this predisposition to thromboembolism may be due to venous stasis secondary to dehydration and immobilization, a tendency toward hypercoagulability has been demonstrated and suggested as a causative factor.

The major complication of ulcerative colitis is the high risk of carcinoma of the colon. This is an especially virulent malignancy that often appears as a filiform stricture and is difficult to detect radiographically at an early stage. Unlike Crohn's colitis, free perforation of the colon and toxic megacolon are relatively common in ulcerative colitis, whereas fistula formation is rare.

RADIOGRAPHIC FINDINGS

In the radiographic evaluation of a patient with known or suspected ulcerative colitis, plain abdominal radiographs are essential (Fig. 48-2). Large nodular protrusions of hyperplastic mucosa, deep ulcers outlined by intraluminal gas, or polypoid

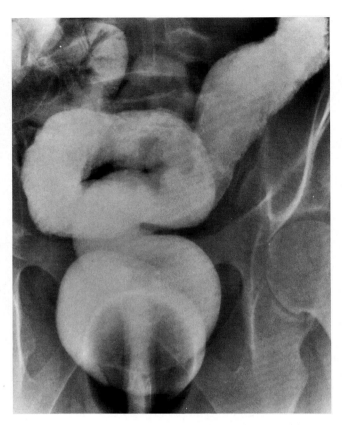

Fig. 48-4.   *Ulcerative colitis with true rectal sparing. In this unusual case, there was no evidence of rectal involvement on barium enema, colonoscopy, or biopsy.*

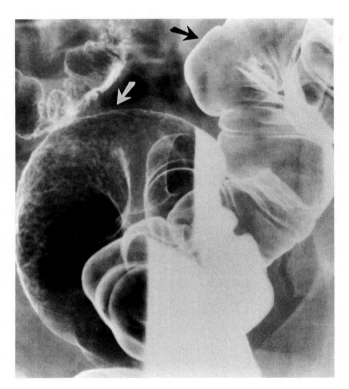

Fig. 48-3.   *Ulcerative colitis primarily involving the rectosigmoid. The distal rectosigmoid mucosa **(white arrow)** is finely granular, compared to the normal-appearing mucosa **(black arrow)** in the more proximal colon.*

changes with a loss of haustral markings suggest the diagnosis. Plain abdominal radiographs can also demonstrate evidence of toxic megacolon or free intraperitoneal gas, contraindications to barium enema examination in patients with acute colitis.

Preparation of the colon prior to a barium enema in a patient with suspected or known ulcerative colitis is controversial. Although a clean colon is desirable, some authors report complications after the use of routine purgatives and sizable enemas. If time permits, the safest preparation is several days of a clear liquid diet with gentle, small-volume enemas the night before and the morning of the examination.

Ulcerative colitis has a strong tendency to begin in the rectosigmoid (Fig. 48-3). Although by radiographic criteria alone the rectum appears normal in about 20% of patients with ulcerative colitis (Fig. 48-4), proctosigmoidoscopy can detect rectosigmoid involvement in about 95% of patients with active disease, especially when minimal or equivocal endoscopic findings are corroborated by rectal biopsy. Therefore, true rectal sparing (no disease seen on barium enema, colonoscopy, or biopsy) should suggest the possibility of another etiology for an ulcerating colitis. Although ulcerative colitis not infrequently spreads to involve the entire colon

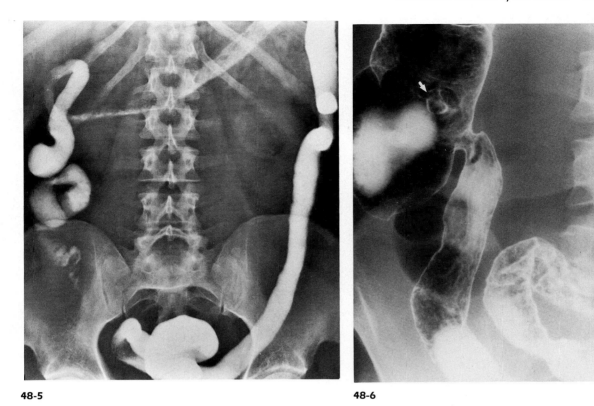

48-5   48-6

Fig. 48-5. Diffuse ulcerative colitis involving the entire colon. Note the gaping ileocecal valve.

Fig. 48-6. Backwash ileitis in ulcerative colitis. The terminal ileum and cecum have lost their normal fold pattern, and the mucosa appears coarsely granular. Note the patulous ileocecal valve and the single large inflammatory polyp **(arrow)**. (Caroline DF, Evers K: Colitis: Radiographic features and differentiation of idiopathic inflammatory bowel disease. Radiol Clin North Am 25:47–66, 1987)

(Fig. 48-5), isolated right colon disease with a normal left colon does not occur.

Terminal ileum involvement can be demonstrated in about 10% to 25% of patients with ulcerative colitis. In this backwash ileitis, minimal inflammatory changes involve a short segment of terminal ileum (Fig. 48-6). In backwash ileitis, unlike Crohn's disease, narrowing and rigidity are almost invariably absent, and sinus tracts or fistulas are very infrequent.

On double-contrast studies, the earliest detectable radiographic abnormality in ulcerative colitis is fine granularity of the mucosa corresponding to the hyperemia and edema seen endoscopically (Figs. 48-7, 48-8). Once superficial ulcers develop, small flecks of adherent barium produce a stippled mucosal pattern (Fig. 48-9).

On full-column examination, an early finding in ulcerative colitis is a hazy or fuzzy quality of the bowel contour that is related to edema, excessive mucus, and tiny ulcerations (Fig. 48-10). Ulcerations can cause the margin of the barium-filled colon to be serrated, or they can appear as small

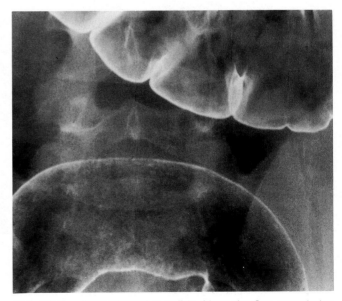

Fig. 48-7. Early ulcerative colitis. Note the fine granularity of the mucosa in the sigmoid (lower loop of bowel) compared to the normal pattern in the upper loop of bowel.

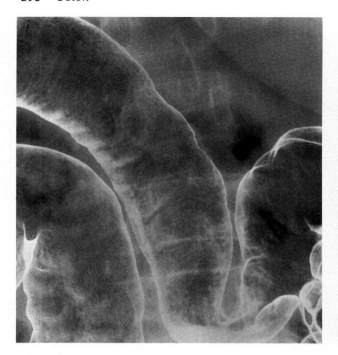

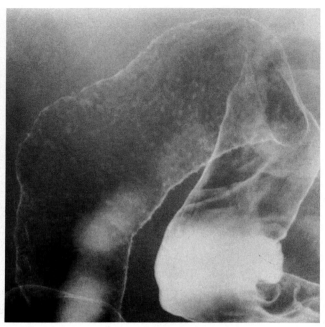

48-8   48-9

Fig. 48-8. Early ulcerative colitis. Fine granularity of the mucosa reflects the hyperemia and edema that are seen endoscopically.

Fig. 48-9. Early ulcerative colitis. Note the stippled mucosal pattern.

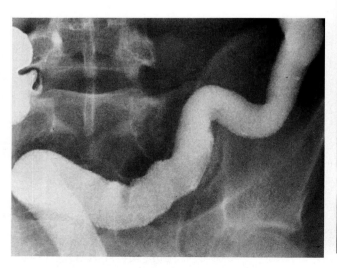

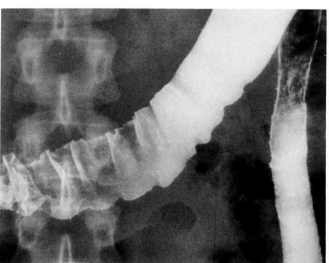

48-10   48-11

Fig. 48-10. Early ulcerative colitis. The hazy quality of the bowel contour is due to edema, excessive mucus, and tiny ulcerations.

Fig. 48-11. Innominate lines. A transient finding, these tiny spicules mimicking ulcerations are symmetric and sharply defined.

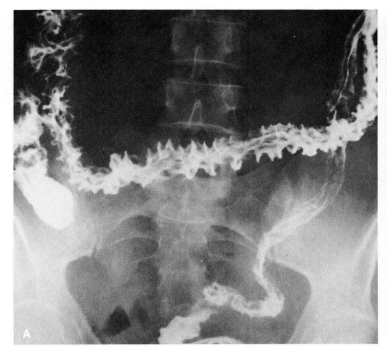

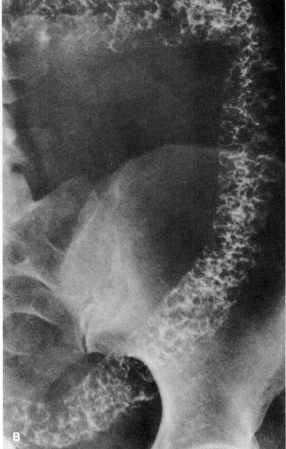

Fig. 48-12. Postevacuation films in two patients with ulcerative colitis. **(A)** The mucosal folds, predominantly in the descending colon, are thickened and indistinct and course in a longitudinal direction. **(B)** Coarse nodular folds.

spicules extending from the mucosa on postevacuation films. It is essential that these hazy, asymmetric, nonuniform ulcerations be distinguished from innominate lines, tiny spicules that mimic ulcerations but are symmetric and sharply defined (Fig. 48-11). These pseudoulcers are a transient finding representing barium penetration into normal grooves that are present on the surface of the colonic mucosa.

Mucosal edema results in thickening of colonic folds and a coarsely granular appearance. There may be flattening and squaring of the normally smoothly rounded haustral markings. Although loss of haustral markings, particularly in the left colon, is often considered a sign of ulcerative colitis, it is a nonspecific appearance that is commonly seen in normal persons.

The postevacuation film is frequently of great value in the detection of early changes of ulcerative colitis. Unlike the fine crinkled pattern of crisscrossing thin mucosal folds seen in the normal colon, the folds in ulcerative colitis become thickened, indistinct, and coarsely nodular and tend to course in a longitudinal direction (Fig. 48-12). The thin coating of barium on the surface appears finely stippled because of countless tiny ulcers, which cause numerous spikelike projections when seen in profile (Fig. 48-13).

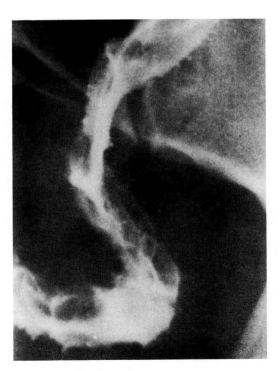

Fig. 48-13. Ulcerative colitis. This postevacuation film shows coarse mucosal folds with numerous spikelike projections causing a finely stippled pattern.

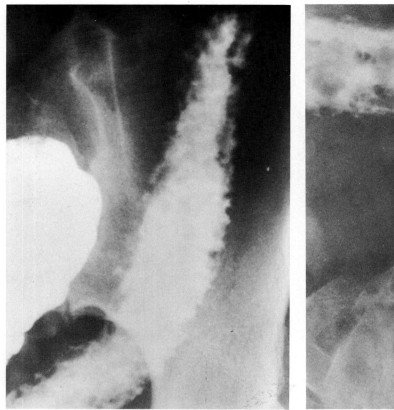
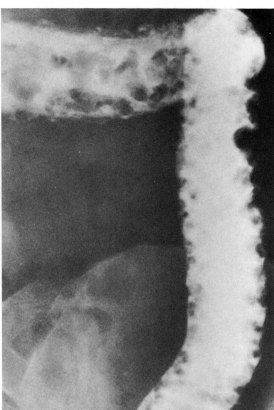

48-14   48-15

Fig. 48-14. *Ulcerative colitis. Progression of the disease results in deep ulceration ("collar-button" ulcers) into the mucosal layer.*

Fig. 48-15. *Ulcerative colitis. Multiple filling defects (pseudopolyps) represent islands of edematous mucosa and re-epithelialized granulation tissue in a sea of ulcerations.*

As the disease progresses, marginal ulcerations become deeper, reflecting penetration into the mucosal layer (Fig. 48-14). Although the ulcers can assume a wide variety of sizes and shapes and be discrete and widely separated, they are usually somewhat monotonous in appearance and symmetrically distributed around the circumference of the bowel wall. The ulcerative process extends into the relatively vulnerable submucosa but is limited by the resistant, more deeply lying muscle. This leads to lateral undermining beneath the relatively resistant mucous membrane and the characteristic radiographic appearance of "collar-button" ulcers, a nonspecific pattern that can be seen in numerous forms of ulcerating colitis. Areas of undermining ulceration eventually join together in an interlacing network. Further extension produces large areas that are essentially denuded of mucosa and submucosa. The remaining scattered islands of edematous mucosa and re-epithelialized granulation tissue cause a pattern of multiple discrete filling defects (pseudopolyps) (Fig. 48-15). As the inflammatory process enters a chronic stage, fibrosis and muscular spasm cause progressive shortening and rigidity of the colon (Fig. 48-16; see also Fig. 48-6). This tubular appearance, combined with atrophy of the colonic mucosa, leads to the characteristic "lead-pipe" configuration of chronic ulcerative colitis.

In patients with mild ulcerative colitis, there is good correlation between the extent of disease on barium enema and clinical severity. In persons with moderate or severe disease, however, the tendency is for fewer radiographic changes to be demonstrated than would be anticipated clinically. With colonoscopy used as a reference standard, the routine barium enema examination clearly underestimates the activity of the inflammatory process.

CROHN'S COLITIS

Crohn's disease of the colon is identical to the same pathologic process involving the small bowel. Therefore, Crohn's colitis is a far better term for the

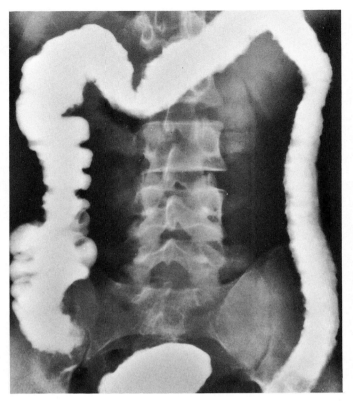

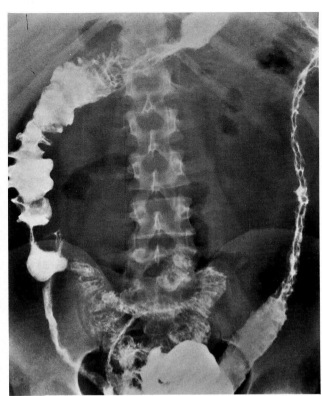

48-16   48-17

Fig. 48-16. Chronic ulcerative colitis. Fibrosis and muscular spasm cause shortening and rigidity of the colon with a loss of haustral markings.

Fig. 48-17. Crohn's colitis. In addition to the diffuse colonic disease, there is severe involvement of much of the distal ileum.

disease than "granulomatous" colitis. In addition, the term granulomatous is imprecise, since about half of patients with Crohn's disease of the colon do not demonstrate granuloma formation.

Crohn's colitis is a chronic inflammatory disease of the colon that occurs primarily in adolescents and young adults. In one series, however, the onset of clinical symptoms of Crohn's disease occurred after the age of 50 in 14% of patients. Although the etiology of the disease is unknown, genetic factors, transmissible infectious agents, and autoimmune phenomena have been suggested as causative factors. The proximal portion of the colon is most frequently involved; concomitant disease of the terminal ileum is seen in up to 80% of patients (Fig. 48-17). Involvement of multiple, noncontiguous segments of colon (skip lesions) not infrequently occurs (Fig. 48-18). Although Crohn's disease is generally considered a disease of the right side of the colon, rectal involvement is not uncommon and can be seen in 30% to 50% of cases. Nevertheless, demonstration of a normal rectal mucosa on sigmoidoscopy in a patient with nonspecific chronic inflammatory bowel disease should suggest Crohn's colitis as a likely diagnosis.

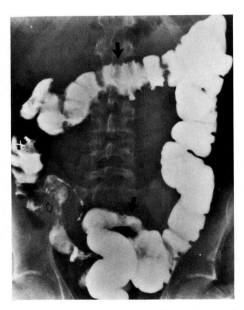

Fig. 48-18. Crohn's colitis. Areas of involved colon in the ascending, transverse, and sigmoid regions **(solid arrows)** are separated by normal-appearing segments. Note the inflammatory changes affecting the distal ileum **(open arrow)**.

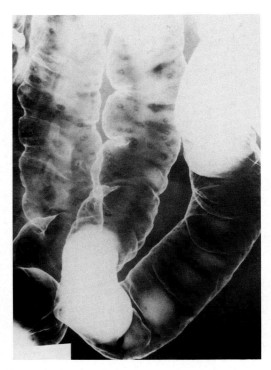

Fig. 48-19. Diffuse aphthous ulcers in early Crohn's colitis. (Caroline DF, Evers K: Colitis: Radiographic features and differentiation of idiopathic inflammatory bowel disease. Radiol Clin North Am 25:47–66, 1987)

The major pathologic abnormalities in Crohn's disease of the colon include penetrating ulcers or fissures, confluent linear ulcers, a discontinuous segmental pattern, and a thickened bowel wall. Microscopically, there is transmural inflammation, in contrast to the inflammation limited to the mucosa and submucosa that is seen in patients with ulcerative colitis. Although granulomas can be demonstrated in only about half of patients with Crohn's disease of the colon, they are virtually a specific histopathologic feature in that they are not seen in patients with ulcerative colitis.

CLINICAL SYMPTOMS

The clinical hallmark of Crohn's disease of the colon is diarrhea, a symptom that is more distressing, more intense, and an earlier complaint in this condition than in ulcerative colitis. Gross bleeding is rare in Crohn's disease of the colon, in contrast to ulcerative colitis. Abdominal pain is a common manifestation of Crohn's colitis; it is generally crampy and colicky and is usually confined to the lower quadrants, particularly on the right side. Insidious weight loss is frequent, presumably due to contiguous ileal disease preventing normal absorption of bile acids. Perianal or perirectal abnormalities (fissures, hemorrhoids, abscesses, fistulas) occur at some point during the course of disease in half of all patients with Crohn's colitis. Indeed,

about 10% of patients first present with one or more of these clinical problems. Enterocutaneous or intestinal fistulas can develop, usually arising from matted or adherent loops of diseased small bowel.

The extraintestinal complications of Crohn's disease of the colon are similar to those of ulcerative colitis but occur less frequently. Concomitant disease of the terminal ileum results in an increased incidence of biliary and renal stones. Deficient absorption of bile salts distorts the ratio of bile salts to cholesterol and predisposes to the development of cholesterol stones in the gallbladder. Excessive oxalate absorption in patients with Crohn's disease leads to hyperoxaluria and a tendency to form oxalate stones in the kidney.

Segmental resection of Crohn's disease of the colon, like that of disease involving the ileum, is associated with a high rate of recurrence (50% or more) at the anastomotic site. Therefore, surgery is usually deferred as long as possible in favor of medical treatment.

RADIOGRAPHIC FINDINGS

The earliest radiographic findings of Crohn's disease of the colon are seen on double-contrast examinations. Isolated, tiny, discrete erosions (aphthoid ulcers) appear as punctate collections of barium with a thin halo of edema around them (Fig. 48-19). Aphthoid ulcers in Crohn's disease have a patchy distribution against a background of normal mucosa, unlike the blanket of abnormal mucosa seen in ulcerative colitis. The ulcers are frequently associated with small, irregular nodules along the contour of the bowel due to submucosal inflammation and mucosal edema. Aphthoid ulcers are not specific for Crohn's disease; morphologically similar lesions can occur in other inflammatory conditions of the colon, such as amebic colitis, tuberculosis, *Yersinia* colitis, and Behcet's syndrome.

As Crohn's colitis progresses, the ulcers become deeper and more irregular (Fig. 48-20). There is great variation in their size, shape, and overall

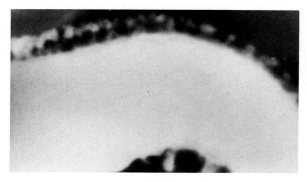

Fig. 48-20. Crohn's colitis. "Collar-button" ulcers are distributed asymmetrically around the circumference of the bowel. This is in contrast to ulcerative colitis, in which the pattern of ulceration is uniform and monotonous.

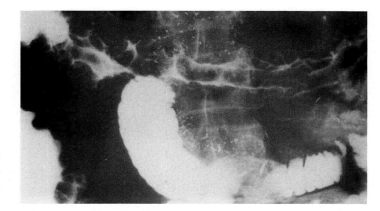

Fig. 48-21. Crohn's colitis. Deep, linear transverse and longitudinal ulcers separate intervening mounds of edematous mucosa, creating a characteristic cobblestone appearance.

appearance. The distribution of ulcers around the circumference of the bowel in Crohn's disease is random and asymmetric, not uniform and monotonous, as it is in ulcerative colitis. Deep, linear transverse and longitudinal ulcers often separate intervening mounds of edematous, but nonulcerated, mucosa, thereby creating a characteristic cobblestone appearance (Fig. 48-21). If the penetrating ulcers extend beyond the contour of the bowel, they can coalesce to form long tracts running parallel to the longitudinal axis of the colon. Penetration of ulcers into adjacent loops of bowel or into the bladder, vagina, or abdominal wall causes fistulas that can be demonstrated radiographically. In late stages of the disease, severe thickening of the colon secondary to intramural fibrosis leads to narrowing of the lumen and stricture formation.

In its pure form, Crohn's disease of the colon can be readily distinguished radiographically from ulcerative colitis. This distinction is of considerable practical importance because of the markedly different diagnostic and therapeutic implications of these disorders. Localized involvement of the ascending or transverse colon and concomitant small bowel disease suggest Crohn's colitis. Skip lesions and segmental involvement with intervening areas of normal-appearing colon are never seen in ulcerative colitis. Extensive inflammatory changes in the terminal ileum, asymmetric ulceration, and the presence of fistulas and sinus tracts are characteristic of Crohn's disease. The finding of an associated anal lesion (ulceration, deep lateral fissures, distortion and nodularity of mucosal folds) is also highly suggestive of Crohn's disease (Fig. 48-22).

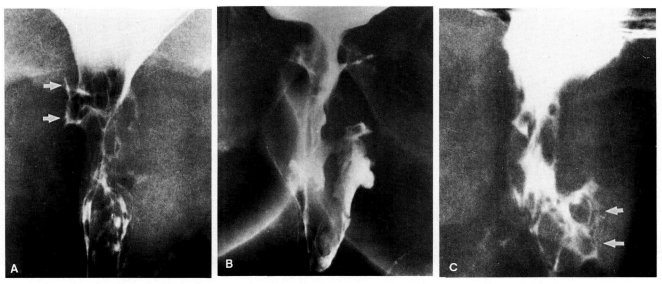

Fig. 48-22. Abnormal anal canals in patients with Crohn's disease. There is distortion of mucosal folds with ulcers or deep lateral fissures **(arrows)** in **A** and **C**. The nodularity of folds is pronounced in **C**. Simple or complex, branching sinus tracts or fistulae are seen in **B**. (DuBrow RA, Frank PH: Barium evaluation of anal canal in patients with inflammatory bowel disease. AJR 140:1151–1157, 1983. Copyright 1983. Reproduced with permission)

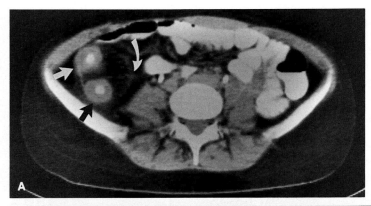

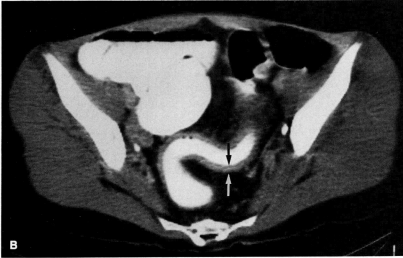

Fig. 48-23. CT of Crohn's disease. **(A)** Homogeneous thickening of the ascending colon **(straight white arrow)** and distal ileum **(black arrow)**. Note the abnormal mesenteric fat **(curved arrow)** and separation of abnormal segments from other small bowel loops. The descending colon has normal mural thickness. **(B)** Homogeneous thickening of the sigmoid colon **(arrows)** imaged longitudinally on a pelvic CT scan in another patient with chronic Crohn's colitis. (Gore RM, Marn CS, Kirby DF et al: CT findings in ulcerative, granulomatous, and indeterminate colitis. AJR 143:279–284, 1984. Copyright 1984. Reproduced with permission)

Computed tomography (CT) has been used to differentiate between Crohn's and ulcerative colitis when the barium examinations were indeterminate. Although there is some overlap, the bowel wall is generally thicker in patients with Crohn's disease (Figs. 48-23, 48-25*A*) and has a more homogeneous attenuation than in patients with ulcerative colitis (Figs. 48-24, 48-25*B*). In addition, the CT demonstration of fistulas (Fig. 48-26), abscess formation, and mesenteric abnormalities strongly suggests Crohn's disease.

ISCHEMIC COLITIS

Although the spectrum of radiographic findings in ischemic colitis broadly overlaps the appearance of other ulcerating diseases of the colon, the classic clinical presentation usually permits a proper diagnosis. Ischemic colitis is characterized by the abrupt onset of lower abdominal pain and rectal bleeding. Diarrhea is common, as is abdominal tenderness on physical examination. Most patients are over the age of 50 and many have a history of prior cardiovascular disease. Ischemic colitis occasionally occurs in persons younger than 50, especially women taking birth control pills. Colonic ischemia is reported to be a complication in about 2% of aortoiliac reconstructions, and it probably affects many more patients who demonstrate only mild or transient symptoms.

The extent and severity of ischemic colitis vary widely. Mesenteric occlusive disease can lead to extensive infarction of the colon with gangrene or perforation. More frequently, there is localized or segmental ischemia with no evidence of large vessel obstruction; in these cases, the pathophysiologic event is presumed to be regional alterations in the vasa recta of the colonic wall. Particularly vulnerable areas of the colon are the "watershed" regions between two adjacent major arterial supplies: the splenic flexure (superior and inferior mesenteric arteries) and the rectosigmoid area (inferior mesenteric and internal iliac arteries) (Fig. 48-27). Because rectal collaterals tend to be extensive, ischemia generally spares the rectum, and proctoscopy is usually negative.

Unlike ulcerative colitis or Crohn's disease of the colon, ischemic colitis (except for the infrequent fulminant variety) tends to follow a short, generally mild clinical course. The radiographic abnormalities often resolve within a few weeks of the

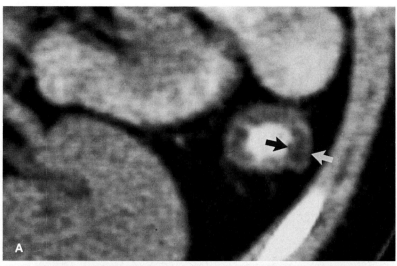

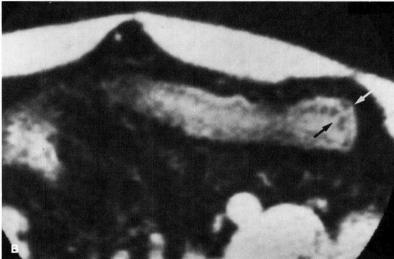

Fig. 48-24. CT of ulcerative colitis. **(A)** Scan at the level of the lower pole of the left kidney shows thickening of the descending colon with several areas of diminished attenuation **(arrows)**. The low-attenuation region measured −5 HU. **(B)** Imaged longitudinally, this section of sigmoid colon in another patient demonstrates inhomogeneous attenuation of thickened bowel wall **(arrows)**. (Gore RM, Marn CS, Kirby DF et al: CT findings in ulcerative, granulomatous, and indeterminate colitis. AJR 143:279–284, 1984. Copyright 1984. Reproduced with permission)

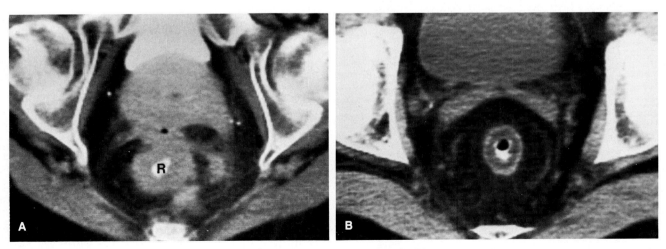

Fig. 48-25. CT of rectal involvement. **(A)** In Crohn's colitis, there is marked homogeneous thickening of the rectum **(R)** with abnormal soft-tissue densities in the left perirectal space. **(B)** In ulcerative colitis, the rectum produces a "target" appearance consisting of contrast- or air-filled lumen surrounded by a ring of soft-tissue density, which in turn is surrounded by a ring of decreased attenuation and finally encompassed by a ring of soft-tissue density. Scattered abnormal streaky densities can be seen in the presacral fat. (Gore RM, Marn CS, Kirby DF et al: CT findings in ulcerative, granulomatous, and indeterminate colitis. AJR 143:279–284, 1984. Copyright 1984. Reproduced with permission)

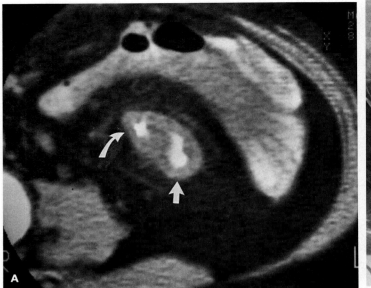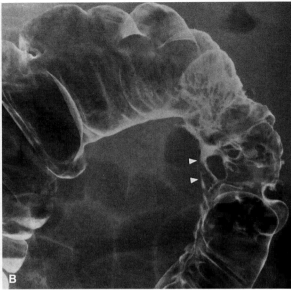

Fig. 48-26. CT of Crohn's disease. **(A)** Scan at the level of a previous ascending colon-splenic flexure anastomosis shows bowel wall thickening with contrast material in both a fistulous tract **(curved arrow)** and the lumen **(straight arrow)**. The small bowel is separated from the colon by abnormal mesenteric fat. **(B)** Barium enema study demonstrates the paracolic fistula **(arrowheads)** and recurrent Crohn's disease. (Gore RM, Marn CS, Kirby DF et al: CT findings in ulcerative, granulomatous, and indeterminate colitis. AJR 143:279–284, 1984. Copyright 1984. Reproduced with permission)

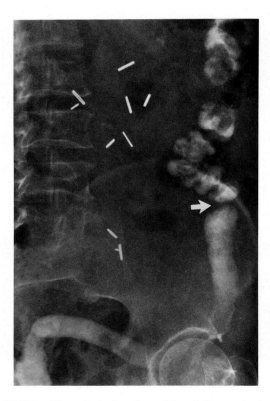

Fig. 48-27. Chronic ischemic colitis of the rectosigmoid and lower descending colon. The condition developed following abdominal aneurysm repair with sacrifice of the inferior mesenteric artery. The pattern is featureless, similar to that in chronic ulcerative colitis. The **arrow** points to the site of abrupt change in the appearance of the colon.

acute onset of abdominal pain, and they rarely recur. Post-ischemic strictures, which are uncommon, tend to develop within a month of the acute event.

RADIOGRAPHIC FINDINGS

The radiographic (and pathologic) appearance of ischemic colitis depends on the phase of the process during which the patient is examined. Because the mucosa is the layer most dependent on intact vascularity, fine superficial ulceration associated with inflammatory edema is the earliest radiographic sign of ischemic colitis. This causes the outer margin of the barium-filled colon to appear serrated, simulating ulcerative colitis (Fig. 48-28). As the disease progresses, longitudinal and deep penetrating ulcers, pseudopolyposis, and "thumbprinting" can be demonstrated. In most cases, the radiographic appearance of the colon returns to normal (Fig. 48-29), though stricturing with proximal dilatation does occur.

In patients with suspected ischemic colitis, mechanical factors such as volvulus and carcinoma must be sought as possible precipitating factors. An extensive ischemic lesion can distract the radiologist, preventing detection of a coexisting malignancy. Bleeding disorders, arteritis, and intravascular occlusion in patients with sickle cell disease can also result in an ischemic colitis pattern.

The differentiation of ischemic colitis from ulcerative colitis and Crohn's disease of the colon can

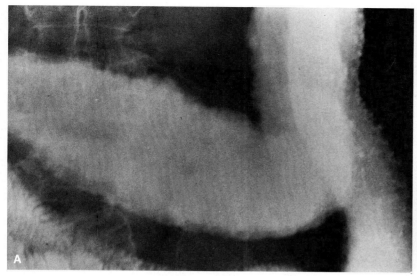

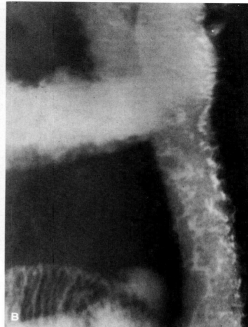

Fig. 48-28. Ischemic colitis. Superficial ulcers and inflammatory edema produce a serrated outer margin of the barium-filled colon simulating ulcerative colitis.

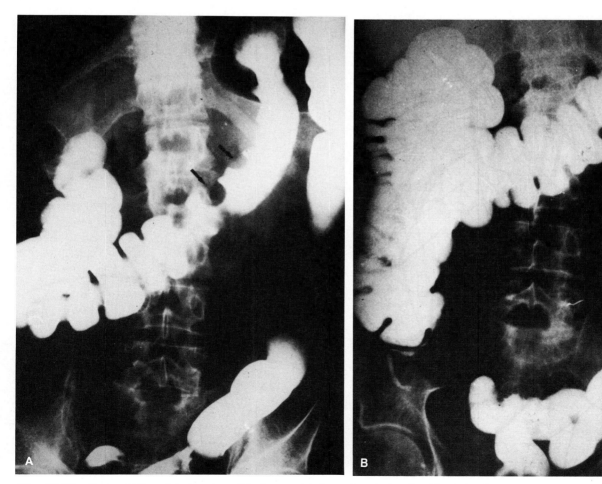

Fig. 48-29. Reversibility of ischemic colitis in an elderly male admitted with abdominal cramps of 3 days' duration and rectal bleeding. **(A)** ''Thumbprinting'' **(arrows)** along the superior aspect of the transverse colon. **(B)** Repeat study 2 days later. The colon now appears normal. (Schwartz S, Boley S, Lash J et al: Roentgenologic aspects of reversible vascular occlusion of the colon and its relationship to ulcerative colitis. Radiology 90:625–635, 1963)

be extremely difficult on radiographic or pathologic examination alone. In such cases, the clinical presentation and subsequent course can be the only basis for making a diagnosis. The characteristic acute episode of abdominal pain and bleeding, the rapid progression of radiographic findings, and the low rate of recurrence usually permit ischemic colitis to be readily distinguished from such conditions as ulcerative colitis and Crohn's disease of the colon, which are typically more indolent, chronic, and recurring.

AMEBIASIS

Infectious diseases involving the colon can present the radiographic pattern of an ulcerating colitis. The most prevalent of these diseases is amebiasis, which is caused by a protozoan that lives and develops in the colon of humans. Amebiasis can present as a segmental process, with skip lesions simulating Crohn's disease, or as a diffuse colitis mimicking ulcerative colitis (Fig. 48-30). It is estimated that 20% of the world's population harbor amebae, though only about 5% of these individuals demonstrate clinical disease. Although the protozoan is most common in tropical countries, it is frequently found in nontropical areas. Indeed, about 5% of the population of the United States is probably infested with the parasite.

Amebiasis begins as a primary infection of the colon that is acquired by the ingestion of food or water contaminated by amebic cysts. The amebae tend to settle in areas of stasis and thus primarily affect the cecum and, to a lesser extent, the rectosigmoid and the hepatic and splenic flexures. The patient is asymptomatic (in a carrier state) until the protozoan actually invades the wall of the colon. Penetration of the bowel wall by the organism incites an inflammatory reaction that leads to a broad clinical spectrum. Some patients, however, remain symptom-free for months or years. Many patients with amebic colitis are acutely ill, complaining of frequent diarrhea, blood and mucus in the stools, and cramping abdominal pain that tends to be located in the right lower quadrant. Others have only mild abdominal discomfort and intermittent diarrhea. The most common extracolonic complication of amebiasis is hepatic abscess, which is seen in about one-third of patients with amebic dysentery. Hepatic abscesses are also frequently found without clinical colonic disease. In about 90% of patients, properly obtained stool specimens are adequate for the diagnosis of amebic colitis. A hemagglutination or ameba precipitin test is positive in a high percentage of patients with the disease.

RADIOGRAPHIC FINDINGS

In the early stages of amebic colitis, superficial ulcerations are superimposed on a pattern of mucosal

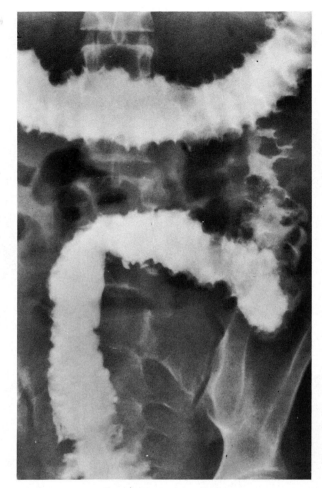

Fig. 48-30. Amebic colitis. Diffuse ulceration and mucosal edema mimic ulcerative colitis.

edema or nodularity, spasm, and loss of the normal haustral pattern (Fig. 48-31). The cecum is the primary site of involvement in up to 90% of patients with clinical disease. Fibrosis due to secondary infection and long-sustained spasm often produces a characteristic cecal deformity (cone-shaped cecum). Scattered areas of segmental involvement can occur, especially in the rectosigmoid, and generalized severe colitis sometimes develops. Deep penetrating ulcers (Fig. 48-32), pseudopolyps, cobblestoning, and thumbprinting can also be demonstrated; multiple skip lesions are frequent. Complications of amebic colitis include perforation, sinuses, fistulas, and pericolic abscesses.

Because amebiasis rarely affects the ileum, the presence of concomitant ileal disease (especially if it is extensive) favors Crohn's disease as the underlying etiology. If disease is limited to the colon, the demonstration of transverse and longitudinal ulcers, eccentric involvement of the colonic wall, or extensive fistula formation should suggest Crohn's disease rather than amebiasis. When colon inflammation is diffuse and simulates ulcerative colitis, the presence of multiple skip areas makes amebic colitis the more likely diagnosis.

SCHISTOSOMIASIS

In schistosomiasis, the sharp terminal or lateral spines of the eggs of the blood flukes, together with the muscular action of the colon wall, permit the parasite to penetrate the colonic mucosa and stimulate an inflammatory response. Because of the predilection of the adult worms to enter the inferior mesenteric vein and discharge their eggs there, the descending and sigmoid colon are most frequently affected. However, any portion of the colon can be involved. The mucosa is edematous and demonstrates tiny ulcerations or mural spiculations that simulate the appearance of ulcerative colitis. On double-contrast studies, a diffuse granular pattern can be seen. Spasm, disturbed motility, and a loss of haustral pattern are common. During this acute stage of the disease, the diagnosis of schistosomiasis is readily made by detection of ova in freshly passed stools. As the disease progresses, formation of discrete granulomas produces the more characteristic radiographic pattern of multiple small filling defects in the barium column.

BACTERIAL INFECTIONS

SHIGELLOSIS/SALMONELLOSIS

Shigellosis (bacillary dysentery) and salmonellosis (food poisoning, typhoid fever) are acute or chronic inflammatory bowel diseases caused by gram-nega-

tive, non-spore-forming bacilli of the *Enterobacteriaceae* family. *Shigella* organisms predominantly involve the colon; salmonellosis mainly affects the terminal ileum, though colon changes are also seen. Although they are generally considered to be tropical diseases, the distribution of *Shigella* and *Salmonella* is worldwide; they not infrequently occur in low socioeconomic groups in the United States (especially in California and Texas). Overcrowding and poor sanitary conditions, particularly in warm, humid climates, predispose to the spread of infection. In well-developed countries with good sanitation, outbreaks of small epidemics of dysentery tend to occur in schools, military barracks, prisons, and mental asylums. Debility, exhaustion, weakness, and malnutrition predispose to development of the disease.

Shigellae and salmonellae enter the bowel in food and drink that have been contaminated by infected fecal material. Acute and chronic carriers serving as cooks or processors of food and milk are important sources of contamination. In tropical countries in which human excrement is used as fertilizer, uncooked vegetables and salads can cause infection. Another major source of infection is flies that have eaten or walked in stools contaminated with the organisms. In addition, many household pets are known to harbor and excrete salmonellae.

Shigella organisms penetrate the colonic mucosa and grow rapidly, liberating exo- and endotoxins that cause inflammation of the colon and rectum. Mucosal edema and submucosal infiltration are associated with an outpouring of mucoid and blood-streaked exudate, which fills the lumen of the gut. As necrotic tissue sloughs, shallow, ragged ulcers remain, partially or completely encircling

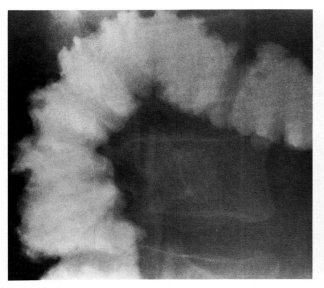

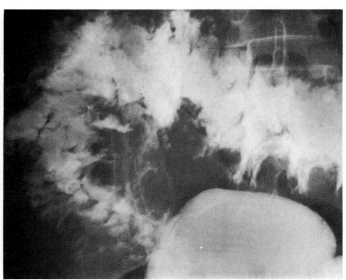

48-31

48-32

Fig. 48-31. Amebic colitis. There is ulceration, mucosal edema, and loss of the normal haustral pattern.

Fig. 48-32. Amebic colitis. Deep, penetrating ulcers produce a bizarre appearance.

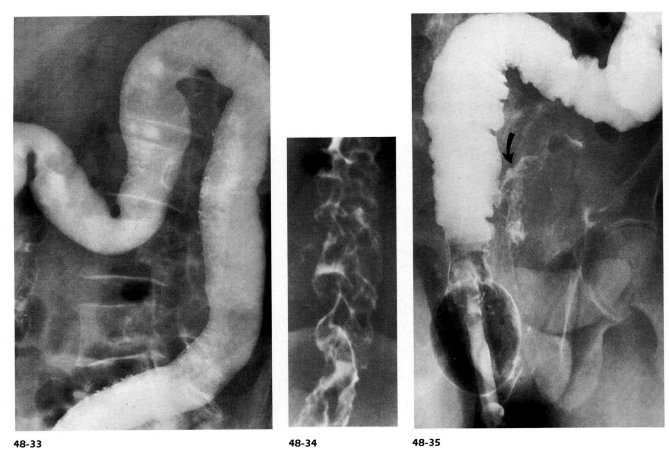

48-33   48-34   48-35

Fig. 48-33. Salmonellosis. Diffuse, fine ulcerations simulate ulcerative colitis.

Fig. 48-34. Salmonellosis. A postevacuation film demonstrates ulceration and irregular thickening of mucosal folds.

Fig. 48-35. Shigellosis. Mucosal edema and ulceration primarily involve the rectosigmoid. Note the fistulous tract **(arrow)**.

the bowel. In salmonellosis, the organisms also penetrate the wall of the small bowel, invading the lymphoid tissues of Peyer's patches and the solitary lymph follicles and thereby gaining access to the blood stream by way of the thoracic duct. The characteristic pathologic lesions of typhoid fever are found primarily in lymphatic tissue of the distal small bowel. Deep ulcerations can cause perforation and peritonitis. The systemic infection in salmonellosis can lead to focal liver necrosis, cholecystitis, and involvement of the lungs and kidney.

Bacillary dysentery has a short incubation period, usually 2 to 3 days but occasionally as long as 1 week. Diarrhea is the most characteristic sign. In acute, fulminating infection, abdominal pain is severe, and profuse diarrhea can result in life-threatening fluid loss and electrolyte imbalance.

The symptoms and signs of salmonellosis vary from acute gastroenteritis to severe septicemia. In typical "food poisoning," there is sudden onset of fever, nausea, vomiting, and diarrhea that occurs

after a very short incubation period, often as little as 12 hr. In most cases, the disease is self-limited, and there is complete recovery in 4 to 5 days. In the classic form of typhoid fever, there is the insidious onset of malaise, frontal headache, muscular aches, and joint pain. After a week, the fever becomes high and continuous; apathy, toxemia, and delirium may become prominent. Complications such as massive intestinal bleeding, perforation, and circulatory failure can be fatal.

Radiographic Findings

Patients with suspected salmonellosis seldom undergo a barium enema examination, since the symptoms are acute and suggest the underlying self-limited condition. However, when performed, the barium enema may demonstrate diffuse, fine ulcerations (Fig. 48-33) and irregular thickening of folds on postevacuation views (Fig. 48-34). In acute bacillary dysentery due to shigellosis, a barium enema examination generally cannot be tolerated. If an examination is performed, severe spasm of the colon may prevent complete filling. When a barium enema examination is successful, the radiographic appearance is related to the severity and stage of colon involvement. The acute, severe form is a pancolitis characterized by deep "collar-button" ulcers, intense spasm, and mucosal edema. In less severe disease, superficial ulcerations with coarse, nodular, edematous folds can involve the entire colon or be segmental in distribution, primarily affecting the rectum and sigmoid and, less commonly, the descending portion (Fig. 48-35). Nonspecific findings, such as spasm, haustral distortion, and excess fluid, usually accompany the mucosal changes.

Radiographic differentiation between salmonellosis and shigellosis is frequently impossible in the colon. Involvement of the terminal ileum, however, strongly suggests salmonellosis as the correct diagnosis. Because it can be impossible to distinguish between these diseases and other forms of ulcerating colitis, bacteriologic investigation is often required for a specific diagnosis. It is critical that the precise causative agent be identified, since steroid therapy, often used to treat noninfectious forms of colitis, is obviously contraindicated in these infectious processes.

TUBERCULOUS COLITIS

Colonic tuberculosis predominantly affects the cecum, and concomitant disease in the distal ileum is usually seen. The ascending and transverse colon can also be involved (Fig. 48-36), though almost invariably in continuity with the cecum. Occasionally,

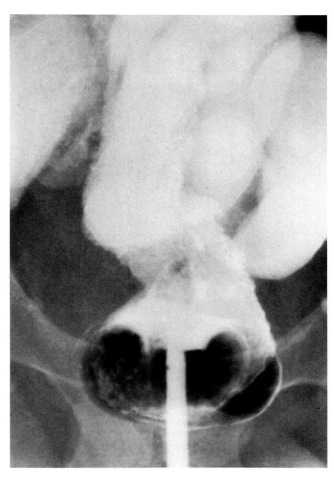

Fig. 48-37. Gonococcal proctitis. There is diffuse rectal ulceration with edematous mucosa. The remainder of the colon was spared. (Eisenberg RL: Diagnostic Imaging in Surgery. New York, McGraw–Hill, 1987)

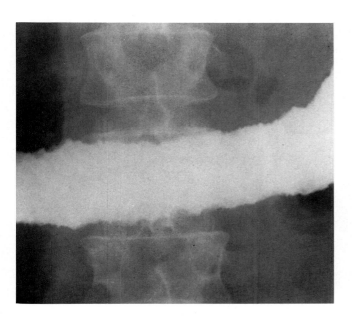

Fig. 48-36. Tuberculosis. Fine ulcerations diffusely involve the transverse colon.

tuberculosis is segmental and occurs elsewhere in the colon, primarily in the sigmoid.

Radiographically, gastrointestinal tuberculosis closely simulates Crohn's disease. The correct diagnosis is often not made before surgery, especially since recognizable pulmonary tuberculosis is frequently not present. In addition, because acutely ill patients can be anergic to skin test antigens, a negative tuberculin skin test is often seen in patients with active gastrointestinal disease.

The majority of cases of tuberculosis of the colon in the United States are caused by *Mycobacterium tuberculosis;* coexistent pulmonary disease can often be demonstrated radiographically. In areas in which cattle are diseased and milk is not pasteurized, *Mycobacterium bovis* can be the etiologic agent. In patients with this form of tuberculosis, intestinal disease is usually associated with a normal chest radiograph.

Tuberculosis of the colon can be asymptomatic or produce a spectrum of nonspecific complaints such as weight loss, fever, anorexia, right lower

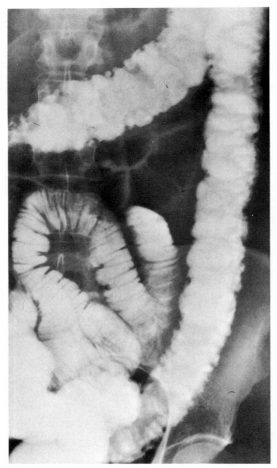

Fig. 48-38. Postantibiotic staphylococcal infection. The features are typical of a severe ulcerating colitis.

quadrant pain, and diarrhea. The primary tuberculous lesion of the gastrointestinal tract originates within the lymphatic structures of the submucosa and is covered by a normal overlying mucosa. A combination of caseous necrosis and ischemia leads to sloughing of the mucosa and development of an ulcer. In early stages of the disease, superficial or deep mucosal ulcerations can sometimes be identified radiographically, though intense spasm and irritability often make adequate filling of the involved portion of the colon impossible. Progressive inflammatory changes, fibrosis, and lymphatic obstruction cause the colon wall to become thickened and rigid.

GONORRHEAL PROCTITIS

Gonorrheal proctitis in men is almost always the result of anal intercourse; in women, most cases are believed to be secondary to genitoanal spread. Most patients with rectal gonorrhea have no symptoms and are discovered only by the meticulous tracing of sexual contacts and a high index of suspicion. To differentiate gonorrheal proctitis from other ulcerative diseases, Gram staining and selective culturing of the purulent exudate must be performed. The symptoms associated with gonorrheal proctitis are similar to those of other forms of ulcerative proctitis and include rectal burning, itching, purulent anal discharge, and blood and mucus in the stools. Barium enema examination is normal in most patients with gonorrheal proctitis. Infrequently, mucosal edema and ulceration confined to the rectum can be demonstrated (Fig. 48-37). Gonorrheal proctitis

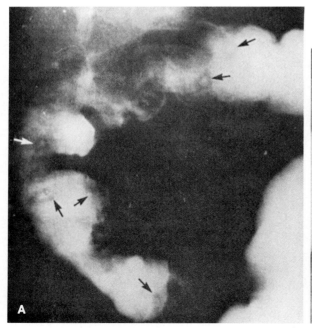
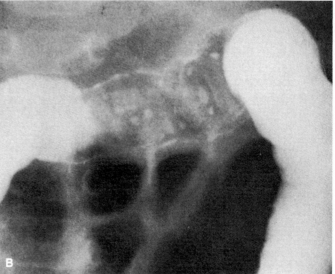

Fig. 48-39. *Yersinia* colitis. **(A)** Magnified spot view of the hepatic flexure and ascending colon and **(B)** magnified spot view of the distal transverse colon show aphthoid ulcers surrounded by rings of edema **(arrows)**. (Atkinson GO, Gay BB, Ball TI et al: *Yersinia enterocolitica* colitis in infants: Radiographic changes. Radiology 148:113–116, 1983)

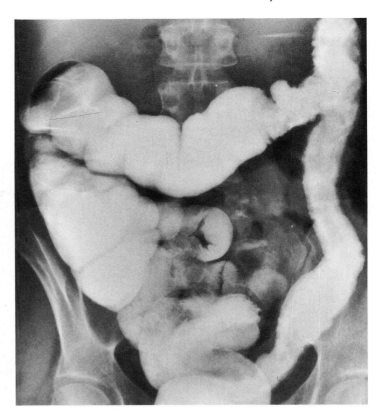

Fig. 48-40. Colitis caused by *Campylobacter fetus*. The radiographic pattern is indistinguishable from ulcerative colitis. Cultures and immunologic studies were necessary for proper diagnosis.

responds promptly to specific antibiotic therapy. Untreated, rectal stricture develops in 20% of patients.

STAPHYLOCOCCAL COLITIS

Postantibiotic staphylococcal diarrhea occurs after a course of orally administered broad-spectrum antibiotics, usually tetracycline. The disease is most common among hospitalized patients and is caused by antibiotic-resistant strains that enter the gastrointestinal tract by way of the nasopharyngeal route and grow profusely in the intestine once the population of normal intestinal flora has been significantly reduced by oral antibiotics. Staphylococcal enteritis can produce only mild, self-limited diarrhea. In severe disease, nausea, vomiting, and profuse diarrhea can occur. Mild staphylococcal enteritis subsides rapidly once the antibiotic to which the organism is resistant is discontinued and the normal intestinal flora is allowed to return. In severe enteritis, it may be necessary to administer an antibiotic to which the *Staphylococcus* is sensitive. Although barium enema examinations are rarely performed in patients with staphylococcal enterocolitis, they can demonstrate the characteristic features of a generalized ulcerating colitis (Fig. 48-38).

YERSINIA COLITIS

Yersinia enterocolitica is a gram-negative bacillus that has been increasingly implicated as a cause of ileitis and colitis in children. Fever, diarrhea, and sometimes blood in the stools are the predominant presentations in infants; a pattern simulating appendicitis can be seen in older children. Barium enema examination can demonstrate multiple small colonic and terminal ileal ulcerations similar to those seen in Crohn's colitis (Fig. 48-39).

CAMPYLOBACTER FETUS COLITIS

Campylobacter fetus, subspecies jejuni, has recently been recognized as a common human enteric pathogen. Indeed, in a recent series, this organism was the most common cause of specific infectious colitis. Patients with this disease typically present with the acute onset of diarrhea, abdominal pain, fever, and constitutional symptoms. Proctoscopy demonstrates an inflamed mucosa with bloody exudate and numerous polymorphonuclear leukocytes on fecal smear. *Campylobacter* colitis is usually self-limited; in protracted or severe cases, antibiotic therapy (erythromycin) may be required.

The radiographic features of *Campylobacter* colitis are nonspecific and may be indistinguishable from other causes of colonic inflammation (Fig. 48-40). The organism may cause a granular mucosal pattern simulating ulcerative colitis or produce multiple aphthoid ulcers of the large bowel mimicking Crohn's colitis (Fig. 48-41). Although generalized involvement of the entire colon is more common, segmental disease has been reported. Edematous narrowing of the terminal ileum and

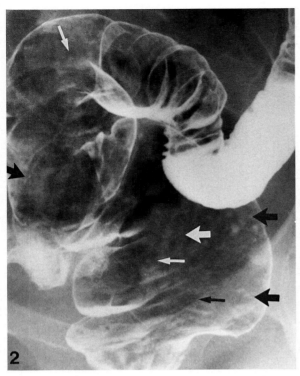

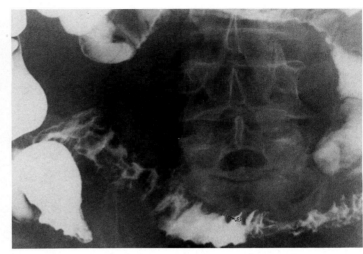

48-41   **48-42**

Fig. 48-41. *Campylobacter* colitis. Multiple mucosal defects, some with edematous halos, in the rectum. **Long arrows** point to aphthous ulcers; **wide arrows** point to mucosal defects without rings of edema. (Tielbeek AV, Rosenbusch G, Muytjens HL et al: Roentgenologic changes of the colon in *Campylobacter* infection. Gastrointest Radiol 10:358–361, 1985)

Fig. 48-42. *Campylobacter* ileitis. The terminal ileum is separated from adjacent loops. Its mucosal folds are thickened and irregular, mimicking Crohn's disease. (Gardiner R, Smith C: Infective enterocolitides. Radiol Clin North Am 25:67–78, 1987)

loss of colonic haustration may also occur (Fig. 48-42).

It has been postulated that single episodes of acute colitis formerly attributed to ulcerative colitis may have been caused by *Campylobacter fetus.* Therefore, in patients presenting with acute colitis, *Campylobacter* infection should be ruled out with appropriate cultures and immunologic studies before the diagnosis of ulcerative colitis is made.

LYMPHOGRANULOMA VENEREUM

Lymphogranuloma venereum is a venereal disease that is especially common in the tropics. It is caused by *Chlamydia trachomatis,* an obligate intracellular parasitic bacterium once believed to be a large virus. The disease is transmitted almost exclusively through sexual contact. The rectal form of the dis-

ease is most prevalent in women, though it is being found with increasing frequency in homosexual men. Lymphogranuloma venereum in men usually appears as a primary genital sore followed by purulent inflammation of inguinal lymph nodes (bubo formation). In women, the primary lesion occurs in the vagina or cervix, where it often goes undetected. In up to 25% of patients, however, the rectum is the predominant site of disease.

The major symptom of lymphogranuloma venereum involving the colon is bleeding. Mucopurulent rectal discharge, diarrhea, low-grade fever, perianal fistulas, and recurrent abscesses can also be present. As rectal stricturing increases, constipation and crampy lower abdominal pain can develop. The diagnosis of lymphogranuloma venereum can be confirmed by the Frei intradermal skin test or the complement fixation test, or by recovery of the virus from the blood, feces, or bubos.

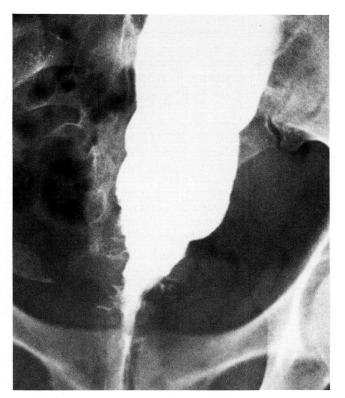

Fig. 48-43. Lymphogranuloma venereum. There is a long rectal stricture with multiple deep ulcers. (Dreyfuss JR, Janower ML: Radiology of the Colon. Baltimore, Williams & Wilkins, 1980)

The rectum is the first and usually the only portion of the colon involved in lymphogranuloma venereum (Fig. 48-43). The pathologic changes result from viral invasion and blockage of the rectal lymphatics which, together with secondary infection, lead to rectal edema and cellular infiltrate in the submucosa and muscularis. In the early stages of lymphogranuloma venereum, as in all forms of ulcerating colitis, the bowel is spastic and irritable with boggy and edematous mucosa and multiple shaggy ulcers. Fistulas and sinus tracts of varying length are frequently present. As the disease progresses, the classic pattern of rectal stricture develops.

FUNGAL INFECTIONS

Histoplasmosis, mucormycosis, actinomycosis, and candidiasis are among the fungal diseases that infrequently involve the colon. They usually occur in chronically ill, debilitated patients and can either arise in the bowel or spread from another site in the body. Fungal invasion of the walls of the bowel and blood vessels produces an intense localized inflammatory reaction. The bowel wall appears irritable and spastic, and the mucosal folds are thickened and irregular. Mucosal ulcerations can occasionally be identified. The correct diagnosis of fungal disease involving the colon is rarely made before operation or postmortem examination.

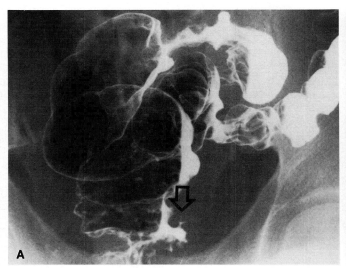
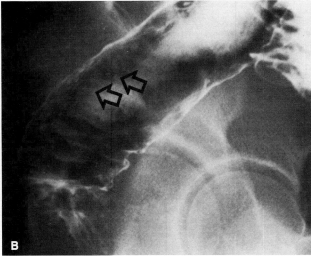

Fig. 48-44. Anorectal herpes. **(A)** Collar-button ulcer **(arrow)** in the rectum just above an area of intense spasm. Note the spasm in the sigmoid colon. **(B)** Lateral radiograph of the rectum shows multiple aphthous ulcers **(arrows)** above the area of rectal spasm. (Shah SJ, Scholz FJ: Anorectal herpes: Radiographic findings. Radiology 147:81–82, 1983)

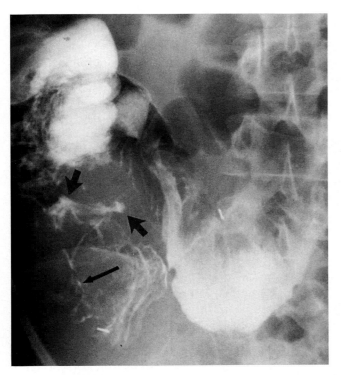

Fig. 48-45. Cytomegalovirus-induced colonic ulceration. A postevacuation film demonstrates a markedly edematous cecum and ascending colon with mucosal irregularity and ulcers in a patient who has undergone a renal transplant. (Cho SR, Tisnado J, Liu CI et al: Bleeding cytomegalovirus ulcers of the colon: Barium enema and angiography. AJR 136:1213–1215, 1981. Copyright 1981. Reproduced with permission)

VIRAL INFECTIONS

HERPES

Anorectal herpes caused by herpes simplex virus (HSV) is now one of the major sexually transmitted infections. On barium examination, aphthous ulcers, plaquelike erosions, and deep collar-button ulcerations may involve the rectum and sigmoid colon (Fig. 48-44). Rarely, herpes zoster causes small ulcerations in a narrowed portion of colon, a radiographic pattern similar to that of a segmental ulcerating colitis. This corresponds to the ulcerative cutaneous changes that sometimes follow the more characteristic vesicular skin lesions. The short length of the colonic lesion and the typical clinical history and skin lesions should suggest the correct diagnosis.

CYTOMEGALOVIRUS

Cytomegalovirus-induced colonic ulcers are the most important cause of severe lower gastrointesti-

nal bleeding in renal transplant recipients in whom immunosuppressive therapy has been initiated (Fig. 48-45). Early diagnosis and prompt surgical intervention are essential in the management of this often fatal complication. Cytomegalovirus infection has become increasingly recognized as a gastrointestinal opportunistic pathogen in patients with AIDS. The radiographic manifestations are nonspecific and usually mimic the appearance of ulcerative colitis with diffuse mucosal ulceration or Crohn's colitis with aphthous ulceration and skip areas (Fig. 48-46). Besides the inflammatory change caused by the cytomegalovirus infection itself, an associated vasculitis contributes to prominent local edema, which can appear radiographically as luminal narrowing, thumbprinting, or even tumorlike defects (Fig. 48-47).

ROTAVIRUS

Rotavirus infections are a common cause of childhood gastroenteritis that is generally mild and self-limited and rarely severe enough to justify radiographic examination. In several patients with

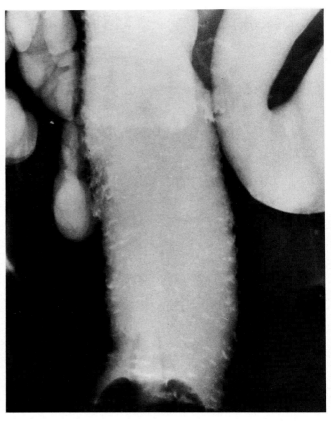

Fig. 48-46. Cytomegalovirus colitis. Superficial ulcers and inflammatory edema produce a serrated outer margin of barium-filled colon in this patient with AIDS.

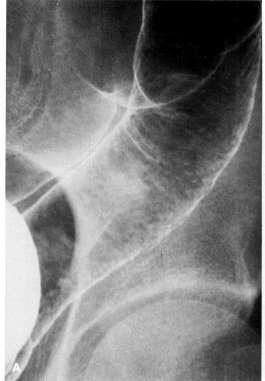
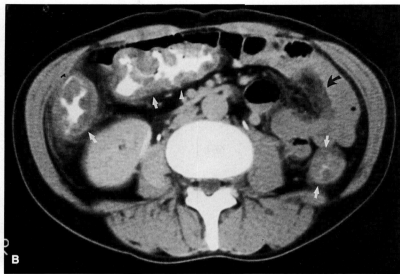

Fig. 48-47. Cytomegalovirus colitis. **(A)** Double-contrast barium enema examination in a patient with AIDS shows numerous mucosal ulcerations in the descending colon. Similar findings were present throughout the large bowel. **(B)** CT scan obtained 12 days later shows marked thickening of the colonic wall **(straight arrows)** and deep ulcers **(arrowheads).** Inflammatory infiltration of the mesentery was also present **(curved arrow).** (Teixidor HS, Honig CL, Norsoph E et al: Cytomegalovirus infection of the alimentary canal: Radiologic findings with pathologic correlation. Radiology 163:317–323, 1987)

rotavirus-induced colitis causing prolonged bloody diarrhea suggesting ulcerative colitis, barium studies showed multiple minute ulcerations involving a segment or all of the colon (Fig. 48-48). Segmental spasm may be prolonged and mimic an area of narrowing.

STRONGYLOIDIASIS

Severe colitis is an extremely unusual manifestation of infestation by *Strongyloides stercoralis.* Invasion of the bowel wall by larvae of this nematode results in a diffuse ulcerating colitis characterized by both small and large ulcers, mucosal edema, and the loss of haustral markings (Fig. 48-49). Colonic infection is often associated with overwhelming sepsis, hemorrhage, and death, though healing with stricture formation can occur.

PSEUDOMEMBRANOUS COLITIS

Pseudomembranous colitis is a spectrum of entities that are potentially serious complications of antibiotic therapy, surgery, uremia, and large bowel obstruction. It most often occurs following the administration of well-established drugs such as tetracycline, penicillin, and ampicillin, or after treatment with newer wide-spectrum antibiotics, such as clindamycin and lincomycin. Pseudomembranous colitis most commonly arises after oral antibiotic therapy, though it can also develop following intravenous administration. Whether the antibiotic-associated pseudomembranous colitis is related to a change in the normal bacterial flora of the colon or to a direct toxic action of the drug itself has been a controversial question. The theory that a resistant strain of a specific organism causes pseudomembranous colitis is supported by recent stud-

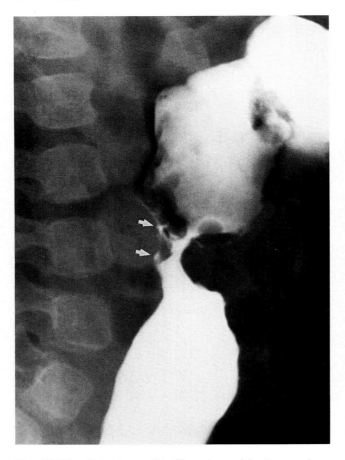

Fig. 48-48. Rotavirus colitis. There is persistent spasm in an area of mucosal edema and ulceration. The arrows point to two ulcerations in the area of stenosis. (Fernbach SK, Lloyd–Still JD: The radiographic findings in severe rotavirus-induced colitis. J Can Assoc Radiol 35:192–194, 1984)

ies demonstrating the presence of *Clostridium difficile* in the stools of a high percentage of patients with this condition. This bacterium elaborates a cytotoxic substance that destroys human cells in culture and produces a severe enterocolitis when injected into the cecum of animals. Clinical symptoms can be identified within 1 day to 1 month (average, 2 weeks) after the initiation of antibiotic therapy. Most patients recover uneventfully after withdrawal of the offending antibiotic and the institution of adequate fluid and electrolyte replacement. However, there is an overall mortality rate in this condition of about 15%.

The clinical hallmark of pseudomembranous colitis is debilitating, severe diarrhea with or without blood. Indeed, this complication should be suspected in any patient receiving antibiotics who suddenly experiences copious diarrhea and signs of abdominal cramps, tenderness, or peritonitis. At proctosigmoidoscopy, there is the characteristic appearance of a friable, edematous mucosa with yellow-green exudate and white, patchy, raised 1-mm to 6-mm plaquelike lesions scattered over the mucosal surface. A confluent, purulent pseudomembrane, histologically composed of mucus, fibrin, leukocytes, and bacteria, can often be observed enveloping the entire mucosal surface.

RADIOGRAPHIC FINDINGS

Plain abdominal radiographs in severe cases of pseudomembranous colitis can demonstrate moderate, diffuse gaseous distention of the colon. The haustral markings are edematous and distorted, with wide transverse bands of thickened colonic

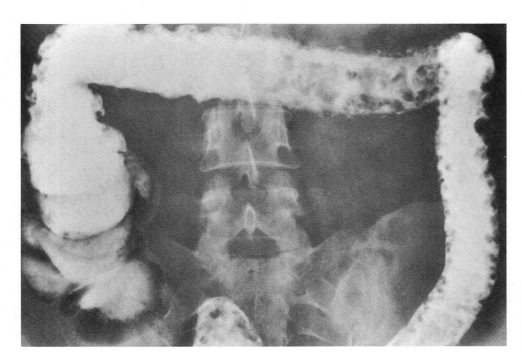

Fig. 48-49. Strongyloidiasis. Diffuse ulcerating colitis is present with deep and shallow ulcers and pronounced mucosal edema.

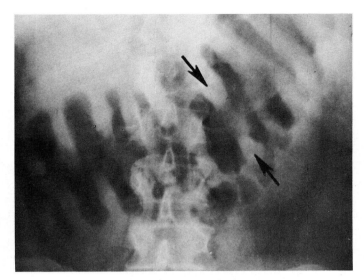

Fig. 48-50. Pseudomembranous colitis. A plain abdominal radiograph demonstrates wide transverse bands of thickened colonic wall **(arrows)**. (Stanley RJ, Melson GL, Tedesco FJ et al: Plain film findings in severe pseudomembranous colitis. Radiology 118:7–11, 1976)

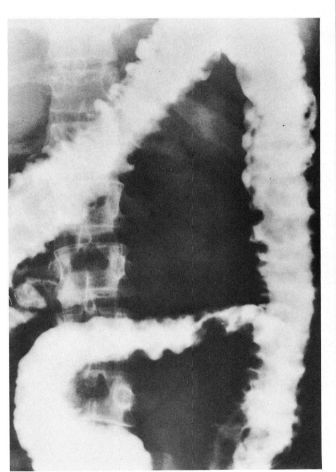

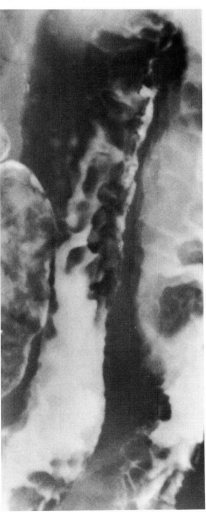

48-51   48-52

Fig. 48-51. Pseudomembranous colitis. The barium column has a shaggy and irregular appearance because of the pseudomembrane and superficial necrosis with mucosal ulceration.

Fig. 48-52. Pseudomembranous colitis. The pseudomembranes appear as multiple flat, raised lesions distributed circumferentially about the margin of the colon.

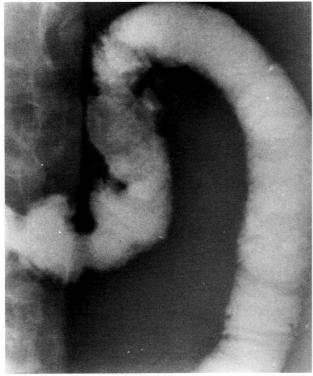
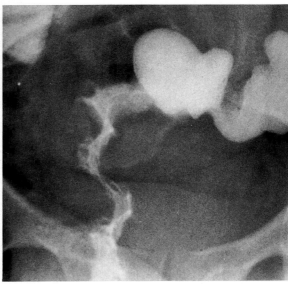

48-53   48-54

Fig. 48-53. Uremic colitis. Diffuse, fine ulceration with mucosal edema simulates ulcerative colitis.

Fig. 48-54. Radiation-induced colitis. Irregularity, spasm, and ulceration produce an appearance similar to other ulcerating diseases of the colon.

wall (Fig. 48-50). Barium enema examination is contraindicated in patients with severe pseudomembranous colitis. In mild cases, or as the condition subsides, a low-pressure barium enema study can be performed with caution. The barium column appears shaggy and irregular because of the pseudomembrane and superficial necrosis (Fig. 48-51). Multiple flat, raised lesions may be distributed circumferentially about the margin of the colon (Fig. 48-52). Mucosal ulcerations simulating other forms of ulcerating colitis are frequently seen. In many cases, however, this serrated outline actually represents barium interposed between the plaquelike membranes rather than true ulceration with surrounding edema.

A fulminant and often fatal type of pseudomembranous colitis characterized by profuse, occasionally bloody diarrhea, dehydration, shock, and toxemia, occasionally occurs in the absence of antibiotic therapy. This nonspecific disorder has multiple etiologies, the most common being postopera-

tive states, uremia (uremic colitis) (Fig. 48-53), colitis proximal to a large bowel obstruction, and any cause of severe hypoxia.

RADIATION INJURY

Transient proctitis manifested as diarrhea, mucoid discharge, tenesmus, or crampy pain occurs in more than half of patients receiving pelvic irradiation for carcinoma of the cervix, endometrium, ovaries, bladder, or prostate. This type of transient radiation injury is benign and self-limited and rarely leads to radiologic investigation.

In patients with more severe acute radiation-induced colitis, barium enema examinations can demonstrate segmental changes of irregularity, spasm, and fine serrations of the bowel wall similar to the appearance of other ulcerating diseases of the colon (Fig. 48-54). Discrete ulceration of the mucosa is frequent and can be superficial or penetrat-

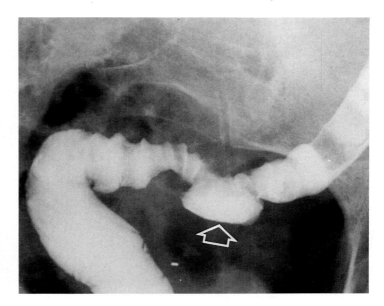

Fig. 48-55. Radiation-induced colitis. A large, discrete penetrating ulcer is visible **(arrow)**. (Rogers LF, Goldstein HM: Roentgen manifestations of radiation injury to the gastrointestinal tract. Gastrointest Radiol 2:281–291, 1977)

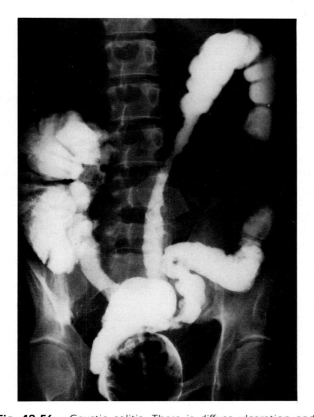

Fig. 48-56. Caustic colitis. There is diffuse ulceration and narrowing of the transverse colon. Note the mild irregularity of the rectal mucosa. (Kim SK, Cho C, Levinsohn EM: Caustic colitis due to detergent enema. AJR 134:397–398, 1980. Copyright 1980. Reproduced with permission)

ing (Fig. 48-55). The anterior rectal wall adjacent to the posterior fornix is usually the site of maximum dosage to the rectum and is the most common site of localized injury. As the condition progresses, strictures and fistulas often develop.

CAUSTIC COLITIS

Transient colitis can develop after a cleansing enema if potentially irritating solutions (soapsuds, detergents) are used (Fig. 48-56). Caustic colitis is rare, since enema solutions are seldom strong enough to cause intestinal injury. In those cases in which colonic injury does occur, the degree of damage depends on the duration of mucosal contact with the caustic agent. An irritant enema tends to produce spasm of the rectosigmoid, which results in rapid expulsion of the solution from this segment. Because fluid trapped in the proximal colon is not promptly expelled, corrosive damage is most severe in this region.

The pathologic and radiographic findings in caustic colitis are identical to those seen in the esophagus following the ingestion of a corrosive agent. In the acute necrotic phase, cellular death is accompanied by an intense inflammatory reaction. After 3 to 5 days, the necrotic mucosa sloughs, and ulcerations can be demonstrated on barium enema examination. Within 3 to 4 weeks, the inflammatory reaction subsides, and scarring leads to the formation of strictures.

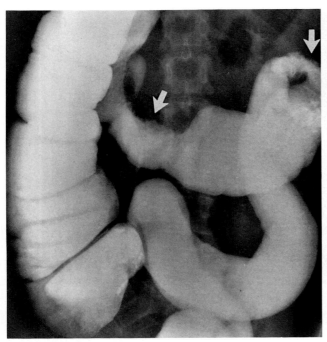

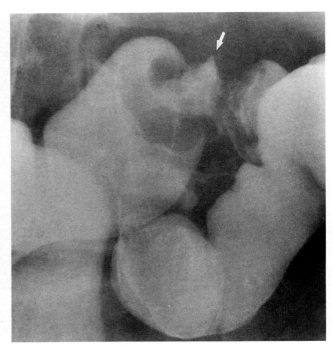

48-57   48-58

Fig. 48-57.   Pancreatitis. Spiculation of the proximal transverse colon and splenic flexure **(arrows)** simulates an ulcerating colitis.

Fig. 48-58.   Ulcerated primary carcinoma of the sigmoid colon **(arrow)**.

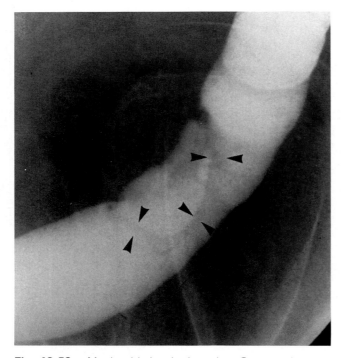

Fig. 48-59.   Meniscoid ulcer in the colon. Compression spot film of the proximal sigmoid shows a lens-shaped ulcer. The inferior border is convex toward the lumen. A semicircular lucency **(arrowheads)** surrounding the ulcer represents the edges of the tumor mass. (Siskind BN, Burrell MI: Intraluminal meniscoid ulcer in the colon: An unusual sign of malignancy. Gastrointest Radiol 11:251–253, 1986)

PANCREATITIS

Pancreatitis can cause spiculation of the mucosa simulating an ulcerating colitis (Fig. 48-57). It usually involves the transverse colon and splenic flexure but can also affect the upper descending colon. The close anatomic relationship between the pancreas and transverse colon provides a pathway for the dissemination of pancreatic inflammatory products. The clinical appearance is usually dominated by the underlying pancreatitis, though in severe cases necrosis of the colon can develop. Radiographic findings include localized perforation, distention with irregular, destroyed mucosa, large penetrating ulcers, and pseudopolyp formation.

MALIGNANT LESIONS

PRIMARY CARCINOMA

Primary carcinoma of the colon must be excluded whenever a solitary ulcerating lesion is detected on barium enema examination (Fig. 48-58). Malignant ulceration can vary from an excavation within a large fungating mass to evidence of mucosal destruction within an annular "apple-core" tumor. Early saddle cancers, flat, plaquelike lesions that involve only one margin of the colon wall, can become centrally ulcerated. An aggressive ulcerating lesion in the colon can rarely produce an intralu-

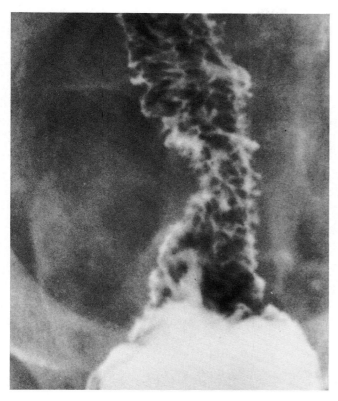

Fig. 48-60. Carcinoma of the prostate metastatic to the rectum and rectosigmoid. The diffuse circumferential ulceration mimics ulcerative colitis.

minal lenticular ulcer surrounded by a meniscoid lucency of tumor, producing an appearance similar to the Carman meniscus sign of gastric malignancy (Fig. 48-59).

METASTASES

Metastatic carcinoma to the colon can occasionally be mistaken, both clinically and radiographically, for a primary ulcerating colitis (Fig. 48-60). Diarrhea, often associated with blood and mucus, can be the predominant clinical presentation. Spiculations of the bowel contour can mimic marginal ulcerations (Fig. 48-61); mucosal thickening, nodular masses, and multiple eccentric strictures can simulate Crohn's colitis (Fig. 48-62). A pattern identical to ulcerating colitis has also been reported in patients with diffuse lymphomatous (Fig. 48-63) or leukemic (Fig. 48-64) infiltration of the colon.

OTHER DISORDERS

AMYLOIDOSIS

Amyloidosis, primarily secondary to connective tissue diseases, lymphoproliferative disorders, or chronic infection, can present as an ulcerating colitis. Histologic material and special amyloid stains (Congo red) are required for the diagnosis.

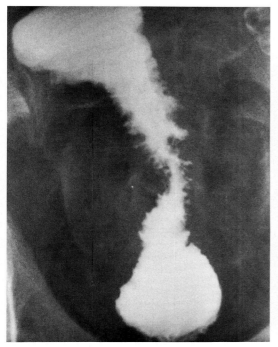

48-61

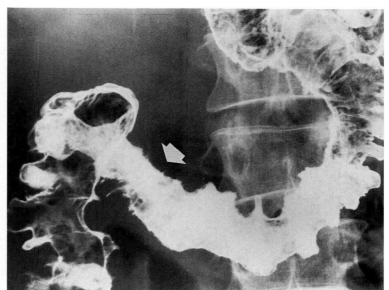

48-62

Fig. 48-61. Carcinoma of the prostate metastatic to the rectum. Spiculations along the bowel wall suggest an ulcerating colitis.

Fig. 48-62. Carcinoma of the stomach metastatic to the transverse colon. Localized right-sided ulceration and narrowing (arrow) simulate Crohn's colitis.

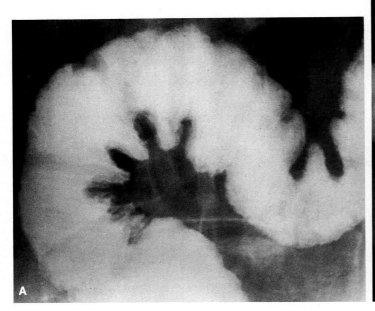

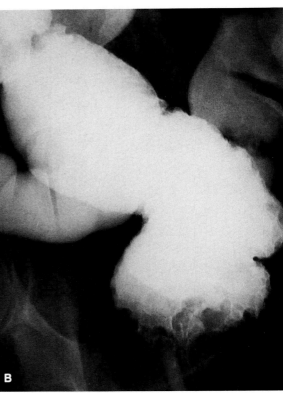

Fig. 48-63. Lymphoma. **(A)** Diffuse, fine ulcerations simulate a non-neoplastic ulcerating colitis. **(B)** Rectal ulcerations with nodular tumor involvement simulate intense inflammatory mucosal edema.

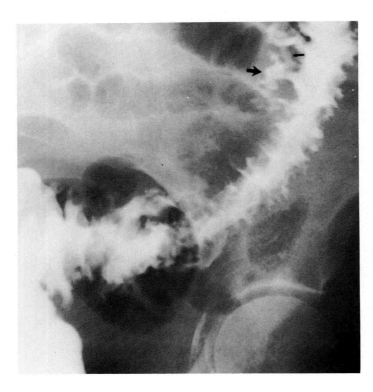

Fig. 48-64. Leukemic infiltration. There is diffuse, deep ulceration with submucosal extension **(arrows)**. (Limberakis AJ, Mossler JA, Roberts L et al: Leukemic infiltration of the colon. AJR 131:725–728, 1978. Copyright 1978. Reproduced with permission)

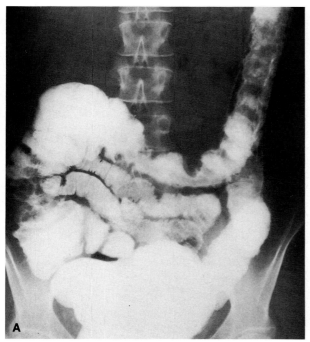
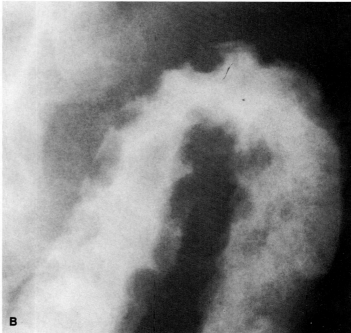

Fig. 48-65.   Colitis in Behcet's syndrome. **(A)** Barium enema examination demonstrates extensive involvement of all of the large bowel except for the rectosigmoid and hepatic flexure regions. The affected mucosa is nodular, ulcerated, and thickened secondary to granulomatous disease. **(B)** Enlarged view of the splenic flexure shows deep, circular ulcerations of uniform size and multiple nodular mucosal lesions. (Goldstein SJ, Crooks DJM: Colitis in Behcet's syndrome. Radiology 128:321–323, 1978)

INORGANIC MERCURY POISONING

Poisoning with inorganic mercury can cause intestinal hemorrhage and ulceration of the colon. The clinical history and concomitant renal involvement should permit differentiation of this condition from other forms of ulcerating colitis.

BEHCET'S SYNDROME

Behcet's syndrome is an uncommon multiple-system disease characterized by ulcerations of the buccal and genital mucosa, ocular inflammation, and a variety of skin lesions. Colonic involvement associated with diarrhea, abdominal pain, and bleeding occasionally occurs. The appearance on barium enema varies from mild proctitis to pancolitis with multiple discrete ulcers and inflammatory polyposis (Fig. 48-65). Aphthous ulcers and skip lesions are common. The appearance of central ringlike collections of barium superimposed on large nodular lesions in the terminal ileum has been reported to be a specific intestinal manifestation of Behcet's syndrome (see Fig. 67-10). The ulcers in Behcet's syndrome tend to be larger and deeper than those in Crohn's colitis, leading to a high incidence of perfo-

ration and hemorrhage, both of which are life-threatening complications.

DIVERTICULOSIS/DIVERTICULITIS

Rarely, small diverticula projecting from the colon are confused with the serrated colonic margin in a patient with ulcerative colitis. In almost every instance, however, the appearance of diverticula as saclike outpouchings with short necks, often associated with deep criss-crossing ridges of thickened circular muscle (sawtooth pattern), is easy to distinguish from true ulceration (Fig. 48-66). In diverticulitis, extravasated contrast material arising as a tiny projection from the top of a perforated diverticulum can simulate an acute ulceration. Ulcerative or Crohn's colitis and diverticular disease of the colon can coexist. In these cases, fine ulcerations within and about the diverticula are often demonstrated.

SOLITARY RECTAL ULCER SYNDROME

The solitary rectal ulcer syndrome is a distinct clinical entity occurring mainly in young patients complaining of rectal bleeding. Constipation or diarrhea

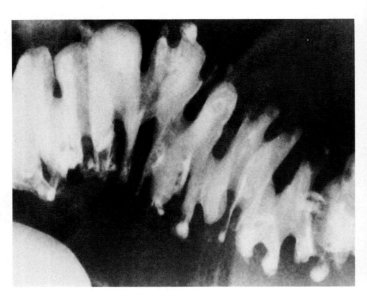

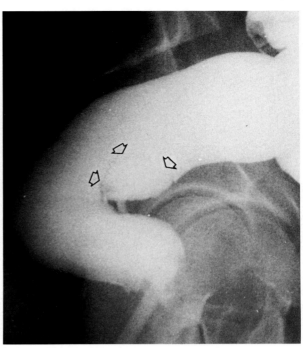

48-66

48-67

Fig. 48-66. Diverticulosis. The small diverticula clearly represent saclike outpouchings with short necks rather than diffuse ulcerations.

Fig. 48-67. Solitary rectal ulcer syndrome. Ill-defined ulcer **(arrows)** on the anterior rectal wall is shown on this single-contrast examination. (Chapa HJ, Smith HJ, Dickinson TA: Benign (solitary) ulcer of the rectum: Another cause for rectal stricture. Gastrointest Radiol 6:85–88, 1981)

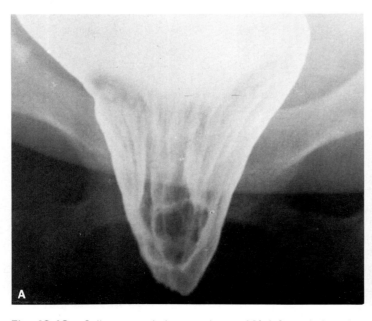

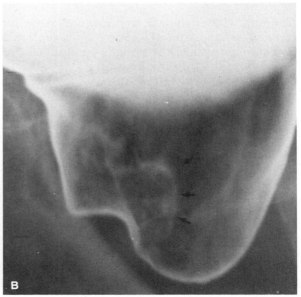

Fig. 48-68. Solitary rectal ulcer syndrome. **(A)** A frontal view demonstrates prolapse of the rectum with a polypoid mass in the posterior aspect. **(B)** An oblique view better defines the polypoid mass. The appearance is that of a submucosal mass lesion without ulceration. (Feczko PJ, O'Connell DJ, Riddell RH et al: Solitary rectal ulcer syndrome: Radiologic manifestations. AJR 135:499–506, 1980. Copyright 1980. Reproduced with permission)

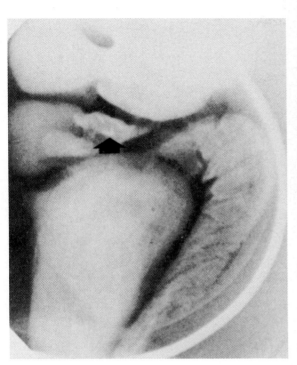
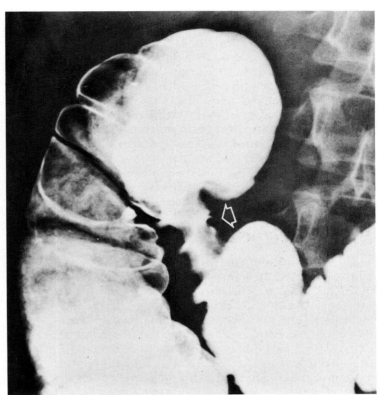

48-69   48-70

Fig. 48-69. Benign cecal ulcer **(arrow)** in the region of the ileocecal valve. (Brodey PA, Hill RP, Baron S: Benign ulceration of the cecum. Radiology 122:323–327, 1977)

Fig. 48-70. Nonspecific ulcer of the colon. A radiograph of the hepatic flexure shows an area of narrowing in the proximal transverse colon with ulceration along its inferior aspect and marginal spiculation **(arrow)**. (Gardiner GA, Bird CR: Nonspecific ulcers of the colon resembling annular carcinoma. Radiology 137:331–334, 1980)

can occur; pain is an inconstant feature. Solitary and occasionally multiple ulcers occur predominantly on the anterior or anterolateral aspects of the rectum (Fig. 48-67). Although the precise etiology is unclear, the ulcers may be secondary to partial rectal mucosal prolapse and traumatic ulceration related to pelvic muscle discoordination during defecation.

The earliest radiographic and pathologic change in this condition is nodularity of the rectal mucosa (preulcerative phase) (Fig. 48-68). This is followed by the development of ulcerations that are usually single but may be of various sizes and shapes and occur within 15 cm of the anal verge and near a thickened, edematous valve of Houston. Long-standing ulceration produces progressive fibrosis leading to rectal stricture. When either ulceration or stricturing is present, differentiation of the solitary rectal ulcer syndrome from inflammatory bowel disease or malignancy can be difficult.

NONSPECIFIC BENIGN ULCERATION OF THE COLON

Nonspecific ulceration of the colon is a diagnosis of exclusion that is rarely made preoperatively. Although several etiologies have been suggested (peptic ulceration, solitary diverticulitis, drugs, mucosal trauma, infection, vascular disease), no precise cause has been identified. The clinical symptoms of nonspecific ulcers depend on their location. Ulcers in the ascending colon usually present acutely, mimicking appendicitis. Nonspecific ulcers of the transverse and descending colon have a more insidious onset and suggest carcinoma, obstruction, or diverticulitis. Severe complications include perforation with secondary peritonitis, frank hemorrhage, and stricture.

More than half of all nonspecific colonic ulcers occur in the cecum and ascending colon in the region of the ileocecal valve (Fig. 48-69). Most are

single, though multiple ulcers are present in up to
20% of cases. The ulcers can be superficial or extend throughout all layers of the colon wall. They
range from small ulcerations, which may be only a
few millimeters in size, to large ulcerations involving the entire circumference of the colon. Nonspecific ulcers usually arise on the antimesenteric wall
of the bowel, in contrast to diverticula, which occur
along the mesenteric border. In most cases, nonspecific benign ulcerations are associated with an intense inflammatory reaction that produces a masslike effect (Fig. 48-70). Based on a barium enema
examination, the preoperative radiographic diagnosis is usually carcinoma of the colon.

DRUG-INDUCED COLITIS

Various drugs and toxins are being increasingly recognized as the cause of colonic damage and should
be included in the differential diagnosis of ulcerating colitis. Among the drugs associated with colitis
are cancer chemotherapeutic agents (cytosine arabinoside, methotrexate, hydroxyurea), methyldopa,
nonsteroidal anti-inflammatory agents, cimetidine,
the antifungal agent flucytosine, and elemental
gold. An appearance mimicking ischemic colitis has
been reported in patients receiving estrogen and
progesterone, vasopressin, and ergot.

DIVERSION COLITIS

Diversion colitis is a nonspecific inflammation in a
segment of colon that has been surgically isolated
from the fecal stream by placement of a proximal
colostomy or ileostomy. It is unknown whether lack

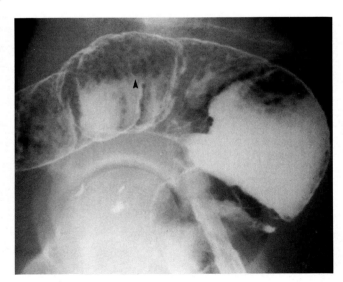

Fig. 48-71. *Diversion colitis. Double-contrast enema of rectosigmoid mucous fistula shows mucosal nodularity and occasional punctate superficial ulceration* **(arrowhead)**. *(Scott RL, Pinstein ML: Diversion colitis demonstrated by double-contrast barium enema. AJR 143:767–768, 1984. Copyright 1984. Reproduced with permission)*

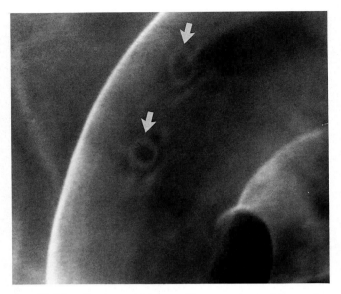

Fig. 48-72. *Post-rectal biopsy. Close-up view of the rectosigmoid shows two shallow, ringlike ulcers* **(arrows)** *with surrounding radiolucent halos. Two other ringlike ulcers were identified more distally in the rectum. These findings were the sites of four rectal biopsies taken from normal-appearing mucosa 4 days earlier. (Lev–Toaff AS, Levine MS, Laufer I et al: Ringlike rectal ulcers after biopsy or polypectomy. AJR 148:285–286, 1987. Copyright 1987. Reproduced with permission)*

of contact of the distal colonic segment to feces
somehow deprives the colonic mucosa of necessary
exposure to enteric bacteria, bacterial byproducts,
or nutrients. Conversely, it is conceivable that diversion colitis results from stasis within the inactive
segment, causing excessive mucosal exposure to
unrecognized intraluminal toxins. Radiographically, diversion colitis resembles ulcerative or
Crohn's colitis with punctate or aphthous ulcerations that may produce a diffuse, granular mucosal
appearance in severe or long-standing cases (Fig.
48-71). Isolated inflammatory polyps or diffuse mucosal nodularity may occur. The proximal colon, up
to the ostomy site, is never involved. Diversion colitis seems to resolve spontaneously when the involved, unused segment is reanastomosed and again
exposed to the fecal stream.

POST-RECTAL BIOPSY

A well-defined ring shadow on a normal background mucosa may be seen on barium enema examinations performed within several days following
rectal biopsy or polypectomy (Fig. 48-72). The shallow, ringlike ulcer is surrounded by a radiolucent
elevation, which is presumably caused by a zone of
edematous mucosa or the re-epithelializing margin
of the mucosal defect. Therefore, it is important that
the radiologist know whether a biopsy or polypectomy has been recently performed on any patient
referred for barium enema examination.

BIBLIOGRAPHY

Annamunthodo H, Marryatt J: Barium studies in intestinal lymphogranuloma venereum. Br J Radiol 34:53–57, 1961

Atkinson GO Jr, Gay BB, Ball TI Jr et al: *Yersinia enterocolitica* colitis in infants: Radiographic changes. Radiology 148:113–116, 1983

Balthazar EJ, Megibow AJ, Fazzini E et al: Cytomegalovirus colitis in AIDS: Radiographic findings in 11 patients. Radiology 155:585–589, 1985

Bjorkengren AG, Resnick D, Sartoris DJ: Enteropathic arthropathies. Radiol Clin North Am 25:189–198, 1987

Brodey PA, Hill RP, Baron S: Benign ulceration of the cecum. Radiology 122:323–327, 1977

Brodey PA, Fertig S, Aron JM: *Campylobacter* enterocolitis: Radiographic features. AJR 139:1199–1201, 1982

Cardoso JM, Kimura K, Stoopen M et al: Radiology of invasive amebiasis of the colon. AJR 128:935–941, 1977

Caroline DF, Evers K: Colitis: Radiographic features and differentiation of idiopathic inflammatory bowel disease. Radiol Clin North Am 25:47–66, 1987

Carrera GF, Young S, Lewicki AM: Intestinal tuberculosis. Gastrointest Radiol 1:147–155, 1976

Chait A: Schistosomiasis mansoni: Roentgenologic observations in a nonendemic area. AJR 90:688–708, 1963

Cho SR, Tisnado J, Liu CI et al: Bleeding cytomegalovirus ulcer of the colon: Barium enema and angiography. AJR 136:1213–1215, 1981

Cole FM: Innominate grooves of the colon: Morphological characteristics and etiologic mechanisms. Radiology 128:41–43, 1978

Dallemand S, Waxman M, Farman J: Radiological manifestations of *Strongyloides stercoralis*. Gastrointest Radiol 8:45–51, 1983

Drasin GF, Moss JP, Cheng SH: *Strongyloides stercoralis* colitis: Findings in four cases. Radiology 126:619–621, 1978

DuBrow RA, Frank PH: Barium evaluation of the anal canal in patients with inflammatory bowel disease. AJR 140:1151–1157, 1983

Eisenberg RL, Montgomery CK, Margulis AR: Colitis in the elderly: Ischemic colitis mimicking ulcerative and granulomatous colitis. AJR 133:1113–1118, 1979

Feczko PJ, Barbour J, Halpert RD et al: Crohn disease in the elderly. Radiology 157:303–304, 1985

Feczko PJ, O'Connell DJ, Riddell RH et al: Solitary rectal ulcer syndrome: Radiologic manifestations. AJR 135:499–506, 1980

Fernbach SK, Lloyd–Still JD: Radiographic findings in severe rotavirus-induced colitis. J Can Assoc Radiol 35:192–194, 1984

Fortson DW, Tedesco FJ: Drug-induced colitis: A review. Am J Gastroenterol 79:878–883, 1984

Frager DH, Frager JD, Wolf EL et al: Cytomegalovirus colitis in acquired immune deficiency syndrome: Radiologic spectrum. Gastrointest Radiol 11:241–246, 1986

Frank DF, Bert RN, Goldstein HM: Pseudoulcerations of the colon on barium enema examination. Gastrointest Radiol 2:129–131, 1977

Gardiner GA, Bird CR: Nonspecific ulcers of the colon resembling annular carcinoma. Radiology 137:331–334, 1980

Gardiner R, Smith C: Infective enterocolitides. Radiol Clin North Am 25:67–78, 1987

Gardiner R, Stevenson GW: Colitides. Radiol Clin North Am 20:797–815, 1982

Gedgaudas–McClees RK: Aphthoid ulcerations in ileocecal candidiasis. AJR 141:973–974, 1983

Gore RM, Morn CS, Kirby DF et al: CT findings in ulcerative, granulomatous, and indeterminate colitis. AJR 143:279–284, 1984

Iida M, Matsui T, Fuchigami T et al: Ischemic colitis: Serial changes on double-contrast barium enema examination. Radiology 159:337–341, 1986

Kim SK, Cho C, Levinsohn EM: Caustic colitis due to detergent enema. AJR 134:397–398, 1980

Lachman R, Soong J, Wishon G et al: *Yersinia* colitis. Gastrointest Radiol 2:133–135, 1977

Lammer J, Dirschmid K, Hugel H: Carcinomatous matastases to the colon simulating Crohn's disease. Gastrointest Radiol 6:89–91, 1981

Levine MS, Piccolello ML, Sollenberger LC et al: Solitary rectal ulcer syndrome: A radiologic diagnosis? Gastrointest Radiol 11:187–193, 1986

Lev–Toaff AS, Levine MS, Laufer I et al: Ringlike rectal ulcers after biopsy or polypectomy. AJR 148:285–286, 1987

Lichtenstein JE: Radiologic-pathologic correlation of inflammatory bowel disease. Radiol Clin North Am 25:3–24, 1987

Limberakis AJ, Mossler JA, Roberts L et al: Leukemic infiltration of the colon. AJR 131:725–728, 1978

Matsuura K, Nakata H, Takeda N et al: Innominate lines of the colon: Radiological-histological correlation. Radiology 123:581–584, 1977

McLean AM, Simms DM, Homer MJ: Ileal ring ulcers in Behcet syndrome. AJR 140:947–948, 1983

Menuck LS, Brahme F, Amberg J et al: Colonic changes of herpes zoster. AJR 127:273–276, 1976

Niv Y, Bat L: Solitary rectal ulcer syndrome: Clinical, endoscopic and histological spectrum. Am J Gastroenterol 81:486–491, 1986

Owen RL, Hill JL: Rectal and pharyngeal gonorrhea in homosexual men. JAMA 220:1315–1318, 1972

Perez CA, Sturim HS, Kouchoukos NT et al: Some clinical and radiolographic features of gastrointestinal histoplasmosis. Radiology 86:482–487, 1966

Rogers LF, Goldstein HM: Roentgen manifestations of radiation injury to the gastrointestinal tract. Gastrointest Radiol 2:281–291, 1977

Rogers LF, Ralls PW, Boswell WD et al: Amebiasis: Unusual radiographic manifestations. AJR 135:1253–1257, 1980

Rubesin SE, Levine MS: Omental cakes: Colonic involvement by omental metastases. Radiology 154:593–596, 1985

Scott RL, Pinstein ML: Diversion colitis demonstrated by double-contrast barium enema. AJR 143:767–768, 1984

Shah SJ, Scholz FJ: Anorectal herpes: Radiographic findings. Radiology 147:81–82, 1983

Siskind BN, Burrell MI: Intraluminal meniscoid ulcer in the colon: An unusual sign of malignancy. Gastrointest Radiol 11:251–253, 1986

Stanley RJ, Melson GL, Tedesco EJ: The spectrum of radiographic findings in antibiotic-related pseudomembranous colitis. Radiology 111:519–524, 1974

Stanley RJ, Tesesco FJ, Melson GL et al: The colitis of Behcet's disease: A clinical-radiographic correlation. Radiology 114:603–604, 1975

Thompson WM, Kelvin FM, Rice RP: Inflammation and necrosis of the transverse colon secondary to pancreatitis. AJR 128:943–948, 1977

Tielbeek AV, Rosenbusch G, Muytjens HL et al: Roentgenologic changes of the colon in *Campylobacter* infection. Gastrointest Radiol 10:358–361, 1985

Williams SM, Harned RK: Hepatobiliary complications of inflammatory bowel disease. Radiol Clin North Am 25:175–188, 1987

49 NARROWING OF THE COLON

Disease Entities

Chronic or healing stage of an ulcerating colitis
  Ulcerative colitis
  Crohn's colitis
  Ischemic colitis
  Specific infections
    Protozoan
      Amebiasis
      Schistosomiasis
    Bacterial
      Bacillary dysentery
      Tuberculosis
      Gonorrheal proctitis
      Lymphogranuloma venereum
    Fungal
    Viral
      Anorectal giant condyloma acuminatum
      Herpes zoster
      Cytomegalovirus
    Helminthic
      Strongyloidiasis
  Radiation injury
  Cathartic colon
  Caustic colitis
  Solitary rectal ulcer syndrome
  Nonspecific benign ulcer of the colon
Malignant lesions
  Primary adenocarcinoma
    "Apple-core"
    Scirrhous

Metastases
  Direct invasion
  Intraperitoneal seeding
  Hematogenous spread
  Lymphangitic spread
Carcinoma developing in an ulcerating colitis
  Ulcerative colitis
  Crohn's colitis
Sigmoid carcinoma following ureterosigmoidostomy
Kaposi's sarcoma
Carcinoid tumor
Lymphoma
Diverticulitis
Miscellaneous disorders
  Pancreatitis
  Amyloidosis
  Endometriosis
  Pelvic lipomatosis
  Retractile mesenteritis
  Adhesive bands
  Typhlitis
  Pseudolymphoma
  Narrowing at the site of surgical anastomosis

The causes of narrowing of the colonic lumen can be conveniently divided into two broad subgroups: a chronic or healing stage of an ulcerating colitis

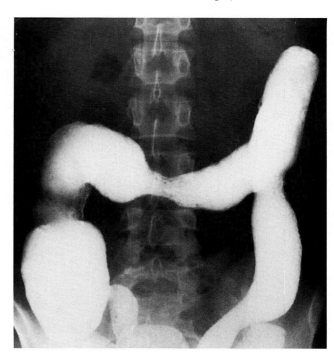

Fig. 49-1. Chronic ulcerative colitis ("lead-pipe" colon). Muscular hypertrophy and spasm cause shortening and rigidity of the colon with a loss of haustral markings.

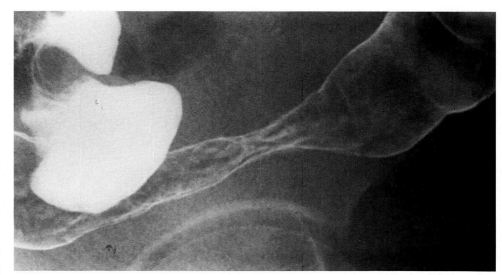

Fig. 49-2. Chronic ulcerative colitis. Smoothly tapered stricture of the sigmoid colon. (Caroline DF, Evers K: Colitis: Radiographic features and differentiation of idiopathic inflammatory bowel disease. Radiol Clin North Am 25:47–66, 1987)

and a malignant lesion. Malignancies of the colon usually arise *de novo*. However, they can represent direct extension or hematogenous spread from an extracolonic primary tumor or be a recognized complication of an ulcerating inflammatory process.

ULCERATIVE COLITIS

The chronic stage of ulcerative colitis is characterized by foreshortening of the colon with depression of the flexures, rigidity, and narrowing of the bowel lumen. The haustral pattern is absent, and the bowel contour is relatively smooth because of healing of ulcerations and re-epithelialization. The colon appears as a symmetric, rigid tubular structure ("lead-pipe" colon) (Fig. 49-1). Although usually considered to be secondary to fibrosis, colonic narrowing can also be due to muscular hypertrophy and spasm. Evidence for the important role of muscular spasm is the occasional demonstration of a narrowed, foreshortened colon reverting to almost normal caliber on follow-up studies. This would not be expected if the narrowing were due solely to fibrosis.

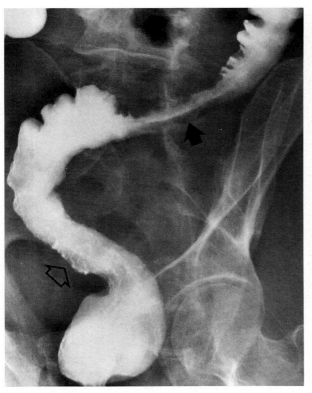
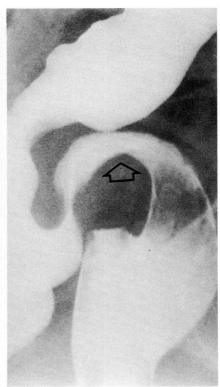

49-3   49-4

Fig. 49-3. Chronic ulcerative colitis. A benign stricture is visible in the sigmoid colon **(solid arrow)**. Note the ulcerative changes in the upper rectum and proximal sigmoid colon **(open arrow)**.

Fig. 49-4. Chronic ulcerative colitis. A benign rectosigmoid stricture with a smooth contour and tapering margins **(arrow)** is evident.

Benign colonic strictures develop in up to 10% of patients with chronic ulcerative colitis (Fig. 49-2). They rarely cause symptoms and are often incidental findings on barium enema examination. Occasionally, they result in partial colonic obstruction. The most common site of benign stricture is the rectum and sigmoid, followed next in frequency by the transverse colon. The strictures are usually short (2–3 cm) but can extend up to 30 cm in length (Fig. 49-3). Although most commonly single, strictures in ulcerative colitis can be multiple, especially in patients with universal colonic disease.

Radiographically, a stricture due to ulcerative colitis has a typically benign appearance with a concentric lumen, smooth contours, and fusiform, pliable, tapering margins (Fig. 49-4). Occasionally, the stricture is somewhat eccentric and has irregular contours, simulating a malignancy. Although the bowel proximal to a benign stricture can be slightly dilated, obstruction is rare, and the colon usually empties well on evacuation. Because carcinoma in patients with ulcerative colitis can have a radiographic appearance indistinguishable from a benign stricture, colonoscopy or surgery is frequently required to make this differentiation.

CROHN'S COLITIS

In Crohn's disease of the colon, deep ulceration and transmural inflammation with thickening of the bowel wall produce multiple irregular stenotic segments and strictures. Narrowing and stricture formation occur frequently and early in the course of Crohn's colitis, in contrast to ulcerative colitis. Patients with chronic disease may develop a "lead-pipe" colon identical to that seen in ulcerative colitis (Fig. 49-5). Occasionally, an eccentric stricture with a suggestion of overhanging edges can make it difficult to exclude the possibility of carcinoma (Fig. 49-6). In most instances, however, characteristic features of Crohn's disease elsewhere in the colon (deep ulcerations, pseudopolyposis, skip lesions, sinus tracts, fistulas) clearly indicate the correct diagnosis.

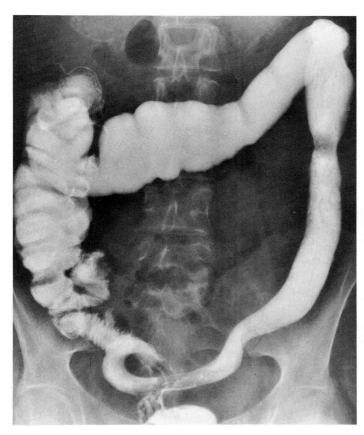

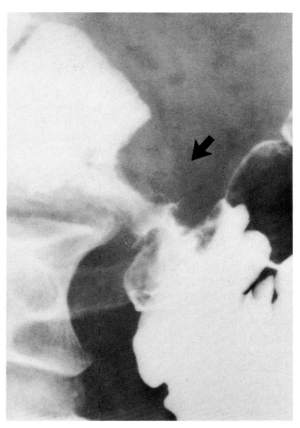

49-5   49-6

Fig. 49-5. Chronic Crohn's colitis. Foreshortening and loss of haustrations involving the colon distal to the hepatic flexure simulate the appearance of chronic ulcerative colitis.

Fig. 49-6. Chronic Crohn's colitis. A benign stricture with overhanging edges in the transverse colon simulates carcinoma **(arrow)**.

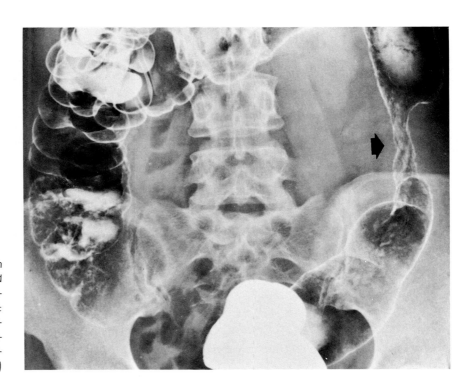

Fig. 49-7. Ischemic colitis. A stricture in the descending colon **(arrow)** followed healing of the ischemic episode. (Eisenberg RL, Montgomery CK, Margulis AR: Colitis in the elderly: Ischemic colitis mimicking ulcerative and granulomatous colitis. AJR 133:1113–1118, 1979. Copyright 1979. Reproduced with permission)

ISCHEMIC COLITIS

During the healing phase of ischemic colitis, marked fibrosis of the submucosal and muscular layers can lead to stricture formation (Fig. 49-7). Flattening and rigidity of the mesenteric border combined with pleating of the antimesenteric margin produce the radiographic appearance of multiple sacculations or pseudodiverticula. Progressive fibrosis causes tubular narrowing and a smooth stricture. Stricture of the rectum rarely occurs because of the excellent collateral blood supply to this segment. Ischemic strictures are generally shorter than the original length of ischemic involvement seen on radiographs obtained during the acute stage of the disease, implying that some of the ischemic bowel has retained sufficient blood supply to permit complete healing. Luminal narrowing due to ischemia can present as an annular constricting lesion. If the history is not typical and no prior radiographs have been obtained, this appearance strongly suggests carcinoma. A repeat examination within 1 week usually permits differentiation between carcinoma and ischemia. An ischemic process often demonstrates an altered appearance or even complete reversion to normal, whereas a malignant lesion is unchanged. At times, bleeding into the colon wall can produce tumorlike masses (thumbprinting) that are so large as to severely encroach upon the lumen and even occlude it.

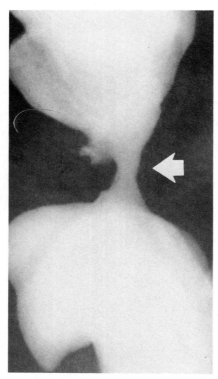

Fig. 49-8. *Ameboma. An eccentric constricting lesion in the cecum* **(arrow)** *simulates malignancy.*

SPECIFIC INFECTIONS

AMEBIASIS

Although patients with acute amebiasis typically have segmental spasm and irritability associated with difficulty in fully distending the colon, chronic benign strictures are uncommon complications if the patients are treated properly. When stenoses occur, they are the result of fibrotic healing of mucosal ulcerations and are most common in the transverse colon, sigmoid colon, and flexures. The strictures are often multiple and long, tapering gradually at both ends into adjacent bowel of normal caliber and mucosal pattern.

Amebomas are localized masses characterized by prominent thickening of the bowel wall due to a granulomatous response to bacterial superinfection in amebiasis. They can present as annular constrictions simulating malignancy (Fig. 49-8). Factors favoring the diagnosis of ameboma rather than a malignant lesion include multiplicity (Fig. 49-9), longer length (Fig. 49-10), and pliability of the lesion, evidence of amebiasis elsewhere in the colon, and rapid improvement on antiamebic therapy.

SCHISTOSOMIASIS

Intense inflammation due to infestation by schistosomiasis can lead to reactive fibrosis, which causes narrowing of the colon, especially the sigmoid portion. This stenosing granulomatous process is often associated with extensive pericolonic infiltration. In nonendemic areas (*e.g.*, among the Puerto Rican population in New York City), this radiographic pattern can be mistaken for Crohn's disease or colonic malignancy.

BACILLARY DYSENTERY

Extensive scarring and fibrosis in chronic bacillary dysentery can cause rigidity, loss of haustration, and tubular narrowing of a segment of the colon. Because repeated episodes of exacerbation and remission are not uncommon, chronic bacillary dysentery can clinically resemble chronic ulcerative colitis.

TUBERCULOSIS

In chronic stages of tuberculosis of the colon, reparative healing with fibrosis leads to distortion, rigidity, and narrowing of the lumen (Fig. 49-11). Segmental involvement can produce an annular ulcerating lesion mimicking colonic carcinoma. Tuberculosis should be considered a strong diagnostic possibility whenever segmental colonic narrowing develops in a young adult who originates from an endemic area, especially if there is chest radiograph or skin test evidence of active or chronic tubercu-

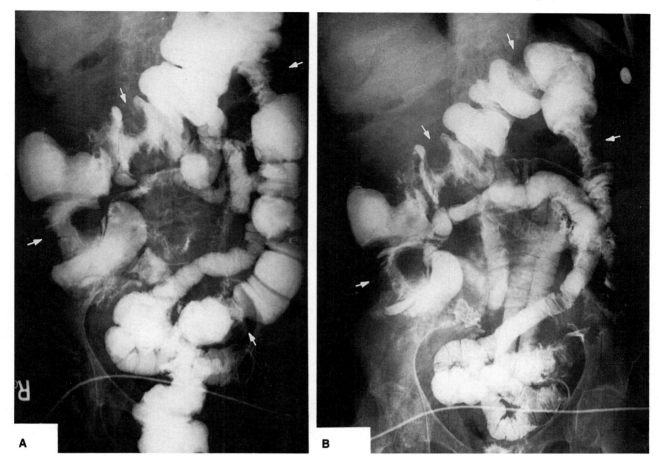

Fig. 49-9. Ameboma. **(A)** Multiple classic "apple-core" lesions with irregular mucosa and overhanging edges. **(B)** Postevacuation film accentuates the constricting lesions and the incompetence of the ileocecal valve. (Messersmith RN, Chase GJ: Amebiasis presenting as multiple apple-core lesions. Am J Gastroenterol 79:238–241, 1984)

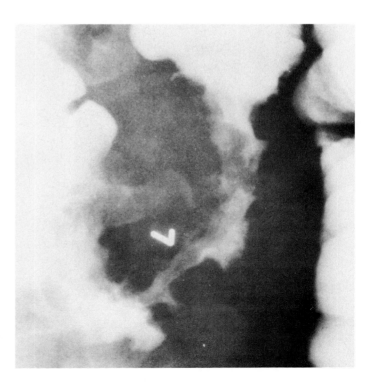

Fig. 49-10. Ameboma. There is an irregular constricting lesion in the transverse colon. The relatively long area of involvement tends to favor an inflammatory etiology.

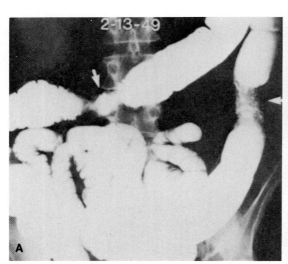 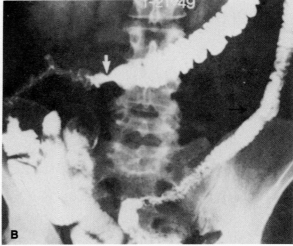

Fig. 49-11. Tuberculosis. **(A)** The patient has ileocecal disease and two sharply demarcated areas of colonic inflammation and narrowing more distally (midtransverse and mid-descending colon; **arrows**). **(B)** After 5 months of streptomycin therapy, the descending colon has healed without scarring. The other areas of involvement remain unchanged. (Carrera GF, Young S, Lewicki AM: Intestinal tuberculosis. Gastrointest Radiol 1:147–155, 1976)

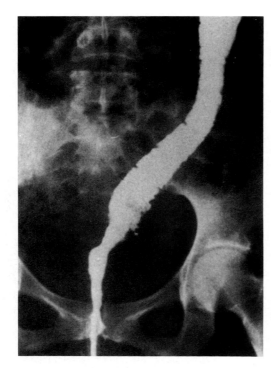

Fig. 49-12. Lymphogranuloma venereum. Long stricture of the rectum and lower sigmoid with shortening and straightening of the more proximal colon. Mucosal ulceration is also seen. (Cockshott WP, Middlemiss H: Clinical Radiology in the Tropics. Edinburgh, Churchill Livingstone, 1979)

losis. In most cases, inflammatory disease in the ileocecal region is also present.

GONORRHEAL PROCTITIS

Anorectal gonorrhea is usually asymptomatic but may produce anal irritation, tenesmus, discharge, or rectal bleeding. Untreated, rectal stricture develops in about 20% of patients.

LYMPHOGRANULOMA VENEREUM

The hallmark of lymphogranuloma venereum is the development of a rectal stricture (Fig. 49-12). These strictures are usually long and tubular, beginning just above the anus and varying in appearance from a short, isolated narrowing to a long, stenotic segment up to 25 cm in length (proctitis obliterans). The mucosa is irregular, with multiple deep ulcers; the lumen can be so narrow that it resembles a thin string. The portion of normal colon proximal to the stricture is usually dilated with loss of haustration and gradually tapers in a smooth, conical fashion. In a patient with a rectal stricture, the demonstration of fistulas and sinus tracts communicating with perirectal abscess cavities, the lower vagina, or perianal skin should suggest the diagnosis of lymphogranuloma venereum (Fig. 49-13).

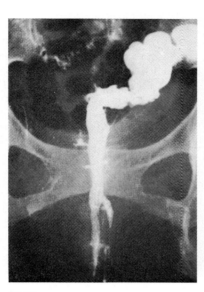
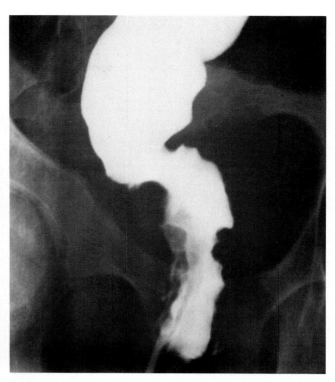

49-13   **49-14**

Fig. 49-13. Lymphogranuloma venereum. Long stricture of the rectum and lower sigmoid with multiple perirectal fistulas and sinuses. (Bockus HL: Gastroenterology. Philadelphia, WB Saunders, 1976)

Fig. 49-14. Anorectal giant condyloma acuminatum. Asymmetric circumferential infiltration of the anal canal and distal rectum for about 8 cm from the anal orifice. There is narrowing, rigidity, and multiple luminal and contour defects. (Balthazar EJ, Streiter M, Megibow AJ: Anal rectal giant condyloma acuminatum [Buschke–Loewenstein tumor]: CT and radiographic manifestations. Radiology 150:651–653, 1984)

FUNGAL DISEASES

An irregular mass of inflammatory tissue due to chronic fungal infestation can produce narrowing of the bowel lumen closely simulating colonic carcinoma.

ANORECTAL GIANT CONDYLOMA ACUMINATUM

Condyloma acuminatum ("venereal wart") is a common papillary epithelial lesion that occurs predominantly in the genital and perianal areas and is caused by a virus from the Papova group. The lesion is typically small, superficial, benign, and noninvasive and responds to topical treatment, though local recurrences are common. Occasionally, a giant form of condyloma develops, possibly associated with homosexual activity. This giant condyloma shows active papillary proliferation leading to local expansion with penetration and invasion of the surrounding tissues. Infiltration of the anal canal and distal rectum causes asymmetric narrowing with thickening of the wall, a pattern that may mimic malignancy (Fig. 49-14). Computed tomography (CT) may be of value to accurately demonstrate the location and extent of the lesion.

OTHER INFECTIOUS CAUSES OF COLITIS

Segmental narrowing with small ulcerations can be a manifestation of colonic involvement with herpes zoster. Although the radiographic appearance can simulate ulcerative or ischemic colitis, the short length of the lesion and the characteristic clinical history should suggest the correct diagnosis. In renal transplant recipients undergoing immunosuppressive therapy, the combination of severe lower gastrointestinal bleeding, colonic ulcers, and intense edema causing luminal narrowing favors the

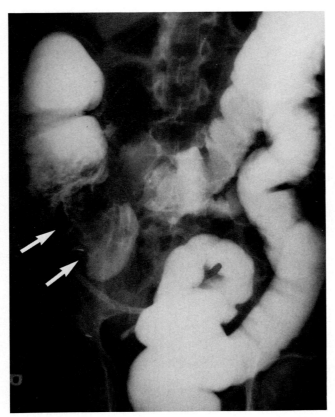

Fig. 49-15. Cytomegalovirus-induced ulcer disease of the colon. Marked intramural swelling of the cecum and proximal ascending colon causes severe narrowing **(arrows)**. (Cho SR, Tisnado J, Liu CI: Bleeding cytomegalovirus ulcers of the colon: Barium enema and angiography. AJR 136:1213–1215, 1981. Copyright 1981. Reproduced with permission)

diagnosis of reactivation of latent cytomegalovirus infection (Fig. 49-15).

Colonic strictures can develop in the late stages of ulcerating colitis caused by the nematode *Strongyloides stercoralis*. The associated loss of normal haustration and mucosal detail can mimic chronic ulcerative colitis.

RADIATION INJURY

The most common manifestation of chronic radiation-induced colitis is a long, smooth stricture of the rectum and sigmoid colon that develops within 6 months to 24 months of irradiation (Fig. 49-16). This complication is probably related to chronic ischemia caused by an obliterative arteritis in the bowel wall; it is therefore most common in patients with diabetes, atherosclerosis, and hypertension, whose vessels are already compromised. Radiation injury to the bowel primarily involves the colon. Although the small intestine is more radiosensitive than the

colon, it is less susceptible to radiation injury from fixed ports because of its inherent mobility. The incidence of radiation injury to the colon depends on the type of radiation, total dose administered, and duration of therapy. In general, radiation colitis is unusual in patients who have received less than 4000 rads. The incidence substantially increases if the dose exceeds 6000 rads or if a second course of irradiation is given for recurrent tumor.

Radiation damage results in mucosal atrophy and fibrous tissue replacement within the bowel wall, leading to narrowing of the lumen. Thickening of the bowel wall and the surrounding pelvic tissues tends to straighten the involved segment, causing it to be elevated out of the pelvis. A short, irregular radiation-induced stricture, especially if it has a relatively abrupt margin of transition, can closely resemble primary or metastatic malignancy. Surgery may be required for a definitive diagnosis to be made.

CATHARTIC COLON

Cathartic colon is due to prolonged use of stimulant/irritant cathartics (*e.g.*, castor oil, phenolphtha-

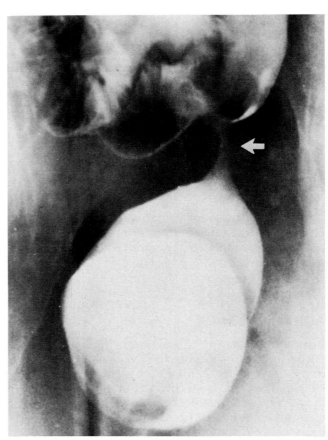

Fig. 49-16. Radiation-induced colitis. This smooth stricture of the rectosigmoid **(arrow)** developed 18 months after irradiation.

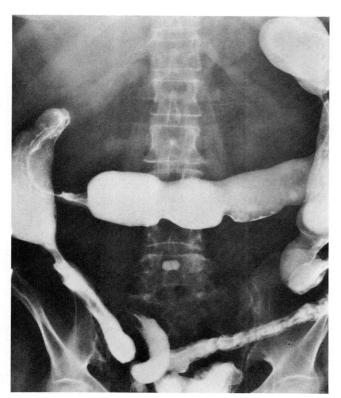

Fig. 49-17. Cathartic colon. Bizarre contractions with irregular areas of narrowing primarily involve the right colon. Although the ileocecal valve is gaping, simulating ulcerative colitis, no ulcerations are identified.

lein, cascara, senna, podophyllum). The typical patient with this condition is a woman of middle age who has habitually used irritant cathartics for more than 15 years. Ironically, the patient often initially denies use of cathartics and complains only of constipation. Because prolonged stimulation of the colon by irritant laxatives results in neuromuscular incoordination and an inability of the colonic musculature to produce adequate contractile force without external stimulants, the patient with cathartic colon is often unable to have a bowel movement without laxative assistance. Cathartic colon can usually be separated clinically from a chronic ulcerating colitis because of the patient's history of life-long constipation and laxative use, in contrast to the complaint of diarrhea in most patients with inflammatory bowel disease.

The radiographic appearance of cathartic colon is similar to that of "burned out" chronic ulcerative colitis (Fig. 49-17). In contrast to ulcerative colitis, however, the absent or diminished haustral markings, bizarre contractions, and inconstant areas of narrowing primarily involve the right colon. In severe cases, the left side of the colon can also be affected, though the sigmoid and rectum usually appear normal. The mucosal pattern is linear or smooth; ulcerations are not seen. The ileocecal valve is frequently flattened and gaping, simulating the backwash ileitis seen in ulcerative colitis. Shortening of the ascending colon can be severe, but, unlike the tubular bowel in chronic ulcerative colitis, which is rigid, the shortened segment in a cathartic colon remains remarkably distensible. Inconstant areas of narrowing of the bowel lumen can be seen at fluoroscopy and on radiographs of patients with cathartic colon. These pseudostrictures primarily involve the hepatic flexure, vary in length, have a concentric lumen with tapering margins, and often disappear during a single examination.

CAUSTIC COLITIS

Luminal narrowing with stricture formation is a late complication of caustic colitis due to detergent enemas (Fig. 49-18). Within 1 month of corrosive damage to the colon, the inflammatory reaction subsides, and scar formation begins. This process eventually results in colonic strictures similar to those caused by caustic agents in the esophagus.

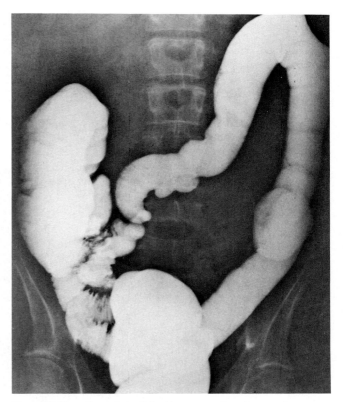

Fig. 49-18. Caustic colitis. Two months after a detergent enema, there is stenosis with irregular sacculations in the midtransverse colon. (Kim SK, Cho C, Levinsohn EM: Caustic colitis due to detergent enema. AJR 134:397–398, 1980. Copyright 1980. Reproduced with permission)

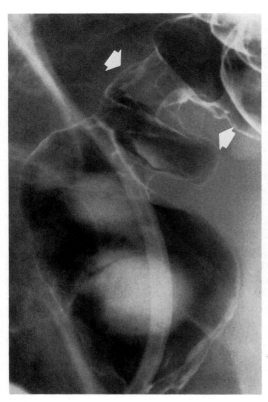
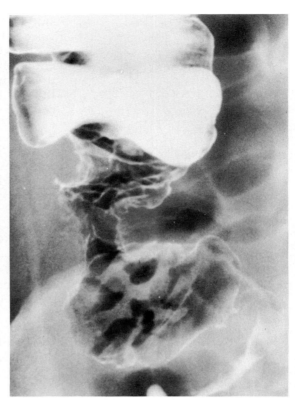

49-19   49-20

Fig. 49-19.   Solitary rectal ulcer syndrome. Steep oblique radiograph of the rectum shows markedly thickened valves of Houston with circumferential narrowing at the level of the second valve or rectosigmoid junction. Proctoscopy in this 57-year-old woman with rectal bleeding and intermittent left lower quadrant abdominal pain confirmed the presence of thickened rectal folds but also revealed multiple superficial ulcerations not seen radiographically in this region. (Levine MS, Piccolello ML, Sollenberger LC: Solitary rectal ulcer syndrome: A radiologic diagnosis? Gastrointest Radiol 11:187–193, 1986)

Fig. 49-20.   Nonspecific ulcer of the cecum. Fibrotic healing has produced an irregular area of narrowing, without visible ulceration, simulating carcinoma.

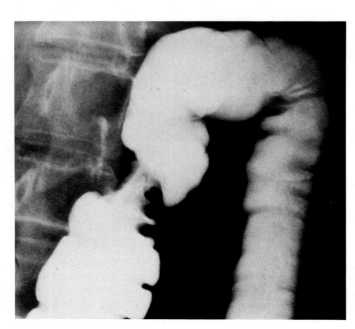

Fig. 49-21.   Nonspecific ulcer of the transverse colon causing irregular narrowing that simulates annular carcinoma. (Gardiner GA, Bird CR: Nonspecific ulcers of the colon resembling annular carcinoma. Radiology 137:331–334, 1980)

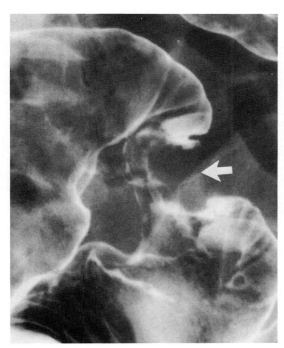

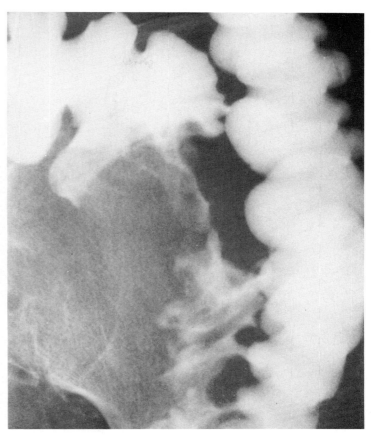

49-22   49-23

Fig. 49-22. Annular carcinoma of the sigmoid colon. A relatively short lesion **(arrow)** is evident with sharply defined proximal and distal margins.

Fig. 49-23. Annular carcinoma of the colon. There is severe narrowing of the bowel lumen with overhanging margins.

SOLITARY RECTAL ULCER SYNDROME

Stricture formation in the final stage of the solitary rectal ulcer syndrome reflects progressive fibrosis due to long-standing ulceration. If there are no previous barium enema examinations demonstrating mucosal nodularity or ulceration, it can be difficult to differentiate a stricture due to the solitary rectal ulcer syndrome from inflammatory bowel disease, lymphogranuloma venereum, or rectal malignancy (Fig. 49-19).

NONSPECIFIC BENIGN ULCER

Fibrotic strictures are a complication of nonspecific benign ulcers of the colon. Most frequently found in the cecum (Fig. 49-20), nonspecific ulcers can be complicated by perforation or hemorrhage. Fibrotic healing can cause smooth or irregular areas of narrowing, often with no visible ulceration, that can be radiographically indistinguishable from carcinoma (Fig. 49-21).

MALIGNANT LESIONS

ANNULAR CARCINOMA

Annular carcinoma ("apple-core," "napkin-ring") is one of the most typical forms of primary malignancy of the colon (Fig. 49-22). The characteristic combination of narrowing of the bowel lumen and abrupt change from tumor to normal bowel ("tumor shelf," "overhanging margins") is caused by extensive tumor infiltration and rigidity of the bowel wall (Fig. 49-23).

Among malignant tumors in the United States, the incidence of carcinoma of the colon is second only to that of skin cancer. This malignancy kills more persons than any malignant tumor other than cancer of the lung in men and breast cancer in

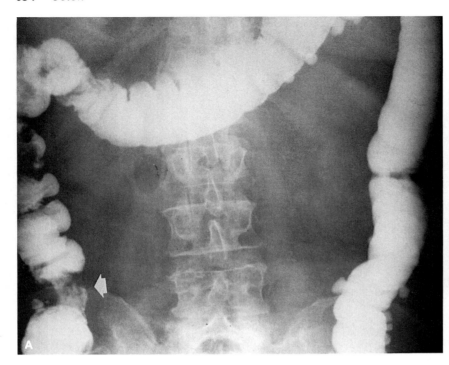

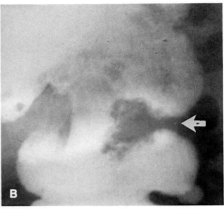

Fig. 49-24. Adenocarcinoma of the right colon. **(A)** Full and **(B)** coned views demonstrate an annular lesion **(arrows)** in a patient with anemia.

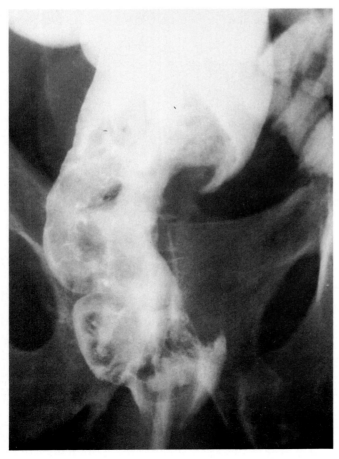

Fig. 49-25. Adenocarcinoma of the rectum. The patient presented with rectal bleeding and change in bowel habits.

women. Even with some improvement in lesion detection and medical and surgical therapy, the 5-year survival rate remains about 40%, having changed little in the last several decades.

Adenocarcinoma of the colon and rectum is primarily a disease of elderly persons, the peak incidence being in the 50- to 70-year range. Nevertheless, the disease occasionally develops in younger persons, in whom it tends to be far more aggressive and is associated with a low survival rate.

The etiology of carcinoma of the colon is unknown. There is considerable evidence to suggest that many, if not most, carcinomas of the colon arise in pre-existing villous or adenomatous polyps. It is unclear and controversial whether cancers arise *de novo* in normal colonic mucosa. Several of the hereditary intestinal polyposis syndromes, as well as ulcerative colitis, are known to have a predilection for secondary development of colon cancer. Because the incidence of the disease is far lower in underdeveloped countries than in the West, diet has been postulated as a possible causative factor. The unrefined high-fiber diet consumed in underdeveloped countries results in bulkier stools and faster fecal transit time, which may diminish the adverse effects of intestinal carcinogens and bacterial flora on the colonic mucosa.

Clinical Presentation

Detection of colonic cancer at an early stage is a difficult clinical problem. When the lesion is small and limited to an insensitive mucosa, cancer of the colon is rarely clinically apparent. Appreciable symptoms develop as the tumor grows and are generally noted earlier in patients with lesions of the left side of the colon. Most patients with right-sided tumors complain of dull abdominal pain or present with symptoms due to bleeding or anemia (Fig. 49-24). Left-sided tumors, in contrast, can be associated with change in bowel habits, crampy abdominal pain, and rectal bleeding (Fig. 49-25). Nonspecific constitutional symptoms, such as weight loss and cachexia, are frequently seen in patients with colonic malignancy. Infrequently, perforation and penetration of adjacent organs with abscess formation may be the initial presentation of carcinoma of the colon.

Extraintestinal abnormalities can be the initial manifestation of an occult carcinoma of the colon. Although acanthosis nigricans is more commonly associated with cancers of the stomach, pancreas, or ovary, it can also be a harbinger of colonic malignancy. The skin lesions are said to regress when the tumor is removed and to reappear when it recurs, presumably because the cancer produces some melanophore-stimulating agent. Neuromyopathy (numbness, paresthesias, muscle weakness) may also occur in patients with colon carcinoma and, similarly, tends to disappear when the tumor is removed. Herpes zoster and dermatomyositis have also been reported as signs of underlying occult colonic malignancy.

Colorectal carcinoma has long been considered a disease affecting primarily the rectum and sigmoid (Fig. 49-26). It has been traditionally emphasized that about 50% of large bowel cancers are detectable by digital examination and that up to 75% are within the reach of the rigid sigmoidoscope. Recent reports have shown a changing site distribution of carcinomas in the colon, with an increased incidence of right-sided lesions for no known reason. In one large retrospective study, cancers involving the cecum, ascending, and transverse colon, which are all beyond the range of the flexible sigmoidoscope, accounted for about one-third of lesions. These data indicate the need for an accurate and inexpensive technique to evaluate the entire colon and suggest that a barium enema examination should be included in the screening of high-risk patients. Nevertheless, since slightly more than one-third of colon cancers in this study were situated in the rectum and apparently within the reach of the examining finger, digital examination of the rectum should still be an essential part of every physical examination, even in asymptomatic persons.

Laboratory Tests

Several laboratory tests have been advocated as screening examinations for occult colonic carcinoma. The most commonly used is the guaiac test for small amounts of blood in the stool. A positive test usually sets in motion a vigorous search for an occult gastrointestinal malignancy. Unfortunately, the guaiac test is an unreliable screening procedure. A negative test does not eliminate the possibility of occult malignancy, and a positive test can be due to a nonmalignant condition, such as a diet high in meat content. The less frequently used Hemoccult slide test is far more effective in detecting occult bleeding. This test has a high degree of accuracy and a low rate of false-positives and thus should be an integral part of any patient workup.

Because carcinoembryonic antigen (CEA) is frequently elevated in patients with carcinoma of the colon, it has been proposed as an effective screening test for colonic malignancy. Unfortunately, elevated CEA levels are nonspecific, since they can be demonstrated in patients with malignancies of the pancreas, breast, lung, genitourinary tract, and bone, as well as in persons with inflammatory bowel disease, cirrhosis, chronic renal disease, and diverticular disease. Heavy smokers with no evidence of organic disease may demonstrate elevated CEA titers. False-negative determinations also occur; normal CEA levels are not uncommon in patients with proved colonic malignancy.

Prognosis

The survival rate of patients with carcinoma of the colon who undergo surgery for curative resection is

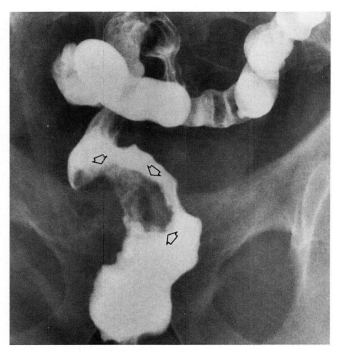

Fig. 49-26. Carcinoma of the rectum. The bulky lesion **(arrows)** could be felt on rectal examination.

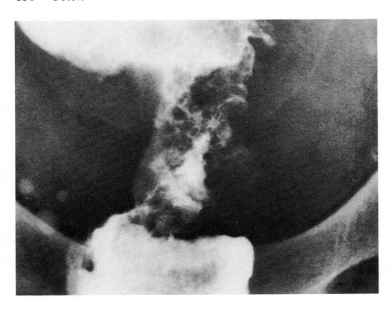

Fig. 49-27. Annular carcinoma of the rectum. Note the diffusely ulcerated mucosa with an overhanging margin.

closely related to the extent of malignant disease. The classic Duke's method of tumor staging is based on the degree of spread of tumor into the bowel wall and regional lymph nodes. In stage A, tumor is limited to the bowel wall without lymph node metastases. In stage B, there is extension through the bowel wall. Stage C implies that lymph node metastases have also occurred. If the tumor is confined to the bowel wall (stage A), there is an 80% to 90% 5-year survival rate; in patients with lymph node metastases (stage C), the 5-year survival rate is about 30%.

The major causes of death in patients with carcinoma of the colon and rectum are due to hematogenous spread of tumor. The liver is the most frequent site of distant metastasis; spread to the lungs is considerably less common.

Radiographic Findings

Annular carcinomas appear to arise from flat plaques of tumor (saddle lesions) that involve only a portion of the circumference of the colon wall. As the tumor grows, it characteristically infiltrates the bowel wall rather than forming a bulky intraluminal mass. This produces a classic bilateral contour defect with ulcerated mucosa, eccentric and irregular lumen, and overhanging margins ("apple-core" lesion) (Fig. 49-27).

Especially in the sigmoid colon, annular carcinoma can be difficult to distinguish from severe narrowing of the bowel lumen caused by diverticulitis. The demonstration of diverticula on barium examination does not establish diverticulitis as the cause of the stenotic segment, since in the sigmoid region almost 30% of colon cancers have associated diverticula, and in 10% the diverticula are adjacent to the carcinoma. Unlike diverticulitis, an annular carcinoma tends to extend over a relatively short segment (rarely more than 5 cm long). The proximal and distal edges of the tumor mass are sharply defined and well demarcated from adjacent normal bowel, in contrast to the tapered margins in diverticulitis (Fig. 49-28). The mucosa through the narrowed segment is intact, though often distorted, in diverticulitis; in carcinoma, the mucosal detail is destroyed. Small fistulous tracts and intramural abscesses are not uncommon in diverticulitis. Significant obstruction to the flow of barium can prevent identification of these distinguishing features; however, intravenous administration of glucagon may relax spasm due to inflammation, thereby permitting differentiation of acute diverticulitis from an annular carcinoma. As the inflammation and edema of diverticulitis subside after a course of therapy, a repeat examination may demonstrate a dramatic decrease in the irritability and irregularity of the affected segment. Nevertheless, colonoscopy or surgery may be required for a definitive diagnosis to be made.

Annular carcinoma can be simulated by an area of transient, localized spasm. This phenomenon can occur anywhere in the colon but is found particularly in the transverse, descending, and sigmoid portions, in which the so-called colonic sphincters are found (Fig. 49-29). These sphincters are areas of spasm that are not due to organic disease but probably reflect localized nerve and muscle imbalance. Unlike the narrowing seen in annular carcinoma, that associated with colon sphincters tends to have tapering margins, changes on sequential films, and is usually relieved by intravenous glucagon. The

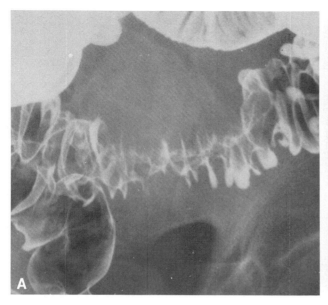

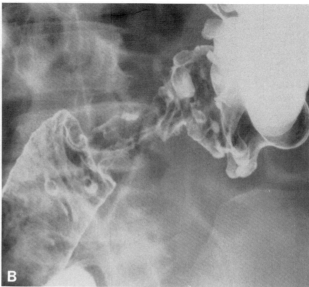

Fig. 49-28. Sigmoid diverticulitis versus carcinoma. Although confident differentiation cannot always be made, a long narrowed colonic segment of distorted but intact mucosa usually indicates diverticular disease **(A)**, whereas a short narrowed segment with abrupt margins and ulcerated mucosa, even in the presence of diverticula, indicates carcinoma **(B)**. (Gardiner R, Smith C: Colon diverticular disease. In Taveras JM, Ferrucci JT [eds]: Radiology: Diagnosis–Imaging–Intervention. Philadelphia, JB Lippincott, 1987)

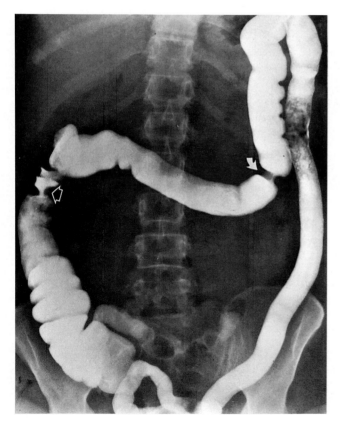

Fig. 49-29. Colonic sphincter (Cannon's point). There is an area of transient, localized spasm in the distal transverse colon **(solid arrow)**. A second area of spasm is seen in the hepatic flexure **(open arrow)**.

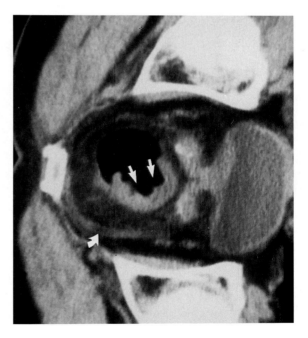

Fig. 49-30. CT of rectal carcinoma. There is a soft-tissue mass on the lateral wall of the rectum containing central ulceration **(straight arrows)**. Thickening of the perirectal fascia **(curved arrow)**, the presence of multiple lymph nodes (on more cephalad images), and increased soft-tissue density of the perirectal fat suggest tumor extension beyond the bowel wall, which was confirmed at surgery. (Butch RJ: Radiology of the rectum. In Taveras JM, Ferrucci JT [eds]: Radiology: Diagnosis–Imaging–Intervention. Philadelphia, JB Lippincott, 1987)

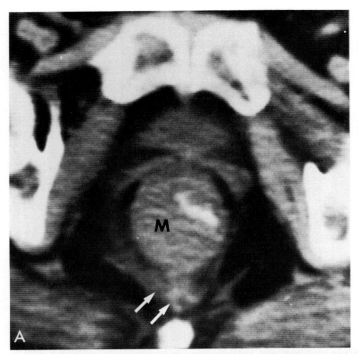

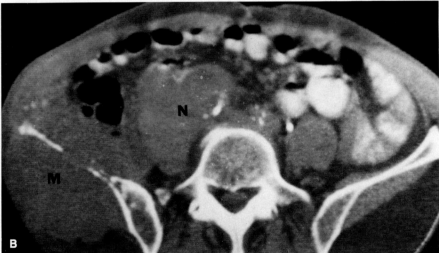

Fig. 49-31. CT of recurrent colon carcinoma. **(A)** A soft-tissue mass extends beyond the bowel wall to invade the mesentery **(arrows)**. **(B)** After a right colectomy, there is a large mass **(M)** destroying the right ilium, and marked retroperitoneal lymph node enlargement **(N)**. ([A] from Moss AA, Thoeni RF: Computed tomography of gastrointestinal tract. In Moss AA, Gamsu G, Genant HK [eds]: Computed Tomography of the Body. Philadelphia, WB Saunders, 1983; [B] from Mauro A, Koehler RE: Alimentary tract. In Lee JKT, Sagel SS, Stanley RJ [eds]: Computed Body Tomography. New York, Raven, 1983)

mucosa running through an area of benign spasm is intact and without ulceration, in contrast to annular carcinoma, in which normal mucosal architecture is destroyed.

Computed tomography is a major modality for staging carcinoma of the colon and in assessing tumor recurrence. In the rectosigmoid region, adenocarcinoma causes asymmetric or circumferential thickening of the bowel wall with narrowing and deformity of the lumen (Fig. 49-30). CT can demonstrate local extension of tumor to the pelvic musculature, bladder, prostate, seminal vesicles, and ovaries by showing the obliteration of fat planes between the colon and the adjacent structures.

Lymphadenopathy, metastases to the adrenals or liver, and masses in the abdominal wall or mesentery can also be detected by this technique. Following surgical resection, CT is the imaging modality of choice for detecting and staging recurrent colorectal cancer (Fig. 49-31). Although endoscopy is very sensitive in the detection of anastomotic recurrences and allows biopsy confirmation of recurrent tumor, this technique (unlike CT) provides no information about the degree of spread of the neoplastic mass. CT can demonstrate tumor recurrence as focal bowel wall thickening that may be accompanied by extension of the mass into adjacent muscles, organs, bone, or the pelvic sidewalls.

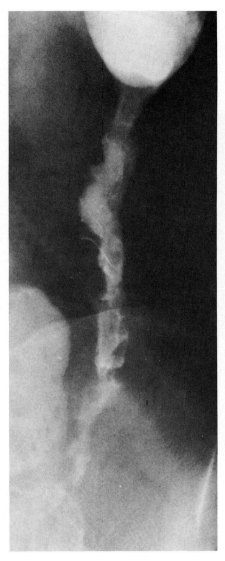

49-32

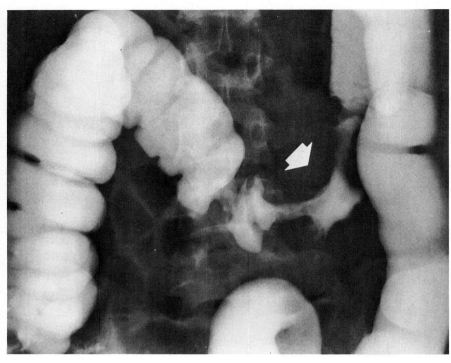

49-33

Fig. 49-32. Scirrhous carcinoma of the colon. There is severe circumferential narrowing of a long segment of descending colon.

Fig. 49-33. Scirrhous carcinoma of the colon. The long, circumferentially narrowed area **(arrow)** simulates segmental colonic encasement due to metastatic disease.

SCIRRHOUS CARCINOMA OF THE COLON

Scirrhous carcinoma is a rare variant of annular carcinoma of the colon in which an intense desmoplastic reaction infiltrates the bowel wall with dense fibrous tissue (Fig. 49-32). As the tumor grows, it spreads circumferentially and longitudinally, producing a long segment of bowel (up to 12 cm) with a luminal diameter of only 1 cm to 3 cm. In scirrhous carcinoma, in contrast to the more common annular form of colon cancer, the mucosa can be partially or completely preserved, and the margins of the lesion tend to taper and fade gradually into normal bowel without the abrupt transition and characteristic "shouldering" often observed in colonic carcinoma.

Scirrhous carcinoma is a particularly virulent form of colonic malignancy with a poor prognosis.

The clinical presentation is insidious, and the relative lack of mucosal destruction makes bleeding an uncommon symptom. Because the tumor grows slowly and only gradually narrows the bowel lumen, the intermittent constipation and progressive decrease in the caliber of the stool may not be readily appreciated by the patient.

Primary scirrhous carcinoma of the colon can be indistinguishable from segmental colonic encasement due either to contiguous spread of carcinoma of the stomach or ovary or to hematogenous metastases from carcinoma of the breast (Fig. 49-33). Patients who develop carcinoma of the colon as a late complication of chronic ulcerative colitis often have a scirrhous type of tumor. This can present a diagnostic dilemma, because the appearance of the tumor often closely simulates a benign stricture or the long, stiff, featureless narrowing that

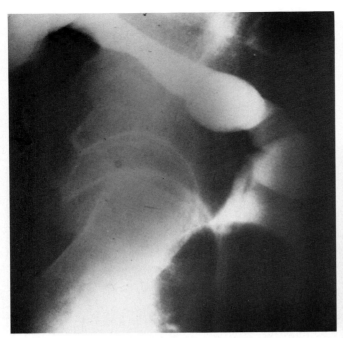

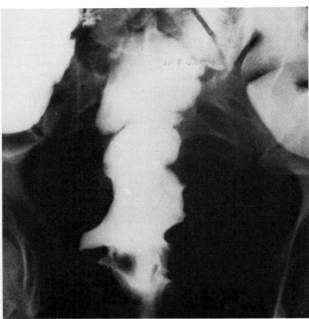

49-34

49-35

Fig. 49-34. *Carcinoma of the prostate involving the colon. The lateral view demonstrates marked anterior compression of the rectosigmoid. (Gengler L, Baer J, Finby N: Rectal and sigmoid involvement secondary to carcinoma of the prostate. AJR 125:910–917, 1975. Copyright 1975. Reproduced with permission)*

Fig. 49-35. *Carcinoma of the prostate involving the colon. The rectum, which has scalloped margins, shows lack of distention and extrinsic infiltration of the bowel wall. (Gengler L, Baer J, Finby N: Rectal and sigmoid involvement secondary to carcinoma of the prostate. AJR 125:910–917, 1975. Copyright 1975. Reproduced with permission)*

is characteristic of the colon in "burned out" ulcerative colitis. Because of this difficulty, the development of scirrhous carcinoma in patients with chronic ulcerative colitis is often not recognized until metastasis or invasion of other organs has occurred.

METASTASES

Metastases to the colon can arise from direct invasion, intraperitoneal seeding, or hematogenous or lymphangitic spread. Rather than a random occurrence, metastases from various primary lesions reflect patterns of spread that are predictable on the basis of anatomic considerations. This is of particular importance, since the site and radiographic appearance of a metastasis can be the foundation for a rational approach to identification of the primary lesion.

Direct Invasion

Direct invasion of the colon from a contiguous primary tumor indicates a locally aggressive lesion that has broken through fascial planes. In men, the most common primary tumor is advanced carcinoma of the prostate gland, which spreads posteriorly across the rectogenital septum (Denonvilliers' fascia) to invade the rectum anteriorly or circumferentially. Because rectal spread of tumor is not infrequent, is often clinically unsuspected, and somewhat alters the therapeutic approach, a barium enema examination is indicated in patients with carcinoma of the prostate.

Spread of carcinoma of the prostate to the rectum can produce one of several radiographic patterns. It can cause a large, smooth, concave pressure defect on the anterior aspect of the rectosigmoid (Fig. 49-34) that is occasionally severe enough to obstruct the colon. Invasion of the anterior rectal wall produces a fungating, ulcerated mass that closely simulates primary rectal carcinoma. The most frequent presentation of prostatic carcinoma metastatic to the colon is a long, asymmetric annular stricture of the proximal rectum or rectosigmoid. The margins of this stricture show irregular scalloping caused either by intramural tumor nodules or by edema infiltrating the bowel wall (Fig. 49-35). Concomitant widening of the retrorectal space is usually seen.

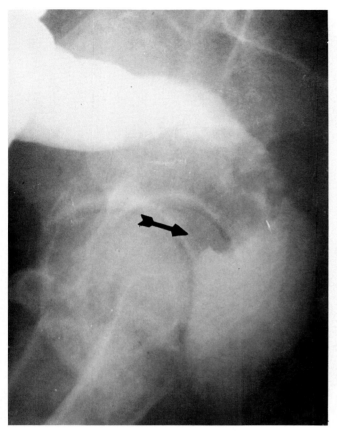

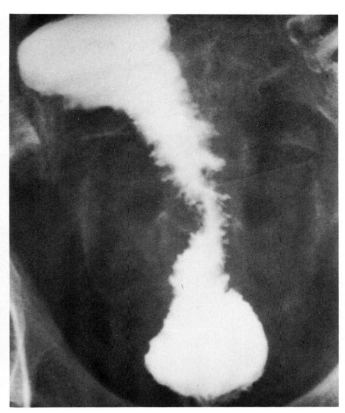

49-36   49-37

Fig. 49-36. *Primary adenocarcinoma of the rectum. Note the tumor shelf at the inferior aspect of the mass* **(arrow)***. Such a shelf is not present in secondary prostatic cancer. (Gengler L, Baer J, Finby N: Rectal and sigmoid involvement secondary to carcinoma of the prostate. AJR 125:910–917, 1975. Copyright 1975. Reproduced with permission)*

Fig. 49-37. *Carcinoma of the prostate involving the rectum. Circumferential involvement causes diffuse rectal narrowing and ulceration. Note the tapered margins of the lesion. There is no evidence of a tumor shelf.*

Differentiation between direct extension of prostatic carcinoma and a primary rectal tumor can be difficult. Primary carcinoma of the colon is usually a less extensive lesion that demonstrates a tumor shelf with overhanging margins (Fig. 49-36), in contrast to a metastatic lesion, which has more tapered edges (Fig. 49-37). Elevated serum acid phosphatase activity indicates extension of prostatic carcinoma beyond its fascia but does not indicate whether such extension represents spread to the rectum or to more remote areas, such as liver or bone.

In women, direct invasion from a noncontiguous primary tumor is usually related to a pelvic tumor arising in the ovary or uterus (Fig. 49-38). Invasion of the bowel wall produces a mass effect that is often of great length and does not demonstrate overhanging margins (Fig. 49-39). An associated desmoplastic reaction causes angulation and

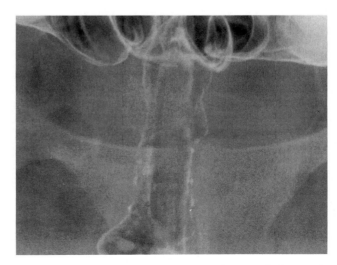

Fig. 49-38. Direct invasion from carcinoma of the cervix concentrically narrowing the rectum.

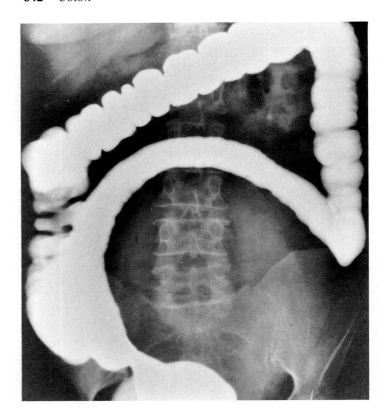

Fig. 49-39. Extrinsic mass effect on the sigmoid colon due to cystadenocarcinoma of the ovary.

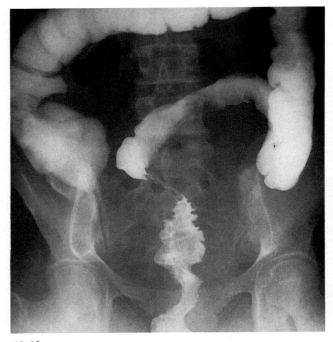

49-40

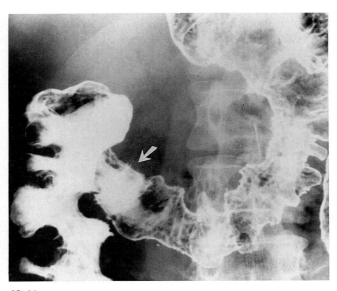

49-41

Fig. 49-40. Metastatic cystadenocarcinoma of the ovary. In addition to the mass effect, an associated desmoplastic reaction causes tethering of mucosal folds and an annular stricture.

Fig. 49-41. Carcinoma of the stomach metastatic to the proximal transverse colon. There is irregular narrowing with marginal spiculation **(arrow)**.

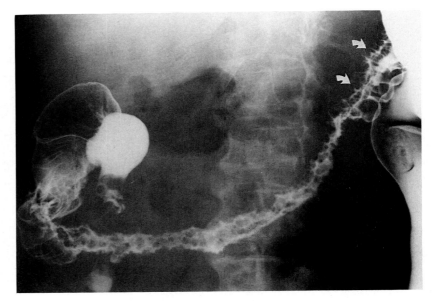

Fig. 49-42. Omental metastases. Diffuse narrowing and fixation of the transverse colon with severely distorted mucosal folds, mimicking the cobblestone appearance of Crohn's colitis. However, there is asymmetric involvement distally, with a mass effect and tethered folds on the superior haustral borders **(arrows)**. These findings are the result of diffuse encasement of the transverse colon by omental metastases from transitional cell carcinoma of the bladder. (Rubesin SE, Levine MS: Omental cakes: Colonic involvement by omental metastases. Radiology 154:593–596, 1985)

tethering of mucosal folds and can even lead to the development of an annular stricture (Fig. 49-40).

Primary renal neoplasms can directly invade adjacent segments of the colon, often resulting in large intraluminal masses with no desmoplastic response or significant obstruction. On the left side, direct spread from a renal primary most commonly involves the distal transverse colon or proximal descending colon.

Carcinomas of the stomach and pancreas are noncontiguous primary tumors that can spread to the colon along mesenteric reflections. Primary carcinoma of the stomach (usually scirrhous) extends down the gastrocolic ligament to involve the transverse colon along its superior haustral border (Fig. 49-41). Contiguous spread of bulky omental metastases from pelvic tumors can produce similar involvement (Fig. 49-42). The tumor incites a desmoplastic reaction that causes the colon wall to become thickened, straightened, and irregular. The mucosal folds become tethered and angulated. The inferior border of the transverse colon is initially uninvolved, so that its haustral contours retain their pliability and produce pseudosacculations. Progressive distortion and fixation of the mucosal pattern eventually cause irregular stenoses and an appearance of cobblestoning that simulates Crohn's disease (Fig. 49-43). However, metastases to the transverse colon can usually be distinguished from inflammatory bowel disease by demonstration of the tethering of mucosal folds and the extent of radiographic abnormality, which is localized specifically to the superior border of the transverse colon and tends to end abruptly at the level of the phrenicocolic ligament (extending from the anatomic

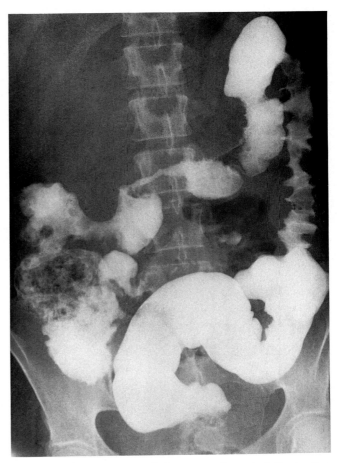

Fig. 49-43. Carcinoma of the stomach metastatic to the colon. Diffuse, irregular narrowing involves the ascending, transverse, and descending portions of the colon, with ulcerations and mucosal edema simulating Crohn's disease.

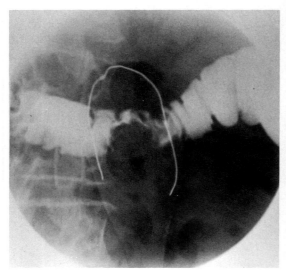

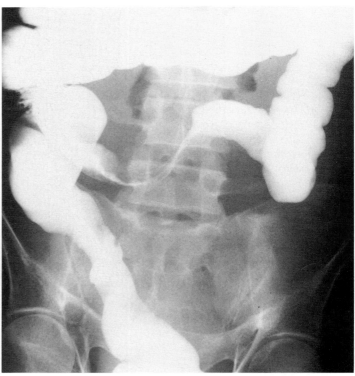

49-44   49-45

Fig. 49-44. Carcinoma of the pancreas with direct extension into the transverse colon. Solitary intramural nonobstructing filling defect typically involving the lower margin of the transverse colon. (Forrest TS, Frick MP: Radiology of the pancreas. In Gedgaudas–McClees RK (ed): Handbook of Gastrointestinal Imaging. New York, Churchill Livingstone, 1987)

Fig. 49-45. Intraperitoneal leiomyosarcoma. Extrinsic narrowing and a mass effect involve the sigmoid colon.

splenic flexure to the diaphragm), where the mesenteric transverse colon continues as the extraperitoneal descending colon.

The pancreas is connected to the transverse colon by the transverse mesocolon. Unlike carcinoma of the stomach, primary malignancy in the pancreas spreads downward through the transverse mesocolon to predominantly involve the inferior aspect of the transverse colon (Fig. 49-44). Thus, fixation and nodularity affect the lower border of the transverse colon, whereas the superior haustral border is uninvolved and can be thrown into pseudosacculations. As metastatic involvement progresses, circumferential narrowing of the colon may develop.

Spread of primary intraperitoneal sarcomas can also involve the colon and present a radiographic appearance of a mass effect with extrinsic luminal narrowing (Fig. 49-45).

Intraperitoneal Seeding

Primary abdominal malignancies can extend into the peritoneal cavity and shed tumor cells into asci-

tic fluid. The serosal bowel metastases caused by this intraperitoneal seeding are not randomly distributed throughout the abdomen. Instead, the ascites containing these malignant cells flows along a predictable course that is determined by mesenteric reflections, peritoneal recesses, and the forces of gravity and negative intra-abdominal pressure.

Intraperitoneal metastases tend to lodge in four specific areas. In more than half of cases, they grow in the region of the pouch of Douglas, the lower extension of the peritoneal reflection between the rectosigmoid and urinary bladder at the level of the lower second to upper fourth sacral segments. Metastatic seeding in this area primarily involves the anterior aspect of the rectosigmoid and produces a characteristic pattern of fixed transverse parallel folds or a nodular mass (Fig. 49-46). If the metastasis incites a desmoplastic response, the resulting mass is often clinically palpable (Blumer's shelf).

The next most common sites of intraperitoneal seeding are the peritoneal recesses along the distal small bowel mesentery in the right lower quadrant. Metastases in this area often produce a smooth or lobulated extrinsic mass indenting the medial and

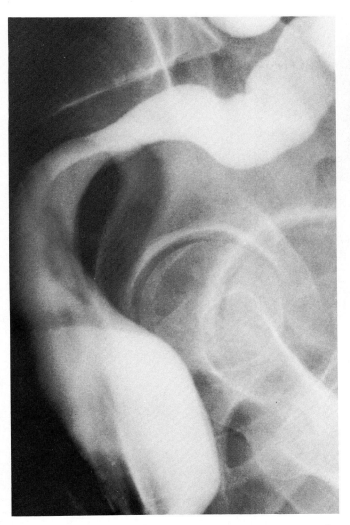

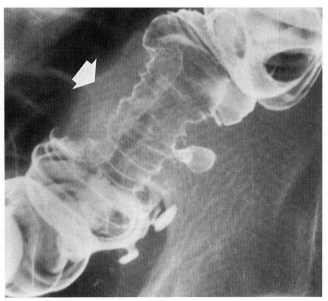

Fig. 49-47. Intraperitoneal seeding of undifferentiated carcinoma involving the sigmoid mesocolon. A mass effect and tethering localized to the superior border of the sigmoid colon **(arrow)** are evident.

Fig. 49-46. Intraperitoneal metastases from carcinoma of the pancreas. The nodular mass in the region of the pouch of Douglas was clinically palpable (Blumer's shelf).

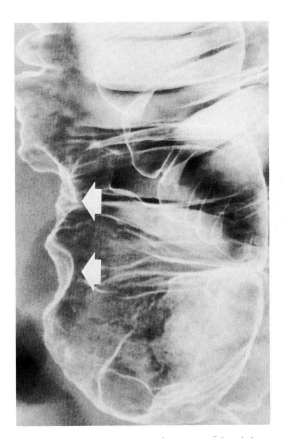

inferior borders of the cecum below the level of the ileocecal valve. In most cases, the cecal mass is associated with evidence of distal mesenteric involvement (fixation, angulation, and separation of loops of the distal ileum) that can simulate Crohn's disease of the ileocecal region.

Intraperitoneal seeding also tends to involve the sigmoid mesocolon and the right paracolic gutter. In the sigmoid mesocolon, radiographic changes are characteristically localized to the superior border (Fig. 49-47). Metastatic spread to the right paracolic gutter involves the lateral and posterior aspects of the cecum and proximal ascending colon (Fig. 49-48).

Metastatic serosal implants incite an intense desmoplastic reaction that appears in profile as characteristic tethering or retraction of folds. When seen *en face* on double-contrast studies, this tethering appears to be projected through the colonic lumen as transverse folds that do not completely

Fig. 49-48. Metastatic spread of tumor to the right paracolic gutter. A lobulated mass **(arrows)** involves the lateral aspect of the cecum.

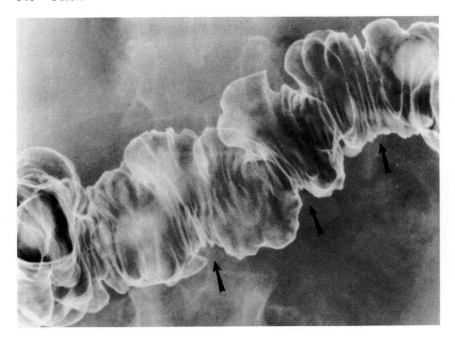

Fig. 49-49. "Striped colon" sign of metastatic serosal implants. A double-contrast barium enema study demonstrates numerous transverse folds of the transverse colon **(arrows)**. (Ginaldi S, Lindell MM, Zornoza J: The striped colon: A new radiographic observation in metastatic serosal implants. AJR 134:453–455, 1980. Copyright 1980. Reproduced with permission)

traverse the lumen of the colon ("striped colon") (Fig. 49-49). This abnormal pattern must be distinguished from the normal double-contrast appearance, in which transverse folds appear to extend around the entire circumference of the bowel wall.

Hematogenous Spread

Carcinoma of the breast is the most common primary tumor causing hematogenous metastases to the colon (Fig. 49-50). In women with breast carcinoma, symptoms of colonic metastases may be the first clinical manifestation of an occult primary or may occur years after mastectomy. The most frequent radiographic appearance is thickening and rigidity of a long segment of colon. This pattern, which is due to densely cellular submucosal metastatic deposits, simulates a primary infiltrating scirrhous carcinoma of the colon. Metastatic breast carcinoma can also mimic primary inflammatory processes such as ulcerative or Crohn's colitis. In these cases, diarrhea, occasionally with bloody mucus, tenesmus, and flatulence, may dominate the clinical presentation. Radiographic findings include mucosal thickening, nodular masses, multiple and eccentric strictures, spiculations, and associated terminal ileal involvement. Other hematogenous metastases to the colon, such as those from primary bronchogenic carcinoma and melanoma, are rare.

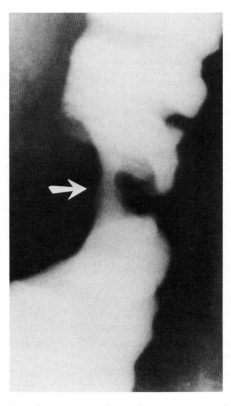

Fig. 49-50. Carcinoma of the breast metastatic to the colon. A relatively short annular lesion **(arrow)** simulates a primary colonic tumor.

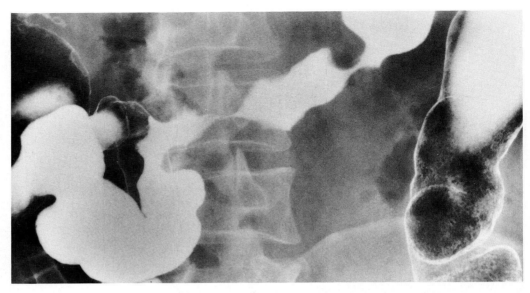

Fig. 49-51. Carcinoma of the colon developing in a patient with long-standing chronic ulcerative colitis. A long, irregular lesion with a bizarre pattern is visible in the transverse colon. Note the pseudopolyposis in the visualized portion of the descending colon.

Lymphangitic Spread

Lymphangitic spread appears to be of little importance in the dissemination of metastases to the colon. Some reports have suggested, however, that lymphatic spread may play a significant role in anastomotic recurrence of tumor after partial colectomy.

CARCINOMA COMPLICATING OTHER CONDITIONS

Ulcerative Colitis

Carcinoma of the colon is about six to ten times more frequent in patients with ulcerative colitis than in the general population. The incidence of cancer is related to the duration of colitis, the age of the patient at the time of onset, and the linear extent of disease; it is not related to the severity or activity of the inflammatory process. During the first 10 years of disease, there is only a small risk of malignancy. Thereafter, however, it is estimated that there is a 25% chance per decade of a patient with ulcerative colitis developing carcinoma. Patients with the onset of ulcerative colitis before the age of 25 are more likely to develop cancer than persons initially affected at a later age. The incidence of malignancy is far higher in patients with universal colitis than in persons with segmental disease. Nevertheless, most carcinomas in patients with ulcerative colitis arise in the distal transverse colon, descending colon, or rectum. Carcinomas of the colon in patients with ulcerative colitis tend to be extremely virulent. Malignant lesions generally occur at a much younger age than in the general population (average of 35 years versus 60 years). Because cancer in ulcerative colitis is multicentric in up to 20% of cases, atypical in its early appearance, and rapidly metastasizing, the diagnosis is often difficult to make, and the prognosis is poor.

Carcinoma of the colon in patients with chronic ulcerative colitis often presents as a filiform stricture rather than having the more characteristic polypoid or "apple-core" appearance of primary colonic malignancy. Initially, the carcinoma is often flat and infiltrating and difficult to detect because of its plaquelike nature. Neoplastic infiltration of the submucosa and adjacent muscular wall typically produces a narrowed segment, usually 2 cm to 6 cm in length, with an eccentric lumen, irregular contours, and margins that are rigid and tapered, simulating primary scirrhous carcinoma of the colon (Fig. 49-51). Although benign strictures in patients with ulcerative colitis tend to have a concentric lumen with smooth contours and pliable tapering margins, eccentric, irregular lesions occasionally occur. Because it is frequently difficult to distinguish carcinoma from benign stricture in these patients, colonoscopy or surgery is often required for an unequivocal diagnosis to be made.

Crohn's Colitis

Patients with Crohn's disease of the colon also appear to have a higher incidence of developing colon cancer than the general population. This risk is less

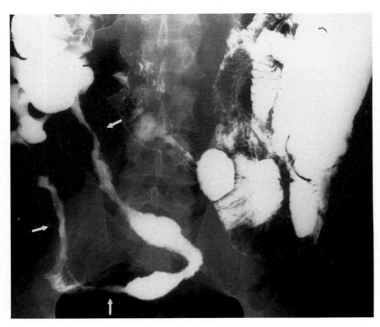

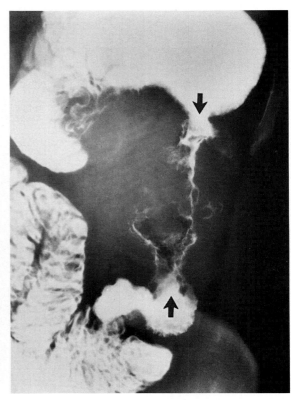

49-52

49-53

Fig. 49-52. Carcinoma of the ileum developing in a patient with long-standing chronic Crohn's colitis. Diffuse irregular luminal narrowing **(arrows)** with an associated soft-tissue mass surrounding the distal ileum. The proximal small bowel is dilated, indicative of a partial obstruction. (Miller TL, Skucas J, Gudex D et al: Bowel cancer characteristics in patients with regional enteritis. Gastrointest Radiol 12:45–52, 1987)

Fig. 49-53. Carcinoma of the jejunum developing in a patient with long-standing chronic Crohn's colitis. Mass **(arrows)** in the proximal jejunum with shouldering, mucosal destruction, and proximal dilatation. (Kerber GW, Frank PH: Carcinoma of the small intestine and colon as a complication of Crohn disease: Radiologic manifestations. Radiology 150:639–645, 1984)

than in a pancolitic patient, but approximately the same as a patient with left-sided ulcerative colitis. Inflamed loops of bowel that have been bypassed are particularly prone to malignant degeneration. Numerous reports of carcinoma developing in chronic fistulas have been described; fistulas that persist for years or develop symptoms of bleeding should be regarded with suspicion.

Carcinoma complicating Crohn's colitis is most common in the proximal portion of the colon. The tumor may appear radiographically as a fungating mass with typical malignant features, or present as an infiltrative or permeative type of carcinoma that spreads both along and through the bowel wall and causes marked luminal narrowing.

Carcinoma of the small intestine has also been reported as a complication of Crohn's disease (Fig. 49-52). Most small bowel carcinomas associated with Crohn's disease occur in grossly diseased seg-

ments of bowel and present as infiltrating and constricting lesions that can be radiographically indistinguishable from long-standing inflammatory disease (Fig. 49-53).

It is interesting to note that a colitis that is histologically and grossly indistinguishable from ulcerative colitis can develop proximal to a carcinoma or other obstructing colonic lesion (Fig. 49-54). The inflammatory bowel disease in this situation is apparently not caused by the tumor itself but is instead a consequence of the elevated intraluminal pressure due to long-standing obstruction, which produces vascular compromise leading to colon ischemia.

Ureterosigmoidostomy

A higher than normal incidence of adenocarcinoma of the sigmoid colon has been reported adjacent to a

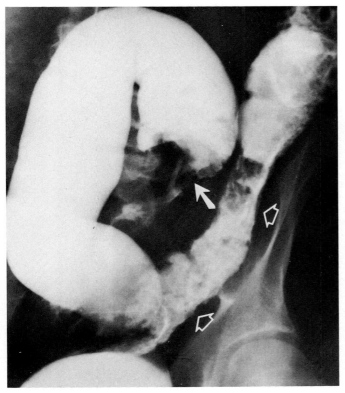
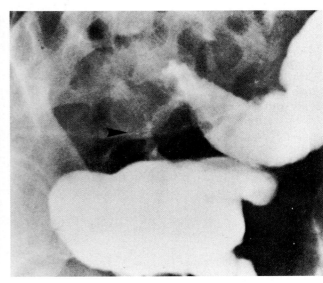

49-54   49-55

Fig. 49-54. Ulcerating colitis **(open arrows)** proximal to a high-grade stenosis **(solid arrow)** caused by carcinoma of the sigmoid.

Fig. 49-55. Adenocarcinoma of the colon as a delayed complication of ureterosigmoidostomy. A typical "apple-core" lesion of the sigmoid colon **(arrow)** may be seen. (Parsons CD, Thomas MH, Garrett RA: Colonic adenocarcinoma: A delayed complication of ureterosigmoidostomy. J Urol 118:31–34, 1977)

ureterosigmoidostomy stoma (Fig. 49-55). Because this urine-diverting procedure is often performed to correct congenital anomalies, patients with this complication are younger than the average patient with cancer of the colon, even though there may be a prolonged delay between the surgical procedure and the appearance of the neoplasm. Postulated mechanisms for development of the carcinoma include the presence of a colon carcinogen in urine and malignant degeneration of an irritation-induced pseudopolypoid mucosal mass.

KAPOSI'S SARCOMA

Kaposi's sarcoma is a systemic, multifocal, steadily progressive tumor of the reticuloendothelial system with a predilection for skin and visceral involvement. In the virulent form that primarily involves immunocompromised patients, especially those with AIDS, individual submucosal nodules within the colon may coalesce and circumferentially infiltrate the wall of the colon, producing a narrowed, nodular, rigid segment.

CARCINOID TUMOR

Although carcinoid tumors of the colon are most often polypoid in nature, they can present as infiltrating, constricting lesions narrowing the lumen of the bowel. Carcinoids tend to be large tumors with a pattern of destruction of mucosal folds, rigidity, and overhanging margins. They can be radiographically indistinguishable from adenocarcinoma.

LYMPHOMA

Lymphoma occasionally appears as an area of localized narrowing simulating annular carcinoma (Fig.

49-56). However, localized lymphoma can also present as an aneurysmal dilatation of a short segment of colon. This dilatation is due both to the absence of a desmoplastic response, which permits a malignant ulcer to greatly increase in size, and to destruction of the muscular layer and nerve plexuses. Both of these manifestations of lymphoma, nevertheless, are much less common than the polypoid or diffuse forms of the disease.

A recent report has shown a statistically significant increase of leukemia in ulcerative colitis and lymphoma in both ulcerative and Crohn's disease. Although the exact etiology is uncertain, there are probably multiple causes including the immunologic deficiencies present in inflammatory bowel disease, the administration of immunosuppressive medications, and the increased exposure to ionizing radiation during diagnostic examinations. Patients with AIDS have been shown to have an increased incidence of intestinal lymphoma, often of the rectum. Although the cause is uncertain, it is postulated

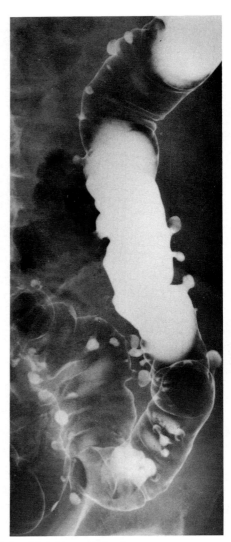

Fig. 49-57. Multiple colonic diverticula.

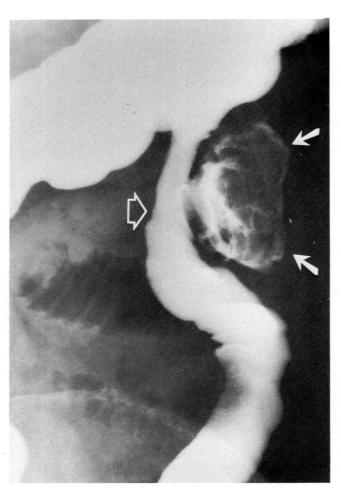

Fig. 49-56. Primary lymphoma of the descending colon. Segmental colonic narrowing **(open arrow)** is complicated by perforation and abscess formation **(solid arrows)** within the tumor mass.

that the underlying mechanism may be a combination of the patient's altered immune status and chronic gut infestation by unusual organisms (*e.g.*, cytomegalovirus) that have oncogenic tendencies.

DIVERTICULAR DISEASE

Colonic diverticula are acquired herniations of mucosa and submucosa through the muscular layers of the bowel wall (Fig. 49-57). The incidence of colonic diverticulosis increases with age. Rare in persons below the age of 30, diverticula can be demonstrated in up to half of people over 60. In about 95% of patients with diverticular disease, the sigmoid is the major segment of colon affected. Proximal colon involvement is much less frequent and is almost always associated with contiguous disease distally. Diverticula usually develop between the mesenteric and lateral tenia at sites of weakness in the

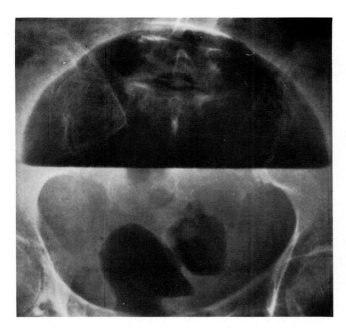

Fig. 49-58. Giant sigmoid diverticulum. A plain abdominal radiograph demonstrates a huge walled-off pelvic abscess with a gas-fluid level.

colon wall, where the longitudinal arteries penetrate the inner circular muscle layer to form the submucosal capillary plexus.

Although the precise pathogenesis of diverticulosis is unclear, increased muscular thickening of the colon wall and abnormally exaggerated intraluminal pressure are thought to be major contributing factors. In response to food, emotional stimuli, or cholinergic drugs, the sigmoid colon in patients predisposed to diverticular disease tends to become segmented, and intraluminal pressure becomes elevated. This exaggerated pressure, combined with prominent muscular thickening, causes herniation of mucosal outpouchings at weak points in the colon wall. The reason for the sigmoid colon being the usual site of diverticulosis can be explained by the law of Laplace, which states that, in a cylindrical structure with a given tension, the pressure is inversely related to the radius. Because the sigmoid has the most narrow caliber of any portion of the colon, the tension generated by circular muscle bundles produces far higher pressures in this region than in more proximal parts of the colon, where the lumen diameter is larger. The elevated pressure causes the mucosa and submucosa to herniate through anatomic weak points in the sigmoid musculature and form diverticula.

Epidemiologic data suggest that diet may play a major role in the development of diverticular disease. Diverticulosis is extremely rare in underdeveloped areas in Africa and Asia. It is postulated that the high fiber content of native diets results in large volumes of semisolid stool, a large-caliber colonic lumen, and a rapid fecal transit time. In contrast, in the United States and Western Europe, the diet is highly refined and low in roughage. This diet tends to cause a small fecal stream, which leads to excessive segmentation of the sigmoid, increased intraluminal pressure, and smooth muscle hypertrophy, all of which combine to produce diverticulosis.

DIVERTICULOSIS

Clinical Symptoms

The majority of patients with diverticulosis have no symptoms. A substantial number, however, have chronic or intermittent lower abdominal pain frequently precipitated by, or related to, meals and emotional stress. Alternating bouts of diarrhea and constipation are common, and a tender, palpable mass may be present in the left lower quadrant. This symptom complex probably represents the altered motor activity of the thickened colonic musculature rather than diverticular inflammation. Evidence for this hypothesis may be seen in the finding that young patients with "prediverticular" muscle dysfunction may have identical symptoms, even when no true diverticula are radiographically detectable. Thus, the degree of pain and altered bowel habits appear to relate to the intensity of segmentation and the degree of increased intraluminal pressure rather than to the presence of diverticula *per se*.

Painless bleeding is a common complication of diverticulosis. It can range from mild hematochezia to massive hemorrhage. Bleeding is caused by inflammatory erosion of penetrating branches of the vasa recta at the base of the diverticulum. For reasons that are not clear, diverticula of the right colon cause significant bleeding more often than those of the left.

Radiographic Findings

Colonic diverticula appear radiographically as round or oval outpouchings of barium projecting beyond the confines of the lumen. They vary in size from barely visible dimples to saclike structures 2 cm or more in diameter. Giant sigmoid diverticula of up to 25 cm in diameter have been reported (Fig. 49-58). Thought to reflect slowly progressing chronic diverticular abscesses, they appear as large, well-circumscribed radiolucent cystic structures in the lower abdomen (Fig. 49-59). Rectal diverticula are rare, presumably because the longitudinal muscle coat completely encircles this portion of the bowel.

Diverticula are usually multiple and tend to occur in clusters, though a solitary diverticulum is occasionally found. Small numbers of diverticula do not distort or alter the configuration of the bowel. With multiple diverticula, however, deep criss-crossing ridges of thickened circular muscle can produce a series of sacculations (sawtooth configuration) (Fig. 49-60). The involved portion of colon may be shortened and relatively fixed, with narrowing of the lumen.

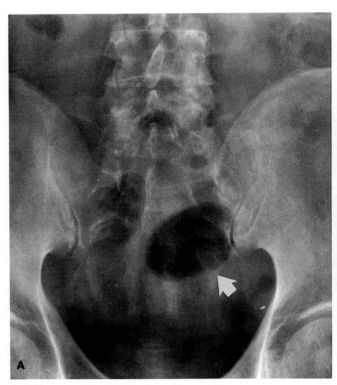

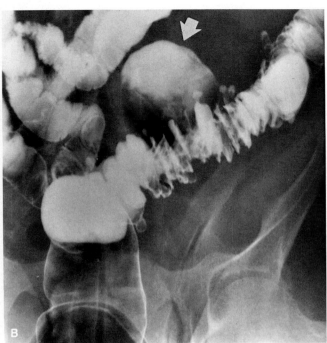

Fig. 49-59. Giant sigmoid diverticulum. **(A)** A plain abdominal radiograph demonstrates a large, well-circumscribed radiolucent structure **(arrow)** in the lower abdomen. **(B)** A barium enema examination demonstrates filling of the giant sigmoid diverticulum with radiopaque contrast **(arrow)**.

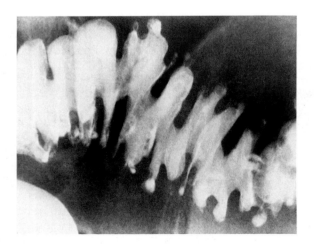

Fig. 49-60. Diverticulosis. Multiple diverticula and deep criss-crossing ridges of thickened circular muscle produce a characteristic sawtooth configuration.

If multiple diverticula are present, the introduction of barium can cause severe sigmoid spasm and complete obstruction to retrograde flow. This is particularly common if the hydrostatic pressure is excessive (because the enema bag is too high) or the enema solution is too cold. Antispasmodic drugs, such as glucagon, usually permit a successful examination.

The postevacuation radiograph can be extremely important in the detection of diverticula, since these outpouchings can be obscured or otherwise not apparent on films of the barium-filled colon. Air-contrast examinations demonstrate more diverticula than single-contrast studies. Because diverticula are dynamic structures during certain phases of their development, they may be evident on one barium examination but not on a second. Barium tends to become trapped within diverticula and

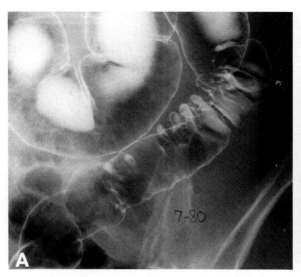 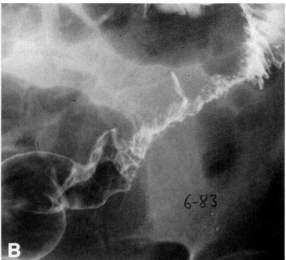

Fig. 49-61. Diverticulitis developing in diverticulosis as seen on barium enema. **(A)** Multiple sigmoid diverticula are present. **(B)** Three years later, acute diverticulitis produces perforation and associated narrowing from the adjacent mass. (Gardiner R, Smith C: Colon diverticular disease. In Taveras JM, Ferrucci, JT (eds): Radiology: Diagnosis–Imaging–Intervention. Philadelphia, JB Lippincott, 1987)

can be retained for long periods following contrast administration.

DIVERTICULITIS

Development

Diverticulitis is a complication of diverticular disease of the colon in which micro- or macroperforation of a diverticulum leads to the development of a peridiverticular abscess (Fig. 49-61). It is estimated that up to 20% of patients with diverticulosis eventually develop acute diverticulitis. The sequence of events begins with inspissation of retained fecal material trapped in a diverticulum by the narrow opening of the diverticular neck. The resultant inflammation of the mucosal lining leads to perforation of the diverticulum, and this usually results in a localized peridiverticular abscess that is walled off by fibrous adhesions. Free intraperitoneal perforation is rare. The inflammatory process may localize within the wall of the colon and produce an intramural mass, or it may dissect around the colon, causing segmental narrowing of the lumen. Subserosal extension of the inflammatory process along the colon can involve adjacent diverticula, resulting

in a longitudinal sinus tract. A common complication of diverticulitis is the development of fistulas to adjacent organs (bladder, vagina, ureter, small bowel, colon). Generalized pelvic inflammation can encase and obstruct the distal left ureter or small bowel. On rare occasions, the inflammatory process in diverticulitis is so extensive that abscesses develop in the thigh, perineum, or anterior abdominal wall.

Clinically, the patient with acute diverticulitis complains of left lower quadrant pain ("left-sided appendicitis") usually associated with fever, a palpable mass, tenderness, and laboratory evidence of infection. If pericolic inflammation causes partial of complete bowel obstruction, constipation, abdominal distention, anorexia, and nausea may result. Extension of the inflammatory process to involve the bladder or ureter can cause symptoms mimicking a urinary tract infection.

Radiographic Findings

The radiographic diagnosis of diverticulitis requires direct or indirect evidence of diverticular perforation. The most specific sign is extravasation, which can appear either as a tiny projection of contrast

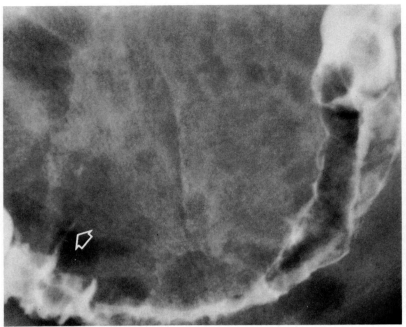

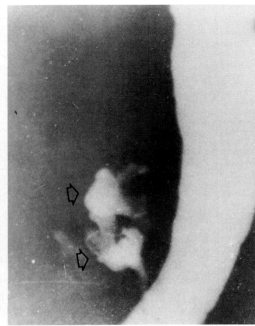

49-62   49-63

Fig. 49-62. Acute sigmoid diverticulitis. A thin projection of contrast **(arrow)** implies extravasation from the colonic lumen. Note the severe spasm of the sigmoid colon due to the intense adjacent inflammation.

Fig. 49-63. Sigmoid diverticulitis. There is obvious contrast filling of a pericolic abscess **(arrows)**.

from the tip of the diverticulum (Fig. 49-62) or as obvious filling of a pericolic abscess (Fig. 49-63). At times, diverticular perforation is not evident on filled radiographs and can be identified only on postevacuation films. In such instances, the increased pressure generated by evacuation is required to demonstrate the extravasation of contrast.

A more common, though somewhat less specific, sign of diverticulitis is the demonstration of a pericolic soft-tissue mass that is due to a localized abscess and represents a walled off perforation. This extraluminal mass appears as a filling defect causing eccentric narrowing of the bowel lumen (Fig. 49-64). Diverticula adjacent to the mass are spastic, irritable, and attenuated and frequently seem to drape over the abscess. It is important to remember, however, that a peridiverticular abscess caused by diverticulitis can occur without radiographically detectable diverticula (Fig. 49-65).

In patients with suspected acute diverticulitis, plain abdominal radiographs often demonstrate large bowel obstruction, and a gas-containing pelvic abscess is occasionally seen. Many radiologists are unwilling to perform a barium enema examination in the case of acute diverticulitis, lest the increased pressure caused by the enema result in additional

bacteria-laden luminal contents being extravasated through the perforated diverticulum. However, after several days of medical management (bowel rest, antibiotics), the inflammatory reaction has usually subsided enough to permit a safe enema examination. If perforation is suspected and an immediate diagnosis is required, a water-soluble contrast agent should be used.

Computed tomography is ideally suited for the evaluation of diverticulitis since it can demonstrate the entire thickness of the colonic wall as well as the pericolic soft tissues (Fig. 49-66). Inflammation of the pericolic fat produces poorly defined areas of increased density paralleling the long axis of the bowel. This early change of diverticulitis may be associated with nonspecific thickening of adjacent fascial planes. Increasing severity of inflammation results in a more definable region of increased density in the pericolic tissues as well as focal fluid collections, which may coalesce and form an abscess. A peridiverticular abscess appears as a mass with a thick wall of soft-tissue density and a low-density center that may contain gas or, if in communication with the lumen, contrast material. Intramural sinus tracts may appear as linear fluid collections within the thickened colon wall. The de-

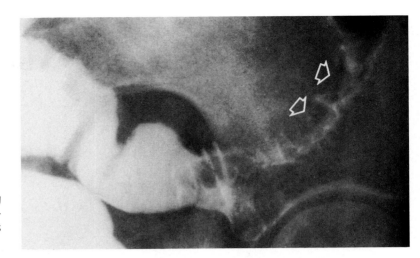

Fig. 49-64. Sigmoid diverticulitis. The resulting localized abscess causes a mass effect on the affected portion of the sigmoid **(arrows)** and incites mucosal spiculation.

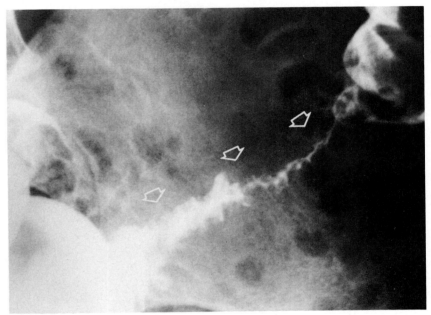

Fig. 49-65. Sigmoid diverticulitis. Severe narrowing of a long, involved portion of the sigmoid colon **(arrows)** in a patient with no radiographically detectable diverticula.

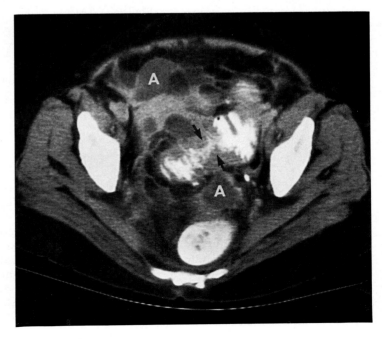

Fig. 49-66. Acute diverticulitis. CT scan demonstrates narrowing of the lumen of the sigmoid colon **(arrows)** and multiple adjacent pericolonic abscesses **(A)**. (Eisenberg RL: Diagnostic Imaging in Surgery. New York, McGraw–Hill, 1987)

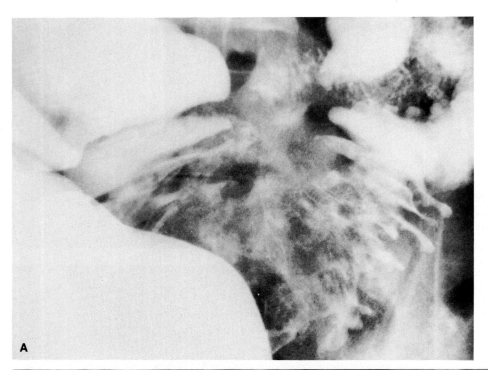

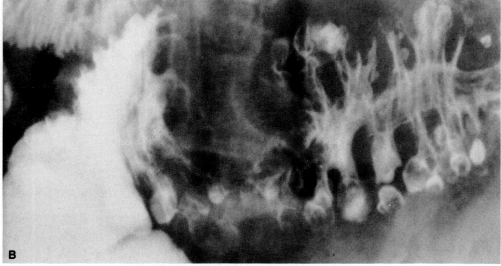

Fig. 49-67. An example of how difficult it is to distinguish diverticulitis from carcinoma. **(A)** Diverticulitis. **(B)** Carcinoma. Surgical resection would be required for a correct diagnosis to be made.

velopment of diffuse inflammatory changes (hazy soft-tissue density, linear strands, and pockets of fluid) scattered throughout the pelvis suggests generalized peritonitis, as does the presence of free ascitic fluid. An extraluminal collection of gas in the bladder, vagina, or abdominal wall indicates an underlying fistula.

Uncomplicated diverticulosis of the colon may appear on CT as thickening of the colonic wall due to circular muscle hypertrophy. The diverticula are often seen in cross section as flask-shaped struc-

tures filled with air, barium, or fecal material and projecting through the wall of the colon.

Diverticulitis can resolve completely following vigorous dietary and antibiotic therapy. However, when treated medically, diverticulitis recurs in about one-third of cases. The vast majority of recurrences occur within the first 5 years; with recurrent attacks, the morbidity is high. About 15% to 30% of patients hospitalized for diverticulitis require surgical intervention for such complications as abscesses, perforation, fistulas, or obstruction.

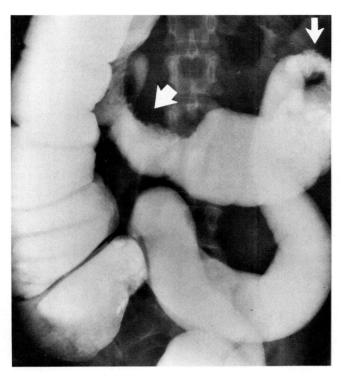

Fig. 49-68. Acute pancreatitis. There is irregular narrowing of the proximal transverse colon and splenic flexure **(arrows)**.

In some patients, the inflammatory process caused by diverticulitis continually worsens. As fibrosis develops, the lumen becomes progressively more stenotic and the bowel more rigid. Extraluminal defects due to walled off abscesses become larger and more constant. As the degree of stenosis increases, differentiation between chronic diverticulitis and carcinoma becomes extremely difficult (Fig. 49-67).

OTHER DISORDERS

PANCREATITIS

Luminal narrowing and stricture formation primarily involving the distal transverse colon and splenic flexure can be demonstrated in patients with pancreatitis (Fig. 49-68). This pattern can be caused by the spread of liberated digestive enzymes along the mesenteric attachments joining the pancreas and transverse colon, or it can be due to a large inflammatory mass in the tail of the pancreas that extends around the colon and produces a radiographic appearance simulating pancreatic or colon carcinoma.

AMYLOIDOSIS

Amyloidosis can cause narrowing and rigidity of the colon, especially in the rectum and sigmoid. It can be due to direct deposition of amyloid within the mucosal and muscular layers of the bowel, or it may be secondary to extensive amyloid deposition in blood vessel walls and subsequent ischemic colitis. The resulting thickening of the bowel with effacement of haustral markings can closely simulate the radiographic appearance of chronic ulcerative colitis.

ENDOMETRIOSIS

In women of child-rearing age, a smooth constricting lesion with intact mucosa and proximal colonic dilatation suggests the possibility of endometriosis (Fig. 49-69). The endometrial implants usually involve the rectosigmoid area and incite a hyperplasia of both smooth muscle and stroma in the affected bowel segment. This results in narrowing of the lumen simulating primary colonic malignancy. Radiographic findings favoring endometriosis are the length and tapered margins of the lesion and the intact mucosa, in contrast to the ulceration and acutely angulated overhanging margins that are seen with carcinoma.

PELVIC LIPOMATOSIS

Pelvic lipomatosis is a benign condition in which there is an increased deposition of normal, mature adipose tissue in the pelvis. Almost all reported cases have been in men. The clinical symptoms are

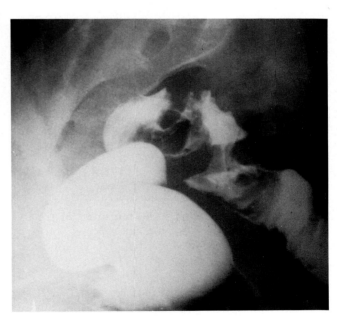

Fig. 49-69. Endometriosis. Areas of stenosis and multiple polypoid lesions are evident in a 7-cm segment of sigmoid colon. The mucosa is intact. The 43-year-old patient had had a previous episode of partial intestinal obstruction. (Spjut HJ, Perkins DE: Endometroisis of the sigmoid colon and rectum. AJR 82:1070–1075, 1959. Copyright 1959. Reproduced with permission)

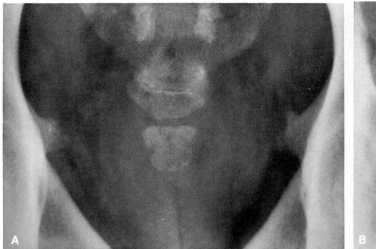
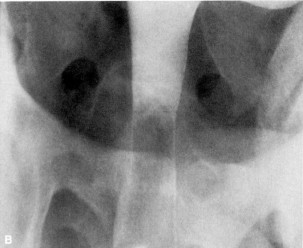

Fig. 49-70. Pelvic lipomatosis. **(A)** A plain abdominal radiograph demonstrates increased radiolucency in the pelvis caused by the excessive deposition of fat. **(B)** Smooth narrowing of the rectum and sigmoid is caused by the extrinsic fatty mass.

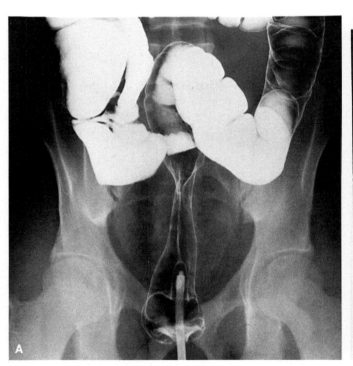
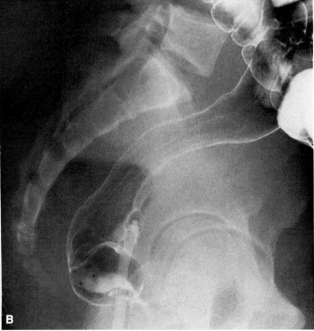

Fig. 49-71. Pelvic lipomatosis. **(A)** Frontal and **(B)** lateral views show smooth narrowing of the rectum and proximal sigmoid colon.

nonspecific and include urinary tract infection, increased frequency of urination, constipation, and low back and abdominal pain. Hypertension is a common presenting symptom, though it may be a fortuitous occurrence.

Plain films of the abdomen in patients with pelvic lipomatosis reveal an increased radiolucency in the pelvis caused by excessive deposition of fat (Fig. 49-70). This radiolucency can be enhanced on low-

kilovoltage films. Barium enema examination demonstrates vertical elongation of the sigmoid colon with narrowing of the rectum and sigmoid by the extrinsic fatty mass (Fig. 49-71). The lumen of the bowel is distensible, and the colonic mucosa remains intact. Pelvic lipomatosis most frequently involves the bladder, which is elongated and compressed into a teardrop or gourd-shaped configuration. Computed tomography can confirm the

fever, nausea, constipation, or diarrhea. The disorder usually involves the small bowel, with resultant distortion of small bowel loops seen on upper gastrointestinal series. The fat necrosis, chronic inflammation, and fibrosis of retractile mesenteritis occasionally is limited to the colonic mesentery, where it causes thickening of mucosal folds and tapered luminal narrowing with a serrated appearance of the stenotic segment, a pattern simulating an inflammatory or neoplastic process (Fig. 49-72).

ADHESIVE BANDS

Adhesive bands can cause narrowing of the colon. Most bands are due to previous abdominal or pelvic surgery; others are secondary to anomalous development of the mesentery or to inflammatory disease of the appendices epiploicae. Adhesive bands usually produce short, smooth areas of circumferential narrowing with normal mucosal contours.

TYPHLITIS

Typhlitis is a necrotizing process of multifactorial origin that may involve the right colon alone or the right colon and other areas of the intestine as well (Fig. 49-73). Initially described as a complication of

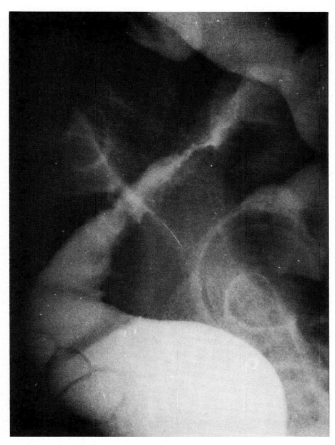

Fig. 49-72. Retractile mesenteritis. Concentric stricture of the rectosigmoid with tapered edges and serration. (Perez–Fontan FJ, Soler R, Sanchez J et al: Retractile mesenteritis involving the colon: The barium enema, sonographic, and CT findings. AJR 147:937–940, 1986. Copyright 1986. Reproduced with permission)

diagnosis of pelvic lipomatosis by demonstrating that the excessive pelvic soft tissue compressing the bladder and rectum have the same attenuation as normal subcutaneous fat.

A major complication of pelvic lipomatosis is urinary tract obstruction, which developed in one study in about 40% of patients followed for 5 years. Pelvic fat accumulating in the peripelvic and periureteric areas elevates and compresses the ureters, causing hydronephrosis and urinary stasis. A permanent urinary diversion procedure must occasionally be performed.

RETRACTILE MESENTERITIS

Narrowing of the rectosigmoid simulating pelvic carcinomatosis has been described as a complication of retractile mesenteritis. In this condition, fibroblastic proliferation and scattered inflammatory cell infiltrate result in thickening and retraction of the mesentery. Patients with retractile mesenteritis can present with a palpable mass, abdominal pain,

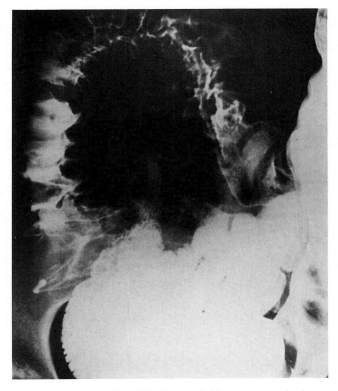

Fig. 49-73. Typhlitis. Thickened folds cause marked narrowing and thumbprinting in the right colon. Dilated loops of small bowel are visible. (Abramson SJ, Berdon WE, Baker DH: Childhood typhlitis: Its increasing association with acute myelogenous leukemia. Radiology 146:61–64, 1983)

acute leukemia in children, typhlitis may also occur in adults with hematologic malignancy or, less commonly, aplastic anemia. On contrast enemas (if colonic perforation, a well-recognized risk, has been excluded), the right colon typically has a rigid, tubular appearance with loss of haustral markings.

PSEUDOLYMPHOMA

Pseudolymphoma may rarely cause irregular narrowing and rigidity of a segment of the colon (Fig. 49-74). Because this appearance cannot be distinguished from that caused by malignant lymphoma, segmental inflammatory bowel disease, or even metastases, surgical resection is usually required.

NARROWING AT THE SITE OF SURGICAL ANASTOMOSIS

Following partial colonic resection for inflammatory or neoplastic disease, narrowing of the colon at the anastomotic site may simulate a malignant process (Fig. 49-75A). Smoothness and distensibility (Fig. 49-75B) of the affected segment, combined with a history of previous surgery, permits a confident diagnosis of benign anastomotic narrowing.

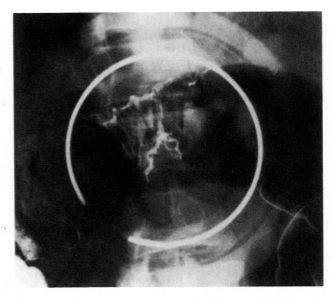

Fig. 49-74. Pseudolymphoma. Irregular area of narrowing in the proximal transverse colon that measures 3 cm and is associated with mucosal nodularity and rigidity. No overhanging margins are identified. (Agha FP, Cooper RF, Strodel W et al: Pseudolymphoma of colon. Gastrointest Radiol 8:81–84, 1983)

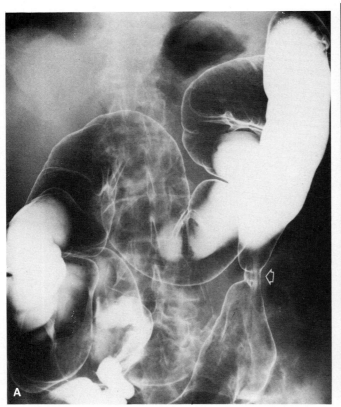

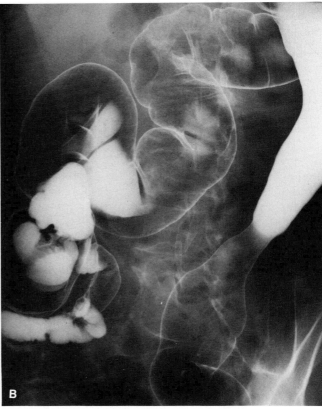

Fig. 49-75. Anastomotic narrowing. **(A)** Short segmental narrowing in the descending colon **(arrow)**. **(B)** A later film from the barium enema examination demonstrates that the narrowed segment is almost fully distensible. In view of the patient's history of previous segmental colonic resection, the diagnosis of benign anastomotic narrowing was made.

BIBLIOGRAPHY

Agha FP, Cooper RF, Strodel WE: Pseudolymphoma of colon. Gastrointest Radiol 8:81–84, 1983

Almy TP, Howell DA: Diverticular disease of the colon. N Engl J Med 302:324–331, 1980

Annamunthodo H, Marryatt J: Barium studies in intestinal lymphogranuloma venereum. Br J Radiol 34:53–57, 1961

Balthazar EJ, Bryk D: Segmental tuberculosis of the colon: Radiographic features in seven cases. Gastrointest Radiol 5:75–80, 1980

Balthazar EJ, Streiter M, Megibow AJ: Anorectal giant condyloma acuminatum (Buschke–Lowenstein tumor): CT and radiographic manifestations. Radiology 150:651–653, 1984

Brandt LJ, Katz HJ, Wolf EL et al: Simulation of colonic carcinoma by ischemia. Gastroenterology 88:1137–1142, 1985

Cardoso JM, Kimura K, Stoopen M et al: Radiology of invasive amebiasis of the colon. AJR 128:935–941, 1977

Caroline DF, Evers K: Colitis: Radiographic features and differentiation of idiopathic inflammatory bowel disease. Radiol Clin North Am 25:47–66, 1987

Carrera GF, Young S, Lewicki AM: Intestinal tuberculosis. Gastrointest Radiol 1:147–155, 1976

Chapa HJ, Smith HJ, Dickinson TA: Benign (solitary) ulcer of the rectum: Another cause for rectal stricture. Gastrointest Radiol 6:85–88, 1981

Crane DB, Smith MJV: Pelvic lipomatosis: Five-year follow-up. J Urol 118:547–550, 1977

Dallemand S, Farman J, Stein D et al: Colonic necrosis complicating pancreatitis. Gastrointest Radiol 2:27–30, 1977

Drasin GF, Moss JP, Cheng SH: *Strongyloides stercoralis* colitis: Findings in four cases. Radiology 126:619–621, 1978

Feczko PJ: Malignancy complicating inflammatory bowel disease. Radiol Clin North Am 25:157–174, 1987

Feczko PJ, O'Connell DJ, Riddell RH et al: Solitary rectal ulcer syndrome: Radiologic manifestations. AJR 135:499–506, 1980

Friedman AC, Hartman DS, Sherman J et al: Computed tomography of abdominal fatty masses. Radiology 139:415–429, 1981

Friedman HB, Silver GM, Brown CH: Lymphoma of the colon simulating ulcerative colitis. Am J Dig Dis 13:910–917, 1968

Gardiner GA, Bird CR: Nonspecific ulcers of the colon resembling annular carcinoma. Radiology 137:331–334, 1980.

Gardiner R, Smith C: Infective enterocolitides. Radiol Clin North Am 25:67–78, 1987

Gardiner R, Stevenson GW: The colitides. Radiol Clin North Am 20:797–816, 1982

Gengler L, Baer J, Finby N: Rectal and sigmoid involvement secondary to carcinoma of the prostate. AJR 125:910–917, 1975

Ginaldi S, Lindell MM, Zornoza J: The striped colon: A new radiographic observation in metastatic serosal implants. AJR 134:453–455, 1980

Greenall MJ, Levine AW, Nolan DJ: Complications of diverticular disease: A review of the barium enema findings. Gastrointest Radiol 8:353–358, 1983

Greenstein AJ, Gennuso R, Sachar DB et al: Extraintestinal cancers in inflammatory bowel disease. Gastroenterology 89:1405, 1985

Kerber GW, Frank PH: Carcinoma of the small intestine and colon as a complication of Crohn disease: Radiologic manifestations. Radiology 150:639–645, 1984

Kim SK, Gerle RD, Rozanski R: Cathartic colitis. AJR 130:825–830, 1978

Kim SK, Cho C, Levinsohn EM: Caustic colitis due to detergent enema. AJR 134:397–398, 1980

Kricun R, Stasik JJ, Reither RD et al: Giant colonic diverticulum. AJR 135:507–512, 1980

Lichtenstein JE: Radiologic-pathologic correlation of inflammatory bowel disease. Radiol Clin North Am 25:3–24, 1987

Maglinte DDT, Keller RE, Miller RE et al: Colon and rectal carcinoma: Spatial distribution and detection. Radiology 147:669–672, 1983

Mauro MA, Koehler RE: Alimentary tract. In Lee JKT, Sagel SS, Stanley RS (eds): Computed Body Tomography. New York, Raven, 1983

Menuck LS, Brahme F, Amberg J et al: Colonic changes of herpes zoster. AJR 127:273–276, 1976

Messersmith RN, Chase GJ: Amebiasis presenting as multiple apple-core lesions. Am J Gastroenterol 79:238–241, 1984

Meyer JE: Radiography of the distal colon and rectum after irradiation of carcinoma of the cervis. AJR 136:691–699, 1981

Meyers MA, Oliphant M, Teixidor H: Metastatic carcinoma simulating inflammatory colitis. AJR 123:74–83, 1975

Meyers MA: Dynamic Radiology of the Abdomen: Normal and Pathologic Anatomy. New York, Springer–Verlag, 1976

Miller TL: Skucas J, Gudex D et al: Bowel cancer characteristics in patients with regional enteritis. Gastrointest Radiol 12:45–52, 1987

Moss AA, Thoeni RF: Computed tomography of the gastrointestinal tract. In Moss AA, Gamsu G, Genant HK (eds): Computed Tomography of the Body. Philadelphia, WB Saunders, 1983

Parsons CD, Thomas MH, Garrett RA: Colonic adenocarcinoma: A delayed complication of ureterosigmoidostomy. J Urol 118:31–34, 1977

Perez–Fontan FJ, Soler R, Sanchez J et al: Retractile mesenteritis involving the colon: Barium enema, sonographic, and CT findings: AJR 147:937–940, 1986

Princenthal RA, Loman R, Zeman RK et al: Ureterosigmoidostomy: The development of tumors, diagnosis and pitfalls. AJR 141:77–81, 1983

Rogers LF, Goldstein HM: Roentgen manifestations of radiation injury to the gastrointestinal tract. Gastrointest Radiol 2:281–291, 1977

Rose HS, Balthazar EJ, Megibow AJ et al: Alimentary tract involvement in Kaposi sarcoma: Radiographic and endoscopic findings in 25 homosexual men. AJR 139:661–666, 1982

Rubesin SE, Levine MS: Omental cakes: Colonic involvement by omental metastases. Radiology 154:593–596, 1985

Smith JH, Vlasak MG: Metastasis to the colon from bronchogenic carcinoma. Gastrointest Radiol 2:393–396, 1978

Spjut HJ, Perkins DE: Endometriosis of the sigmoid colon and rectum. AJR 82:1070–1075, 1959

Taylor AJ, Dodds WJ, Gonyo JE et al: Typhlitis in adults. Gastrointest Radiol 10:363–369, 1985

Thompson WM, Halvorsen RA: Computed tomographic staging of gastrointestinal malignancies. Part II. The small bowel, colon, and rectum. Invest Radiol 22:96–105, 1987

Thompson WM, Kelvin FM, Rice RP: Inflammation and necrosis of the transverse colon secondary to pancreatitis. AJR 128:943–948, 1977

Urso FP, Urso JM, Lee CH: The cathartic colon: Pathological findings and radiological/pathological correlation. Radiology 116:557–559, 1975

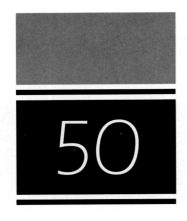

50

SINGLE FILLING DEFECTS IN THE COLON

Disease Entities

Neoplastic disorders
  Benign tumors
    Hyperplastic polyp
    Adenomatous polyp
    Hamartoma
    Peutz-Jeghers polyp
    Juvenile polyp
    Villous adenoma
    Villoglandular polyp
    Spindle cell tumor (lipoma, leiomyoma,
      fibroma, neurofibroma, cystic lymph-
      angioma)
    Traumatic neuroma
  Tumors of intermediate potential
    Carcinoid tumor
  Malignant tumors
    Carcinoma
    Sarcoma
    Metastases
    Lymphoma
    Extramedullary plasmacytoma
Inflammatory disorders
  Ameboma
  Crohn's colitis
  Giant inflammatory pseudopolyp
  Schistosomiasis (polypoid granuloma)
  Tuberculosis
  Ascaris lumbricoides (bolus of worms)

Mucormycoma
Periappendiceal abscess
Diverticular abscess
Nonspecific benign ulceration
Foreign-body perforation and abscess
    (chicken bone)
Miscellaneous disorders
  Fecal impaction
  Endometrioma
  Intussusception
  Foreign body
  Gallstone
  Hypertrophied anal papilla
  Pseudotumors
    Adhesions
    Superimposed sacral foramen
  Amyloidosis
  Suture granuloma
  Colitis cystica profunda
  Solitary rectal ulcer syndrome
  Bezoar

BENIGN TUMORS

Polypoid lesions arising from the colonic mucosa
are the most common causes of solitary filling defects in the colon. The word polyp refers to any
small mass of tissue, with or without a stalk, that
arises from the mucosa and projects into the lumen
of the bowel (Fig. 50-1). The true incidence of co-

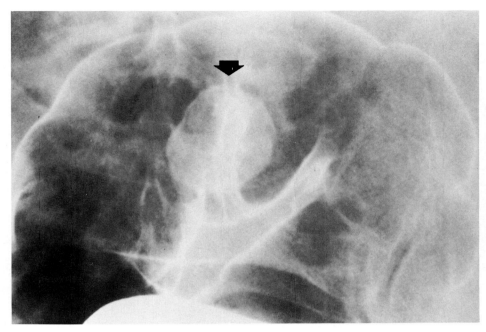

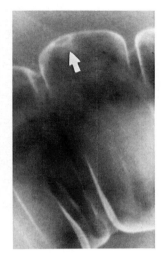

50-1   50-2

Fig. 50-1. Colonic polyp. The mass of tissue arises from the mucosa and projects into the lumen of the bowel **(arrow)**.

Fig. 50-2. Hyperplastic (metaplastic) colonic polyp. This smooth, sessile mucosal elevation **(arrow)** 2 mm in size was seen on double-contrast examination.

lonic polyps in the general population is difficult to determine, since various clinical and autopsy series differ widely. The best statistics have been reported from Malmo, Sweden, where both autopsy and double-contrast enema studies yielded a 12.5% incidence of polyps of all sizes.

HYPERPLASTIC POLYP

The hyperplastic (metaplastic) polyp is a focal epithelial proliferation of colonic mucosa that appears as a smooth, sessile mucosal elevation less than 5 mm in size (Fig. 50-2). Hyperplastic polyps arise from excessive cellular proliferation in the crypts of Lieberkuhn but maintain their cellular differentiation and have no dysplastic features or malignant potential. More than three-quarters of hyperplastic polyps are located from the splenic flexure distally; more than half arise in the rectosigmoid area. They are typically sessile and project off the apex of colonic folds. The cause of hyperplastic polyps is unclear, but trauma, inflammation, degeneration, or ischemia may play a role in their genesis.

Hyperplastic polyps were previously considered the most common colonic polyp, representing more than 90% of these lesions. However, more recent studies suggest that hyperplastic polyps may be second in prevalence to adenomas. Even in the case of diminutive polyps (<5 mm in size), a recent colonoscopic study showed that almost half the polyps were neoplastic with only 37% hyperplastic and the remainder proving to be either inflammatory masses or normal mucosa.

ADENOMATOUS POLYP

Adenomatous polyps are true neoplasms composed of branching glandular tubules lined by well-differentiated mucus-secreting goblet cells (Fig. 50-3). About 5% to 10% of people over age 40 have colonic adenomas, and the frequency rises with increasing age. Although traditionally it has been believed that more than 75% of colonic polyps occur in the rectum and sigmoid, recent studies have shown a more general distribution of polyps throughout the colon. More adenomas are found in the distal than in the proximal portion of the large bowel in patients less than 60 years old, though in patients over age 70 there seems to be a preponderance of right-sided adenomatous polyps. The sampling process could

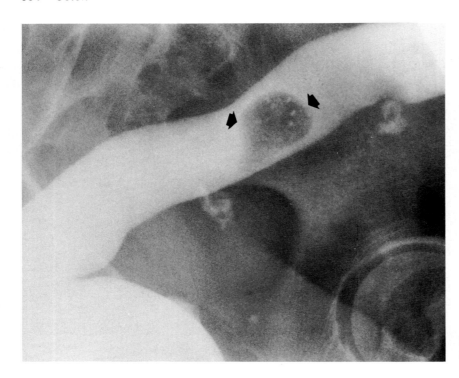

Fig. 50-3. Adenomatous polyp **(arrows)** in the sigmoid colon.

account for some of this proximal shift, because there is now better detection of lesions within the proximal colon. Large adenomatous polyps are reported to occur more frequently in the right colon. The reason for this predominance of right-sided lesions may be related to the fact that small masses in the right colon are not readily detected and, because most patients are not examined until they become symptomatic, right-sided polyps may not cause symptoms until they are much larger than symptomatic left-sided lesions.

The majority of colonic polyps, even diminutive ones (<5 mm in size) are adenomatous rather than hyperplastic. Although adenomas are benign, by definition they show dysplasia and may carry a malignant potential. This precancerous nature of an adenoma is related to several factors, including the degree of dysplasia, the size of the adenoma, the number of concurrent adenomas (probability of a polyposis syndrome), and the proportion of villous structures.

The most common symptom of adenomatous polyps is bleeding, though this occurs in only a minority of patients. Right-sided polyps tend to produce melena or guaiac-positive stools; left-sided lesions more often cause bright red blood to streak the surface of the stool or be mixed with it. Malignant polyps are more likely to bleed than benign ones, though, in the individual patient, this is of little diagnostic significance. Patients with polyps larger than 1 cm may complain of intermittent or alternating constipation and diarrhea, decreased caliber of stools, crampy abdominal pain, and mucus discharge.

Radiographic Demonstration

The radiographic detection of small polypoid lesions requires meticulous colon preparation and examination. Several studies have reported that 10% to 20% of colon carcinomas are missed on initial barium examination, primarily because poor prepa-

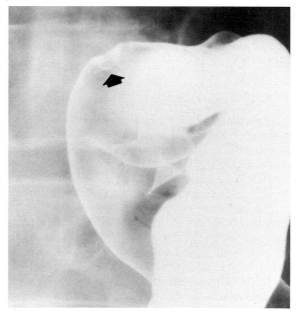

Fig. 50-4. Small polyp **(arrow)** in the splenic flexure seen with the double-contrast technique. The polyp was not visualized on a single-contrast study performed 1 week earlier.

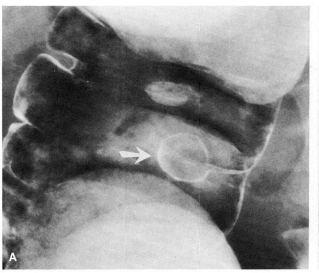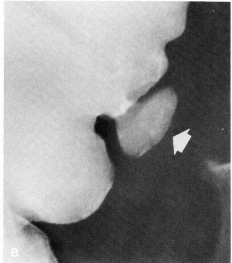

Fig. 50-5. Diverticulum mimicking a colonic polyp. **(A)** On the *en face* projection, the barium-coated diverticulum simulates a polyp **(arrow)** lying within the lumen. **(B)** A radiograph obtained after rotation of the patient demonstrates that the diverticulum fills with barium **(arrow)** and clearly extends beyond the colonic lumen.

ration results in the tumor being overlooked or confused with fecal material. Proper cleansing of the colon (laxatives, dietary restrictions, cleansing enemas in the radiology department) should improve these dismal statistics.

The double-contrast barium enema appears to have greater sensitivity in detecting polyps than the single-contrast technique (Fig. 50-4; see also Fig. 50-2). This is especially true in the case of small colonic lesions. Nevertheless, reports of polyps that were missed on double-contrast studies but identified with single-contrast techniques indicate that the two procedures have complementary value.

Fecal material, air bubbles, oil droplets, and intraluminal-appearing diverticula can be confused with adenomatous polyps. All of these artifacts, except for diverticula, usually move freely with the flow of barium or can be dislodged by palpation. Fecal material, however, can be adherent; a repeat examination may be necessary for definite diagnosis. Diverticula seen *en face* rather than in profile can appear to lie within the lumen, rather than projecting beyond it, and may be difficult to distinguish from polyps (Fig. 50-5*A*). Rotation of the patient usually demonstrates that the diverticulum truly extends beyond the colonic lumen (Fig. 50-5*B*). At times, the barium-coated, air-filled diverticulum remains superimposed on the lumen of the bowel on multiple projections. Demonstration of an air-fluid level clearly excludes the diagnosis of a polypoid lesion. Polyps and diverticula can sometimes be differentiated by an evaluation of the quality of the barium coating them. The ring of barium coating a diverticulum has a smooth, well-defined outer border (where it is in contact with the diverticular mucosa) but an irregular inner surface. In contrast, the barium coating a polyp is smooth on its inner border (where it abuts the mucosal surface of the polyp) but is poorly defined on its outer surface (where it is in contact with the fecal stream). Nevertheless, a small adenomatous polyp can easily be

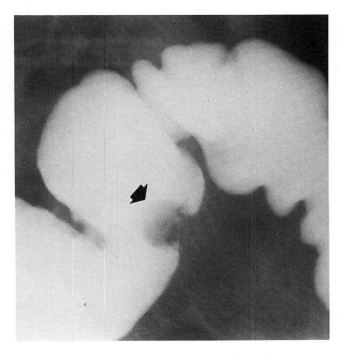

Fig. 50-6. Benign sessile colonic polyp **(arrow)**.

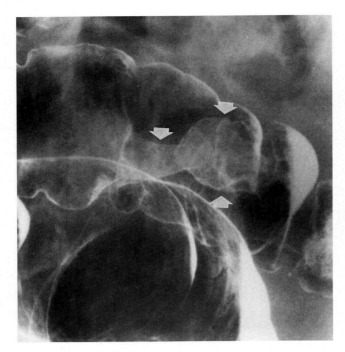

Fig. 50-7. Pedunculated colonic polyp **(arrows)**.

hidden in a patient with a large number of diverticula, and a diverticulum filled with fecal material may simulate a polyp.

There are three major morphologic types of polypoid tumor: sessile, intermediate or protuberant, and pedunculated. The earliest stage is the sessile polyp, a flat lesion attached to the mucosa by a broad base (Fig. 50-6). On *en face* views, the sessile polyp appears rounded. In profile, it may protrude only slightly into the lumen of the colon and may therefore be difficult to differentiate from the normal mucosa of the colon wall. Although the sessile polyp has a central fibrovascular core arising from the submucosa, this potential stalk is not yet detectable radiographically.

Peristaltic waves and the flow of the fecal stream cause traction on a sessile polyp, and this can force the underlying normal mucosa to be drawn out into a pedicle (stalk) (Fig. 50-7). In profile view, the pedicle may appear as a linear lucency in the barium-filled colon (Fig. 50-8*A*) or be thinly coated by barium in an air-contrast examination (Fig. 50-8*B*). When seen *en face* (with the central beam parallel to the long axis of the pedicle), the

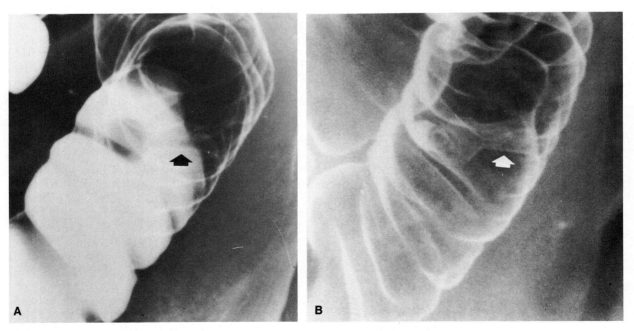

Fig. 50-8. Pedunculated colonic polyp. **(A)** On single-contrast examination, the stalk appears as a linear lucency in the barium-filled colon **(arrow)**. **(B)** On the double-contrast examination, the stalk of the polyp is thinly coated by barium **(arrow)**.

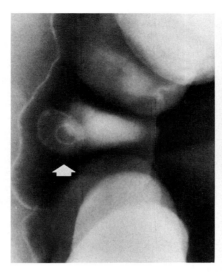

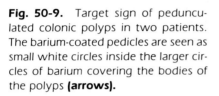

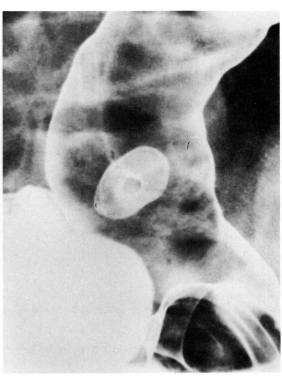

Fig. 50-9. Target sign of pedunculated colonic polyps in two patients. The barium-coated pedicles are seen as small white circles inside the larger circles of barium covering the bodies of the polyps **(arrows).**

barium-coated pedicle is seen as a small white circle within a larger circle of barium covering the body of the polyp (target sign; Fig. 50-9).

The radiographic demonstration of a thin pedicle of 2 cm or more in length is virtually pathognomonic of a benign polyp (see Fig. 50-8). This is true regardless of the presence of focally invasive carcinoma in the head of the polyp. Malignant sessile polyps that have invaded deep into the mucosa will not develop long stalks. When these polypoid carcinomas are pedunculated, the stalks are usually short, thick, and irregular.

Relationship Between Adenomatous Polyps and Carcinoma

The precise relationship between adenomatous polyps and carcinoma has created considerable controversy. Most authorities believe that the vast majority of adenocarcinomas of the colon arise in pre-existing benign adenomas. Evidence for this theory includes the well-documented coexistence of invasive carcinoma and benign-appearing adenomas, the rare demonstration of *de novo* carcinomas of less than 5 mm in size in otherwise normal colons, and the fact that almost all patients with familial intestinal polyposis who do not have surgery develop colon cancer. It is estimated that the evolution of cancer of the colon from a benign adenomatous polyp requires at least 5 years and may take as many as 20 years. Though it is difficult to establish a true malignancy rate, it is believed that about 5% of adenomatous polyps eventually transform into malignant lesions.

There is a close correlation between the size of adenomatous polyps of the colon and the incidence of invasive carcinoma within them. Adenomas measuring 5 mm to 9 mm in diameter have about a 1% probability of containing an invasive malignancy; those under 5 mm have less than a 0.5% incidence. Adenomatous polyps between 1 cm and 2 cm in size have been reported to have a 10% incidence of malignancy, whereas those greater than 2 cm in diame-

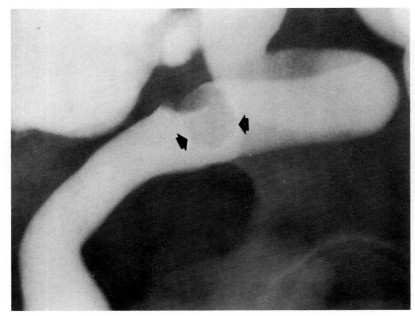

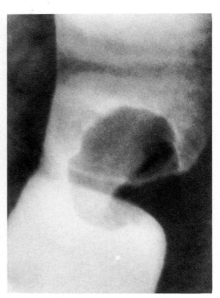

50-10   50-11

Fig. 50-10.   Malignant polyp **(arrows)** in the sigmoid colon. Although the lesion is smooth, its 4-cm diameter makes malignancy likely.

Fig. 50-11.   Malignant sessile colonic polyp. This large sessile mass has an irregular, lobulated surface.

ter are reported to have a malignancy rate of up to 46% (Fig. 50-10).

Radiographic Differentiation Between Benign and Malignant Polyps

Carcinomatous degeneration of an adenomatous polyp can be suggested by several radiographic criteria: surface characteristics; change in size, shape, or appearance of an associated pedicle; puckering of the base of the tumor; and interval growth on sequential examination.

Benign sessile polyps tend to have a smooth surface and a normal adjacent colon wall. An irregular or lobulated surface suggests malignancy (Fig. 50-11), as does a flat lesion whose base is longer than its height (Fig. 50-12).

Pedunculated polyps with long, thin stalks that move freely on palpation are almost always benign. Carcinomatous transformation in the head of a pedunculated polyp not only enlarges the head but also grows into the stalk. This causes gradual shortening and obliteration of the pedicle and can eventually produce a sessile lesion (Fig. 50-13). It is extremely rare for carcinoma developing in a pedunculated polyp to metastasize to adjacent tissues prior to invading its stalk.

Retraction or indentation (puckering) of the colon wall seen on profile view at the site of origin of a sessile polyp has traditionally been considered

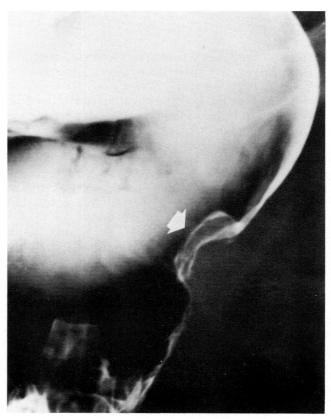

Fig. 50-12.   Malignant sessile rectal polyp **(arrow)**. Note that the base of this flat lesion is longer than its height.

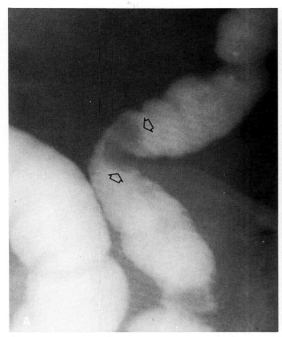

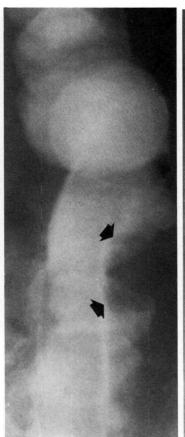

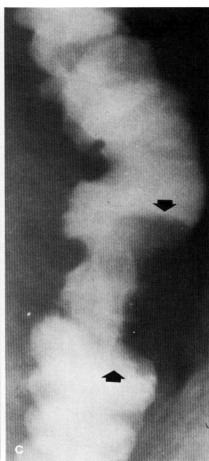

Fig. 50-13. Sessile malignant lesion developing from a pedunculated polyp. **(A)** Large pedunculated polyp **(arrows)**. **(B)** Four years later, the mass has become sessile **(arrows)**. **(C)** One year after **(B)**, an annular constricting lesion has formed **(arrows)**.

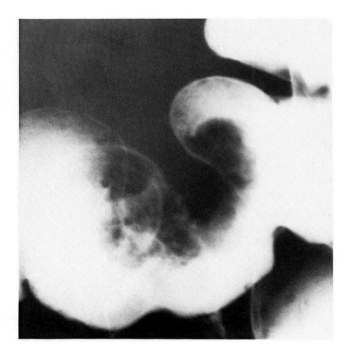

Fig. 50-14. Malignant sessile colonic polyp. Retraction or indentation (puckering) of the colon wall is seen on profile view.

as an almost invariable indication that the polyp is malignant (Fig. 50-14). However, recent studies have suggested that smooth basal indentation may be a projectional artifact related to the geometry at the junction of the base of the polyp and colonic wall. This consideration is especially important in evaluating smaller polyps with smooth, minimal indentation. Among larger malignant polyps, the basal indentation tends to be more prominent and irregular, and on pathologic examination it represents carcinomatous infiltration. Benign pedunculated polyps may also demonstrate a puckered appearance, which represents tugging of the stalk rather than malignant invasion of the bowel wall.

Sudden or steady interval growth of a polyp on sequential examinations strongly suggests malignancy. Although a benign polyp can grow slowly, it tends to maintain its initial configuration. Carcinomatous proliferation alters the growth of a polyp and can change its shape from round or elliptical to a variety of bizarre configurations (*e.g.,* triangular, rectangular, polyhedral).

Another form of carcinoma of the colon is a flat, centrally ulcerated plaque involving a segment of the bowel wall. As the tumor enlarges, it appears to sit on the barium column, much like a saddle on a horse (saddle lesion; Fig. 50-15). Unless they are demonstrated in tangent, saddle carcinomas can be easily overlooked on barium enema examination. These lesions are extremely virulent and grow rapidly, eventually spreading circumferentially about the bowel to become annular carcinomas (Fig. 50-16).

Saddle cancer has been described as analogous to a malignant Carman ulcer of the stomach. Spot-films with compression can demonstrate trapping of barium within a centrally ulcerated lesion with heaped up edges, producing a true Carman meniscus sign.

Because saddle cancers ulcerate at an early stage of development, rectal bleeding is usually the only symptom. Only by meticulous searching for an area of minimal straightening or slight contour defect can these small and subtle, but lethal, lesions be detected.

Diagnostic Management of Colonic Polyps

Because of the high likelihood of cure with removal of small adenomas, and because it is difficult to dis-

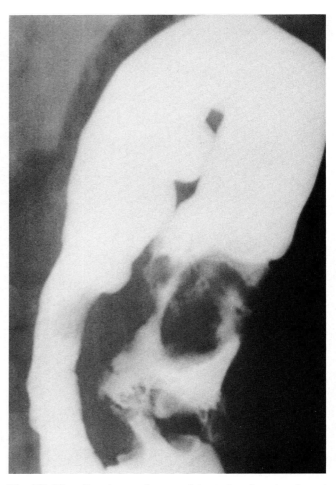

Fig. 50-16. Annular carcinoma of the colon that developed from circumferential spread of a saddle lesion.

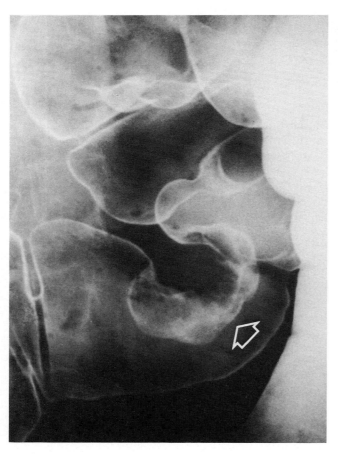

Fig. 50-15. Saddle cancer of the colon. The tumor **(arrow)** appears to sit on the upper margin of the distal transverse colon like a saddle on a horse.

tinguish neoplasms (adenomas) from nonneoplastic polyps, all detected polyps should be removed and analyzed. If this procedure is followed, many neoplastic lesions will be removed when they are benign or when carcinoma is limited to the mucosa (carcinoma *in situ*), thus resulting in a complete cure. About half the patients who have had one adenoma will develop another adenoma within 4 years. Therefore, periodic surveillance of the colon is essential, and the degree of follow-up depends on the size, number, villous content, and degree of dysplasia of the initial adenoma. Hyperplastic polyps also should be removed endoscopically when found since their gross and radiographic appearances closely resemble the small adenoma. However, no specific follow-up is necessary after the removal of a simple hyperplastic polyp.

HAMARTOMA

A hamartoma is a nonneoplastic tumorlike lesion composed of abnormal quantities of normal elements. There are two types of colonic hamartomas, the Peutz–Jeghers polyp and the juvenile polyp, both of which can occur singly or as multiple lesions.

The Peutz–Jeghers polyp is composed of branching bands of smooth muscle covered by colonic epithelium. Both grossly and radiographically, the Peutz–Jeghers polyp has a complex nodular surface reflecting its arborizing infrastructure and frequently looks like the head of a cauliflower. Although solitary colonic polyps of this type may occur, they are much more frequently multiple and seen in association with multiple small bowel polyps in the Peutz–Jeghers syndrome.

The juvenile polyp is composed of an expanded lamina propria containing glands but without muscularis mucosae. Because the colonic glands are often dilated and appear as large cystic spaces filled with mucus, the mass may be termed "retention polyp." The juvenile polyp is usually smooth, round, almost always pedunculated, and cherry red in gross appearance. Its surface is frequently eroded. About 70% of juvenile polyps are solitary; in most of the remaining cases, the polyps number three to five. The occurrence of numerous polyps (juvenile polyposis syndromes) is rare. The "solitary" juvenile polyp is generally seen in children under age 10, but can occur occasionally in adolescents and adults. The patient can present with rectal bleeding, cramping, abdominal pain, and prolapse of the

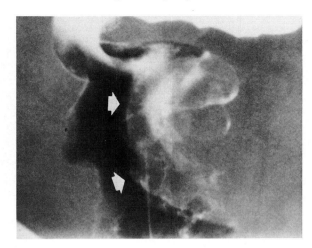

Fig. 50-18. Benign villous adenoma of the rectum **(arrows)**. Barium can be seen entering the interstices of the tumor.

polyp. Juvenile polyps average 1 cm to 2 cm in diameter (range, 2 mm to 5 cm) and about 70% are situated in the rectum.

Carcinomatous transformation in the solitary Peutz-Jeghers type polyp is exceedingly rare. Thus, a totally hamartomatous polyp of this type can be simply removed with no subsequent follow-up. Juvenile polyps are also benign, have no malignant potential, and tend to autoamputate or regress. Therefore, surgical removal of juvenile polyps is indicated only if there are significant or repeated episodes of rectal bleeding or intussusception.

VILLOUS ADENOMA

Villous adenomas of the colon are benign exophytic tumors consisting of innumerable villous fronds that give the surface a corrugated appearance (Fig. 50-17). Most are solitary and are located in the rectosigmoid area (Fig. 50-18). However, they can be found anywhere in the colon, particularly in the cecum. Villous adenomas are usually sessile but can be pedunculated (Fig. 50-19). Although they constitute only 10% of all benign neoplastic polyps of the colon, they are of great importance because of their high malignant potential. In contrast to the far more numerous adenomatous polyps, which have a low malignancy rate, about 40% of villous adenomas demonstrate infiltrating carcinoma, usually at the base. Villous adenomas also tend to be much larger than adenomatous polyps; about 75% exceed 2 cm in diameter, whereas only 5% of adenomatous polyps reach this size.

Villous adenomas are often asymptomatic and are frequently an unexpected finding on barium enema examination performed for another purpose. Extremely large tumors (10–15 cm) can produce obstructive symptoms. Large amounts of mucus are occasionally secreted into the lumen

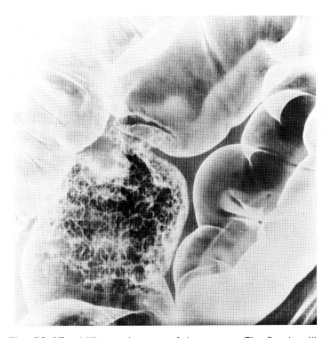

Fig. 50-17. Villous adenoma of the rectum. The fine lacelike pattern results from seepage of barium into interstices between individual tumor fronds. The bulk of the tumor expands the lumen, and there is a notch on the right superolateral aspect representing the point of attachment. (Margulis AR, Burhenne HJ, [eds]: Alimentary Tract Radiology. St. Louis, CV Mosby, 1983)

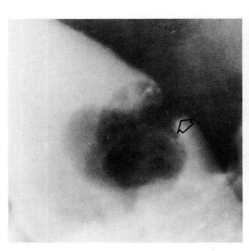

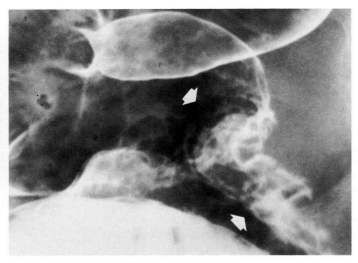

50-19   50-20

Fig. 50-19.   Benign villous adenoma of the transverse colon. Note the short stalk **(arrow)** leading to the lobulated mass.

Fig. 50-20.   Benign villous adenoma of the rectum **(arrows).** Barium is seen filling the deep clefts between the multiple fronds.

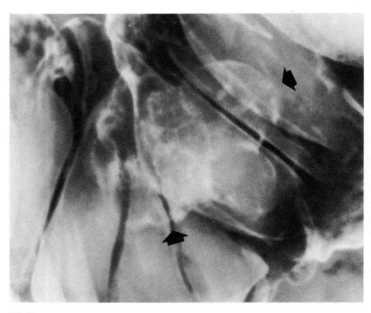

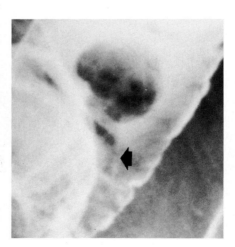

50-21   50-22

Fig. 50-21.   Villous adenocarcinoma. The large size of the mass **(arrows)** suggests malignancy. Barium is seen entering the interstices of the mass, suggesting that the lesion represents a villous tumor.

Fig. 50-22.   Villoglandular polyp. This benign lesion is composed of mixed adenomatous and villous elements and has a relatively long stalk **(arrow)**.

across the papillary surface of a villous adenoma. This mucus diarrhea causes severe fluid, protein, and electrolyte (especially potassium) depletion. Rectal bleeding is unusual, since the mucosal surface of a villous adenoma is usually intact and not ulcerated.

Radiographically, villous adenomas classically present as bulky tumors with a spongelike pattern ("bouquet of flowers") caused by barium filling of deep clefts between the multiple fronds (Fig. 50-20). This radiographic feature is best demonstrated on the postevacuation view, in which barium remains within the interstices of the villous tumor. Because the lobular, irregular tumor has a soft consistency, its appearance can change on serial films and with palpation. The adjacent bowel wall is pliable and distensible, since the tumor does not incite a desmoplastic response.

Large size (Fig. 50-21), ulceration, and indentation of the tumor base have been suggested as radiographic signs of malignancy in villous adenomas. Nevertheless, no radiographic finding in villous adenoma is sufficient to exclude malignant degeneration. Because invasive carcinoma in villous adenoma is usually found at the base of a lesion rather than on the surface, biopsies can be unreliable as a result of inadequate tissue sampling. Therefore, even a benign-appearing villous adenoma should be totally excised.

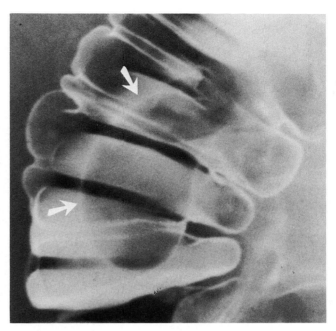

Fig. 50-24. Lipoma of the ascending colon. An extremely lucent mass with smooth margins and a tear-drop shape **(arrows)** is visible.

VILLOGLANDULAR POLYP

Villoglandular polyps are composed of mixed adenomatous and villous elements (Fig. 50-22). Although they tend to be pedunculated and grossly simulate adenomatous polyps, villoglandular polyps have an intermediate malignant potential (about 20%) that is higher than that of adenomatous polyps but less than that of villous adenomas.

LIPOMA

Lipomas are the second most common benign tumors of the colon. Submucosal in origin, lipomas grow slowly, rarely cause symptoms, and generally are incidental findings on barium enema examination. The tumors are usually single and occur most commonly in the right colon (Fig. 50-23). Because of the motor activity of the colon and the soft consistency of the tumor, a lipoma tends to protrude into the bowel lumen. The resulting polyp often seems to have a stalk, but this actually represents a thick pseudopedicle of normal mucosa rather than the true pedicle of an adenomatous polyp. Stretching of the epithelium over the lipoma can result in ulceration and continued oozing of blood. Intermittent episodes of intussusception are not uncommon.

On barium studies, lipomas are typically circular or ovoid, sharply defined, smooth filling defects (Fig. 50-24). In comparison with other colon

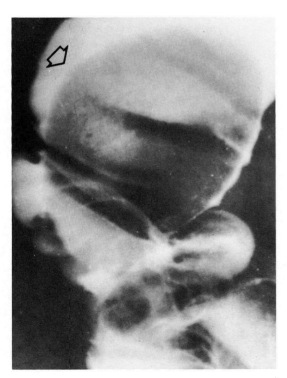

Fig. 50-23. Lipoma. A large, smooth mass **(arrow)** is visible in the ascending colon.

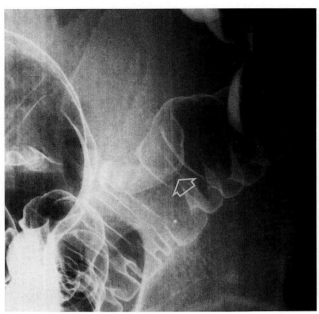 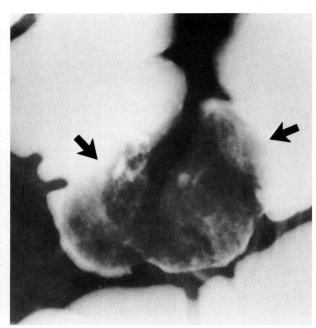

50-25   50-26

Fig. 50-25.   Hemangioma of the sigmoid colon. A large, smooth intramural mass **(arrow)** may be seen.

Fig. 50-26.   Leiomyoma of the transverse colon. A large mass protrudes into the lumen and appears as a sessile, polypoid filling defect **(arrows)**.

tumors, lipomas have an unusually lucent appearance. This is due both to the fat content of the lesion and to the very smooth surface of the mucosa stretched over the mass, which does not permit as good barium coating as does the more irregular surface of an adenomatous polyp. The adjacent bowel wall is normally distensible, with intact mucosa. If the tumor has an associated pseudopedicle, it generally appears short and thick. The pathognomonic diagnostic feature of lipomas is their changeability in size and shape during the course of barium enema examination. Because these tumors are extremely soft, their configuration can be altered by palpation and extrinsic pressure. Although a lipoma can appear round or oval on filled films, the malleable tumor characteristically becomes elongated (sausage or banana-shaped) on postevacuation films in which the colon is contracted.

OTHER SPINDLE CELL TUMORS

Other spindle cell tumors (leiomyoma, fibroma, neurofibroma, hemangioma, cystic lymphangioma) are rare. They tend to remain more intramural than lipomas (Fig. 50-25), though large lesions can protrude into the lumen and appear as sessile, polypoid tumors mimicking carcinoma (Fig. 50-26). The overlying mucosa tends to be stretched but intact.

Unlike lipomas and cystic lymphangioma, other spindle cell tumors do not change shape in response to extrinsic pressure or during various phases of filling and emptying of the colon.

Malignant spindle cell tumors are extremely rare (Fig. 50-27). They tend to be much larger and more irregular than their benign counterparts, though differentiation between benign and malignant submucosal tumors can be extremely difficult.

TRAUMATIC NEUROMA

Traumatic neuroma, or amputation neuroma, is a nonneoplastic proliferative mass of Schwann's cells that may develop at the proximal end of a severed or injured nerve, most commonly in an extremity following amputation. Very rarely, traumatic neuromas develop in the nerves innervating the digestive tract after surgery in this region. One case report has described a traumatic neuroma arising at the site of a previous ileocolic anastomosis (see Fig. 39-19). Barium enema examination showed an extramucosal mass in a patient who presented with abdominal pain, rectal bleeding, and anemia. Obstructive symptoms due to luminal narrowing have occurred with traumatic neuromas of the esophagus and biliary tree.

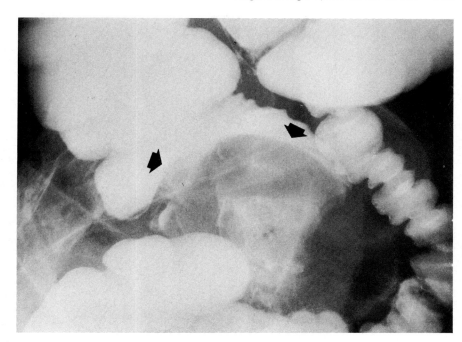

Fig. 50-27. Leiomyosarcoma. Although the mass **(arrows)** is large, the malignant nature of the lesion cannot be determined radiographically, and a biopsy specimen is required.

TUMORS WITH INTERMEDIATE MALIGNANT POTENTIAL

CARCINOID TUMOR

Almost all nonappendiceal carcinoid tumors of the colon arise in the rectum (Fig. 50-28). The vast majority are small (under 1 cm in size), solitary, and asymptomatic. Most are found only incidentally on barium enema or sigmoidoscopic examination. Rectal carcinoids are slow-growing tumors that are much less malignant than carcinomas; metastases develop in about 10% of cases. They have a significantly better prognosis than the more proximal colonic lesions and are usually cured by simple local excision. The size of the lesion is closely correlated with the aggressiveness of the tumor, and the survival rate is associated with the size. Small colonic carcinoids (<1 cm) rarely invade locally or metastasize to the liver. In contrast, larger lesions (>2 cm) are often locally aggressive and invade the muscularis, extending beyond the serosa into adjacent tissues and metastasizing in more than 80% of cases (Fig. 50-29). Unlike ileal tumors, carcinoids of the colon and rectum rarely give rise to the carcinoid syndrome.

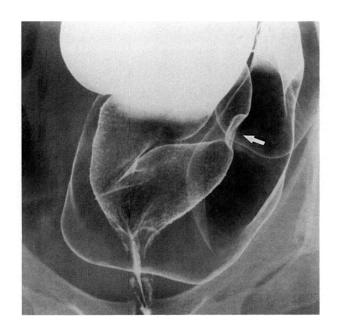

Fig. 50-28. Rectal carcinoid. Small sessile tumor with a broad base **(arrow)** arising on the left side of the rectum. (Sato T, Sakai Y, Sonoyama A et al: Radiologic spectrum of rectal carcinoid tumors. Gastrointest Radiol 9:23–26, 1984)

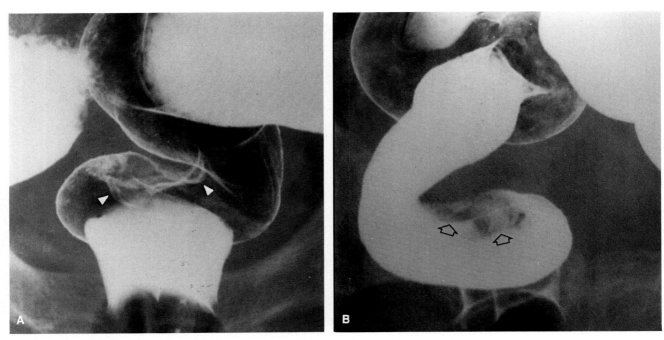

Fig. 50-29. Invasive rectal carcinoid. **(A)** Irregular tumor invading the muscular layer **(arrows)**. **(B)** On a film taken with the patient in the prone position, there is a deep crater with nodular edge **(arrows)**. (Sato T, Sakai Y, Sonoyama A et al: Radiologic spectrum of rectal carcinoid tumors. Gastrointest Radiol 9:23–26, 1984)

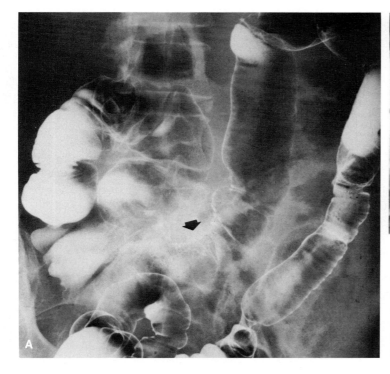

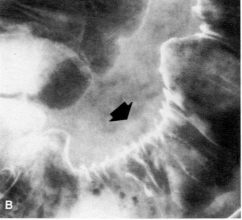

Fig. 50-30. Carcinoma of the pancreas metastatic to the transverse colon. **(A)** Full and **(B)** coned views reveal a shallow extrinsic pressure defect with multiple spiculations **(arrows)**.

Although colonic carcinoids arise from the submucosa, they most frequently present radiographically as solitary, smooth, round polypoid protrusions into the lumen. Large ulcerating lesions can produce rectal bleeding, intussusception, or obstruction. Rarely, rectal carcinoids appear as infiltrating or annular lesions indistinguishable from adenocarcinoma.

Colonic carcinoids elsewhere than in the appendix and rectum are extremely rare. These tumors tend to be relatively large, often have a prominent extramural component, and have a higher malignant potential than rectal carcinoids.

MALIGNANT TUMORS

METASTASES

Metastases to the colon can produce shallow extrinsic pressure defects along the contour of the barium column (Fig. 50-30). A similar appearance may be caused by omental metastases involving the transverse colon (Fig. 50-31). When the impression involves the transverse colon, proximal descending colon, or the medial aspect of the cecum, spread of inflammation from pancreatitis must be excluded

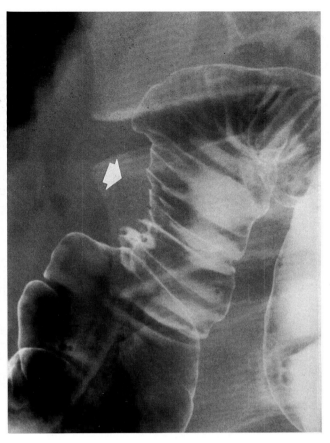

Fig. 50-32. Pancreatitis. A shallow extrinsic pressure defect with spiculations involves the splenic flexure **(arrow)**. The appearance is radiographically indistinguishable from a metastatic serosal implant.

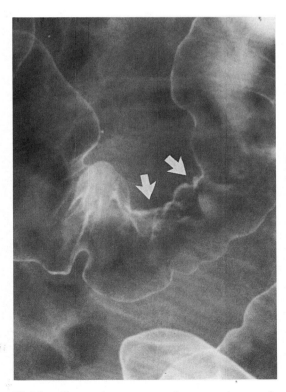

Fig. 50-31. Omental metastases from ovarian carcinoma. Mass effect with slight tethering of mucosal folds on the superior border of the transverse colon **(arrows)**, due to contiguous spread of tumor from the greater omentum. (Rubesin SE, Levine MS: Omental cakes: Colonic involvement by omental metastases. Radiology 154:593–596, 1985)

(Fig. 50-32). Larger lesions cause smooth or lobulated masses mimicking intramural, extramucosal tumors (Fig. 50-33). In contrast to primary carcinoma, metastases to the colon often occur at multiple sites.

LYMPHOMA

Localized lymphoma can appear as a single smooth (Fig. 50-34) or lobulated (Fig. 50-35) polypoid mass that is radiographically indistinguishable from carcinoma. Unlike carcinoma, localized lymphoma tends to be unusually bulky and to extend over a longer segment of the colon. Polypoid lymphoma is seen most frequently in the cecum. As lymphoma extends through the bowel wall, it can develop a large extracolonic component that displaces adjacent abdominal structures.

EXTRAMEDULLARY PLASMACYTOMA

Extramedullary plasmacytomas of the colon are rare tumors that may precede, accompany, or fol-

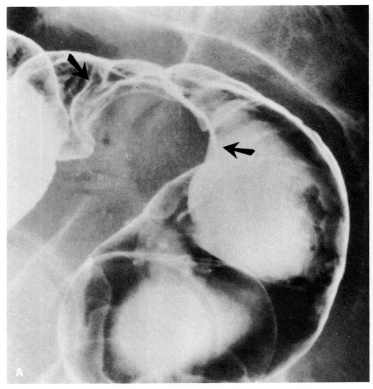

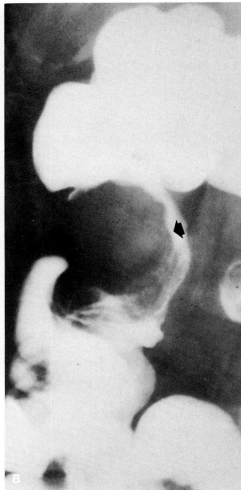

Fig. 50-33. Two examples of metastatic carcinoma producing large masses that mimic intramural, extramucosal tumors. **(A)** Colon carcinoma metastatic to the cul-de-sac **(arrow)**. **(B)** Carcinoma of the ovary metastatic to the ascending colon **(arrow)**.

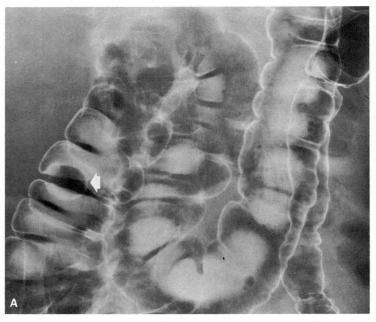

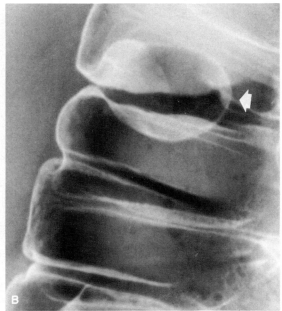

Fig. 50-34. Lymphoma. **(A)** Full and **(B)** coned views reveal a smooth polypoid mass **(arrows)**.

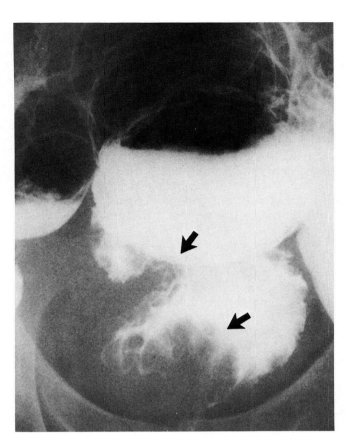

Fig. 50-35. Lymphoma. This bulky, irregular, ulcerated mass involves much of the rectum **(arrows)**.

low the onset of multiple myeloma or may occur as isolated lesions. Over three-fourths of these extraosseous plasmacytomas occur in the head and neck, especially the nasal cavity, paranasal sinuses, and upper airway. Plasmacytomas of the colon have a variable clinical presentation, but there is usually some degree of rectal bleeding. The most frequent radiographic pattern is a polypoid mass or constricting lesion, which may show mucosal or submucosal infiltration. Less common appearances include superficial ulcers, complete colonic obstruction, and even intussusception.

AMEBOMA

An ameboma is a focal hyperplastic granuloma caused by secondary bacterial infection of an amebic abscess in the bowel wall. The lesion has a core of acute and chronic inflammation and necrosis surrounded by a peripheral rim of dense fibrosis.

Amebomas have been reported in 1.5% to 8.5% of patients with amebic colitis. Almost half are multiple; most are associated with evidence of disease elsewhere in the colon. Amebomas are most common in the cecum and ascending colon but can be found anywhere in the large bowel. Most patients with amebomas present with acute or chronic amebic dysentery. Abdominal or rectal examination occasionally demonstrates a large, firm mass that is relatively fixed and tender to palpation.

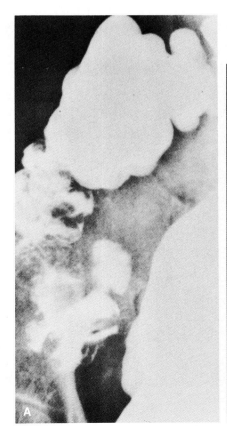
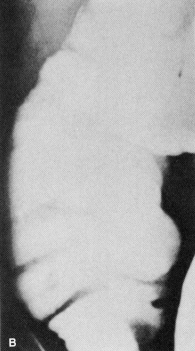

Fig. 50-36. Ameboma. **(A)** Irregular mass in the cecum and ascending colon. **(B)** Rapid regression of the lesion following antiamebic therapy. (Cardosa JM, Kimura K, Stoopen M et al: Radiology of invasive amebiasis of the colon. AJR 128:935–941, 1977. Copyright 1977. Reproduced with permission)

Radiographically, amebomas are characterized by eccentric or concentric thickening of the entire circumference of the bowel wall. They can appear as discrete luminal masses or as annular, nondistensible lesions with irregular mucosa that simulate colonic carcinoma (Fig. 50-36*A*).

The differential diagnosis between ameboma and carcinoma can be extremely difficult. The most reliable features of ameboma are multiplicity of lesions, lack of a shelving deformity, and rapid improvement with antiamebic therapy (Fig. 50-36*B*). Less important findings suggesting ameboma are long length of the lesion, tapered ends, and concentricity of the narrowing. Evidence of mucosal ulcerations elsewhere in the colon, especially in the cecum, strongly suggests amebiasis as the underlying etiology. If a colonic filling defect or annular lesion is suspected to represent an ameboma (especially in a young patient with a history of having lived in or traveled through an endemic area), a trial with antiamebic therapy is essential. Shrinkage of an ameboma in response to antiamebic therapy is often achieved in less than 1 month. In addition,

there is a high rate of postoperative morbidity and mortality (over 50% in one series) if a colostomy or other surgical procedure is performed without adequate antiamebic therapy beforehand.

INFLAMMATORY MASSES

Single or multiple small (1–1.5 cm) localized eccentric contour defects have been reported to be an early manifestation of Crohn's disease of the colon. These focal lesions may occur as the only abnormal radiographic finding or may appear in association with more obvious segmental disease elsewhere in the colon. Surface irregularity of the contour defects can suggest the presence of ulceration. These focal lesions seen on barium enema examination correspond pathologically to sharply localized ulcers of variable depth that are associated with pronounced edema and inflammation of the adjacent mucosa and submucosa.

Individual inflammatory pseudopolyps usually measure less than 1.5 cm in diameter and appear as

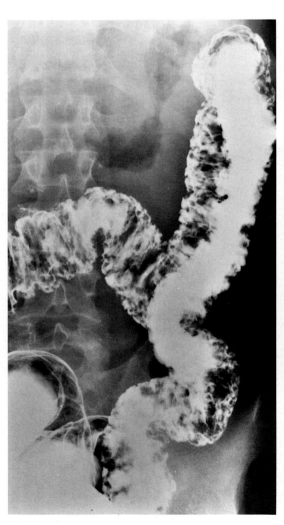

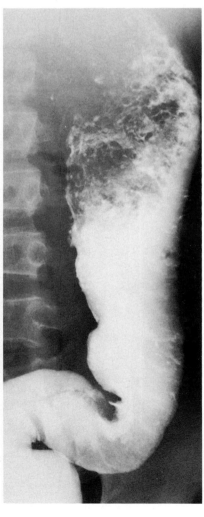

Fig. 50-37. Inflammatory pseudopolyps in Crohn's disease. Multiple nodular filling defects, each less than 1 cm in diameter, are scattered throughout the colon.

Fig. 50-38. Localized giant pseudopolyposis in ulcerative colitis. Barium enema examination shows obstruction of the splenic flexure by a bulky mass with a nodular surface. Superficial mucosal ulcerations are present in the descending colon. (Bernstein JR, Ghahremani GG, Paige ML et al: Localized giant pseudopolyposis of the colon in ulcerative and granulomatous colitis. Gastrointest Radiol 3:431–435, 1978)

50-37   50-38

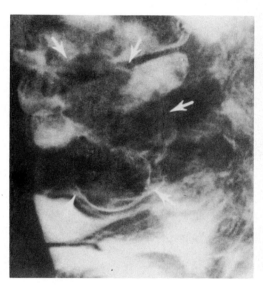

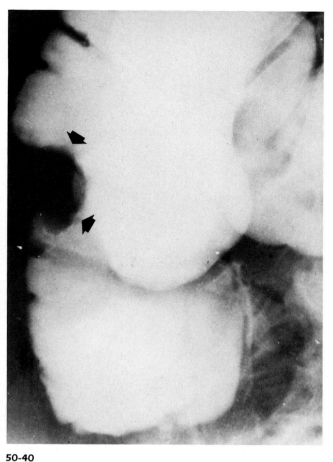

50-39   50-40

Fig. 50-39. Mucormycoma. Compression spot film of the cecum shows a large polypoid mass **(arrows)** with smooth inferior margin and poorly defined superior aspect. (Agha FP, Lee HH, Boland CR: Mucormycoma of the colon: Early diagnosis and successful management. AJR 145: 739–741, 1985. Copyright 1985. Reproduced with permission)

Fig. 50-40. Periappendiceal abscess. Perforation of a retrocecal appendix has produced an inflammatory mass that has caused an extrinsic impression on the lateral margin of the proximal ascending colon **(arrows)**.

discrete masses scattered throughout involved segments of the colon (Fig. 50-37). A localized giant cluster of pseudopolyps occasionally develops in patients with ulcerative or Crohn's colitis (Fig. 50-38). Adherence and retention of fecal particles within the hyperplastic mass further contribute to the bulk of the lesion. The resultant localized giant pseudopolyp can obliterate the lumen of the colon and simulate a malignant tumor or colonic intussusception.

Although polypoid granulomas caused by schistosomiasis usually present as multiple filling defects in the rectosigmoid, they can occur singly and simulate adenocarcinoma. These masses sometimes become so large that obstruction or intussusception results. A primary submucosal epithelioid tubercule can present radiographically as a sharply outlined contour defect mimicking an intramural

tumor; however, because lesions at this stage of development are asymptomatic, this radiographic pattern is rarely seen. Tuberculosis can also cause an intraluminal mass simulating carcinoma. Rarely, large numbers of *Ascaris lumbricoides* organisms clump together to form a bolus of worms that appears as a polypoid filling defect in the colon. In patients with chronic debilitating disease or immunosuppression, the nonspecific finding of a polypoid pedunculated lesion may represent a rare mucormycoma, which tends to involve the colon and stomach (Fig. 50-39). The fungal infection may extend from the lumen of the gut and cause bowel obstruction or perforation. Whenever an intramural or extrinsic filling defect is seen in the cecum (even if on the lateral margin), the possibility of rupture of the appendix and formation of a periappendiceal abscess must be considered (Fig. 50-40). Diverticuli-

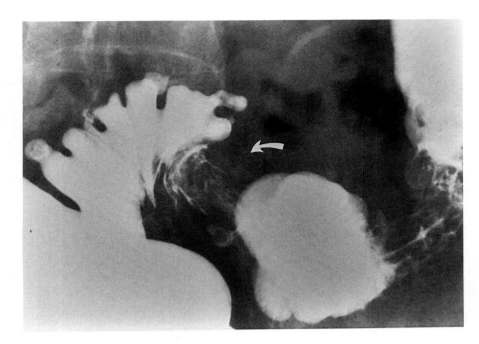

Fig. 50-41. Diverticulitis. The resulting pericolic abscess has caused a large extrinsic filling defect on the sigmoid colon **(arrow)**.

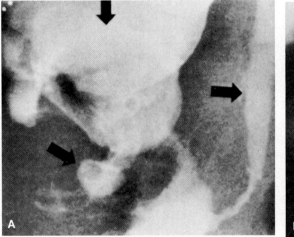 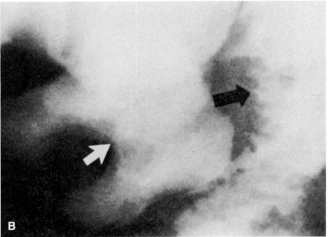

Fig. 50-42. Benign ulceration of the cecum. **(A)** This distorted and incompletely distended cecum is not fixed in appearance, despite its masslike effect [see **(B)**]. The **upper arrow** points to the superior surface of the inflammatory mass. The **slanted arrow** points to the persistent collection of barium representing an ulcer. The **horizontal arrow** points to the partially filled appendix, the base of which is narrowed and irregular. **(B)** The cecum is more distended than in **(A)**, indicating that the distortion is not fixed. The **white arrow** points to the same collection of barium in the ulcer as in **(A)**. The **black arrow** points to the normal terminal ileum with no adjacent mass effect. (Brodey PA, Hill RP, Baron S: Benign ulceration of the cecum. Radiology 122:323–327, 1977)

tis can appear as a broad intramural or extrinsic colonic filling defect almost always involving the sigmoid (Fig. 50-41). The presence of multiple diverticula intimately associated with the mass, especially if they are deformed, suggests a diverticular abscess. Nonspecific benign ulceration of the colon, which predominantly occurs in the cecum, can present as a large filling defect with or without radiographically demonstrable ulceration (Fig. 50-42). Foreign body perforation with abscess formation, most commonly due to a chicken bone, can also appear as a colonic mass.

MISCELLANEOUS DISORDERS

FECAL IMPACTION

Fecal impactions are large, firm, immovable masses of stool in the rectum that produce filling defects on barium enema examination. They develop whenever there is incomplete evacuation of feces over an extended period. Fecal impactions occur in elderly, debilitated, or sedentary persons, in narcotic addicts and patients receiving large doses of tranquilizers, and in children who have undiagnosed megacolon or psychogenic problems. Institutionalized patients, especially those of geriatric age, are prone to the development of fecal impactions.

The symptoms of fecal impaction usually consist of vague rectal fullness and nonspecific abdominal discomfort. A common complaint is overflow diarrhea, the uncontrolled passage of small amounts of watery and semiformed stool around a large obstructing impaction. In elderly, bedridden patients, it is essential that this overflow phenomenon be recognized as secondary to fecal impaction rather than perceived as true diarrhea.

Plain radiographs of the pelvis are usually diagnostic of fecal impaction (Fig. 50-43). Typically, there is a soft-tissue density in the rectum containing multiple small, irregular lucent areas that reflect pockets of gas within the fecal mass. Barium studies demonstrate a large, irregular intraluminal mass.

ENDOMETRIOSIS

Endometriosis is the presence of heterotopic foci of endometrium in an extrauterine location. Although tissues in proximity to the uterus (ovaries, uterine ligaments, rectovaginal septum, pelvic peritoneum) are most frequently involved in endometriosis, the colon and even the small bowel can be affected.

Endometriosis primarily involves those parts of the bowel that are situated in the pelvis. In most instances, the rectosigmoid colon is affected, though endometrial implants can be found in the appendix, cecum, ileum, and even jejunum. The heterotopic endometrium initially invades the subserosal layer of the bowel. Under hormonal influence, the surface epithelium matures and finally sloughs, resulting in bleeding similar to that which occurs in endometriosis in the uterine cavity. If bleeding occurs in an enclosed cystic area, expansion of the lesion can cause necrosis of adjacent tissues. Cyclic repetition of this process causes dissection through the subserosal and muscular layers to the submucosa. Because the spread of endometriosis rarely involves the mucosa, cyclic bleeding into the intestinal lumen is uncommon.

Endometriosis is usually clinically apparent only when ovarian function is active. Although symptoms have been reported in teenagers and even in postmenopausal females, most women who are symptomatic from endometriosis are between 20 and 45 years of age. The typical gastrointestinal complaint is abdominal cramps and diarrhea during the menstrual period. Each exacerbation of disease provokes hyperplasia of smooth muscle and fibrous stroma, which, if sufficiently extensive, can narrow the lumen and cause symptoms of partial colonic or small bowel obstruction. On rare occasions, hemoperitoneum arising from eroded or ruptured endometrial implants can cause acute, intense abdominal pain.

An isolated endometrioma typically presents as an intramural defect involving the sigmoid colon (Fig. 50-44). There can be pleating or crenulation of the adjacent mucosa due to secondary fibrosis (Fig. 50-45). The sharply defined, eccentric defect simulates a flat saddle cancer. In contrast to the mucosa in primary colonic malignancy, the mucosal pattern underlying and adjacent to an endometrioma usually remains intact. Less frequently, endometriosis involving the colon presents as an intralu-

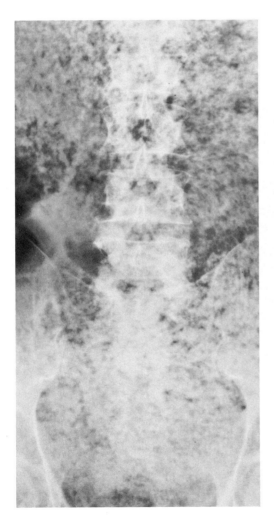

Fig. 50-43. *Fecal impaction. This large rectal mass has multiple irregular lucent areas reflecting pockets of gas within the fecal mass.*

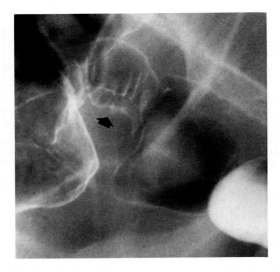

Fig. 50-44. *Endometriosis. There is an intramural mass in the proximal sigmoid near the rectosigmoid junction* **(arrow)***. The sharply defined, eccentric defect simulates a flat saddle cancer. Pleating of the adjacent mucosa is due to secondary fibrosis.*

minal polypoid mass with little distortion of the bowel wall (Fig. 50-46).

Endometriosis can also present as a constricting lesion simulating annular carcinoma. Radiographic findings favoring endometriosis are an intact mucosa, a long lesion with tapered margins, and the absence of ulceration within the mass. Repeated shedding of endometrial tissue and blood into the peritoneal cavity can lead to the development of dense adhesive bands causing extrinsic obstruction of the bowel.

INTUSSUSCEPTION

Intussusception, the telescoping of a segment of bowel into the lumen of a contiguous distal portion, produces an intraluminal filling defect that is often associated with intestinal obstruction and vascular compromise. Most intussusceptions occur in children under the age of two and consist of invagination of the ileum into the colon (ileocolic intussusception). Colocolic intussusceptions are much less common. In children, a specific cause of intussus-

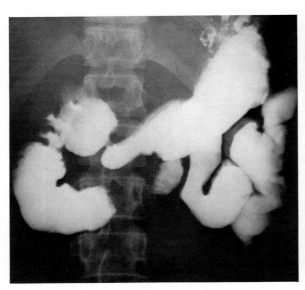

50-45

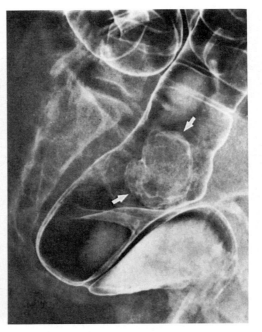

50-46

Fig. 50-45. *Endometriosis. Large extramucosal deposit at the rectosigmoid junction with tethering of overlying mucosa* **(arrows)** *and crenulation. (Gordon RL, Evers K, Kressel HY et al: Double-contrast enema in pelvic endometriosis. AJR 138:549–552, 1982. Copyright 1982. Reproduced with permission)*

Fig. 50-46. *Endometriosis. Lobulated polypoid mass that appears entirely intraluminal. (Bashist B, Forde KA, McCaffrey RM: Polypoid endometrioma of the rectosigmoid. Gastrointest Radiol 8:85–88, 1983)*

ception is infrequently demonstrated; the process is most likely a functional disturbance of bowel motility resulting from an increased deposition of fat and lymphoid tissue within the bowel. In older children and adults, however, a specific causative lesion can be demonstrated in more than half of all intussusceptions. Common leading points of intussusception are Meckel's diverticula, Peyer's patches, lymphoma, large mesenteric nodes, duplications, and polyps (Fig. 50-47).

Patients with intussusception typically present with recurrent crampy abdominal pain and vomiting. A palpable mass and thick, bloody stools ("currant-jelly" stools) are not uncommon.

Plain abdominal radiographs can reveal a soft-tissue mass with gas in the distal colon outlining the intussuscepting bowel (Fig. 50-48A). A proximal obstructive pattern can often be demonstrated. On barium enema examination, contrast flows in a retrograde fashion through the colon until it reaches the leading point of the intussusception, where it may stop abruptly and produce a concave configuration about the edge of the mass (Fig. 50-48B). Streaks of barium can extend around the mass in a spiral, ringlike fashion to produce a characteristic coiled-spring appearance (Fig. 50-49A). Many intussusceptions can be reduced by increased hydrostatic pressure of a barium enema examination (Fig. 50-49B, C). Reduction of intussusceptions by rectal insufflation of air has recently been reported as a substitute for hydrostatic reduction in children. In older children and adults, it is recommended that the radiologist carry out a repeat barium enema

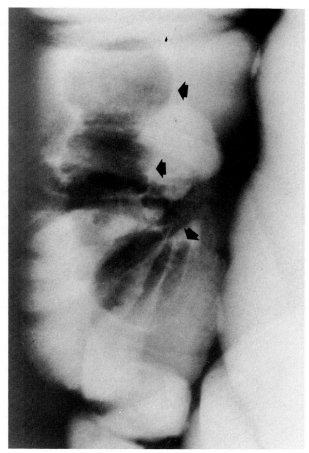

Fig. 50-47. Large polypoid carcinoma intussuscepting into the ascending colon **(arrows)**.

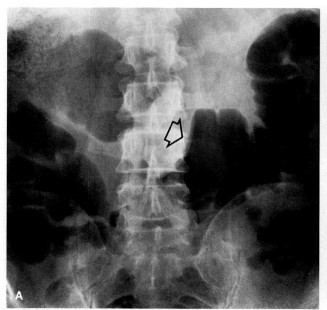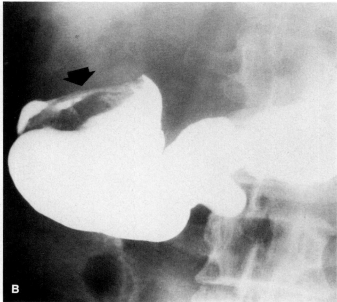

Fig. 50-48. Intussusception. **(A)** A plain abdominal radiograph demonstrates a soft-tissue mass **(arrow)** with gas in the distal colon outlining the intussuscepted bowel. **(B)** Barium enema examination demonstrates obstruction at the level of the intussusception **(arrow)**.

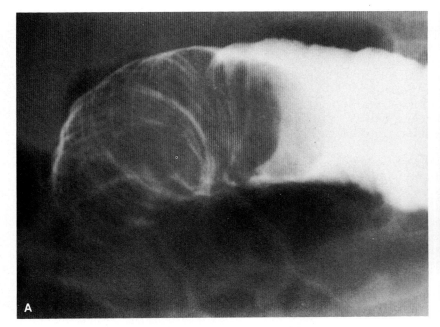

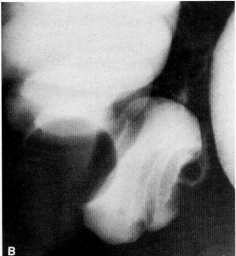

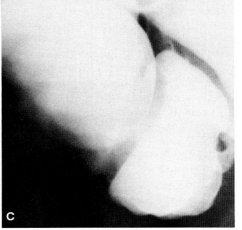

Fig. 50-49. Intussusception. **(A)** Obstruction of the colon at the hepatic flexure. The intussuscepted bowel has a characteristic coiled-spring appearance. **(B)** Partial and **(C)** complete reduction of the intussusception by careful barium enema examination.

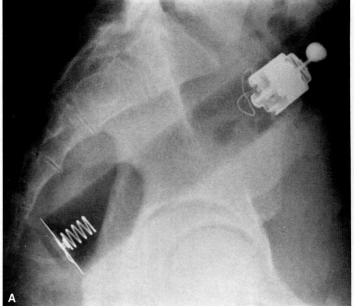

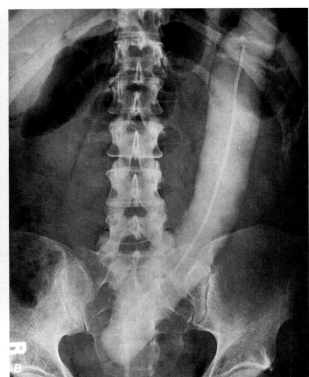

Fig. 50-50. Foreign body. **(A)** Vibrator in the rectum. **(B)** Double-headed dildo in the left colon.

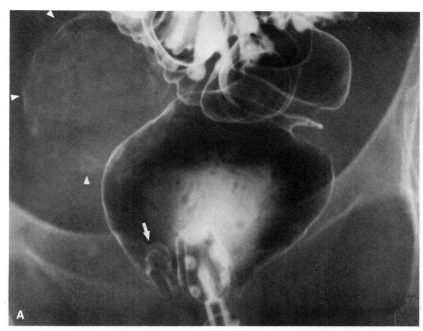

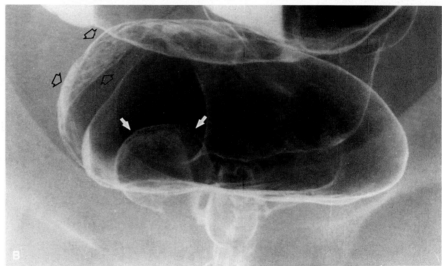

Fig. 50-51. Hypertrophied anal papilla. **(A)** Small polyp **(arrow)** arising just inside the anal verge. At surgery, the calcified right pelvic mass **(arrowheads)** proved to be a necrotic ovarian cyst. **(B)** In another patient, there is a much larger though still smooth mass **(white arrows)** arising just inside the anal verge. The area of irregular mucosa on the right lateral wall of the rectum **(black arrows)** was shown at biopsy to represent acute and chronic inflammation. (Heiken JP, Zuckerman GR, Balfe DM: The hypertropied anal papilla: Recognition on air–contrast barium enema examinations. Radiology 151:315–318, 1984)

after reduction to search for a specific etiology for the intussusception.

FOREIGN BODY

Rarely, foreign bodies produce intraluminal filling defects in the colon. Round, undigestable material that reaches the colon from above generally passes without difficulty. Sharp objects (pins, needles, nails) occasionally perforate the rectum at sites of vigorous perstalsis and narrowed lumen caliber. However, even these foreign bodies usually pass without difficulty, presumably because they are coated by semisolid stool and thus are unable to lacerate the bowel wall.

A varied array of foreign bodies have been in-serted into the colon from below, usually in homosexuals seeking sexual gratification. These foreign bodies are generally radiopaque and present no diagnostic difficulty (Fig. 50-50). However, foreign bodies inserted into the rectum from below have a higher likelihood of causing perforation or obstruction.

GALLSTONE

On rare occasions, gallstones that have entered the bowel by way of cholecystoduodenal fistulas pass through the terminal ileum and become trapped within the distal sigmoid colon, where they must be differentiated from polypoid filling defects. Rare cases of gallstones lodged in the colon have been

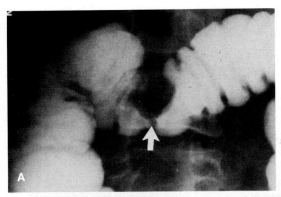

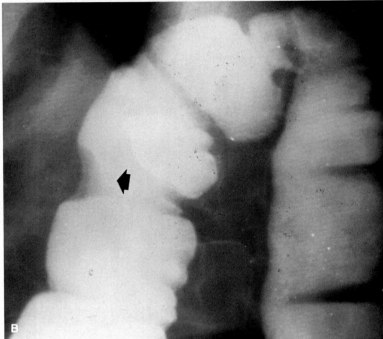

Fig. 50-52. Colonic pseudotumors due to adhesions. Examples of filling defects **(arrows)** in the **(A)** proximal and **(B)** distal portions of the transverse colon. (Kyaw MM, Koehler PR: Pseudotumors of the colon due to adhesions. Radiology 103:597–599, 1972)

reported in patients with fistulas between the gallbladder and the colon and in patients with fistulas between the proximal small bowel and colon that bypass the ileocecal valve.

HYPERTROPHIED ANAL PAPILLA

Anal papillae are acquired structures that arise from the base of the rectal columns of Morgagni at the dentate line. They enlarge in response to congestion, irritation, injury, or infection. Although anal papillae are seen in almost 50% of the patients undergoing proctoscopic examination, radiographic demonstration of a hypertrophied anal papilla is uncommon and occurs only when it becomes large enough to prolapse into the rectum. When it is identified on barium enema examination, an enlarged anal papilla appears as a smooth polyp arising just inside the anal verge (Fig. 50-51). Although the radiographic appearance may simulate internal hemorrhoid, rectal polyp, anal carcinoma, or submucosal anorectal tumor, the location of a smooth mass just inside the anal verge should suggest the possibility of a hypertrophied anal papilla, especially in a patient with a history of chronic anal irritation or infection.

PSEUDOTUMORS

Intraluminal or intramural polypoid masses in the colon that closely simulate primary or metastatic tumors can be due to pseudotumors caused by adhesions or fibrous bands (Fig. 50-52). In most patients, these fibrous bands are secondary to previous abdominal surgery. Less frequently, they are the result of changes in the appendices epiploicae secondary to ischemia or to an inflammatory process arising in the bowel wall or adjacent organs. Pseudotumors are usually located in the transverse

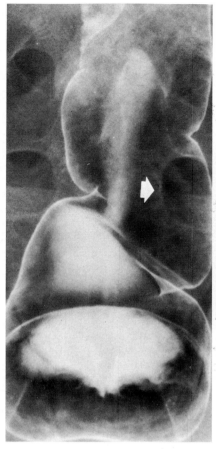

50-53

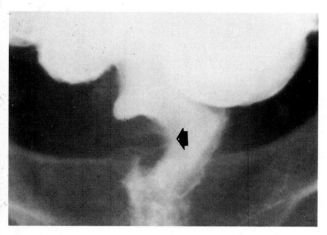

50-54

Fig. 50-53. Colonic pseudotumor **(arrow)** due to fortuitous superimposition of a sacral foramen over the rectosigmoid lumen.

Fig. 50-54. Rectal amyloid presenting as a localized filling defect **(arrow)**.

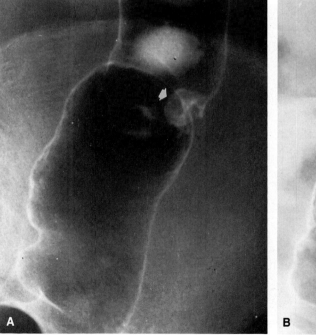

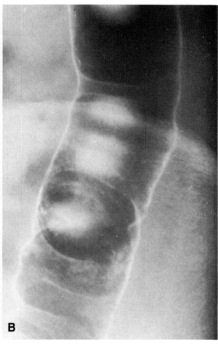

Fig. 50-55. Suture granuloma simulating recurrent carcinoma. **(A)** Barium enema examination 5 months after resection of a well-differentiated adenocarcinoma clearly shows the mass **(arrow)** at the anastomotic site. **(B)** Repeat examination 2½ years after surgery shows an entirely normal colon. (Shauffer IA, Sequeira J: Suture granuloma simulating recurrent carcinoma. AJR 128:856–857, 1977. Copyright 1977. Reproduced with permission)

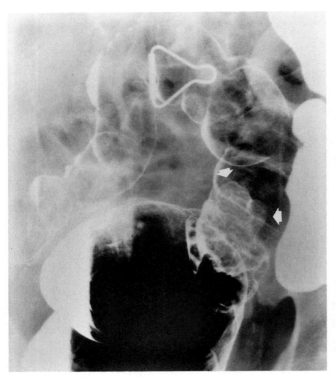

or sigmoid colon (the distribution of appendices epiploicae) and have an intact mucosa overlying the intraluminal or intramural mass. Nevertheless, these tumorlike lesions may be indistinguishable from colonic neoplasms and require surgical intervention. Another pseudotumor that can be mistaken for a true colonic filling defect is the fortuitous superimposition of a sacral foramen over the rectosigmoid lumen (Fig. 50-53).

OTHER CAUSES OF FILLING DEFECTS

Rarely, a localized collection of amyloid appears as a filling defect in the rectum (Fig. 50-54). Edematous granulation tissue can develop following surgery and present as a distinct mass at the anastomotic site (Fig. 50-55). However, unlike a true neoplastic process, these suture granulomas eventually resolve and disappear. Although usually multiple, colitis cystica profunda can present as a single filling defect mimicking a neoplasm (Fig. 50-56). In a patient with the solitary rectal ulcer syndrome, the relatively shallow ulcer may be undetectable and the only radiographic finding may be a lobulated submucosal mass in the distal rectum adjacent to the anal verge (Fig. 50-57*A*) or to thickened, edematous valves of Houston (Fig. 50-57*B*). Rarely, be-

Fig. 50-56. *Colitis cystica profunda. A single filling defect* **(arrows)** *simulates a neoplasm.*

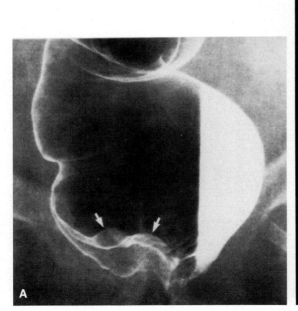

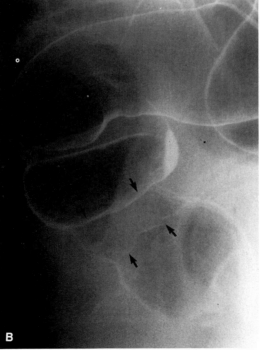

Fig. 50-57. *Solitary rectal ulcer syndrome.* **(A)** *Left lateral decubitus radiograph in an asymptomatic elderly man shows a slightly lobulated submucosal-appearing mass in the distal rectum* **(arrows)** *adjacent to the anal verge.* **(B)** *Lateral view of the rectum in a young man with rectal bleeding shows a markedly thickened, edematous first valve of Houston* **(arrows)** *without ulceration. At proctoscopy, however, a shallow ulcer was also detected anteriorly 8 cm from the anal verge. (Levine MS, Piccolello ML, Sollenberger LC et al: Solitary rectal ulcer syndrome: A radiologic diagnosis? Gastrointest Radiol 11:187–193, 1986)*

zoars may cause filling defects in the colon or even large bowel obstruction. Primary colonic bezoars are extremely rare; most bezoars are formed in the stomach, and the colonic lesions are secondary to breakup and migration of a gastric mass.

BIBLIOGRAPHY

Agha FP, Francis IR, Simms SM: Cystic lymphangioma of the colon: AJR 141:709–710, 1983

Agha FP, Lee HH, Boland CR et al: Mucormycoma of the colon: Early diagnosis and successful management. AJR 145:739–741, 1985

Agha FP, Nostrant TT, Fiddian–Green RG: "Giant colonic bezoar": A medication bezoar due to psyllium seed husks. Am J Gastroenterol 79:319–321, 1984

Ament AE, Alfidi RJ, Rao PS: Basal indentation of sessile polypoid lesions: A function of geometry rather than a sign of malignancy. Radiology 143:341–344, 1982

Balthazar EJ, Bryk D: Segmental tuberculosis of the distal colon: Radiographic features in seven cases. Gastrointest Radiol 5:75–80, 1980

Bashist B, Forde KA, McCaffrey RM: Polypoid endometrioma of the rectosigmoid. Gastrointest Radiol 8:85–88, 1983

Baumgartner BR, Hartmann TM: Extramedullary plasmacytoma of the colon. Am J Gastroenterol 80:1017–1019, 1985

Bernstein JR, Ghahremani GG, Paige ML et al: Localized giant pseudopolyposis of the colon in ulcerative and granulomatous colitis. Gastrointest Radiol 3:431–435, 1978

Bernstein MA, Feczko PJ, Halpert RD et al: Distribution of colonic polyps: Increased incidence of proximal lesions in older patients. Radiology 155:35–38, 1985

Brodey PA, Hill RP, Baron S: Benign ulceration of the cecum. Radiology 122:323–327, 1977

Chandrasoma P, Wheeler D, Radin DR: Traumatic neuroma of the intestine. Gastrointest Radiol 10:161–162, 1985

Delamarre J, Descombes P, Marti R et al: Villous tumors of the colon and rectum: Double-contrast study of 47 cases. Gastrointest Radiol 5:69–73, 1980

de Roos A, Hermans J, Shaw PC et al: Colon polyps and carcinomas: Prospective comparison of the single- and double-contrast examinations in the same patient. Radiology 154:11–13, 1985

Dreyfuss JR, Benacerraf B: Saddle cancers of the colon and their progression to annular carcinomas. Radiology 129:289–293, 1978

Feczko PJ, Bernstein MA, Halpert RD et al: Small colonic polyps: A reappraisal of their significance. Radiology 152:301–303, 1984

Ferin P, Skucas J: Inflammatory fibroid polyp of the colon simulating malignancy. Radiology 149:55–56, 1983

Gordon RL, Evers K, Kressel HY et al: Double-contrast enema in pelvic endometriosis. AJR 138:549–552, 1982

Gu L, Alton DJ, Daneman A et al: Intussusception reduction in children by rectal insufflation of air. AJR 150:1345–1348, 1988

Harned RK, Williams SM, Maglinte DDT: Clinical application of *in vitro* studies for barium-enema examinations following colorectal biopsy. Radiology 154:319–321, 1985

Heiken JP, Zuckerman GR, Balfe DM: The hypertrophied anal papilla: Recognition on air–contrast barium enema examinations. Radiology 151:315–318, 1984

Keller CE, Halpert RD, Feczko PJ et al: Radiologic recognition of colonic diverticula simulating polyps. AJR 143:93–97, 1984

Kelvin FM, Maglinte DDT: Colorectal carcinoma: A radiologic and clinical review: Radiology 164:1–8, 1987

Kyaw MM, Koehler PR: Pseudotumors of colon due to adhesions. Radiology 103:597–599, 1972.

Lane N, Fenoglio CM: Observations on the adenoma as precursor to ordinary large bowel carcinoma. Gastrointest Radiol 1:111–119, 1976

Levine MS, Piccolello ML, Sollenberger LC et al: Solitary rectal ulcer syndrome: A radiologic diagnosis? Gastrointest Radiol 11:187–193, 1986

Lockhart–Mummery HE: Diffuse conditions of the large bowel which are premalignant. Br J Surg 55:735–738, 1968

Maglinte DDT, Keller KJ, Miller RE et al: Colon and rectal carcinoma: Spatial distribution and detection. Radiology 147:669–672, 1983

Morson BC: The polyp cancer sequence in large bowel. Proc R Soc Med 67:451–457, 1974

Morson BC, Konishi F: Contribution of a pathologist to the radiology and management of colorectal polyps. Gastrointest Radiol 7:275–281, 1982

Muto T, Bussey HJR, Morson BC: The evolution of cancer of the colon and rectum. Cancer 36:2251–2270, 1975

O'Connell DJ, Thompson AJ: Lymphoma of the colon. The spectrum of radiologic changes. Gastrointest Radiol 2:377–385, 1978

Olmsted WW, Ros PR, Sobin LH: The solitary colonic polyp: Radiologic-histologic differentiation and significance. Radiology 160:9–16, 1986

Ott DJ, Chen YM, Gelfand DW et al: Single-contrast vs double-contrast barium enema in the detection of colonic polyps. AJR 146:993–996, 1986

Ott DJ, Gelfand DW, Chen YM et al: Colonoscopy and the barium enema: A radiologic viewpoint. South Med J 78:1033–1035, 1985

Ott DJ, Gelfand DW, Wu WC et al: Colon polyp morphology on double-contrast barium enema: Its pathologic predictive value. AJR 141:965–970, 1983

Ott DJ, Gelfand DW, Wu WC et al: How important is radiographic detection of diminutive polyps of the colon? AJR 146:876–878, 1986

Sato T, Sakai Y, Sonoyama A et al: Radiologic spectrum of rectal carcinoid tumors. Gastrointest Radiol 9:23–26, 1984

Shauffer IA, Sequeira J: Suture granuloma simulating recurrent carcinoma. AJR 128:856–857, 1977

Tedesco FJ, Hendrix JC, Pickens CA et al: Diminutive polyps: Histopathology, spatial distribution, and clinical significance. Gastrointest Endosc 28:1–5, 1982

Wolf BS: Lipoma of the colon. JAMA 235:2225–2226, 1976

51
MULTIPLE FILLING DEFECTS IN THE COLON

Disease Entities

Neoplasms
  Multiple adenomatous polyps
  Intestinal polyposis syndromes
    Familial polyposis
    Gardner's syndrome
    Peutz-Jeghers syndrome
    Disseminated gastrointestinal polyposis
    Turcot syndrome
    Juvenile polyposis coli
    Generalized gastrointestinal juvenile
      polyposis
    Cronkhite-Canada syndrome
    Neurocrest and colonic tumors
    Ruvalcaba–Myhre–Smith syndrome
  Multiple juvenile polyps
  Multiple adenocarcinomas
  Metastases
  Lymphoma
  Leukemic infiltration
  Neurofibromatosis
  Lipomatosis
  Hemangiomas
  Multiple hamartoma syndrome (Cowden's
    disease)
Inflammatory diseases
  Ulcerative colitis
  Crohn's colitis
  Ischemic colitis
  Amebiasis
  Schistosomiasis

Trichuriasis
Strongyloidiasis
Cytomegalovirus colitis
Yersinia colitis
Pseudomembranous colitis
Diversion colitis
Artifacts
  Feces
  Air bubbles
  Oil droplets
  Mucus strands
  Ingested foreign bodies
Miscellaneous disorders
  Hemorrhoids
  Diverticula
  Pneumatosis intestinalis
  Colitis cystica profunda
  Nodular lymphoid hyperplasia
  Lymphoid follicular pattern
  Cystic fibrosis
  Submucosal edema pattern
    Colonic urticaria
    Herpes zoster/*Yersinia*
    Ischemia
    Colonic obstruction
  Ulcerative pseudopolyps proximal to an
    obstruction
  Endometriosis
  Malacoplakia
  Colonic varices
  Amyloidosis

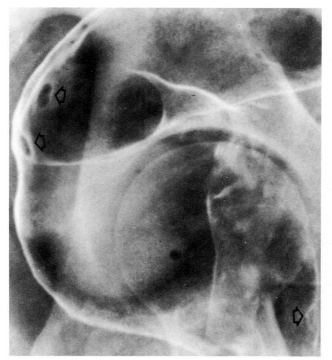

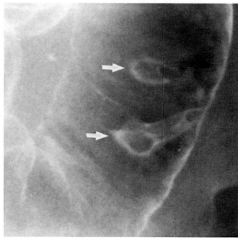

51-1   51-2

Fig. 51-1. Multiple small adenomatous polyps of the colon **(arrows).** There was no recognized polyposis syndrome.

Fig. 51-2. Two benign adenomatous polyps **(arrows).**

MULTIPLE ADENOMATOUS POLYPS

Multiple adenomatous polyps of the colon can occur as an isolated event without a recognized polyposis syndrome (Fig. 51-1). In the Malmo series of more than 3000 double-contrast enemas, 12.5% of patients had radiographically demonstrated polyps in the colon. Among those patients with polyps, 24% had multiple polyps (17% had 2 polyps [Fig. 51-2], and 7% had 3 or more polyps [Fig. 51-3]). According to these statistics, therefore, multiple polyps should be expected in about 3% of barium enema examinations. There is an increased incidence of multiple adenomas in older patients. As the number of adenomas increase, there is also a trend toward a higher percentage of the adenomas having severe dysplasia and thus a consequently greater risk of the patient developing cancer.

INTESTINAL POLYPOSIS SYNDROMES

The intestinal polyposis syndromes are a diverse group of conditions that differ widely in the histology of the polyps, the incidence of extracolonic polyps, extra-abdominal manifestations, and the potential for developing malignant disease. An intestinal polyposis disorder should be suspected when a polyp is demonstrated in a young person, when multiple polyps are found in any person, or when carcinoma of the colon is found in a patient under 40 years of age. In these situations, extraintestinal manifestations of the polyposis syndromes should be carefully sought. If one of the hereditary forms of intestinal polyposis is diagnosed, the patient's immediate family should be studied so that a potentially fatal disease is not missed in its premalignant stage.

FAMILIAL POLYPOSIS

Familial polyposis is an inherited disease (autosomal dominant) with multiple adenomatous polyps almost exclusively limited to the colon and rectum (Fig. 51-4). Scattered cases of associated adenomas of the stomach and duodenum have also been reported. Small polypoid lesions similar to colonic polyps can be present in the terminal ileum, but these are histologically lymphoid hyperplasia rather than true polyps.

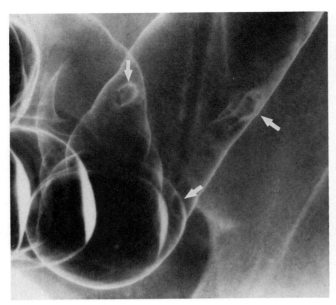

51-3

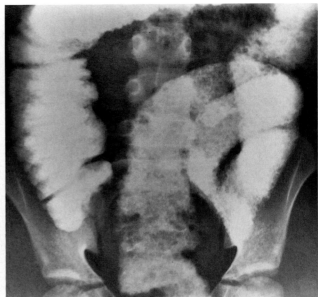

51-4

Fig. 51-3. Three benign adenomatous polyps **(arrows)**.

Fig. 51-4. Familial polyposis.

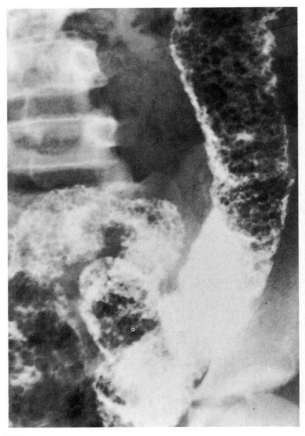

51-5

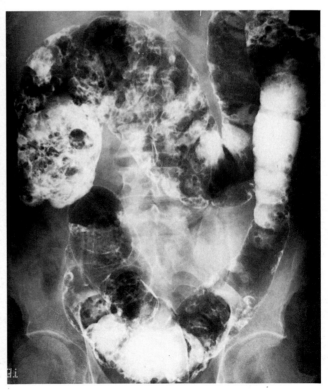

51-6

Fig. 51-5. Familial polyposis.

Fig. 51-6. Familial polyposis. Innumerable adenomatous polyps blanket the entire length of the colon. The overall pattern simulates diffuse fecal material in a ''poorly prepared'' colon.

The colonic polyps in this syndrome are not present at birth and tend to arise around puberty. Clinical symptoms, which usually do not develop until the third or fourth decade of life, are confined to the gastrointestinal tract (intermittent rectal bleeding and diarrhea, abdominal pain, mucus discharge) with no evidence of extraintestinal involvement. Many patients with familial polyposis are asymptomatic and are discovered during routine investigation of relatives of a patient known to have the disease.

On barium enema examination, the polyps appear as sessile or pedunculated lesions (0.5–1 cm in size) scattered throughout the colon (Fig. 51-5). Although the rectum and left colon are involved more frequently than the right, myriads of polyps often blanket the entire length of the colon (Fig. 51-6). With diffuse disease, the colon can appear to be "poorly prepared"; however, in familial polyposis, the true adenomatous polyps remain fixed in position with palpation, unlike retained fecal material, which is usually freely movable. The distinction between familial polyposis and multiple adenomas can be made on the absolute number of polyps present in the large bowel. It is very rare for more than 50 adenomas to be present in multiple adenomatosis. Careful pathologic studies have shown that if fewer than 70 polyps are present, the condition is simply multiple adenomas, whereas if more than 100 polyps are found, it is familial polyposis.

Patients with familial polyposis have virtually a 100% risk of developing carcinoma of the colon or rectum by age 50 (Fig. 51-7); 40% of patients with

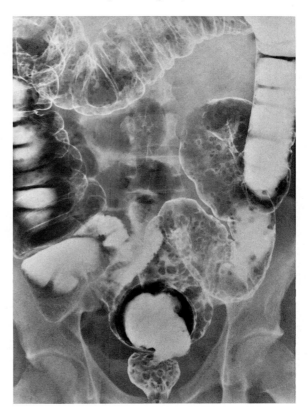

Fig. 51-8. *Gardner's syndrome. Innumerable adenomatous polyps throughout the colon present a radiographic appearance indistinguishable from familial polyposis.*

this syndrome have colon carcinoma when the colonic polyposis is initially diagnosed. If untreated, the average patient with this syndrome will be dead by age 45 from metastatic colon carcinoma. Like colonic carcinoma in patients without this genetic disorder, malignant lesions complicating familial polyposis can be lobulated or plaquelike or have an annular configuration. Because of the extremely high risk of malignancy, total colectomy is usually recommended at the time of diagnosis. An earlier mode of treatment, subtotal colectomy with ileorectal anastomosis, was based on the assumption that any recurrent polyp could be easily excised during proctoscopy. However, the risk of a patient developing carcinoma within the retained rectum has proved so unacceptably high that subtotal colectomy is now indicated only in a select group of patients with minimal or no rectal polyposis who are willing to subject themselves to meticulous follow-up.

GARDNER'S SYNDROME

Gardner's syndrome is an inherited disorder (autosomal dominant) in which diffuse colonic polyposis is associated with bony abnormalities and soft-tissue tumors (Fig. 51-8). These extraintestinal signs often develop earlier than intestinal polyposis and suggest the need for a barium enema for further evaluation.

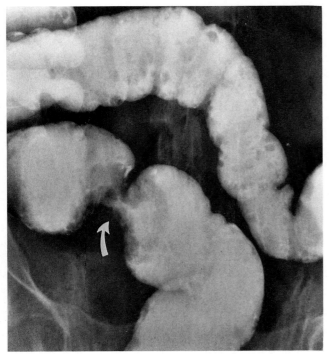

Fig. 51-7. *Carcinoma of the sigmoid* **(arrow)** *developing in a patient with long-standing familial polyposis.*

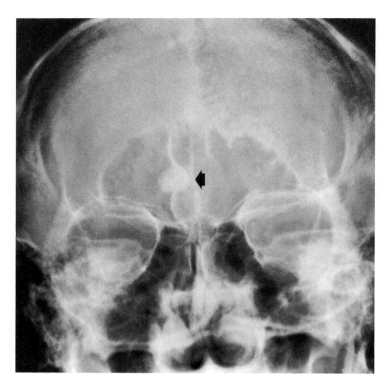

Fig. 51-9. Gardner's syndrome. An osteoma **(arrow)** is present in the frontal sinus.

Patients with Gardner's syndrome often present with cosmetic deformities. Localized bony overgrowth in the skull can cause excessive prominence of the jaw, entrapment of cranial nerves, or osteomas in the sinuses (Fig. 51-9). Exostoses and cortical thickening can involve the long bones and ribs. Dental abnormalities are not infrequent and include odontomas, extra teeth, unerupted teeth, and a propensity toward numerous caries.

Soft-tissue lesions associated with Gardner's syndrome include sebaceous cysts of the face, scalp, and back, as well as subcutaneous fibromas, leiomyomas, and lipomas. These tumors tend to progress in number and size regardless of whether colonic polyps are present or the colon has been resected. An increased incidence of adenomas occurs in the upper gastrointestinal tract, especially in the periampullary region. The fibrous tissue in patients with Gardner's syndrome has a marked tendency to proliferate, resulting in dense scars or keloids after surgery. In the abdomen, this excessive fibrosis can produce adhesions that may even cause small bowel obstruction. Up to 30% of patients with Gardner's syndrome develop a desmoid tumor, a nonencapsulated, locally invasive form of fibromatosis that is believed to be associated with prior surgery. The lesion most commonly involves the anterior abdominal wall, may arise in a prior laparotomy scar, and tends to recur after local excision. Desmoid tumors infrequently arise in the mesentery, where they are best detected by CT.

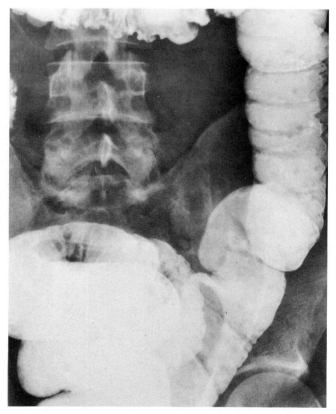

Fig. 51-10. Peutz-Jeghers syndrome. Multiple colonic hamartomas are evident in this patient, who also demonstrated abnormal mucocutaneous pigmentation.

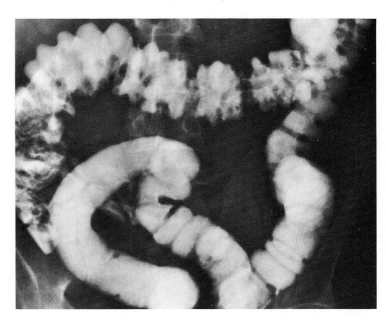

Fig. 51-11. Turcot syndrome. Multiple colonic adenomatous polyps were found in this young patient, who died of a malignant glioma.

The distribution and appearance of the adenomatous polyps in Gardner's syndrome are indistinguishable from the pattern in familial polyposis. The polyps are almost always limited to the colon and rectum; extracolonic polyps occasionally occur in the small bowel and stomach. Like patients with familial polyposis, patients with Gardner's syndrome have almost a 100% risk of developing carcinoma of the colon or rectum. Therefore, total colectomy is recommended. In addition, patients with Gardner's syndrome appear to have a predilection toward small bowel malignancies, particularly in the pancreaticoduodenal region.

PEUTZ–JEGHERS SYNDROME

Peutz–Jeghers syndrome is an inherited disorder (autosomal dominant) in which multiple gastrointestinal polyposis is associated with mucocutaneous pigmentation (Fig. 51-10). The syndrome usually develops during childhood or adolescence. The excessive melanin deposits characteristic of Peutz–Jeghers syndrome are flat and small (1–5 mm in size) and occur predominantly on the lips and buccal mucosa. They can also be seen on the face, abdomen, genitalia, hands, and feet. The most common clinical symptom is intermittent colicky pain caused by small bowel intussusception led by one of the polyps. Rectal bleeding or melena is not infrequent, though massive gastrointestinal bleeding is rare.

The polyps in Peutz–Jeghers syndrome are hamartomas, masses of cell types normally present in the bowel, but mixed in abnormal proportions. The polyps are primarily found in the small bowel (especially the jejunum and ileum) but can also occur in the stomach, colon, and rectum. The polypoid lesions in Peutz–Jeghers syndrome are benign and apparently do not undergo malignant transformation. However, in a recent study of 31 patients with Peutz–Jeghers syndrome, 15 (48%) developed carcinoma within 12 years or less (gastrointestinal carcinomas in 4; nongastrointestinal carcinomas in 10; multiple myeloma in 1). This incidence is far greater than expected in the general population and suggests that patients with the Peutz–Jeghers syndrome may have an increased risk for development of cancer at both gastrointestinal and nongastrointestinal sites.

DISSEMINATED GASTROINTESTINAL POLYPOSIS

Disseminated gastrointestinal polyposis refers to a condition in which multiple adenomatous polyps involve the stomach or small bowel as well as the colon, but in which the extraintestinal stigmata of the Gardner's or Peutz–Jeghers syndrome are absent. This very rare condition, which has an extremely high risk of gastrointestinal carcinoma, may be a variant of familial polyposis rather than a discrete clinical entity.

TURCOT SYNDROME

Turcot syndrome (glioma-polyposis syndrome) is the association of multiple colonic adenomatous polyps with malignant tumors of the central nervous system (Fig. 51-11). Patients with this extremely rare syndrome usually present in the sec-

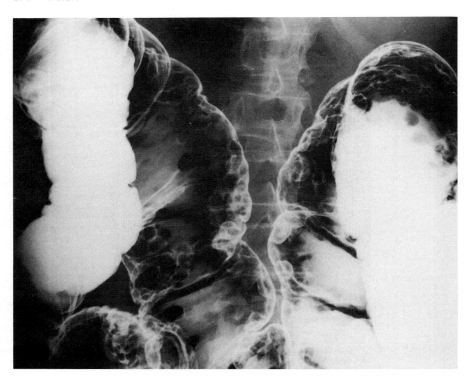

Fig. 51-12. Cronkhite-Canada syndrome. Multiple polypoid lesions simulate familial polyposis. (Dodds WJ: Clinical and roentgen features of the intestinal polyposis syndromes. Gastrointest Radiol 1:127–142. 1976)

ond decade of life with neurologic complaints caused by a brain tumor (usually supratentorial glioblastoma) or diarrhea due to colonic polyposis. Because neither brain tumors nor colonic polyps have been noted in the parents of afflicted patients, it seems likely that the disorder is inherited as an autosomal recessive. An increased incidence of colorectal carcinoma has been reported in patients with Turcot syndrome. However, the precise malignant potential of the colonic polyps is unknown, since most patients with this syndrome have died of central nervous system tumors at a very young age.

JUVENILE POLYPOSIS SYNDROMES

There are three rare, but distinct, syndromes associated with juvenile polyps of the colon. These polyps are hamartomatous lesions that are sometimes referred to as retention or inflammatory polyps. Although almost always found in children, juvenile polyps are occasionally first detected in adults. *Juvenile polyposis coli* is probably an inherited disorder in which multiple hamartomatous polypoid lesions can be associated with a variety of congenital anomalies. Juvenile polyps can involve the stomach and small bowel as well as the colon, and if this occurs without any extraintestinal manifestations, it is termed *generalized gastrointestinal juvenile polyposis*. If there is associated hyperpigmentation, alopecia, and atrophy and subsequent loss of fingernails and toenails, the condition is called the *Cronkhite-Canada syndrome* (Fig. 51-12). The latter disorder presents much later in life than other intestinal polyposis syndromes (average age of

onset, over 50) and may be accompanied by malabsorption and severe diarrhea resulting in substantial electrolyte and protein loss (Fig. 51-13). Although spontaneous remissions occur, the disease is usually relentlessly progressive (especially in women) and leads to death within 1 year of diagnosis.

The hamartomatous (inflammatory) juvenile polyps are not premalignant in any of these three diseases. Several instances of gastrointestinal carcinoma have been described in patients with generalized gastrointestinal juvenile polyposis and the Cronkhite-Canada syndrome, but these may represent merely chance occurrences.

NEUROCREST AND COLONIC TUMORS

A new syndrome has been recently reported in which multiple colonic adenomatous polyps are associated with malignant tumors of neurocrest origin (pheochromocytoma, carcinoid tumor, multiple endocrine neoplasia syndrome type IIB with malignant medullary thyroid carcinoma) (Fig. 51-14). This entity differs from familial polyposis by the lack of a family history of polyps and by the fewer number of polyps and somewhat older age of presentation.

RUVALCABA–MYHRE–SMITH SYNDROME

This rare syndrome (autosomal dominant) consists of macrocephaly, pigmented genital lesions, and intestinal polyposis (Fig. 51-15). Other reported

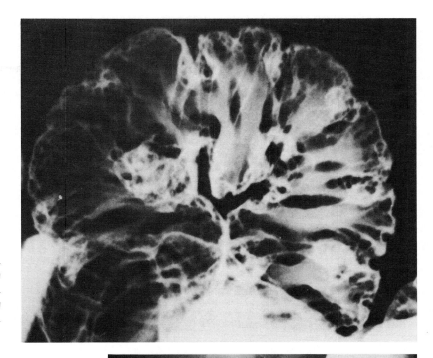

Fig. 51-13. Cronkhite-Canada syndrome. This coned view of the sigmoid colon demonstrates multiple small polyps in a 55-year-old man. (Koehler PR, Kyaw MM, Fenlon JW: Diffuse gastrointestinal polyposis with ectodermal changes: Cronkhite-Canada syndrome. Radiology 103:589–594, 1972)

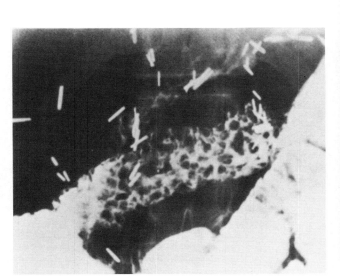

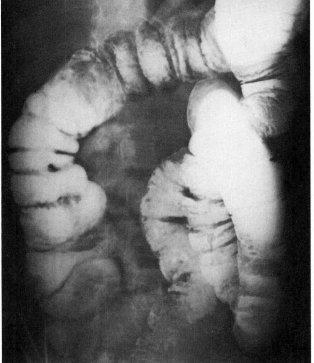

51-14   **51-15**

Fig. 51-14. Neurocrest and colonic tumors. Carpeting of the colon with small polyps in a young man with previously diagnosed multiple endocrine neoplasia type IIB (locally invasive medullary thyroid carcinoma, adrenal pheochromocytcma, vocal cord neurofibromas). Biopsy specimens of three of the polyps showed tubular adenomas. (Shapir J, Frank P: Radiologic manifestations of the syndrome of neurocrest and colonic tumors. Gastrointest Radiol 10:383–386, 1985)

Fig. 51-15. Ruvalcaba–Myhre–Smith syndrome. Multiple polypoid filling defects throughout the colon (and terminal ileum). (Foster MA, Kilcoyne RF: Ruvalcaba–Myhre–Smith syndrome: A new consideration in the differential diagnosis of intestinal polyposis. Gastrointest Radiol 11:349–350, 1986)

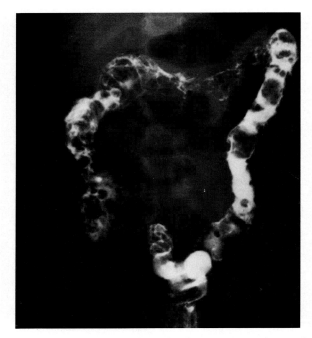

Fig. 51-16. *Juvenile polyposis. A postevacuation radiograph demonstrates many filling defects of various sizes throughout the colon. (Schwartz AM, McCauley RGK: Juvenile gastrointestinal polyposis. Radiology 121:441–444, 1976)*

anomalies include delayed psychomotor development in childhood, prominent corneal nerves, lipid storage myopathy, and subcutaneous lipomas. The polyps in this condition are primarily hamartomas, which seem to involve the gastrointestinal tract diffusely and appear to have no malignant potential.

MULTIPLE JUVENILE POLYPS

The presence of one or more juvenile polyps in the colon of a young child (2–5 years of age) is not uncommon without an inherited disorder and with no evidence of extraintestinal manifestations or associated intestinal malignancy (Fig. 51-16). These juvenile polyps have a smooth, round contour and contain multiple mucin-filled cysts and an abundant connective tissue stroma. Hemorrhage and ulceration are common, leading to symptoms of rectal bleeding, mucus discharge, diarrhea, and, occasionally, abdominal pain. Juvenile polyps are almost always solitary, though multiple polyps (rarely more than a few) do occur. The polyps are benign, have no malignant potential, and tend to autoamputate or regress. Therefore, surgical removal of juvenile polyps is indicated only if there are significant or repeated episodes of rectal bleeding or intussusception.

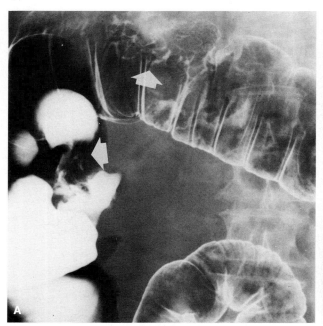
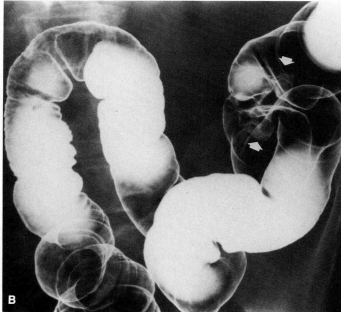

Fig. 51-17. Multiple synchronous carcinomas of the colon. **(A)** Carcinomas of the ascending and transverse portions of the colon **(arrows)**. **(B)** Carcinoma **(arrows)** within a tortuous descending colon.

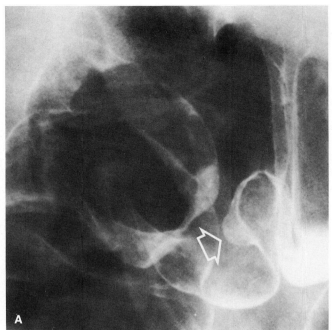

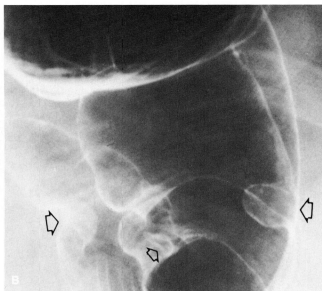

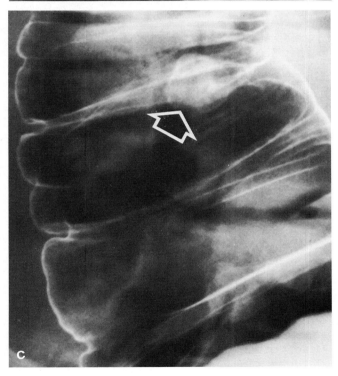

Fig. 51-18. Melanoma metastatic to the colon. **(A)** Double-contrast view of the hepatic flexure showing a single sessile polyp **(arrow)**. **(B)** View of the splenic flexure showing at least three sessile polyps **(arrows)**. **(C)** View of the ascending colon showing a sessile polyp **(arrow)**. (Sacks BA, Jaffe N, Antonioli DA: Metastatic melanoma presenting clinically as multiple colonic polyps. AJR 129:511–513, 1977. Copyright 1977. Reproduced with permission)

MULTIPLE ADENOCARCINOMAS

A patient with carcinoma of the colon has a 1% risk of having multiple synchronous colon cancers, which can produce the radiographic pattern of multiple filling defects in the colon (Fig. 51-17). In addition, such a patient has a 3% risk of developing additional metachronous cancers at a later date. Colon carcinomas can also coexist with benign adenomatous polyps (of which there was a 20% inci-

dence in the Malmo series), again presenting the radiographic appearance of multiple colonic filling defects.

METASTASES

Hematogenous metastases to the colon can produce multiple filling defects. Major primary sites include the breast, lung, stomach, ovary, pancreas, and

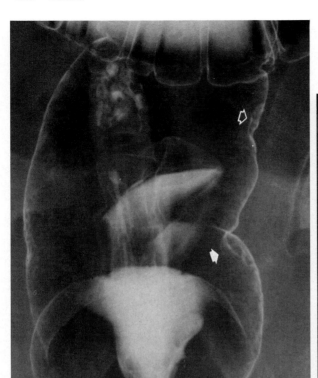
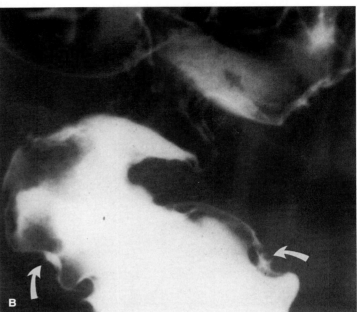

Fig. 51-19.   Kaposi's sarcoma. **(A)** Early submucosal nodular deposits **(arrows)**. **(B)** In another patient with more advanced disease, there is central umbilication **(arrows)** within the nodular filling defects. ([**B**] from Wall SN: Abdominal radiology of AIDS. Contemp Diag Radiol 9:1–6, 1986)

uterus, as well as other primary locations in the colon. Although the colon is the least common site for gastrointestinal metastases from melanoma, single or multiple colonic metastases can represent the initial manifestation of malignant melanoma and can occur without a clinically obvious primary lesion (Fig. 51-18). In addition to discrete masses that mimic intramural, extramucosal tumors, metastases to the colon can also produce thickening of the colon wall, diffuse nodularity, and mesenteric involvement leading to a fibrotic reaction with fixation and acute angulation of the bowel.

In patients with AIDS, Kaposi's sarcoma may produce multiple discrete, nodular, submucosal colonic defects ranging in size from a few millimeters to 3 cm (51-19). In more advanced disease, the individual submucosal nodules may coalesce and circumferentially infiltrate the wall of the colon to produce one or more narrowed, rigid segments.

LYMPHOMA

Although the gastrointestinal tract is the most common location of primary extranodal lymphoma, the colon is the segment of gut that is least often affected. Lymphoma of the colon can appear as a single (rarely multiple) relatively large lesion (see Fig. 50-34) or as an extensive infiltrating tumor that extends over long segments of bowel (see Fig. 49-56). Multiple lymphomatous nodules may appear as variable-sized, closely spaced, smooth, sessile masses throughout the colon (Fig. 51-20). Multiple large masses may also develop (Fig. 51-21). Umbilication of the nodules may occur, representing both smooth surface depressions resulting from flattening or atrophy of villi at the apex of some lymph follicles or instances of true superficial mucosal erosions. At times, diffuse lymphoma may mimic Crohn's disease, with filiform nodules simulating

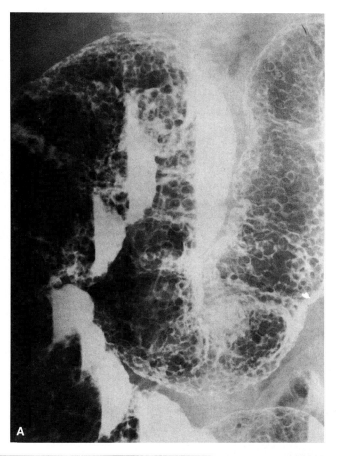

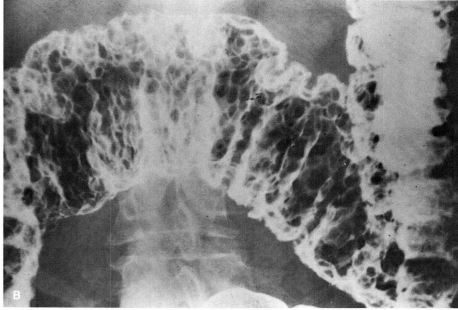

Fig. 51-20. Multinodular lymphoma. Two views of the colon show multiple smooth sessile, closely spaced nodules of varying size throughout the colon. (Williams FM, Berk RN, Harned RK: Radiologic features of multinodular lymphoma of the colon. AJR 143:87–91, 1984. Copyright 1984. Reproduced with permission)

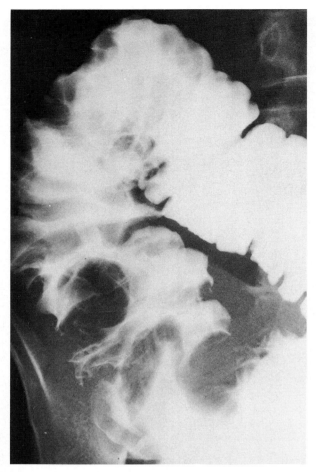

Fig. 51-21. *Lymphoma of the colon presenting as multiple irregular nodular filling defects.*

pseudopolyps and umbilicated nodules mimicking aphthous ulcers. In contrast to familial polyposis, simultaneous extensive involvement of the ileum is not uncommon in lymphoma. According to one report, multinodular colonic lymphoma is frequently associated with a cecal mass and evidence of incomplete evacuation of the barium, which may occur as a result of lymphomatous infiltration of the muscularis propria, preventing normal contraction, or infiltration of the wall, preventing complete collapse.

LEUKEMIC INFILTRATION

Leukemic infiltration of the gastrointestinal tract, even when extensive, is usually asymptomatic. Reported clinical complaints range from nonspecific nausea, mild abdominal pain, and diarrhea to severe necrotizing enterocolitis, bowel hemorrhage, and perforation. In lymphocytic lymphoma, involvement is usually confined to the mucosa and submucosa and can produce a radiographic pattern of diffuse interlacing filling defects in the colon. In myelogenous leukemia, the infiltrate can cause localized or diffuse plaques, nodules, or masses. In addition to colonic lesions, leukemic infiltration can present as intraluminal defects in the esophagus or as an infiltrative process in the stomach that may be indistinguishable from carcinoma.

MULTIPLE SPINDLE CELL TUMORS

Colonic neurofibromatosis associated with von Recklinghausen's disease can produce multiple dif-

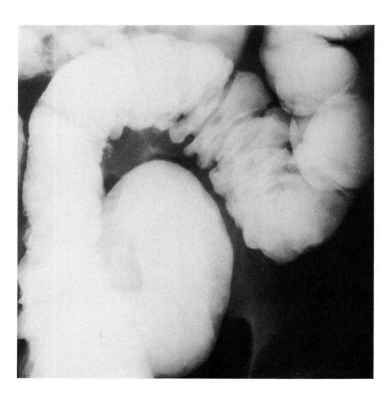

Fig. 51-22. *Segmental polypoid lipomatosis presenting as multiple filling defects in the sigmoid colon. (Danoff DM, Nisenbaum HL, Stewart WB et al: Segmental polypoid lipomatosis of the colon. AJR 128:858–860, 1977. Copyright 1977. Reproduced with permission)*

fuse intraluminal and intramural defects. These masses, which tend to be larger than the defects seen in the hereditary intestinal polyposis syndromes, are usually detected in patients with characteristic skin lesions.

Colonic lipomatosis can present as multiple filling defects in the colon (Fig. 51-22). This rare lesion can be segmental or diffuse and tends to primarily involve the right colon.

Hemangiomas are a rare cause of multiple intraluminal and intramural filling defects in the colon. The correct diagnosis requires demonstration of characteristic phleboliths associated with the lesions.

MULTIPLE HAMARTOMA SYNDROME (COWDEN'S DISEASE)

The multiple hamartoma syndrome (Cowden's disease) is a rare hereditary disorder associated with

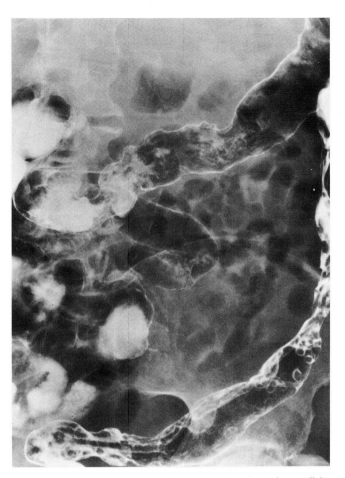

Fig. 51-24. Pseudopolyposis in chronic ulcerative colitis. There was no evidence of acute ulceration.

multiple malformations, tumors, and various involvement of different organs. The most characteristic clinical features are circumoral papillomatosis and nodular gingival hyperplasia. Several patients with this disorder have demonstrated single or multiple polyps of varied morphology along the gastrointestinal tract (Fig. 51-23). Although there is no convincing evidence of a predisposition to colonic malignancy, the multiple hamartoma syndrome does appear to be associated with an increased incidence of malignant tumors of the thyroid and breast.

INFLAMMATORY PSEUDOPOLYPOSIS

ULCERATIVE AND CROHN'S COLITIS

Pseudopolyps are islands of hyperplastic, inflamed mucosa that remain between areas of ulceration in inflammatory bowel disease (Fig. 51-24). They vary in size, shape, and pattern in relation to the degree and position of the ulceration and the inflammatory response of the bowel. In contrast to the otherwise normal appearance of the bowel in familial poly-

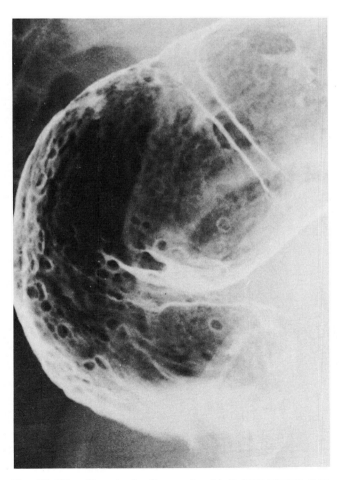

Fig. 51-23. Cowden's disease (multiple hamartoma syndrome). Numerous round, sessile polyps are spread over the entire rectum. (Hauser H, Ody B, Plojoux O et al: Radiological findings in multiple hamartoma syndrome [Cowden's disease]. Radiology 137:317–323, 1980)

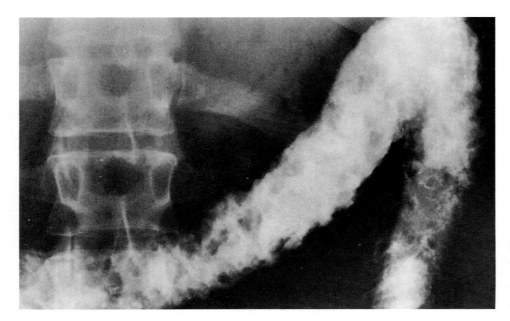

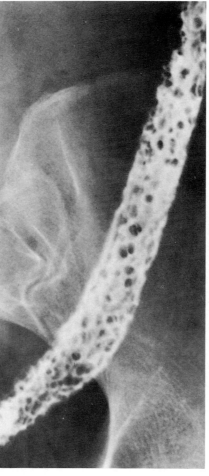

Fig. 51-25. *Pseudopolyposis in acute ulcerative colitis. The irregular filling defects are associated with radiographic evidence of a severe ulcerating process.*

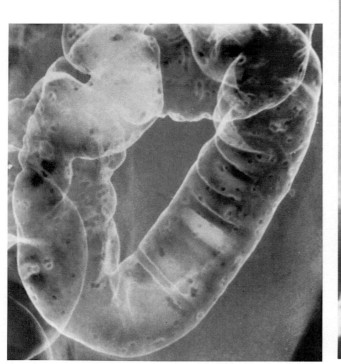

51-26

51-27

Fig. 51-26. Pseudopolyposis in chronic ulcerative colitis. If there is no radiographic evidence of inflammatory disease, the pattern is indistinguishable from familial polyposis.

Fig. 51-27. Pseudopolyposis in Crohn's colitis. The swollen and edematous mucosa surrounded by long, deep, linear ulcers and transverse fissures produces a coarsely nodular cobblestoning appearance.

posis, pseudopolyps in ulcerative and Crohn's colitis are usually associated with radiographic evidence of an inflammatory process (ulceration, absence or irregularity of haustral folds, narrowing of the lumen) and a history of chronic diarrhea (Fig. 51-25). However, in an occasional case of ulcerative colitis in which the inflammatory process has healed and the only residual radiographic abnormality is a large number of pseudopolyps, it can be impossible to distinguish this appearance from familial polyposis (Fig. 51-26).

The inflammatory pseudopolyps in ulcerative colitis tend to occur in those areas of the colon where inflammation was most active and severe, and their appearance generally correlates with periods of clinical remission. The pseudopolyps are usually small and uniform in appearance, producing a somewhat nodular pattern. On rare occasions, however, the mucosa can undergo such extreme hyperplasia that the pseudopolyps appear as large masses simulating fungating polypoid tumors.

When Crohn's disease involves the colon, long, deep linear ulcers and transverse fissures surrounding swollen and edematous mucosa result in a coarsely nodular appearance (cobblestoning) (Fig. 51-27). These irregular pseudopolyps can produce the radiographic appearance of multiple filling defects, simulating the intestinal polyposis syndromes (Fig. 51-28). Patients with pseudopolyposis of the colon due to Crohn's disease usually have concomitant disease of the terminal ileum, unlike patients with ulcerative colitis, in whom ileal involvement is absent or minimal.

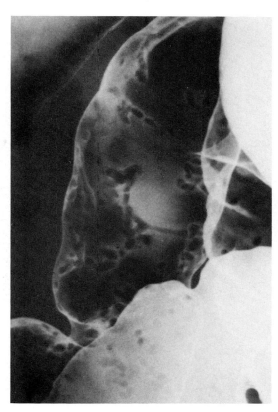

Fig. 51-29. Filiform polyposis with a characteristic branching pattern.

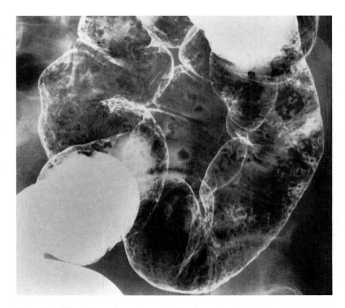

Fig. 51-28. Pseudopolyposis in chronic Crohn's colitis. Multiple filling defects without radiographic evidence of inflammatory changes simulate familial polyposis.

Filiform polyposis is a benign, nonspecific sequela of diffuse, severe mucosal inflammation that is seen in both ulcerative and Crohn's colitis. Filiform polyps usually appear as thin, straight filling defects resembling the stalks of polyps without the heads. In some cases, a radiating pattern of filling defects can be seen; in others, there is a branching pattern, particularly at the tip of the polyp (Fig. 51-29). These small lesions can be easily hidden if the barium column is underpenetrated; they can also be mistaken for mucus threads. In most cases, there is no radiologic evidence of acute colitis when filiform polyps are discovered; indeed, the finding of filiform polyposis may be the first clue to the presence of inflammatory bowel disease. Filiform polyps are not associated with the development of carcinoma and therefore should not be mistaken for a neoplastic polyposis syndrome.

Mucosal dysplasia is a precancerous histologic change that is frequently present in the colons of patients with ulcerative colitis at high risk for developing cancer. A similar pattern has also recently been recognized in patients with Crohn's disease who develop malignancies. Most dysplasia occurs in flat or low villous mucosa and thus cannot be detected on barium studies. Radiographically visible dysplasia most commonly appears as a group of

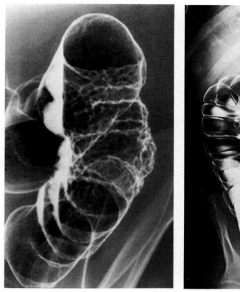 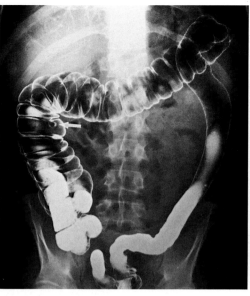 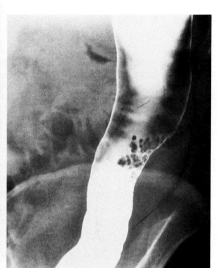

51-30   **51-31**   **51-32**

Fig. 51-30. Dysplasia in ulcerative colitis. Multiple adjacent nodules with apposed, flattened borders. (Hooyman JR, MacCarty RL, Carpenter HA et al: Radiographic appearance of mucosal dysplasia associated with ulcerative colitis. AJR 149:47–51, 1987. Copyright 1987. Reproduced with permission)

Fig. 51-31. Dysplasia in ulcerative colitis. Diffuse symmetric narrowing of much of the left colon, consistent with inflammatory bowel disease. A solitary nodule is present in the ascending colon **(arrow)**. Random colonoscopic biopsies of flat mucosa in the left colon showed widespread mild and moderate dysplasia. The nodule in the ascending colon also contained moderate dysplasia. (Hooyman JR, MacCarty RL, Carpenter HA et al: Radiographic appearance of mucosal dysplasia associated with ulcerative colitis. AJR 149:47–51, 1987. Copyright 1987. Reproduced with permission)

Fig. 51-32 Dysplasia in ulcerative colitis. Close grouping of dysplasia-containing nodules in the descending colon. (Hooyman JR, MacCarty RL, Carpenter HA et al: Radiographic appearance of mucosal dysplasia associated with ulcerative colitis. AJR 149:47–51, 1987. Copyright 1987. Reproduced with permission)

multiple adjacent nodules with apposed, sharply angulated borders producing a coarse or fine mosaic tile appearance (Fig. 51-30). Another radiographic form of dysplasia consists of a solitary nodule (Fig. 51-31) or several separate nodules (Fig. 51-32) that may be indistinguishable from an adenomatous polyp or inflammatory pseudopolyps, respectively.

Dysplasia is thought to be a risk indicator for subsequent or concurrent malignancy, in part because of the frequent finding of dysplasia in resected colons containing cancer. Thus, there is a great interest in detecting dysplasia, and the presence of this condition in a colitic colon is a factor favoring prophylactic colectomy.

ISCHEMIC COLITIS

In an elderly patient with the acute onset of severe abdominal pain and rectal bleeding and no history of inflammatory bowel disease, diffuse pseudopolyposis should suggest the possibility of ischemic colitis (Fig. 51-33). The radiographic appearance can be indistinguishable from ulcerative or Crohn's colitis; often, only the clinical picture permits differentiation.

AMEBIASIS

The granulomatous reaction that occurs in areas of amebic infestation can produce large, hard masses

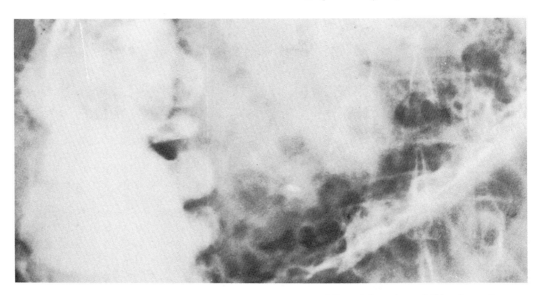

Fig. 51-33. *Pseudopolyposis in ischemic colitis. Multiple filling defects are visible along the lower margin of the transverse colon. The diagnosis was suggested by the clinical presentation of acute, severe abdominal pain and rectal bleeding in a patient with no history of inflammatory bowel disease.*

(amebomas) that are fixed and tender to palpation and can appear as filling defects within the lumen of the bowel. Amebomas can occur anywhere in the colon, though they are most common in the cecum and, to a lesser degree, in the rectosigmoid. They are usually solitary but can be multiple. Amebic infection can also result in a pattern of pseudopolyposis simulating ulcerative colitis or Crohn's disease, giving the radiographic appearance of multiple filling defects in the colon (Fig. 51-34).

SCHISTOSOMIASIS

Schistosomiasis is an infectious disease caused by a blood fluke that inhabits the portal venous system in humans and certain animals. More than 100 million people are infected worldwide, especially in tropical and subtropical countries. After partially maturing in the body of a suitable snail host, the schistosoma organism emerges into the water and enters its human host by penetrating the unbroken skin or buccal membrane. Those larvae that make their way to the liver develop into adult worms, which can reside within the portal venous bed for 20 to 30 years. The mature worms then migrate against the flow of portal venous blood into the smaller venules

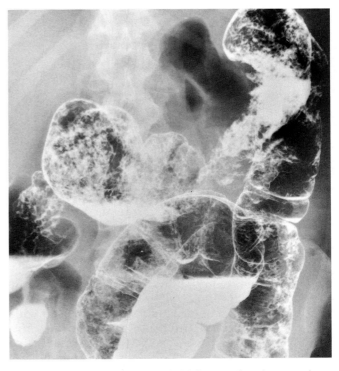

Fig. 51-34. *Amebic colitis. Multiple pseudopolyps produce a pattern identical to ulcerative or Crohn's colitis.*

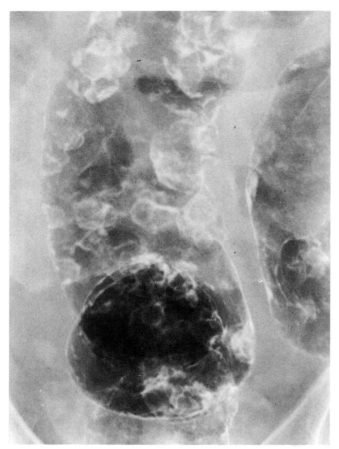

Fig. 51-35. *Schistosomiasis. Multiple filling defects represent polypoid granulomas.*

ations and edema of the mucosa, as well as narrowing and areas of stricture formation due to reactive fibrosis.

TRICHURIASIS

Trichuris trichiura (whipworm) is a ubiquitous parasite that is primarily found in warm, moist tropics. Humans become infested by ingesting whipworm ova from contaminated soil or vegetables. The ova hatch into larvae that migrate down to the cecum, where they develop into adult worms. Whipworms become attached to the colon and lie embedded between intestinal villi, coiled upon themselves with their blunt caudal portions projecting into the bowel lumen. Mild infections are usually asymptomatic, but heavy infestation, especially in children, can result in chronic diarrhea, abdominal pain, dehydration, weight loss, rectal prolapse, eosinophilia, and anemia.

The radiographic findings in trichuriasis are similar to the appearance in mucoviscidosis (cystic fibrosis) of the colon (Fig. 51-36). There is a diffuse

of the inferior mesenteric vein, where the females deposit their eggs. Those ova that penetrate into the lumen of the bowel are passed from the body and continue the life cycle.

The irritative effect of the ova that pass through or lodge in the bowel wall stimulates an inflammatory response with granuloma formation and progressive fibrosis. Because the adult worm has a predilection for entering the inferior mesenteric vein, the sigmoid colon is most commonly involved. In severe infestation, the proximal colon can also be affected. The most characteristic radiographic appearance in schistosomiasis is multiple filling defects (usually 1–2 cm large) due to the development of polypoid granulomas (Fig. 51-35). These masses are friable and vascular, and they bleed easily with the passage of feces, which explains the frequently bloody stools associated with severe infestation. Other radiographic findings include ragged ulcer-

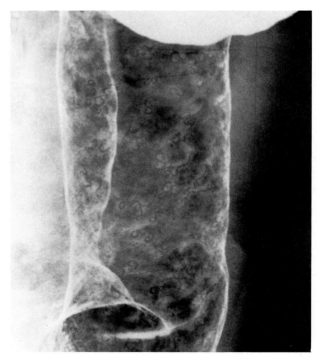

Fig. 51-36. *Trichuriasis. Double-contrast enema shows the multiple worms outlined in the descending colon. (Margulis AR, Burhenne HJ (eds): Alimentary Tract Radiology. St. Louis, CV Mosby, 1983)*

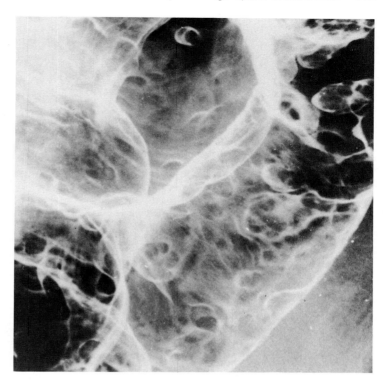

Fig. 51-37. *Strongyloidiasis. Multiple hyperplastic pseudopolyps simulate ulcerative or Crohn's colitis.*

granular mucosal pattern throughout the colon with considerable flocculation of barium due to abundant mucus secretions surrounding the tiny whipworms. In addition, multiple filling defects are produced by the individual outlines of the innumerable worms, which are attached to the mucosa with their posterior portions either tightly coiled or unfurled in a whiplike configuration.

OTHER COLITIS

Localized or diffuse pseudopolyps or pseudomembranes producing multiple colonic filling defects may occur in strongyloidiasis (Fig. 51-37), cytomegalovirus colitis, *Yersinia* colitis, pseudomembranous colitis (Fig. 51-38), and diversion colitis (nonspecific inflammatory bowel disease occurring in patients in whom parts of the large intestine are excluded from the fecal stream by placement of a proximal colostomy or ileostomy) (see Fig. 48-71).

ARTIFACTS

Although the material most commonly confused with polypoid tumors on barium enema examination is feces, the radiographic features of retained fecal material are usually distinctive and should

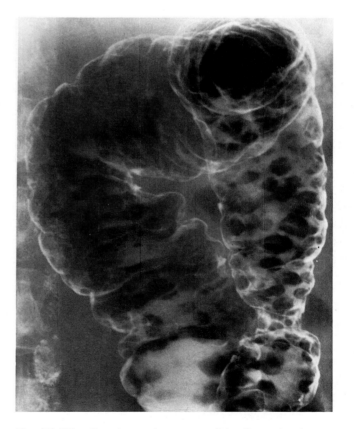

Fig. 51-38. *Pseudomembranous colitis. Extensive hyperplastic pseudopolyposis produces a pattern of multiple colonic filling defects.*

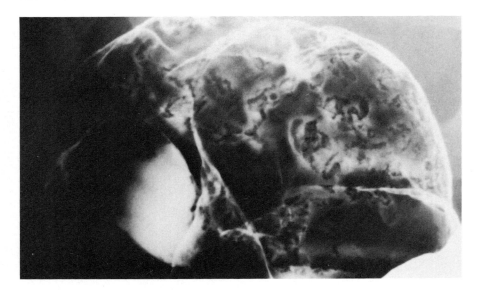

Fig. 51-39. Retained fecal material. There are multiple freely moving colonic filling defects.

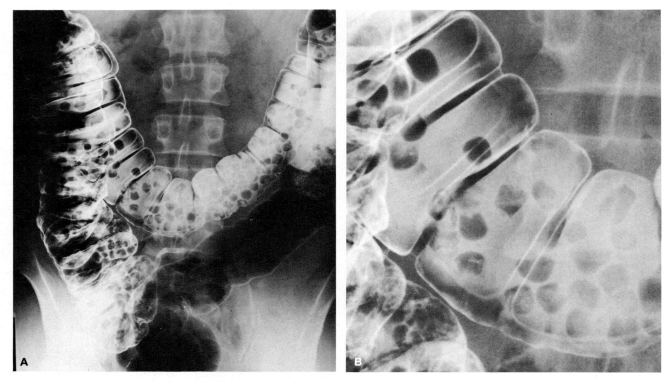

Fig. 51-40. Ingested corn kernels simulating multiple polyposis in the colon. **(A)** Full and **(B)** coned views. (Press HC, Davis TW: Ingested foreign bodies simulating polyposis: Report of six cases AJR 127:1040–1042. 1976. Copyright 1976. Reproduced with permission)

pose no diagnostic problems (Fig. 51-39). A "fecaloma" is generally freely movable, though it occasionally adheres so firmly to the bowel mucosa that it resembles a broad-based polyp. Fecal material tends to be irregular in shape, with an uneven barium coating; barium can usually be seen interposed between the fecal mass and the mucosa. The inability to demonstrate the point of attachment of a "polypoid mass" to the wall of the colon should suggest an intraluminal fecal mass rather than a discrete colonic lesion. Complications of fecalomas include ulceration, perforation, and obstruction.

Radiolucent air bubbles surrounded by thin, gradually fading barium margins can simulate multiple colonic filling defects. They frequently appear as several very small air bubbles clustered around a larger one. Oil bubbles from excessive castor oil or mineral oil used as a laxative in preparation for barium enema examination can produce a similar radiographic pattern.

Long, slender lucent strands within the barium column usually represent mucus. They are generally irregular branching defects, are often seen in association with retained fecal material, and are easily differentiated from pathologic lesions.

FOREIGN BODIES

Ingested foreign bodies, especially kernels of corn, can simulate multiple polyposis in the colon (Fig. 51-40). Intact corn kernels have thin outer coverings composed of cellulose that are not digested in the human gastrointestinal tract. These cellulose coverings are normally disrupted by mastication, which permits digestion of the corn by enzymes in the stomach and duodenum. However, in edentulous patients who chew poorly, corn kernels can be swallowed whole, remain undigested, and appear intact in the colon, where they mimic polyps.

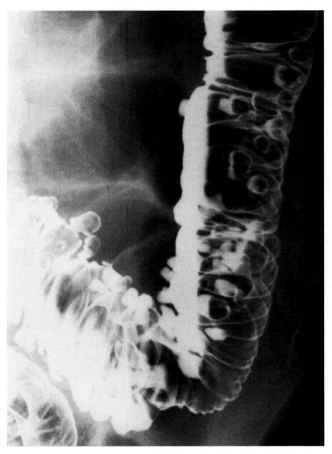

Fig. 51-42. Diverticula simulating colonic filling defects. Multiple barium-coated, air-filled diverticula superimposed on the lumen of the bowel mimic discrete colonic filling defects.

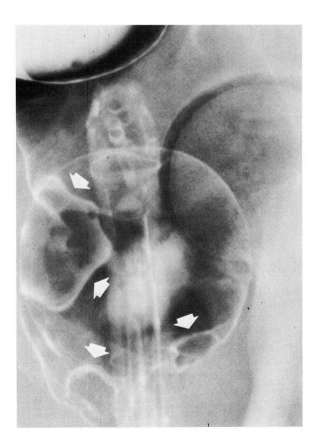

Fig. 51-41. Internal hemorrhoids. Multiple rectal filling defects **(arrows)** simulate polyps.

MISCELLANEOUS DISORDERS

HEMORRHOIDS

Internal hemorrhoids can produce multiple rectal filling defects that simulate polyps (Fig. 51-41). In most cases, however, hemorrhoids are associated with the linear shadows of the veins from which they arise.

DIVERTICULA

Barium-coated, air-filled diverticula superimposed on the lumen of the bowel sometimes mimic multiple colonic filling defects (Fig. 51-42). However, close attention to the inner and outer borders of the filling defects may permit the distinction to be made between diverticula and polypoid tumors. The ring of barium coating a diverticulum has a smooth, well-defined outer border and a blurred, irregular inner border. Conversely, barium coating a polyp

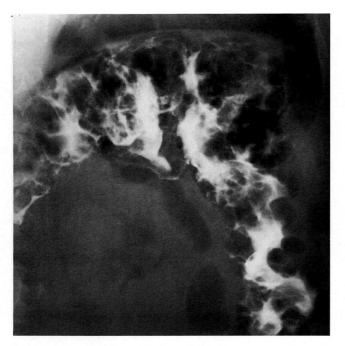

Fig. 51-43. *Pneumatosis intestinalis in an asymptomatic person. The intramural collections of gas simulate multiple colonic filling defects. Note that the filling defects in this condition appear to be more radiolucent than the soft-tissue masses in the intestinal polyposis syndromes.*

tends to be smooth on its inner border and poorly defined on its outer margin. It is usually necessary, however, to carefully evaluate multiple films in various obliquities to be certain that all of the "filling defects" can be projected clear of the colonic lumen and thus be seen to represent multiple diverticula.

PNEUMATOSIS INTESTINALIS

Intramural collections of gas can simulate multiple colonic filling defects. In contrast to true colonic polyps, the filling defects in pneumatosis intestinalis appear to be more radiolucent and to have broader bases (Fig. 51-43). When the abdomen is palpated, cysts of pneumatosis intestinalis are compressed, and the radiographic defects change shape.

COLITIS CYSTICA PROFUNDA

In colitis cystica profunda, large mucus epithelium-lined cysts up to 2 cm in diameter form in the submucosal layer of the colon. These submucosal cysts are most commonly seen in the pelvic colon and rectum. The disorder almost always involves a short segment of bowel; infrequently, the colon is diffusely affected. Although the pathogenesis of the

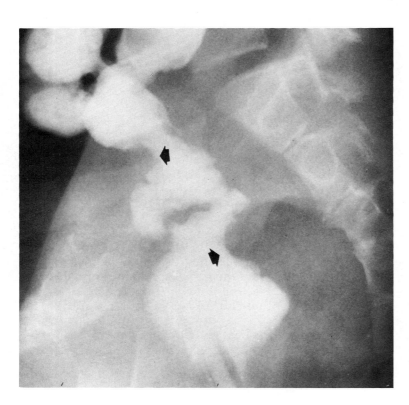

Fig. 51-44. *Colitis cystica profunda. There are multiple intraluminal filling defects* **(arrows)** *in the rectum. (Ledesma-Medina J, Reid BS, Girdany BR: Colitis cystica profunda. AJR 131:529–530, 1978. Copyright 1978. Reproduced with permission)*

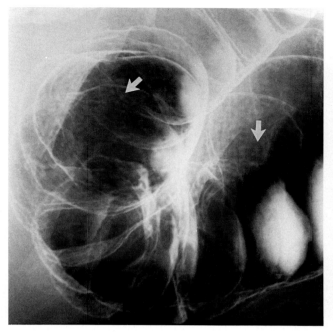

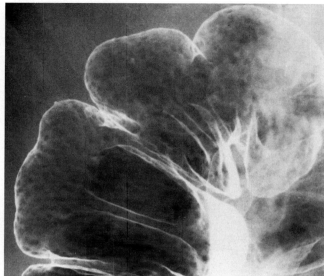

51-45

51-46

Fig. 51-45. Diffuse nodular lymphoid hyperplasia of the colon. **Arrows** point to characteristic flecks of barium in the centers of several of the lymphoid masses.

Fig. 51-46. Lymphoid follicular pattern of the colon in an adult. (Kelvin FM, Max RJ, Norton GA et al: Lymphoid follicular pattern of the colon in adults. AJR 133:821–825, 1979. Copyright 1979. Reproduced with permission)

disease is obscure, its frequent association with proctitis or colitis suggests that the cysts are formed when surface mucosa is implanted into the colonic submucosa during the healing phase of an ulcerative inflammatory process. Since the cells cannot be shed into the lumen and mucus cannot be discharged, a cystic mass develops. Bright red rectal bleeding, mucus discharge, and diarrhea are the most common presenting clinical symptoms; a rubbery or hard polypoid mass simulating carcinoma can sometimes be felt on rectal examination.

Colitis cystica profunda usually presents as multiple, irregular colonic filling defects suggesting adenomatous polyps (Fig. 51-44). Barium filling of the clefts between these nodular polypoid lesions can mimic ulceration. If sufficient scalloping of the colon is produced, the appearance may simulate ischemic colitis. Occasionally, only a single rectal mass mimicking a sessile polyp is seen. Colitis cystica profunda is a benign condition with no malignant potential; surgery is indicated only in patients in whom there is significant bleeding or associated rectal prolapse.

Colitis cystica superficialis is a rare condition in which minute cysts are diffusely distributed throughout the entire colon. This disorder is almost always associated with pellagra, though a few cases have been described in patients with tropical sprue or leukemia.

NODULAR LYMPHOID HYPERPLASIA/ LYMPHOID FOLLICULAR PATTERN

Early studies reported that a characteristic finding of nodular lymphoid hyperplasia was a fleck of barium in the center of the "polyps" (Fig. 51-45), representing umbilication at the apex of the lymphoid nodule. However, an identical appearance may be produced by the aphthous ulcers of inflammatory bowel disease and by occasional umbilication in nodular colonic lymphoma. This umbilicated appearance must be distinguished from the lymphoid follicular pattern, which is now recognized as a frequent, normal feature of the pediatric colon and can even be seen in 10% to 15% of adults on double-contrast examinations (Fig. 51-46). In normal adults, radiographically apparent lymphoid follicles are smooth and round, 1 mm to 3 mm in size, are generally limited to one or two segments of the bowel (usually the right colon), and are unusual in patients over age 60. In a recent report, four elderly patients with colonic carcinoma had associated dif-

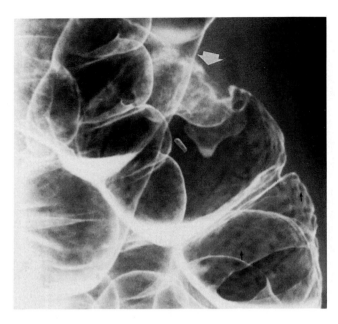

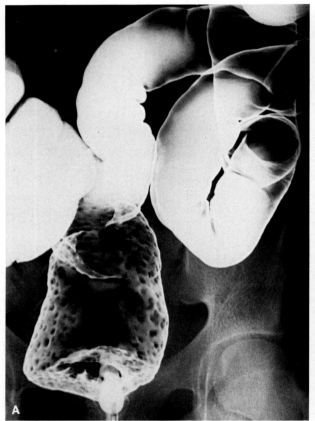

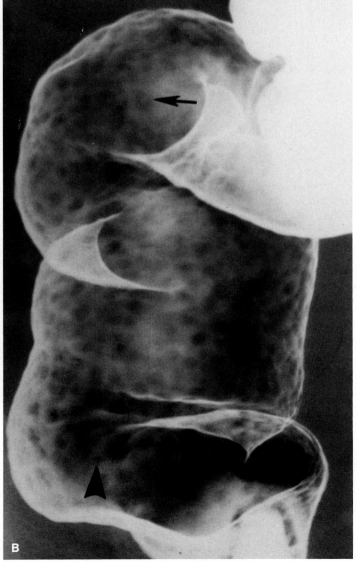

Fig. 51-47. Colon carcinoma associated with diffuse lymphoid follicles. Flat, 3 × 4 cm, nodular carcinoma **(arrow)** associated with prominent lymphoid follicles **(arrowheads)**. Lymphoid follicles were also present from the sigmoid to ascending colon. (Bronen RA, Glick SN, Teplick SK: Diffuse lymphoid follicles of the colon associated with colonic carcinoma. AJR 142:105–109, 1984. Copyright 1984. Reproduced with permission)

Fig. 51-48. Large colonic lymphoid follicles in inflammatory bowel disease. **(A)** Girl, aged 12, with painless rectal bleeding for 3 months due to nonspecific proctitis. The lymphoid follicles (confirmed by biopsy) ranged up to 6 mm and were confined to the rectosigmoid region. **(B)** Boy, aged 12, with lymphadenopathy, abdominal pain, and frequent bowel movements for 5 years. Lymphoid follicles ranging from 2 mm **(arrowhead)** to 5 mm **(arrow)** throughout the colon. (Kenney PJ, Koehler RE, Shackelford GD: The clinical significance of large lymphoid follicles of the colon. Radiology 142:41–46, 1982)

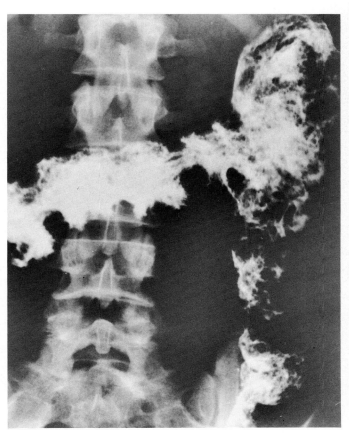

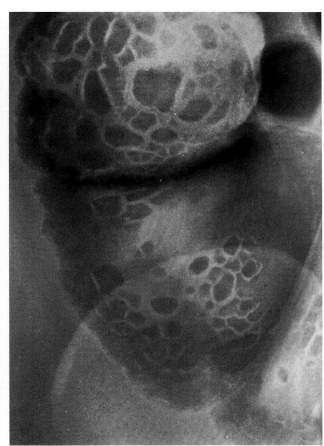

51-49   51-50

Fig. 51-49.   Cystic fibrosis. These multiple, poorly defined filling defects are caused by residual thick secretions.

Fig. 51-50.   Colonic urticaria. Large polygonal, raised plaques are visible in a dilated cecum and ascending colon.

fuse lymphoid follicles in the colon (Fig. 51-47). Large colonic lymphoid follicles (>4 mm), which are predominantly located in the rectosigmoid region, have been reported in patients with hypogammaglobulinemia, familial polyposis, sarcoidosis, infectious mononucleosis, inflammatory bowel disease (Fig. 51-48), and lymphoma.

CYSTIC FIBROSIS

Cystic fibrosis in adolescents can produce a striking radiographic appearance of the colon. Because of adherent collections of viscid mucus, adequate cleansing prior to barium enema examination is rarely achieved. The residual thick secretions can cause multiple, poorly defined filling defects that give the colonic mucosa a hyperplastic appearance simulating polyposis (Fig. 51-49).

SUBMUCOSAL EDEMA PATTERN

A characteristic mucosal pattern of large, round or polygonal, raised plaques in a grossly dilated bowel (Fig. 51-50) was first described as an allergic reaction of the colonic mucosa to medication. This "colonic urticaria" predominantly involves the right colon, can be seen without concomitant cutaneous lesions, and regresses once the offending medication is withdrawn. A pattern similar to colonic urticaria has been reported in several other conditions for which the common denominator seems to be submucosal edema. In herpes zoster, an exanthematous neurocutaneous disorder secondary to reactivation or reinfection by a large pox virus, colonic mucosal blebs infrequently appear as multiple small, discrete, polygonal filling defects with sharp

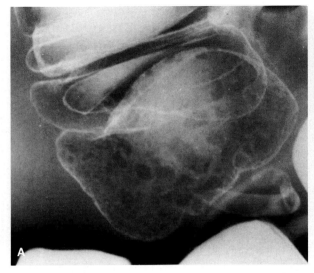

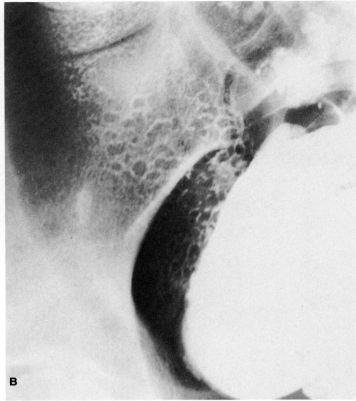

Fig. 51-51. Herpes zoster. Polygonal filling defects with sharp angular margins are evident in two patients with this disease.

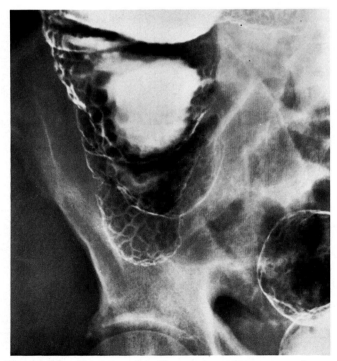

Fig. 51-52. *Yersinia* colitis. Coned view of the cecum demonstrates the characteristic urticarial pattern of submucosal edema. (Miller VE, Han SY, Witten DM: Reticular mosaic (urticarial) pattern of the colonic mucosa in *Yersinia* colitis. Radiology 146:307–308, 1983)

angular margins (Fig. 51-51). These blebs correspond morphologically and temporally to the vesicular phase of the cutaneous lesion and are segmentally arrayed in a corresponding or noncorresponding dermatome. In *Yersinia* colitis, submucosal edema is caused by an alteration in vascular permeability (Fig. 51-52). A similar radiographic pattern has also been observed in patients with submucosal colonic edema secondary to obstructing carcinoma, cecal volvulus, ischemia, colonic ileus, and benign colonic obstruction.

ULCERATIVE PSEUDOPOLYPS PROXIMAL TO AN OBSTRUCTION

Ulcerative disease has been described proximal to partial or complete obstruction of the lumen of the esophagus, stomach, small bowel, or colon. In all reported cases, the bowel was normal distal to the point of obstruction. The pathogenesis of ulcerative disease proximal to an obstructing bowel lesion appears to be a function of ischemia caused by distention of the bowel, with decreased blood flow through the vessels extending from the mesenteric border to the bowel wall. In the colon, this process often presents radiographically as prominent nodularity with pseudopolyp formation simulating the appearance of an ulcerating colitis.

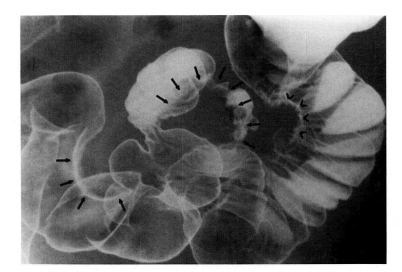

Fig. 51-53. Endometriosis. Three separate endometrial implants **(arrows** and **arrowheads)** in the sigmoid colon. The most distal lesion has a smooth interface with the bowel wall, indicating no intramural invasion. The two more proximal lesions demonstrate crenulations indicating intramural or submucosal invasion. (Gedgaudas RK, Kelvin FM, Thompson WM et al: Value of the preoperative barium enema examination in the assessment of pelvic masses. Radiology 146:609–616, 1983)

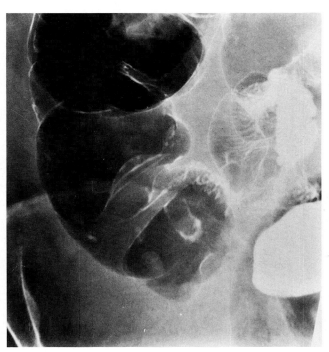

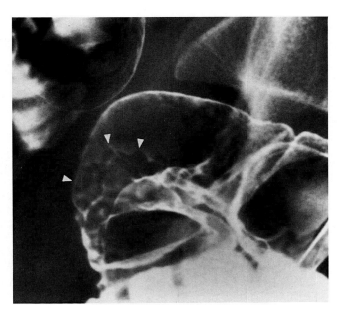

51-54

51-55

Fig. 51-54. Malacoplakia. Coned view of the cecum demonstrates several small polypoid filling defects. (Radin DR, Chandrasoma P, Halls JM: Colonic malacoplakia. Gastrointest Radiol 9:359–361, 1984)

Fig. 51-55. Colonic varices. Multiple serpiginous tubular lesions **(arrowheads)** in the sigmoid colon. (Deutsch AL, Davis GB, Berk RN: Diagnosis of colonic varices by air-contrast barium enema examination: Report of a case. Gastrointest Radiol 6:336–338, 1981)

ENDOMETRIOSIS

A pattern of multiple colonic filling defects is one of the many manifestations of heterotopic foci of endometrial tissue involving the bowel (Fig. 51-53). More commonly, endometriosis presents as either an isolated intramural defect with pleating of crenulation of the adjacent mucosa due to secondary fibrosis (see Fig. 50-45) or as a constricting lesion that typically has an intact mucosa, tapered margins, and no ulceration within it (see Fig. 49-69).

MALACOPLAKIA

Malacoplakia is a chronic granulomatous reaction characterized by the accumulation of distinctive macrophages that ingest microorganisms and cel-

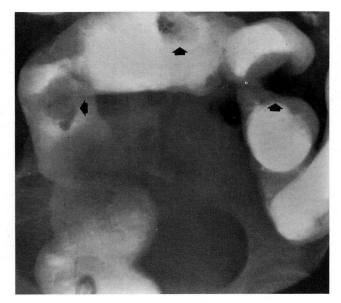

Fig. 51-56. *Amyloidosis. Multiple discrete filling defects* **(arrows)** *represent localized deposition of amyloid in the sigmoid colon.*

lular debris but are unable to digest them. The colon is the most common site of malacoplakia outside the urogenital tract. Malacoplakia may involve the colon segmentally or diffusely, with the rectosigmoid and cecum being most frequently involved. Radiographically, colonic malacoplakia typically presents as one or more polypoid lesions (Fig. 51-54); there occasionally may be associated ulceration and fistulas simulating Crohn's disease. Abdominal pain, diarrhea, rectal bleeding, and fever are the most common symptoms. In cases of limited involvement of the colon, surgical resection is usually curative. With more extensive lesions, however, intractable diarrhea, bowel obstruction, and fistulization produce significant morbidity and even death.

COLONIC VARICES

Colonic varices represent collateral pathways between the inferior mesenteric vein and the left iliac vein that may develop in patients with portal hypertension. The rarity of colonic varices is primarily a reflection of the preferential development of esophageal varices through the rich coronary–azygos system. However, in patients with isolated inferior mesenteric vein occlusion or congenital venous anomalies, additional blood flow through venous collateral channels in the colon results in colonic varices. Colonic varices appear as serpiginous and tubular submucosal lesions in the sigmoid colon (Fig. 51-55). They are reported to be best seen on double-contrast studies, since on solid-column examinations the varices are often misinterpreted as air bubbles or fecal material.

AMYLOIDOSIS

Rarely, extensive deposition of amyloid in the colon produces a pattern of multiple discrete filling defects (Fig. 51-56).

BIBLIOGRAPHY

Bartram CI, Thornton A: Colonic polyp patterns in familial polyposis. AJR 142:305–308, 1984

Berk RN, Millman SJ: Urticaria of the colon. Radiology 99:539–540, 1971

Bronen RA, Glick SN, Teplick SK: Diffuse lymphoid follicles of the colon associated with colonic carcinoma. AJR 142:105–109, 1984

Childress MH, Martel W: Fecaloma simulating colonic neoplasm. Surg Gynecol Obstet 142:664–666, 1976

Denzler TB, Harned RK, Pergam CJ: Gastric polyps in familial polyposis coli. Radiology 130:63–66, 1979

Deutsch AL, Davis GB, Berk RN: Diagnosis of colonic varices by air-contrast barium enema examination: Report of a case. Gastrointest Radiol 6:336–338, 1981

Dodds WJ: Clinical roentgen features of intestinal polyposis syndromes. Gastrointest Radiol 1:127–142, 1976

Dolan KD, Seibert J, Seibert RW: Gardner's syndrome. AJR 119:359–364, 1973

Foster MA, Kilcoyne RF: Ruvalcaba–Myhre–Smith syndrome: A new consideration in the differential diagnosis of intestinal polyposis. Gastrointest Radiol 11:349–350, 1986

Gardiner R, Smith C: Infective enterocolitides. Radiol Clin North Am 25:67–78, 1987

Gedgaudas RK, Kelvin FM, Thompson WM et al: The value of the preoperative barium-enema examination in the assessment of pelvic masses. Radiology 146:609–613, 1983

Giardiello FM, Welsh SB, Hamilton SR et al: Increased risk of cancer in the Peutz–Jeghers syndrome. New Engl J Med 316:1511–1514, 1987

Glick SN, Teplick SK, Goren RA: Small colonic nodularity and the double contrast barium enema. RadioGraphics 1:73–86, 1981

Godard JE, Dodds WJ, Phillips JC et al: Peutz–Jeghers syndrome: Clinical and roentgenographic features. AJR 113:316–324, 1971

Hauser H, Ody B, Plojoux O et al: Radiological findings in multiple hamartoma syndrome (Cowden disease). Radiology 137:317–323, 1980

Hooyman JR, MacCarty RL, Carpenter HA et al: Radiographic appearance of mucosal dysplasia associated with ulcerative colitis. AJR 149:47–51, 1987

Kagan AR, Steckel RJ: Colon polyposis and cancer. AJR 131:1065–1067, 1978

Kelvin FM, Max RJ, Norton GA et al: Lymphoid follicular pattern of the colon in adults. AJR 133:821–825, 1979

Kenney PJ, Koehler RE, Shackelford GD: The clinical significance of large lymphoid follicles of the colon. Radiology 142:41–46, 1982

Khilnani MT, Marshak RH, Eliasoph J et al: Roentgen features of metastases of the colon. AJR 96:302–310, 1966

Koehler PR, Kyaw MM, Fenlon JW: Diffuse gastrointestinal polyposis with ectodermal changes. Cronkhite–Canada syndrome. Radiology 103:589–594, 1972

Laufer I, de Sa D: Lymphoid follicular pattern: A normal feature of the pediatric colon. AJR 130:51–55, 1978

Ledesma–Medina J, Reid BS, Girdany BR: Colitis cystica profunda. AJR 131:529–530, 1978

Magid D, Fishman EK, Jones B et al: Desmoid tumors in Gardner syndrome: Use of computed tomography. AJR 142:1141–1145, 1984

Manzano C, Thomas MA, Valenzuela C: Trichuriasis: Roentgenographic features and differential diagnosis with lymphoid hyperplasia. Pediatr Radiol 8:76–78, 1979

McCartney WH, Hoffer PB: The value of carcinoembryonic antigen (CEA) as an adjunct to the radiological colon examination in the diagnosis of malignancy. Radiology 110:325–328, 1974

Meyers MA, McSweeny J: Secondary neoplasms of the bowel. Radiology 105:1–11, 1972

Miller VE, Han SY, Witten DM: Retricular mosaic (urticarial) pattern of the colon mucosa in *Yersinia* colitis. Radiology 146:307–308, 1983

Moertel CG, Schutt AJ, Go VLW: Carcinoembryonic antigen test for recurrent colorectal carcinoma: Inadequacy for early detection. JAMA 329:1065–1066, 1978

Munyer TP, Montgomery CK, Thoeni RF et al: Postinflammatory polyposis (PIP) of the colon: The radiologic-pathologic spectrum. Radiology 145:607–614, 1982

Nebel OT, Masry NA, Castell DO et al: Schistosomal disease of the colon: A reversible form of polyposis. Gastroenterology 67:939–943, 1974

Press HC, Davis TW: Ingested foreign bodies simulating polyposis: Report of six cases. AJR 127:1040–1042, 1976

Pochaczevsky R, Sherman RS: Diffuse lymphomatous disease of the colon: Its roentgen appearance. AJR 87:670–683, 1962

Rabin MS, Bledin AG, Lewis D: Polypoid leukemic infiltration of the large bowel. AJR 131:723–724, 1978

Radin DR, Fortgang KC, Zee CS et al: Turcot syndrome: A case with spinal cord and colonic neoplasms. AJR 142:475–476, 1984

Reeder MM, Hamilton LC: Tropical diseases of the colon. Semin Roentgenol 3:62–80, 1968

Rubesin SE, Saul SH, Laufer I et al: Carpet lesions of the colon. RadioGraphics 5:537–552, 1985

Sacks BA, Joffe N, Antonioli DA: Metastatic melanoma presenting clinically as multiple colonic polyps. AJR 129:511–513, 1977

Schwartz AM, McCauley RGK: Juvenile gastrointestinal polyposis. Radiology 121:441–444, 1976

Scott RL, Pinstein ML: Diversion colitis demonstrated by double-contrast barium enema. AJR 143:767–768, 1984

Seaman WB, Clements JL: Urticaria of the colon: A nonspecific pattern of submucosal edema. AJR 138:545–547, 1982

Shapir J, Frank P: Radiologic manifestations of the syndrome of neurocrest and colonic tumors. Gastrointest Radiol 10:383–386, 1985

Simpson S, Traube J, Riddell RH: The histologic appearance of dysplasias (precancerous change) in Crohn's disease of the small and large intestine. Gastroenterology 81:492–501, 1981

Stevenson GW, Goodacre R, Jackson R et al: Dysplasia to carcinoma transformation in ulcerative colitis. AJR 143:108–110, 1984

Strada M, Meregaglia D, Donzelli R: Double-contrast enema in antibiotic-related pseudomembranous colitis. Gastrointest Radiol 8:67–69, 1983

Williams SM, Berk RN, Harned RK: Radiologic features of multinodular lymphoma of the colon. AJR 143:87–91, 1984

Yatto RP: Colonic lipomatosis. Am J Gastroenterol 77:436–437, 1982

Zegel HG, Laufer I: Filiform polyposis. Radiology 127:615–619, 1978

LARGE BOWEL OBSTRUCTION

Large bowel obstructions differ greatly from obstructions involving the small bowel. The majority of small bowel obstructions are caused by adhesions; in colonic obstructions, adhesions are rarely the cause. The major sites of obstruction in the large bowel are the cecal region, the flexures, the sigmoid colon, and the upper part of the rectum. Colonic obstructions occur far more frequently on the left side than on the right. They generally produce less fluid and electrolyte disturbances than small bowel obstructions. Colonic obstructions also tend to be more subacute, with symptoms developing more slowly.

The radiographic appearance of colonic obstruction depends on the competency of the ileocecal valve. If the ileocecal valve is competent, obstruction causes a large, dilated colon with a markedly distended, thin-walled cecum and little small bowel gas (Fig. 52-1). If the ileocecal valve is incompetent, however, there is distention of gas-filled loops of both colon and small bowel (Fig. 52-2), often with cecal hypertrophy and thickening of the haustra and colon wall.

It is sometimes very difficult to distinguish between a low colonic obstruction and colon ileus. In proximal colonic obstruction, the abnormal distention ends abruptly at the level of the lesion; the colon distal to it is free of gas. This transition is often impossible to detect in low colonic obstructions. In the case of such an obstruction, radiographs should be obtained with the patient in the lateral decubitus position (right-side down). This position facilitates the entry of gas into the rectosigmoid and rectum,

unless there is mechanical obstruction at or above this level. Distention of the rectum implies colonic ileus; a collapsed rectum suggests mechanical obstruction. If there is doubt, a barium enema is required to demonstrate either the presence of an obstructing lesion or the patency of the colonic lumen.

The major danger in colonic obstruction is perforation. If the ileocecal valve is competent, the colon behaves like a closed loop, and the increased pressure due to the obstruction cannot be dissipated. If the colon is massively distended by gas, perforation can occur. Because the cecum is spherical in shape and has a large diameter, it is the most likely site for perforation. In acute colonic obstruction, the possibility of perforation is very likely if the cecum distends to more than 10 cm. In intermittent or chronic obstruction, however, the cecal wall can become hypertrophied and the diameter greatly exceed 10 cm without perforation (Fig. 52-3). If colonic obstruction is due to a malignant neoplasm, the most common site of perforation is adjacent to the tumor rather than in the cecum. Massive distention of the colon can compromise the mesenteric vascular supply, leading to strangulation and bowel necrosis.

Causes of Large Bowel Obstruction

Malignant lesions
Inflammatory strictures
   Diverticulitis
   Inflammatory bowel disease
   Infectious granulomatous disease

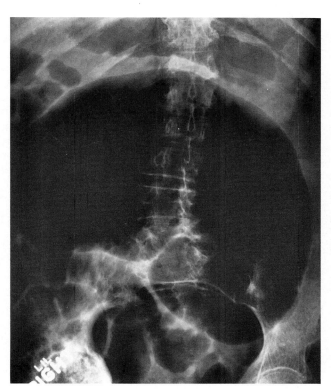

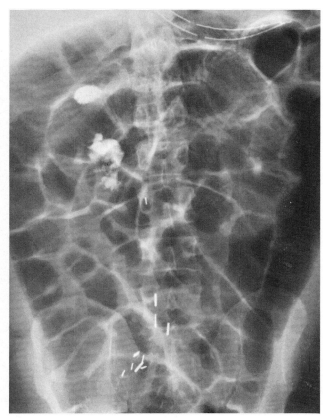

52-1   52-2

Fig. 52-1. Cecal volvulus. The thin-walled cecum is markedly distended. Because the ileocecal valve is competent, there is little small bowel gas.

Fig. 52-2. Large bowel obstruction due to torsion of the splenic flexure entering a traumatic diaphragmatic hernia. Because of the incompetent ileocecal valve, there is diffuse dilatation of gas-filled loops of both colon and small bowel producing a radiographic pattern that suggests adynamic ileus.

Parasitic disease
Ischemia
Extrinsic bowel lesions
   Volvulus
   Hernias
   Neoplasms/abscesses/distended bladder
   Endometriosis
Fecal impaction
Intussusception
Aganglionosis of the colon (Hirschsprung's
   disease)
Imperforate anus
Meconium plug syndrome
Adhesions
Retractile mesenteritis
Bezoar
Colonic pseudo-obstruction

MALIGNANT LESIONS

Almost 70% of large bowel obstructions are secondary to primary colonic carcinoma (Fig. 52-4). The sigmoid region is the site of obstruction in a majority of cases. Carcinomas frequently encircle the colon over a short segment, producing a classic "napkin-ring" or "apple-core" lesion characterized by luminal narrowing and overhanging margins (Fig. 52-5). As the mass of the tumor increases, progressive constriction of the bowel can cause complete colonic obstruction (Fig. 52-6).

INFLAMMATORY STRICTURES

Diverticulitis is the second most common cause of large bowel obstruction. Severe spasm, an adjacent

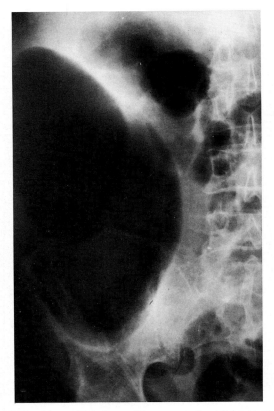

Fig. 52-3. Huge dilatation of the cecum (to 13 cm in diameter) without perforation.

walled off abscess, and fibrous scarring can produce marked narrowing of the lumen of the colon (Fig. 52-7).

Inflammatory bowel disease, such as chronic ulcerative colitis or Crohn's disease, can produce colonic narrowing and obstruction as a result of thickening of the bowel wall by the inflammatory process or of subsequent healing with fibrosis. Colonic obstruction can rarely be caused by a giant pseudopolyp in inflammatory bowel disease (Fig. 52-8). Infectious granulomatous processes (actinomycosis, tuberculosis, lymphogranuloma venereum) and parasitic diseases (amebiasis, schistosomiasis) can also result in luminal narrowing and colonic obstruction. In Chagas' disease, destruction of the colonic myenteric plexuses by the protozoan *Trypanosoma cruzi* causes striking elongation and dilatation, especially of the rectosigmoid and descending colon (Fig. 52-9). During the healing phase of mesenteric ischemia, intense fibrosis can produce large bowel obstruction.

VOLVULUS

Volvulus of the large bowel is the third most common cause of colonic obstruction. Because torsion of the bowel usually requires a long, movable mesentery, volvulus of the large bowel most frequently involves the cecum and sigmoid colon. The trans-

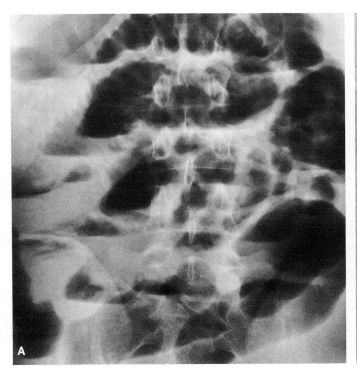

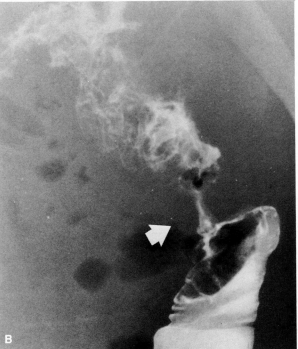

Fig. 52-4. Large bowel obstruction secondary to primary colonic carcinoma. **(A)** A plain abdominal radiograph demonstrates gas-fluid levels in multiple loops of small bowel. Although the transverse colon is dilated, no gas can be identified in the descending colon or rectosigmoid. **(B)** A barium enema demonstrates a small amount of contrast passing the high-grade malignant obstruction **(arrow)**.

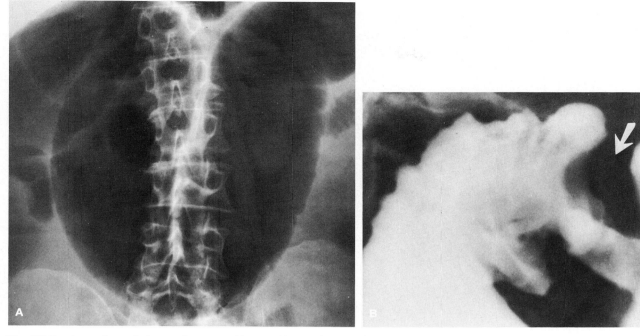

Fig. 52-5. Large bowel obstruction caused by annular carcinoma of the sigmoid. **(A)** A plain abdominal radiograph demonstrates pronounced dilatation of the gas-filled transverse and ascending colon. **(B)** A barium enema demonstrates a typical "apple-core lesion" **(arrow)** producing the colonic obstruction.

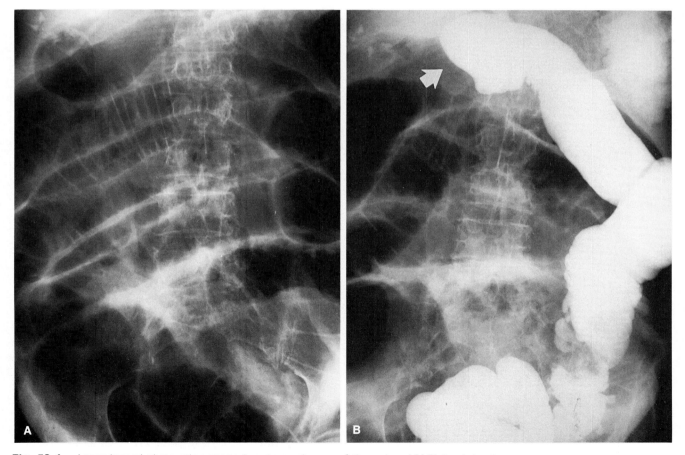

Fig. 52-6. Large bowel obstruction secondary to carcinoma of the colon. **(A)** Plain abdominal radiograph demonstrating massively dilated loops of small and proximal large bowel. **(B)** Complete obstruction to the flow of barium at the site of the malignant lesion **(arrow)**.

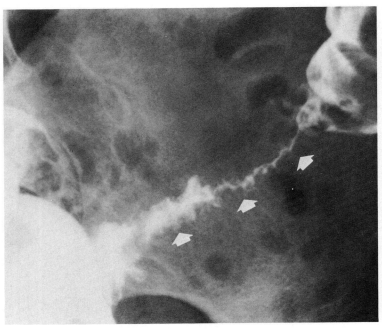

52-7

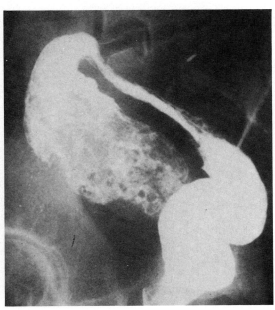

52-8

Fig. 52-7. Diverticulitis. Severe spasm and an adjacent walled off abscess cause marked narrowing of the colonic lumen **(arrows)**.

Fig. 52-8. Giant pseudopolyp in ulcerative colitis. Retrograde obstruction to the flow of barium by the large inflammatory mass in the sigmoid colon. (Solomon A, Stadler J, Goland L: Giant pseudopolypoidal retrograde obstruction in ulcerative colitis. Am J Gastroenterol 78:248–250, 1983)

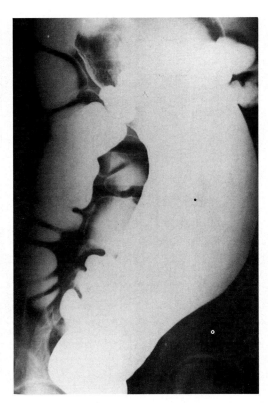

Fig. 52-9. Large bowel obstruction due to Chagas' disease. There is striking elongation and dilatation of the rectosigmoid.

verse colon, which has a short mesentery, is rarely affected by volvulus.

CECAL VOLVULUS

The ascending colon and cecum may have a long mesentery as a fault of rotation and fixation during development of the gut (Fig. 52-10). This situation predisposes to volvulus, with the cecum twisting on its long axis. It should be stressed, however, that only a few patients with a hypermobile cecum ever develop cecal volvulus. Other factors (colon ileus, distal obstruction as in sigmoid carcinoma, pregnancy, and chronic fecal retention) have been implicated as precipitating causes.

In cecal volvulus, the distended cecum tends to be displaced upward and to the left (Fig. 52-11), though it can be found anywhere within the abdomen. A pathognomonic sign of cecal volvulus is the twisted cecum appearing as a kidney-shaped mass with the torqued and thickened mesentery mimicking the renal pelvis (Fig. 52-12A). A barium enema examination is usually required for definite confirmation of the diagnosis. This study demonstrates obstruction of the contrast column at the level of the stenosis, with the tapered edge of the column pointing toward the site of torsion (Fig. 52-12B).

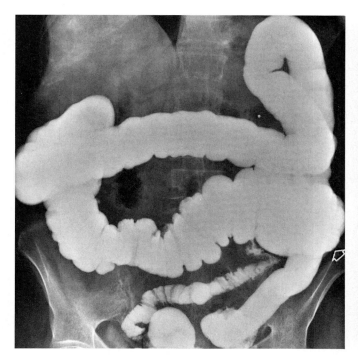

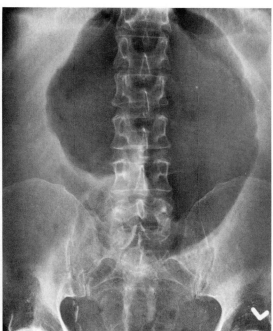

52-10

52-11

Fig. 52-10. Mobile cecum. The unusually long mesentery permits the cecum and ascending colon to course horizontally with the tip of the cecum **(arrow)** near the left wall of the abdomen.

Fig. 52-11. Cecal volvulus. The distended, gas-filled cecum is displaced upward and to the left.

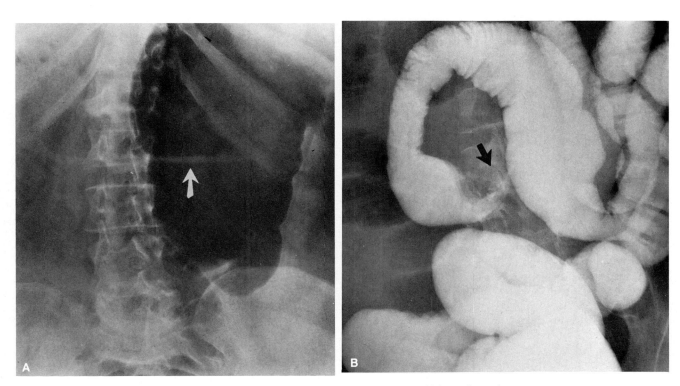

Fig. 52-12. Cecal volvulus. **(A)** The dilated, gas-filled cecum appears as a kidney-shaped mass with the torqued and thickened mesentery **(arrow)** mimicking the renal pelvis. **(B)** A barium enema examination demonstrates obstruction of the contrast column at the level of the stenosis, with the tapered edge of the column pointing toward the site of torsion **(arrow)**.

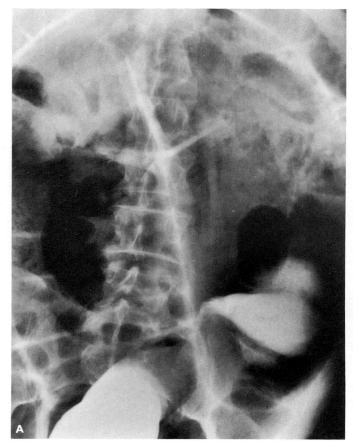

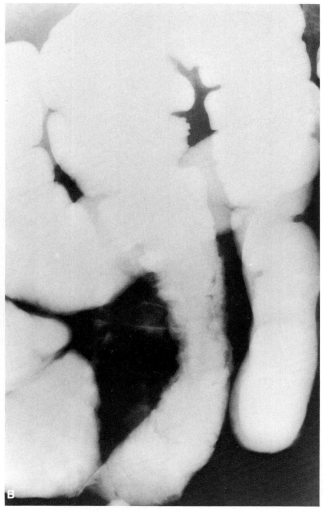

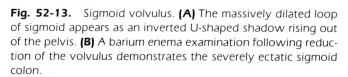

Fig. 52-13. *Sigmoid volvulus.* **(A)** The massively dilated loop of sigmoid appears as an inverted U-shaped shadow rising out of the pelvis. **(B)** A barium enema examination following reduction of the volvulus demonstrates the severely ectatic sigmoid colon.

SIGMOID VOLVULUS

A long, redundant loop of sigmoid colon can undergo a twist on its mesenteric axis and form a closed-loop obstruction. In sigmoid volvulus, the greatly inflated sigmoid loop appears as an inverted U-shaped shadow that rises out of the pelvis in a vertical or oblique direction and can even reach the level of the diaphragm (Fig. 52-13). The affected loop appears devoid of haustral markings and has a sausage or balloon shape. On supine radiographs, there are often three dense, curved lines running downward and converging toward the point of stenosis (Fig. 52-14). These lines appear to end in a small tumorlike density that corresponds to the twisted mesenteric root. The central and most constant line is a dense midline crease produced by the two walls of the torqued loop lying pressed together. The other two lines, less frequently seen, are made up of the outer margins of the closed loop joined with the medial walls of the cecum on the right and the descending colon on the left. When a barium enema is performed in a patient with sigmoid volvulus, the flow of contrast ceases at the obstruction, and the rectum becomes distended. The lumen tapers toward the site of stenosis and a pathognomonic "bird's beak" is produced (Fig. 52-15).

As with any colonic obstruction, prompt decompression of sigmoid volvulus is necessary to prevent bowel ischemia and perforation. Fluoroscopic or sigmoidoscopic guidance of a rectal tube is often therapeutic and is the preferred form of initial treatment if there are no signs of vascular compromise (Fig. 52-16). Tube decompression allows time for medical stabilization of the patient and is the only viable approach to the patient who is at high risk for surgery. Because there is a high recurrence rate of sigmoid volvulus (up to 80%), resection of the redundant sigmoid is often necessary.

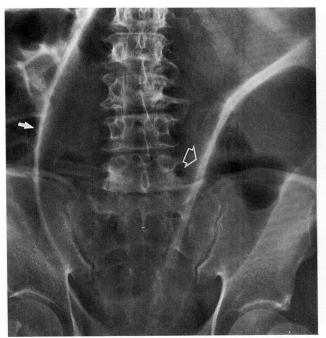 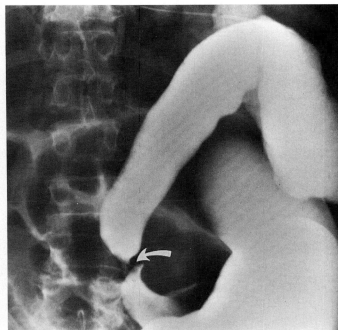

52-14   52-15

Fig. 52-14. Sigmoid volvulus. Two of the characteristic three dense lines are seen running downward and converging toward the point of stenosis. The central line **(open arrow)** is produced by the two walls of the torqued loop lying pressed together. The right line **(solid arrow)** consists of the outer margin of the closed loop joined with the medial wall of the cecum. The left line is not clearly seen, because there is no gas within the lower descending colon.

Fig. 52-15. Sigmoid volvulus. A barium enema demonstrates luminal tapering at the site of stenosis producing the characteristic "bird's-beak" configuration.

TRANSVERSE COLON VOLVULUS

Transverse colon volvulus is unusual because the normal fixation of the colon at the flexures and the relatively short mesentery of the transverse colon makes torsion of this segment unlikely. Causative factors are thought to include malrotation, chronic constipation with subsequent redundancy of the bowel, previous surgery with adhesions, and distal obstructing lesions.

Both acute and chronic forms of transverse colon volvulus have been described. A patient with acute volvulus typically presents with a history of sudden abdominal pain and rapid deterioration. The chronic form has a more gradual onset of symptoms and a history of previous similar episodes. Women are more commonly affected than men. Transverse colon volvulus tends to occur at a younger average age than sigmoid or cecal volvulus and has a higher mortality rate.

The diagnosis of transverse colon volvulus is not commonly made preoperatively. Supine films generally reveal a large bowel obstruction with a dilated loop of colon in the upper abdomen (Fig. 52-17). Although the appearance of two air–fluid levels on upright or lateral decubitus views has been described as characteristic, plain abdominal radiographs are less diagnostic in transverse colon volvulus than in the other types. A barium enema examination demonstrates the typical "bird beak" of a volvulus at the level of the transverse colon, thus establishing the diagnosis. The treatment is surgical detorsion and should be immediate, as opposed to sigmoid volvulus which can be reduced by a rectal tube with surgery performed electively at a later date.

HERNIAS

Large bowel obstruction can be caused by displacement of colon into an inguinal, femoral, umbilical, incisional (Fig. 52-18), or diaphragmatic (congenital or post-traumatic) hernia. Internal colonic hernias through the foramen of Winslow also occur. As with small bowel herniation producing obstruction, strangulation of bowel is a frequent complication.

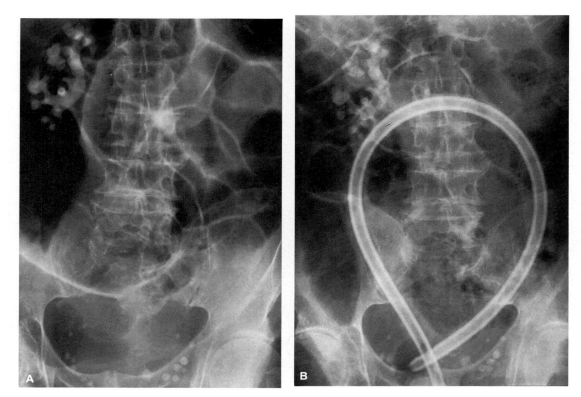

Fig. 52-16. *Sigmoid volvulus with decompression.* **(A)** *Plain abdominal radiograph demonstrating pronounced dilatation of the sigmoid.* **(B)** *Following the insertion of a rectal tube, there is resolution of the sigmoid volvulus.*

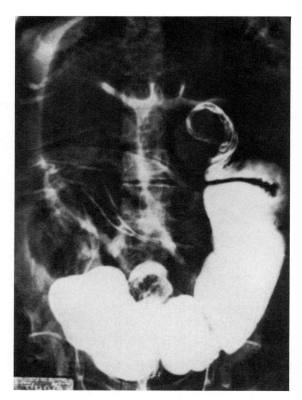

Fig. 52-17. Transverse colon volvulus. Single-contrast barium enema demonstrates an obstruction at the splenic flexure with characteristic twisting of bowel mucosa due to the volvulus. (Wolf EL, Frager B, Beneventano TC: Volvulus of the transverse colon. Am J Gastroenterol 79:797–798, 1984)

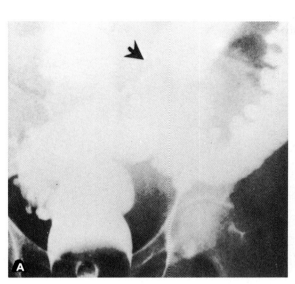

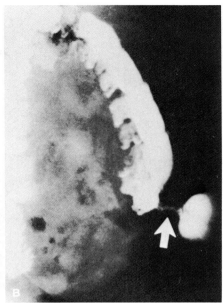

Fig. 52-18. Incisional hernia. **(A)** A barium enema shows that the obstruction to flow is at the level of the midtransverse colon **(arrow)**. **(B)** A lateral film reveals constriction of the transverse colon **(arrow)** as it enters a midline anterior incisional hernia. (Love L: Large bowel obstruction. Semin Roentgenol 8:299–322, 1973)

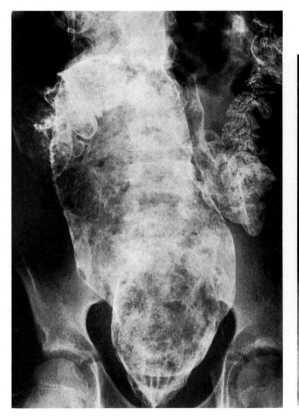

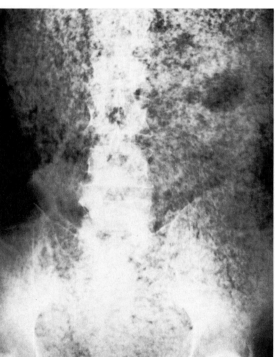

52-19

52-20

Fig. 52-19. Psychogenic megacolon in a child. There is huge dilatation of the feces-filled rectum.

Fig. 52-20. Fecal impaction. The characteristic mottled density of feces throughout the colon is diagnostic on this plain abdominal radiograph.

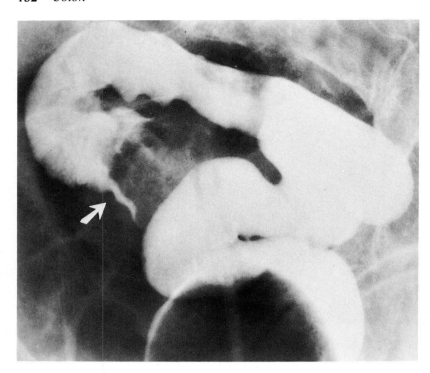

Fig. 52-21. Inspissated fecalith obstructing the sigmoid colon **(arrow).** The radiographic appearance simulates a primary colonic malignancy.

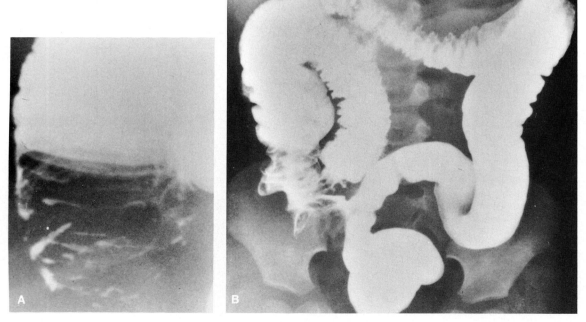

Fig. 52-22. Ileocolic intussusception in a child. **(A)** Characteristic coiled-spring appearance at the point of obstruction. **(B)** Partial reduction of the intussusception by barium enema.

EXTRINSIC PROCESSES

Tumors and abscesses adjacent to the colon occasionally lead to large bowel obstruction. Similar effects can be caused by extracolonic structures, such as a hugely distended bladder or a large tumor mass situated within the pelvis.

ENDOMETRIOSIS

Endometriosis is the presence of islands of endometrial tissue in an extrauterine location. A fibrotic reaction to cyclical activity of these endometrial implants can produce symptoms and radiographic findings of large bowel obstruction. Endometriosis should be considered a possible etiology whenever colonic obstruction develops in a young woman with a history of menstrual irregularities, especially if she has had episodic symptoms of obstruction with exacerbations at the time of menstruation.

FECAL IMPACTION

Incomplete evacuation of feces over a prolonged period can result in the formation of a fecal impac-tion, a large, firm, immovable stool in the rectum that causes large bowel obstruction. Fecal impactions are most commonly seen in elderly, debilitated, or sedentary persons. They can develop in patients who have been inactive for long periods (because of myocardial infarction, traction), in narcotic addicts and patients on large doses of tranquilizers, and in children with megacolon or psychogenic problems (Fig. 52-19). The characteristic mottled density of feces within the rectum is usually diagnostic on plain abdominal radiographs (Fig. 52-20). Occasionally, large fecal masses (fecalomas) in the rectum can be confused with colonic malignancy (Fig. 52-21). For fecal impaction to be confirmed as the cause of large bowel obstruction, an enema of water-soluble contrast should be used instead of barium; hypertonic contrast will draw fluid into the bowel and can aid in breaking up the fecal mass.

INTUSSUSCEPTION

Colonic obstruction due to intussusception is much more common in infants and children than in adults (Fig. 52-22A). Almost all intussusceptions in children are ileoileal or ileocolic (Fig. 52-23; see also

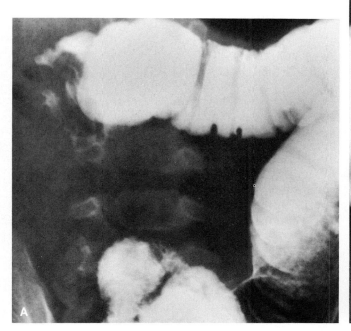
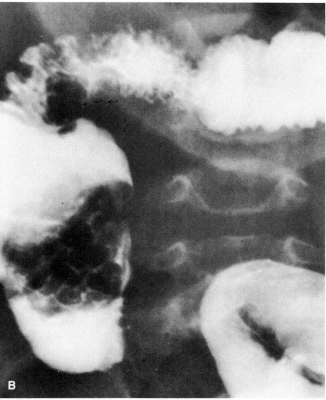

Fig. 52-23. Ileocolic intussusception in a child. **(A)** Complete obstruction in the region of the hepatic flexure. **(B)** A gentle barium enema, which has succeeded in reducing the intussusception, reveals a multilobulated mass in the region of the ileocecal valve.

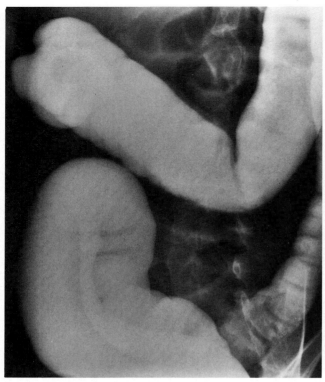

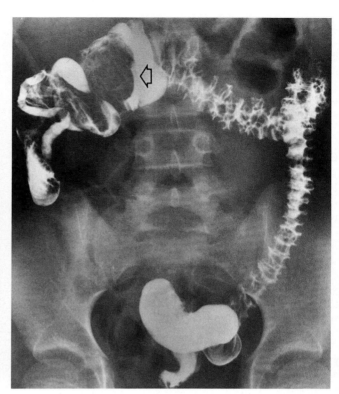

52-24   52-25

Fig. 52-24. Colocolic intussusception in an adult. Complete obstruction in the region of the hepatic flexure is due to a polypoid carcinoma.

Fig. 52-25. Ileocolic intussusception in an adult caused by intussusception of a pseudolymphomatous mass **(arrow)**.

Fig. 52-22); often, no specific cause can be demonstrated. In adults, colocolic intussusceptions are much more common, and the leading edge is frequently shown to be a mucosal or mural colonic lesion (*e.g.* carcinoma, benign polyp, inflammatory disease) (Figs. 52-24, 52-25). Reduction of an intussusception can sometimes be accomplished by barium enema examination or rectal insufflation of air, though great care must be exercised to prevent excessive intraluminal pressure and consequent colonic perforation (Figs. 52-23*B*). An indication to discontinue hydrostatic reduction and to institute surgical treatment, especially in patients under age 2, is the dissection sign (Fig. 52-26). This occurs when barium tracks between the intussusceptum and intussuscipiens, resulting in loss of hydrostatic pressure for retrograde propulsion by the barium column.

If a colonic intussusception is reduced in an adult, a repeat barium enema examination is necessary to determine whether an underlying polyp or tumor is present.

AGANGLIONOSIS (HIRSCHSPRUNG'S DISEASE)

Aganglionosis of the colon (Hirschsprung's disease) can cause massive dilatation of the large bowel and prolonged retention of fecal material within the colon. This congenital form of megacolon, which is most common in males, usually becomes evident in infancy. Clinical symptoms include constipation, abdominal distention and vomiting. The distention can be relieved initially by enemas; eventually, enemas become ineffective. Perforation of the bowel is a serious complication, especially in infants with long segment or total colonic Hirschsprung's disease. Occasional cases of congenital megacolon are first discovered in late childhood or early adulthood.

The diagnosis of Hirschsprung's disease can often be made from a plain abdominal radiograph. Fecal matter and gas within a severely dilated colon produce the typical mottled shadow of fecal impaction (Fig. 52-27). On lateral view, the rectum or rec-

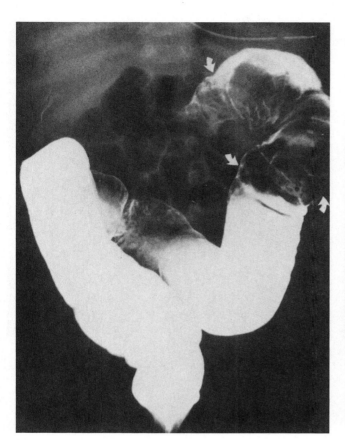

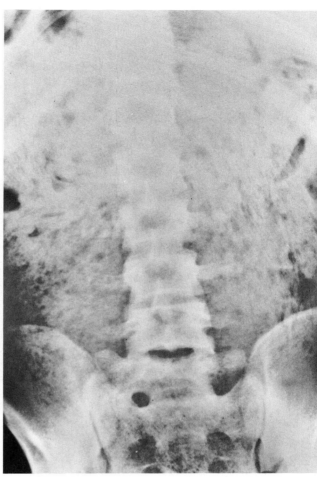

52-26   **52-27**

Fig. 52-26.   Dissection sign of nonreducible ileocolic intussusception. Barium enema in a 7-month-old boy after 18 hours of rectal bleeding, vomiting, and irritability. Despite three attempts at hydrostatic reduction, the intussusception stalled in the proximal left colon as barium outlined the dissection **(arrows)**. At surgery, the intussusception was reduced manually with difficulty. (Fishman MC, Borden S, Cooper A: The dissection sign of nonreducible ileocolic intussusception. AJR 143:5–8, 1984. Copyright 1984. Reproduced with permission)

Fig. 52-27.   Hirschsprung's disease. A plain abdominal radiograph reveals fecal matter and gas within a severely dilated colon.

tosigmoid is not distended and contains little or no gas or feces. On barium enema examination, the rectum appears to be of essentially normal caliber. At some point in the upper rectum or distal sigmoid, there is an abrupt transition to an area of grossly dilated bowel (Fig. 52-28). It is important to remember that the narrowed, relatively normal-appearing distal colon is actually the abnormal segment in which there is marked diminution or complete absence of ganglion cells in the myenteric plexuses. In contrast, the severely dilated proximal colon has a normal pattern of innervation.

Rarely, aganglionosis involves the entire colon. This condition is associated with a very high mortality rate, possibly because the frequently normal ap-

pearance of the colon on barium enema examination makes early diagnosis difficult. In total colonic aganglionosis, the small bowel can be markedly distended, far exceeding the diameter of the colon.

In the infrequent cases of adult Hirschsprung's disease, the principal radiographic findings include a cone- or funnel-shaped zone of transition with a narrowed rectum (Fig. 52-29) and a markedly dilated, feces-filled colon proximally (Fig. 52-30). A mosaic colonic pattern is caused by collapsed redundant mucosa after colon cleaning (Fig. 52-31). Complications of adult Hirschsprung's disease include severe fecal impaction leading to obstruction, hemorrhage, volvulus of the colon secondary to an elongated colonic mesentery, ischemia due to com-

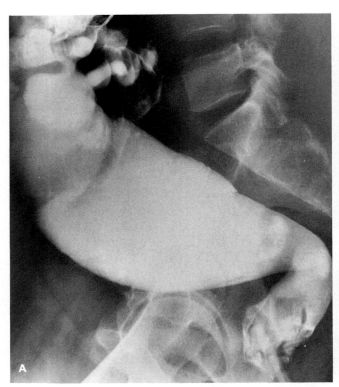 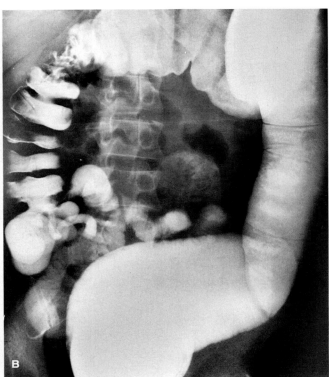

Fig. 52-28. Hirschsprung's disease in an adult. **(A)** The abrupt transition between normal caliber and massive dilatation of the bowel is evident. **(B)** A frontal view demonstrates severe dilatation of the descending and transverse portions of the colon.

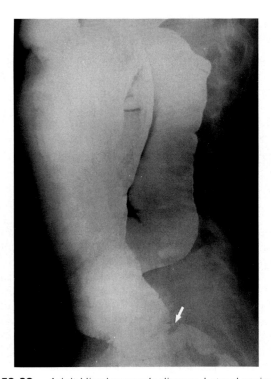

Fig. 52-29. Adult Hirschsprung's disease. Lateral projection from a barium enema examination shows the narrowed rectum with an abrupt, coned-shaped transitional zone **(arrow)**. Note the marked distention of the proximal colon. (Mindelzun RE, Hicks SM: Adult Hirschsprung's disease: Radiographic findings. Radiology 160:623–625, 1960)

promise of the vasculature by colonic distention, perforation, colonic ulceration, and decreased diaphragmatic excursion leading to pulmonary atelectasis.

IMPERFORATE ANUS

Imperforate anus refers to the blind ending of the terminal bowel with no opening or fistula to the skin surface. This is one facet of a spectrum of disorders that includes ectopic anus (hindgut opening ectopically at an abnormally high location, such as the perineum, vestibule, bladder, urethra, vagina, or cloaca), rectal atresia, and anal and rectal stenosis. Plain abdominal radiographs demonstrate a pattern of low colonic obstruction. Upside-down films (invertograms) have traditionally been the major diagnostic study in the assessment of an imperforate anus (Fig. 52-32). If the patient is in this position, gas outlines the distal rectum and thus demonstrates the level of termination of the hindgut. Separation between the end of the gas shadow and a coin placed on the skin in the region of the anal dimple has been considered pathognomic of imperforate anus. However, because the distal colon may not always be filled with gas (because films are taken too early, before gas reaches the distal colon) or because impacted meconium, normal mobility of the hindgut pouch, or distal rectal spasm may pro-

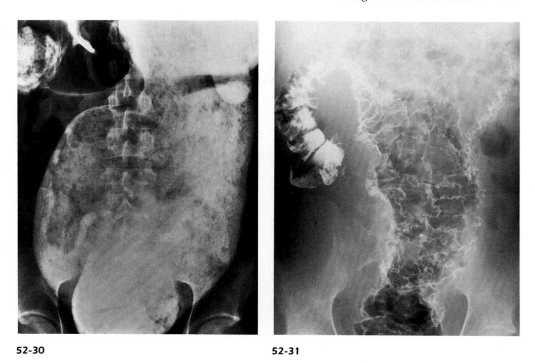

52-30   52-31

Fig. 52-30. Adult Hirschsprung's disease. Massively dilated, feces-filled colon proximal to the zone of transition.

Fig. 52-31. Adult Hirschsprung's disease. There is marked redundancy of the mucosa of the sigmoid colon, resulting in a mosaic pattern. On sigmoidoscopy, there was no evidence of mucosal inflammation. (Mindelzun RE, Hicks SM: Adult Hirschsprung's disease: Radiographic findings. Radiology 160:623–625, 1960)

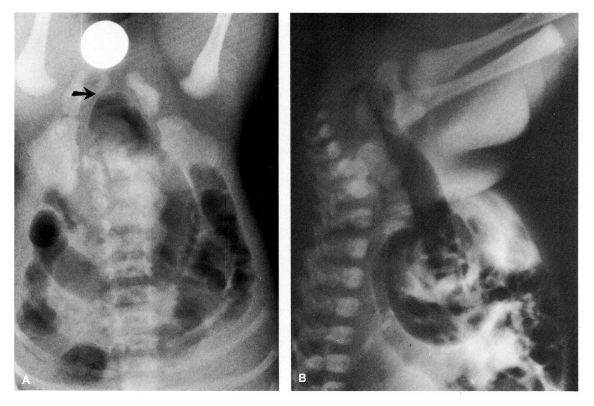

Fig. 52-32. Imperforate anus. **(A)** Frontal and **(B)** lateral views of the abdomen obtained with the infant in an upside-down position demonstrate a wide separation between the end of the gas shadow **(arrow)** and the metallic-density coin placed on the skin.

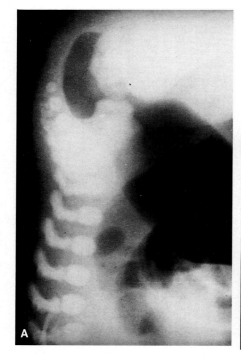

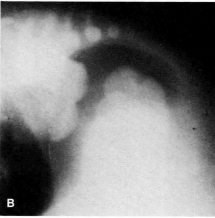

Fig. 52-33. Imperforate anus. **(A)** Invertogram shows a low anorectal anomaly. The rectal gas shadow extends distal to the ischial line. **(B)** The prone lateral view also shows the low anomaly, but the level of the gas shadow is 4 mm caudal to that shown in the invertogram. (Narasimharao KL, Prasad GR, Katariya S et al: Prone cross-table lateral view: An alternative to the invertogram in imperforate anus. AJR 140:227–229, 1983. Copyright 1983. Reproduced with permission)

duce a false appearance of the distal hindgut, results of the upside-down technique are currently viewed with some skepticism.

The prone cross-table lateral radiograph has been recommended as providing equal or sometimes better information compared to the upside-down film in a patient with suspected imperforate anus (Fig. 52-33). Easy positioning, better cooperation of the patient, elimination of the effect of gravity, and better delineation of the rectal gas shadow are advantages of the prone lateral view. Since the rectum is the highest part of the bowel in the prone position, gas may be seen more caudally than in the upside-down position, and it may be easier to distinguish supralevator from translevator lesions.

MECONIUM PLUG SYNDROME

The term meconium plug syndrome refers to local inspissation of meconium causing a low colonic obstruction during the neonatal period. Plain abdominal radiographs in infants with this condition demonstrate dilatation of the small bowel and proximal colon, mottled and bulky colonic masses, and, rarely, an intracolonic soft-tissue mass of meconium outlined by rectal gas on lateral projection. As soon as the meconium is passed, the obstructive symptoms disappear. This can occur spontaneously

or be aided by rectal examination or insertion of a thermometer. If the meconium plug is more persistent, a water-soluble enema can dislodge it, presumably because of the hypertonic nature of the contrast and its stimulation of peristalsis. It must be remembered, however, that the use of such hypertonic contrast tends to draw water into the colon and can lead to severe dehydration. Although the initial radiographic appearance can be difficult to differentiate from aganglionosis of the colon, the clinical course is usually that of a normal, healthy infant once the plug is expelled.

ADHESIONS

Postsurgical, postinflammatory, or congenital adhesions involving the ascending colon can present clinically as acute intestinal obstruction (Fig. 52-34). Such an adhesion causes only partial obstruction, resulting in cecal distention. If there is also an anomaly of mesenteric fixation and therefore a mobile cecum, the distended cecum can become folded anteriorly on the ascending colon over the adhesive band, causing an acute obstruction. This cecal bascule appears radiographically as anterior positioning of the cecum relative to the ascending colon and a folding rather than twisting of the mucosa at the site of obstruction.

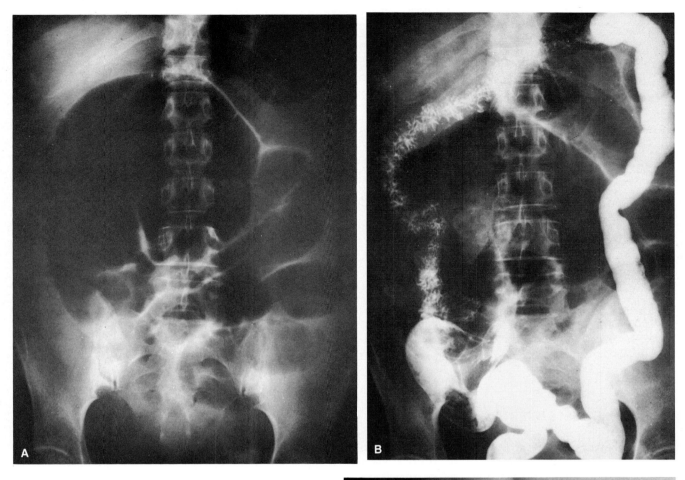

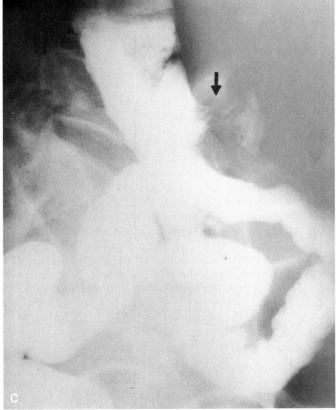

Fig. 52-34. Right colonic adhesions causing bowel obstruction. **(A)** A markedly dilated cecum occupies the midabdomen. There is small bowel dilatation. **(B)** A small amount of contrast material has entered the distended cecum. The remainder of the colon is normal in caliber. **(C)** A lateral view reveals the constricted area **(arrow)**. There is no twisting of mucosal folds. (Twersky J, Himmelfarb E: Right colonic adhesions. Radiology 120:37–40, 1976)

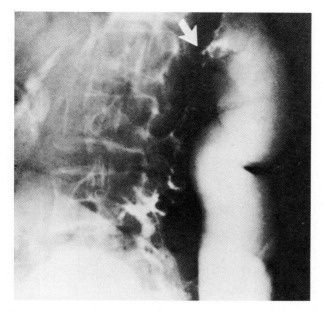

Fig. 52-35. *Retractile mesenteritis. There is almost complete obstruction at the level of the splenic flexure* **(arrow)***. (Williams RG, Nelson JA: Retractile mesenteritis: Initial presentation as colonic obstruction. Radiology 126:35–37, 1978)*

RETRACTILE MESENTERITIS

Colonic obstruction can dominate the initial clinical picture in patients with retractile mesenteritis (Fig. 52-35). Although this fibrotic process predominantly involves the mesentery of the small intestine and associated vessels, the mesocolon and colon can also be affected. Colonic obstruction in patients with retractile mesenteritis may be due to luminal obliteration or vascular compromise.

BEZOAR

Colonic bezoars can rarely cause large bowel obstruction. Primary colonic bezoars are extremely rare. Most bezoars in the colon are formed in the stomach and may cause colonic obstruction after breakup and migration of the gastric masses. Obstruction of the colon and other portions of the alimentary tract can occasionally be caused by the medication-induced bezoar (see Fig. 20-15). These iatrogenic gastrointestinal lesions have been reported in association with hygroscopic bulk laxatives, cholestyramine, nonabsorbable antacids, and vitamin C tablets, all of which should be used with caution in patients with prolonged colonic transit.

COLONIC PSEUDO-OBSTRUCTION

Colonic pseudo-obstruction is a clinical syndrome in which the patient has signs and symptoms of colonic obstruction without any obstructing lesion (see "colonic ileus" in Chapter 34).

BIBLIOGRAPHY

Agha FP: Intussusception in adults. AJR 146:527–531, 1986

Berdon WE, Baker DH: The roentgenographic diagnosis of Hirschsprung's disease in infancy. AJR 93:432–446, 1965

Bobroff LM, Messinger NH, Subbarao K et al: The cecal bascule. AJR 115:249–252, 1972

Byrk D, Soong KY: Colonic ileus and its differential diagnosis. AJR 101:329–337, 1967

Fishman MC, Borden S, Cooper A: The dissection sign of nonreducible ileocolic intussusception. AJR 143:5–8, 1984

Gu L, Alton DJ, Daneman A et al: Intussusception reduction in children by rectal insufflation of air. AJR 150:1345–1348, 1988

Hope JW, Borns PF, Berg PK: Radiologic manifestations of Hirschsprung's disease in infancy. AJR 95:217–229, 1965

Kerry RL, Lee F, Ransom HK: Roentgenologic examination in the diagnosis and treatment of colon volvulus. AJR 113:343–348, 1971

Love L: Large bowel obstruction. Semin Roentgenol 8:299–322, 1973

Mindelzun RE, Hicks SM: Adult Hirschsprung's disease: Radiographic features. Radiology 160:623–625, 1986

Narasimharao KL, Prasad GR, Katariya S et al: Prone cross-table lateral view: An alternative to the invertogram in imperforate anus. AJR 140:227–229, 1983

Pochachevsky R, Leonidas JC: Meconium plug syndrome. AJR 120:342–352, 1974

Reeder MM, Hamilton LC: Radiologic diagnosis of tropical diseases of the gastrointestinal tract. Radiol Clin North Am 7:57–81, 1969

Rosenfield NS, Ablow RC, Markowitz RK et al: Hirschsprung's disease: Accuracy of the barium enema examination. Radiology 150:393–400, 1984

Siroospour D, Berardi RS: Volvulus of the sigmoid colon: A ten-year study. Dis Colon Rectum 19:535–541, 1976

Solomon A, Stadler J, Goland L: Giant pseudopolypoidal retrograde obstruction in ulcerative colitis. Am J Gastroenterol 78:248–250, 1983

Twersky J, Himmelfarb E: Right colonic adhesions. Radiology 120:37–40, 1976

Williams RG, Nelson JA: Retractile mesenteritis: Initial presentation as colonic obstruction. Radiology 126:35–37, 1978

Wolf EL, Frager D, Beneventano TC: Volvulus of the transverse colon. Am J Gastroenterol 79:797–798, 1984

TOXIC MEGACOLON

53

Disease Entities

Ulcerative colitis
Crohn's colitis
Ischemic colitis
Amebic colitis
Bacillary dysentery
Typhoid fever
Cholera
Strongyloidiasis
Campylobacter colitis
Pseudomembranous colitis
Behçet's syndrome

Toxic megacolon is a dramatic and ominous complication of fulminant ulcerating diseases of the colon, primarily ulcerative colitis (Fig. 53-1). It is characterized by extreme dilatation of a segment of colon, or an entire diseased colon, combined with systemic toxicity (abdominal pain and tenderness, tachycardia, fever, and leukocytosis). The prominent dilatation is most commonly observed in the transverse colon, and to a lesser extent, in the sigmoid and ascending colon.

Up to 75% of episodes of toxic megacolon develop during relapses of chronic, intermittent ulcerative colitis. In many of the remaining cases, toxic megacolon constitutes the acute initial manifestation of ulcerative colitis. Toxic megacolon, however, can occur during any stage of ulcerative colitis; there is an overall incidence of up to 10% in patients with this disease. Toxic megacolon has been reported to develop in about 2% of patients with Crohn's colitis (Fig. 53-2). Infrequently, toxic megacolon complicates other ulcerating diseases of the colon, such as ischemic colitis (Fig. 53-3), Behcet's syndrome, and infectious colitis due to amebiasis (Fig. 53-4), shigellosis (bacillary dysentery), salmonellosis (typhoid fever) (Fig. 53-5), cholera, strongyloidiasis, or *Campylobacter* colitis. It is seldom seen in pseudomembranous colitis, because use of the offending antibiotic is generally terminated once the symptoms are sufficiently severe.

Surgical or autopsy specimens from patients with toxic megacolon show extensive, deep ulcerations with marked muscle destruction and serosal inflammation. No evidence of organic obstruction can be demonstrated. The wall of the colon is extremely thin and friable, predisposing to perforation.

The precise pathogenesis of toxic megacolon is not well understood, though it appears that severe inflammatory colitis is a prerequisite for its development. A major hypothesis is that widespread inflammation and destruction of colonic musculature, combined with edema and distortion of the myenteric plexus, lead to disturbed motility, loss of the colon's ability to contract, and a dilated atonic bowel. The metabolic derangements of severe colitis lead to electrolyte imbalance (especially hypokalemia), hypoalbuminemia, metabolic alkalosis, and volume alterations that may lead to severe hypotension.

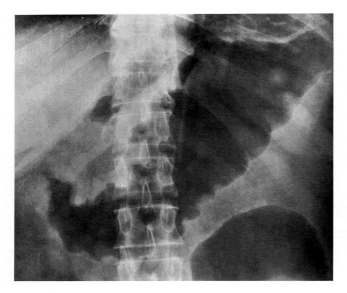

Fig. 53-1. Ulcerative colitis. There is dilatation of the transverse colon with multiple pseudopolypoid projections extending into the lumen.

Increased intraluminal pressure during barium enema examination has been implicated as a precipitating factor in the development of toxic megacolon. Thus, some authors have recommended that this procedure be deferred in acutely ill patients with documented or suspected inflammatory bowel disease. More recent reports have noted a wide variation in the amount of time (ranging from 1 to 9 days) between barium enema and the subsequent development of toxic megacolon and have concluded that the relationship may be more temporal than a cause-and-effect phenomenon. Nevertheless, because patients with signs of acute exacerbation of ulcerative colitis (abdominal pain, tenderness, fever) are particularly prone to the development of toxic megacolon following barium enema, the radiologist must evaluate carefully the plain radiographs in such patients and, if a barium enema is to be performed, filling should be largely passive under low pressure, using gravity to a much greater extent and hydrostatic pressure to a much lesser extent during the course of the examination. Over-

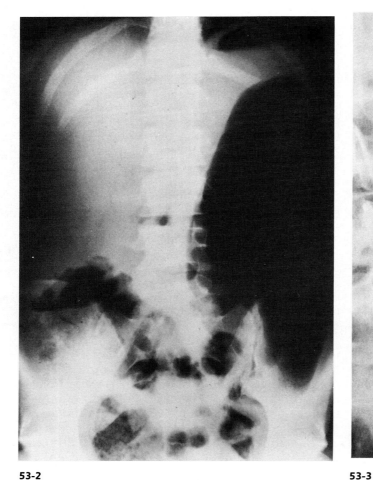

53-2

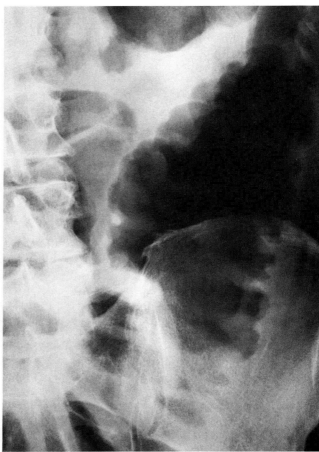

53-3

Fig. 53-2. Crohn's disease causing toxic megacolon.

Fig. 53-3. Ischemic colitis presenting as toxic megacolon.

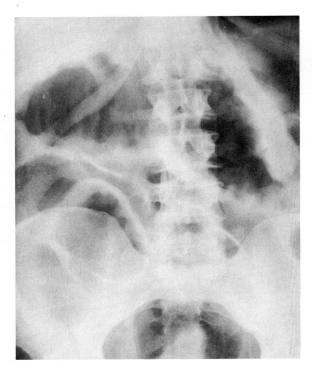

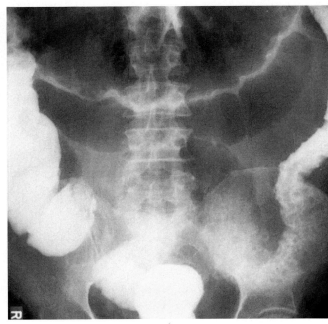

53-4   53-5

Fig. 53-4. Amebiasis causing toxic megacolon.

Fig. 53-5. Salmonellosis presenting as toxic megacolon. Note the thickened folds and ulceration involving the descending and sigmoid colon.

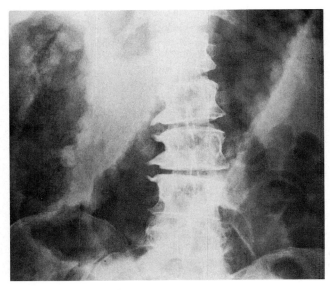

Fig. 53-6. Ulcerative colitis. Acute dilatation (7 cm) and mucosal islands are evident in the transverse colon. (Bartram CI: Radiology in the current assessment of ulcerative colitis. Gastrointest Radiol 1:383–392, 1977)

distention should be avoided in all cases where inflammatory changes are evident within the colon. The progression of both barium and air proximally can be facilitated greatly by positioning.

Other causes of increased intraluminal pressure reportedly associated with toxic megacolon include aerophagia and the use of hydrophilic agents, which produce a bulky fecal bolus that can cause relative impaction. Decreased colonic muscle tone secondary to hypokalemia or to the excessive use of opiates or anticholinergic drugs has also been related to toxic megacolon.

The abdomen is often obviously distended in patients with toxic megacolon. Tenderness varies from minimal to extreme, perhaps in relation to the degree of distention and peritoneal irritation. Bowel sounds are characteristically infrequent and less intense than normal.

RADIOGRAPHIC FINDINGS

In most patients with toxic megacolon, a simple plain film of the abdomen demonstrating marked

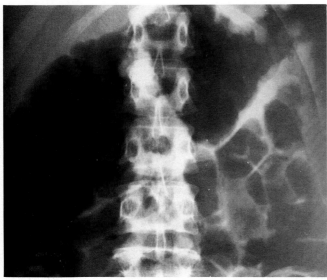 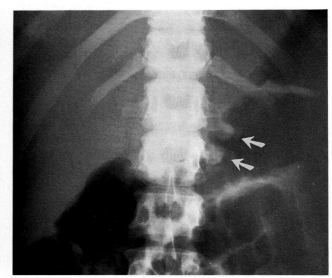

53-7   **53-8**

Fig. 53-7. Ulcerative colitis. With the patient supine, colonic gas rises to the transverse colon, the highest segment, which is the most prominently distended.

Fig. 53-8. Ulcerative colitis. Multiple nodular pseudopolypoid projections **(arrows)** extend into the lumen.

distention of the colon (>6 cm) is diagnostic (Fig. 53-6). Because patients with toxic megacolon are usually severely ill and bedridden and the radiographic examination almost invariably occurs in the supine position, the transverse colon is the portion most prominently distended (since colonic gas rises to the most anterior and thus the highest segment) (Fig. 53-7). The distal descending colon and sigmoid are less frequently dilated; distention of the rectum is uncommon. By repositioning the patient and changing the position of the air column, other colonic segments may be displayed and, if present, the typical changes of toxic megacolon may be observed elsewhere in the colon. Decubitus as well as prone and upright positioning, if possible, provides valuable information on the extent of disease in these patients in whom barium enema examination is contraindicated.

In itself, dilatation of the colon is a nonspecific radiographic finding and can be seen in any number of patients with causes ranging from distal colonic obstruction to generalized motility disorders. In terms of the radiologic diagnostic criteria for toxic megacolon, the appearance of the bowel wall is of greater significance than the presence of increased colon caliber. In involved colonic segments, the normal haustral pattern is markedly edematous or absent. Gas in the dilated segment of colon is frequently sufficient to silhouette the mucosa and often reveals multiple broad-based, nodular pseudopolypoid projections extending into the lumen (Fig. 53-8). There may also be gas-filled crevices, which probably represent deep ulcers between the nodular masses. In patients with massive colonic dilatation, it is important to distinguish between toxic megacolon and mechanical obstruction of the distal colon. In patients with toxic megacolon, decubitus views (right-side down) demonstrate gas distending the descending colon, sigmoid colon, and rectum, thereby eliminating the possibility of distal mechanical obstruction. Dissection of gas into deep ulcers occasionally produces a radiolucent line that parallels the colon, representing gas in the bowel wall.

An unusual presentation of toxic megacolon is the patient with typical clinical manifestations but whose radiographic evaluation shows little or no colonic dilatation. In this particular setting, the first consideration should be spontaneous decompression of the colon as a result of perforation, and abdominal radiographs should be evaluated carefully for free air. If there is no evidence of perforation, the demonstration of a continuous column of gas involving all or a large portion of the colon, usually

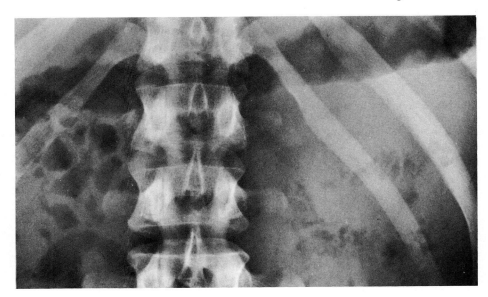

Fig. 53-9. "Toxic dilatation" without bowel distention. There is a continuous column of colonic gas with absent haustral markings and irregular contours secondary to pseudopolyp formation.

in association with absent haustral markings and irregular nodular contours secondary to pseudopolyp formation, should be considered as an indication of toxic megacolon despite the lack of classic dilatation (Fig. 53-9).

CLINICAL COURSE

The major complication of toxic megacolon is spontaneous perforation, which is reported to occur in up to 50% of cases. The event can be dramatic and sudden, and the associated shock can be irreversible. Because there is such a high danger of spontaneous perforation, barium enema examination is contraindicated during a recognized attack of toxic megacolon. Other complications of toxic megacolon include multiple walled-off perforations and pericolic abscesses, gram-negative bacteremia, acute renal tubular necrosis (from shock, sepsis, and prolonged fluid and electrolyte depletion), and cardiac arrhythmias (from hypokalemia, acid–base imbalance, and shock). Occasionally, massive colonic hemorrhage requires total colectomy.

The mortality rate from toxic megacolon is extremely high (20%–30%), although it has been somewhat reduced by early diagnosis and aggressive surgical therapy. The extent of inflammatory involvement of the colon and the presence or absence of perforation are probably the most significant risk factors. Even in patients who survive, a severe inflammatory process involving the entire thickness of the bowel permanently alters the colon so that it never returns to a normal state.

BIBLIOGRAPHY

Binder SD, Patterson JF, Glotzer DJ: Toxic megacolon in ulcerative colitis. Gastroenterology 66:909–915, 1974

Buzzard AJ, Baker WNM, Needham PRG et al: Acute toxic dilatation of the colon in Crohn's colitis. Gut 15:416–419, 1974

Caprilli R, Vernia P, Colaneri O et al: Risk factors in toxic megacolon. Dig Dis Sci 25:817–822, 1980

Diner WC, Barnhard JH: Toxic megacolon. Semin Roentgenol 8:433–436, 1973

Goldberg HI: The barium enema and toxic megacolon: Cause–effect relationship? Gastroenterology 68:617–618, 1975

Greenstein AJ, Sachar DB, Gibas A et al: Outcome of toxic dilatation in ulcerative colitis and Crohn's colitis. J Clin Gastroenterol 7:137–144, 1985

Halpert RD: Toxic dilatation of the colon. Radiol Clin North Am 25:147–155, 1987

Hill MC, Goldberg HI: Roentgen diagnosis of intestinal amebiasis. AJR 99:77–83, 1967

Hoogland T, Cooperman AM, Farmer RG et al: Toxic megacolon: Unusual complication of pseudomembranous colitis. Cleve Clin Q 44:149–155, 1977

Kalkay MN, Ayanian ZS, Lehaf EA et al: *Campylobacter*-induced toxic megacolon. Am J Gastroenterol 78:557–559, 1983

Kramer P, Wittenberg J: Colonic gas distribution in toxic megacolon. Gastroenterology 80:433–437, 1981

Scholfield PF, Mandal BK, Ironside AG: Toxic dilatation of the colon in *Salmonella* colitis and inflammatory bowel disease. Br J Surg 66:5–8, 1979

Torsoli A: Toxic megacolon. Clin Gastroenterol 10:117–121, 1981

54

THUMBPRINTING OF THE COLON

Disease Entities

Ischemic colitis
    Occlusive vascular disease
    Hemorrhage into the bowel wall (bleeding diathesis, anticoagulants)
    Traumatic intramural hematoma
Ulcerative colitis
Crohn's colitis
Infectious colitis
    Amebiasis
    Schistosomiasis
    Strongyloidiasis
    Cytomegalovirus
Pseudomembranous colitis
Malignant lesions
    Lymphoma
    Metastases
Endometriosis
Amyloidosis
Pneumatosis intestinalis
Diverticulosis/diverticulitis
Hereditary angioneurotic edema
Typhlitis
Retractile mesenteritis
Hemolytic-uremic syndrome

Thumbprinting refers to sharply defined, fingerlike marginal indentations along the contours of the colon wall. Although these well-circumscribed fill-ing defects are generally considered to be manifestations of colon ischemia or hemorrhage, thumbprinting can occur in any inflammatory or neoplastic disease that produces polypoid masses or substantial enlargement of mucosal folds.

ISCHEMIC COLITIS

In patients with occlusive vascular disease or a hypercoagulability state, thumbprinting can be the result of ischemia. After vascular occlusion, the endothelial cells in the damaged distal capillary bed no longer adhere to one another properly. Collateral blood flowing into the area can thus pass between the endothelial cells into the interstitial portion of the bowel, where it produces an intramural hematoma. An identical radiographic pattern can be caused by direct hemorrhage into the bowel (due to a bleeding diathesis or an anticoagulant overdose) or post-traumatic hematoma.

Plain abdominal radiographs demonstrate thumbprinting in about 20% of patients with ischemic colitis (Fig. 54-1). In an elderly person presenting with abdominal pain and rectal bleeding, the detection of multiple smooth soft-tissue densities protruding into the lumen of the bowel permits a provisional diagnosis of ischemic colitis (Fig. 54-2). On barium studies, these rounded masses indent the contrast column (Fig. 54-3); when seen *en face,* they simulate polypoid filling defects. Obliteration of thumbprinting has been noted during the double-contrast barium enema examination when the

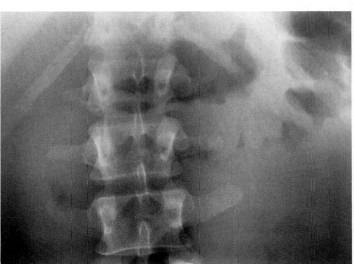

54-1

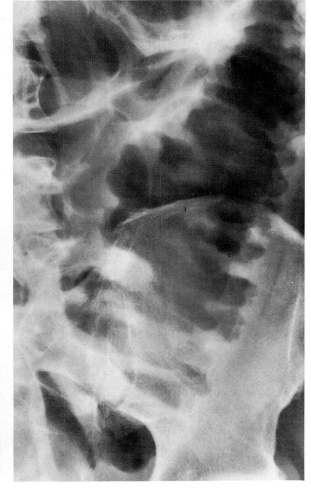

54-2

Fig. 54-1. Ischemic colitis. A plain abdominal radiograph demonstrates well-circumscribed filling defects along the wall of the transverse colon.

Fig. 54-2. Ischemic colitis. Soft-tissue polypoid densities protrude into the lumen of the descending colon in a patient with acute abdominal pain and rectal bleeding.

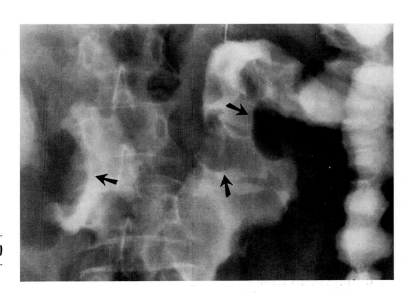

Fig. 54-3. Ischemic colitis. A barium enema examination demonstrates multiple filling defects **(arrows)** indenting the margins of the transverse and descending portions of the colon.

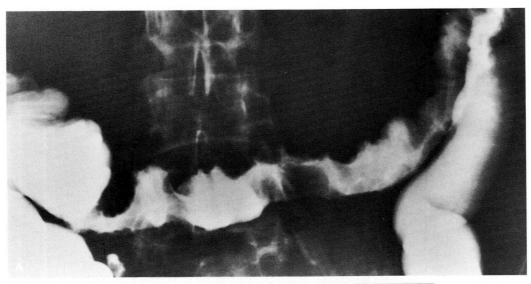

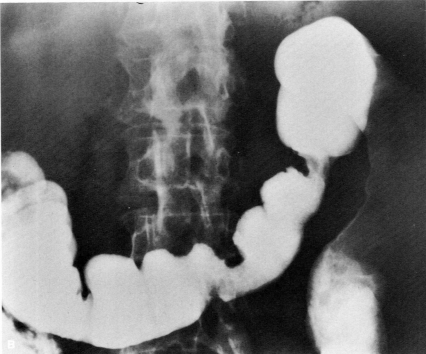

Fig. 54-4. Reversibility of ischemic colitis. **(A)** Thumbprinting involves the transverse colon during an acute ischemic attack. **(B)** One week later, the ischemic changes have reversed, and the patient has clinically recovered.

colon is fully distended by air insufflation. Therefore, thumbprinting is usually most apparent on postevacuation films, when the reduced intraluminal pressure is less likely to efface the soft mural masses. Localized or diffuse ulcerations superimposed on ischemia-induced thumbprinting can mimic an inflammatory colitis. Although the thumbprinting in ischemic colitis tends to be more smoothly defined and symmetric, it can sometimes be distinguished from an inflammatory colitis only by the mode of presentation and the clinical course.

Thumbprinting due to colonic ischemia usually reverts to a normal radiographic appearance if good collateral circulation is established (Fig. 54-4). Ischemic colitis can heal by stricture formation; if blood flow is insufficient, acute bowel necrosis and perforation may result.

The prompt recognition of ischemia as the probable causative factor of thumbprinting can permit expectant watching rather than operative treatment. However, if ischemia is extensive and signs of irreversible bowel necrosis develop (unre-

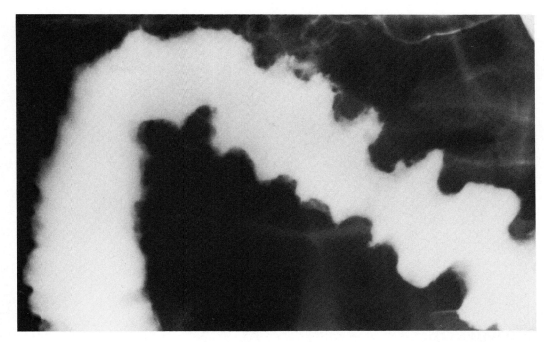

Fig. 54-5. Ulcerative colitis. Multiple filling defects indent the barium-filled transverse colon.

lenting abdominal pain, rapidly rising polymor-phonuclear leukocytosis, shock) in response to sup-portive measures, surgery may become necessary to avoid a fatal outcome.

It must be remembered that ischemic colitis can develop proximal to a colonic carcinoma. Al-though the mechanism is unclear, malignant ob-struction of the colon appears to interfere with the transmural blood supply to the bowel proximal to the lesion. It is therefore essential that the possibil-ity of malignancy be excluded once the acute isch-emic episode has subsided.

ULCERATIVE AND CROHN'S COLITIS

The intense mucosal inflammation and edema in patients with ulcerative (Fig. 54-5) and Crohn's co-litis (Fig. 54-6) can produce multiple symmetric contour defects closely resembling the characteris-tic thumbprinting of ischemic disease. Ulcerative colitis usually involves the rectum, unlike ischemic colitis, in which rectal involvement is infrequent. Demonstration of transverse linear ulcerations, skip areas, and concomitant disease of the small bowel favors the diagnosis of Crohn's colitis.

INFECTIOUS COLITIS

Thumbprinting is an unusual manifestation of acute amebiasis (Fig. 54-7). In this disease, the pattern is

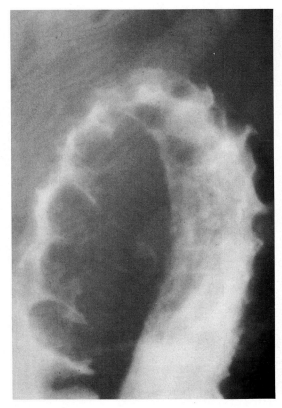

Fig. 54-6. Crohn's colitis. Postevacuation view of the splenic flexure shows a thumbprinting pattern related to in-tense inflammatory edema. (Lichtenstein JE: Radiologic-pathologic correlation of inflammatory bowel disease. Radiol Clin North Am 25:3–24, 1987)

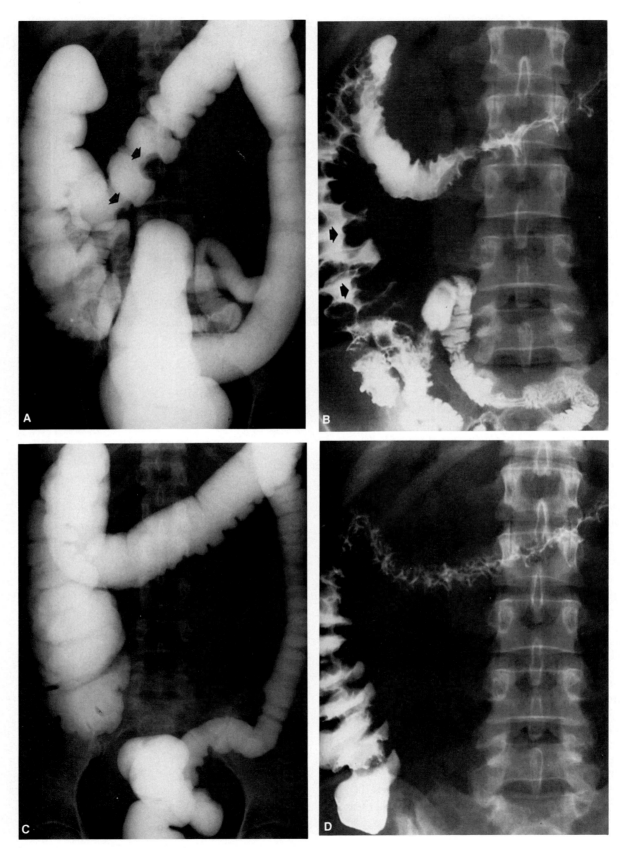

Fig. 54-7.   Amebic colitis. **(A)** Filled and **(B)** postevacuation films demonstrate marginal filling defects **(arrows)** and overlying mucosal abnormalities. Post-treatment **(C)** filled and **(D)** post-evacuation films illustrate return of the colon to normal. (Hardy R, Scullin DR: Thumbprinting in a case of amebiasis. Radiology 98:147–148, 1971)

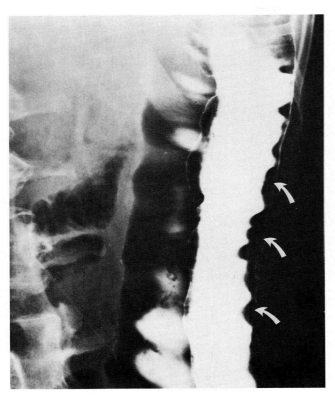

Fig. 54-8. Cytomegalovirus. Thumbprinting in the descending colon **(arrows)**. (Frager DH, Frager JD, Wolf EL et al: Cytomegalovirus colitis in acquired immune deficiency syndrome: Radiologic spectrum. Gastrointest Radiol 11:241–246, 1986)

caused by extensive necrosis and segmental thickening of the bowel wall due to submucosal and mucosal edema. Thumbprinting can be segmental or generalized but is most frequently seen in the transverse colon. Although the appearance can be similar to that of ischemic colitis, deep ulcerations and a long segment of bowel involvement favors amebiasis or another inflammatory etiology. A similar pattern has been reported in a patient infested by schistosomiasis and strongyloidiasis and in renal transplant patients on immunosuppressive therapy or patients with AIDS infected with cytomegalovirus (Fig. 54-8).

PSEUDOMEMBRANOUS COLITIS

A radiographic pattern similar to thumbprinting is a manifestation of pseudomembranous colitis (Fig. 54-9). Although most prominent in the transverse colon, the "thumbprinting" in pseudomembranous colitis is usually generalized rather than segmental, as it is in ischemic disease. In contrast to ischemic colitis, in which thumbprinting reflects submucosal

collections of blood or edema fluid, the radiographic pattern in pseudomembranous colitis is due to marked thickening of the bowel wall, which can be so severe that the lumen of the colon is nearly obliterated by the touching surfaces of the haustra on opposite walls of the colon. Wide transverse bands of thickened colonic wall are usually seen. Unlike ischemic colitis, pseudomembranous colitis generally develops after a course of antibiotic therapy and is rarely associated with significant rectal bleeding.

MALIGNANT LESIONS

Localized primary lymphoma of the colon can cause a submucosal cellular infiltrate that produces the radiographic pattern of thumbprinting (Fig. 54-10). A similar appearance can be secondary to hematogenous metastases. In these conditions, the thumbprinting is usually not as symmetric or regular as in ischemic colitis. The clinical onset of colonic lymphoma and metastases to the colon is insidious, unlike the presentation of ischemic colitis, which is acute. In addition, the reversibility of thumbprinting, which is frequently demonstrated in patients with ischemic colitis, does not occur with malignant disease.

OTHER CAUSES

Nonmalignant infiltrative processes can produce a radiographic appearance of thumbprinting that simulates ischemic disease. In women of child-bearing age, the detection of multiple intramural defects suggests endometriosis. Deposition of amyloid in the submucosal layer can present a similar pattern. Pneumatosis intestinalis can be diagnosed as the cause of thumbprinting by the demonstration that the polypoid masses indenting the barium column are composed of air rather than soft-tissue density (Fig. 54-11).

The extensive muscle hypertrophy of the bowel wall that accompanies diverticulosis can cause accentuation of haustral markings and shortening of the colon. This produces an accordionlike effect that can simulate the radiographic pattern of thumbprinting. Although the muscular thickening and spasm in diverticulosis can in some cases be more striking than the actual presence of diverticula, it is generally easy to distinguish this appearance from true thumbprinting due to intramural hemorrhage or an infiltrative process. Walled-off abscesses secondary to diverticulitis can also produce discrete masses that indent the barium column and mimic thumbprinting.

Patients with hereditary angioneurotic edema may demonstrate thumbprinting on barium enema examinations performed during acute attacks (Fig.

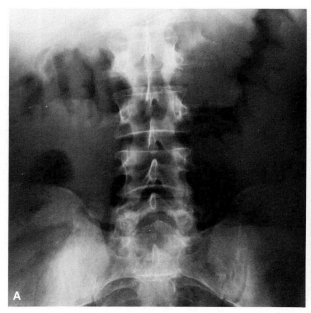

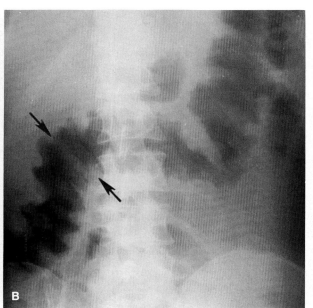

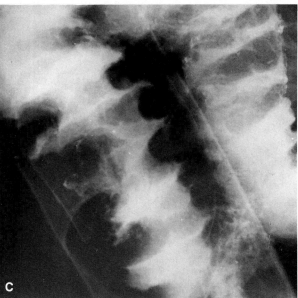

Fig. 54-9. Pseudomembranous colitis. **(A)** Polypoid projections into the lumen of the transverse colon simulating the thumbprinting seen in ischemic disease. **(B)** Wide transverse bands of thickened colonic wall **(arrows)**. **(C)** Film from a barium enema demonstrates wide transverse bands of mural thickening identical to the zones of mural thickening visible on plain abdominal radiographs. (Stanley RJ, Nelson GL, Tedesco FJ et al: Plain-film findings in severe pseudomembranous colitis. Radiology 118:7–11, 1976)

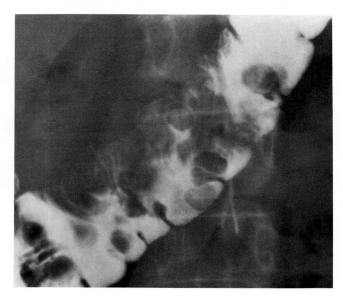

Fig. 54-10. Lymphoma. Submucosal cellular infiltrate produces the radiographic pattern of thumbprinting.

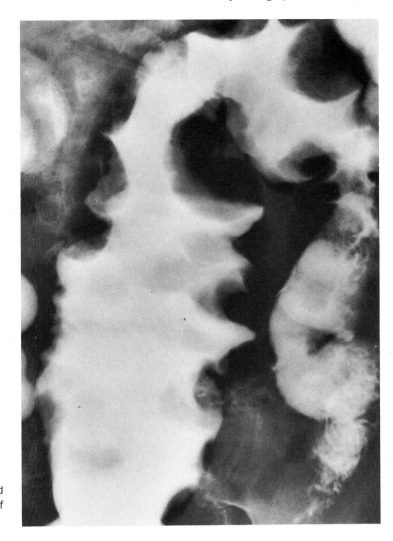

Fig. 54-11. Pneumatosis intestinalis. The polypoid masses indenting the barium column are composed of air rather than soft-tissue density.

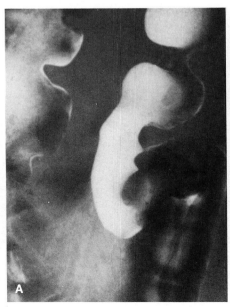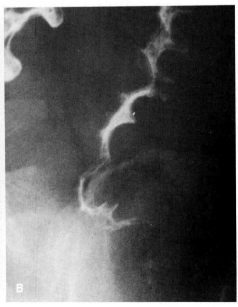

Fig. 54-12. Hereditary angioneurotic edema. Persistent, localized thumbprinting is demonstrated in the descending colon. The remainder of the colon appears within normal limits. (Pearson KD, Buchignani JS, Shimkin PM et al: Hereditary angioneurotic edema of the gastrointestinal tract. AJR 116:256–261, 1972. Copyright 1972. Reproduced with permission)

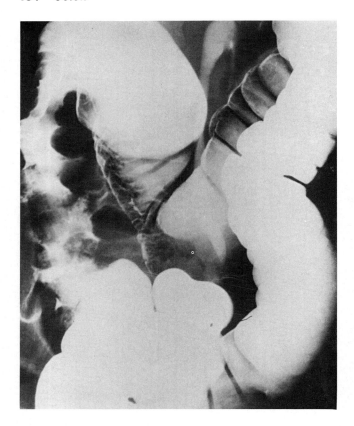

Fig. 54-13. Typhlitis. Thumbprinting with irregular mucosal folds in the right colon. (Abramson SJ, Berdon WE, Baker DH: Childhood typhlitis: Its increasing association with acute myelogenous leukemia. Radiology 146:61–64, 1983)

54-12). The radiographic appearance of the colon rapidly reverts to normal once the acute episode subsides.

Thumbprinting due to submucosal edema or hemorrhage that primarily involves the cecum and right colon may develop in patients with typhlitis (Fig. 54-13), a necrotizing inflammatory process that most commonly develops in leukemic children on chemotherapy in the terminal stages of the disease.

In the rare cases of retractile mesenteritis involving the sigmoid colon, an appearance of thumbprinting may be produced by edema and desmoplastic reaction and highlighted by associated lymphatic and vascular congestion (Fig. 54-14).

Ischemic enterocolitis with thumbprinting and ulceration typically occurs 3 to 16 days before the renal manifestations of the hemolytic-uremic syndrome, the most common cause of acute renal failure in infants and children (Fig. 54-15). The intestinal prodrome of this entity is caused by fibrin thrombi in the colonic microvasculature similar to those that occur in the kidneys. Symptoms and signs may include cramping abdominal pain and tenderness, vomiting, diarrhea with or without blood, low-grade fever, and leukocytosis. The usually self-limited and reversible ischemic lesion may occasionally progress to toxic megacolon, bowel necrosis, or perforation. When the intestinal prodrome precedes the development of characteristic laboratory findings or oliguria, the diagnosis of the hemolytic-uremic syndrome may be delayed. Find-

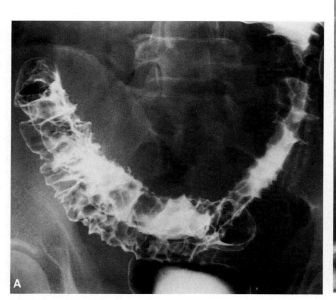
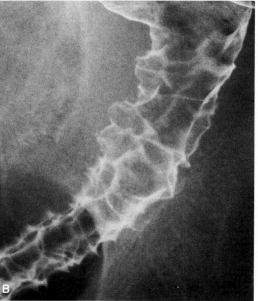

Fig. 54-14. Retractile mesenteritis. **(A)** Extensive edema of the submucosa produces a thumbprinting pattern. **(B)** In this coned view, note the sharp demarcation of diseased from normal bowel. (Thompson GT, Fitzgerald EF, Somers SS: Retractile mesenteritis of the sigmoid colon. Br J Radiol 58:266–267, 1985)

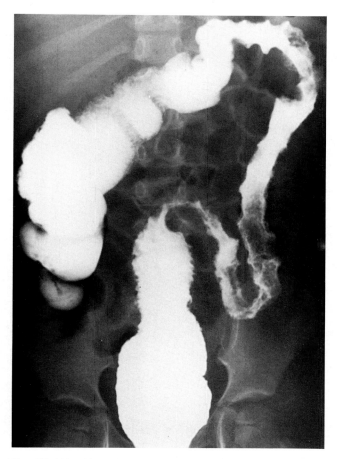

Fig. 54-15. Hemolytic-uremic syndrome. In addition to thumbprinting (best seen in the splenic flexure), there is spasticity of the colon with effacement of normal haustral markings, serrations, spiculations, and mucosal irregularity in the distal half of the colon. (Kawanami T, Bowen A, Girdany BR: Enterocolitis: Prodrome of the hemolytic-uremic syndrome. Radiology 151:91–92, 1984)

ings of thumbprinting on plain radiographs or on barium enema examination permit the radiologist to suggest the hemolytic-uremic syndrome as a possible cause before renal or hematologic abnormali-

ties become manifest. This is important because prompt diagnosis and supportive treatment, including transfusion and dialysis, have reduced mortality from 50% to 15% or less in this condition.

BIBLIOGRAPHY

Abramson SJ, Berdon WE, Baker DH: Childhood typhlitis: Its increasing association with acute myelogenous leukemia. Radiology 146:61–64, 1983

Bartram CI: Obliteration of thumbprinting with double-contrast enemas in acute ischemic colitis. Gastrointest Radiol 4:85–88, 1979

Cardoso JM, Kimura K, Stoopen M et al: Radiology of invasive amebiasis of the colon. AJR 128:935–941, 1977

Cho SR, Tisnado J, Liu CI: Bleeding cytomegalovirus ulcers of the colon: Barium enema and angiography. AJR 136:1213–1215, 1981

Gardiner R, Stevenson GW: The colitides. Radiol Clin North Am 20:797–816, 1982

Hardy R, Scullin DR: Thumbprinting in a case of amebiasis. Radiology 98:147–148, 1971

Hyson EA, Burrell M, Toffler R: Drug-induced gastrointestinal disease. Gastrointest Radiol 2:183–212, 1977

Kawanami T, Bowen AD, Girdany BR: Enterocolitis: Prodrome of the hemolytic-uremic syndrome. Radiology 151:91–92, 1984

Lichtenstein JE: Radiologic-pathologic correlation of inflammatory bowel disease. Radiol Clin North Am 25:3–24, 1987

Loughran CF, Tappin JA, Whitehouse GH: The plain abdominal radiograph in pseudomembranous colitis due to *Clostridium difficile*. Clin Radiol 33:277–281, 1982

Pearson KD, Buchignani JS, Shimkin PM et al: Hereditary angioneurotic edema of the gastrointestinal tract. AJR 116:256–261, 1972

Schwartz S, Boley S, Lash J et al: Roentgenologic aspects of reversible vascular occlusion of the colon and its relationship to ulcerative colitis. Radiology 80:625–635, 1963

Stanley RJ, Melson GL, Tedesco FJ et al: Plain-film findings in severe pseudomembranous colitis. Radiology 118:7–11, 1976

Thompson GT, Fitzgerald EF, Somers SS: Retractile mesenteritis of the sigmoid colon. Br J Radiol 58:266–267, 1985

Williams LF, Bosniak MA, Wittenberg J et al: Ischemic colitis. Am J Surg 117:254–264, 1969

55

DOUBLE TRACKING IN THE SIGMOID COLON

Double tracking is the presence of longitudinal extraluminal tracts of barium paralleling the lumen of the sigmoid colon.

Disease Entities

Diverticulitis
Crohn's colitis
Carcinoma of the colon

In diverticulitis, double tracking reflects focal mucosal perforation of the extramural portion of a diverticulum producing a dissecting sinus tract that extends through paracolonic tissues along the axis of the bowel (Fig. 55-1). Multiple communications to the bowel lumen by way of additional perforated diverticula are often seen (Fig. 55-2). Although these may represent independent, coincidental diverticular perforations, the fistulous communications at multiple sites are probably due to a paracolic abscess arising from a single diverticulum that then dissects longitudinally and serially involves adjacent diverticula (Fig. 55-3).

Extraluminal longitudinal sinus tracts of 10 cm or more in length have been considered pathognomonic of Crohn's disease of the colon (Fig. 55-4), in contrast to the shorter tracts (3–6 cm) seen in patients with diverticulitis. However, several examples of double tracking of longer than 10 cm have been reported with diverticulitis.

Differentiation between diverticulitis and Crohn's disease can be difficult. Not only can the two conditions coexist, but diverticulitis can be a complication of Crohn's colitis (Fig. 55-5). The characteristic deep fissuring of Crohn's disease can communicate with one or several diverticula, leading to peridiverticulitis or abscess formation. The resulting abscess can then penetrate through the domes of adjacent diverticula, thereby extending the extraluminal longitudinal sinus tract.

Clinically, both diverticulitis and Crohn's disease can present with pain, partial obstruction, a lower abdominal mass, rectal bleeding, fever, and leukocytosis. Radiographically, they can be indistinguishable. However, the demonstration of ulceration, edematous and distorted folds, and other sites of colon involvement should suggest the diagnosis of Crohn's disease.

The radiographic pattern of double tracking can also be demonstrated in patients with primary carcinoma of the sigmoid colon (Fig. 55-6). Transmural ulceration can lead to perforation with abscess formation in the pericolic fat (Fig. 55-7). A superimposed inflammatory reaction simulating diverticulitis (thickened mucosal folds, colonic muscle spasm) can be seen. Although the sinus tracts in carcinoma have been reported to be wider and more irregular in caliber than those in diverticulitis, it can be extremely difficult to distinguish these two entities by their radiographic appearances alone. Regardless of whether diverticula are visible, the demonstration of double tracking in the sigmoid colon without clear radiographic evidence of inflammatory bowel disease may require surgical intervention to exclude the possibility of primary colon carcinoma and allow a definitive diagnosis to be made.

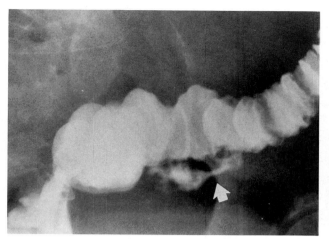

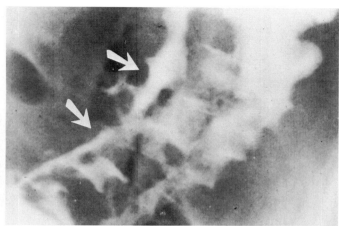

55-1   **55-2**

Fig. 55-1. Dissecting peridiverticulitis. There is a short extraluminal track **(arrow)** along the antimesocolic border of the sigmoid colon. Note the apparent absence of other demonstrable diverticula.

Fig. 55-2. Dissecting peridiverticulitis. The extraluminal tract **(arrows)** extends along the mesocolic border of the sigmoid colon.

Fig. 55-3. Dissecting peridiverticulitis. There is diffuse sigmoid involvement with extraluminal tracks extending along both the mesocolic **(upper arrows)** and antimesocolic **(lower arrow)** borders.

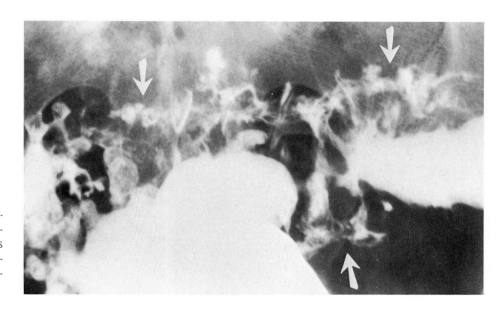

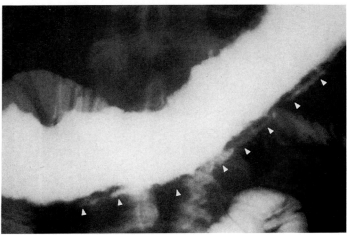

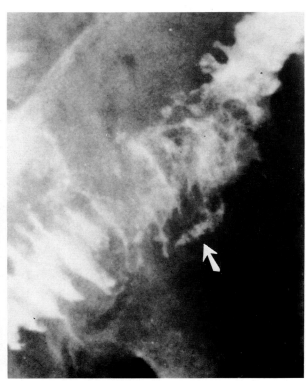

55-4

55-5

Fig. 55-4. Crohn's colitis. Long intramural fistula **(arrows)** in the transverse colon. (Lichtenstein JE: Radiologic-pathologic correlation of inflammatory bowel disease. Radiol Clin North Am 25:3–23, 1987)

Fig. 55-5. Crohn's colitis grafted on diverticulosis. A short (1.5-cm) track of barium **(arrow)** is visible along the antimesocolic border of the sigmoid. The mucosal fold pattern appears granular and ulcerated, and multiple diverticula are apparent. (Ferrucci JT, Ragsdale BD, Barrett PJ et al: Double tracking in the sigmoid colon. Radiology 120:307–312, 1976)

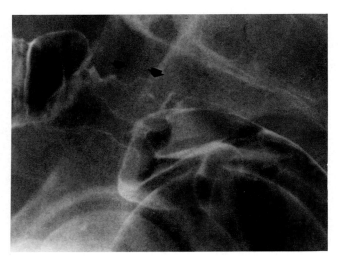

Fig. 55-6. Primary carcinoma of the rectosigmoid associated with the radiographic appearance of double tracking **(arrows)**.

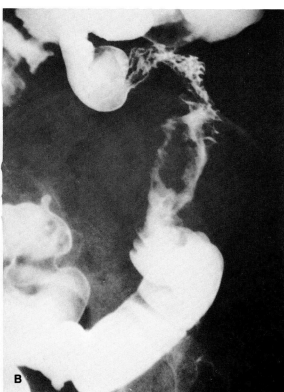

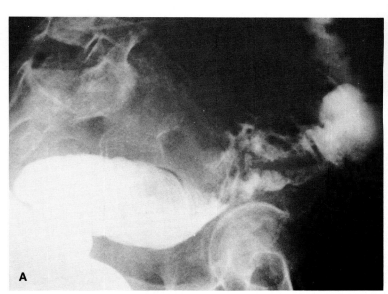

Fig. 55-7. Primary carcinomas of **(A)** the sigmoid and **(B)** the distal descending colon producing a double-track appearance due to transmural perforation. (Ferrucci JT, Ragsdale BD, Barrett PJ et al: Double tracking in the sigmoid colon. Radiology 120:307–312, 1976)

BIBLIOGRAPHY

Berman LG, Burdick D, Heitzman ER et al: A critical reappraisal of sigmoid peridiverticulitis. Surg Gynecol Obstet 127:481–491, 1968

Ferrucci JT, Ragsdale BD, Barrett PJ et al: Double tracking in the colon. Radiology 120:307–312, 1976

Fleischner FG, Ming SC: Revised concepts on diverticular disease of the colon. Radiology 84:599–609, 1965

Greenall MJ, Levine AW, Nolan DJ: Complications of diverticular disease: A review of the barium enema findings. Gastrointest Radiol 8:353–358, 1983

Loeb PM, Berk RN, Saltzstein SL: Longitudinal fistula of the colon in diverticulitis. Gastroenterology 67:720–724, 1974

Marshak RH: Granulomatous disease of the intestinal tract. Radiology 114:3–22, 1975

Marshak RH, Janowitz HD, Present DH: Granulomatous colitis in association with diverticula. N Engl J Med 283:1080–1084, 1970

Marshak RH, Lindner AE, Pochaczevsky R et al: Longitudinal sinus tracts in granulomatous colitis and diverticulitis. Semin Roentgenol 11:101–110, 1976

Meyers MA, Alonso DR, Morson BC et al: Pathogenesis of diverticulitis complicating granulomatous colitis. Gastroenterology 74:24–31, 1978

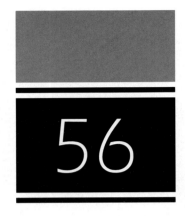

56

ENLARGEMENT OF THE RETRORECTAL SPACE

Disease Entities

Normal variant
Inflammatory conditions
  Ulcerative colitis
  Crohn's disease
  Infectious proctitis
    Tuberculosis
    Amebiasis
    Lymphogranuloma venereum
  Radiation proctitis
  Ischemic colitis
  Presacral abscess
  Diverticulitis
  Perforated appendix
  Idiopathic proctosigmoiditis
Tumors
  Developmental cysts
    Dermoid cyst
    Duplication cyst
    Postanal (tail gut) cyst
  Lipoma and hemangioendothelioma
  Primary rectal tumors
    Adenocarcinoma
    Lymphoma
    Sarcoma
    Cloacogenic carcinoma
  Secondary rectal tumors (contiguous spread)
    Prostate
    Bladder

    Ovary
    Uterus
  Neurogenic tumors
    Chordoma
    Neurofibroma
    Schwannoma
  Primary sacral tumors
    Osteogenic sarcoma
    Chondrosarcoma
    Giant cell tumor
  Metastases to the sacrum
  Teratoma
  Anterior sacral meningocele
  Multiple myeloma and solitary plasmacytoma
Miscellaneous lesions
Inguinal hernias containing segments of colon
  Amyloidosis
  Pelvic lipomatosis
  Cushing's disease
  Inferior vena cava obstruction
  Postsurgical lesions (partial sigmoid
    resection)
  Fracture of the sacrum
  Colitis cystica profunda

The retrorectal area is a potential space bounded in front by the posterior wall of the rectum and behind by the ventral surface of the sacrum. It lies between

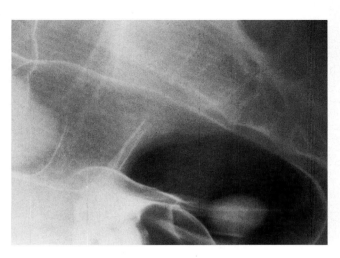

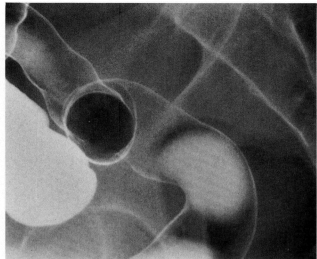

56-1

56-2

Fig. 56-1. Normal retrorectal space.

Fig. 56-2. "Enlarged" retrorectal space, measuring 2 cm, representing a normal variant. The patient had no abnormality by clinical history, digital rectal examination, or proctoscopy.

two fascial layers, the fascia of Waldeyer, which covers the anterior sacral surface, and the fascia propria, which covers the posterior rectum. The lower margin of the retrorectal space is formed by the pelvic floor, which is composed mainly of the levator ani and coccygeus muscles. The upper margin of the space is limited by the peritoneal reflection at the rectosigmoid junction, at the level of the third sacral segment.

The rectum is fixed as it forms the anterior border of the retrorectal space. Only at the rectosigmoid junction is there some mobility of the bowel, the degree of which depends on the extent of the pelvic mesocolon. Closely related to the retrorectal space are the presacral lymph nodes and the superior rectal vessels that lie within the fascia propria of the rectum. Fat and areolar tissues are also included in the retrorectal space.

The retrorectal space is normally very small, because the barium-filled rectum balloons out to closely parallel the hollow of the sacrum (Fig. 56-1). Measurement of the retrorectal space is based on the shortest distance between the posterior rectal wall and the anterior sacral surface at the third to the fifth sacral segments. Measurements at the S5 level are considered more accurate than those at the S3 level, since there is less of a chance at the lower level that the rectum will be displaced from the midline, thereby giving the false impression of an enlarged retrorectal space. Care should be taken to measure the retrorectal space when the rectum is well filled, since an underfilled normal rectum appears to fall away from the sacral concavity and may falsely seem to widen the space.

NORMAL VARIANT

In about 95% of normal patients, the retrorectal space measures 0.5 cm or less. In the past, measurements greater than 1 cm or 1.5 cm were considered to be probably abnormal; measurements greater than 2 cm were deemed definitely abnormal. However, a recent study demonstrated that 38% of patients with an "enlarged" retrorectal space (≥1.5 cm) had no abnormality by clinical history, digital rectal examination, or proctoscopy and therefore represented normal variants (Fig. 56-2). Although the majority of these patients were large or obese, more than one-quarter were normal-sized individuals. Therefore, it appears that increased width of the retrorectal space *per se* is not necessarily an abnormal finding. True pathologic widening of the retrorectal space is usually associated with changes in the contour of the rectum, abnormalities of the sacrum, or other alterations of the presacral soft tissues.

INFLAMMATORY DISEASES OF THE BOWEL

Inflammatory diseases of the bowel, especially ulcerative colitis, are the most common causes of pathologic enlargement of the retrorectal space. Generalized widening of the space without evidence of a focal mass is common in patients with ulcerative colitis, presumably because of a combination of thickening of the bowel wall, inflammatory edema

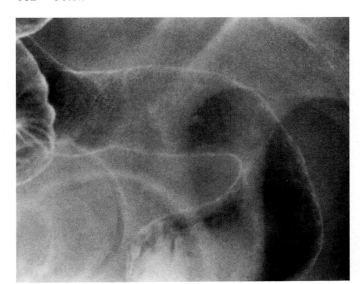

Fig. 56-3. Ulcerative colitis. Granularity of the rectal mucosa is associated with widening of the retrorectal space.

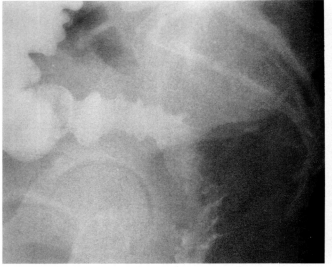

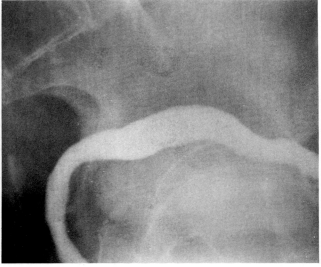

56-4   56-5

Fig. 56-4.   Acute ulcerative colitis. Widening of the retrorectal space with diffuse ulceration and mucosal thickening that primarily involve the posterior wall of the rectum.

Fig. 56-5.   Crohn's disease. Severe fibrotic narrowing of the rectosigmoid causes widening of the retrorectal space.

of the presacral soft tissues, and rigidity of the bowel, which together prevent the rectum from distending and filling the sacral concavity (Fig. 56-3). In chronic ulcerative colitis, shortening of the colon and rectum tends to draw the rectum away from the sacrum and enlarge the retrorectal space. Radiographically, irregularity and ulceration of the posterior wall of the rectum reflect acute or chronic inflammatory changes (Fig. 56-4).

Widening of the retrorectal space is more prevalent in elderly than in young patients and in persons with severe, chronic, and extensive colitis. The precise size of the retrorectal area is not of diagnostic significance, though an increasing width indicates progression of the disease. Once enlargement of the retrorectal space has occurred in a patient with ulcerative colitis, the space either remains unchanged or enlarges further during the course of the

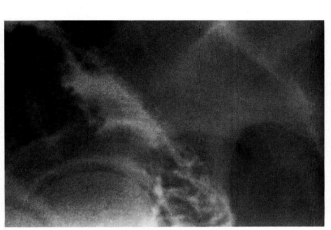

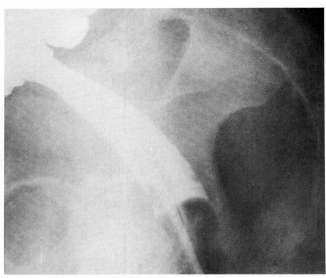

56-6

56-7

Fig. 56-6. Amebiasis. A widened retrorectal space is associated with diffuse ulceration and mucosal edema.

Fig. 56-7. Lymphogranuloma venereum. There is characteristic smooth narrowing of the rectum with widening of the retrorectal space.

disease. The retrorectal space does not become smaller even during remission, probably because of permanent damage of the bowel wall beneath the mucosa.

Crohn's disease involving the rectum can diffusely widen the retrorectal space because of fatty deposition, fibrosis, edema, and lymph node enlargement (Fig. 56-5). At times, widening of the retrorectal space is seen in Crohn's disease even without direct rectal involvement. In contrast to that in ulcerative colitis, this widening may decrease during remission. The demonstration of rectal fistulas or sinus tracts should suggest the possibility of Crohn's disease as a cause of widening of the retrorectal space. Perirectal abscesses can produce focal presacral masses and, on rare occasions, even cause osteomyelitis of the sacrum.

Inflammatory widening of the retrorectal space can be caused by proctitis due to infections (tuberculosis, amebiasis [Fig. 56-6], lymphogranuloma venereum [Fig. 56-7], cytomegalovirus in AIDS [Fig. 56-8]), radiation (Fig. 56-9), or ischemia. Retrorectal abscesses causing widening of the retrorectal space can be secondary to infected developmental cysts. Such a lesion can present with a draining sinus opening onto the perianal skin between the anus and coccyx or as a communication by way of a fistulous tract between the cyst and the anus, rectum or, very rarely, the vagina. Injection of contrast material into the sinus tract can outline a cystic cavity lying anterior to the coccyx or demonstrate a fistulous connection between the cyst and the rectum or anus. Other causes of retrorectal abscess producing widening of the retrorectal space include diverticulitis (Fig. 56-10), perforated appendix, and perforation due to carcinoma.

BENIGN RETRORECTAL TUMORS

Benign retrorectal tumors that widen the retrorectal space are frequently asymptomatic and are discovered incidentally during routine physical examination or childbirth. In some patients, enlargement of the tumor causes pressure symptoms, such as a feeling of fullness in the pelvis, constipation, and difficulty in urinating. Low back pain is common, and pressure on nerves can lead to pain and numbness in the perineum and legs, as well as to fecal and urinary incontinence.

The most common benign tumors of the retrorectal space are developmental cysts. Most of these are dermoid cysts that are lined by stratified squamous epithelium and contain dermal appendages (hair follicles, sebaceous glands, sweat glands). Less common congenital developmental cysts are enteric cysts (duplications) or postanal (tail gut) cysts. Enteric cysts are lined by squamous or glandular epithelium of the intestinal type; they contain one or

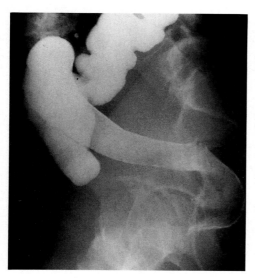

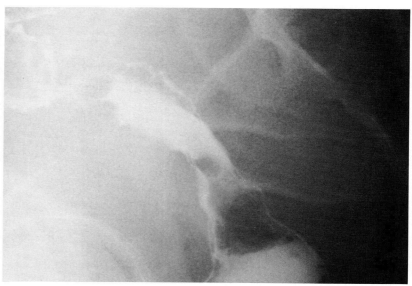

56-8   56-9

Fig. 56-8. Cytomegalovirus rectosigmoiditis in a homosexual man with AIDS. In addition to widening of the retrorectal space, there is symmetric narrowing of the rectum and sigmoid colon, which have a slightly granular mucosal surface. (Balthazar EJ, Megibow AJ, Fazzini E et al: Cytomegalovirus colitis in AIDS: Radiographic findings in 11 patients. Radiology 155:585–589, 1985)

Fig. 56-9. Radiation changes. Widening of the retrorectal space is evident 1 year following radiation for carcinoma of the cervix.

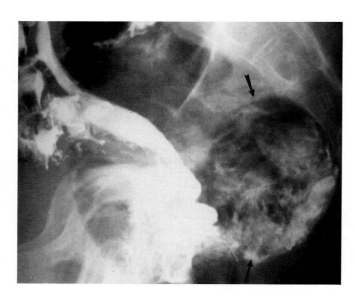

Fig. 56-10. Diverticulitis with a presacral abscess. There is marked widening of the retrorectal space with a large collection of barium in an abscess **(arrows)**. The site of perforation was clearly demonstrated on other projections. (Teplick SK, Stark P, Clark RE et al: The retrorectal space. Clin Radiol 29:177–184, 1978)

more layers of smooth muscle in their wall. Post-anal cysts appear to originate from persistent remnants of the embryonic postanal or tail gut. They are lined by squamous or columnar epithelium and contain mucin-secreting goblet cells.

Uncomplicated developmental cysts appear as soft-tissue masses in the retrorectal space. They produce a smooth, extrinsic pressure indentation on the posterior wall of the barium-filled rectum. The overlying rectal mucosa remains intact. The sacrum is usually normal, though smooth, bony erosions due to pressure have been described. Retrorectal developmental cysts often become infected and can present as recurrent retrorectal abscesses

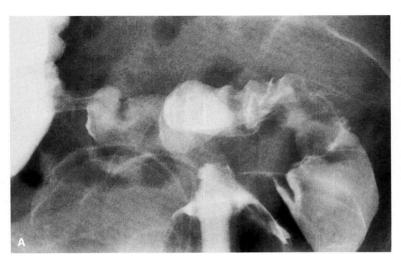

Fig. 56-11. Adenocarcinoma of the rectum causing irregular narrowing of the rectum and widening of the retrorectal space in two patients. (**B** is from Craig JOMC, Highman JH, Palmer FJ: The lateral view in the radiology of the rectum and rectosigmoid. Br J Surg 58:908–912, 1971)

with draining sinuses and fistulas to adjacent organs. Sacral osteomyelitis occasionally occurs.

Rare benign retrorectal tumors include lipomas (large, soft, palpable masses) and hemangioendotheliomas.

PRIMARY AND METASTATIC MALIGNANCIES

Primary malignant tumors of the rectum that widen the retrorectal space can be readily diagnosed on barium enema examination. Although most are adenocarcinomas (Fig. 56-11), lymphoma (Fig. 56-12), sarcoma, and cloacogenic carcinoma can produce a similar radiographic pattern.

Carcinoma of the prostate can extend posteriorly to involve the rectum and widen the retrorectal space (Fig. 56-13). The tumor tends to encircle the rectum, causing narrowing and, occasionally, obstruction (Fig. 56-14). At times, carcinoma of the prostate simulates primary rectal carcinoma with

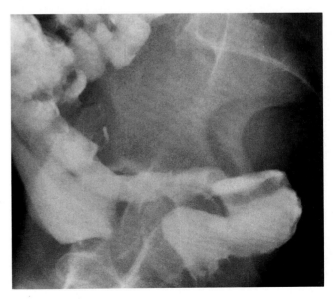

Fig. 56-12. Lymphoma. There is marked widening of the retrorectal space with narrowing of a long segment of the rectosigmoid.

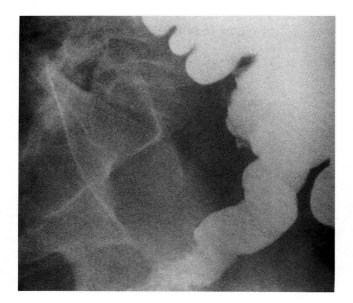

Fig. 56-13.   Carcinoma of the prostate. Posterior extension causes an extrinsic mass with spiculation and widening of the retrorectal space.

mucosal destruction and shelf formation. Because of the presence of bone metastases and urinary tract involvement by the time spread to the rectum has occurred, the correct diagnosis of carcinoma of the prostate can usually be made. Direct infiltration of perirectal tissue causing widening of the retrorectal space can be secondary to tumors of the bladder, cervix (Fig. 56-15), or ovary. Following radiation therapy for pelvic carcinoma, it can be difficult to distinguish between a widened retrorectal space caused by radiation effects (Fig. 56-16) and that due to recurrence of tumor (Fig. 56-17). Computed tomography or magnetic resonance imaging may permit differentiation between retrorectal inflammation (Fig. 56-18) or fibrosis and a recurrent tumor mass (Fig. 56-19). Metastases to lymph nodes in the presacral region can also increase the distance between the rectum and the sacrum.

NEUROGENIC/SACRAL TUMORS

Neurogenic tumors tend to displace the rectum anteriorly without invading the bowel wall. Chor-

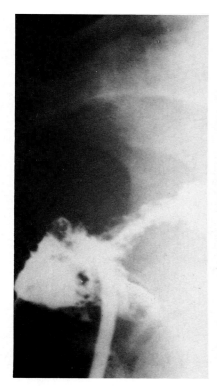

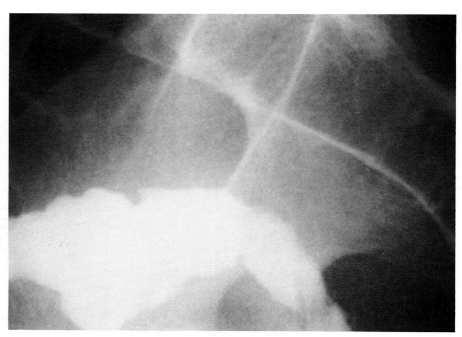

56-14   **56-15**

Fig. 56-14.   Carcinoma of the prostate. The tumor is encircling the rectosigmoid and extending into the presacral area. The rectal mucosa is normal. The bones are dense from skeletal metastases. (Teplick SK, Stark P, Clark RE et al: The retrorectal space. Clin Radiol 29:177–184, 1978)

Fig. 56-15.   Carcinoma of the cervix. Direct infiltration of the perirectal tissues causes irregular narrowing of the rectosigmoid and widening of the retrorectal space.

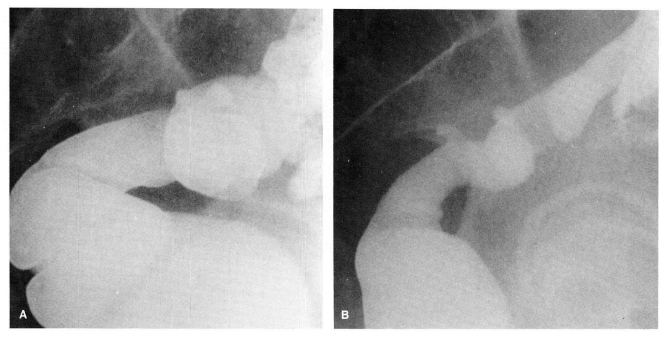

Fig. 56-16. Moderate radiation effect. **(A)** Pretreatment barium examination. **(B)** Ten months after radiation treatments for stage II carcinoma of the cervix, mild rectal bleeding prompted re-examination. An increase in the retrorectal space and moderate foreshortening of the rectosigmoid are evident. Bleeding subsided after stool softeners and a low-roughage diet were instituted. (Meyer JE: Radiography of the distal colon and rectum after irradiation of carcinoma of the cervix. AJR 136:691–699, 1981. Copyright 1981. Reproduced with permission)

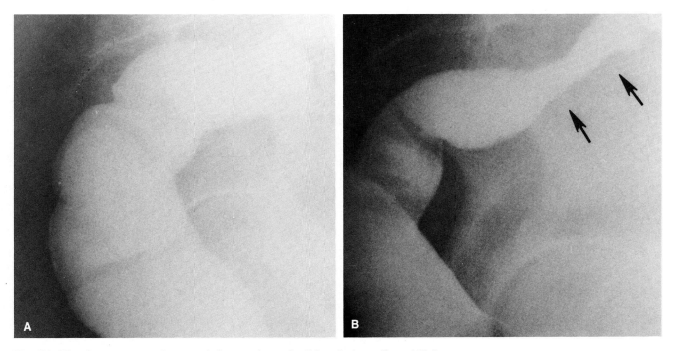

Fig. 56-17. Recurrent carcinoma of the cervix and mild radiation effect. **(A)** Pretreatment barium examination. **(B)** Fifteen months after radiotherapy for a stage II carcinoma of the cervix, diarrhea and weight loss developed. A loss of volume and increase in the retrorectal space secondary to radiation are evident. The sigmoid is irregularly narrowed and elevated by an adjacent mass, suggesting tumor involvement **(arrows)**. Extensive tumor recurrence was documented at surgical exploration. (Meyer JE: Radiography of the distal colon and rectum after irradiation of carcinoma of the cervix. AJR 136:691–699, 1981. Copyright 1981. Reproduced with permission)

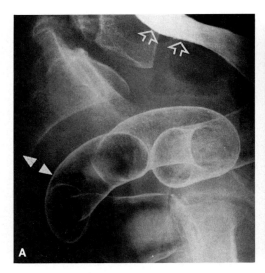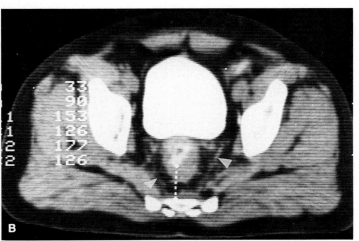

Fig. 56-18. Ulcerative colitis. **(A)** Double-contrast barium enema shows diffuse enlargement **(arrowheads)** of the retrorectal space (2.6 cm) without evidence of ulceration of the rectal mucosa, but clearly visible spicules of the distal sigmoid **(open arrows)**. **(B)** CT scan shows thickening of the rectal wall and perirectal fascia with edema of the perirectal tissues **(arrowheads)**. (Krestin GP, Beyer D, Steinbrich W: Computed tomography in the differential diagnosis of the enlarged retrorectal space. Gastrointest Radiol 11:364–369, 1986)

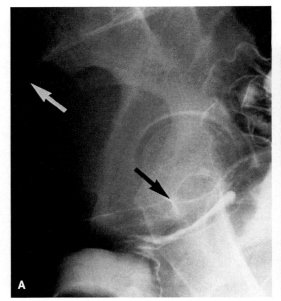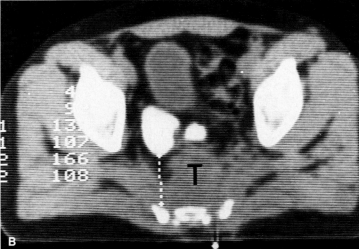

Fig. 56-19. Recurrent retroperitoneal fibrosarcoma. **(A)** Double-contrast barium enema shows an extremely enlarged retrorectal space (11 cm) **(arrows)** and a double contour of the rectal wall. **(B)** CT scan shows the large space-occupying tumorous mass **(T)**. (Krestin GP, Beyer D, Steinbrich W: Computed tomography in the differential diagnosis of the enlarged retrorectal space. Gastrointest Radiol 11:364–369, 1986)

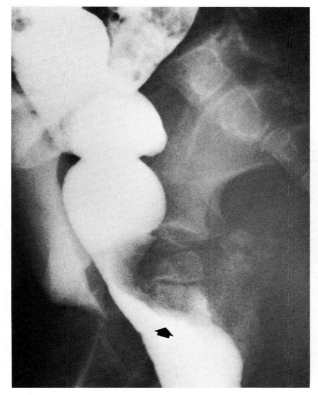

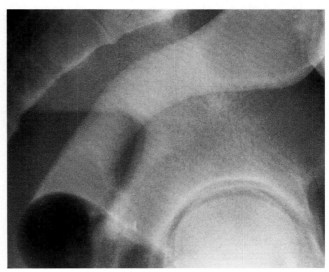

56-20   56-21

Fig. 56-20. Sacrococcygeal teratoma. There has been contrast filling of rectum and bladder. The large intrapelvically growing tumor mass widens the retrorectal space and compresses the rectal lumen. The **arrow** indicates calcifications within the tumor. (Eklof O: Roentgenologic findings in sacrococcygeal teratoma. Acta Radiol [Diagn] (Stockh), 3:41–48, 1965)

Fig. 56-21. Pelvic lipomatosis. Widening of the retrorectal space is due to massive deposition of fat in the pelvis.

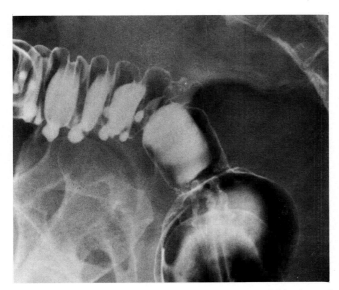

Fig. 56-22. Sigmoid resection for carcinoma. Widening of the retrorectal space is due to operative trauma altering the normal anatomic relationships in the pelvis.

domas arising in the sacrococcygeal region are slow-growing tumors that originate from remnants of the primitive notochord. The lesions commonly cause expansion and destruction of the sacrum and can extend anteriorly to produce a soft-tissue mass that displaces the rectum. Amorphous calcifications are present in about 50% of sacrococcygeal chordomas. Neurofibromas arising in a sacral foramen can enlarge and distort the foramen in addition to causing widening of the retrorectal space.

Primary and secondary malignancies of the sacrum can widen the retrorectal space. These lesions are associated with bone destruction and can usually be diagnosed on the basis of clinical findings and plain radiographs of the sacrum and coccyx.

Sacrococcygeal teratomas (Fig. 56-20) and anterior sacral meningoceles are causes of widening of the retrorectal space in the pediatric age group. Teratomas frequently contain calcification; anterior sacral meningoceles are readily diagnosed by myelography and can be suspected on the basis of an anomalous sacrum.

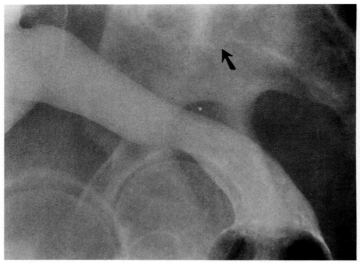

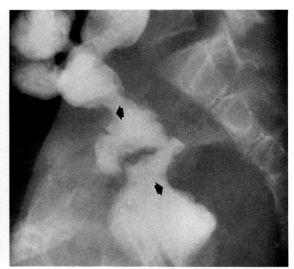

56-23   56-24

Fig. 56-23. Previous sacral fracture **(arrow)**. Bleeding into the presacral soft tissues causes widening of the retrorectal space.

Fig. 56-24. Colitis cystica profunda. Widening of the retrorectal space accompanies multiple intraluminal filling defects **(arrows)** in the rectum. (Ledesma-Medina J, Reid BS, Girdany BR: Colitis cystica profunda. AJR 131:529–530, 1978. Copyright 1978. Reproduced with permission)

OTHER CAUSES

A widened retrorectal space can sometimes be demonstrated in patients with inguinal hernias containing a segment of colon. Constant pulling on the rectum by a portion of the sigmoid within left-sided hernia sacs may be the cause of enlargement of the retrorectal space; the widening associated with right-sided hernias is probably coincidental. Extensive deposition of amyloid in rectal and perirectal tissues can also widen the retrorectal space. In patients with pelvic lipomatosis (Fig. 56-21) or Cushing's disease, massive deposition of fat in the pelvis can widen the retrorectal space; the surrounding soft tissues often demonstrate excessive lucency. Because the major constituent of the retrorectal space is fatty areolar tissue that can be swollen by edema, widespread venous thrombosis or inferior vena cava obstruction can lead to widening of the space. In patients who have undergone partial sigmoid resection, operative trauma can alter the normal anatomic relationships in the pelvis and produce the radiographic pattern of enlargement of the retrorectal space (Fig. 56-22). A previous sacral fracture (Fig. 56-23) can cause bleeding into the presacral soft tissues and widening of the retrorectal space. Finally, in colitis cystica profunda, cystic dilatation of the mucous glands of the colon can cause widening of the retrorectal space (Fig. 56-24) in addition to multiple intraluminal filling defects.

BIBLIOGRAPHY

Becker JA: Prostatic carcinoma involving the rectum and sigmoid colon. AJR 94:421–428, 1965

Campbell WL, Wolff M: Retrorectal cysts of developmental origin. AJR 117:307–313, 1973

Craig JOMC, Higham JH, Palmer FJ: The lateral view in the radiology of the rectum and rectosigmoid. Br J Surg 58:908–912, 1971

Eklof O: Roentgenologic findings in sacrococcygeal teratoma. Acta Radiol [Diagn] (Stockh) 3:41–48, 1965

Jackman RJ, Clark RLM, Smith ND: Retrorectal tumors. JAMA 145:956–961, 1951

Kattan KR, King AY: Presacral space revisited. AJR 132:437–439, 1979

Krestin GP, Beyer D, Steinbrich W: Computed tomography in the differential diagnosis of the enlarged retrorectal space. Gastrointest Radiol 11:364–369, 1986

Mather BS: Presacral dermoid cyst. Br J Surg 52:198–200, 1965

Old WL, Stokes TL: Pelvic lipomatosis. Surgery 83:173–180, 1978

Seliger G, Krassner RL, Beranbaum ER et al: The spectrum of roentgen appearance in amyloidosis of the small and large bowel: Radiologic pathologic correlation. Radiology 100:63–70, 1971

Teplick SK, Stark P, Clark RE et al: The retrorectal space. Clin Radiol 29:177–184, 1978

PART EIGHT

BILIARY SYSTEM

NONVISUALIZATION OF THE GALLBLADDER

57

Disease Entities

Extrabiliary causes of nonvisualization
  Failure of patient to ingest contrast material
  Fasting
  Failure of contrast material to reach
      absorptive surface of small bowel
    Vomiting
    Nasogastric suction
    Diarrhea
    Obstruction
      Esophageal
      Gastric outlet
    Diverticula
      Zenker's diverticulum
      Epiphrenic diverticulum
      Gastric diverticulum
      Duodenal diverticulum
      Multiple jejunal diverticulosis
    Hernias
      Hiatal
      Umbilical
      Inguinal
    Gastric ulcer crater
    Gastric bezoar
    Gastrocolic fistulas (inflammatory,
      neoplastic, surgical)
    Malabsorption diseases
  Postoperative ileus
  Severe trauma

Inflammatory disease of the abdomen
  Acute pancreatitis
  Acute peritonitis
    Peptic ulcer disease
    Appendicitis
    Diverticulitis
  Deficiency of bile salts
    Crohn's disease
    Surgical resection of a large portion of
      terminal ileum
    Cholestyramine therapy
  Age of patient under 6 months
  Pregnancy
  Pernicious anemia
Liver disease
Abnormal communication between biliary
    system and gastrointestinal tract
Intrinsic gallbladder disease
  Previous cholecystectomy
  Anomalous position of gallbladder (apparent
    nonvisualization)
  Obstruction of cystic duct or neck of
    gallbladder
  Chronic cholecystitis

ABSORPTION AND EXCRETION OF ORAL CHOLECYSTOGRAPHIC CONTRAST AGENTS

Oral cholecystographic contrast agents are absorbed from the proximal small intestine. With fat-soluble media (*e.g.*, Telapaque [iopanoic acid]), the presence of bile salts in the intestinal lumen promotes the formation of micelles, which increase the water solubility of the contrast. The bile salts are excreted by the liver, stored in the gallbladder, and emptied into the small bowel under the influence of cholecystokinin, a hormone that is secreted by the duodenal and jejunal mucosa in response to the presence of fat and peptides in the intestinal lumen. The bile salts are then reabsorbed in the terminal ileum and returned to the liver. Water-soluble contrast agents (*e.g.*, Bilopaque [tyropanoate]) dissolve more rapidly in the intestinal lumen. Once they are in aqueous solution, however, they are not absorbed across the mucosa as rapidly as fat-soluble contrast media.

The oral cholecystographic contrast next enters the portal circulation and flows to the liver, where it passes through the hepatic sinusoids and is taken up by the hepatocytes across the sinusoidal hepatic cell membrane. Within the liver, oral contrast media are conjugated with glucuronic acid and converted into more water-soluble substances. The conjugated contrast is then excreted into the bile by a process mediated by active transport involving liver enzymes. With fat-soluble media, an increased rate of excretion of bile salts into bile directly influences the biliary excretion rate, possibly by enhancing bile flow.

Bile normally flows from the liver down the hepatic and common bile ducts into the ampulla of Vater. If the sphincter of Oddi is closed, bile backs up to the level of the opening of the cystic duct. When the cystic duct is patent, most of the contrast enters the gallbladder, and only a small amount is lost in the bile that flows to the duodenum. Once in the gallbladder, reabsorption of water by the gallbladder mucosa concentrates the contrast material. Because the contrast-laden bile entering the gallbladder is diluted by the nonopaque bile already present in the organ, there is a time delay before sufficient radiographic opacification is achieved. With fat-soluble contrast agents, peak opacification of the gallbladder does not occur until 14 hr to 21 hr after ingestion. It should therefore be expected that radiographs obtained 12 hr or less after the ingestion of contrast (as is frequently the case) often result in poor visualization of the gallbladder, even without any gallbladder pathology. In contrast, with water-soluble agents, maximum radiographic opacification occurs 10 hr after ingestion; radiographs should therefore be obtained at about that time.

EXTRABILIARY CAUSES OF NONVISUALIZATION OF THE GALLBLADDER

Probably the most frequent extrabiliary cause of nonvisualization of the gallbladder is simply that the patient either received no contrast material or failed to properly ingest the contrast that was given. A full abdominal radiograph should be obtained in the patient with a nonvisualized gallbladder. This will usually reveal scattered traces of unabsorbed Telapaque in the intestine. The absence of these bits of amorphous density within the bowel suggests that no contrast agent was taken.

In patients who have been fasting, stagnation of concentrated nonopaque bile in the gallbladder due to the lack of fat stimulation can prevent filling of the gallbladder with contrast-laden bile. In addition, patients who are fasting or on a low-fat, low-protein diet tend to sequester their bile salt pool in the gallbladder, resulting in a reduction in biliary excretion of bile salts and consequently decreased absorption and biliary excretion of oral cholecystographic contrast media. Feeding the patient a high-fat lunch the day before the examination (to rid the gallbladder of residual bile) may alleviate this problem.

Any cause of contrast material not reaching the absorptive surface of the proximal small bowel can ultimately result in nonvisualization of the gallbladder. Because Telapaque is an irritant to the gastrointestinal tract, it often provokes vomiting and diarrhea, which decrease the amount of contrast that is absorbed from the small bowel. This most commonly occurs when more than the recommended dose of Telepaque is given. Obstruction of the esophagus (due to malignancy, achalasia, stricture) or gastric outlet obstruction (Fig. 57-1) can prevent

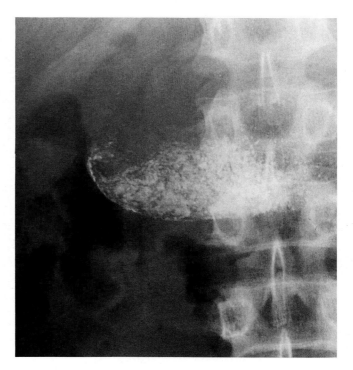

Fig. 57-1. *Gastric outlet obstruction. The Telepaque has been trapped in the stomach proximal to the obstruction and therefore has not reached the absorptive surfaces in the small bowel.*

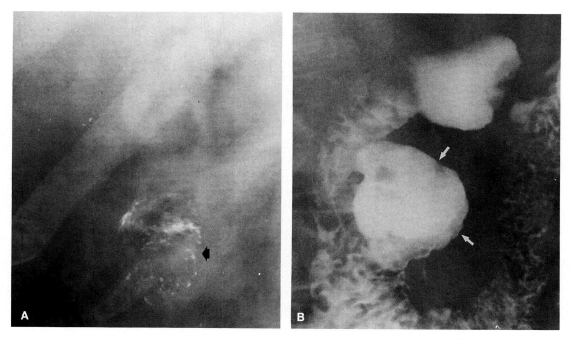

Fig. 57-2.   **(A)** Retained Telepaque within **(B)** a large duodenal diverticulum **(arrows)**.

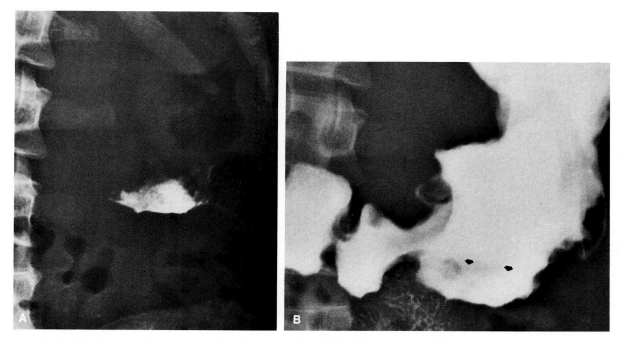

Fig. 57-3.   **(A)** Retained Telepaque within **(B)** a large ulcer **(arrows)** in an adenocarcinoma of the stomach.

contrast material from reaching the small bowel. Similarly, oral cholecystographic contrast can be retained in large diverticula (Zenker's, epiphrenic, gastric, duodenal diverticula [Fig. 57-2], multiple jejunal diverticulosis) or within a hernia sac (hiatal, umbilical, inguinal). Contrast can also be trapped within a gastric ulcer crater (Fig. 57-3) or coat a large gastric bezoar (Fig. 57-4). In patients with gastrocolic fistulas (inflammatory, neoplastic, surgical), oral cholecystographic contrast can circumvent the absorptive surface of the small bowel. Intrinsic small bowel diseases causing malabsorption can also result in poor opacification of the gallbladder.

In persons who have undergone surgery or severe trauma to any part of the body, reflex-induced impairment of gastrointestinal function can lead to decreased absorption of oral cholecystographic agents and impaired gallbladder visualization. In most of these patients, intravenous cholangiography successfully reveals the common bile duct and gallbladder.

After an attack of acute pancreatitis, an intrinsically normal gallbladder may not be visualized on oral cholecystography. This may be due to diminished secretion of pancreatic juices and consequently poor absorption of contrast. In addition, pancreatic secretions may play a role in controlling the tone and absorptive function of the gallbladder itself. Hypotonicity of the gallbladder may lead to decreased water absorption, poor concentration of contrast, and nonvisualization.

Decreased gallbladder visualization can be demonstrated in patients with peritonitis associated with pancreatitis, a perforated ulcer, appendicitis,

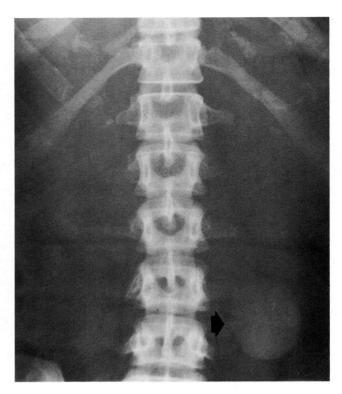

Fig. 57-5. *No visualization of the gallbladder in the right upper quadrant. A full abdominal radiograph demonstrates that the functioning gallbladder is situated in an anomalous position in the left lower quadrant* **(arrow)**. *On oblique views, the lucencies projected over the gallbladder were shown to represent gas in overlying loops of bowel.*

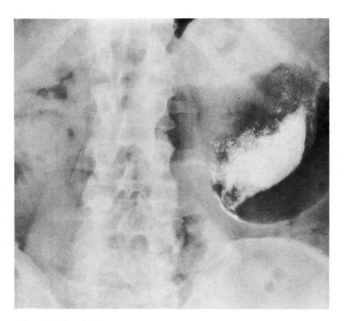

Fig. 57-4. *Telepaque retained in the stomach coating a large gastric bezoar.*

or diverticulitis. Nonvisualization of the gallbladder can also occur in patients with acute duodenal ulcers and peritoneal irritation without perforation, presumably because of the proximity of the inflammatory process to the gallbladder. In patients with these abdominal inflammatory diseases, oral cholecystography is usually normal once the acute symptoms have subsided.

In patients with Crohn's disease or surgical resection of large portions of the terminal ileum, nonvisualization of the gallbladder is probably secondary to a deficiency of bile salts (normally reabsorbed in the distal ileum), which impairs intestinal absorption of oral cholecystographic contrast media. A similar mechanism is presumably responsible for nonvisualization of the gallbladder in patients being treated with cholestyramine. This medication is prescribed for the relief of pruritus associated with partial biliary obstruction or as adjunctive therapy to diet in the management of patients with elevated levels of serum cholesterol. Cholestyramine is an anion exchange resin that strongly binds bile acids in the intestine to form an insoluble complex that is excreted in the feces. The resulting partial removal of bile acids from the enterohepatic circulation decreases the absorption of oral cholecystographic contrast agents and leads to nonvisualization of the gallbladder.

Nonvisualization of the gallbladder has also been reported in infants under 6 months of age, in women in the last months of pregnancy, and in patients with pernicious anemia.

Liver disease with disturbed hepatocellular function can result in nonvisualization of the gallbladder either because of an inability of the patient to properly conjugate the oral cholecystographic contrast agent or because of insufficient production and flow of bile. The liver abnormalities that most commonly produce nonvisualization of the gallbladder are hepatitis and cirrhosis. Serum bilirubin determination is the laboratory test that best reflects the ability of the liver to excrete an oral cholecystographic contrast agent. Because bilirubin and Telepaque compete for the same hepatic excretion mechanism, opacification of the gallbladder after administration of oral contrast rarely occurs if the serum bilirubin level is more than 3.5 mg/dl.

Abnormal communication between the biliary system and the gastrointestinal tract is a cause of nonvisualization of the gallbladder on both oral cholecystography and intravenous cholangiography. A fistula due to surgery or a pathologic process permits bile to flow directly and continuously into the intestine, resulting in nonfilling of the gallbladder.

The radiographic demonstration of surgical clips in the right upper quadrant or the identification of a right upper abdominal scar on physical examination should suggest the possibility of previous cholecystectomy as a cause for nonvisualization of the gallbladder. Nonvisualization on coned views of the right upper quadrant may be due to the gallbladder being in an anomalous position (even if there is not situs inversus) outside the margins of the film. A full abdominal radiograph should be obtained in such a case to show the position of the gallbladder (Fig. 57-5).

BILIARY TRACT CAUSES OF NONVISUALIZATION OF THE GALLBLADDER

If extrabiliary and hepatocellular causes of nonvisualization can be excluded, failure of the gallbladder to opacify after the administration of two doses of oral cholecystographic contrast medium is highly reliable evidence of gallbladder disease. The major causes of nonvisualization intrinsic to the gallbladder are obstruction of the cystic duct or neck of the gallbladder and chronic cholecystitis. Obstruction of the cystic duct prevents contrast-containing bile from reaching the gallbladder and opacifying the organ. In chronic cholecystitis, nonvisualization can be due to obliteration of the gallbladder lumen by chronic inflammatory changes, inability of the inflamed gallbladder mucosa to absorb and concentrate water, or diffusion of contrast through the diseased mucosa of the gallbladder and into the blood stream.

In patients with nonvisualization of the gallbladder, the presence of conjugated oral cholecystographic contrast material in the small bowel and colon is an excellent radiographic sign of intrinsic gallbladder disease with normal liver function and patent bile ducts. Conjugated contrast appears radiographically as a homogeneous, uniform density (Fig. 57-6) that is easily distinguished from the dense, granular, particulate pattern of unabsorbed, unconjugated contrast material (Fig. 57-7). The finding of conjugated contrast medium in the small bowel or colon indicates that the opaque medium was adequately absorbed from the small bowel and properly excreted by the liver. Therefore, its appearance in combination with nonvisualization of the

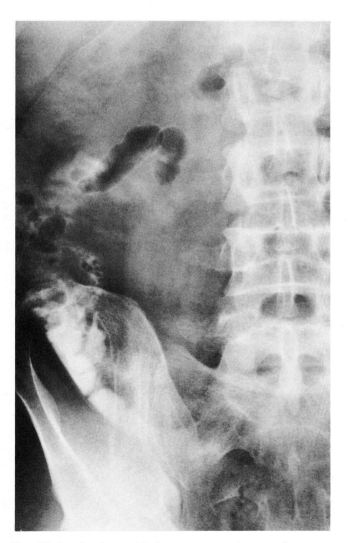

Fig. 57-6. Conjugated Telepaque appearing as a homogeneous, uniform density.

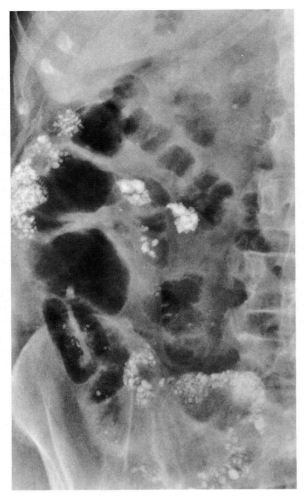

Fig. 57-7. Unconjugated Telepaque producing a dense, granular, particulate pattern.

gallbladder implies intrinsic gallbladder disease (obstruction of the cystic duct or neck of the gall-bladder, severe chronic cholecystitis).

BIBLIOGRAPHY

Berk RN, Clemett AR: Radiology of the Gallbladder and Bile Ducts. Philadelphia, WB Saunders, 1977

Goldberg HI: Small bowel disease and oral cholecystography. Gastroenterology 71:529, 1976

Howard JM: Gallbladder function (cholecystographic studies) following nonspecific trauma. Surgery 36:1051–1055, 1953

L'Heureux PR, Isenberg JN, Sharp HL et al: Gallbladder disease in cystic fibrosis. AJR 128:953–956, 1977

Low-Beer TS, Heaton KW, Roylance J: Oral cholecystography in patients with small bowel disease. Br J Radiol 45:427–428, 1972

Mujahed Z: Nonopacification of the gallbladder and bile ducts: A previously unreported cause. Radiology 112:297–298, 1974

Mujahed Z: Factors interfering with the opacification of a normal gallbladder. Gastrointest Radiol 1:183–185, 1976

Mujahed Z, Evans JA, Whalen JP: The nonopacified gallbladder on oral cholecystography. Radiology 112:1–3, 1974

Nathan MH, Newman A: Conjugated iopanoic acid (Telepaque) in the small bowel: An aid in the diagnosis of gallbladder disease. Radiology 109:545–548, 1973

Ochsner SF, Buchtel BC: Nonvisualization of the gallbladder caused by hiatus hernia. AJR 101:589–591, 1967

Sanchez-Ubeda R, Ruzicka FF, Rousselot LM: Effect of peritonitis of nonbiliary origin on the function of the gallbladder as measured by cholecystography, its frequency and its duration. N Engl J Med 257:389–394, 1957

Shehadi WH: Radiologic examination of the biliary tract: Oral cholecystography. Radiol Clin North Am 4:463–482, 1966

Sparkman RF, Jernigan CR: Visualization of gallbladder and bile ducts following trauma. Surgery 41:595–604, 1957

Teplick JG, Adelman BP: Retention of the opaque medium during cholecystography. AJR 74:256–261, 1955

ALTERATIONS IN GALLBLADDER SIZE

Disease Entities

Enlarged gallbladder
    Courvoisier phenomenon
    Hydrops
    Empyema
    Vagotomy
    Diabetes mellitus
Small gallbladder
    Chronic cholecystitis
    Cystic fibrosis
    Multiseptate gallbladder
    Hypoplasia

ENLARGED GALLBLADDER

COURVOISIER PHENOMENON

The gallbladder is generally considered to be enlarged when the body of the organ measures 5 cm or more in width. In the presence of jaundice, enlargement of the gallbladder usually indicates the Courvoisier phenomenon secondary to extrahepatic neoplastic disease arising in the head of the pancreas, duodenal papilla, ampulla of Vater, or lower common bile duct (Fig. 58-1). The law of Courvoisier is based on the fact that most patients with malignant biliary obstruction have intrinsically normal gallbladders that can be distended; in contrast, persons with jaundice due to an impacted common duct stone usually have chronically inflamed, scarred, shrunken gallbladders. Gallbladder enlargement is seen in about 90% of patients undergoing surgery for carcinoma of the head of the pancreas, though it is an uncommon finding in patients with common duct stones.

It should be stressed that, although the presence of a nontender, palpable gallbladder is a highly reliable indicator of a malignant cause of obstructive jaundice, the converse is certainly not true. Enlargement of the gallbladder may be undetectable on physical examination because hepatomegaly prevents palpation. Simultaneous cystic duct obstruction, even without gallstones, can prevent the gallbladder from distending with bile. In addition, obstructive jaundice caused by a tumor located in the common hepatic duct proximal to the entrance of the cystic duct into the common bile duct is not associated with gallbladder enlargement.

HYDROPS/EMPYEMA

If the gallbladder is enlarged but jaundice is not present, hydrops and empyema are the most likely diagnoses. Hydrops is distention of the gallbladder with clear mucoid fluid secondary to persistent cystic duct obstruction after the inflammation of acute cholecystitis has subsided. Empyema of the gallbladder, also a complication of acute cholecystitis, is accompanied by severe pain and tenderness, fever, chills, leukocytosis, and the finding of pus in the gallbladder. Because these conditions are associated with nonvisualization of the gallbladder, they can be identified radiographically only by the demonstration of a large soft-tissue mass in the right

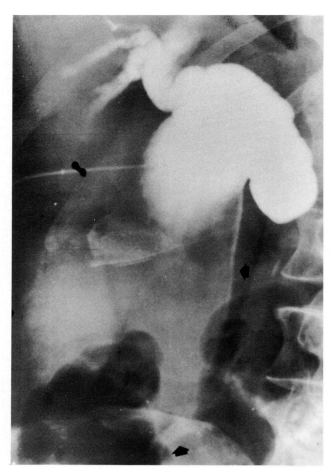

Fig. 58-1. *Courvoisier phenomenon. Huge gallbladder* **(arrows)** *injected by error at percutaneous transhepatic cholangiography. The patient had carcinoma of the pancreas and presented with painless jaundice.*

DIABETES MELLITUS

Up to 20% of patients with diabetes mellitus have enlarged gallbladders. Gallbladder enlargement in this condition is most likely related to an autonomic neuropathy, possibly due to interference with the vagus nerve. Other suggested mechanisms for gallbladder enlargement in diabetes are an abnormality of gallbladder musculature, a change in the physical and chemical characteristics of bile, and an alteration in function of the valves of Heister. There is no correlation between the degree of gallbladder enlargement and other manifestations of diabetes, the severity of the disease, or the mode of therapy. The impaired function of the gallbladder in diabetics leads to stasis of bile and an increased incidence of gallstones.

RADIOGRAPHIC FINDINGS WITH ENLARGED GALLBLADDERS

In most patients with gallbladder enlargement secondary to obstruction, there is nonvisualization of the gallbladder following the administration of oral cholecystographic contrast media. However, gallbladders enlarged because of vagotomy or diabetes

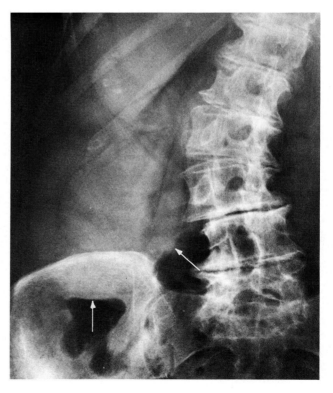

Fig. 58-2. *Empyema of the gallbladder. The hepatic flexure* **(arrows)** *is indented by the large supramesocolic mass. The right kidney is seen through the mass. (Margulis AR, Burhenne HJ (eds): Alimentary Tract Radiology. St. Louis, CV Mosby, 1983)*

upper quadrant (Fig. 58-2) or an impression on adjacent barium-filled loops of bowel (Fig. 58-3).

VAGOTOMY

Enlargement of the gallbladder without obstruction of the biliary tract can be seen after vagotomy. The size of the gallbladder in the resting state is reported to approximately double after truncal vagotomy. However, if the patient undergoes a selective vagotomy with sparing of the hepatic vagal branch, no gallbladder enlargement is noted. Emptying of the gallbladder in response to a fatty meal is decreased after vagotomy (especially the truncal type). Although gallbladder enlargement following vagotomy should theoretically lead to stasis of bile and an increased likelihood of gallstone formation, the relationship of gallstones to vagotomy is still very controversial.

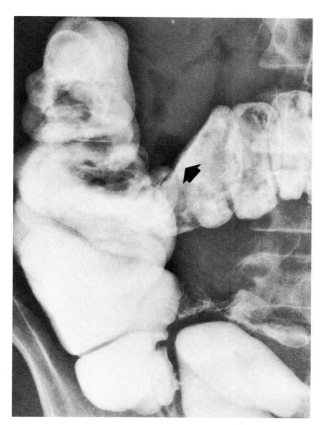

Fig. 58-3. Hydrops of the gallbladder. Marked enlargement of the gallbladder causes an extrinsic impression **(arrow)** on the adjacent barium-filled colon.

generally may be visualized to some extent. Gallbladder enlargement after vagotomy is usually associated with enlargement of the biliary tree; in diabetics, concomitant common bile duct dilatation does not occur.

SMALL GALLBLADDER

CHRONIC CHOLECYSTITIS

The most common cause for a small, shrunken gallbladder is chronic cholecystitis (Fig. 58-4). After repeated attacks of biliary colic and acute cholecystitis, the gallbladder wall can become greatly thickened and undergo fibrous constriction, resulting in decreased gallbladder size on oral cholecystography.

CYSTIC FIBROSIS

A small, contracted, poorly functioning gallbladder can be seen in 30% to 50% of patients with cystic fibrosis of the pancreas (Fig. 58-5). The microgallbladders in children and young adults with this disorder have marginal irregularities and multiple weblike trabeculations and are filled with thick, tenacious, colorless bile and mucus. Gallstones are frequently seen in these patients. In view of the high incidence of cholecystographic abnormalities in

Fig. 58-4. Chronic cholecystitis. Multiple radiolucent stones **(arrow)** fill the small, shrunken gallbladder.

Fig. 58-5. Cystic fibrosis. Diminutive microgallbladder in a 10-year-old boy. (L'Heureux PR, Isenberg JN, Sharp HL et al: Gallbladder disease in cystic fibrosis. AJR 128:953–956, 1977. Copyright 1977. Reproduced with permission)

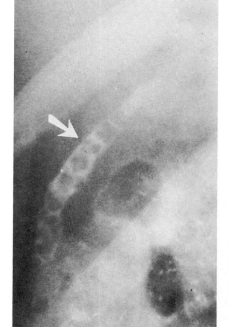

58-4

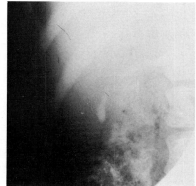

58-5

asymptomatic patients with cystic fibrosis, it is unclear to what extent gallbladder disease is responsible for the frequent attacks of abdominal pain experienced by patients with this condition.

CONGENITAL ANOMALIES

Congenital multiseptate gallbladder is a hyperplastic structure with multiple intercommunicating septa dividing the lumen of the gallbladder. This rare anomaly generally appears on oral cholecystography as a small gallbladder with a honeycomb pattern. The stasis of bile in a multiseptate gallbladder predisposes to infection and gallstone formation.

Infants and children occasionally demonstrate hypoplasia of the gallbladder, which appears as little more than a small, rudimentary pouch at the end of the cystic duct.

BIBLIOGRAPHY

Amberg JR, Jones RS, Mass A et al: Effect of vagotomy on gallbladder size and contractility in the dog. Invest Radiol 8:371–376, 1973

Berk RN, Clemett AR: Radiology of the Gallbladder and Bile Ducts. Philadelphia, WB Saunders, 1977

Bloom AA, Stachenfeld R: Diabetic cholecystomegaly. JAMA 208:357–359, 1969

Bouchier IAD: The vagus, the bile, and gallstones. Gut 11:799–803, 1970

Eaton SB, Ferrucci JT, Margulis AR et al: Unfamiliar roentgen findings in pancreatic disease. AJR 116:396–405, 1972

Fagerberg S, Grevsten S, Johansson H et al: Vagotomy and gallbladder function. Gut 11:789–793, 1970

Harris RC, Caffey J: Cholecystography in infants. JAMA 153:1333–1337, 1953

Hopton DS: The influence of the vagus nerves on the biliary system. Br J Surg 60:216–218, 1973

L'Heureux PR, Isenberg JN, Sharp HL et al: Gallbladder disease in cystic fibrosis. AJR 138:953–956, 1977

Rovsing H, Sloth K: Micro-gallbladder and biliary calculi in mucoviscidosis. Acta Radiol [Diagn] (Stockh) 14:588–592, 1973

DISPLACEMENT OR DEFORMITY OF THE GALLBLADDER

Disease Entities

Normal structures
    Duodenum
    Colon
Liver masses
    Hepatoma
    Hemangioma
    Regenerating nodule
    Metastases
    Polycystic liver
    Hydatid cyst
    Hepar lobatum (tertiary syphilis)
    Granuloma
    Abscess
Extrahepatic masses
    Retroperitoneal tumors (renal, adrenal)
    Polycystic kidney
    Lymphoma/metastases to lymph nodes of
        the porta hepatis
    Pancreatic pseudocyst

The gallbladder normally lies in a fossa on the inferior surface of the liver and is covered to some extent with peritoneum. It has a smooth contour and a generally pear-shaped configuration. The gallbladder can lie as high as the level of the first lumbar vertebra in a hypersthenic patient and as low as the fourth lumbar vertebra in an asthenic person.

Mass lesions in the right upper quadrant (primarily in the liver or in the region of the porta hepatis; Fig. 59-1), as well as dilatation of adjacent structures (duodenum [Fig. 59-2], colon [Fig. 59-3]), can displace or deform the soft, compressible gallbladder. At times, a contour deformity of the contrast-filled gallbladder on an abdominal radiograph can be the first sign of the presence of a lesion in a nearby organ.

Deformity of the gallbladder secondary to distention of the gas-filled duodenum or the gas- and feces-filled colon is generally variable and inconstant in appearance, changing with the position of the patient. In contrast, mass lesions in the liver produce discrete, localized extrinsic impressions on the gallbladder that are persistent and reproducible and tend not to vary when the patient assumes a different position (Fig. 59-4). Deformities due to hepatic masses also remain constant in radiographs obtained before and after the administration of a fatty meal. Enlarging hepatic masses generally displace the gallbladder downward in relation to the bile ducts or the usual skeletal levels (Fig. 59-5). Depending on its position in the liver, the mass can

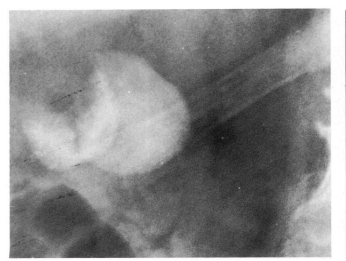

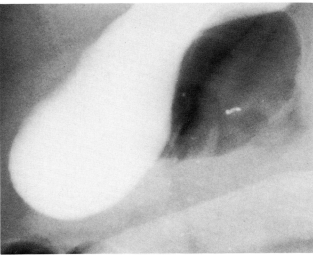

59-1

59-2

Fig. 59-1. Hepatoma invading the gallbladder and causing a fixed impression on the superolateral aspect.

Fig. 59-2. Indentation of the gallbladder by the gas-filled duodenum.

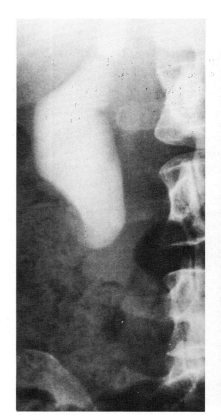

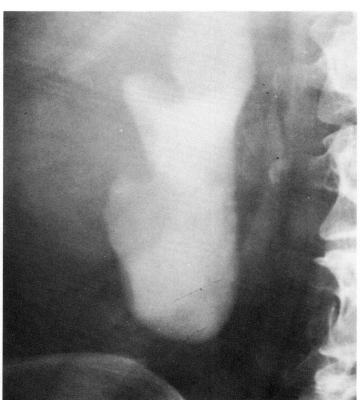

59-3

59-4

Fig. 59-3. Indentation and compression of the lateral aspect of the gallbladder by the colon, which is distended with feces. (Ochsner SF: Extrinsic abnormalities affecting the biliary system. Semin Roentgenol 11:283–287, 1976. Reproduced with permission)

Fig. 59-4. Polycystic liver causing persistent round filling defects on the lateral aspect of the gallbladder. (Hedgcock MW, Shanser JD, Eisenberg RL et al: Polycystic liver and other hepatic masses mimicking gallbladder disease. Br J Radiol 52:897–899, 1979)

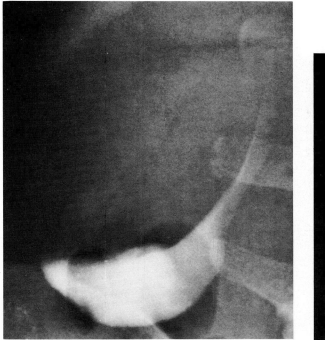

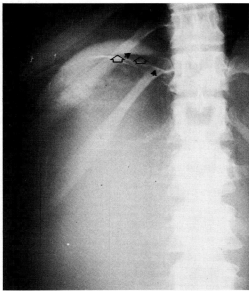

59-5   59-6

Fig. 59-5. Massively enlarged liver causing extrinsic compression and downward displacement of the gallbladder.

Fig. 59-6. Huge, partly calcified renal cyst **(closed arrows)** with mural renal cell carcinoma causing upward displacement of the gallbladder and compression of its inferior contour **(open arrows)**. (Ochsner SF: Extrinsic abnormalities affecting the biliary system. Semin Roentgenol 11:283–287, 1976. Reproduced with permission)

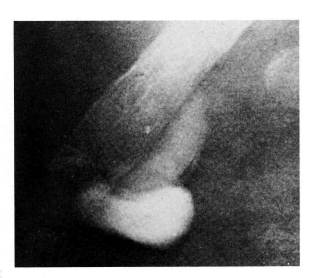

Fig. 59-7. Large lymph nodes (lymphoma) impressing the gallbladder. (Fisher MS: Hepar lobatum and other less exotic causes of gallbladder deformity. Radiology 91:308–309, 1968)

push the gallbladder laterally or medially as well as downward.

Localized pressure defects of the gallbladder caused by hepatic masses can usually be easily differentiated from intrinsic gallbladder lesions. An exception is the sharply circumscribed impression of a hepatic mass on the fundus of the gallbladder, which simulates an adenomyoma (adenomyomas almost invariably occur at this site).

Radionuclide scanning of the liver provides a simple method for identifying the presence of a hepatic mass. A normal scan, however, does not entirely exclude a hepatic cause for gallbladder deformity, especially when the lesion arises from the inferior aspect of the liver surface. Ultrasound and computed tomography can better characterize a hepatic lesion compressing the gallbladder.

Upward displacement of the gallbladder suggests a neoplasm originating below the liver, such as a renal (Fig. 59-6) or adrenal tumor. Polycystic kidneys, pancreatic pseudocysts, and enlarged lymph nodes in the porta hepatis (lymphoma [Fig. 59-7],

metastases) can also displace or deform the gallbladder.

BIBLIOGRAPHY

Berk RN, Clemett AR: Radiology of the Gallbladder and Bile Ducts. Philadelphia, WB Saunders, 1977

Brust RW, Conlon PC: Roentgenologic manifestations of primary hepatoma with particular reference to some unusual cholecystographic findings. AJR 87:777–786, 1962

Caplan LH, Simon M: Nonparasitic cyst of liver. AJR 96:421–428, 1966

Conlon PC, Brust RW: Cholecystography as an aid in the localization of upper abdominal masses. AJR 88:756–767, 1962

Fisher MS: Hepar lobatum and other less exotic causes of gallbladder deformity. Radiology 91:308–309, 1968

Hedgcock MW, Shanser JD, Eisenberg RL et al: Polycystic liver and other hepatic masses mimicking gall-bladder disease. Br J Radiol 52:897–899, 1979

Joffe N, Babenco GO: Localized deformity of the gallbladder secondary to hepatic mass lesions. AJR 121:412–419, 1974

Ochsner SF: Extrinsic abnormalities affecting the biliary system. Semin Roentgenol 11:283–287, 1976

FILLING DEFECTS IN AN OPACIFIED GALLBLADDER

60

Movable filling defects
  Gallstones
Fixed filling defects
  Cholesterolosis
  Adenomyomatosis
  Gallstone adherent to the gallbladder wall
  Inflammatory polyp
  Mucosal adenoma
    Glandular adenoma (adenomatous polyp)
    Papillary adenoma (villous adenoma,
      papilloma)
    Fibroadenoma
    Cystadenoma
  Unusual benign tumors
    Neurinoma
    Carcinoid
    Hemangioma
    Mixed tumor
  Malignant tumors
    Carcinoma of the gallbladder
    Leiomyosarcoma
    Metastases
  Parasite granuloma
  Metachromatic leukodystrophy
  Fibroxanthogranulomatous inflammation
  Intramural epithelial cyst
  Pseudopolyps
    Pseudodefect in the neck of the gallbladder
    Congenital fold, septum, or multiseptate
      gallbladder

Heterotopic gastric or pancreatic tissue
Postoperative defect of the gallbladder wall
Vascular lesion (varices, arterial tortuosity
  or aneurysm)

GALLSTONES

The large majority of filling defects in an opacified gallbladder represent gallstones. Gallstones can develop whenever bile contains insufficient bile salts and lecithin in proportion to cholesterol to maintain the cholesterol in solution. This situation can result from a decrease in the amount of bile salts present (because of decreased reabsorption in the terminal ileum secondary to inflammatory disease or surgical resection) or can be caused by increased hepatic synthesis of cholesterol. Because cholesterol is not radiopaque, most gallstones are radiolucent and visible only on contrast examination. In up to 20% of patients, however, gallstones are composed of calcium bilirubinate or are of mixed composition and contain sufficient calcium to be radiographically detectable. Bilirubin stones are less common and occur in patients with excessive red blood cell destruction (*e.g.,* in persons with hemolytic anemias, such as sickle cell disease or congenital spherocytosis).

Because gallstones are seen with increased frequency in certain disease states, additional signs on plain radiographs should be sought. These include the characteristic thickened trabeculae and "fish-mouth" vertebrae in sickle cell disease, ascites in patients with cirrhosis, abnormal gas-filled loops of bowel in persons with Crohn's disease, severe vascular calcification in patients with diabetes mellitus, and pancreatic calcification in persons with pancreatic disease or hyperparathyroidism. Other conditions apparently associated with a higher than normal incidence of gallstones include prolonged use of estrogen or progesterone, hypothyroidism, hypercholesterolemia, hepatitis, muscular dystrophy, parasitic infestation, and obesity.

RADIOGRAPHIC FINDINGS

The size, shape, number, and degree of calcification of gallstones are extremely varied. Gallstones can be lucent (Fig. 60-1), contain a central nidus of calcification (Fig. 60-2), be laminated (Fig. 60-3), or have calcification around the periphery (Fig. 60-4). They can be as large as 4 cm to 5 cm, or as small as 1 mm to 2 mm. Large numbers of stones can have a sand- or gravel-like consistency and be visible only on radiographs taken with a horizontal beam (upright or lateral decubitus) (Fig. 60-5). Gallstones are almost always freely movable and fall by gravity to the de-

pendent portion of the gallbladder. They frequently layer out at a level that depends on the relation of the specific gravity of the stone to that of the surrounding bile (Fig. 60-6). Occasionally, gallstones of different densities can be seen to lie at separate levels on upright views (Fig. 60-7). Infrequently, a gallstone is coated with tenacious mucus and adheres to the gallbladder wall (Fig. 60-8); this appearance can be impossible to differentiate from the extensive differential diagnosis of fixed filling defects in the opacified gallbladder. Stones can also become trapped in the neck of the gallbladder (Fig. 60-9) or cystic duct (Fig. 60-10).

Though infrequently seen, a characteristic finding of gallstones is the "Mercedes–Benz" sign. Stellate radiolucencies reflecting gas-containing fissures or faults within the gallstone produce a triradiate pattern similar to the German automobile trademark (Fig. 60-11). Linear radiating deposits of calcium in the fissures within a gallstone have been reported as the "reversed Mercedes–Benz" sign.

Ultrasound is now the major imaging modality for demonstrating gallstones. This noninvasive technique is equal in accuracy to oral cholecystography, is independent of hepatic function, and does not

Text continues on page 792

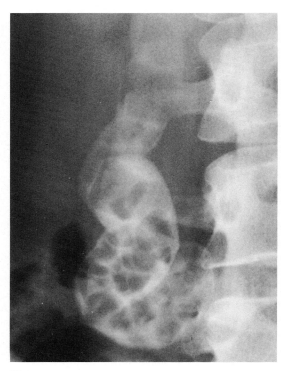

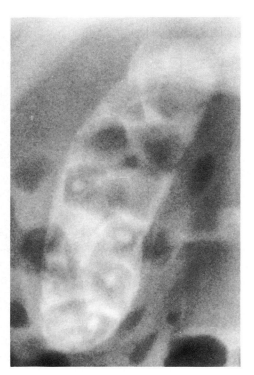

60-1

60-2

Fig. 60-1. *Multiple lucent gallstones.*

Fig. 60-2. *Multiple lucent gallstones, many of which contain a central nidus of calcification.*

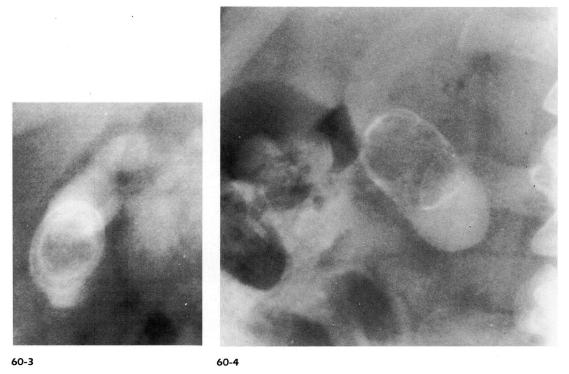

60-3   60-4

Fig. 60-3. Laminated gallstone with alternating lucent and opaque layers.

Fig. 60-4. Gallstone with peripheral rim of calcification.

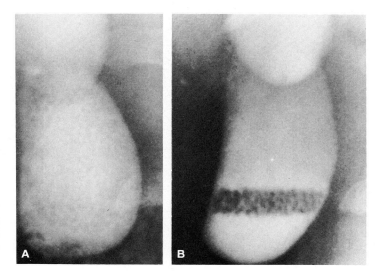

Fig. 60-5. Multiple gallstones. **(A)** With the patient supine, the stones are poorly defined and have a gravel-like consistency. **(B)** On an erect film taken with a horizontal beam, the innumerable gallstones layer out and are easily seen.

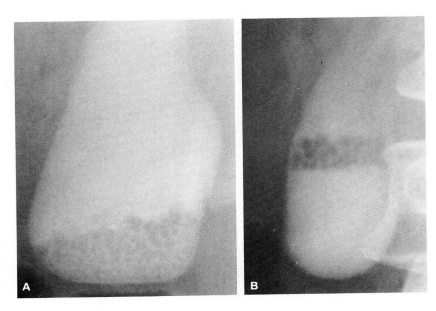

Fig. 60-6. Layering of gallstones in two patients. **(A)** Gallstones fall to the base of the gallbladder on upright film. **(B)** Gallstones layer out at a level in the midportion of the gallbladder.

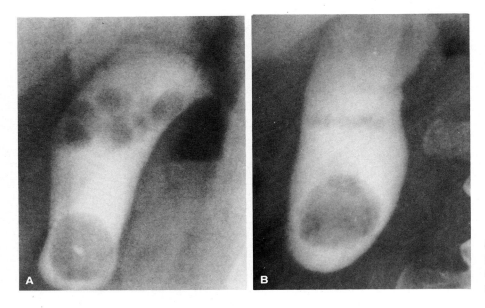

Fig. 60-7. Two examples of patients with gallstones of different densities lying at separate levels on upright views.

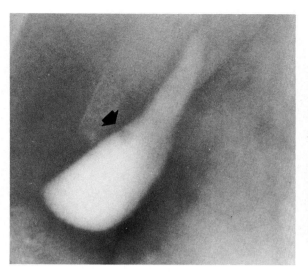

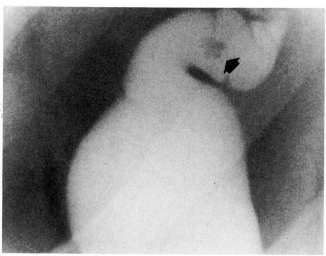

60-8

60-9

Fig. 60-8. Stone **(arrow)** impacted in the wall of the gallbladder mimicking a polypoid lesion.

Fig. 60-9. Gallstone located at the junction of the neck of the gallbladder and cystic duct **(arrow)**.

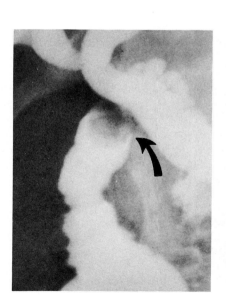

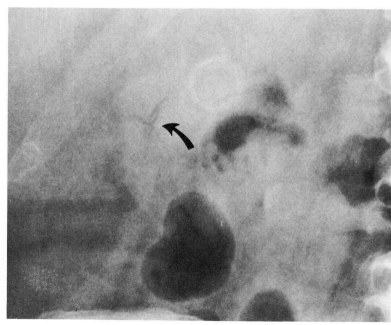

60-10

60-11

Fig. 60-10. Gallstone trapped in the cystic duct **(arrow)**. Contrast has been introduced by way of a catheter in the base of the gallbladder.

Fig. 60-11. Mercedes–Benz sign of fissuring in a gallstone **(arrow)**. Note the adjacent gallstone with a radiopaque rim.

rely on patient compliance in taking oral contrast agents. In addition to imaging the gallbladder, ultrasound can provide important additional information by effectively demonstrating the biliary tree and hepatic parenchyma.

The classic sonographic appearance of a gallstone is a high-amplitude intraluminal echo (reflecting from the surface of the stone) that is associated with posterior acoustic shadowing (Fig. 60-12). This finding can be demonstrated in about two-thirds of patients with gallstones and is virtually 100% specific for the diagnosis of cholelithiasis. The mobility of free-floating gallstones may be demonstrated by performing the examination with the patient in various positions. Most stones gravitate to the dependent portion of the gallbladder (Fig. 60-13). However, gallstones may float if they contain gas or if the bile is highly viscous or has a high specific gravity (as in the presence of cholecystographic contrast material; Fig. 60-14). A calculus impacted in the gallbladder neck does not move (Fig. 60-15), nor does a gallstone adherent to or embedded within the gallbladder wall (Fig. 60-16). The demonstration of a posterior acoustic shadow caused by a gallstone may be difficult and requires high-frequency transducers and optimal focusing, and fine adjustment of the time-gain compensation. The chemical compensation of gallstones does not affect their shadowing characteristics. However, the size of a gallstone is important, because small stones (<5 mm) usually do not produce an acoustic shadow. Another cause for absent posterior acoustic shadowing is sludge, which represents echogenic bile that is situated in a dependent position within the gallbladder below the normal echo-free bile and may produce a fluid–fluid level with it (Fig. 60-17). Sludge may move slowly with changes in the patient's position, indicating that it is viscous, or may settle focally within the gallbladder to simulate a

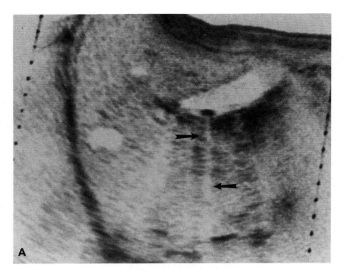

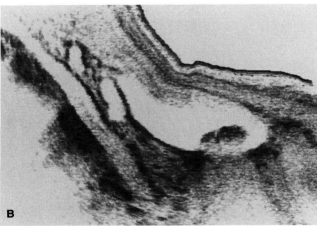

Fig. 60-13.   *Ultrasound of movable gallstones.* **(A)** *High-intensity intraluminal echoes with posterior acoustic shadowing* **(arrows)** *on routine supine projection.* **(B)** *With the patient in a sitting position, the gallstones roll to the dependent portion of the gallbladder fundus.* (Harned RK, Williams FM, Anderson JC: Gallbladder disease. In Eisenberg RL (ed): Diagnostic Imaging: An Algorithmic Approach. Philadelphia, JB Lippincott, 1988)

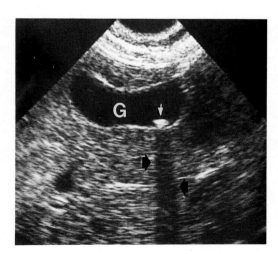

Fig. 60-12.   *Ultrasound of gallstones. The anechoic gallbladder* **(G)** *contains an echogenic focus representing a large gallstone* **(white arrow)**. *Note the acoustic shadowing immediately inferior to the stone* **(black arrows)**.

mass (Fig. 60-18). At times, a high-amplitude echo caused by a small calculus may emanate from within the sludge layer (see Fig. 60-16).

The sonolucent lumen of the gallbladder cannot be identified in about 20% of patients with gallstones because it is completely filled with calculi. In such cases, the diagnosis of cholelithiasis is made by demonstrating a high-amplitude echo in the gallbladder fossa associated with a posterior acoustic shadow (Fig. 60-19). It is often difficult to differentiate the calculus-filled gallbladder from surrounding gas-containing bowel. Demonstration of the double-arcuate echo sign with posterior shadowing can aid in identifying the stone-filled gallbladder (Fig. 60-20). In addition, the characteristics of the shadow are important, because shadows caused by

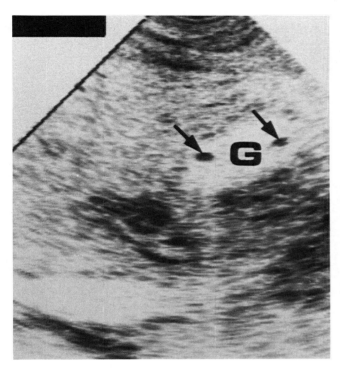

Fig. 60-14. Floating calculi **(arrows)** in the gallbladder **(G)**. (Harned RK, Williams FM, Anderson JC: Gallbladder disease. In Eisenberg RL (ed): Diagnostic Imaging: An Algorithmic Approach. Philadelphia, JB Lippincott, 1988)

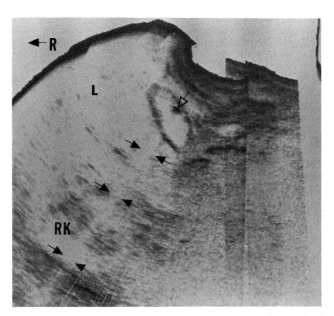

Fig. 60-16. Gallstone adherent to the gallbladder wall. A prominent echo **(open arrow)** is seen adjacent to the anterior wall of the gallbladder. Note the prominent acoustic shadow (between **closed arrows**). **L,** liver; **RK,** right kidney. (Margulis AR, Burhenne HJ (eds): Alimentary Tract Radiology. St. Louis, CV Mosby, 1983)

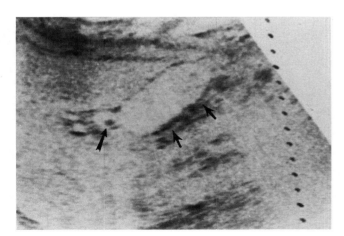

Fig. 60-15. Impacted stone **(arrow)** in the neck of the gallbladder. Note also the thin layer of nonshadowing tiny gallstones **(arrowheads)** along the posterior wall of the gallbladder. (Harned RK, Williams FM, Anderson JC: Gallbladder disease. In Eisenberg RL (ed): Diagnostic Imaging: An Algorithmic Approach. Philadelphia, JB Lippincott, 1988)

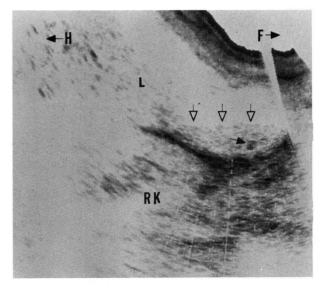

Fig. 60-17. Sludge. In addition to the sludge **(open arrows)** layered in the dependent portion of the gallbladder, there is also a small calculus **(closed arrow)**. Close attention to machine settings was necessary to avoid obscuring the stones. **L,** liver; **RK,** right kidney. (Margulis AR, Burhenne HJ (eds): Alimentary Tract Radiology. St. Louis, CV Mosby, 1983)

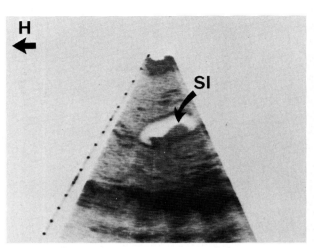

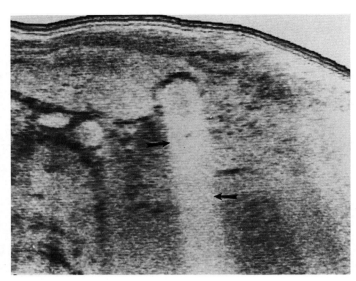

60-18   60-19

Fig. 60-18. Sludge. Focal rounded accumulation of sludge **(SI)** within the gallbladder of a young girl with right upper quadrant pain. No posterior acoustic shadow could be demonstrated emanating from this focus. (Margulis AR, Burhenne HJ (eds): Alimentary Tract Radiology. St. Louis, CV Mosby, 1983)

Fig. 60-19. Nonvisualization of the gallbladder lumen. The echogenic contour with posterior shadowing **(arrows)** from the gallbladder fossa is diagnostic of cholelithiasis. (Harned RK, Williams FM, Anderson JC: Gallbladder disease. In Eisenberg RL (ed): Diagnostic Imaging: An Algorithmic Approach, Philadelphia, JB Lippincott, 1988)

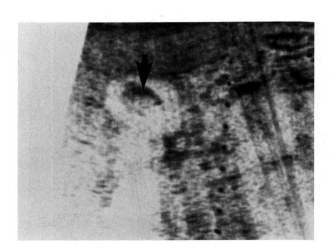

Fig. 60-20. Double-arcuate echo sign in nonvisualization of the gallbladder lumen. The outer arcuate contour is from the gallbladder wall, and the inner echogenic arc with acoustic shadowing is from gallstones **(arrow)**. (Harned RK, Williams FM, Anderson JC: Gallbladder disease. In Eisenberg RL (ed): Diagnostic Imaging: An Algorithmic Approach. Philadelphia, JB Lippincott, 1988)

gallstones are usually free of reverberations, whereas those caused by bowel gas are cluttered with reverberation artifacts. The differential diagnosis of the gallbladder without a sonolucent lumen includes previous cholecystectomy, gas in the gallbladder from biliary surgery or fistula, emphysematous cholecystitis, gallbladder wall calcification, nonfasting status, and extreme obesity.

Small gallstones (and occasionally large ones) can spontaneously disappear. This phenomenon is most likely due to the passage of gallstones through the cystic and common bile ducts into the duodenum without the production of symptoms of biliary colic. Stone dissolution and fistulous communication with the gastrointestinal tract are possible alternative mechanisms.

The optimal treatment of patients with asymptomatic gallstones is controversial. In general, surgeons have advocated early removal of the gallbladder because of the higher mortality and morbidity rates of cholecystectomy in the older age group and in patients with acute cholecystitis and common duct obstruction. Internists, confronted with the patient with silent stones, usually do not recommend operation since, in many patients, cholecystectomy will never prove necessary. In a recent long-term study of asymptomatic patients with asymptomatic gallstónes, only 10% developed symptoms and 7% required biliary tract operations. These data suggest that patients with asymptomatic gallstones can be followed by their physicians with reasonable safety.

HYPERPLASTIC CHOLECYSTOSES

The hyperplastic cholecystoses, noninflammatory disordersthatconsistofbenignproliferationofnormal tissue elements, include cholesterolosis and adenomyomatosis. Radiographically, cholesterolosis and adenomyomatosis have traditionally been associated with functional abnormalities of the gallbladder, such as hyperconcentration, hypercontractility, and hyperexcretion. In response to a fatty meal, gallbladder contraction in patients with these conditions has been reported to be hyperactive, with

rapid evacuation of the contrast-laden bile. However, these observations are anecdotal and have not been proven in any controlled study. The density of contrast material in the normal gallbladder is extremely variable, depending on the extent of the intestinal absorption of the contrast agent, and the rate and amount of emptying of the gallbladder in healthy individuals also varies over a wide range. Consequently, it is impossible to determine the concentration and rate and amount of emptying that are abnormal, and thus these features are not useful in establishing the diagnosis of either cholesterolosis or adenomyomatosis.

CHOLESTEROLOSIS

Cholesterolosis ("strawberry" gallbladder) is characterized by normal deposits of triglycerides, cholesterol precursers, and cholesterol esters in fat-laden macrophages in the lamina propria layer of the gallbladder wall. This fatty material causes coarse, yellow, speckled masses on the surface of a

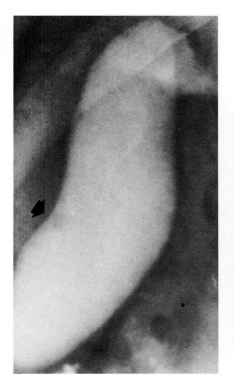
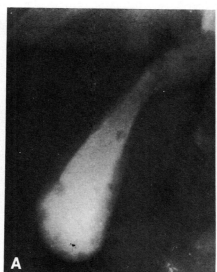
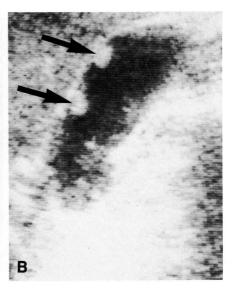

60-21   60-22

Fig. 60-21. *Cholesterol polyp* **(arrow)**.

Fig. 60-22. *Cholesterolosis.* **(A)** *Oral cholecystogram and* **(B)** *ultrasound show multiple discrete small polypoid defects adherent to the gallbladder wall. There was no movement with change in position in either study. No shadowing is present by ultrasound. (Simeone JF: The gallbladder: Pathology. In Taveras JM, Ferrucci JT (eds): Radiology: Diagnosis—Imaging—Intervention. Philadelphia, JB Lippincott, 1987)*

reddened, hyperemic gallbladder mucosa, an appearance resembling strawberry seeds.

Cholesterolosis can produce single or multiple small polypoid filling defects in the opacified gallbladder (Fig. 60-21). These lesions can occur in any portion of the gallbladder and have no malignant potential. The filling defects in cholesterolosis (as well as in adenomyomatosis) are best seen on radiographs made after partial emptying of the gallbladder. Compression or a fatty meal can also be employed to demonstrate the lesions to better advantage. The filling defect of cholesterolosis or adenomyomatosis is fixed in position with respect to the gallbladder wall, in contrast to gallstones, which move freely in response to gravity with changes in patient position. Cholesterol polyps are often attached to the gallbladder wall by delicate stalks. Spontaneous detachment of a cholesterol polyp can provide a nidus for gallstone formation.

On sonography, cholesterol polyps appear as nonshadowing, single or multiple fixed echoes that project into the lumen of the gallbladder (Fig. 60-22).

ADENOMYOMATOSIS

Adenomyomatosis is a proliferation of surface epithelium with glandlike formations and outpouchings of the mucosa into or through the thickened muscular layer. The sinuses (Rokitansky–Aschoff) associated with this form of intramural diverticulosis can be limited to a single segment (Fig. 60-23) or be scattered diffusely throughout the gallbladder (Fig. 60-24).

Radiographically, the Rokitansky–Aschoff sinuses appear as single or multiple oval collections of contrast material projected just outside the lumen of the gallbladder (Fig. 60-25). These opaque dots range in diameter from pinpoint size to 10 mm. When multiple and viewed tangentially, they resemble a string of beads closely applied to the circumference of the opacified gallbladder lumen. The clear line separating the opaque sacs from the gallbladder cavity represents the thickness of the mucosa and muscularis.

Adenomyomatosis is often associated with a focal circumferential narrowing of the lumen of the gallbladder caused by a septum or annular thicken-

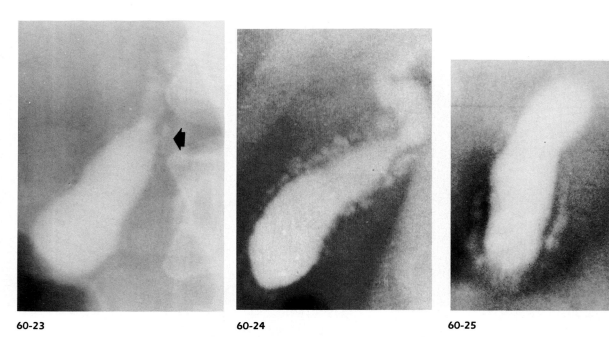

60-23   60-24   60-25

Fig. 60-23. Adenomyomatosis. Rokitansky-Aschoff sinuses are limited to the neck and upper body of the gallbladder **(arrow)**.

Fig. 60-24. Adenomyomatosis. Rokitansky–Aschoff sinuses are scattered diffusely throughout the gallbladder. (Berk RN, van der Vegt JH, Lichtenstein JE: The hyperplastic cholecystosis: Cholesterolosis and adenomyomatosis. Radiology 146:593–601, 1983)

Fig. 60-25. Rokitansky-Aschoff sinuses in adenomyomatosis. Collections of intramural contrast appear to parallel the opacified gallbladder lumen, from which they are separated by a lucent space representing the thickness of the mucosa and muscularis.

ing in the gallbladder wall (Fig. 60-26). Annular thickening can result in a pattern of multiple septal folds. The circumferential luminal narrowing in adenomyomatosis must be differentiated from a congenital infolding of the gallbladder wall, such as the Phrygian cap (see Fig. 60-39), which is usually thinner and smoother and involves only the fundus, whereas adenomyomatosis may affect any portion of the gallbladder. Gallstones are often present in patients with adenomyomatosis; they can be seen in a diverticular sinus or in the fundal portion of a septated gallbladder.

An adenomyoma is a single filling defect in the gallbladder that reflects a localized form of adenomyomatosis rather than a true neoplasm. It is almost invariably situated in the tip of the fundus. Radiographically, an adenomyoma is seen as an intramural mass projecting into the gallbladder (Fig. 60-27), often with an opaque central speck of contrast medium representing umbilication of the mound. Opaque dots representing intramural diverticula can often be seen at the periphery of the nodule. Overdistention of the gallbladder can camouflage the mass so that only the central area of umbilication is seen. When compression is applied, both the mass of the adenomyoma and the surrounding contrast-filled intramural diverticula can be visualized.

Sonography may demonstrate adenomyomatosis as focal (Fig. 60-28) or diffuse (Fig. 60-29) thickening of the gallbladder wall in association with anechoic cystic spaces. A repeat examination obtained after contraction of the gallbladder may be useful to distinguish adenomyomatosis from an abscess or perforation adjacent to the fundus or neck of the gallbladder. Anecdotal experience suggests that sonography is considerably less sensitive than oral cholecystography for the detection of adenomyomatosis.

Most patients with cholesterolosis or adenomyomatosis are asymptomatic, and the detection of these conditions on oral cholecystography may be entirely coincidental. Those symptoms that may be experienced are commonly vague and nondescript; classical biliary colic occurs only infrequently. Nevertheless, an appreciable proportion of patients with symptomatic cholesterolosis or adenomyomatosis improve after cholecystectomy, especially when the symptoms include recurrent biliary colic. Therefore, the presence of symptoms in these pa-

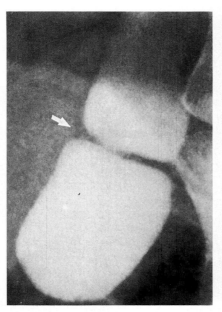
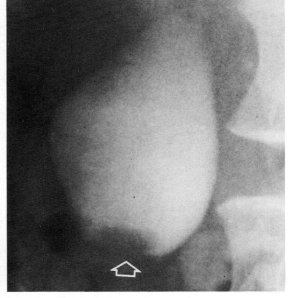

60-26   **60-27**

Fig. 60-26. *Segmental adenomyomatosis. Compartmentalization of the gallbladder produced by a thin septum* **(arrow)**. *(Berk RN, van der Vegt JH, Lichtenstein JE: The hyperplastic cholecystoses: Cholesterolosis and adenomyomatosis. Radiology 146:593–601, 1983)*

Fig. 60-27. *Solitary adenomyoma. A broad mass* **(arrow)** *is evident at the tip of the fundus of the gallbladder.*

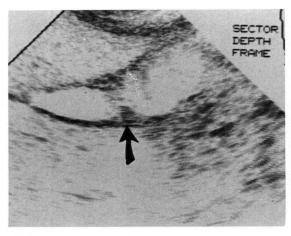

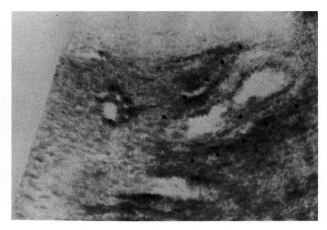

60-28   **60-29**

Fig. 60-28. Segmental adenomyomatosis. Localized circumferential thickening **(arrow)** of the gallbladder wall. (Harned RK, Williams FM, Anderson JC: Gallbladder disease. In Eisenberg RL (ed): Diagnostic Imaging: An Algorithmic Approach, Philadelphia, JB Lippincott, 1988)

Fig. 60-29. Diffuse adenomyomatosis. Generalized thickening of the gallbladder wall **(arrows)** with an area of focal prominence **(*)**. (Margulis AR, Burhenne HG (eds): Alimentary Tract Radiology, St. Louis, CV Mosby, 1983)

tients is usually considered an indication for surgical removal of the gallbladder, even if there are no demonstrable gallstones.

INFLAMMATORY POLYP

Inflammatory polyps are single or multiple localized projections of inflammatory tissue that occasionally develop during the course of chronic cholecystitis. In this condition, hyperplastic mucosa is associated with glandular proliferation, inflammatory cellular infiltrate, thickening of the wall of the gallbladder, prominence of Rokitansky–Aschoff sinuses, and intramural or luminal calculi. Chronic cholecystitis is clearly evident in the adjacent gallbladder mucosa.

BENIGN TUMORS

True benign neoplasms of the gallbladder are rare. Adenomatous polyps are composed primarily of glandular structures with a vascular stroma and minimal inflammatory change. Papillary adenomas (papillomas) have fine villous processes and a loose connective tissue stroma covered by columnar epithelium similar to that of the normal gallbladder (Fig. 60-30). Adenomatous polyps occur throughout the gallbladder, most commonly in or near the fundus. They are generally small and are often best seen on compression films or after a fatty meal. Adenomas are usually pedunculated and often multiple,

and they are commonly associated with gallstones and chronic cholecystitis. On oral cholecystography, an adenoma can present on tangential view

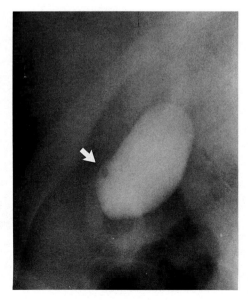

Fig. 60-30. Papillary adenoma **(arrow)**. (Ochsner SF: Solitary polypoid lesions of the gallbladder. Radiol Clin North Am 4:501–510, 1966)

as a notch in the contour of the gallbladder. The tumor appears as a round, fixed radiolucent filling defect on the *en face* projection.

An adenoma can produce symptoms if a small portion breaks off into the gallbladder and causes intermittent cystic duct obstruction. The tumor can also intussuscept and block the cystic duct; spontaneous reduction usually follows.

The report of several cases of carcinoma, usually *in situ*, arising in adenomas of the gallbladder has raised the possibility that these lesions are premalignant. This has created a controversy as to the proper approach to patients with fixed radiolucent filling defects in the gallbladder. Because the risk of carcinoma in a patient with a gallbladder tumor but no calculi is extremely small, the majority opinion holds that, if there are no significant symptoms, there is no indication for cholecystectomy.

Other rarely reported benign tumors of the gallbladder include fibroadenoma, cystadenoma, neurinoma, carcinoid, hemangioma, and tumors of mixed cellular elements.

MALIGNANT TUMORS

CARCINOMA OF THE GALLBLADDER

Carcinoma of the gallbladder usually causes nonvisualization of the organ on oral cholecystography. This is due to obstruction of the cystic duct by an invasive tumor or to the presence of associated chronic cholecystitis or cholelithiasis, which almost invariably accompanies gallbladder cancer. On rare occasions, noninvasive carcinoma appears as a solitary, fixed polyp (Fig. 60-31) or an irregular mural filling defect in a well-opacified gallbladder (Fig. 60-32).

Carcinoma of the gallbladder primarily affects the elderly. Like cholelithiasis, it has a high predominance in women. Cholelithiasis is present in about 80% to 90% of patients with gallbladder carcinoma and is widely considered to be an important predisposing condition.

Most primary carcinomas of the gallbladder are adenocarcinomas; squamous tumors also occur oc-

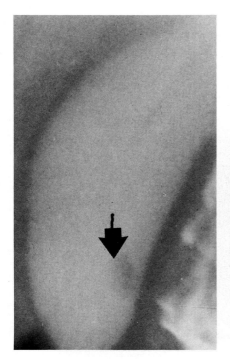

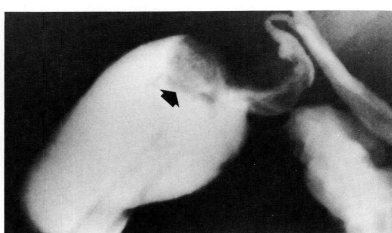

60-31   60-32

Fig. 60-31. Carcinoma of the gallbladder appearing as a discrete filling defect **(arrow)** in a well-opacified gallbladder. (Cimmino CV: Carcinoma in a well-functioning gallbladder. Radiology 71:563–564, 1958)

Fig. 60-32. Carcinoma of the gallbladder. There is an irregular mural mass **(arrow)** with tumor growth extending into the cystic duct.

casionally. In its early stages, carcinoma of the gallbladder is nearly always asymptomatic; if symptoms do occur, they are secondary to coexisting cholecystitis or cholelithiasis. More severe symptoms, such as obstructive jaundice; right upper quadrant pain, anorexia, weight loss, and fatigue, do not appear until the tumor is well advanced and has spread beyond the gallbladder. Carcinoma of the gallbladder is usually rapidly progressive and almost invariably fatal. Death occurs within 1 year of diagnosis in 80% of patients; the 5-year survival rate is a dismal 1% to 5%.

Carcinomas of the gallbladder tend to arise in the body of the organ. The tumor can appear as a bulky mass within or around the gallbladder; scirrhous reaction resulting in thickening and rigidity of the wall can produce a contracted, fibrotic gallbladder. Carcinoma occasionally arises in the cystic duct. Regardless of the site of origin, obstruction of the cystic duct is common and is due either to direct extension of the tumor or to extrinsic compression by spread to adjacent lymph nodes. Local metastases to the porta hepatis and liver are frequent.

The detection of extensive calcification in the wall of the gallbladder ("porcelain gallbladder") should suggest the possibility of carcinoma (Fig. 60-33). Although porcelain gallbladder is uncommon in cases of carcinoma of the gallbladder, the incidence of carcinoma in porcelain gallbladders (up to 60% of cases) is striking. It is generally agreed that carcinoma occurs in the porcelain gallbladder with sufficient frequency to warrant prophylactic

cholecystectomy in patients with this condition, even when the disease is asymptomatic.

If a carcinoma of the gallbladder contains mucinous elements, plain abdominal radiographs occasionally demonstrate fine punctate calcifications in the right upper quadrant similar to the calcifications caused by tumors of the same cell type in the colon. Another plain radiographic sign of carcinoma of the gallbladder is the presence of a local, irregular accumulation of gas in the center of the tumor mass (not in the biliary tree). Such gas accumulation is due to a fistulous connection between the gallbladder and the intestinal tract (usually transverse colon or duodenum) and has been considered almost diagnostic of carcinoma of the gallbladder.

Both ultrasound and computed tomography may be valuable in demonstrating carcinoma of the gallbladder and the extent of tumor spread. The most common manifestation of carcinoma of the gallbladder on ultrasound or CT is a mass in the gallbladder fossa with extension into the liver (Fig. 60-34). Frequently associated findings include thickening of the gallbladder wall, a fixed intraluminal gallbladder mass (Fig. 60-35), gallstones, biliary obstruction, nodal involvement (Fig. 60-36), and hematogenous metastases. Percutaneous transhepatic cholangiography can permit biliary decompression and localize the point of bile duct obstruction secondary to direct tumor extension or nodal involvement (if neither CT nor ultrasound can provide this information).

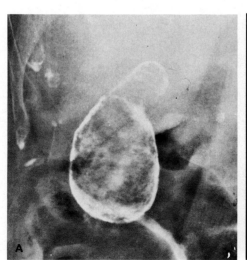
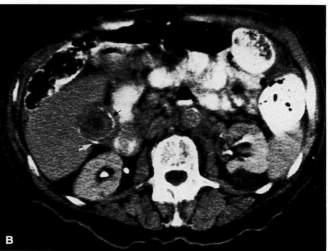

Fig. 60-33. Porcelain gallbladder. **(A)** Plain radiograph demonstrates extensive mural calcification around the perimeter of the gallbladder. **(B)** CT scan in another patient shows calcification of the gallbladder wall **(arrows)**.

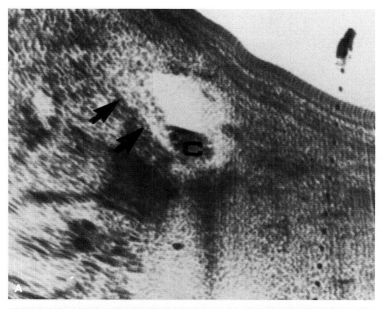

Fig. 60-34. Carcinoma of the gallbladder. **(A)** Ultrasound shows cholelithiasis **(C)** and asymmetric thickening of the posterior gallbladder wall **(arrows)**. **(B)** CT shows an irregular mass **(arrows)** arising from the wall of the contrast-filled gallbladder **(arrowheads)**. (Harned RK, Williams FM, Anderson JC: Gallbladder disease. In Eisenberg RL (ed): Diagnostic Imaging: An Algorithmic Approach, Philadelphia, JB Lippincott, 1988)

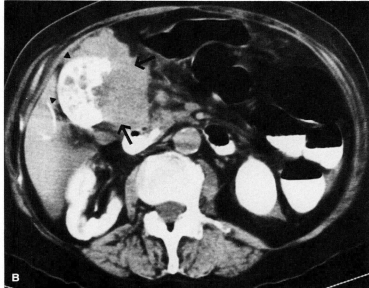

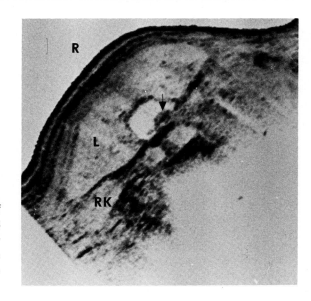

Fig. 60-35. Carcinoma of the gallbladder. Transverse sonogram of the right upper abdomen demonstrates a focal gallbladder mass **(arrow)** that was not dependent or associated with acoustic shadowing. **RK,** right kidney. (Courtesy Dr. James Waskey). (Margulis AR, Burhenne HG (eds): Alimentary Tract Radiology, St. Louis, CV Mosby, 1983)

Other malignant neoplasms of the gallbladder (carcinoid, leiomyosarcoma) very rarely occur. They have no distinctive clinical or radiographic features.

METASTASES

Radiographically apparent hematogenous metastases to the gallbladder are rare and are almost always secondary to metastatic melanoma. Metastases to the gallbladder, however, are not rare in melanoma, occurring in about 15% of patients with the disease (Fig. 60-37). These lesions are usually flat subepithelial nodules that can become polypoid and even pedunculated in the gallbladder lumen. On oral cholecystography, they can occasionally be identified as single or multiple fixed filling defects in an opacified gallbladder. The largest defect is frequently more than 10 mm in diameter, in contrast to most benign lesions, which seldom exceed 7 mm. The "bull's-eye" appearance (large central ulceration) that is characteristic of metastatic melanoma to the bowel is rarely seen when this tumor involves the gallbladder. At times, a large, bulky filling defect in the gallbladder is the first clinical manifestation of melanoma. Metastases to the gallbladder from carcinomas of the lung, kidney, and esophagus have been reported.

OTHER DISORDERS

PARASITE GRANULOMA

Parasitic infestations of the gallbladder very rarely form tumorlike nodules. In patients with *Ascaris lumbricoides* and *Paragonimus westermanii*, eggs deposited in the wall of the gallbladder incite an intense inflammatory cell infiltration (parasite granuloma) that can appear as a filling defect in an opacified gallbladder.

METACHROMATIC LEUKODYSTROPHY

In patients with metachromatic leukodystrophy, a deficiency of the enzyme arylsulfatase-A permits metachromatic sulfatides to deposit in various organs, especially in the central nervous system. Deposition of this substance in macrophages in the mucosa of the gallbladder leads to a progressive inability of the gallbladder to concentrate bile and, rarely, to the formation of single or multiple filling defects.

FIBROXANTHOGRANULOMATOUS INFLAMMATION

Tumorlike nodules of gray-yellow, fat-containing tissue with ulceration of the overlying gallbladder

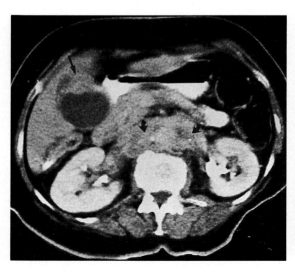

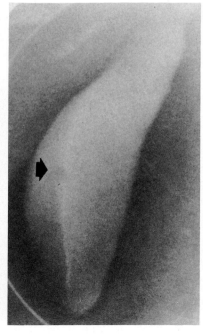

Fig. 60-36. Carcinoma of the gallbladder. CT scan demonstrates a soft-tissue mass along the anterior wall of the gallbladder **(straight arrow)**. Note the para-aortic nodal metastases **(curved arrow)**.

Fig. 60-37. Melanoma metastatic to the gallbladder. A sessile lesion appears as a single fixed filling defect **(arrow)** within the opacified gallbladder.

60-36

60-37

mucosa can be seen in fibroxanthogranulomatous inflammation. This diffuse inflammatory reaction of the gallbladder is very rare and is always associated with acute or chronic cholecystitis, usually with cholelithiasis.

INTRAMURAL EPITHELIAL CYST

Intramural epithelial cysts of the gallbladder are extremely rare. They are reported to present on oral cholecystography as large, smooth intramural defects (Fig. 60-38).

PSEUDOPOLYPS

A variety of pseudopolyps can appear on oral cholecystography as fixed filling defects that simulate true tumors of the gallbladder. A projectional artifact due to folding or coiling of the junction between the neck of the gallbladder and the cystic duct can produce a pseudodefect. A similar defect is occasionally seen when the cystic duct is viewed *en face*, superimposed on the neck of the gallbladder. The cystic duct orifice appears radiolucent because it is not distended at the time the radiograph is made, thereby creating a summation artifact. Placing the patient in a variety of positions will cause this false filling defect to disappear, thereby differentiating it from a true lesion.

Congenital folds or septa within the gallbladder can simulate the appearance of polypoid lesions. The Phyrgian cap is a developmental anomaly in which an incomplete septum extends across the fundus of the gallbladder, partially separating it from the body (Fig. 60-39). Although of no clinical

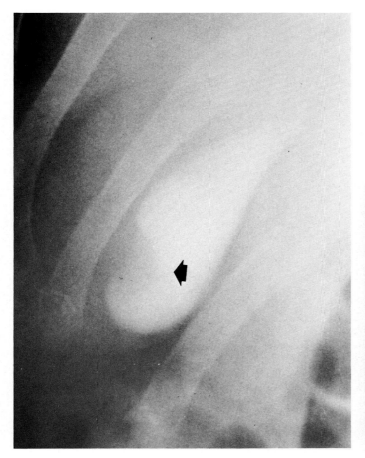

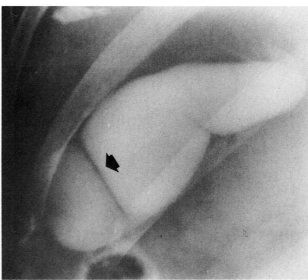

60-38

60-39

Fig. 60-38. Epithelial cyst of the gallbladder appearing as a large marginal filling defect **(arrow)** on cholecystography. (Ochsner SF, Blalock JB: Epithelial cyst of the gallbladder. Am J Surg 108:419–420, 1964)

Fig. 60-39. Phyrgian cap. An incomplete septum **(arrow)** extends across the fundus of the gallbladder, partially separating it from the body.

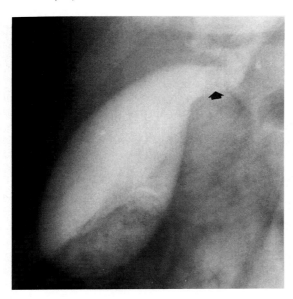

Fig. 60-40. Heterotopic pancreatic tissue implanted intramurally appearing as ill-defined lucencies **(arrow)** in the neck of the gallbladder.

significance, this congenital deformity must be differentiated from localized adenomyomatosis. In a multiseptate gallbladder, the organ is divided into a variable number of intercommunicating chambers. These are lined by mucosa with an underlying muscular coat that may contain Rokitansky–Aschoff sinuses. This anomaly appears to arise during the embryonic stage from persistence of a folding mechanism in the formation of the gallbladder. The gallbladder is usually shrunken and has a characteristic multicystic, honeycomb appearance. The mechanically obstructive features of this anomaly predispose to bile stasis and stone formation.

A rare cause of filling defects in the gallbladder is heterotopic gastric or pancreatic tissue implanted in the gallbladder wall. This condition is usually associated with nonvisualization of the gallbladder on oral cholecystography. Intermittent obstruction due to a ball-valve action of the polyp of heterotopic tissue presumably allows mucus secretions to pass out of the gallbladder but does not permit contrast-laden bile to enter. This partial or intermittent obstruction accounts for the typical symptoms of episodic right upper quadrant pain, nausea, vomiting, and fatty food intolerance that simulate acute cholecystitis. When the gallbladder is opacified, heterotopic gastric or pancreatic tissue can appear as single or multiple mural nodules, most frequently in the neck of the gallbladder or cystic duct (Fig. 60-40).

BIBLIOGRAPHY

Becker CD, Hassler H, Terrier F: Preoperative diagnosis of the Mirizzi syndrome: Limitations of sonography and computed axial tomography. AJR 143:591–596, 1984

Bentivegna S, Hirschl S: Heterotopic gastric mucosa in the gallbladder presenting as a symptom-producing tumor. Am J Gastroenterol 57:423–428, 1972

Berk RN, Armbuster TG, Saltzstein SL: Carcinoma in the porcelain gallbladder. Radiology 106:29–31, 1973

Berk RN, Clemett AR: Radiology of the Gallbladder and Bile Ducts. Philadelphia, WB Saunders, 1977

Berk RN, van der Vegt JH, Lichtenstein JE: The hyperplastic cholecystoses: Cholesterolosis and adenomyomatosis. Radiology 146:593–601, 1983

Christensen AH, Ishak KG: Benign tumors and pseudotumors of the gallbladder. Report of 180 cases. Arch Pathol 90:423–432, 1970

Cooperberg PL, Burhenne HJ: Real-time ultrasonography: Diagnostic techniques of choice in calculous gallbladder disease. N Engl J Med 300:1277–1278, 1980

Croce EJ: The multiseptate gallbladder. Arch Surg 107:104–105, 1973

Evans RC, Kaude JV, Steinberg W: Spontaneous disappearance of large stones from the common bile duct. Gastrointest Radiol 5:47–48, 1980

Harned RK, Babbitt DP: Cholelithiasis in children. Radiology 117:391–393, 1975

Jutras JA: Hyperplastic cholecystoses. AJR 83:795–827, 1960

Jutras JA, Levesque HP: Adenomyoma and adenomyomatosis of the gallbladder: Radiologic and pathologic correlations. Radiol Clin North Am 4:483–500, 1966

Kleinman P, Winchester P, Volberg F: Sulfatide cholecystosis. Gastrointest Radiol 1:99–100, 1976

Krook PM, Allen FH, Bush WH et al: Comparison of real-time cholecystosonography and oral cholecystography. Radiology 135:145–153, 1980

Martinez LO, Gregg M: Aberrant pancreas in the gallbladder. J Can Assoc Radiol 24:234–235, 1973

McGregor JC, Cordiner JW: Papilloma of the gallbladder. Br J Surg 61:356–358, 1974

McSherry CK, Ferstenberg H, Calhoun WF et al: The natural history of diagnosed gallstone disease in symptomatic and asymptomatic patients. Ann Surg 202:59–63, 1985

Melson GL, Reiter F, Evens RG: Tumorous conditions of the gallbladder. Semin Roentgenol 11:269–282, 1976

Meyers MA, O'Donohue N: The Mercedes–Benz sign: Insight into the dynamics of formation and disappearance of gallstones. AJR 119:63–70, 1973

Niv Y, Kosakov K, Shcolnik B: Fragile papilloma (papillary adenoma) of the gallbladder. Gastroenterology 91:999–1001, 1986

Ochsner SF: Solitary polypoid lesions of the gallbladder. Radiol Clin North Am 14:501–510, 1966

Ochsner SF: Intramural lesions of the gallbladder. AJR 113:1–9, 1971

Rice J, Sauerbrei EE, Semogas P et al: Sonographic appearance of adenomyomatosis of the gallbladder. J Clin Ultra 9:336–337, 1981

Shimkin PM, Soloway MS, Jaffe E: Metastatic melanoma of the gallbladder. AJR 116:393–395, 1972

Yeh HC: Ultrasonography and computed tomography of carcinoma of the gallbladder. Radiology 133:167–173, 1979

FILLING DEFECTS IN THE BILE DUCTS

61

Disease Entities

Biliary calculi
  Mirizzi syndrome
Artifacts (Pseudocalculi)
  Contraction of the sphincter of Oddi
  Air bubble
  Blood clot
  Right hepatic artery
  Bile duct varices
Neoplasms
  Malignant tumors
    Cholangiocarcinoma
    Ampullary carcinoma
    Hepatoma
    Villous adenoma
    Metastases
    Sarcoma botryoides
    Tumor-induced mucus/floating tumor debris
  Benign tumors
    Adenoma
    Papilloma
    Fibroma
    Lipoma
    Neuroma
    Cystadenoma
    Hamartoma
    Carcinoid

Parasites
  Clonorchis sinensis
  Ascaris lumbricoides
  Fasciola hepatica
  Echinococcus
Oriental cholangiohepatitis

BILIARY CALCULI

Biliary calculi are the most common filling defects seen in the opacified bile duct (Fig. 61-1). They usually arise in the gallbladder and reach the bile duct either by passage through the cystic duct or by fistulous erosion through the wall of the gallbladder (Fig. 61-2). Calculi rarely originate in either the extrahepatic or the intrahepatic bile ducts, except in patients with congenital or acquired cystic dilatation of bile ducts or strictures due to biliary obstruction (Fig. 61-3). Stones in the extrahepatic bile ducts tend to move freely and change location with alteration in patient position. However, a calculus can become impacted in the distal common duct and cause obstruction (Fig. 61-4). The impacted stone can usually be diagnosed with confidence because of the characteristic appearance of a smooth, sharply defined meniscus (Fig. 61-5). Occasionally, an irregular stone ("mulberry stone") simulates a polypoid tumor.

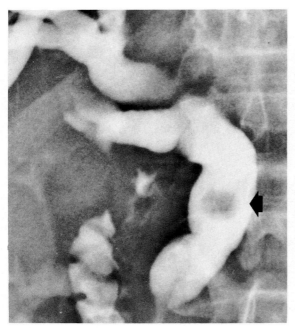

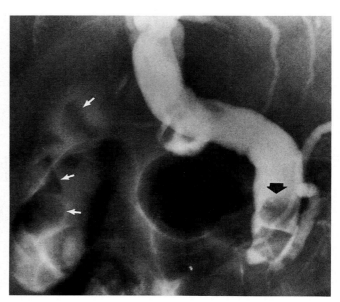

61-1

61-2

Fig. 61-1. Common bile duct stone **(arrow)**.

Fig. 61-2. Calculi seen within both the common bile duct **(black arrow)** and the gallbladder **(white arrows)**.

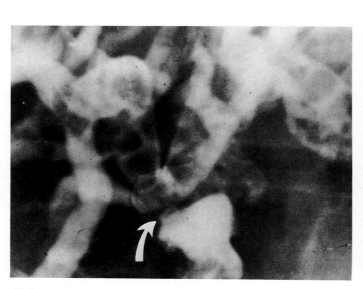

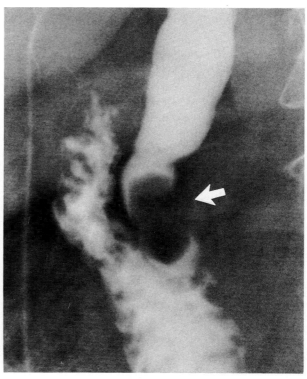

61-3

61-4

Fig. 61-3. Multiple hepatic duct stones in a patient who developed a stricture at the junction of the left and right hepatic ducts **(arrow)**. This juncture was the site of an anastomosis with the jejunum for a previous distal bile duct stricture.

Fig. 61-4. Impacted ampullary stone **(arrow)** with an unusual peanut-shaped configuration.

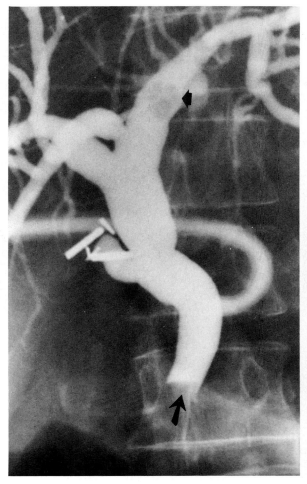

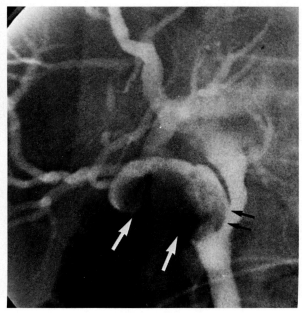

61-5   61-6

Fig. 61-5.   Impacted ampullary stone producing the characteristic appearance of a smooth, sharply defined meniscus in the distal common bile duct **(long arrow).** Note the second large stone **(short arrow)** in the left hepatic duct.

Fig. 61-6.   Mirizzi syndrome. ERCP demonstrates a stone **(white arrows)** that has penetrated into the common hepatic duct causing obstruction with stenosis. The shrunken gallbladder is opacified by a cholecystobiliary fistula **(black arrows).** The cystic duct was not identified at surgery. (Becker CD, Hassler H, Terrier F: Preoperative diagnosis of the Mirizzi syndrome: Limitations of sonography and computed tomography. AJR 143:591–596, 1984. Copyright 1984. Reproduced with permission)

MIRIZZI SYNDROME

The Mirizzi syndrome refers to partial obstruction of the common hepatic duct resulting from inflammation associated with an impacted stone in the cystic duct or neck of the gallbladder. This uncommon condition has been reported to occur most frequently in patients who have a cystic duct running a parallel course (up to 3 cm in length) with the common hepatic duct. The lumens of the cystic and common hepatic ducts can share a common outer sheath and be separated by only a thin septum. With chronic inflammation of the gallbladder, progressive foreshortening of the gallbladder neck and cystic duct eventually causes compression and partial obstruction of the adjacent common duct (Fig. 61-6). The impression on the common duct is usually noted on its lateral aspect (Fig. 61-7), though medial impressions and concentric narrowing have been reported. Continued inflammation and pressure necrosis can permit a stone in the neck of the gallbladder or cystic duct to erode into the common

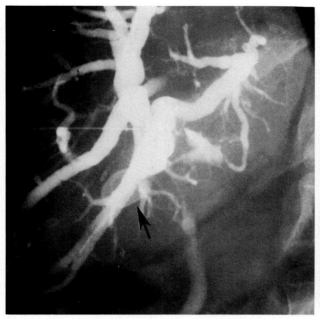

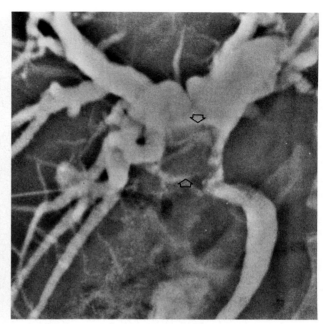

61-7   61-8

Fig. 61-7. Mirizzi syndrome. Transhepatic cholangiogram shows a dilated intrahepatic ductal system and pronounced narrowing of the common hepatic duct by a calcified impacted gallstone **(arrow).** (Cruz FO, Barriga P, Tocornal J et al: Radiology of the Mirizzi syndrome: Diagnostic importance of the transhepatic cholangiogram. Gastrointest Radiol 8:249–253, 1983)

Fig. 61-8. Mirizzi syndrome. Transhepatic cholangiogram shows a filling defect in the common hepatic duct **(arrows)** due to a large gallstone penetrating from the cystic duct. At surgery, this jaundiced patient was shown to have a fistula from the neck of the gallbladder to the common hepatic duct. (Cruz FO, Barriga P, Tocornal J et al: Radiology of the Mirizzi syndrome: Diagnostic importance of the transhepatic cholangiogram. Gastrointest Radiol 8:249–253, 1983)

hepatic duct (Fig. 61-8), producing a single cavity with diffuse mural inflammation and some degree of duct obstruction.

The diagnosis of Mirizzi syndrome is difficult to make preoperatively by radiographic studies. The gallbladder is usually not visualized on oral cholecystography in patients with this syndrome and may be only faintly opacified on intravenous cholangiography. The diagnosis of Mirizzi syndrome should be suggested whenever narrowing or a compression defect is seen in the common bile duct at or just above the level at which the cystic duct is thought to insert. On rare occasions, multiple filling defects representing small stones can be radiographically demonstrated in a single large cavity in a patient with the Mirizzi syndrome.

A major complication of the Mirizzi syndrome is the danger that, at operation, the surgeon can be confused by the altered anatomy and consider a single large cavity consisting of the gallbladder or cystic duct and the common hepatic duct to represent the gallbladder itself. If this occurs, the surgeon may inadvertently ligate and transect the common bile duct, thinking it to be the cystic duct draining a large gallbladder. If the common duct is ligated, obstructive jaundice rapidly ensues. Transection of the duct results in a persistent biliary fistula.

The Mirizzi syndrome can also occur in patients with large cystic duct remnants after cholecystectomy. This is most frequent in patients in whom the cystic duct has a long course parallel with the common bile duct and a low insertion into it. The cystic duct remnant can gradually increase in size and become a site of bile stasis, chronic inflammation, and stone formation; occasionally, it obstructs the adjacent common bile duct.

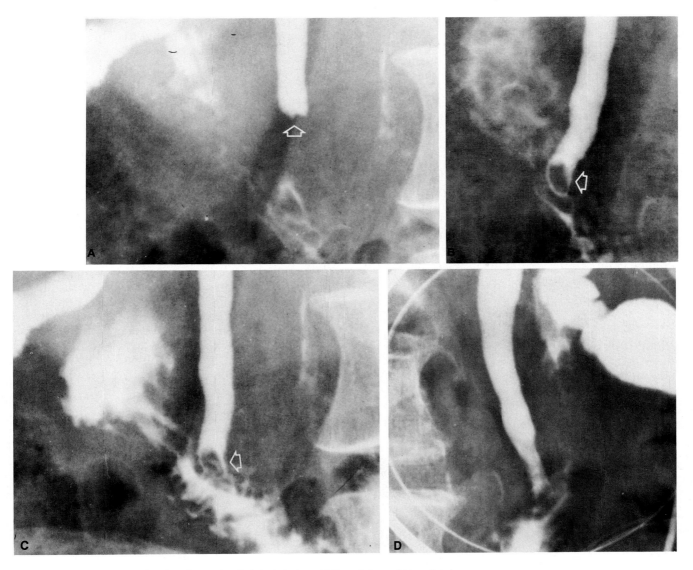

Fig. 61-9. Pseudocalculus. **(A)** Smooth, slightly lobulated filling defect of the distal common bile duct simulating an impacted stone **(arrow)**. Note, however, that some contrast has already flowed into the duodenum. **(B)**, **(C)** Contrast has encircled the stonelike filling defect **(arrows)** in two projections. **(D)** Following relaxation of the sphincter of Oddi, the distal common bile duct appears normal, and contrast flows freely into the duodenum.

ARTIFACTS (PSEUDOCALCULI)

CONTRACTION OF THE SPHINCTER OF ODDI

Cyclic contraction of the sphincter of Oddi can produce a smooth, arcuate filling defect in the distal portion of the common bile duct that closely simulates an impacted gallstone (Fig. 61-9A). This pseudocalculus effect is often seen on operative cholangiograms after surgical manipulation or instrumentation of the common bile duct. Occasion-

ally, it can be demonstrated on intravenous cholangiography. Unlike an impacted stone, the pseudocalculus never obstructs the bile duct, and some contrast flows into the duodenum when the sphincter relaxes or after glucagon has been administered. Serial radiographs or cine examination may be necessary to demonstrate the cyclic, phasic contraction and relaxation of the sphincter (Fig. 61-9B, C, D); the pseudocalculus appears during the contracted phase and disappears as the sphincter relaxes.

AIR BUBBLE

Air bubbles are a particularly vexing cause of artifactual filling defects in the bile duct during T-tube cholangiography. They are smooth, round, and generally multiple, unlike biliary calculi, which are frequently faceted and have a straight border. For an air bubble artifact to be distinguished from a stone in the bile duct, the patient should be raised toward an upright position. Air bubbles are lighter than contrast-laden bile and tend to rise toward the proximal portion of the biliary tree; however, true calculi tend to remain in a stationary position or fall with gravity. If the nature of the lucent filling defect remains in doubt, the examination should be repeated on the following day. Careful prefilling of the injection syringe and tubing should decrease the chance of air bubbles being introduced into the biliary tree during T-tube cholangiography.

BLOOD CLOT

Blood clots are an unusual cause of filling defects in the bile ducts. The margins of blood clots are generally not as smooth as those of biliary calculi. Clots are softer and more easily molded and thus tend to elongate within the duct, rather than having the generally spheroid configuration of stones in the bile ducts.

RIGHT HEPATIC ARTERY

Extrinsic pressure by the right hepatic artery on the posterior aspect of the common hepatic duct immediately distal to the confluence of the right and left hepatic ducts may be the cause of a pseudocalculus in the biliary tree (Fig. 61-10A). The eccentric nature of this vascular impression can be demonstrated when the patient is placed in the lateral position (Fig. 61-10B).

BILE DUCT VARICES

Following extrahepatic obstruction of the portal vein, multiple collateral veins may develop within the hepatoduodenal ligament around the common bile duct. These collateral veins anastomose with the cystic and pyloric veins, which drain into the main portal vein. Radiographically, these variceal channels produce smooth extrinsic impressions

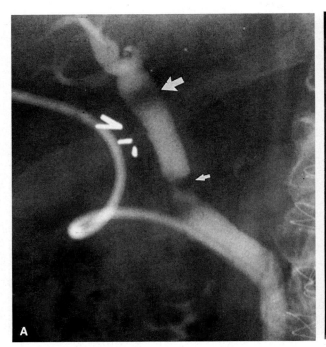 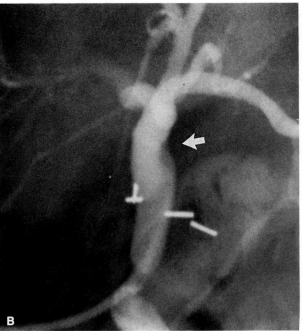

Fig. 61-10. *Pseudocalculus due to the right hepatic artery.* **(A)** Frontal view of a T-tube cholangiogram shows a deformity at the site of T-tube insertion **(small arrow)**. A defect with indistinct borders is noted proximal to the bifurcation of the common bile duct **(large arrow)**. **(B)** The latter defect becomes eccentric with sloping margins when the patient is in the lateral position, indicating an extrinsic pressure defect caused by the right hepatic artery. (Baer JW, Adiri M: Right hepatic artery as a cause of pseudocalculus in the biliary tree. Gastrointest Radiol 7:269–273, 1982)

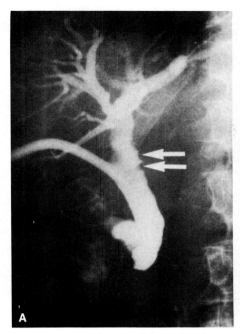

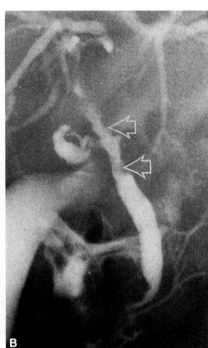

Fig. 61-11. Bile duct varices. **(A)** T-tube cholangiogram shows scalloped defects **(arrows)** representing varices in the common hepatic and common bile ducts. **(B)** ERCP shows a similar pattern of scalloped defects representing varices **(arrows)**. (Spira R, Widrich WC, Keusch KD et al: Bile duct varices. Arch Surg 120:1194–1196, 1985)

along the common bile duct or nodular defects that may simulate calculi adherent to the wall (Fig. 61-11). Recognition of choledochal varices is important because they may cause partial obstruction of the bile duct or excessive bleeding during biliary surgery.

NEOPLASMS

MALIGNANT TUMORS

Primary malignant lesions of the bile duct (cholangiocarcinoma) occasionally present as filling defects within the common hepatic or bile ducts (Fig. 61-12). However, due to the intense ductal fibrosis that often accompanies the carcinoma, these tumors more typically appear as irregular strictures. A carcinoma of the ampulla that abruptly occludes the common bile duct can be associated with a markedly irregular intraluminal polypoid mass. One manifestation of hepatoma is a bulky intraluminal filling defect in a proximal extrahepatic duct that often causes obstructive jaundice. In the rare villous tumor arising in the common bile duct (Fig. 61-13), or extending into it from the duodenum (Fig. 61-14), contrast enters the interstices of the lesion,

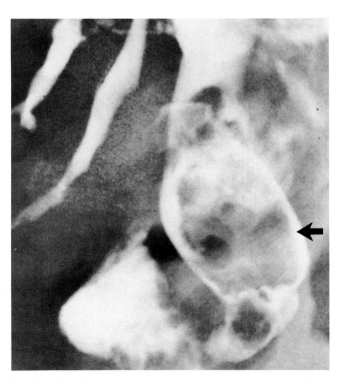

Fig. 61-12. Cholangiocarcinoma presenting as a large filling defect **(arrow)** in the common bile duct.

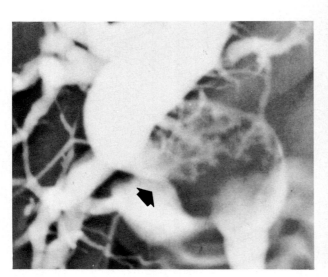

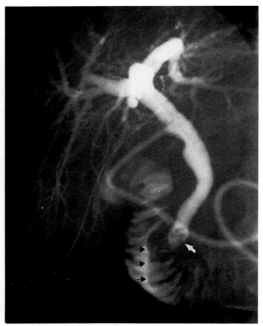

61-13   61-14

Fig. 61-13. Villous adenocarcinoma of the common bile duct **(arrow)**. Contrast is seen entering the interstices of the lesion.

Fig. 61-14. Duodenal villous tumor. There is an obstructing lesion **(white arrow)** characterized by fronds projecting into the bile duct lumen and producing a feathery margin. Note the large mass in the duodenum **(black arrows)**. (Janes JO, Laughlin CL, Goldberger LE et al: Differential features of some unusual biliary tumors. Gastrointest Radiol 7:341–348, 1982)

as it does also in neoplasms of this cell type elsewhere in the gastrointestinal tract.

Autopsy series of patients with various neoplasms (lung, melanoma, lymphoma) have shown secondary metastatic deposits in extrahepatic ducts in approximately 1% to 2% of cases. Metastases to the bile ducts can produce single (Fig. 61-15) or multiple (Fig. 61-16) intraluminal filling defects of various sizes.

The sarcoma botryoides variant of rhabdomyosarcoma can rarely develop as a primary neoplasm in the biliary tree in young children. The slow-growing lesion infiltrates along the wall of the bile ducts and produces grapelike intraluminal projections that may eventually become large enough to cause biliary obstruction (Fig. 61-17). Early diagnosis of biliary sarcoma botryoides is important because the tumor is responsive to both radiation and chemotherapy.

Tumor-induced mucus (Fig. 61-18) and floating tumor debris (Fig. 61-19) can also cause filling defects in the biliary tree. Masses of thick mucus in the

bile duct may be produced by benign or malignant tumors of the pancreas, gallbladder, or liver. Tumor debris may arise from a neoplasm that directly invades the bile duct or from necrosis of a tumor mass that is adjacent to a major bile duct. Free-floating debris is a cause of intermittent biliary obstruction, the site of which may be in close proximity to or quite distant from the main tumor mass depending both on the size of the duct and the tumor fragments.

BENIGN TUMORS

Benign tumors of the extrahepatic biliary ducts are rare. Most of the lesions that have been reported are primarily adenomas (Fig. 61-20) and papillomas. They usually appear as small polypoid filling defects, often with some element of obstruction. Extremely rare tumors of the bile duct include fibromas, lipomas, neuromas, cystadenomas (Fig. 61-21), hamartomas, and carcinoids.

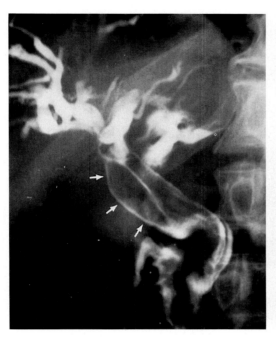

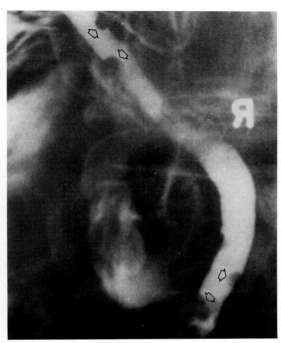

61-15   61-16

Fig. 61-15. Metastasis from carcinoma of the colon. Transhepatic cholangiogram shows contrast material streaming around a large defect that fills virtually all the lumen of the common bile duct **(arrows)**. Note also the elevation of the right hepatic duct by an intrahepatic secondary lesion. (Gray RR, Mackenzie RL, Alan KP: Cholangiographic demonstration of carcinoma of the colon metastatic to the lumen of the common bile duct. Gastrointest Radiol 7:71–72, 1982)

Fig. 61-16. Metastatic melanoma. Multiple small, round smooth intraluminal defects **(arrows)** in the common hepatic and bile ducts. (Janes JO, Laughlin CL, Goldberger LE et al: Differential features of some unusual biliary tumors. Gastrointest Radiol 7:341–348, 1982)

PARASITES

ASCARIS LUMBRICOIDES

The migration of *Ascaris lumbricoides* from the intestines to the biliary tract can result in partial obstruction complicated by cholangitis, cholecystitis, and liver abscess. Biliary ascariasis can also cause pancreatitis either by the mechanical effect of the worm in the common duct or by its migration into the main pancreatic duct. As in *Ascaris* infestation of the intestine, worms in the biliary system produce characteristic long, linear filling defects with tapering ends (Fig. 61-22). At times, the filling defect caused by the worm can be seen extending through the papilla of Vater into the proximal descending duodenum. Worms coiled in the bile duct may appear as more discrete masses.

LIVER FLUKES

Liver flukes (*Clonorchis sinensis* and *Fasciola hepatica*) can produce filling defects in the biliary system (Fig. 61-23). *Clonorchis* has two intermediate

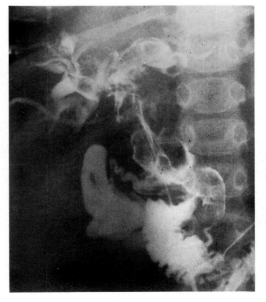

Fig. 61-17. Sarcoma botryoides. There are grapelike projections from a large bulky intraluminal mass. (Janes JO, Laughlin CL, Goldberger LE et al: Differential features of some unusual biliary tumors. Gastrointest Radiol 7:341–348, 1982)

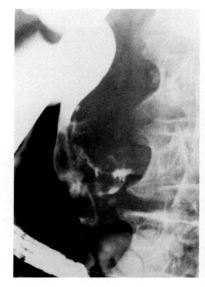
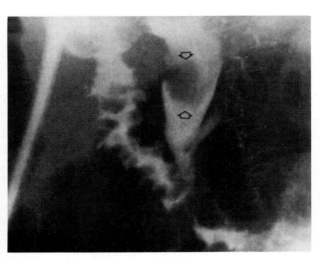

61-18   **61-19**

Fig. 61-18.   Tumor-induced mucus. ERCP shows a diffuse filling defect in the biliary tree and pancreatic duct due to a large mass of mucinous material produced by a benign cystic tumor in the head of the pancreas. (Smith E, Matzen P: Mucus-producing tumors with mucinous biliary obstruction causing jaundice: Diagnosed and treated endoscopically. Am J Gastroenterol 80:287–289, 1985)

Fig. 61-19.   Floating tumor debris. Intraoperative cholangiogram shows a large filling defect **(arrows)** in the distal common bile duct due to metastases from colon carcinoma. (Roslyn JJ, Kuchenbecker S, Longmier WP et al: Floating tumor debris: A cause of intermittent biliary obstruction. Arch Surg 119:1312–1315, 1984)

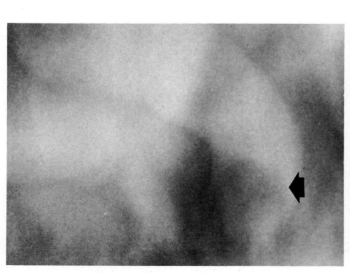
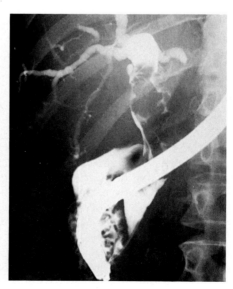

61-20   **61-21**

Fig. 61-20.   Adenomatous polyp **(arrow)** of the common bile duct seen on intravenous cholangiography.

Fig. 61-21.   Cystadenoma. ERCP demonstrates a large, multilobular tumor mass in the common bile duct that extends proximally to the hilum and distally to about 2 cm from the papilla. (van Steenbergen W, Ponette E, Marchal G et al: Cystadenoma of the common bile duct demonstrated by endoscopic retrograde cholangiopancreatography: An uncommon cause of extrahepatic obstruction. Am J Gastroenterol 79:466–470, 1984)

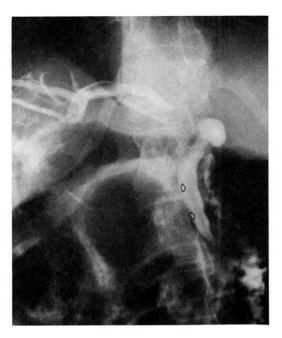

Fig. 61-22. Ascariasis. A worm in the biliary system produces a characteristic long, linear filling defect **(arrows)**.

hosts, a snail and then a freshwater fish. Humans acquire the infection by eating the raw or partially cooked fish. *Fasciola* infects persons in sheep-growing areas who ingest pond water or watercress contaminated with the metacercarial form of the fluke life cycle. The adult worms in both these conditions reside in the small intrahepatic bile ducts, where they produce epithelial hyperplasia and periductal fibrosis. These parasites can cause cholangitis, liver abscess, or hepatic duct stones (with ova or adult flukes forming the nidus) and even common duct obstruction. When viewed *en face*, the worms produce smooth filling defects simulating calculi, which also frequently coexist in these patients. When seen in profile, however, the typical linear filling defects readily permit the diagnosis of a parasitic infection (Fig. 61-24). *Clonorchis* infestation has also been associated with a higher than normal incidence of carcinoma of the intrahepatic bile ducts.

HYDATID CYSTS

Hydatid cysts (*Echinococcus*) of the liver can communicate with the biliary tree (Fig. 61-25). Periodic

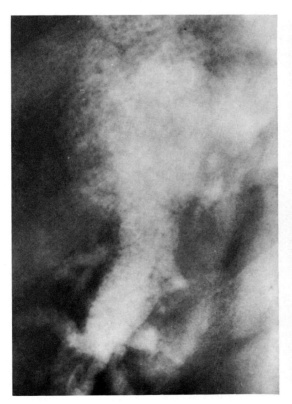

61-23

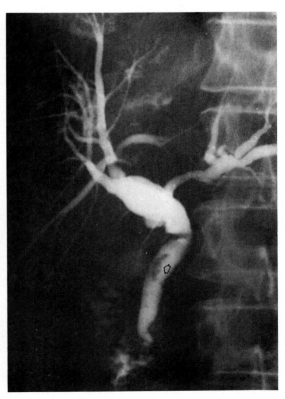

61-24

Fig. 61-23. Liver fluke (*Clonorchis sinensis*) causing multiple filling defects in the biliary system. Many of the filling defects represent coexistent calculi, which are often seen in this condition.

Fig. 61-24. Liver fluke (*Fasciola hepatica*). A radiolucent, somewhat crescent-shaped filling defect **(arrow)** is seen in the common bile duct. (Condomies J, Rene–Espinet JM, Espinos–Perez JC et al: Percutaneous cholangiography in the diagnosis of hepatic fascioliasis. Am J Gastroenterol 80:384–386, 1985)

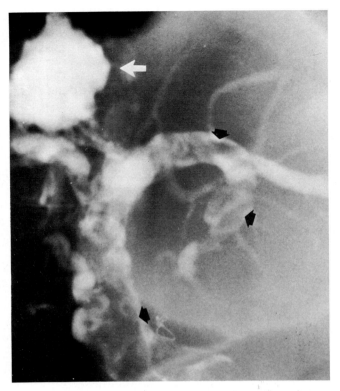

Fig. 61-25. Hydatid disease of the liver and biliary tree. Multiple cysts present as filling defects in the bile ducts **(black arrows)**. Note contrast filling a large communicating cystic cavity in the liver parenchyma **(white arrow)**.

discharge of cyst membranes, daughter cysts, or scolices causes recurrent episodes of biliary colic and can produce round or irregular filling defects in the bile duct or cyst cavity. On rare occasions, intact daughter cysts completely obstruct the common bile duct.

ORIENTAL CHOLANGIOHEPATITIS (RECURRENT PYOGENIC CHOLANGITIS)

Oriental cholangiohepatitis (recurrent pyogenic hepatitis) is a major cause of an acute abdomen in the Far East and is occasionally seen in Asian immigrants in the United States. The hallmark of the disease is the development of soft pigmented bilirubinate stones within markedly dilated intra- and extrahepatic ducts (Fig. 61-26). These stones have a claylike consistency and often fill the ducts with casts. Recent reports have indicated the value of percutaneous interventional procedures for removal of biliary stones and dilatation of the strictures that often develop in this condition.

BIBLIOGRAPHY

Baer JW, Abiri M: Right hepatic artery as a cause of pseudocalculus in the biliary tree. Gastrointest Radiol 7:269–273, 1982

Berk RN, Clemett AR: Radiology of the Gallbladder and Bile Ducts. Philadelphia, WB Saunders, 1977

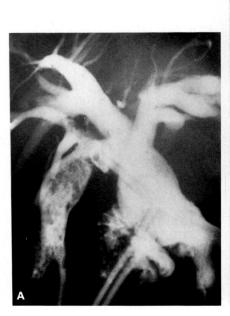

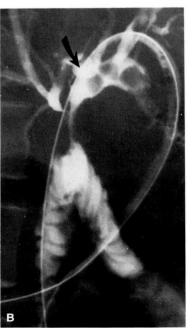

Fig. 61-26. Oriental cholangiohepatitis. **(A)** Numerous calculi within a dilated right intrahepatic duct. **(B)** In a different patient with recurrent cholangitis following choledochal jejunostomy, there are mutiple calculi **(arrow)** within the left ductal system. (Kerlan RK, Pogany AC, Goldberg HI et al: Radiologic intervention in oriental cholangiohepatitis. AJR 145:809–813, 1985. Copyright 1985. Reproduced with permission)

Condomines J, Rene–Espinet JM, Espinos–Perez JC et al: Percutaneous cholangiography in the diagnosis of hepatic fascioliasis. Am J Gastroenterol 80:384–386, 1985

Cruz FD, Barriga P, Tocornal J et al: Radiology of the Mirizzi syndrome: Diagnostic importance of the transhepatic cholangiogram. Gastrointest Radiol 8:249–253, 1983

Evans JA, Mujahed Z: Percutaneous transhepatic cholangiography. Semin Roentgenol 11:219–222, 1976

Gerlock AJ, Muhletaler CA: Primary common bile duct carcinoid. Gastrointest Radiol 4:263–264, 1979

Goldberg H: Operative and postoperative cholecystocholangiography. Semin Roentgenol 11:203–211, 1976

Gray RR, Mackenzie RL, Alan KP: Cholangiographic demonstration of carcinoma of the colon metastatic to the lumen of the common bile duct. Gastrointest Radiol 7:71–72, 1982

Janes JO, Laughlin CL, Goldberger LE et al: Differential features of some unusual biliary tumors. Gastrointest Radiol 7:341–348, 1982

Kerlan RK Jr, Pogany AC, Goldberg HI et al: Radiologic intervention in Oriental cholangiohepatitis. AJR 145:809–813, 1985

Khuroo MS, Zargar SA: Biliary ascariasis: A common cause of biliary and pancreatic disease in an endemic area. Gastroenterology 88:416–423, 1985

Koehler RE, Melson GL, Lee JKT et al: Common hepatic duct obstruction by cystic duct stone: Mirizzi syndrome AJR 132:1007–1009, 1979

Larsen CR, Scholz FJ, Wise RE: Diseases of the biliary ducts. Semin Roentgenol 11:259–267, 1976

Lewall DB, McCorkell SJ: Rupture of echinococcal cysts: Diagnosis, classification and clinical implications. AJR 146:391–394, 1986

May GR, James EM, Bender CE et al: Diagnosis and treatment of jaundice. RadioGraphics 6:847–890, 1986

McCorkell SJ: Echinococcal cysts in the common bile duct: An uncommon cause of obstruction. Gastrointest Radiol 10:390–393, 1985

Mujahed Z, Evans JA: Pseudocalculus defect in cholangiography. AJR 116:337–341, 1972

Roslyn JJ, Kuchenbecker S, Longmire WP Jr et al: Floating tumor debris: A cause of intermittent biliary obstruction. Arch Surg 119:1312–1315, 1984

Smith E, Matzen P: Mucus-producing tumors with mucinous biliary obstruction causing jaundice: Diagnosed and treated endoscopically. Am J Gastroenterol 80:287–289, 1985

Spira R, Widrich WC, Keusch KD et al: Bile duct varices. Arch Surg 120:1194–1196, 1985

Styne P, Warren GH, Kumpe DA et al: Obstructive cholangitis secondary to mucus secreted by a solitary papillary bile duct tumor. Gastroenterology 90:748–753, 1986

Thompson WM, Halvorsen RA, Foster WL et al: Optimal cholangiographic technique for detecting bile duct stones. AJR 146:537–541, 1986

Uflacker R, Wholey MH, Amaral NM et al: Parasitic and mycotic causes of biliary obstruction. Gastrointest Radiol 7:173–179, 1982

van Sonnenberg E, Casola G, Cubberley DA et al: Oriental cholangiohepatitis: Diagnostic imaging and interventional management. AJR 146:327–331, 1986

van Sonnenberg E, Ferrucci JT: Bile duct obstruction in hepatocellular carcinoma (hepatoma)–Clinical and cholangiographic characteristics. Radiology 130:7–13, 1979

van Steenbergen W, Ponette E, Marchal G et al: Cystadenoma of the common bile duct demonstrated by endoscopic retrograde cholangiopancreatography: An uncommon cause of extrahepatic obstruction. Am J Gastroenterol 79:466–470, 1984

Watanabe H, Matsumoto T, Maekawa T: Filling defects at the hepatic hilum due to compression by the right hepatic artery in cholangiography. Gastrointest Radiol 7:263–267, 1982

Way LW: Retained common duct stones. Surg Clin North Am 53:1169–1190, 1973

Williams SM, Burnett DA, Mazer MJ: Radiographic demonstration of common bile duct varices. Gastrointest Radiol 7:69–70, 1982

62

BILE DUCT NARROWING/OBSTRUCTION

Disease Entities

Neoplastic lesions
    Malignant tumors
        Carcinoma of the common bile duct
            (cholangiocarcinoma)
        Ampullary carcinoma
        Carcinoma of the pancreas
        Carcinoma of the duodenum
        Carcinoma of the gallbladder
        Hepatoma
        Metastases to lymph nodes in the porta
            hepatis
        Lymphoma
        Villous tumor
        Tumor-induced mucus/floating tumor
            debris
    Benign tumors
        Papilloma
        Adenoma
        Neurinoma of the cystic duct
        Granular cell tumor
        Fibroma
        Leiomyoma
        Cystadenoma
Inflammatory disorders
    Primary sclerosing cholangitis
    Oriental cholangiohepatitis
    Cholangiolitic hepatitis
    Chronic pancreatitis
    Acute pancreatitis

Pancreatic pseudocyst
Duodenal ulcer disease
Papillary stenosis
Parasites
    Ascaris lumbricoides
    Clonorchis sinensis
    Fasciola hepatica
    Echinococcus granulosis
    Amebiasis
    Shistosomiasis
AIDS-related cholangitis
Granulomatous disease in adjacent lymph
      nodes
    Tuberculosis
    Sarcoidosis
Bile duct calculi
    Impacted stone in ampulla of Vater
    Papillary edema secondary to recent passage
      of biliary stone
    Mirizzi syndrome
Traumatic stricture
Congenital/neonatal anomalies
    Biliary atresia/hypoplasia
    Congenital membranous diaphragm
    Duodenal diverticulum
Vascular impressions
    Calcified portal vein
    Aortic aneurysm
Hepatic cysts (simple, polycystic)
Cirrhosis

In the patient with jaundice, ultrasound is usually the initial procedure of choice in differentiating biliary obstruction from hepatocellular disease (Fig. 62-1*A*). Although computed tomography (CT) is as sensitive as ultrasound in demonstrating a dilated biliary system in patients with obstructive jaundice (Fig. 62-1*B*), ultrasound is generally the first imaging study since it is substantially less expensive and involves no ionizing radiation. However, CT is much more accurate than ultrasound in determining the level and cause of biliary obstruction. In patients with malignant biliary obstruction, CT is of considerable value in detecting intra-abdominal nodal metastases as well as in the preoperative assessment of the extent of local invasion.

If ultrasound and CT fail to define precisely the exact site and cause of biliary obstruction, direct cholangiography is indicated (Fig. 62-1*C*). This is most often accomplished by the percutaneous transhepatic approach with a thin needle; if available, endoscopic retrograde cholangiopancreatography (ERCP) can be used, especially when abnormal bleeding parameters make the percutaneous approach too risky.

It should be noted that the absence of bile duct dilatation does not completely exclude obstruction, since intermittent obstruction (*e.g.*, choledocholithiasis) or disease causing diffuse bile duct stenosis (*e.g.*, sclerosing cholangitis) may produce obstruction without bile duct dilatation. Conversely, bile duct dilatation may occur in the absence of obstruction (*e.g.*, residual duct dilatation after a previous episode of obstruction).

MALIGNANT TUMORS

CHOLANGIOCARCINOMA

Primary carcinomas of the bile ducts (cholangiocarcinoma) are almost invariably adenocarcinomas. They have a wide range of histologic appearances, depending on the amount of fibrous stroma present between cells. Because of their strategic location, obstructive jaundice is usually the first clinical manifestation. Pain, weight loss, and other constitutional symptoms are common. In contrast to cancer of the gallbladder, bile duct carcinoma occurs more frequently in men than in women. The peak incidence of cholangiocarcinoma is during the sixth decade of life. Most patients have hepatomegaly; about one-third have a palpable gallbladder (Courvoisier phenomenon). Ulcerative colitis and antecedent inflammatory disease of the biliary tree, particularly primary sclerosing cholangitis, seem to predispose to the development of bile duct carcinoma. The relatively high incidence of biliary carcinoma in the Orient is thought to be related in part to chronic infestation by *Clonorchis sinensis*. A recent report has described the development of cholangiocarcinoma as a late complication of choledochoenteric anastomoses.

Carcinoma can occur at any site along the bile ducts. The most common locations are in the retroduodenal or supraduodenal segments of the common bile duct and in the common hepatic duct at the carina (Fig. 62-2). Because of their infiltrative nature, most bile duct carcinomas are far advanced

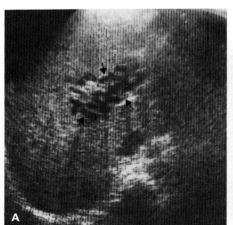
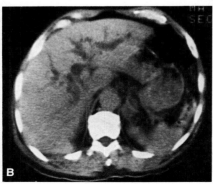
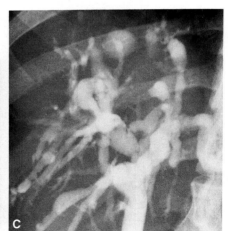

Fig. 62-1. Dilated bile ducts in obstructive jaundice. **(A)** Ultrasound. **(B)** Computed tomography. **(C)** Percutaneous transhepatic cholangiography.

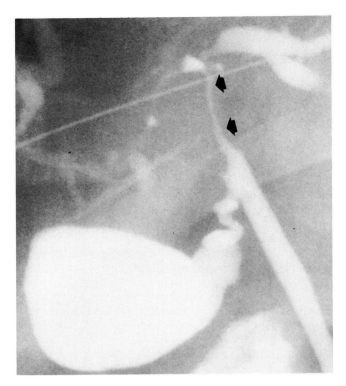

Fig. 62-2. Cholangiocarcinoma presenting as a smooth stricture **(arrows)** extending from the carina to the junction of the cystic duct. Areas of relative narrowing of the right and left hepatic ducts may represent additional sites of tumor involvement.

at the time of diagnosis, with regional lymph node metastases and extension along the bile ducts. Tumors arising at the junction of the right and left hepatic ducts (Klatskin tumors) behave as distinct clinical entities (Fig. 62-3). They tend to grow slowly and to be late to metastasize.

Cholangiocarcinoma most commonly presents radiographically as a short, well-demarcated segmental constriction (Fig. 62-4). The tumor usually begins as a plaquelike lesion of the wall that infiltrates and spreads along the duct in both directions. An extensive desmoplastic response tends to produce diffuse narrowing of the duct (Fig. 62-5); little intraluminal extension of tumor is seen. An obstructing tumor most often causes abrupt occlusion of the common bile duct with proximal dilatation. Passage of contrast through the lesion can demonstrate the site of occlusion to be smooth or to contain small, irregular polypoid masses protruding into the lumen. Cholangiocarcinoma occasionally appears as a discrete, bulky polypoid tumor with a large intraluminal component. If the mass is relatively smooth, it may resemble a biliary calculus. An annular infiltrating lesion with ulceration and overhanging edges is much less commonly seen. Cholangiocarcinoma may be multicentric (Fig. 62-6) and, because of the fibrosing nature of the disease, can produce an appearance of stricture-like narrowing with proximal dilatation that is indistinguishable from sclerosing cholangitis.

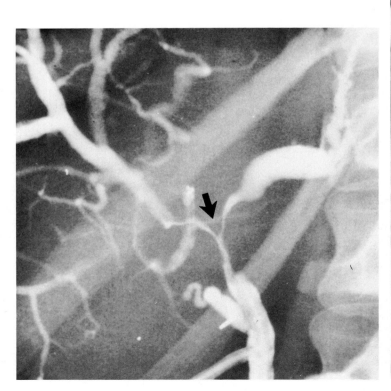

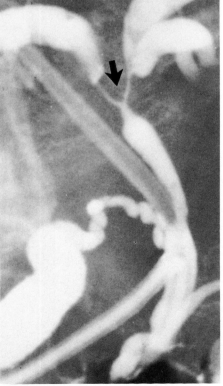

Fig. 62-3. Klatskin tumor. Sclerosing cholangiocarcinomas **(arrows)** in two patients are visible arising at the junction of the right and left hepatic ducts.

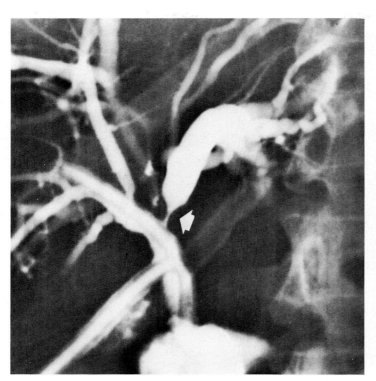

62-4

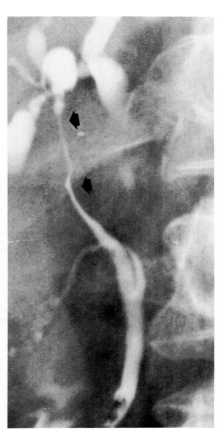

62-5

Fig. 62-4. Cholangiocarcinoma primarily involving the origin of the left hepatic duct and presenting as a short, well-demarcated segmental constriction **(arrow)**.

Fig. 62-5. Cholangiocarcinoma causing severe narrowing of a long segment of the common hepatic duct **(arrows)**.

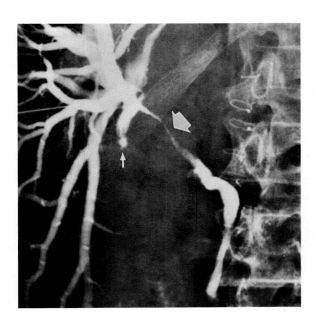

Fig. 62-6. Multicentric cholangiocarcinoma. In addition to severe narrowing of the common hepatic duct **(thick arrow)**, there is obstruction of a branch of the right hepatic duct **(thin arrow)** and poor filling of the left hepatic radicles.

AMPULLARY CARCINOMA

When the bile duct is obstructed at its distal end, the possibility of carcinoma of the ampulla of Vater should be considered (Fig. 62-7). These small neoplasms can appear as irregular or polypoid masses or merely cause distal common bile duct obstruction without a demonstrable tumor mass (Fig. 62-8). The prognosis for carcinoma of the ampulla is much better than that for carcinoma of the common bile duct, since the more localized ampullary neoplasms are more amenable to surgical resection (radical pancreaticoduodenectomy).

OTHER ADJACENT PRIMARY MALIGNANCIES

Carcinoma of the head of the pancreas can encircle and asymmetrically narrow the common bile duct (Fig. 62-9). Complete obstruction can develop (Fig. 62-10); ductal invasion and mucosal destruction can also occur. These tumors are often relatively large and are associated with a mass effect on barium studies of the upper gastrointestinal tract. Primary

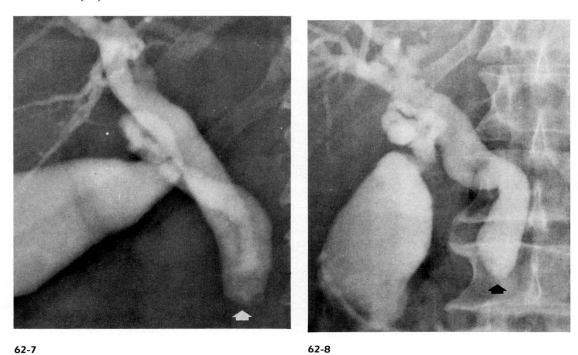

62-7

62-8

Fig. 62-7. Villous adenocarcinoma of the ampulla of Vater causing lobulated obstruction of the distal common bile duct **(arrow)**.

Fig. 62-8. Adenocarcinoma of the ampulla causing an abrupt occlusion **(arrow)** of the distal common bile duct.

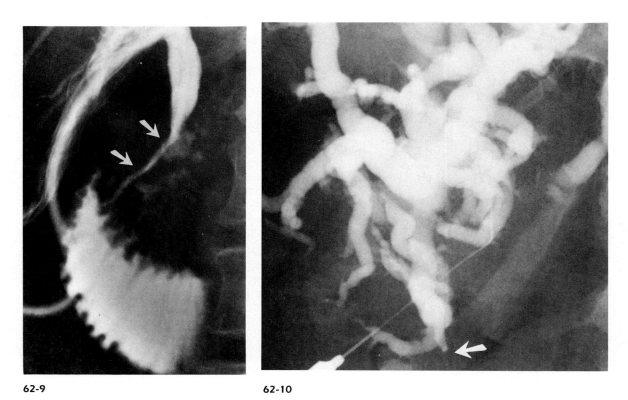

62-9

62-10

Fig. 62-9. Carcinoma of the head of the pancreas. There is irregular narrowing of the common bile duct **(arrows)**. The calcifications reflect underlying chronic pancreatitis.

Fig. 62-10. Carcinoma of the pancreas causing complete obstruction of the bile duct **(arrow)**.

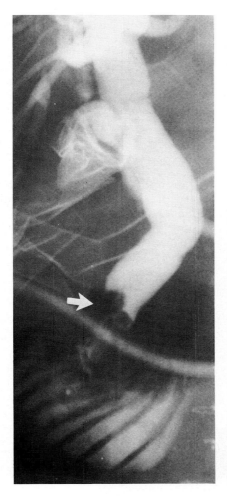

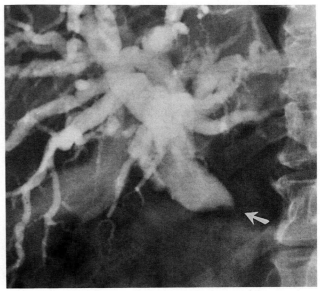

62-11 **62-12**

Fig. 62-11. Adenocarcinoma arising in the second portion of the duodenum and causing an irregular mass in the distal common bile duct **(arrow)** with a high-grade biliary stenosis.

Fig. 62-12. Extrinsic obstruction of the common bile duct **(arrow)** due to nodal metastases from carcinoma of the colon.

carcinoma of the duodenum in the region of the papilla of Vater can extend to involve the distal common bile duct and cause obstructive jaundice (Fig. 62-11). A mass in the gallbladder fossa with simultaneous obstruction of the common hepatic and cystic ducts suggests direct spread of carcinoma of the gallbladder. Extension of a strategically placed hepatoma very rarely produces bile duct obstruction and jaundice. Hepatomas tend to undergo necrosis and degeneration, especially in a large tumor nodule. Necrosis and degeneration of a hepatoma contiguous with a bile duct may conceivably permit a large tumor fragment to enter the biliary tree and flow distally until it becomes lodged in the common bile duct.

METASTASES

Metastases to lymph nodes in the porta hepatis or along the medial margin of the descending duodenum can cause extrinsic obstruction of the main hepatic or common bile ducts (Fig. 62-12). These metastases are usually secondary to primary malignancies of the gastrointestinal tract but can also represent spread from carcinoma of the lung or breast. In these conditions, the diffuse desmoplastic response evoked by the metastasis can simulate the appearance of primary cholangiocarcinoma. Multiple sites of mucosal destruction and luminal narrowing may occur, reflecting the multiplicity of deposits characteristic of metastatic disease (Fig.

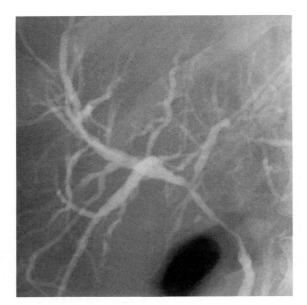

Fig. 62-13. Metastatic breast carcinoma. There are multiple areas of irregularity and narrowing of the common bile duct and left hepatic duct. (Janes JO, Laughlin CL, Goldberger LE et al: Differential features of some unusual biliary tumors. Gastrointest Radiol 7:341–348, 1982)

62-13). However, this is not a pathognomonic finding since multiple areas of narrowing not infrequently occur with primary cholangiocarcinoma. It must be remembered that involvement of the extrahepatic biliary tree by metastatic carcinoma is not common. The usual cause of jaundice in these patients is massive liver replacement by metastatic tumor.

LYMPHOMA

Lymphoma involving nodes in the porta hepatis can also produce obstructive jaundice. Whenever the bile duct is deviated as well as obstructed, the possibility of lymph node metastases should be considered.

VILLOUS TUMOR

Villous tumors causing distal common bile duct obstruction may arise from the duodenum and grow through the ampulla of Vater (Fig. 62-14) or, very rarely, arise primarily from the ampulla of Vater itself. The tumors are composed of fronds that project into the lumen of the duodenum or common

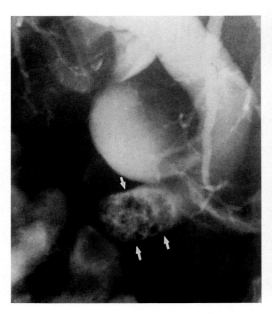

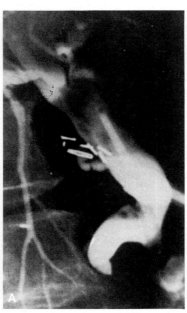

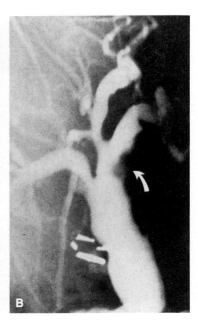

62-14   62-15

Fig. 62-14. Duodenal villous tumor. Contrast material fills the interstices of this large mass **(arrows)** that grew into the distal common bile duct and caused a high-grade obstruction. (Janes JO, Laughlin CL, Goldberger LE et al: Differential features of some unusual biliary tumors. Gastrointest Radiol 7:341–348, 1982)

Fig. 62-15. Tumor-induced mucus. **(A)** Initial T-tube cholangiogram shows multiple large filling defects in the common hepatic and left hepatic ducts due to mucus. **(B)** After multiple saline irrigations clear mucus from the duct, there is a persistent filling defect representing a benign papilloma on the anteromedial surface of the origin of the left hepatic duct. (Styne P, Warren GH, Kumpe DA et al: Obstructive cholangitis secondary to mucus secreted by a solitary papillary bile duct tumor. Gastroenterology 90:748–753, 1986)

bile duct. If the tumor obstructs the bile duct, its feathery margin may be outlined by contrast material. As with these tumors in the colon, villous adenomas in the periampullary region have a high incidence of malignant degeneration; however, they infrequently are associated with mucorrhea or potassium loss.

TUMOR-INDUCED MUCUS/FLOATING TUMOR DEBRIS

Masses of thick mucus causing obstruction of the bile duct may be produced by benign or malignant tumors of the pancreas, gallbladder, or liver (Fig. 62-15). Tumor debris may arise from a neoplasm that directly invades the bile duct or from necrosis of a tumor mass that is adjacent to a major bile duct. Free-floating debris is a cause of intermittent biliary obstruction, the site of which may be in close proximity to or quite distant from the main tumor mass depending both on the size of the duct and the tumor fragments.

BENIGN TUMORS

Benign neoplasms of the bile ducts are extremely rare. Most appear radiographically as small polypoid filling defects associated with some degree of obstruction. Because their margins tend to be smoothly rounded, these benign tumors often closely resemble biliary stones. About 75% of benign neoplasms of the bile ducts are located in the distal portion of the biliary tree. They are rare in the

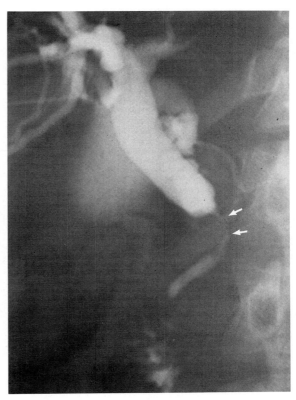

Fig. 62-17. *Granular cell tumor. There is smooth, eccentric narrowing of the common bile duct with proximal ductal dilatation. (Mauro MA, Jaques PF: Granular-cell tumors of the esophagus and common bile duct. J Can Assoc Radiol 32:254–256, 1981)*

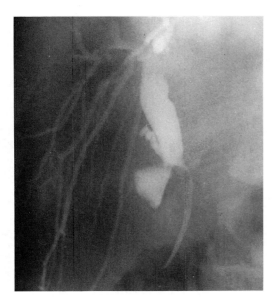

Fig. 62-16. *Granular cell tumor. There is smooth eccentric narrowing with partial obstruction of the common bile duct. (Janes JO, Laughlin CL, Goldberger LE et al: Differential features of some unusual biliary tumors. Gastrointest Radiol 7:341–348, 1982)*

proximal extrahepatic ducts and even less frequent in the intrahepatic ducts.

Most benign neoplasms of the bile ducts are papillomas or adenomas. Adenomas are usually single, whereas papillomas are not uncommonly of multifocal origin. Because papillomas often have cellular atypia and tend to recur if they are not widely excised, it has been suggested (without definite evidence) that they may be precancerous lesions.

Cystic duct neurinomas occasionally develop after cholecystectomy at the site of ligation and transection of the cystic duct. These are not true neoplasms but rather consist of regenerating nerve trunks and scar tissue. Granular cell tumor (granular cell myoblastoma) is a small benign lesion, probably of mesenchymal and Schwann cell origin, that tends to cause ductal obstruction (Fig. 62-16). When the tumor involves the cystic duct, it causes pain and hydrops of the gallbladder; involvement of the common hepatic or common bile duct produces obstructive jaundice. Almost all patients who present clinically with this rare tumor are young black women. On cholangiography, granular cell tumor causes a smooth, eccentric narrowing of a bile duct (Fig. 62-17). Other rare benign tumors of the bile

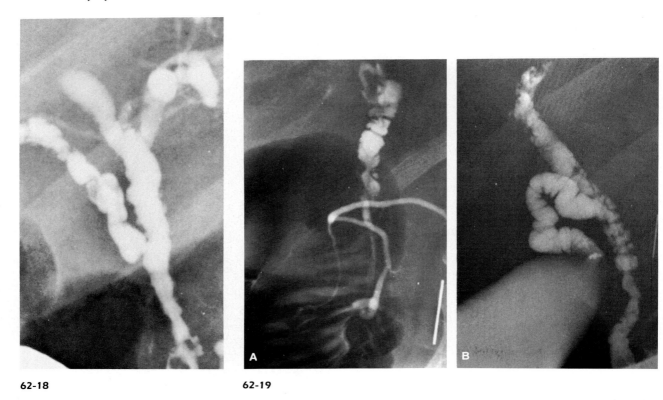

62-18   **62-19**

Fig. 62-18.   Primary sclerosing cholangitis in a patient with chronic ulcerative colitis.

Fig. 62-19.   Primary sclerosing cholangitis. **(A)** Multiple short, bandlike strictures involving the common hepatic duct alternate with protruding, diverticulum-like outpouchings. Portions of the main and accessory pancreatic ducts are superimposed on a long stricture of the lower common bile duct. **(B)** Extensive, complex band strictures with "diverticula" involving the common hepatic and bile ducts. Note the normal valves of Heister in the cystic duct. (Mac-Carty RL, LaRusso NF, Wiesner RH et al: Primary sclerosing cholangitis: Findings on cholangiography and pancreatography. Radiology 149:39–44, 1983)

ducts include fibromas, leiomyomas, and cystadenomas.

INFLAMMATORY DISORDERS

CHOLANGITIS

Cholangitis is usually secondary to long-standing partial obstruction of the common bile duct, which can be due to biliary calculi, parasitic infestation, malignancy, or prior surgery. Primary sclerosing cholangitis is a rare disease in which diffuse thickening and stenosis of the bile ducts develop without calculi in the gallbladder or common duct (unless clearly a coincidental finding), a history of previous operative trauma, or evidence of malignant disease. Many cases of primary sclerosing cholangitis occur in patients with inflammatory bowel disease (both Crohn's disease and chronic ulcerative colitis), though the precise incidence and cause of this relationship are unclear (Fig. 62-18). This and other forms of hepatic pathology (cirrhosis, fatty degeneration, chronic active hepatitis, pericholangitis) usually arise 8 to 10 years after the onset of inflammatory bowel disease, though the liver disease is occasionally noted before the intestinal changes. There does not appear to be any relationship between the severity of the liver disease and that of the biliary tract disease; the liver disease may be progressive when the bowel disease is clinically in remission or even following total colectomy. The presence of diverticula or saccular outpouchings of the common or hepatic ducts, in addition to mural irregularities and stenoses, appears to be specific for the sclerosing cholangitis seen with inflammatory bowel disease (Fig. 62-19). A higher than normal incidence of primary sclerosing cholangitis has

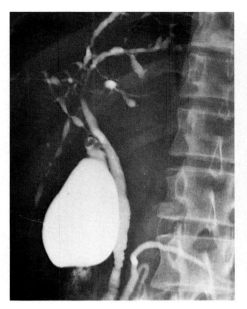 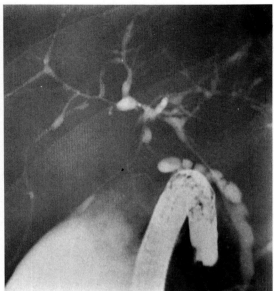

62-20   62-21

Fig. 62-20. *Primary sclerosing cholangitis. Typical diffuse annular strictures of the intrahepatic ducts combined with relatively distensible intervening ductal segments results in a characteristic beaded appearance. (MacCarty RL, LaRusso NF, Wiesner RH et al: Primary sclerosing cholangitis: Findings on cholangiography and pancreatography. Radiology 149:39–44, 1983)*

Fig. 62-21. *Primary sclerosing cholangitis. Confluent stricutres, several centimeters in length, involve the intrahepatic ducts and common hepatic duct. The diminished arborization of the intrahepatic ducts results in a classic pruned-tree appearance. (MacCarty RL, LaRusso NF, Wiesner RH et al: Primary sclerosing cholangitis: Findings on cholangiography and pancreatography. Radiology 149:39–44, 1983)*

also been described in patients with retroperitoneal fibrosis, mediastinal fibrosis, Reidel's thyroiditis, and retroorbital tumors.

The diffuse periductal fibrosis in patients with sclerosing cholangitis leads to biliary strictures that are usually multiple and of variable length. Beading of the ducts occurs between the narrowed segments; the degree of dilatation varies (Fig. 62-20). The extrahepatic ducts are almost always involved, often with progressive involvement of the intrahepatic ducts. The smaller radicles are obliterated, resulting in a pruned-tree appearance (Fig. 62-21). It is sometimes very difficult, both radiographically and histologically, to distinguish between sclerosing cholangitis and diffuse sclerosing carcinoma of the bile ducts, especially when the periductal glands are distorted by fibrosis and inflammation. Consequently, patients with the diagnosis of sclerosing cholangitis should be followed regularly to exclude

a misdiagnosed common duct carcinoma. The presence of an associated fibrosing disease (fibrosing mediastinitis, fibrosing mesenteritis, retroperitoneal fibrosis) supports the diagnosis of sclerosing cholangitis.

Primary sclerosing cholangitis has a strong tendency to undergo malignant degeneration. Cholangiographic findings that suggest malignant degeneration include markedly dilated ducts or ductal segments, the presence of a polypoid mass 1 cm or greater in diameter, and progressive stricture formation or ductal dilatation.

A radiographic appearance similar to that of primary sclerosing cholangitis has been reported in patients receiving hepatic arterial chemotherapy, primarily with Floxuridine (FUDR). The spectrum of radiographic abnormalities has varied from minimal luminal irregularity of the ductal contour to near obliteration of the ductal lumen with proximal

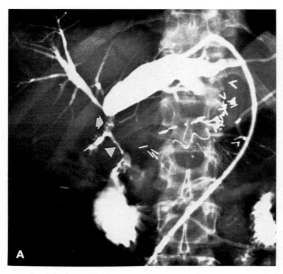
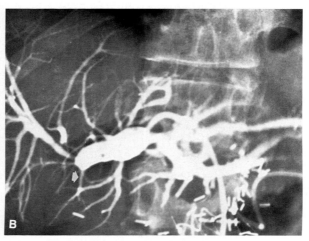

Fig. 62-22.   Cholangitis complicating intra-arterial chemotherapy. **(A)** Cholangiogram shows a narrowed common hepatic duct **(arrow)**, common bile duct **(arrowhead)**, and proximal right hepatic radicles. **(B)** Cholangiogram obtained 6 months later shows complete obliteration of the common hepatic and common bile duct **(arrow)**. (Botet JF, Watson RC, Kemeny N et al: Cholangitis complicating intraarterial chemotherapy and liver metastasis. Radiology 156:335–337, 1985)

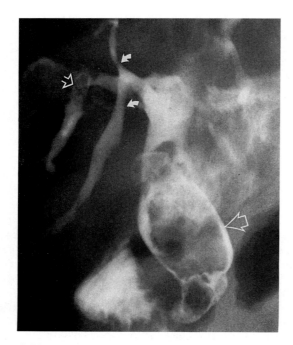

Fig. 62-23.   Oriental cholangiohepatitis. Transhepatic cholangiogram demonstrates gross dilatation of the common bile duct and less striking dilatation of the hepatic ducts, with irregular areas of stenosis **(curved arrows)** and the rapid tapering characteristic of the disease. The left ductal system is incompletely filled. Large, amorphous filling defects form a virtual cast of the common duct **(large open arrow)** and are present in the intrahepatic ducts as well **(small open arrow)**. At surgery, the ducts were filled with soft, pigmented calculi, sludge, and mudlike pus. (Federle MP, Cello JP, Laing FC et al: Recurrent pyogenic cholangitis in Asian immigrants. Radiology 143:151–156, 1982)

dilatation (Fig. 62-22). In all cases, the bifurcation of the common bile duct has been involved, though the distal common bile duct has been spared. A similar appearance of cholangitis has been reported as a complication of transcatheter hepatic arterial embolization for hepatoma and liver metastases.

ORIENTAL CHOLANGIOHEPATITIS

Oriental cholangiohepatitis (recurrent pyogenic cholangitis) is the most common benign bile duct pathology in Asia and is now being seen with increasing frequency in Asian immigrants to the United States. The syndrome is characterized by recurrent right upper quadrant pain, fever, and jaundice. Multiple pigmented biliary stones form in both the intra- and extrahepatic biliary tree in association with bile stasis and recurrent infection with gram-negative bacteria. Cholangiography shows a typical pattern of marked ductal dilatation, multiple stones, and areas of stricturing (Fig. 62-23). Recently, interventive radiographic procedures have been used for dilatation of bile duct strictures and removal of biliary stones.

CHOLANGIOLITIC HEPATITIS

Cholangiolitic hepatitis is a chronic, slowly progressive intrahepatic disease of unknown etiology. This rare condition is characterized by diffuse and focal narrowing or shortening and diminished branching of the intrahepatic biliary ductal system (Fig. 62-24). The extrahepatic biliary ducts are not involved in

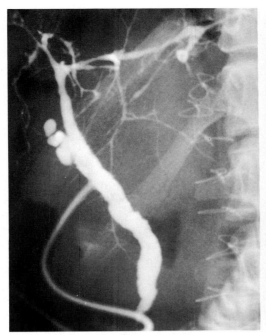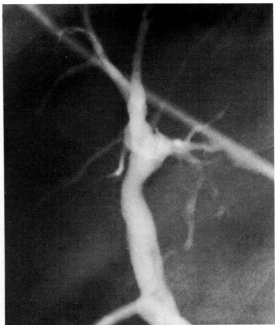

Fig. 62-24. Cholangiolitic hepatitis. T-tube cholangiograms in two patients demonstrate decreased branching of the intrahepatic ducts with associated diffuse and focal narrowing. The hepatic bile ducts are normal in both patients. (Legge DA, Carlson HC, Dickson ER et al: Cholangiographic findings in cholangiolitic hepatitis. AJR 113:16–20, 1971. Copyright 1971. Reproduced with permission)

cholangiolitic hepatitis, in contrast to sclerosing cholangitis.

CHRONIC PANCREATITIS

Because of the intimate relationship of the pancreas to the distal common bile duct, chronic fibrotic changes in the pancreas can lead to inflammatory strictures of the common bile duct (Fig. 62-25). Radiographically, inflammatory and fibrotic changes in the periductal tissues cause smooth, concentric, gradual tapering of the common bile duct with moderate dilatation of the proximal extrahepatic ducts and mild dilatation of intrahepatic ducts. Associated pancreatic calcification is seen not infrequently (Fig. 62-26). Complete common duct obstruction is rare. The stricture involves that portion of the bile duct that lies in the pancreatic tissue. There is often an abrupt transition between the encased "pipe-stem" segment and the dilated suprapancreatic portion of the duct (Fig. 62-26). Although the strictured bile duct can be tortuous, the smooth margins and relative lack of dilatation of the intrahepatic ducts serve to differentiate this appearance from that of pancreatic carcinoma.

ACUTE PANCREATITIS/ULCER DISEASE

In acute pancreatitis, the enlarged edematous pancreas can circumferentially narrow the common bile duct (Fig. 62-27). This appearance is often re-

versible when the acute inflammatory process subsides. A strategically located pseudocyst in the head of the pancreas can also displace and narrow the bile duct, producing obstructive jaundice. An unusual cause of benign stricture is a penetrating duodenal ulcer in the region of the bile duct.

PAPILLARY STENOSIS

Papillary stenosis (stenosis of the sphincter of Oddi) is an ill-defined and controversial entity for which the surgical criterion is failure to pass a dilator larger than a Bakes No. 3 from the common bile duct into the duodenum. Papillary stenosis is associated with chronic inflammatory disease of the biliary tract and pancreas. It appears pathologically as an inflammatory process consisting of mucosal ulceration, granulation tissue, and fibrosis. Papillary stenosis has been suggested as the cause of postcholecystectomy symptoms resembling biliary colic. It can be successfully treated by surgical relief of the obstruction at the choledochoduodenal junction. Radiographically, there is smooth stenosis of the terminal portion of the bile duct with prolonged retention of contrast material in dilated proximal bile ducts.

PARASITIC INFESTATION

Obstructive jaundice can be secondary to parasitic infestation of the biliary tree. The larvae of the liver fluke *Clonorchis sinensis*, ingested by humans who

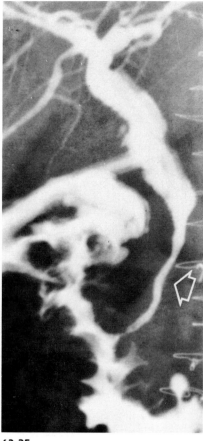

62-25

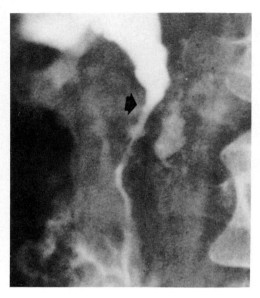

62-26

Fig. 62-25. Chronic pancreatitis causing smooth narrowing of the intrapancreatic portion of the common bile duct **(arrow)**. Note the associated irregular thickening of folds in the adjacent second portion of the duodenum.

Fig. 62-26. Chronic pancreatitis causing severe narrowing of the common bile duct. Note the abrupt transition between the encased "pipestem" segment and the dilated suprapancreatic portion of the common bile duct **(arrow)**. Calcification suggestive of chronic pancreatitis can also be seen.

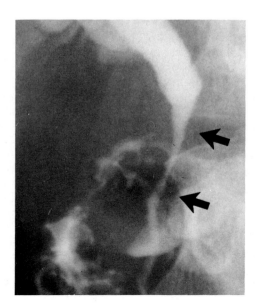

Fig. 62-27. Acute pancreatitis. Enlargement of the edematous pancreas circumferentially narrows the common bile duct **(arrows)**.

eat uncooked fish in endemic areas in the Orient, enter the biliary tree by passing through the ampulla of Vater. Most of the organisms migrate into the peripheral branches of the bile duct, though some may remain in the larger ducts. The larvae burrow into the duct walls and incite a diffuse inflammatory reaction leading to biliary stricture and stone formation, which, in addition to causing conglomerations of the worms themselves, can result in obstructive jaundice (Fig. 62-28). *Fasciola hepatica* can produce a similar radiographic appearance. In endemic areas of the United States, *Ascaris lumbricoides* infects up to 30% of the population. Although primarily a disease of the bowel, the worms can cross the sphincter of Oddi and cause partial or complete obstruction of bile ducts with resultant cholangitis, cholecystitis, and stone formation.

Many parasites indirectly affect the bile ducts by inhabiting the liver. In patients with *Echinococcus* infestation, large parent cysts can communicate with the biliary tree. Daughter cysts shed into the bile ducts can be trapped in the region of the ampulla and obstruct the common bile duct (Fig.

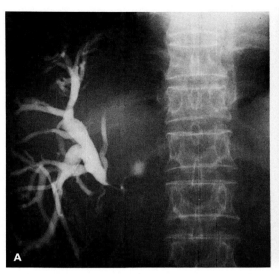
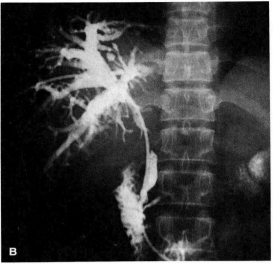

Fig. 62-28. Liver fluke (*Clonorchis sinensis*). **(A)** Obstruction of the common bile duct with severe stenosis of the right and left hepatic ducts at the bifurcation. **(B)** In another patient, there is total segmental stenosis of the common bile duct through which a catheter was inserted percutaneously down to the duodenum. Note the multiple small liver abscesses that communicate with the bile ducts. (**[A]** Lin AC, Chapman SW, Turner HR et al: Clonorchiasis: An update. South Med J 80:919–922, 1987; **[B]** Uflacker R, Wholey MH, Amaral NM et al: Parasitic and mycotic causes of biliary obstruction. Gastrointest Radiol 7:173–179, 1982)

Fig. 62-29. *Echinococcus* infestation. **(A)** ERCP shows dilatation of the common bile duct with diffuse changes of cholangitis. Note the contrast material entering the infected echinococcal cyst **(arrows)** and the filling defect in the biliary system **(arrowhead)** due to a daughter cyst. **(B)** Spot film shows a single small echinococcal cyst **(arrows)** obstructing the distal common bile duct. (McCorkell SJ: Echinococcal cyst in the common bile duct: An uncommon cause of obstruction. Gastrointest Radiol 10:390–393, 1985)

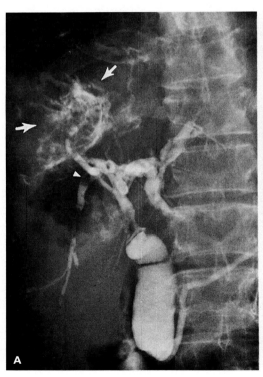
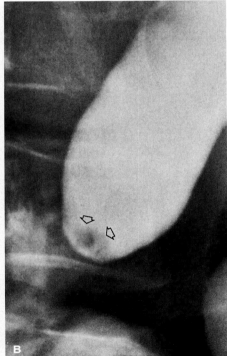

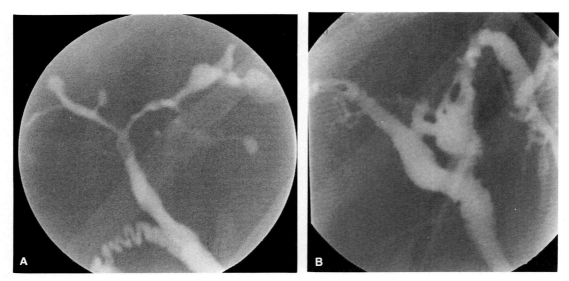

Fig. 62-30. AIDS-related cholangitis. **(A)** Irregular narrowing with pruning of the intrahepatic bile ducts resembles the findings of sclerosing cholangitis. **(B)** In this patient, there is marked irregularity of the intrahepatic bile ducts with areas of both focal narrowing and dilatation. (Dolmatch BL, Laing FC, Federle MP et al: AIDS-related cholangitis: Radiographic findings in nine patients. Radiology 163:313–316, 1987)

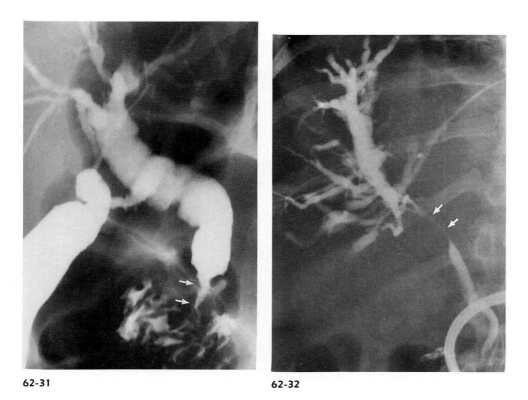

62-31   62-32

Fig. 62-31. Cytomegalovirus cholangitis. Fixed, irregular narrowing of the distal 2 cm of the common bile duct **(arrows)** with associated dilatation and irregularity of the more proximal portions of the biliary tree. (Teixidor HS, Honig CL, Norsoph E et al: Cytomegalovirus infection of the alimentary canal: Radiologic findings with pathologic correlation. Radiology 163:317–323, 1987)

Fig. 62-32. Nonspecific inflammatory mass in the porta hepatis causing narrowing of the common bile duct **(arrows)**.

62-29). Both echinococcal cysts and amebic abscesses can displace and narrow bile ducts. Fibrosis of the periportal connective tissue and contraction of the liver in patients with schistosomiasis can cause irregular narrowing and tortuosity of intrahepatic bile ducts simulating the pattern in cirrhosis.

Biliary tract obstruction or filling defects within the biliary tree due to parasitic or mycotic diseases is rare in developed countries, compared to the incidence of stones and neoplasms. However, the increasing movement and migration of the world population from endemic areas to other countries make it necessary for general radiologists to be aware of the radiographic presentation of these entities.

AIDS-RELATED CHOLANGITIS

Acalculous inflammation of the biliary tract is a recently reported complication of the acquired immunodeficiency syndrome (AIDS). Cholangitis caused by cytomegalovirus or *Cryptosporidium* infection is the proposed pathophysiologic mechanism. The cholangiographic findings are identical to those seen in sclerosing cholangitis and include strictures, focal dilatation, and mural thickening of both intra- and extrahepatic bile ducts (Fig. 62-30). Isolated distal common duct strictures have been described that are indistinguishable from papillary stenosis seen in immunocompetent hosts (Fig. 62-31). The combination of papillary stenosis and intrahepatic ductal strictures has been described as unique to AIDS-related cholangitis.

GRANULOMATOUS DISEASE

Inflammatory processes occurring in lymph nodes adjacent to the common bile duct and porta hepatis can result in biliary obstruction (Fig. 62-32). Tuberculosis (Fig. 62-33), sarcoidosis, and other chronic granulomatous diseases involving periductal lymph nodes can cause compression, narrowing, and even secondary invasion of the hepatic or common bile ducts.

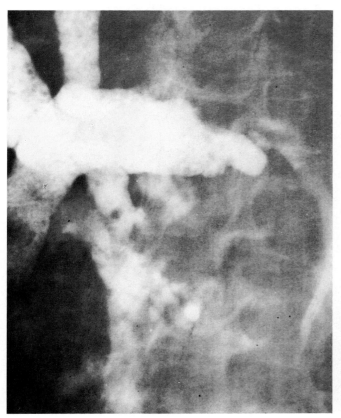

62-33

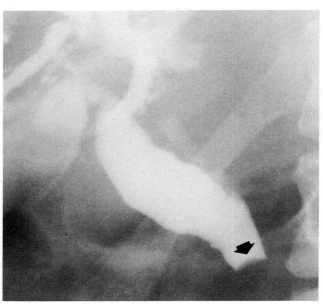

62-34

Fig. 62-33. Tuberculous involvement of the biliary ductal system. There is severe stenosis near the junction of the right and common hepatic ducts with innumerable calculi in the intrahepatic ducts.

Fig. 62-34. Impacted stone in the ampulla producing common duct obstruction proximal to a characteristic smooth, concave intraluminal filling defect **(arrow)**.

BILIARY CALCULI

A common duct stone impacted in the ampulla or edema of the papilla secondary to a recently passed stone is a relatively common cause of bile duct obstruction. On cholangiography, an impacted stone in the ampulla appears as a characteristic smooth, concave intraluminal filling defect (Fig. 62-34). In some instances, other radiolucent stones can be identified in proximal segments of the dilated ductal system. An impacted stone or edema following passage of a stone can cause swelling of the papilla that is detectable on an upper gastrointestinal series.

Calculi in the biliary ducts are almost always secondary to gallstones that enter the common bile duct by way of the cystic duct or by erosion. True primary common duct stones arising in the intrahepatic or extrahepatic biliary tree are unusual and tend to occur proximal to a pre-existing stricture or narrowing of the common bile duct. "Common duct stones" in patients who have had their gallbladders removed usually represent retained intrahepatic or extrahepatic duct stones that were not identified at the time of cholecystectomy. After cholecystectomy, stones can develop secondary to stasis in a large cystic duct remnant.

In the Mirizzi syndrome, a stone impacted in the cystic duct or neck of the gallbladder erodes into the adjacent common hepatic duct and can result in inflammatory or machanical obstruction of the biliary tree. This characteristically produces narrowing of the ductal lumen as a result of a broad extrinsic impression on the lateral aspect of the common hepatic duct (Fig. 62-35).

SURGICAL/TRAUMATIC STRICTURES

The overwhelming majority of benign strictures of the common bile duct are related to previous biliary tract surgery (Fig. 62-36). They can be caused by severing, clamping, or excessive probing of the common bile duct during the operative procedure. In many cases, the operation is completed without

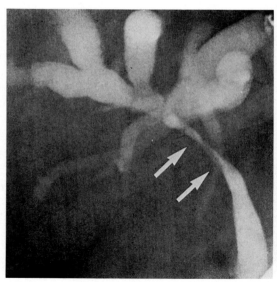

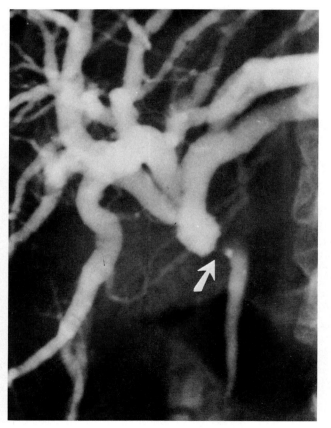

62-35   62-36

Fig. 62-35. Mirizzi syndrome. Long, smooth stenosis of the common hepatic duct **(arrows)**. (Becker CD, Hassler H, Terrier F: Preoperative diagnosis of the Mirizzi syndrome: Limitations of sonography and computed tomography. AJR 143:591–596, 1984. Copyright 1984. Reproduced with permission)

Fig. 62-36. Benign stricture of the common bile duct **(arrow)** related to previous biliary tract surgery.

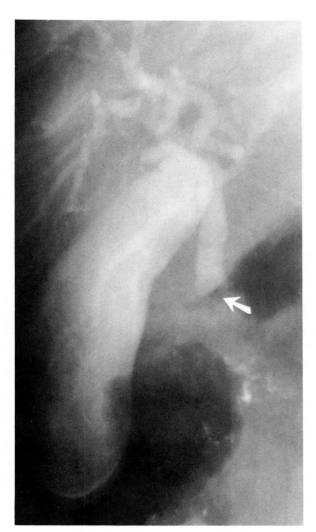

Fig. 62-37. Benign stricture of the common bile duct **(arrow)** following blunt abdominal trauma.

the surgeon being aware that an accident to a major bile duct has occurred. Postoperatively, stricture of the bile duct can be secondary to a suture, biliary leakage, or prolonged T-tube placement. Tearing of a major bile duct can cause a biliary fistula. If the common bile duct or common hepatic duct has been ligated, the patient becomes obviously jaundiced within a few days of surgery. There is often considerable drainage of bile from the T-tube; the volume varies inversely with the degree of jaundice. Infrequently, biliary strictures can be secondary to blunt abdominal trauma with torsion injuries to the common bile duct (Fig. 62-37).

Radiographically, the postoperative stricture is generally smooth and concentric, with the obstructed end appearing funnel-shaped or convex distally, in contrast to the concave margin produced by an obstructing calculus. Unlike malignant lesions, benign strictures tend to involve long segments of the bile duct without total obstruction; there is usually a gradual transition to normal segments of the duct.

CONGENITAL/NEONATAL ANOMALIES

BILIARY ATRESIA

The most common cause of persistent neonatal jaundice is biliary atresia. Rather than representing a congenital defect, biliary atresia probably develops postpartum as a complication of a chronic inflammatory process that causes ductal lumen obliteration, which is often segmental and irregular in distribution. Indeed, this condition and neonatal hepatitis may represent opposite extremes of the same disease, with biliary atresia reflecting hepatitis with a component of sclerosing cholangitis of the extrahepatic ducts. The entire extrahepatic biliary ductal system usually is atretic, though the common hepatic duct or common bile duct may be individually involved. Children with this anomaly generally have an unfavorable prognosis. However, in patients with some types of extrahepatic atresia and in persons with biliary hypoplasia, biliary-intestinal anastomosis can result in a cure rate of up to 30% if the diagnosis is made before liver damage progresses to an advanced stage.

MEMBRANOUS DIAPHRAGM

Congenital membranous diaphragm of the common bile or hepatic duct is an extremely rare lesion that is usually not diagnosed until early adult life (Fig. 62-38). The diaphragm can cause chronic partial bil-

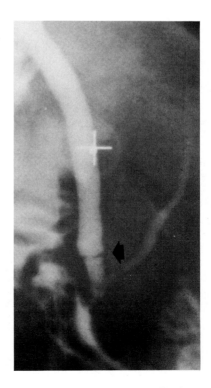

Fig. 62-38. Congenital membranous diaphragm (web) of the common bile duct **(arrow)**.

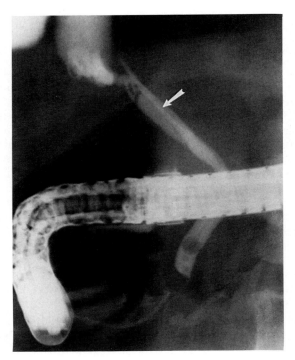

Fig. 62-39. Hepatic artery aneurysm. The common hepatic duct **(arrow)**, seen overlying the cystic duct, demonstrates smooth, gradual tapering with failure of opacification of the intrahepatic bile ducts. Although the preoperative diagnosis was bile duct carcinoma, at surgery a huge hepatic artery aneurysm was found to be obstructing the common hepatic duct. (Lewis RD, Kung H, Connon JJ: Biliary obstruction secondary to hepatic artery aneurysm: Cholangiographic appearance and diagnostic considerations. Gastroenterology 82:1446–1451, 1982)

iary obstruction resulting in bile stasis, stone formation, and recurring cholangitis.

DUODENAL DIVERTICULUM

Most duodenal diverticula arise within 1 cm to 2 cm of the ampulla. Infrequently, the common duct empties directly into a duodenal diverticulum. When this occurs, the duodenal diverticulum may obstruct the common duct because of anatomic distortion of its entry into the duodenum, diverticulitis, or the presence of an enterolith (of bile acids) within the sac.

OTHER CAUSES OF BILE DUCT NARROWING/OBSTRUCTION

VASCULAR IMPRESSIONS

An extremely rare cause of obstructive jaundice is benign vascular compression of the common bile duct. This mechanism has been reported in associa-

tion with hepatic artery aneurysm (Fig. 62-39), aortic aneurysm, or calcified portal vein compressing and occluding the common bile duct.

HEPATIC CYSTS

Rarely, obstructive jaundice is produced by nonparasitic cysts of the liver. Strategically positioned simple cysts or cysts in a polycystic liver can cause a mass effect in the porta hepatitis that narrows the common or hepatic ducts. Decompression of the liver cysts at surgery or under ultrasound guidance results in rapid clearing of jaundice.

CIRRHOSIS

Cirrhosis of any etiology is characterized by progressive destruction of liver cells associated with regeneration of liver substance and fibrosis. During its early stages, the disease usually has little or no effect on the biliary ductal system. Fatty infiltration can cause straightening, elongation with separation, and occasional dilatation of the intrahepatic ducts. As the disease progresses, extrinsic pressure of the regenerating nodules can displace ductal structures. As the liver shrinks with increasing fibrosis, the intrahepatic ducts become crowded together and often assume an irregular tortuous or corkscrew appearance, with or without changes in caliber, that simulates the pattern seen on angiography.

BIBLIOGRAPHY

Becker CD, Hassler H, Terrier F: Preoperative diagnosis of the Mirizzi syndrome: Limitations of sonography and computed tomography. AJR 143:591–596, 1984

Botet JF, Watson RC, Kemeny N et al: Cholangitis complicating intra-arterial chemotherapy in liver metastasis. Radiology 156:335–337, 1985

Buonocore E: Transhepatic percutaneous cholangiography. Radiol Clin North Am 14:527–542, 1976

Chang SF, Burrell MI, Brand MH et al: The protean gastrointestinal manifestations of metastatic breast carcinoma. Radiology 126:611–617, 1978

Cruz FO, Barriga P, Tocornal J et al: Radiology of the Mirizzi syndrome: Diagnostic importance of the transhepatic cholangiogram. Gastrointest Radiol 8:249–253, 1983

Dolmatch BL, Laing FC, Federle MP et al: AIDS-related cholangitis: Radiographic findings in nine patients. Radiology 163:313–316, 1987

Ergun H, Wolf BH, Hissong SL: Obstructive jaundice caused by polycystic liver disease. Radiology 136:435–436, 1980

Geisse G, Melson GL, Tedesco FJ et al: Stenosing lesions of the biliary tree. Evaluation with endoscopic retrograde cholangiopancreatography (ERC) and percutaneous transhepatic cholangiography (PTC). AJR 123:378–385, 1975

Herba MJ, Casola G, Bret PM et al: Cholangiocarcinoma as a late complication of choledochoenteric anastomoses. AJR 147:513–515, 1986

Ho CS, Wesson DE: Recurrent pyogenic cholangitis in Chinese immigrants. AJR 122:368–374, 1974

Janes JO, Laughlin CL, Goldgerger LE et al: Differential features of some unusual biliary tumors. Gastrointest Radiol 7:341–348, 1982

Kerlan RK Jr, Pogany AC, Goldberg HI et al: Radiologic intervention in Oriental cholangiohepatis. AJR 145:809–813, 1985

Klatskin G: Adenocarcinoma of the hepatic duct at its bifurcation within the porta hepatis: An unusual tumor with distinctive clinical and pathological features. Am J Med 38:241–256, 1965

Larsen CR, Scholz FJ, Wise RE: Diseases of the biliary ducts. Semin Roentgenol 11:259–267, 1976

Legge DA, Carlson HC, Dickson ER et al: Cholangiographic findings in cholangiolitic hepatitis. AJR 113:16–20, 1971

Lewis DR Jr, Kung H, Connon JJ: Biliary obstruction secondary to hepatic artery aneurysm: Cholangiographic appearance and diagnostic considerations. Gastroenterology 82:1446–1451, 1982

Lin AC, Chapman SW, Turner HR et al: Clonorchiasis: An update. South Med J 80:919–922, 1987

Li–Yeng C, Goldberg HI: Sclerosing cholangitis: Broad spectrum of radiographic features. Gastrointest Radiol 9:39–47, 1984

MacCarty RL, LaRusso NF, May GR et al: Cholangiocarcinoma complicating primary sclerosing cholangitis: Cholangiographic appearances. Radiology 156:43–46, 1985

MacCarty RL, LaRusso NF, Wiesner RH et al: Primary sclerosing cholangitis: Findings on cholangiography and pancreatography. Radiology 149:39–44, 1983

Makuuchi M, Sukigara M, Mori T et al: Bile duct necrosis: Complication of transcatheter hepatic arterial embolization. Radiology 156:331–334, 1985

Mauro MA, Jaques PF: Granular-cell tumors of the esophagus and common bile duct. J Can Assoc Radiol 32:254–256, 1981

May GR, James EM, Bender CE et al: Diagnosis and treatment of jaundice. RadioGraphics 6:847–890, 1986

McCorkell SJ: Echinococcal cysts in the common bile duct: An uncommon cause of obstruction. Gastrointest Radiol 10:390–393, 1985

Menuck L, Amberg J: The bile ducts. Radiol Clin North Am 14:499–523, 1976

Mujahed Z, Evans JA: Pseudocalculus defect in cholangiography. AJR 116:337–341, 1972

Nichols DA, MacCarty RL, Gaffey TA: Cholangiographic evaluation of bile duct carcinoma. AJR 141:1291–1294, 1983

Roslyn JJ, Kuckenbecker S, Longmire WP et al: Floating tumor debris. Arch Surg 119:1312–1315, 1984

Shea WJ Jr, Demas BE, Goldberg HI et al: Sclerosing cholangitis associated with hepatic arterial FUDR chemotherapy: Radiographic-histologic correlation. AJR 146:717–721, 1986

Shingleton WW, Gamberg D: Stenosis of the sphincter of Oddi. Am J Surg 119:35–37, 1970

Smith E, Matzen P: Mucus-producing tumors with mucinous biliary obstruction causing jaundice: Diagnosed and treated endoscopically. Am J Gastroenterol 80:287–289, 1985

Styne P, Warren GH, Kumpe DA et al: Obstructive cholangitis secondary to mucus secreted by a solitary papillary bile duct tumor. Gastroenterology 90:748–753, 1986

Trambert JJ, Bron KM, Zajko AB et al: Percutaneous transhepatic dilatation of benign biliary strictures. AJR 149:945–948, 1987

Uflacker R, Wholey MH, Amaral NM et al: Parasitic and mycotic causes of biliary obstruction. Gastrointest Radiol 7:173–179, 1982

Van Sonnenberg E, Casola G, Cubberley DA et al: Oriental cholangiohepatitis: Diagnostic imaging and interventional management. AJR 146:327–331, 1986

Van Steenbergen W, Ponette E, Marchal G et al: Cystadenoma of the common bile duct demonstrated by endoscopic retrograde cholangiography: An uncommon cause of extrahepatic obstruction. Am J Gastroenterol 79:466–470, 1984

Williams SM, Harned RK: Hepatobiliary complications of inflammatory bowel disease. Radiol Clin North Am 25:175–188, 1987

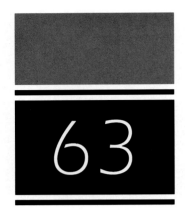

CYSTIC DILATATION OF THE BILE DUCTS

Disease Entities

General bile duct dilatation (see Chap. 62)
Dilatation of extrahepatic bile ducts
    Choledochal cyst
    Choledochocele
    Hepatic duct diverticulum
Dilatation of intrahepatic bile ducts
    Congenital anomalies
        Caroli's disease
        Congenital hepatic fibrosis
    Neoplastic disease
        Papillomatosis
        Epithelioma
    Choledocholithiasis
        Western type
        Oriental type
    Cholangitis
    Oriental cholangiohepatitis (recurrent
        pyogenic cholangitis)
    Secondary involvement
        Benign tumors
        Malignant tumors
        Parasites (hydatid cysts, *Clonorchis
            sinensis, Ascaris lumbricoides*)
        Liver infarcts after transcatheter emboliza-
            tion of hepatic artery branches

The diameter of the common bile duct on cholangiography should measure 11 mm or less. General dilatation of the bile ducts is usually secondary to an obstructing lesion in the distal common duct. This may be due to an inflammatory or neoplastic process or to an impacted or recently passed biliary calculus (see Chap. 62). It is controversial whether the common bile duct dilates after cholecystectomy because it must assume a reservoir function. It is generally agreed that, unless bile duct pathology (*e.g.*, stenosis, stones, cancer) develops, an extrahepatic system that is normal before gallbladder removal will remain normal in most cholecystomized patients. In most cases, the finding of an enlarged common bile duct after cholecystectomy merely reflects dilatation that was already present, but possibly not appreciated, before surgery. This interpretation is supported by the fact that the common bile duct frequently does not return to a normal caliber after the operative relief of biliary obstruction.

CHOLEDOCHAL CYST

A choledochal cyst is a cystic or fusiform dilatation of the common bile duct and adjacent portions of the common hepatic and cystic ducts (Fig. 63-1) that is typically associated with localized constriction of the distal common bile duct (Fig. 63-2). Concomitant dilatation of intrahepatic bile ducts has recently been recognized with increasing frequency (Fig. 63-3). Although usually considered to be a congenital, developmental abnormality, many choledochal cysts are probably acquired lesions caused by re-

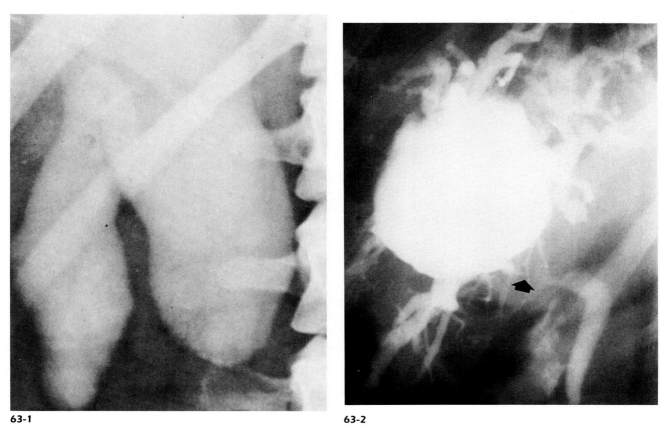

63-1

63-2

Fig. 63-1. Choledochal cyst. There is fusiform dilatation of the common bile duct and adjacent portions of the common hepatic and cystic ducts.

Fig. 63-2. Choledochal cyst. Note the localized constriction **(arrow)** separating the cyst from the normal-caliber distal duct.

gurgitation of pancreatic secretions into the distal common bile duct. This regurgitation, which causes cholangitis, gradual stricture formation, and ductal dilatation over a long period of time, is apparently due to a minor variation in the anatomic development of the confluence of the common bile and pancreatic ducts.

Choledochal cysts are classically described as presenting with a triad of upper abdominal pain, mass, and jaundice. Although the presence of all three is relatively unusual, most patients have at least one of these clinical manifestations. Jaundice is the most common presenting symptom, seen in about 70% of patients. Cholangitis is a frequent complication, and biliary stones may develop (Fig. 63-4). Very large cysts can compress neighboring organs, such as the duodenal sweep and head of the pancreas. Rarely, choledochal cysts perforate and cause biliary peritonitis. Carcinoma is a recognized complication of choledochal cysts, with a reported frequency of 3% to 28%. The risk of cholangiocarcinoma increases with age and is reported to be increased in patients whose cysts have been decompressed by internal drainage.

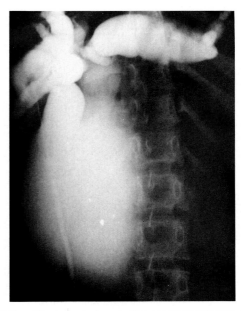

Fig. 63-3. Choledochal cyst. The intrahepatic bile ducts are also involved in the generalized dilatation of the biliary system.

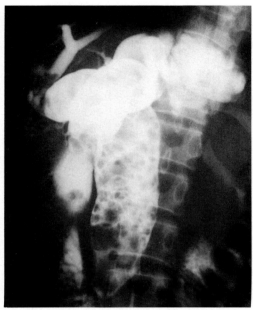

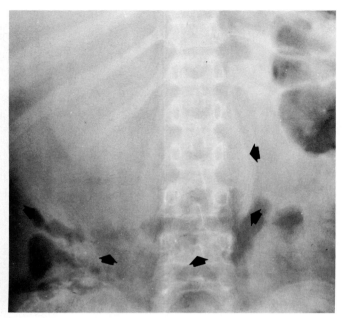

63-4   **63-5**

Fig. 63-4.   Choledochal cyst. Multiple lucent biliary stones can be seen within the markedly dilated extra- and intrahepatic bile ducts.

Fig. 63-5.   Choledochal cyst. A huge soft-tissue mass in the right upper quadrant **(arrows)** displaces gas-filled loops of bowel.

A soft-tissue mass representing the markedly dilated bile duct is often seen on plain abdominal radiographs (Fig. 63-5). Upper gastrointestinal examination can demonstrate displacement of the duodenum anteriorly, inferiorly, and to the left. Oral cholecystography and intravenous cholangiography can opacify the choledochal cyst if they are performed between attacks of hepatic dysfunction, but are usually unsuccessful when there is jaundice or distal obstruction. Ultrasound, computed tomography, and radionuclide scanning permit specific preoperative diagnosis of a choledochal cyst (Fig. 63-6).

CHOLEDOCHOCELE

A choledochocele is a cystic dilatation of the intra-duodenal portion of the common bile duct in the region of the ampulla of Vater. The "cyst" communicates with the duodenal lumen through a small opening and is the terminus of the pancreatic duct. The major radiographic abnormality caused by a choledochocele is a well-defined, smooth filling defect that projects into the duodenal lumen on upper gastrointestinal series (Fig. 63-7A). At cholangiography, the bulbous terminal portion of the common bile duct projects into the duodenal lumen and is separated from contrast in the duodenum by a radiolucent membrane (Fig. 63-7B). This cholangiographic appearance of a choledochocele is similar to that of a ureterocele on excretory urography.

HEPATIC DUCT DIVERTICULUM

Diverticulum-like cysts can arise from the common bile duct or hepatic ducts. These extremely rare lesions are associated with jaundice and displacement of adjacent organs and can be indistinguishable from choledochal cysts.

CONGENITAL ANOMALIES

CAROLI'S DISEASE

Caroli's disease is an extremely rare disorder characterized by segmental saccular dilatation of the intrahepatic bile ducts throughout the liver (Fig.

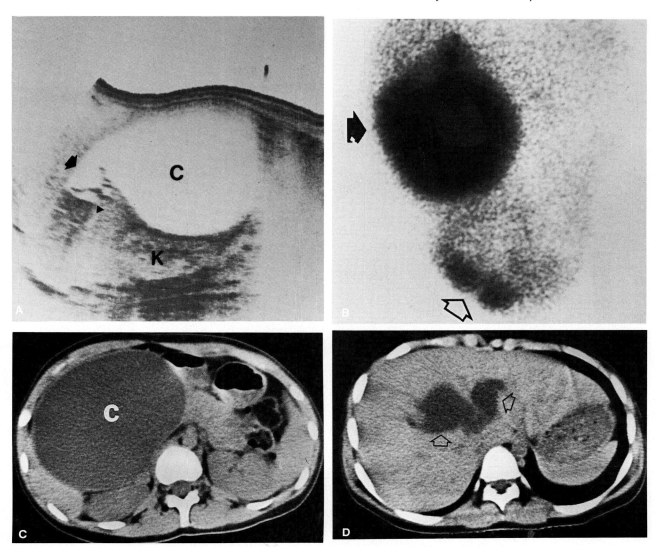

Fig. 63-6. Choledochal cyst. **(A)** Longitudinal sonogram 4 cm to the right of the midline shows a large choledochal cyst **(C)** located in the region of the hilum of the liver and extending down to the area of the pancreatic head. Note the dilated proximal common hepatic duct **(arrow)** branching off from the cystic mass, with dilated central intrahepatic bile ducts **(arrowhead)**. **(B)** A delayed film from a hepatic scintigram shows a large amount of isotope uptake within the choledochal cyst **(closed arrow)**. There is also isotope activity within the intestines **(open arrow)**. **(C)** A CT scan shows a 15-cm choledochal cyst **(C)**. **(D)** A more cephalad scan shows cystic dilatation of the right and left main hepatic ducts **(arrows)**. The peripheral intrahepatic ducts are not dilated. [**(A,B** from Han BK, Babcock DS, Gelfand MH: Choledochal cyst with bile duct dilatation: Sonography and ^{99m}Tc IDA cholescintigraphy. AJR 136:1075–1079, 1981; **C,D** from Araki T, Itai Y, Tasaka A: Computed tomography of choledochal cyst. AJR 135:729–734, 1980. Copyright 1981, 1980. Reproduced with permission)]

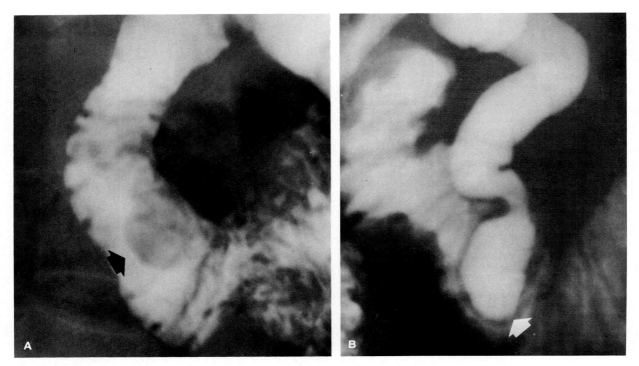

Fig. 63-7.   Choledochocele. **(A)** A well-defined, smooth filling defect **(arrow)** projects into the duodenal lumen on upper gastrointestinal series. **(B)** At cholangiography, the bulbous terminal portion of the common bile duct fills with contrast and projects into the duodenal lumen **(arrow)**. It is separated from contrast in the duodenum by a radiolucent membrane.

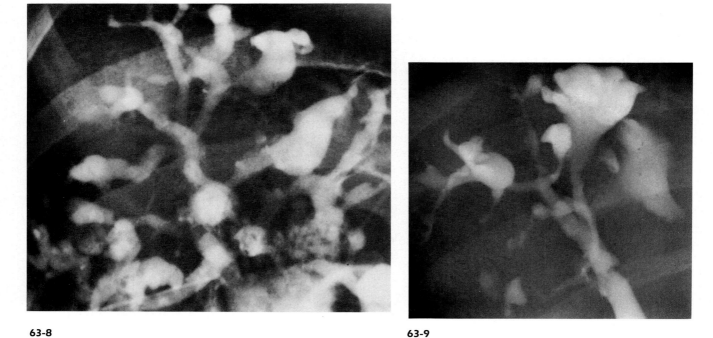

63-8

63-9

Fig. 63-8.   Caroli's disease. Segmental saccular dilatation of the intrahepatic bile ducts throughout the liver.

Fig. 63-9.   Congenital hepatic fibrosis. An operative cholangiogram demonstrates a "lollipop-tree" appearance of the biliary system. (Unite I, Maitem A, Bagnasco SM et al: Congenital hepatic fibrosis associated with renal tubular ectasia. Radiology 190:565–570, 1973)

63-8). The dilated cystic segments contain bile and communicate freely with the biliary tree and with each other. This is in contrast to polycystic liver disease, in which the cysts contain a clear serous fluid, rather than bile, and do not communicate with the biliary tree or other cysts. Although this familial disease is congenital (autosomal recessive), it is frequently not discovered until the patient is a young adult. The patient usually experiences crampy abdominal pain and fever secondary to a marked stasis-induced predisposition to biliary calculus disease, cholangitis, and liver abscesses. About 80% of patients with Caroli's disease have associated medullary sponge kidney.

CONGENITAL HEPATIC FIBROSIS

Congenital hepatic fibrosis is a rare disease in which there is excessive proliferation of the small intrahepatic bile ducts that form cystlike structures, which occasionally enlarge (possibly because of blockage of outflow of bile) and simulate the cysts encountered in Caroli's disease (Fig. 63-9). A far more severe disorder than Caroli's disease, congenital hepatic fibrosis is usually seen in children and is complicated by massive periportal fibrosis leading to portal hypertension, liver decompensation, and gastrointestinal bleeding. Death occurs at an early age as a result of liver failure and portal hypertension.

RADIOGRAPHIC FINDINGS

In both Caroli's disease and congenital hepatic fibrosis, T-tube or operative cholangiography demonstrates large or small cystic spaces communicating with the intrahepatic bile ducts. This produces a "lollipop-tree" appearance of the biliary system (Fig. 63-10). On ultrasound, the dilated ducts may mimic multiple small cysts and are often associated with stones (Fig. 63-11*A*). Computed tomography demonstrates multiple low-density branching tubular structures reflecting dilated bile ducts communicating with focal areas of increased ectasia (Fig. 63-11*B*).

BENIGN TUMORS

Papillomas are fairly common neoplasms of the extrahepatic biliary tract that are most frequently found at the ampulla, where the tumor represents only hypertrophy of a normal anatomic structure. Papillomatosis of the intrahepatic biliary ducts is a rare disease that has been associated with similar tumors in the extrahepatic biliary system and has been described to occur after resection of the ampulla for a papilloma. Colicky right upper abdominal pain and intermittent jaundice, often dating from childhood, is caused by biliary obstruction due

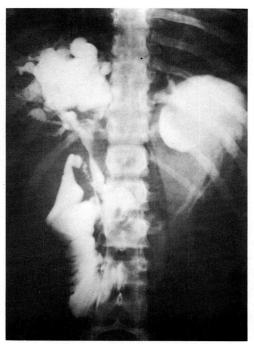

Fig. 63-10. *Caroli's disease. An operative cholangiogram demonstrates diffuse dilatation of the intrahepatic biliary tree. (Lucaya J, Gomez JL, Molino C et al: Congenital dilatation of the intrahepatic bile ducts (Caroli's disease). Radiology 127:746, 1978)*

to thick mucus material produced by the villous tumors, by fragmentation of the papillary fronds, or by amputation of entire polyps into the biliary tract. Bleeding into the bile ducts from intrahepatic papillomatosis can present as upper gastrointestinal hemorrhage. Radiographically, multiple rounded filling defects resembling nonopaque calculi are evident in the bile ducts. When intrahepatic or extrahepatic ducts are obstructed by large tumors, proximal bile duct dilatation occurs. A high incidence of carcinoma has been reported in patients with this disorder.

Primary epitheliomas of the intrahepatic bile duct are rare. Secondary epitheliomas, also uncommon, can be caused by hepatomatous nodules, which are often large and extend into the biliary ducts, where they obliterate the lumen and cause proximal cystic dilatation.

CHOLEDOCHOLITHIASIS

In Western countries, intrahepatic calculi are almost invariably associated with either extrahepatic calculi or an obstruction in the hilum of the liver. In Oriental countries, intrahepatic lithiasis and cystic dilatation of bile ducts are frequently complications of parasitic infestation. Ascariasis and the liver fluke

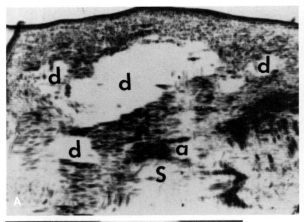

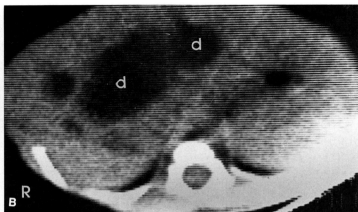

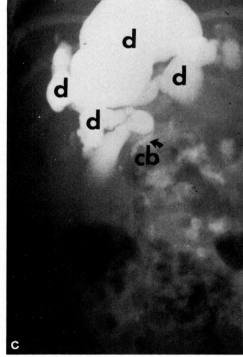

Fig. 63-11. Caroli's disease. **(A)** Transverse supine sonogram demonstrates multiple dilated bile ducts **(d)** as sonolucent spaces within the liver. **S,** spine; **a,** aorta. **(B)** CT scan at the same level shows the dilated duct as low-density areas **(d)** that appear larger in the central part of the liver. **(C)** Frontal view of a transhepatic cholangiogram in a projection corresponding to **A** shows cystic dilatation of the distal intrahepatic ducts **(d)** with a normal-sized common bile duct **(cb)**. (Mittelstaedt CA, Volberg FM, Fischer GJ et al: Caroli's disease: Sonographic findings. AJR 134:585–587, 1980. Copyright 1980. Reproduced with permission)

Clonorchis sinensis can cause large, round filling defects in a dilated intrahepatic ductal system. *Clonorchis* infestation is associated with an increased frequency of intrahepatic bile duct carcinoma.

CHOLANGITIS

Cholangitis of any etiology causes diffuse periductal inflammatory fibrosis leading to strictures of varying length and areas of cystic dilatation of the bile ducts. In patients with severe acute suppurative cholangitis, single or multiple small liver abscesses can communicate with the biliary tree and enhance the radiographic appearance of cystic dilatation of intrahepatic bile ducts (Fig. 63-12).

ORIENTAL CHOLANGIOHEPATITIS

Oriental cholangiohepatitis (recurrent pyogenic hepatitis) is a major cause of an acute abdomen in

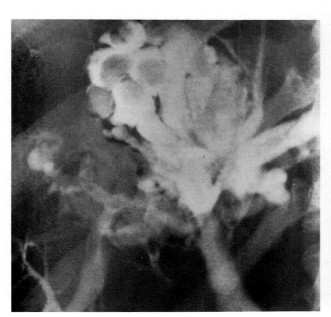

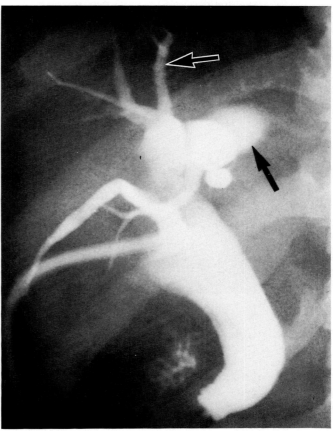

63-12   63-13

Fig. 63-12. Communicating hepatic abscess simulating localized cystic dilatation of an intrahepatic bile duct.

Fig. 63-13. Cholangiohepatitis (recurrent pyogenic cholangitis). A T-tube cholangiogram demonstrates that the common bile duct and intrahepatic duct **(lower arrow)** are dilated. The **upper arrow** shows a moderately dilated bile duct with short branches arising at right angles to the duct. (Ho CS, Wesson DE: Recurrent pyogenic cholangitis in Chinese immigrants. AJR 122:368–374, 1974. Copyright 1974. Reproduced with permission)

the Far East and is occasionally seen in Asian immigrants in the United States (Fig. 63-13). It is unclear whether the disease is secondary to *Clonorchis sinensis* infestation causing stone formation, biliary obstruction, stasis, and superimposed infection or whether it is related to portal septicemia resulting from poor eating habits. Cholangiohepatitis is characterized clinically by episodic attacks of right upper quadrant pain, fever, chills, and jaundice; patients may develop severe septicemia and obstructive jaundice requiring immediate surgical or percutaneous catheter drainage of the common bile duct. Radiographic findings include a decreased and abnormal arborization pattern of intrahepatic radicles and segmental dilatation of bile ducts along with areas of rapid peripheral tapering (arrowhead sign). Radiolucent calculi and dilatation of the common bile duct (up to 3–4 cm in diameter) are usually present.

SECONDARY INVOLVEMENT OF THE BILIARY SYSTEM

If large enough, any intrahepatic growth (benign or malignant tumor, parasitic infestation) will distort the segmental biliary ducts of the affected lobe, causing partial obstruction and cystic dilatation of portions of the intrahepatic biliary tree. In patients with hydatid cysts, fistulous communications between the cysts and the bile ducts can mimic intrahepatic bile duct dilatation (Fig. 63-14).

Improvements in transcatheter embolization techniques have permitted superselective occlusion of hepatic artery branches for control of hepatic bleeding and for palliative treatment of liver tumors. Rarely, this procedure leads to irreversible ischemia, infarction, and the development of bile cysts that communicate with the biliary tree (Fig. 63-15).

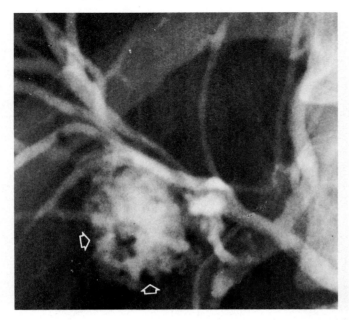
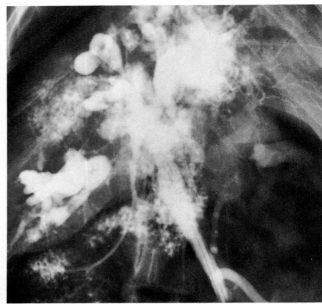

63-14   **63-15**

Fig. 63-14. Hydatid disease (echinococcosis). Fistulous communications between the cysts and the bile ducts mimic intrahepatic bile duct dilatation.

Fig. 63-15. Bile duct cysts secondary to liver infarcts. (Doppman JL, Dunnick NR, Girton M et al: Bile duct cysts secondary to liver infarcts: Report of a case and experimental production by small vessel hepatic artery occlusion. Radiology 130:1–5, 1979)

BIBLIOGRAPHY

Araki T, Itai Y, Tasaka A: Computed tomography of choledochal cyst. AJR 135:729–734, 1980

Babitt DP, Starshak RJ, Clemett AR: Choledochal cyst: A concept of etiology. AJR 119:57–62, 1973

Belamaric J: Intrahepatic bile duct carcinoma and *C. sinensis* infection in Hong Kong. Cancer 31:468–473, 1973

Berk RN, Clemett AR: Radiology of the Gallbladder and Bile Ducts. Philadelphia, WB Saunders, 1977

Caroli J: Diseases of the intrahepatic biliary tree. Clin Gastroenterol 2:147–161, 1973

Doppman JL, Dunnick NR, Girton M et al: Bile duct cysts secondary to liver infarcts. Report of a case and experimental production by small vessel hepatic artery occlusion. Radiology 130:1–5, 1979

Federle MP, Cello JP, Laing FC et al: Recurrent pyogenic cholangitis in Asian immigrants: Use of ultrasonography, computed tomography, and cholangiography. Radiology 143:151–156, 1982

Han BK, Babcock DS, Gelfand MH: Choledochal cyst with bile duct dilatation: Sonography and ^{99m}Tc IDA cholescintigraphy. AJR 136:1075–1079, 1981

Hatfield PM, Scholtz FJ, Wise RE: Congenital disease of the gallbladder and bile ducts. Semin Roentgenol 11:235–243, 1976

Ho CS, Wesson DE: Recurrent pyogenic cholangitis in Chinese immigrants. AJR 122:368–374, 1974

Kaiser JA, Mall JC, Salmen BJ et al: Diagnosis of Caroli's disease by computed tomography. Radiology 132:661–664, 1979

Li–Yeng C, Goldberg HI: Sclerosing cholangitis: Broad spectrum of radiographic findings. Gastrointest Radiol 9:39–47, 1984

MacCarty RL, LaRusso NF, Wiesner RH et al: Primary sclerosing cholangitis: Findings on cholangiography and pancreatography. Radiology 149:39–44, 1983

Mall JC, Ghahremani GG, Boyer JL: Caroli's disease associated with congenital hepatic fibrosis and renal tubular ectasia. Gastroenterology 66:1029–1035, 1974

Mittelstaedt CA, Volberg FM, Fischer GJ et al: Caroli's disease: Sonographic findings. AJR 134:585–587, 1980

Montana MA, Rohrmann CA: Cholangiocarcinoma in a choledochal cyst: Preoperative diagnosis. AJR 147:516–517, 1986

Moreno AJ, Parker AL, Spicer MJ et al: Scintigraphic and radiographic findings in Caroli's disease. Am J Gastroenterol 79:299–303, 1984

Mueller PR, Ferrucci JT, Simeone JF et al: Postcholecystectomy bile duct dilatation. Myth or reality? AJR 136:355–358, 1981

Mujahed Z, Glenn F, Evans JA: Communicating cavernous ectasia of the intrahepatic ducts (Caroli's disease). AJR 113:21–26, 1969

Reeder MM, Hamilton LC: Radiologic diagnosis of tropical diseases of the gastrointestinal tract. Radiol Clin North Am 7:57–81, 1969

Rosenfield N, Griscom NT: Choledochal cysts: Roentgenographic techniques. Radiology 114:113–119, 1975

Rosewarne MD: Cystic dilatation of the intrahepatic bile duct. Br J Radiol 45:825–827, 1972

Schey WL, Pinsky SM, Lipschutz HS et al: Hepatic duct diverticulum simulating a choledochal cyst. AJR 128:318–320, 1977

Scholz FJ, Carrera GF, Larsen CR: The choledochocele: Correlation of radiological, clinical and pathological findings. Radiology 118:25–28, 1976

Unite I, Maitem A, Bagnasco FM et al: Congenital hepatic fibrosis associated with renal tubular ectasia: A report of three cases. Radiology 109:565–570, 1973

ENLARGEMENT OF THE PAPILLA OF VATER

Disease Entities

Normal variant
Papillary edema
   Impacted common duct stone
   Pancreatitis
   Acute duodenal ulcer
Perivaterian neoplasms
   Carcinoma
   Adenomatous polyp
Papillitis
Lesions simulating enlarged papilla
   Benign spindle cell tumor
   Ectopic pancreas

The papilla of Vater is an elevated mound of tissue which projects into the duodenal lumen and into which opens the common bile duct. It can be identified radiographically in about 60% of barium upper gastrointestinal series. It appears as a small, regular indentation surrounded by normal mucosal folds. The papilla is most frequently situated on the inner border of the second portion of the duodenum at or just below the promontory (Fig. 64-1). In about 8% of patients, it is located in the third portion of the duodenum.

The papilla is generally considered to be enlarged whenever the greatest dimension seen radiographically exceeds 1.5 cm. In about 1% of examinations, however, the papilla appears to be larger than 1.5 cm (up to 3 × 1.2 cm) without there being any

disease process (Fig. 64-2). This normal variant is a diagnosis of exclusion; all other causes of an enlarged papilla must be ruled out before a normal variant can be seriously considered.

PAPILLARY EDEMA

An enlarged papilla is most commonly due to edema secondary to an impacted stone in the distal common duct, pancreatitis, or acute duodenal ulcer disease. Regardless of the cause, an edematous papilla has a characteristic smooth, semilunar configuration that can become more spherical when papillary swelling is severe (more than 3 cm in length). This is distinct from the usual pattern of perivaterian carcinoma, in which the filling defect is generally irregular or nodular and can ulcerate. Occasionally, however, perivaterian malignancy produces a smooth, rounded enlargement of the duodenal papilla that is indistinguishable from benign papillary edema.

An impacted common bile duct stone is a much more frequent cause of obstructive jaundice in adults than is neoplastic disease. When a calculus lodges in the distal common bile duct (where the lumen abruptly narrows as the duct passes through the duodenal wall), the impacted stone causes mechanical irritation of the mucus lining of the duct. This incites an inflammatory reaction, which frequently spreads to the duodenal papilla. The resulting congestion and swelling cause the papilla to en-

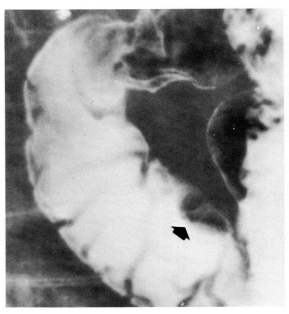
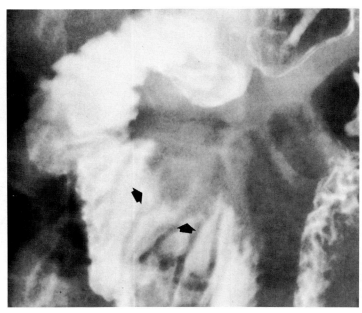

64-1   64-2

Fig. 64-1. Normal papilla. There is a small, regular indentation on the inner border of the second portion of the duodenum **(arrow)**.

Fig. 64-2. Normal variant of the papilla **(arrows)**. Although the papilla measured 2.5 × 1 cm, all pathologic entities causing enlargement of the papilla were excluded.

large to a diameter several times that of the impacted stone (Fig. 64-3). An identical phenomenon can occur in the urinary tract when a stone impacted at the ureterovesical junction produces a filling defect in the bladder as a result of edema of the interureteric ridge. An enlarged papilla secondary to an impacted common duct stone occasionally is irregular and mimics a perivaterian neoplasm. However, differentiation between these two entities is usually not difficult in view of the typical clinical symptoms of acute biliary colic.

Edematous swelling of the papilla can be seen in acute pancreatitis (Poppel's sign; Fig. 64-4). In patients who are known to have chronic pancreatitis, edematous enlargement of the papilla indicates acute or subacute exacerbation of the disease (Fig. 64-5). This is a very early sign that is usually present before pancreatic swelling can be detected. Papillary edema reflects the activity of the underlying pathologic process; it can increase or decrease almost daily in response to the degree of pancreatic inflammation. When pancreatitis is severe, edema can spread from the papilla and cause associated duodenal changes, such as mucosal fold thickening and atony.

Differentiation of papillary enlargement due to an impacted common duct stone from papillary enlargement secondary to pancreatitis can be difficult, especially since choledocholithiasis and pancreatitis are so frequently associated with each other. Although edema of the duodenal folds or gross pan-

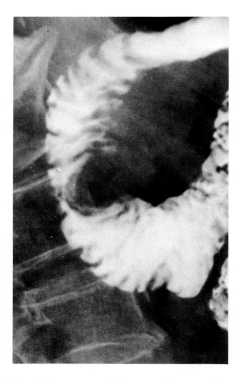

Fig. 64-3. Enlargement of the papilla caused by impacted common bile duct stone. The smooth, round to oval filling defect is caused by marked inflammatory edema of the papilla. (Ferrucci JT: The postbulbar duodenum. In Taveras JM, Ferrucci JT (eds): Radiology: Diagnosis—Imaging—Intervention. Philadelphia, JB Lippincott, 1987)

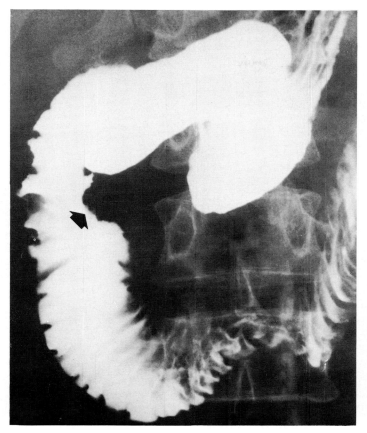

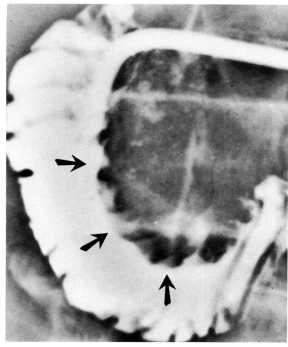

64-4

64-5

Fig. 64-4. Enlargement of the papilla **(arrow)** in acute pancreatitis.

Fig. 64-5. Enlargement of the papilla **(arrows)** in a patient who had chronic pancreatitis and was experiencing an acute exacerbation of the disease.

creatic enlargement indicates the presence of pancreatitis, it does not exclude the possibility of an impacted biliary stone. However, given that pancreatic calcification develops only infrequently in pancreatitis secondary to gallstones, the presence of such calcification in a patient with an enlarged papilla makes an impacted common duct stone an unlikely diagnosis.

In patients with acute duodenal ulcer disease, diffuse enlargement of the duodenal mucosal folds can occur. When the second portion of the duodenum is involved, maximum fold thickening tends to occur at the apex of the bulb, with the enlarged folds gradually decreasing in size distally. This enlargement of folds extends to and beyond the region of the papilla. The papillary fold can participate in this generalized edema and, because the papilla is larger than other duodenal folds, can become especially prominent (Fig. 64-6). If enlargement of the papilla

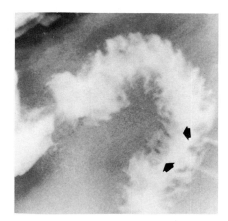

Fig. 64-6. Enlargement of the papilla in a patient with diffuse peptic ulcer disease **(arrows)**. There is generalized thickening of folds throughout the first and second portions of the duodenum.

is due to acute duodenal ulcer disease, a bulbar ulcer crater can almost invariably be demonstrated.

In patients with an impacted common duct stone, the papilla is primarily enlarged; duodenal fold thickening gradually decreases away from the papilla. In pancreatitis, the pattern of papilla enlargement and thickening of duodenal folds can appear identical to that seen in peptic ulcer disease. However, associated pancreatic swelling or calcification is usually also seen.

PERIVATERIAN NEOPLASMS

Perivaterian carcinomas (a collective term for malignancies arising in the duodenum, head of the pancreas, distal common bile duct, and ampulla of Vater) can protrude into the duodenal lumen and give the radiographic appearance of enlargement of the papilla (Fig. 64-7). In addition to the tumor mass, papillary enlargement can reflect malignant lymphatic obstruction with secondary papillary edema. In patients with perivaterian neoplasms, the surface of the papilla is often irregular and can demonstrate local erosion (Fig. 64-8). There is no thickening of surrounding duodenal folds, as may be seen in enlargement of the papilla due to edema. Perivaterian carcinoma occasionally has a smooth surface and appears identical to a benign edematous process.

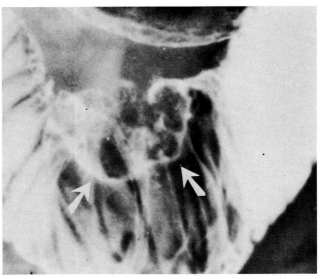

Fig. 64-8. Villous adenocarcinoma of the ampulla producing irregular enlargement of the papilla **(arrows)**.

Adenomatous polyps of the papilla of Vater can have a radiographic appearance simulating enlargement of the papilla. These tumors often have considerable inflammatory hyperplasia. Because evidence of foci of low-grade malignancy is usually histologically detectable, these adenomatous polyps of the papilla are generally considered to be premalignant lesions.

PAPILLITIS

Periductal inflammation and hyperplastic ductal proliferation can result in papillary "polyps." Rather than being a true neoplasm, this process is more likely an inflammatory reaction (papillitis) that eventually produces sphincter stenosis because of the formation of exuberant fibrosis.

LESIONS SIMULATING AN ENLARGED PAPILLA

A benign spindle cell tumor situated on the inner aspect of the second portion of the duodenum can mimic an enlarged papilla and, unless the papilla itself is clearly demonstrated, can be difficult to distinguish from papillary enlargement. Similarly, ectopic pancreatic tissue in the descending duodenum can simulate papillary edema. The presence of a central barium collection (ulcer or rudimentary duct) in what appears to be an enlarged papilla should suggest the possibility of a spindle cell tumor (especially leiomyoma) or ectopic pancreas.

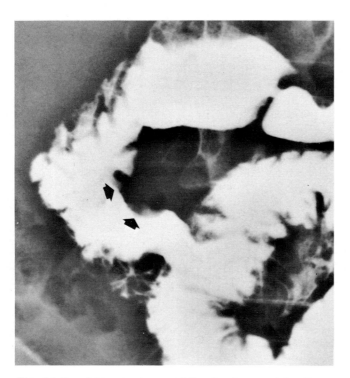

Fig. 64-7. Adenocarcinoma of the duodenum giving the radiographic appearance of enlargement of the papilla **(arrows)**.

DIFFERENTIAL DIAGNOSIS

Because a variety of entities can produce an almost identical radiographic pattern of enlargement of the papilla, clinical and laboratory data are essential to the proper diagnosis. Whenever an enlarged papilla is seen without jaundice, the most likely cause is ectopic pancreas, duodenal leiomyoma, or a large normal papilla. If jaundice, inflammatory manifestations, or clinical signs of malignancy are present, papillary enlargement suggests an impacted common duct stone, pancreatitis, duodenal ulcer disease, or perivaterian carcinoma. Jaundice is usually progressive in patients with malignancy; it can subside or fluctuate in patients with impacted common duct stones and is generally mild in persons with pancreatitis.

Patients with impacted common duct stones frequently have a previous history of cholelithiasis or biliary colic. Persons with pancreatitis causing papillary enlargement report similar episodes of abdominal pain and a history of alcohol abuse. In both of these benign conditions, the abdominal pain usually has an abrupt onset; in contrast, the pain associated with malignancy is generally more insidious. Fever and leukocytosis are frequently noted in patients with impacted common duct stones or acute pancreatitis; weight loss is more likely to reflect a malignant tumor or chronic pancreatitis. Guaiac-positive stools are fairly common in patients with perivaterian malignancy but rare in persons with impacted stones or pancreatitis. A palpable gallbladder can be felt in about one-fourth of patients with perivaterian malignancy but is rare in persons with papillary enlargement due to pancreatitis or an impacted common duct stone. Serum amylase or lipase levels are almost universally elevated in patients with pancreatitis. Transient elevation of these enzymes can be seen in about one-third of patients with impacted common duct stones but is unusual in persons with malignant perivaterian neoplasms.

BIBLIOGRAPHY

Berk RN, Clemett AR: Radiology of the Gallbladder and Bile Ducts. Philadelphia, WB Saunders, 1977

Bree RL, Flynn RE: Hypotonic duodenography in the evaluation of choledocholithiasis and obstructive jaundice. AJR 116:309–319, 1972

Eaton SB, Ferrucci JT, Benedict KT et al: Diagnosis of choledocholithiasis by barium duodenal examination. Radiology 102:267–273, 1972

Eaton SB, Ferrucci JT, Margulis AR et al: Unfamiliar roentgen findings in pancreatic disease. AJR 116:396–405, 1972

Griffen WO, Schaefer JW, Schindler S et al: Ampullary obstruction by benign duodenal polyps. Arch Surg 97:444–449, 1968

Jacobson HG, Shapiro JH, Pisano D et al: The vaterian and perivaterian segments in peptic ulcer. AJR 79:793–798, 1958

Oh C, Jemerin EE: Benign adenomatous polyps of the papilla of Vater. Surgery 57:495–503, 1965

Poppel MH: The roentgen manifestations of relapsing pancreatitis. Radiology 62:514–521, 1954

Poppel MH, Jacobson HG, Smith RW: The Roentgen Aspects of the Papilla and Ampulla of Vater. Springfield, IL, Charles C Thomas, 1953

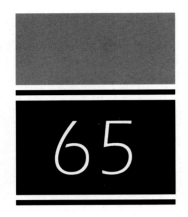

65

GAS IN THE BILIARY SYSTEM (PANCREATICOBILIARY REFLUX)

Disease Entities

Surgery
    Sphincterotomy
    Biliary–intestinal anastomosis
        Choledochoduodenostomy
        Cholecystoduodenostomy
        Cholecystojejunostomy
Inflammatory diseases
    Cholecystitis
    Recently passed common duct stone
    Perforated ulcer
    Pancreatitis
    Diseases associated with chronic scarring
        Crohn's disease
        Strongyloidiasis
        Clonorchis sinensis
        Ascaris lumbricoides
Neoplastic infiltration
    Primary carcinoma of the ampulla,
        duodenum, or pancreas
    Metastatic malignancy
Emphysematous cholecystitis
Anomalous insertion of common bile duct
    into a duodenal diverticulum
Pseudopneumobilia

The sphincter of Oddi is a complex of smooth muscle fibers surrounding the intraduodenal portions of the common bile duct, pancreatic duct (in 80% of persons), and ampulla of Vater. It regulates the flow of bile into the small bowel, inhibits entry of bile into the pancreatic duct, and prevents reflux of intestinal contents into both the bile and pancreatic ducts. Any disruption of the normal sphincter mechanism (*e.g.*, postsurgical, inflammatory, neoplastic) permits reflux of gas from the gastrointestinal tract into the biliary tree, and this can be detected on plain abdominal radiographs. Similarly, contrast material from an upper gastrointestinal series can be seen to reflux into the biliary ductal system (pancreaticobiliary reflux).

Reflux of barium into the bile duct or main pancreatic duct is definitely abnormal and indicates dysfunction of the sphincteric fibers in the duodenal wall or in the supraduodenal portions of the ducts. A distinction must be made between the normal finding of barium visualization of the ampulla of Vater and pathologic reflux filling of the biliary or pancreatic ducts. Barium occasionally fills the ampulla, especially during hypotonic duodenography, in which the spasmolytic effect of the drug causes relaxation of the lower portion of the sphincter of Oddi. The ampulla is seen radiographically as a short, truncated, conical or pyramidal projection that usually arises from the promontory and extends 7 mm to 10 mm in length. It must be differentiated from diverticula of the mid-descending duodenum, which are usually larger, more spherical, have a visible neck, and empty more slowly.

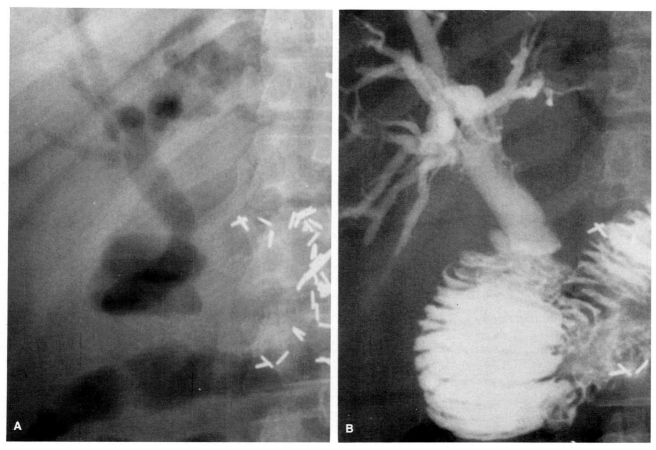

Fig. 65-1. **(A)** Gas in the biliary tree and **(B)** pancreaticoduodenal reflux of barium in a patient who had undergone a surgical procedure to relieve biliary obstruction.

SURGERY

The most common cause of gas in the biliary tree or pancreaticobiliary reflux is prior surgery, usually performed for biliary obstruction (Fig. 65-1). This is most frequently secondary to sphincterotomy, though an identical appearance can be seen in any biliary–intestinal anastomosis (Fig. 65-2).

INFLAMMATORY DISEASES

Inflammatory processes can lead to the presence of gas in the biliary tree and pancreaticobiliary reflux, either by fistulization between the biliary system and intestinal tract (Fig. 65-3) or by anatomic distortion and resultant incompetence of the sphincter of Oddi. In 90% of cases, this pattern is due to fistula formation between the gallbladder and an adjacent organ, primarily the duodenum (Fig. 65-4). A stone passing into the duodenum can produce mechanical obstruction if it becomes impacted in the small

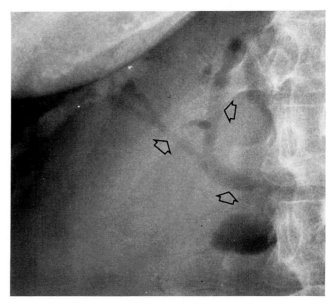

Fig. 65-2. Gas in the biliary tree **(arrows)** following cholecystoduodenostomy for stricture of the common bile duct.

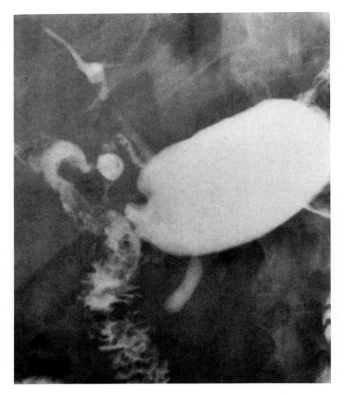

Fig. 65-3. Pancreaticobiliary reflux in a patient with gallstone ileus. Note that barium fills the tract extending from the gallbladder to the duodenal bulb. The distal common bile duct and region of the papilla are normal.

bowel (gallstone ileus; Fig. 65-5). Uncomplicated cholecystointestinal fistulas rarely cause significant complications and are often asymptomatic. Indeed, deliberate surgical anastomosis from the gallbladder to the intestinal tract is frequently performed to bypass an obstructed common bile duct. A recently passed common duct stone can distort the sphincteric architecture, resulting in gas in the biliary tree and pancreaticobiliary reflux.

Fistulas between the biliary system and duodenum are occasionally present without gas in the biliary tree. This occurs in the patient with a cholecystoduodenal fistula in whom the cystic duct is obstructed by a stone or tumor. In this situation, gas is unable to enter the biliary tree, though it is often present in the gallbladder.

In patients with severe peptic ulcer disease, fistulas can extend from the duodenum or stomach into the gallbladder or bile duct. Jaundice or cholangitis can develop in these patients, but biliary involvement is often asymptomatic and is usually only incidentally discovered on plain abdominal radiographs or on an upper gastrointestinal series. Acute spasm or fibrous healing of a postbulbar ulcer adjacent to the papilla or acute inflammation of the head of the pancreas can deform the orifice of the ampulla and lead to incompetence of the

sphincter of Oddi and pancreaticobiliary reflux (Fig. 65-6).

Rigidity of the duodenal wall, caused by the diffuse cicatrization that is associated with granulomatous disease of the duodenum, can result in gas in the biliary tree and pancreaticobiliary reflux. In Crohn's disease, reflux is postulated to occur either by fistula formation or through a damaged ampulla of Vater. In strongyloidiasis, periampullary scarring and incompetence of the sphincter of Oddi can produce a similar radiographic appearance.

Gas in the biliary tree and pancreaticobiliary reflux can be due to biliary infestation by *Clonorchis sinensis* or *Ascaris lumbricoides*. *Clonorchis* is a parasitic fluke that is acquired by the ingestion of raw freshwater fish. The parasite migrates from the duodenum into the biliary tree, where it may live for many years and incite an inflammatory reaction. This inflammation predisposes to stone formation, obstruction, secondary bacterial infection, and scarring. Recurrent attacks of abdominal pain and cholangitis are common. *Clonorchis* should be considered a possible cause of gas in the biliary tree and pancreaticobiliary reflux in patients with the appro-

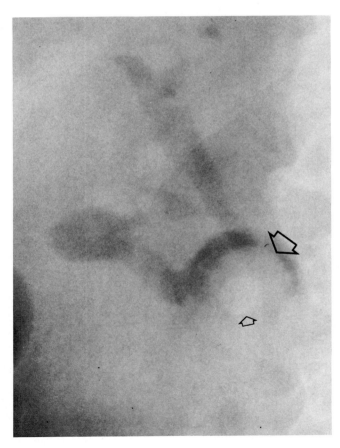

Fig. 65-4. Gas in the biliary tree due to fistulization between the gallbladder and duodenum. Note the central calcification **(small arrow)** within the offending gallstone **(large arrow)**, which is situated in the duodenum.

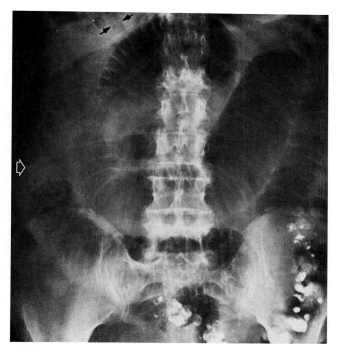

Fig. 65-5. Gallstone ileus. An obstructing stone **(open arrow)** causes dilatation of proximal small bowel loops. Note the gas in the biliary tree **(solid arrow)**.

priate clinical symptomatology who have spent a long time in the Orient. *Ascaris* invades the bile ducts by passing through the sphincter of Oddi from the duodenum. Migration of the worms can disrupt the normal sphincter architecture and permit reflux into the common bile duct. Once in the biliary system, the worms or their ova induce an inflammatory response that can lead to progressive cholangitis and bile duct obstruction.

MALIGNANT DISEASES

Gas in the biliary tree and pancreaticobiliary reflux can be seen in patients with primary or metastatic lesions involving the ampulla of Vater or perivaterian region. Indeed, the appearance of biliary reflux in a patient without a history of surgery or known Crohn's disease points to perivaterian malignancy as the most likely etiology.

EMPHYSEMATOUS CHOLECYSTITIS

Gas in the bile ducts is an infrequent occurrence in patients with emphysematous cholecystitis (Fig.

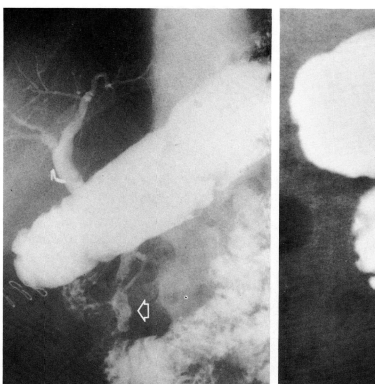

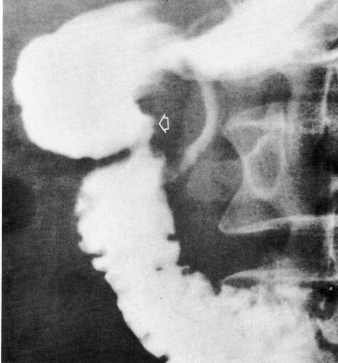

Fig. 65-6. Two patients with pancreaticobiliary reflux associated with postbulbar peptic ulcers **(arrows)**.

65-7). Its presence suggests that the cystic duct is patent, allowing gas to escape from the gallbladder lumen. If gas is not also identified in the wall of the gallbladder, the diagnosis of emphysematous cholecystitis may not even be considered.

CONGENITAL ANOMALY

Spontaneous reflux from the duodenum into the pancreatic or common bile duct can occur without any duodenal or pancreaticobiliary disease. This is a rare occurrence that is usually associated with the anomalous insertion of one or both of these ducts into a duodenal diverticulum.

PSEUDOPNEUMOBILIA

An appearance simulating gas in the biliary tree (pseudopneumobilia) is occasionally produced by the normal periductal fat that surrounds and parallels the course of the major bile ducts (Fig. 65-8). This lucent band is continuous with the extraperitoneal fat outlining the visceral border of the liver. It is typically wider than a nonobstructed ductal system, is not as radiolucent as gas in the bile ducts, and does not involve the intrahepatic portion of the biliary tree. The true nature of pseudopneumobilia is readily apparent on intravenous cholangiography.

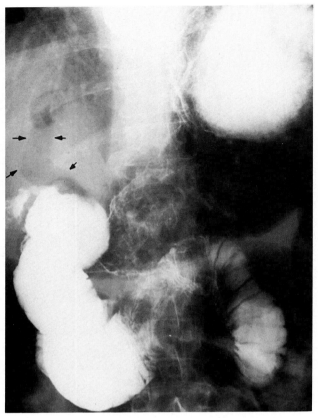

Fig. 65-7. Gas in the biliary tree **(arrows)** in a patient with phlegmonous emphysematous gastritis.

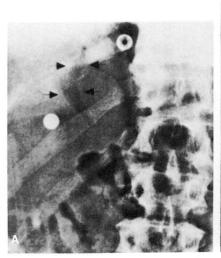

Fig. 65-8. Pseudopneumobilia. **(A)** On a plain abdominal radiograph, the curved tubular radiolucent band **(arrows)** projecting over the upper renal pole (together with the liver shadow) was interpreted as "air in the biliary system." An upper gastrointestinal series showed no fistulous communication. **(B)** An intravenous cholangiogram demonstrates the shape and position of the normal common bile ducts, particularly the sleevelike lucent periductal fat paralleling their contours **(arrows)**. Extraperitoneal fat outlining the visceral border of the liver is continuous with the periductal hilar fat. (Govoni AF, Meyers MA: Pseudopneumobilia. Radiology 118:536, 1976)

BIBLIOGRAPHY

Berk RN, Clemett AR: Radiology of the Gallbladder and Bile Ducts. Philadelphia, WB Saunders, 1977

Dallemand S, Waxman M, Farman J: Radiological manifestations of *Strongyloides stercoralis*. Gastrointest Radiol 8:45–51, 1983

Eaton SB, Ferrucci JT, Margulis AR et al: Unfamiliar roentgen findings in pancreatic disease. AJR 116:396–405, 1972

Govoni AF, Meyers MA: Pseudopneumobilia. Radiology 118:526, 1976

Haff RC, Wise L, Ballinger WF: Biliary–enteric fistulas. Surg Gynecol Obstet 133:84–88, 1971

Harley WD, Kirkpatrick RH, Ferrucci JT: Gas in the bile ducts (pneumobilia) in emphysematous cholecystitis. AJR 131:661–663, 1978

Legge DA, Carlson HC, Judd ES: Roentgenolgic features of re-gional enteritis of the upper gastrointestinal tract. AJR 110:355–360, 1970

Lewandowski BJ, Withers C, Winsberg F: The air-filled left hepatic duct: The saber sign as an aid to the radiographic diagnosis of pneumobilia. Radiology 153:329–332, 1984

Michowitz M, Farago C, Lazarovici I et al: Choledochoduodenal fistula: A rare complication of duodenal ulcer. Am J Gastroenterol 79:416–420, 1984

Mindelzun R, McCort JJ: Hepatic and perihepatic radiolucencies. Radiol Clin North Am 18:221–238, 1980

Poppel MH, Jacobson HG, Smith RW: The Roentgen Aspects of the Papilla and Ampulla of Vater. Springfield, IL, Charles C. Thomas, 1953

Rice RP, Thompson WM, Gedgaudas RK: The diagnosis and significance of extraluminal gas in the abdomen. Radiol Clin North Am 20:819–837, 1982

Shehadi WH: Radiologic examination of the biliary tree. Radiol Clin North Am 4:463–482, 1966

66 GAS IN THE PORTAL VEINS

Disease Entities

Childhood disorders
   Necrotizing enterocolitis
   Neonatal gastroenteritis
   Erythroblastosis fetalis
   Surgery for congenital intestinal obstruction
      Esophageal atresia
      Duodenal atresia
      Imperforate anus
   Umbilical venous catheterization
Adult disorders
   Mesenteric arterial occlusion and bowel
      infarction
   Diabetes mellitus
   Mesenteric vein thrombosis secondary
      to peritonitis
   Hemorrhagic pancreatitis
   Diverticulitis
   Pelvic abscess
   Perforated gastric ulcer
   Necrotic colon cancer
   Ingestion of corrosive substances
   Hydrogen peroxide gastric lavage
   Emphysematous cholecystitis
   Barium enema or colonoscopy in a patient
      with inflammatory bowel disease
      (ulcerative or Crohn's colitis)
   Overinflation of rectal balloon catheter
   Gastric emphysema

Except when it is associated with umbilical venous catheterization in children and in rare instances in adults, the presence of gas in the portal venous system is of grave prognostic significance and a sign of imminent death. Two major mechanisms are postulated to result in the radiographic appearance of gas in the portal veins. Mechanical intestinal obstruction or mesenteric artery occlusion may lead to loss of intestinal mucosal integrity (necrosis), permitting intraluminal bowel gas to penetrate vessel walls and flow to the liver. A second mechanism suggests either that local intestinal necrosis is followed by infection of the bowel wall by gas-producing organisms or that bowel necrosis is initially caused by an overwhelming enterocolitis. In either situation, gas in the bowel wall enters the portal venous system and lodges peripherally in the liver.

Gas in the portal veins must be distinguished from gas in the biliary system secondary to fistula formation between the bile duct and gastrointestinal tract. When gas embolizes into the portal venous system, bubbles are carried into the fine peripheral radicles in the liver by the centrifugal flow of portal venous blood. This presents a characteristic radiographic appearance of radiating tubular radiolucencies branching from the porta hepatis to the edge of the liver (Fig. 66-1). Visualization of gas in the outermost 2 cm of the liver is considered presumptive evidence of portal vein gas. In contrast, gas in the biliary tree is found in the larger, more centrally situated bile ducts; it is prevented from entering finer radicles by the continuous centripetal

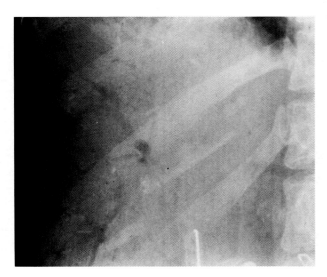

Fig. 66-1. Portal vein gas. Characteristic radiographic appearance of tubular lucencies extending to the edge of the liver. In this elderly woman, the portal venous gas resulted from ischemic disease and infarction of the small bowel. (Rice RP: The plain film of the abdomen. In Taveras JM, Ferrucci JT (eds): Radiology: Diagnosis—Imaging—Intervention. Philadelphia, JB Lippincott, 1987)

flow of the secreted bile. If it is difficult to distinguish between peripherally located gas in the portal venous system and the more central appearance of gas in the biliary tree, oral contrast can be administered in an attempt to delineate an intestinal–biliary fistula.

CHILDHOOD DISORDERS

NECROTIZING ENTEROCOLITIS

The most common cause of gas in the portal veins in children is necrotizing enterocolitis, an often fatal clinical syndrome characterized by abdominal distention, bloody vomitus and stools, and shock (Fig. 66-2). In this condition, the intestinal mucosa is so severely ulcerated and damaged that gas-producing organisms proliferate and penetrate the bowel wall, frequently producing pneumatosis intestinalis. Pre- and postmortem cultures are often positive for gas-forming organisms. If there is sepsis, severe distention alone can force gas into the submucosa, even without overt evidence of mucosal damage.

ERYTHROBLASTOSIS FETALIS

Erythroblastosis fetalis (hemolytic disease of the newborn) usually results from Rh incompatibility, in which there is isoimmunization of an Rh-negative pregnant woman by Rh-positive fetal erythrocytes. Maternal anti-Rh agglutinins cross the placenta to

the fetal circulation, where they cause hemolysis of fetal red blood cells. This hemolysis of fetal cells before birth causes jaundice, anemia, edema, splenomegaly, and hepatomegaly in the newborn infant. The presence of gas in the portal veins is a dire prognostic sign.

UMBILICAL VEIN CATHETERIZATION

In relatively asymptomatic infants, the presence of an umbilical vein catheter in association with portal vein gas excludes most serious illnesses (Fig. 66-3). Portal vein gas in these infants is caused by inadvertent injection of air during umbilical venous catheterization or during drug administration through the catheter and does not reflect a potentially fatal disorder. Umbilical venous catheterization offers a simple pathway through which to give fluids and medications to infants with respiratory distress and other medical problems. The tip of the catheter should be positioned in the inferior vena cava, just below the right hemidiaphragm. To reach this point, the catheter must pass through the umbilical vein and cross the ductus venosus before entering the inferior vena cava. If the catheter lodges in the umbilical vein or ductus venosus, or if it reaches the portal sinus, any gas inadvertently administered

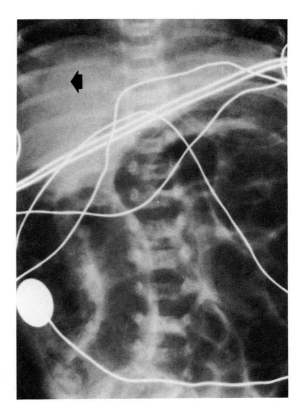

Fig. 66-2. Portal vein gas **(arrow)** in an infant who died of necrotizing enterocolitis.

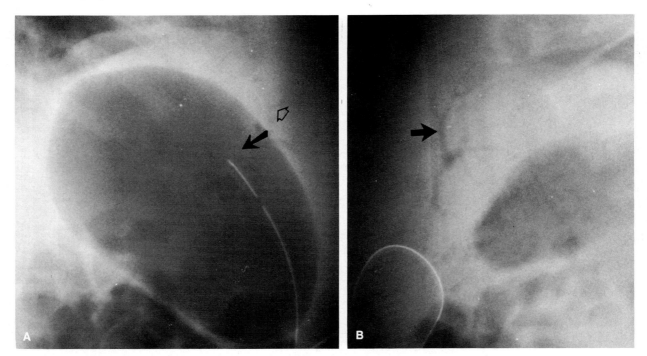

Fig. 66-3. Portal vein gas related to umbilical catheterization. **(A)** This newborn male infant was noted to have "grunting respirations." The symptoms rapidly cleared. Note the portal vein gas **(open arrow)** and the tip of the catheter in the umbilical vein **(solid arrow). (B)** This newborn male infant had mild respiratory distress, which cleared rapidly. Note the portal vein gas **(arrow)** and the umbilical catheter, its tip (not identified in this picture) in the umbilical vein. (Swaim TJ, Gerald B: Hepatic portal venous gas in infants without subsequent death. Radiology 94:343–345, 1970)

through it is injected almost directly into the hepatic portal venous system.

ADULT DISORDERS

In adults, most cases of gas in the portal veins are associated with mesenteric arterial occlusion and bowel infarction. Gas in the portal veins has also been described in patients with diabetes, mesenteric vein thrombosis, hemorrhagic pancreatitis, diverticulitis, pelvic abscesses, perforated gastric ulcers, necrotic colon carcinoma, and emphysematous cholecystitis (Fig. 66-4), and after acute necrotizing gastroenteritis following the ingestion of corrosive substances or hydrogen peroxide colon lavage. Portal vein gas has been demonstrated in a few patients with ulcerative or Crohn's colitis after barium enema examination or colonoscopy. An interplay of factors—damaged mucosa, bowel disten-

tion, sepsis—may be responsible for the passage of gas into the portal venous system. A single case of portal venous air associated with a barium enema examination has been reported in a patient with diverticulosis. This probably represented a complication of overinflation of the rectal balloon catheter, which led to a rectal mucosal laceration that allowed colonic gas to gain entrance into the rich submucosal venous plexus and eventually through the inferior mesenteric vein to the portal venous system. Unless associated with free perforation, portal venous gas following barium enema examination or colonoscopy is not associated with symptoms or complications and resolves within 2 days. Another rare benign cause of portal venous gas is acute gastric dilatation with air in the wall of the stomach (gastric emphysema) (Fig. 66-5). The few patients reported with this condition have been bedridden young people who recovered completely after decompression of the stomach with a nasogastric tube.

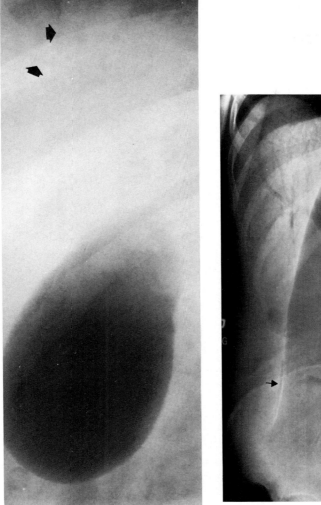

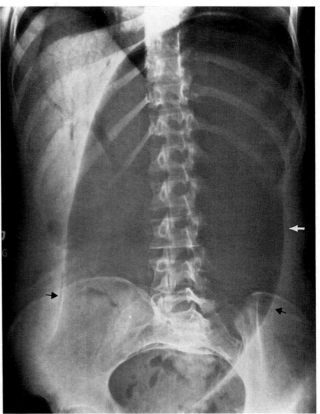

66-4   66-5

Fig. 66-4. Portal vein gas **(arrows)** associated with emphysematous cholecystitis.

Fig. 66-5. Portal venous gas associated with acute gastric dilatation. The branching radiolucencies in the right upper quadrant extend to within 2 cm of the liver capsule. There is massive gastric dilatation with lucent streaks in the wall of the stomach **(arrows).** (Radin DR, Rosen RS, Halls JM: Acute gastric dilatation: A rare cause of portal venous gas. AJR 148:279–280, 1987. Copyright 1987. Reproduced with permission)

PROGNOSIS OF PORTAL VEIN GAS

On rare occasions, the discovery of gas in the portal veins has led to immediate surgery and patient survival. Nevertheless, except in the case of the asymptomatic infant with an umbilical venous catheter, the patient with ulcerative or Crohn's colitis following barium enema examination or colonoscopy, or the bedridden young adult with acute gastric dilatation and gastric emphysema, gas in the portal veins is generally associated with an extremely dismal prognosis.

BIBLIOGRAPHY

Berk RN, Clemett AR: Radiology of the Gallbladder and Bile Ducts. Philadelphia, WB Saunders, 1977

Fink DW, Boyden FM: Gas in the portal veins. A report of two cases due to ingestion of corrosive substances. Radiology 87:741–743, 1966

Gold RP, Seaman WB: Splenic flexure carcinoma as a source of hepatic portal venous gas. Radiology 122:329–330, 1977

Graham GA, Bernstein RB, Gronner AT: Gas in the portal and inferior mesenteric veins caused by diverticulitis of the sigmoid colon: Report of a case with survival. Radiology 114:601–602, 1975

Huycke A, Moeller DD: Hepatic portal venous gas after colonoscopy in granulomatous colitis. Am J Gastroenterol 80:637–638, 1985

Liebman PR, Pattern MT, Manny J et al: Hepatic–portal venous gas in adults: Etiology, pathophysiology and clinical significance. Ann Surg 187:281–287, 1978

Paciulli J, Jacobson G: Survival following roentgenographic demonstration of gas in the hepatic portal venous system. AJR 99:629–631, 1967

Pappas D, Romeu J, Tarkin N et al: Portal vein gas in a patient with Crohn's colitis. Am J Gastroenterol 79:728–730, 1984

Radin DR, Rosen RD, Halls JM: Acute gastric dilatation: A rare cause of portal venous gas. AJR 148:279–280, 1987

Rice RP, Thompson WM, Gedgaudas RK: The diagnosis and significance of extraluminal gas in the abdomen. Radiol Clin North Am 20:819–837, 1982

Sisk PB: Gas in the portal venous system. Radiology 77:103–107, 1961

Stein MG, Crues JV, Hamlin JA: Portal venous air associated with barium enema. AJR 140:1171–1172, 1983

Susman N, Senturia HR: Gas embolization of the portal venous system. AJR 83:847–850, 1960

Swaim TJ, Gerald B: Hepatic portal venous gas in infants without subsequent death. Radiology 94:343–345, 1970

Wiot JF, Felson B: Gas in the portal venous system. AJR 86:920–929, 1961

Wolfe JN, Evans WA: Gas in the portal veins of the liver in infants: A roentgenographic demonstration with postmortem anatomical correlation. AJR 74:486–489, 1955

PART NINE

MISCELLANEOUS

BULL'S-EYE LESIONS IN THE GASTROINTESTINAL TRACT

67

Disease Entities

Metastatic melanoma
Primary neoplasms
    Spindle cell tumor (benign or malignant)
    Lymphoma
    Carcinoid
    Carcinoma
Hematogenous metastases
    Breast cancer
    Lung cancer
    Renal cancer
    Kaposi's sarcoma
Peptic ulcer disease/superficial erosions
Eosinophilic granuloma
Ectopic pancreas
Mastocytosis
Behcet's syndrome

Bull's-eye or target lesions of the gastrointestinal tract reflect ulceration or umbilication of mass lesions. The ulceration can cause gastrointestinal hemorrhage and, if the underlying mass lesion is sufficiently large, can be associated with intestinal obstruction.

METASTATIC MELANOMA

Multiple bull's-eye lesions in the gastrointestinal tract are highly suggestive of metastatic melanoma (Fig. 67-1). This tumor metastasizes widely and frequently involves the gastrointestinal tract, usually sparing the large bowel. Metastases of melanoma can be well-circumscribed round or oval nodules, plaques, or sessile or pedunculated polypoid masses. As the metastasis outgrows its blood supply, central ulceration is common (Fig. 67-2). The borders of the filling defect are sharply defined, and the ulcer is quite large relative to the size of the metastatic mass. Some nodules of metastatic melanoma can be centrally umbilicated without there being actual ulceration. Metastatic melanoma in the form of an enlarging pedunculated mass projecting into the bowel lumen can lead to intussusception. Gastrointestinal metastases can be the first clinical manifestation of metastatic melanoma; at times, it can be impossible to identify the primary tumor site. In a patient with a known primary melanoma, the presence of multiple bull's-eye gastrointestinal lesions is virtually pathognomonic of metastatic melanoma.

PRIMARY NEOPLASMS

Spindle cell tumors of the bowel (especially leiomyoma) can demonstrate central necrosis and ulceration of the overlying mucosal surface, which give rise to gastrointestinal hemorrhage and the radiographic appearance of a single bull's-eye lesion (Fig. 67-3). Central ulceration of a discrete mass (occasionally multiple) is one of the many manifestations of gastrointestinal lymphoma (Fig. 67-4). In-

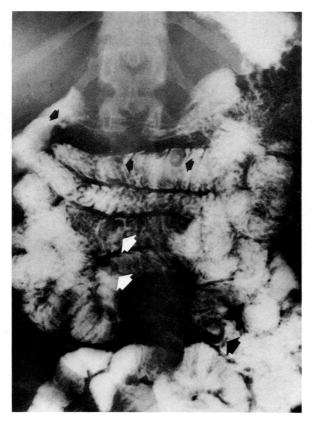

Fig. 67-1. Metastatic melanoma. Multiple nodular filling defects **(arrows)** varying from 6 mm to 2 cm in diameter are present throughout the small bowel. Central ulceration can be identified in most of the lesions; in some, the central ulcer is large in relation to the size of the mass, causing a bull's-eye appearance. At least ten separate discrete nodular lesions could be identified on the complete series of original radiographs. Except for the isolated lesions, the small bowel is normal in appearance. (Cavanagh RC, Buchignani JS, Rulon DB: RPC of the month from the AFIP. Radiology 101:195–200, 1971)

frequently, an ulcerated carcinoid tumor or primary carcinoma of the small bowel can present as an isolated bull's-eye lesion.

HEMATOGENOUS METASTASES

Hematogenous metastases can cause multiple ulcerating mass lesions of the bowel (Fig. 67-5). Breast cancer metastasizes to the gastrointestinal tract, especially the stomach and duodenum, in about 15% of cases. Although this tumor does not elicit a desmoplastic response, the highly cellular deposits can narrow and deform the lumen, causing a scirrhous appearance. Metastases to the small bowel usually produce large mesenteric masses, with infiltration of the bowel wall, fixation, and angulation. Occasionally, there are discrete submucosal masses that may have central ulceration (Fig. 67-6).

KAPOSI'S SARCOMA

Kaposi's sarcoma is a systemic disease that characteristically affects the skin and causes an ulcerated hemorrhagic dermatitis. The typical nodules or pigmented patches initially involve the extremities and are frequently associated with intense edema, which causes the limbs to become firm, thick, and heavily pachydermatous. Biopsy and histologic studies show that the Kaposi's lesions are composed of capillaries that sometimes anastomose freely. The space between the blood vessels is filled with spindle-shaped cells and reticulin fibers resembling a well-differentiated fibrosarcoma. The lesions are sensitive to irradiation and have a low-grade malignant course.

There are three distinct types of clinical presentation of Kaposi's sarcoma. A relatively benign form

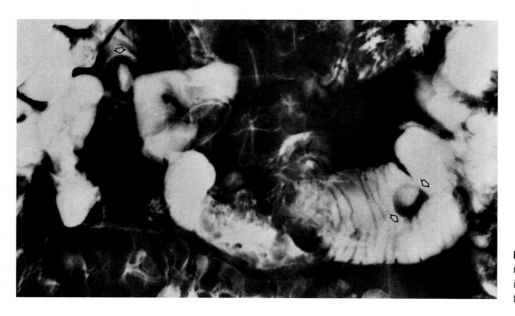

Fig. 67-2. Metastatic melanoma. Large central ulcerations in two sharply defined filling defects **(arrows)**.

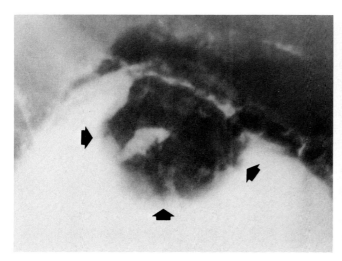

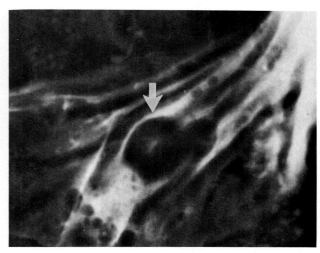

67-3

67-4

Fig. 67-3. Ulcerated leiomyoma of the fundus of the stomach **(arrows)** causing a bull's-eye appearance.

Fig. 67-4. Lymphoma of the stomach **(arrow)** with central ulceration presenting as a bull's-eye lesion.

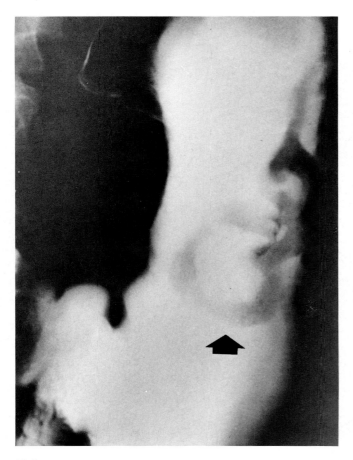

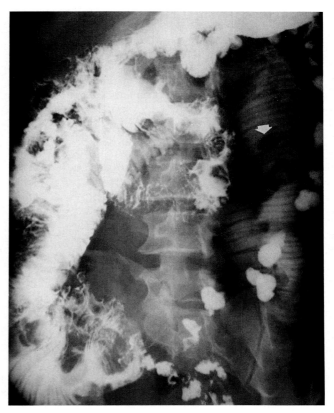

67-5

67-6

Fig. 67-5. Carcinoma of the breast metastatic to the stomach. There is a huge, centrally ulcerated lesion **(arrow)**.

Fig. 67-6. Mesothelioma (lung primary) metastatic to small bowel and mesentery. Several of the multiple submucosal masses demonstrate central ulceration and a bull's-eye pattern **(arrow)**.

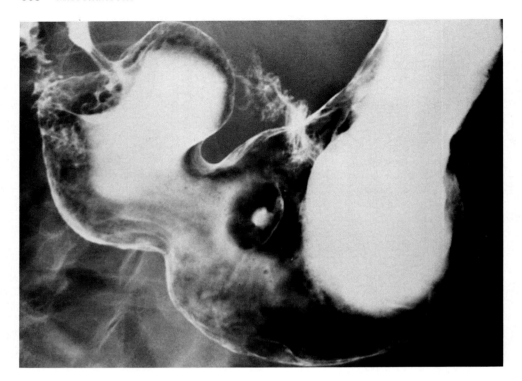

Fig. 67-7. Peptic ulcer disease. Discrete benign ulcer sitting on a distinct mound of inflammatory edema. The smooth character of the mucosal surface surrounding the ulcer is indicative of its benign nature. (Gelfand DW: Gastrointestinal Radiology. New York, Churchill Livingstone, 1984)

primarily involves middle-aged or elderly men originally from southeastern Europe and northern Italy. The lesions in this group develop slowly over many years, and visceral involvement is uncommon. The second form is prevalent in parts of central and southern Africa, where it accounts for up to 10% of all malignant neoplasms. The average age of affected patients is significantly lower, and the disease exhibits a virulent, aggressive biologic behavior associated with a poor prognosis. The disease presents systemically with generalized lymphadenopathy, hepatosplenomegaly, anemia, and usually without skin manifestations.

Most recently, a systemic and virulent form of Kaposi's sarcoma has become more widespread in patients with immunologic compromise, especially AIDS. In addition to extensive hemorrhagic skin lesions, these patients demonstrate constitutional symptoms and peripheral adenopathy and suffer a poor prognosis similar to that in the African form of the disease. There is a 50% incidence of retroperitoneal and mesenteric lymphadenopathy, reflecting the high malignant potential of this form of disease.

Metastases of Kaposi's sarcoma to the small bowel are relatively common and consist of multiple reddish or bluish-red nodules that intrude into the lumen of the bowel and frequently produce central ulceration. Although infrequently seen radiographically, metastases of Kaposi's sarcoma to the small bowel characteristically appear as multiple bull's-eye lesions containing central collections of barium.

PEPTIC ULCER

Intense inflammatory edema incited by a benign peptic ulcer of the stomach or duodenum can cause a smooth elevated soft-tissue mound around the ulcer, producing a bull's-eye appearance (Fig. 67-7). In an aphthous ulcer of any etiology, a small central collection of barium is surrounded by a halo of adjacent inflammation (see Chapter 15).

EOSINOPHILIC GRANULOMA

Eosinophilic granuloma is a sharply localized polypoid lesion that can demonstrate central ulceration. It is most frequently seen in the stomach but can occur in the small bowel, colon, or rectum. Unlike eosinophilic gastroenteritis, eosinophilic granuloma is a discrete lesion that is not associated with specific food intolerance or peripheral blood eosinophilia.

ECTOPIC PANCREAS

Ectopic pancreatic tissue can form a polypoid mass in the stomach or duodenum. The bull's-eye radiographic appearance frequently seen with these solitary lesions represents umbilication of a central rudimentary pancreatic duct rather than necrotic ulceration (Fig. 67-8).

MASTOCYTOSIS

Multiple bull's-eye lesions have been reported in a case of systemic mastocytosis (Fig. 67-9), a rare disorder characterized by mast cell proliferation in the skin, bones, lymph nodes, and parenchymal organs. More common types of gastrointestinal involvement in mastocytosis include sandlike lucencies and irregular thickening of folds in the small bowel as well as an increased incidence of peptic ulcers and malabsorption. In the case presented, the central umbilication seen radiographically could not be explained by either the endoscopic or histologic findings.

BEHÇET'S SYNDROME

The hallmark of intestinal involvement in Behçet's disease is ulceration, which may involve any part of the gastrointestinal tract but predominantly affects the terminal ileum, ileocecal region, and proximal ascending colon. Central ringlike barium collections within multiple large, discrete nodular lesions in the terminal ileum has been reported as a specific gastrointestinal manifestation of Behçet's disease (Fig. 67-10). The ulcers tend to penetrate deeply to the muscular or serosal layer, resulting in a high incidence (up to 40%) of perforation.

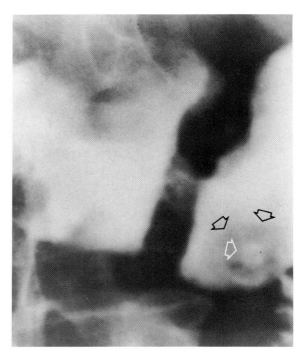

Fig. 67-8. Ectopic pancreas. Umbilication of a rudimentary pancreatic duct, rather than necrotic ulceration, causes central opacification **(white arrow)** within the soft-tissue mass **(black arrows)** in the distal antrum, producing a bull's-eye pattern.

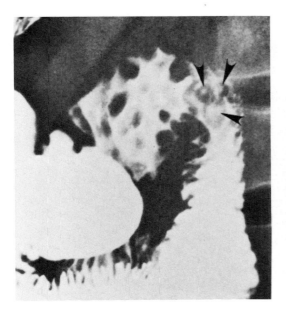

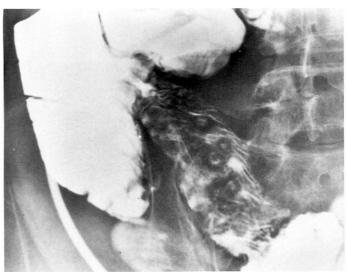

67-9

67-10

Fig. 67-9. Mastocytosis. Several of the duodenal nodules have central barium collections **(arrowheads).** (Quinn SF, Shaffer HA, Willard MR et al: Bull's-eye lesions: New gastrointestinal presentation of mastocytosis. Gastrointest Radiol 9:13–15, 1984)

Fig. 67-10. Behçet's syndrome. Coned view of the terminal ileum shows multiple, large, discrete, nodular lesions with central ringlike barium collections. The remainder of the small bowel appeared normal. (McLean AM, Simms DM, Homer MJ: Ileal ring ulcers in Behçet's syndrome. AJR 140:947–948, 1983. Copyright 1983. Reproduced with permission.

BIBLIOGRAPHY

Asch MJ, Wiedel PD, Habif DV: Gastrointestinal metastases from carcinoma of the breast: Autopsy study and 18 cases requiring operative intervention. Arch Surg 96:840–843, 1968

Balthazar EJ, Megibow A, Bryk D et al: Gastric carcinoid tumors: Radiographic features in eight cases. AJR 139:1123–1127, 1982

Bryk D, Farman J, Dallemand S et al: Kaposi's sarcoma of the intestinal tract: Roentgen manifestations. Gastrointest Radiol 3:425–430, 1978

Cavanagh RC, Buchignani JJ Jr, Rulon DB: Metastatic melanoma of the small intestine. Radiology 101:195–200, 1971

Farmer RG, Hawk WA: Metastatic tumors of the small bowel. Gastroenterology 47:496–504, 1964

Goldstein HM, Beydoun MT, Dodd, GD: Radiologic spectrum of melanoma metastatic to the gastrointestinal tract. AJR 129:605–612, 1977

Graham WP: Gastrointestinal metastases from carcinoma of the breast. Ann Surg 159:477–480, 1964

Khilnani MT, Wolf BS: Late involvement of the alimentary tract by carcinoma of the kidney. Am J Dig Dis 5:529–540, 1960

McLean AM, Simms DM, Homer MJ: Ileal ring ulcers in Behcet's syndrome. AJR 140:947–948, 1983

Meyers MA, McSweeney J: Secondary neoplasms of the bowel. Radiology 105:1–11, 1972

Oddson TA, Rice RP, Seigler HR et al: The spectrum of small bowel melanoma. Gastrointest Radiol 3:419–423, 1978

Quinn SF, Shaffer HA, Willard MR et al: Bull's-eye lesions: A new gastrointestinal presentation of mastocytosis. Gastrointest Radiol 9:13–15, 1984

Rose HS, Balthazar EJ, Megibow AJ et al: Alimentary tract involvement in Kaposi sarcoma: Radiographic and endoscopic findings in 25 homosexual men. AJR 139:661–666, 1982

Simmons JD: Solitary or multiple nodular lesions in the gastrointestinal tract with central ulceration (bull's-eye or target lesions). Semin Roentgenol 15:267, 1980

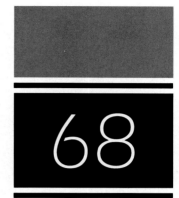

NONDIAPHRAGMATIC HERNIAS

Sites of Herniation

Paraduodenal hernia (duodenal–jejunal flexure)
Lesser sac hernia (foramen of Winslow)
Paracecal hernia
Small bowel mesentery hernia
Sigmoid mesentery hernia
Pelvic hernia (broad ligament)
Lumbar hernia
External hernias
  Inguinal
  Femoral
  Obturator
  Umbilical
  Ventral
  Incisional
  Omphalocele
  Spigelian

Internal hernias are rare congenital lesions in which herniation of a viscus occurs through a normal or abnormal aperture within the confines of the peritoneal cavity. Some result from anomalous intestinal rotation causing various defects in the developing peritoneum and mesenteries. The potential fossae containing the herniated viscera become enlarged, and a portion of the developing bowel elongates within them. Bowel can also herniate through a rent in the mesentery or peritoneum following trauma or a surgical procedure. Internal hernias can contain a few loops or almost the entire small bowel. Clinically, they can present as acute or chronic intermittent small bowel obstructions, sometimes associated with strangulation or a palpable upper abdominal mass.

PARADUODENAL HERNIA

More than half of all internal hernias are paraduodenal, resulting from failure of the mesentery to fuse with the parietal peritoneum at the ligament of Treitz (mesentericoparietal hernia). Depending on the position of the duodenum and the orientation of the opening of the paraduodenal fossa, either left or right paraduodenal hernias can result. Paraduodenal hernias occur about 3 to 4 times more frequently on the left than on the right.

Clinical findings in patients with paraduodenal hernias vary from mild, intermittent gastrointestinal complaints to acute intestinal obstruction with volvulus and infarction. A paraduodenal hernia is best demonstrated by an upper gastrointestinal series performed during a period of acute symptoms, since examination during an asymptomatic interval can fail to show the hernia or merely demonstrate nonspecific dilatation, stasis, and edematous mucosal folds. Even at surgery, a paraduodenal hernia may not be evident, either because of spontaneous resolution of the hernia or because of inadvertent operative reduction due to traction on small bowel loops. In addition, the extent of potential space in a peritoneal fossa seen at exploratory laparotomy is generally not evident from the relatively small size of the orifice of the fossa.

The small intestine generally fills the lower half of the abdomen, extending laterally into each flank, where it is bounded by the colon, and downward into the true pelvis. The jejunum chiefly occupies the left side of the abdomen, and the ileum the right. Dilated loops of jejunum or ileum extending beyond the midline are strong presumptive signs of the presence of an internal hernia, torsion, or adhesions. In both types of paraduodenal hernia, the principal radiographic finding is that of displaced, bunched loops of small bowel that appear to be confined in a sac (Fig. 68-1). If there is partial obstruction, dilatation and delay in transit time can be noted. In the more common left paraduodenal hernia, small bowel loops pass into the paraduodenal fossa posteriorly and into the left mesocolon, producing dilated loops of small bowel clustered in the left upper quadrant of the abdomen lateral to the fourth portion of the duodenum (Fig. 68-2). Paraduodenal hernias occurring on the right side are associated with incomplete intestinal rotation. The junction of the duodenum and jejunum has a low, right paramedian position. The duodenum is dilated, and the jejunal loops are situated on the right side of the abdomen, extending into the right transverse mesocolon. In both types of paraduodenal

hernia, the transverse colon tends to be depressed inferiorly by the mass.

Repeated episodes of paraduodenal herniation can increase the size of the defect and lead to adhesions between the intestinal loops or between the trapped bowel and hernia sac. This process can result in obstruction or circulatory compromise. Therefore, even a small paraduodenal hernia is potentially dangerous and is usually considered an operable condition.

LESSER SAC HERNIA

Herniation into the lesser peritoneal sac through the foramen of Winslow is a rare condition that typically presents as an acute abdominal emergency. Unless promptly relieved by surgery, it can rapidly lead to intestinal strangulation and death. The lesser sac is a potential space bounded anteriorly by the caudate lobe of the liver, the lesser omentum, the posterior wall of the stomach, and the anterior layer of the greater omentum. The posterior border includes the left kidney and adrenal gland, pancreas, transverse colon and mesocolon, and posterior layer of the greater omentum. The lateral margin consists of the spleen and the phrenicolienal and

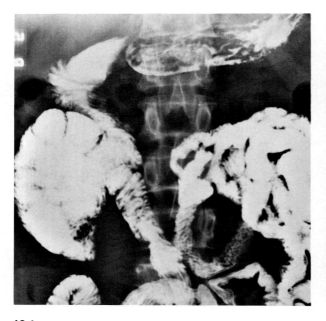

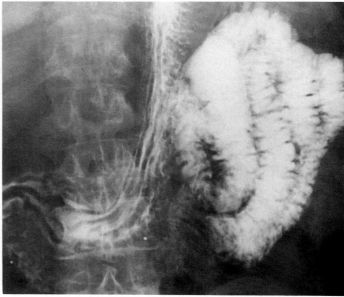

68-1

68-2

Fig. 68-1. *Right paraduodenal hernia. The jejunal loops are bunched together on the right side of the abdomen, and the junction of the duodenum and jejunum has a low right paramedian position.*

Fig. 68-2. *Left paraduodenal hernia. Small bowel loops are clustered in the left upper quadrant lateral to the fourth portion of the duodenum and the stomach.*

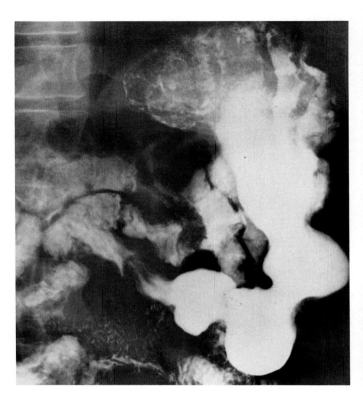

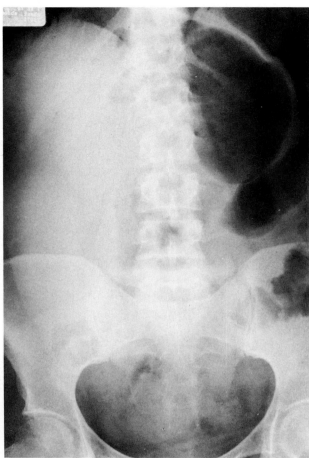

68-3   68-4

Fig. 68-3.   Herniation through the foramen of Winslow into the lesser sac. Loops of small bowel are seen in an abnormal position along the lesser curvature medial and posterior to the stomach.

Fig. 68-4.   Cecal herniation through the foramen of Winslow. Gas in the cecum is seen medial and posterior to the stomach. There is no gas or fecal material in the right lower quadrant. (Henisz A, Matesanz J, Westcott JL: Cecal herniation through the foramen of Winslow. Radiology 112:575–578, 1974)

gastrolienal ligaments. The free edge of the hepatoduodenal ligament (containing the bile duct, hepatic arteries, and portal vein) forms the right border of the lesser sac and the anterior margin of the foramen of Winslow. The posterior margin of the foramen is the anterior surface of the inferior vena cava.

Lesser sac hernias can contain small bowel, colon, gallbladder, or merely omentum. Radiographically, abnormal gas-filled loops of bowel can be seen along the lesser curvature medial and posterior to the stomach. The herniated bowel and omentum displace the stomach and transverse colon anteriorly, inferiorly, and to the left. Oral contrast reveals bunched and dilated bowel confined, as if in a bag, in the left upper and midabdomen (Fig. 68-3). If incarceration occurs, multiple fluid levels can be seen within the limits of the lesser sac. Dilatation, stretching, and medial displacement of the duodenum are commonly seen. This finding is of value in the differentiation of an intestinal hernia from a lesser sac abscess, which displaces the descending duodenum laterally rather than medially. If large bowel (especially cecum) protrudes into the lesser sac, the presence of gas medial and posterior to the stomach is associated with an absence of gas and fecal material in the right lower quadrant (Fig. 68-4). A barium enema examination in this condition can demonstrate compression of the colon as it passes through the foramen of Winslow, or tapering of a contrast-filled segment pointing to the opening of the lesser peritoneal sac.

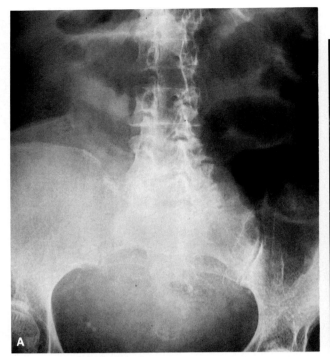

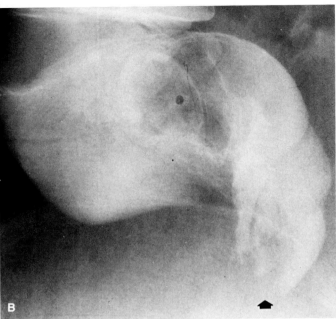

Fig. 68-5. Internal hernia of the ileum. **(A)** A plain abdominal radiograph demonstrates a large soft-tissue mass (pseudotumor) in the right lower quadrant. **(B)** A barium enema examination demonstrates obstruction to flow in the distal ileum **(arrow)** as it enters the internal hernia.

OTHER INTERNAL HERNIAS

Very rarely, internal hernias occur in one of the four principal fossae located in the region of the cecum (ileocolic, ileocecal, retro-appendiceal, and retrocecal; Fig. 68-5). Herniation through the small bowel mesentery (Fig. 68-6), sigmoid mesentery, or broad ligament is also extremely rare. Posterolateral herniation of colon or small bowel with bowel gas overlying the posterior portion of the spine (lumbar hernia) is an uncommon lesion that usually follows trauma but occasionally occurs spontaneously.

INGUINAL/FEMORAL HERNIAS

Herniation of loops of bowel into an inguinal or femoral hernia sac is relatively frequent. When this occurs, gas-filled loops of bowel can be seen to extend beyond the normal pelvic contour on plain abdominal radiographs or may be filled with barium during contrast examination. Left-sided hernias

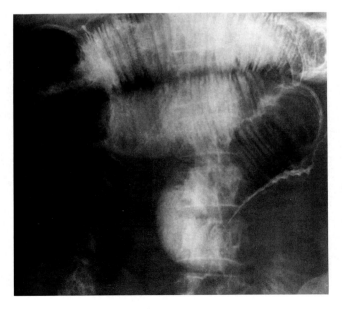

Fig. 68-6. Herniation of small bowel through a hole in the mesentery. Note the marked dilatation of small bowel proximal to the point of obstruction.

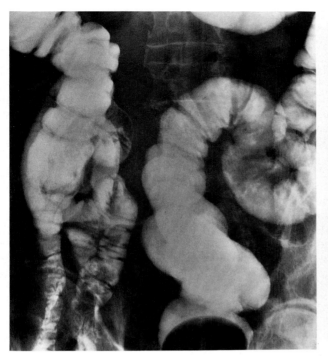

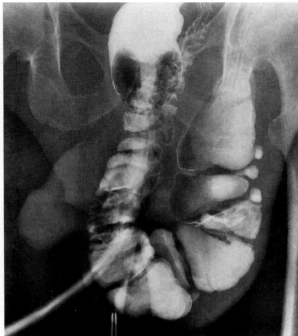

68-7   68-8

Fig. 68-7. Right inguinal hernia containing distal ileum.

Fig. 68-8. Large scrotal hernia containing sigmoid colon.

tend to involve the sigmoid colon. Right-sided hernia sacs usually contain small bowel (Fig. 68-7); infrequently, the cecum is present in the hernia. A long segment of bowel occasionally extends into a large scrotal hernia (Fig. 68-8). Although inguinal hernias tend to be larger than femoral ones, it is usually difficult to distinguish between them radiographically.

Plain radiographs can suggest incarceration and strangulation of inguinal or femoral hernias. Massively distended small bowel loops may appear to converge toward the region of herniation, with the afferent loop of the hernia tapering toward the groin and being relatively fixed in position on serial films. A gas-filled loop overlying the obturator foramen with associated bowel distention also suggests strangulation of an incarcerated hernia.

OBTURATOR HERNIA

Obturator hernias are rare lesions that are far more common in females than males and occur most often on the right side (Fig. 68-9). An obturator hernia can contain any or all of the internal female genital organs, urinary bladder, variable segments of small and large bowel, appendix, and omentum. Early diagnosis is imperative, because the signs of

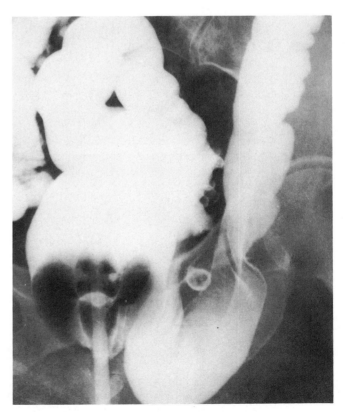

Fig. 68-9. Obturator hernia containing sigmoid colon.

small bowel obstruction in an obturator hernia are more apt to become manifest after strangulation or other complication occurs. A positive Howship-Romberg sign, although not always present, is highly indicative of this condition. The sign consists of pain along the inner aspect of the thigh to the knee or below and is due to compression of the obturator nerve by the hernial contents. Although the hernia is infrequently palpable externally, it can often be felt by vaginal or rectal examination. Radiographic examination may demonstrate gas or contrast agent within a herniated segment of bowel confined to the region of the obturator canal.

On computed tomography, an obturator hernia first increases the separation of the muscular bands of the internal obturator muscle and later separates the external obturator muscle. Eventually, the hernia passes through the obturator canal and emerges between the pectineus and obturator externus muscles (Fig. 68-10).

HERNIATION THROUGH THE ANTERIOR ABDOMINAL WALL

Herniation of bowel occurs not uncommonly through the anterior abdominal wall (umbilical hernia, ventral hernia, postoperative incisional hernia). Because this is essentially a clinical diagnosis, radiographic examination is used only to demonstrate the nature of the herniated contents (Fig. 68-11) and to determine whether there is evidence of bowel obstruction (Fig. 68-12). On the anteroposterior view, bowel loops herniated into an anterior abdominal wall sac are superimposed on normal intraperitoneal loops (Fig. 68-13*A*). Therefore, oblique or lateral radiographs of the abdomen are required for optimum evaluation (Fig. 68-13*B*). Contrast studies of the small and large bowel can confirm the clinical diagnosis and demonstrate sharp constriction of bowel loops as they enter and exit from the hernia sac.

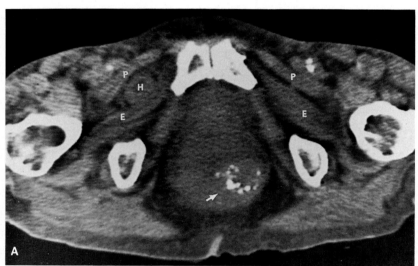

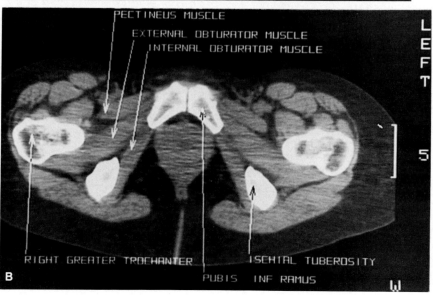

Fig. 68-10. Obturator foramen hernia. **(A)** CT scan through the level of the symphysis shows a small bowel loop **(H)** herniated through the right obturator foramen between the pectineus and external obturator muscles. Of incidental note is calcification within a uterine fibroid **(arrow)**. **(B)** CT scan illustrating the normal anatomy at the level of the symphysis pubis. (Meziane MA, Fishman EK, Siegelman SS: Computed tomographic diagnosis of obturator foramen hernia. Gastrointest Radiol 8:375–377, 1983)

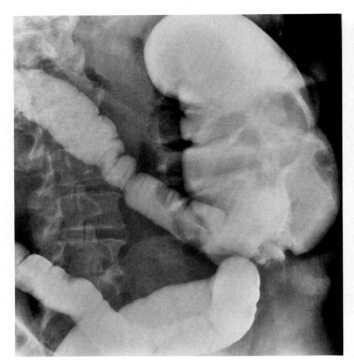

68-11

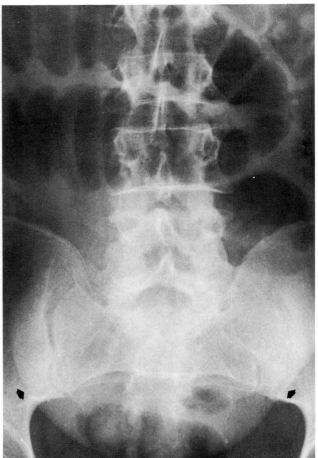

Fig. 68-11. Umbilical hernia. A barium enema examination demonstrates a dilated cecum in the hernia sac.

Fig. 68-12. Umbilical hernia. A large soft-tissue mass **(arrows)** in the midabdomen and upper pelvis is clearly demonstrated on a plain abdominal radiograph. The loops of small bowel proximal to the obstruction are dilated.

68-12

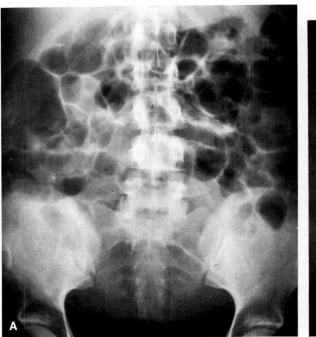

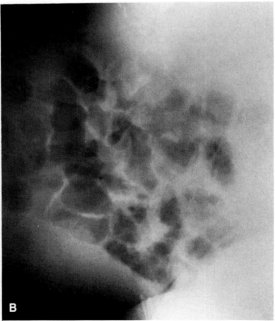

Fig. 68-13. Umbilical hernia. **(A)** On the frontal view, bowel loops within the hernia sac are superimposed on normal intraperitoneal loops. **(B)** A lateral radiograph clearly shows that the bowel loops are in the hernia sac.

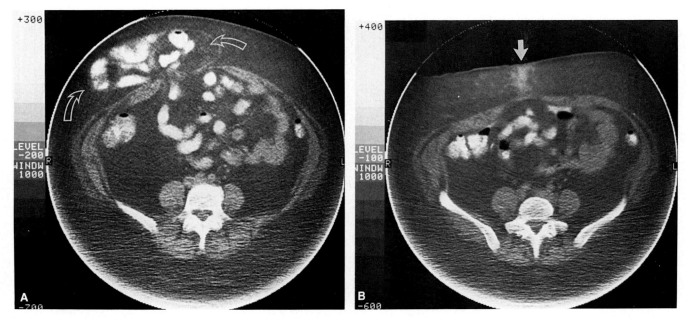

Fig. 68-14. *Occult incisional hernia. **(A)** CT scan at the level of the iliac crest shows several small bowel loops deeply imbedded within the subcutaneous fat **(arrows)**. This large, nonpalpable hernia was a complication of a right paramedial incision in an obese woman who presented with postprandial cramps in the periumbilical region. **(B)** Another section 4 cm caudad after abdominal compression with a sponge shows that the rest of the paramedian incision has healed completely **(arrow)**. (Ghahremani GG, Jimenez MA, Rosenfeld M et al: CT diagnosis of occult incisional hernias. AJR 148:139–142, 1987. Copyright 1987. Reproduced with permission)*

Postoperative incisional hernias are among the most frequent complications following abdominal surgery. They may occasionally cause symptoms of partial small bowel obstruction, but may be impossible to palpate because of the patient's obesity or abdominal pain or distention and be undetectable on radiographic studies because of their easy reducibility and intermittent occurrence. Computed tomography is an accurate method for demonstrating these nonpalpable incisional hernias (Fig. 68-14). At times, occult incisional hernias may be shown on barium studies by placing the patient in the lateral or steep oblique position and then asking the patient to cough or strain (Fig. 68-15). If enteroclysis is performed, the same maneuver should be done after the tube has been removed and the small bowel is in a state of collapse, since the hernia may not be seen when the bowel loops are distended.

OMPHALOCELE

An omphalocele is a protrusion of the abdominal viscera into the base of the umbilical cord with an associated defect in the abdominal wall. It represents persistence of normal fetal herniation with failure of complete withdrawal of the midgut from the umbilical cord during the tenth fetal week. The hernia contains loops of small bowel, which are usually filled with gas and are readily seen on plain abdominal films (Fig. 68-16). Liver, colon, spleen, and pancreas can also be trapped in the hernia sac. Complications of an omphalocele include infection, rupture, and obstruction of loops of bowel entering or exiting from the hernia sac.

SPIGELIAN HERNIA

An interesting form of ventral hernia is the lateral spigelian hernia, a spontaneous defect of the abdominal wall that arises along the linea semilunaris (Fig. 68-17). This curved depression runs just lateral to the outer border of the rectus abdominis muscle, extending from the tip of the costal cartilage of the ninth rib to the symphysis pubis. Spigelian hernias pass through the fibers of the transverse and internal oblique muscles but stay beneath the intact ex-

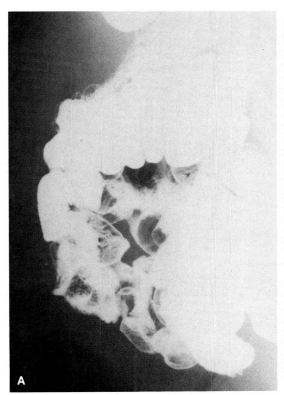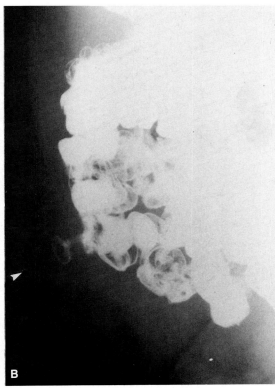

Fig. 68-15. Occult incisional hernia. Lateral radiographs of the anterior abdomen after removal of the enteroclysis tube. **(A)** During normal respiration, no hernia is seen. **(B)** During coughing or straining, a small incisional hernia is demonstrated. The distance between the hernia and the skin **(arrowhead)** precludes clinical confirmation. The site of the hernia should be marked on the skin under fluoroscopy to guide the surgical incision. (Maglinte DDT, Miller RE, Lappas JC: Radiologic diagnosis of ocult incisional hernias of the small intestine. AJR 142:931–932, 1984. Copyright 1984. Reproduced with permission)

ternal oblique aponeurosis and can therefore be difficult to palpate. Although the precise etiology of spigelian hernias is unclear, they tend to occur more frequently in persons with greater than normal intra-abdominal pressure, such as heavy laborers, and in persons with urinary retention, chronic lung disease, and gastric outlet obstruction. They can also be seen in multiparous women and in patients who have recently lost large amounts of weight.

Intermittent abdominal pain with point tenderness or a mass in the region of the semilunar line should suggest the possibility of spigelian hernia. Small bowel, colon, or omentum can be trapped in the narrow-necked hernia sac. Incarceration of herniated bowel can present with symptoms simulating gallbladder disease, acute appendicitis, or intermittent small bowel obstruction. Radiographically, gas- or contrast-filled bowel can be found laterally, outside the confines of the peritoneal cavity. Bowel loops often appear sharply constricted as they enter and exit from the hernia sac.

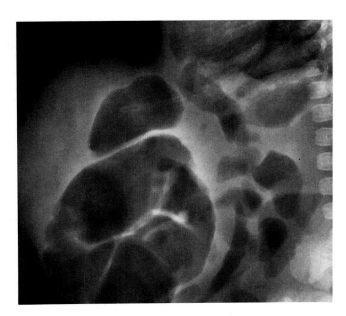

Fig. 68-16. Omphalocele containing loops of gas-filled small bowel.

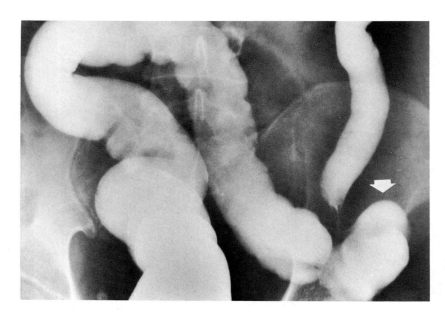

Fig. 68-17. Spigelian hernia. Small bowel is trapped in the hernia sac **(arrow)** that arises along the left semilunar line.

BIBLIOGRAPHY

Back DB, Satin R, Palayew M et al: Herniation and strangulation of the gallbladder through the foramen of Winslow. AJR 142:541–542, 1984

Bartlett JD, Martel W, Lindenauer SM: Right paraduodenal hernia. Surg Gynecol Obstet 132:443–449, 1971

Frimann–Dahl J: Roentgen examination in acute abdomen diseases. Springfield, IL, Charles C. Thomas, 1974

Ghahremani GG, Jimenez MA, Rosenfeld M et al: CT diagnosis of occult incisional hernias. AJR 148:139–142, 1987

Gibson LD, Gaspar MR: A review of 606 cases of umbilical hernia. Surg Gynecol Obstet 109:313–322, 1959

Goldberger LE, Berk RN: Cecal hernia into the lesser sac. Gastrointest Radiol 5:169–172, 1980

Henisz A, Matesanz J, Westcott JL: Cecal herniation through the foramen of Winslow. Radiology 112:575–578, 1974

Holder LE, Schneider HJ: Spigelian hernias: Anatomy and roentgenographic manifestations. Radiology 112:309–313, 1974

Lawler RE, Duncan TR: Retrocecal hernia. Radiology 87:1051–1052, 1966

Maglinte DDT, Miller RE, Lappas JC: Radiologic diagnosis of occult incisional hernias of the small intestine. AJR 142:931–932, 1984

Meyers MA: Paraduodenal hernias: Radiologic and arteriographic diagnosis. Radiology 95:29–37, 1970

Meziane MA, Fishman EK, Siegelman SS: Computed tomographic diagnosis of obturator foramen hernia. Gastrointest Radiol 8:375–377, 1983

Schaefer C, Waugh D: Mesentericoparietal hernia. Am J Surg 116:847–852, 1968

Williams AJ: Roentgen diagnosis of intra-abdominal hernia. Radiology 59:817–825, 1952

Zausner J, Dumont AE, Ring SM: Obturator hernia. AJR 115:408–410, 1972

GAS IN THE BOWEL WALL (PNEUMATOSIS INTESTINALIS)

69

Gas in the bowel wall (pneumatosis intestinalis) can exist as an isolated entity or in conjunction with a broad spectrum of diseases of the gastrointestinal tract or respiratory system. In primary pneumatosis (about 15% of cases), no respiratory or other gastrointestinal abnormality is present. Primary pneumatosis usually occurs in adults and mainly involves the colon. Secondary pneumatosis intestinalis (about 85% of cases) more commonly involves the small bowel and is associated with a wide variety of pre-existing disorders. In the primary form, gas collections usually appear cystic; in the secondary type, a linear distribution of gas is generally seen.

Disease Entities

Primary (idiopathic)
Secondary
    Gastrointestinal disease with bowel necrosis
        Necrotizing enterocolitis in infants
        Ischemic necrosis due to mesenteric vascular disease
        Intestinal obstruction (especially if there is strangulation)
        Primary infection of the bowel wall
        Ingestion of corrosive agents
    Gastrointestinal disease without associated necrosis of the bowel wall
        Pyloroduodenal peptic ulcer disease
        Bowel obstruction
        Adynamic ileus

Inflammatory bowel diseases (*e.g.*, ulcerative colitis, Crohn's disease, tuberculosis)
        Connective tissue disease
        Gastrointestinal endoscopy/colonoscopy
        Jejunoileal bypass surgery
        Transcutaneous feeding jejunostomy tube
        Obstructive lesions of the colon in children (*e.g.*, imperforate anus, Hirschsprung's disease, meconium plug)
        Leukemia
        Steroid therapy
        Graft-vs-host disease
        Perforated jejunal diverticulum
        Whipple's disease
        Intestinal parasites
    Obstructive pulmonary disease
        Pulmonary emphysema
        Bullous disease of the lung
        Chronic bronchitis
        Asthma
    Conditions mimicking pneumatosis intestinalis

PRIMARY PNEUMATOSIS INTESTINALIS

Primary pneumatosis intestinalis is a relatively rare benign condition characterized pathologically by multiple thin-walled, noncommunicating, gas-filled cysts in the subserosal or submucosal layer of the bowel. The overlying mucosa is entirely normal, as is the muscularis. The disorder primarily involves the colon (particularly the left side), is usually segmental in distribution, and rarely affects the rectum. Because patients with primary pneumatosis intestinalis have no associated gastrointestinal or respiratory abnormalities, symptoms are infrequent, and gas in the bowel wall is usually an unexpected finding on plain abdominal radiographs or barium studies.

The appearance of radiolucent clusters of cysts along the contours of the bowel is diagnostic of primary pneumatosis intestinalis (Fig. 69-1). On barium examinations, the filling defects are seen to lie between the lumen (outlined by contrast) and the water density of the outer wall of the bowel. The radiographic pattern of pneumatosis can simulate more severe gastrointestinal conditions. Small cysts may be confused with tiny polyps. Larger cysts can produce scalloped defects simulating inflammatory pseudopolyps or the thumbprinting seen with intramural hemorrhage (Fig. 69-2). At times, the cysts of pneumatosis intestinalis concentrically compress the lumen, causing gas shadows that extend on either side of the bowel contour surrounding a thin, irregular stream of barium and mimicking the appearance of an annular carcinoma. To differentiate pneumatosis intestinalis from these other conditions, it is important to note the striking lucency of the gas-filled cysts in contrast to the soft-tissue density of an intraluminal or intramural lesion. In areas of obstruction, the overhanging edges are relatively lucent, in contrast to the soft-tissue density of tumors. Other distinguishing factors are the compressibility of the cysts on palpation and the not infrequent occurrence of asymptomatic pneumoperitoneum. The large amount of extraluminal gas within the peritoneal cavity can present a spectacular radiographic appearance and suggest a perforated viscus. However, the discovery of pneumoperitoneum in an apparently healthy patient with no peritoneal signs should make pneumatosis intestinalis the likely diagnosis. If the amount of gas that is absorbed by the peritoneum (about 100 ml/day) equals the amount that enters daily from ruptured cysts, a "balanced" pneumoperitoneum is the result, and large amounts of free intraperitoneal gas may be continuously present for months or years.

Before assuming that pneumatosis intestinalis is benign, the radiologist and clinician must review all of the pertinent findings to ensure that the patient does not have bowel necrosis. This mandatory review includes repeat films and close monitoring of clinical parameters until any possibility of infarcted bowel is excluded. In patients receiving steroids, immunosuppressive agents, or chemotherapy, the problem can be particularly difficult

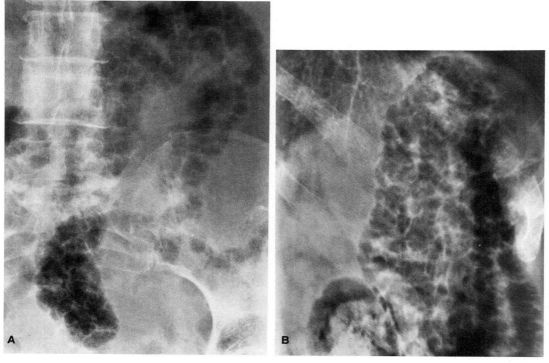

Fig. 69-1. *Primary pneumatosis intestinalis in an asymptomatic man. Radiolucent clusters of gas-filled cysts are seen along the contours of the bowel in* **(A)** *the rectosigmoid and* **(B)** *the splenic flexure.*

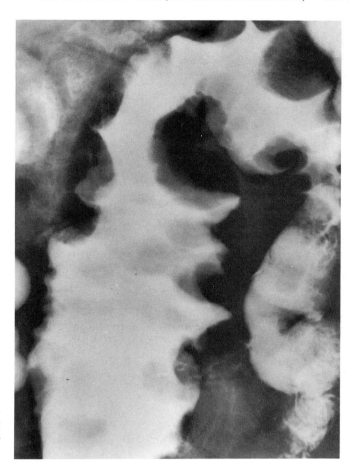

Fig. 69-2. *Primary pneumatosis intestinalis in an asymptomatic elderly man. The large gas-filled cysts produce scalloped defects in the colon simulating inflammatory pseudopolyps or the thumbprinting seen with intramural hemorrhage.*

because these patients may have very few signs of an intra-abdominal catastrophe even when bowel necrosis is present.

Primary pneumatosis intestinalis usually requires no treatment and resolves spontaneously. Surgery is required only in the very rare case of a patient with hemorrhage, obstruction, or perforation. In some severe cases, oxygen breathing (70% for 6 days) has been reported to be effective in decompressing the gas-filled cysts. Breathing high concentrations of oxygen alters the balance of diffusion of gases between the cysts and venous blood in favor of absorption of gases in the cysts, thereby causing cyst decompression.

GASTROINTESTINAL DISEASE WITH BOWEL NECROSIS

NECROTIZING ENTEROCOLITIS

Pneumatosis intestinalis in infants is usually associated with an underlying necrotizing enterocolitis, for which there is a very low survival rate (Fig. 69-3).

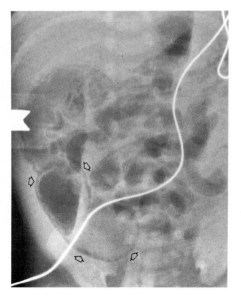

Fig. 69-3. *Pneumatosis intestinalis in a premature infant with underlying necrotizing enterocolitis. Intramural gas* **(arrows)** *parallels the course of the bowel loops.*

The disease primarily occurs in premature or debilitated infants, who apparently have a decreased ability to fight infection. Gas-forming bacteria from the lumen invade the bowel wall through an insufficiently resistant mucosa, leading to a fulminant necrotizing cellulitis and septicemia. Necrotizing enterocolitis most commonly affects the ileum and right colon, though total gut involvement may occur. There is variable mucosal destruction, and a dirty brown pseudomembrane often covers the denuded areas. The bowel wall tends to be thickened and friable; multiple perforations can be present.

Babies who develop necrotizing enterocolitis are usually asymptomatic during the first 48 hr to 72 hr of life. On the third or fourth day, the infant begins to vomit bile-tinged material and develops mild to severe abdominal distention and respiratory distress. About half of the infants with this condition have a few loose blood-streaked stools; severe diarrhea, however, is infrequent. Clinical deterioration is usually progressive and rapid. Unless vigorous therapeutic measures are instituted, the infant can suffer spells of apnea, jaundice, and shock before succumbing.

Radiographic Findings

Pneumatosis intestinalis in infants suffering from necrotizing enterocolitis is characterized by a frothy or bubbly appearance of gas in the wall of diseased bowel loops (Fig. 69-4). The appearance often resembles fecal material in the right colon. However, it must be remembered that, although this feces-like appearance is perfectly normal in adults, it is always abnormal in premature infants. The gas in the wall of the colon in necrotizing enterocolitis is probably related to mucosal necrosis and subsequent passage of intraluminal gas into the bowel wall. This is complicated by the presence of intraluminal gas-forming organisms that also penetrate the diseased mucosa to reach the inner layers of the bowel wall. Gas entering the damaged intestinal capillary bed can spread to the intrahepatic branches of the portal vein. The radiographic detection of this appearance is an ominous sign. Extensive necrosis can result in perforation of the bowel wall and pneumoperitoneum. In contrast to pneumatosis intestinalis in adults, in whom cyst rupture and pneumoperitoneum are usually asymptomatic, bowel perforation

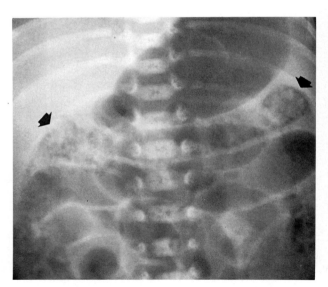

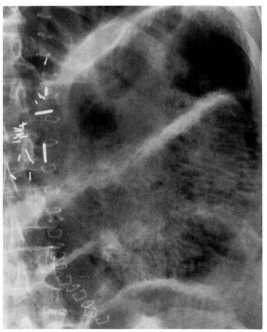

69-4   69-5

Fig. 69-4.   Pneumatosis intestinalis in a premature infant with necrotizing enterocolitis. The bubbly appearance of gas in the wall of diseased colon resembles fecal material **(arrows)**; although this appearance is normal in adults, it is always abnormal in premature infants.

Fig. 69-5.   Pneumatosis intestinalis in an adult secondary to a fatal necrotizing enterocolitis that developed following a motor vehicle accident and partial colon resection.

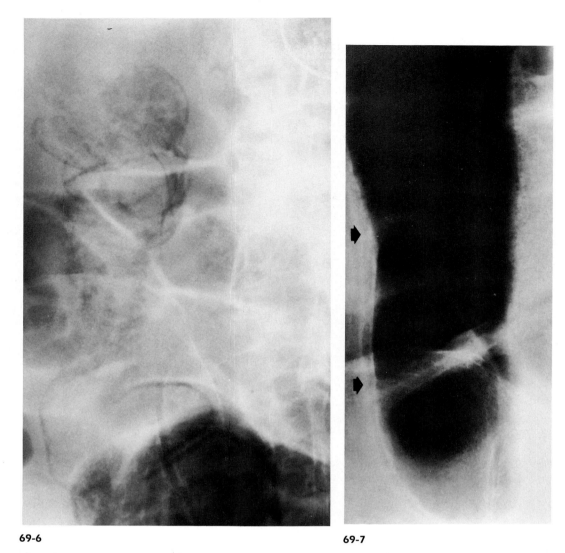

69-6   69-7

Fig. 69-6. Pneumatosis intestinalis due to mesenteric arterial thrombosis. Crescentic linear gas collections are seen in the wall of ischemic bowel loops.

Fig. 69-7. Pneumatosis intestinalis in the cecum and ascending colon **(arrows)** secondary to large bowel obstruction (adenocarcinoma of the rectum).

in infants with necrotizing enterocolitis results in peritonitis and usually a fatal outcome.

The radiographic appearance of pneumatosis in a child with necrotizing enterocolitis is pathognomonic, especially if it is associated with pneumoperitoneum or portal vein gas. A barium enema examination is rarely needed for diagnosis; indeed, in view of the friable consistency of the colon, this procedure is hazardous.

Several cases have been reported of pneumatosis in neonates with a "benign" form of necrotizing enterocolitis. This relatively mild inflammatory process may be related to transient intestinal hypoxia; it does not progress to significant bowel necrosis.

MESENTERIC VASCULAR DISEASE

Two basic mechanical factors are implicated in the development of most cases of secondary pneumatosis intestinalis in adults. Regardless of the underlying etiology, most patients with gas in the bowel wall have loss of mucosal integrity and/or increased intraluminal pressure in the bowel. In those with ischemic, infectious, or traumatic damage to the mucosa, pneumatosis intestinalis can reflect a potentially fatal bacterial invasion (Fig. 69-5).

Peripheral occlusion of mesenteric vascular branches results in a transient ischemic break in the integrity of the highly sensitive mucosa and intramural extension of bowel gas. Although mesenteric

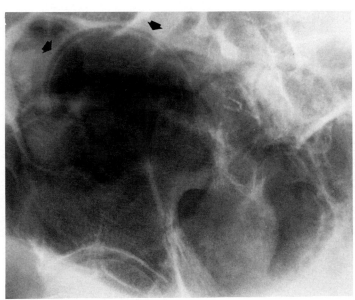

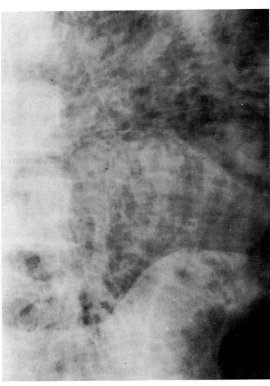

69-8   69-9

Fig. 69-8. Pneumatosis intestinalis involving the colon **(arrows)** in a patient with severe pyloric stenosis.

Fig. 69-9. Pneumatosis intestinalis developing proximal to carcinoma of the colon. The linear streaks of gas that appear to cross the bowel loops represent gas in the retroperitoneal space.

vascular disease most commonly occurs in elderly persons, it occasionally arises in younger patients with conditions predisposing to the premature onset of occlusive disease (*e.g.,* diabetes, hypercholesterolemia, hypothyroidism). Bowel ischemia can be produced by an aneurysm of the abdominal aorta or be a complication of reconstructive surgery of the cardiac valves or the aorta.

Pneumatosis intestinalis secondary to mesenteric arterial (or venous) thrombosis presents as crescentic linear gas collections in the wall of ischemic bowel loops (Fig. 69-6). When gas is present in the bowel wall without intestinal necrosis, signs of severe peritoneal irritation are absent, and pneumatosis typically disappears once blood flow to the affected segment of bowel improves. The concomitant finding of gas in the portal vein, however, is a reliable indicator of irreversible intestinal necrosis and a poor prognostic sign.

Mucosal ischemia can be secondary to strangulating obstructions, such as volvulus or incarcerated hernia. Even if strangulation has not occurred, markedly increased intraluminal pressure proximal to an obstruction can compress the intramural cir-

culation and lead to vascular compromise and ischemic necrosis (Fig. 69-7). Mucosal necrosis can also be caused by infectious organisms that invade the bowel wall or by powerful corrosive agents (*e.g.,* lye, hydrochloric acid, formalin) that have been ingested accidentally or intentionally in a suicide attempt.

GASTROINTESTINAL DISEASE WITHOUT BOWEL NECROSIS

Even if there is no necrosis of the bowel wall, any gastrointestinal tract lesion that results in mucosal ulceration or intestinal obstruction may be associated with gas in the bowel wall. The most common of these conditions is obstructive peptic ulcer disease of the pyloroduodenal region. In severe pyloric stenosis, the increase in intraluminal pressure proximal to the obstructing lesion apparently forces intraluminal gas either through an intact mucosa or through small breaks in the mucosa into the wall of the bowel. From this site proximal to the obstruction, the gas penetrates the wall to reach the subse-

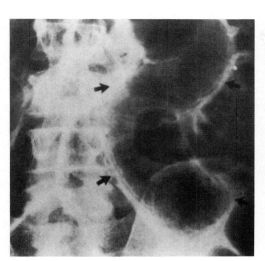

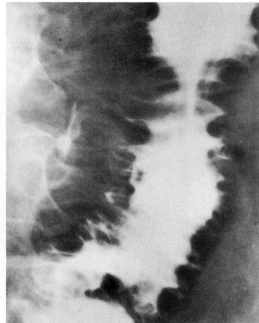

69-10   **69-11**

Fig. 69-10. "Benign" linear pneumatosis intestinalis. Supine film of the abdomen demonstrates extensive linear pneumatosis of the small bowel **(arrows)** in a 70-year-old man with postoperative ileus. The pneumatosis was not associated with any acute abdominal complaints and resolved over several days. (Rice RP, Thompson WM, Gedgaudas RK: The diagnosis and significance of extraluminal gas in the abdomen. Radiol Clin North Am 20:819–837, 1982)

Fig. 69-11. Pneumatosis intestinalis in a patient with scleroderma. The pattern could be mistaken for inflammatory disease causing deep ulcerations in the colon if the extremely lucent outline of the gas-filled cysts in the bowel wall were not appreciated.

rosal layer. It can then dissect and extend to points far distal to the primary obstructing lesion (Fig. 69-8). Gas can also dissect along interstitial tissues of the mesentery or by way of lymphatics to the bowel. This relatively benign process can cause short, sharply defined intramural gas collections parallel to the wall of the stomach. It is essential to differentiate this interstitial gastric emphysema in relatively asymptomatic patients from extensive, bubbly collections of gas in acutely ill patients with emphysematous gastritis. The intramural gas in interstitial gastric emphysema almost always disappears spontaneously within a few days or once the gastric outlet obstruction is relieved.

Pneumatosis arising proximal to an obstructing lesion has also been reported in patients with esophageal stenosis secondary to lye stricture and in persons with ulcerative disease developing above an obstructing carcinoma of the colon (Fig. 69-9). A benign self-limited linear pneumatosis intestinalis has been reported in patients with nonobstructive ileus causing dilatation of the bowel (Fig. 69-10).

Chronic inflammatory diseases, such as ulcerative colitis, Crohn's disease, or tuberculosis, can

lead to the development of pneumatosis intestinalis. In toxic megacolon (most commonly associated with acute ulcerative colitis), the presence of subserosal gas can reflect abnormal permeability of the bowel wall. This can be complicated by the presence of gas-forming organisms and can indicate an impending colonic perforation. In Crohn's disease, mucosal ulcerations, fistulas, and stenotic segments lead to increased intraluminal pressure, which can predispose to the development of pneumatosis intestinalis. Gas in the serosal layers is characteristically seen in stenotic, chronically inflamed regions in which marked scarring of the submucosa makes the serosa the only portion of the bowel capable of expansion. In contrast, submucosal collections of gas tend to develop in the intervening portions of dilated bowel and are probably related to mucosal ulcerations.

Pneumatosis intestinalis can develop in patients with connective tissue diseases. In scleroderma, the underlying mechanism is probably chronic intestinal distention and increased intraluminal pressure (Fig. 69-11). Overgrowth of bacterial flora and electrolyte disturbances due to stasis and

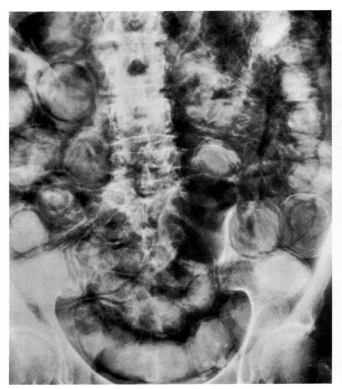

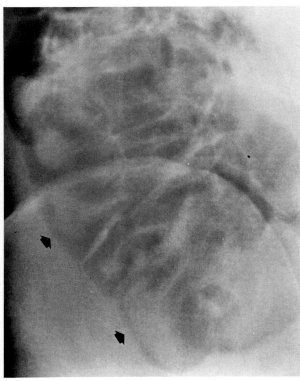

69-12   69-13

Fig. 69-12.   *Pneumatosis intestinalis secondary to primary amyloidosis of the small bowel. Linear collections of gas are seen to parallel essentially the entire course of the small bowel.*

Fig. 69-13.   *Pneumatosis intestinalis of the colon* **(arrows)** *that developed following gastrointestinal endoscopy.*

malabsorption may play a contributing role. The development of pneumatosis is less common in patients with dermatomyositis or rheumatoid arthritis. In persons with systemic lupus erythematosus, polyarteritis nodosa, or amyloidosis, a vasculitis of small and medium-sized arteries and arterioles causes mucosal ischemia, which can lead to ulceration, infarction, and perforation (Fig. 69-12). This loss of mucosal integrity can permit gas and enteric organisms to gain access to the bowel wall and cause a necrotizing enterocolitis. In some cases, intramural gas develops because of structural changes in the supporting connective tissue within the bowel wall without intestinal ischemia.

Pneumatosis intestinalis is an uncommon complication of gastrointestinal endoscopy (Fig. 69-13). In the performance of colonoscopy, distention of the colon by gas insufflation facilitates passage of the colonoscope and visualization of the mucosa. However, the resultant increase in intraluminal pressure occasionally causes the colon to rupture in an area of anatomic weakness, such as a diverticulum. A pre-existing break in the integrity of the co-

lonic mucosa due to ulceration or a recent biopsy site enhances this dissection of intraluminally introduced gas in the wall of the colon. Colonoscopy can result in localized or generalized pneumatosis primarily affecting the left side of the colon.

Elevated intraluminal pressure may be responsible for the development of pneumatosis intestinalis as a complication of the jejunoileal bypass procedure for morbid obesity (Fig. 69-14). This procedure involves an end-to-end anastomosis of the defunctionalized small bowel with the sigmoid colon. Pneumatosis has been demonstrated from 2 weeks to 30 months after surgery. It can be confined to the colon, primarily on the right, or also involve the defunctionalized small bowel. The large difference in intraluminal pressure between the sigmoid colon and the ileum is thought to permit dissection of gas into the bowel wall. It is also possible that pneumatosis in the bypassed small bowel segment may be due to bacterial overgrowth, particularly anaerobic organisms.

Following the intraoperative placement of a transcutaneous feeding jejunostomy tube, extensive

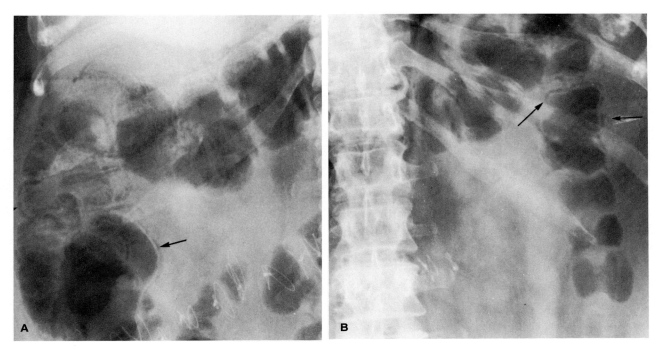

Fig. 69-14. Pneumatosis intestinalis as a complication of jejunoileal bypass. **(A)** Four weeks after surgery, pneumatosis intestinalis involves the cecum, ascending colon, and portions of the transverse colon **(arrow)**. **(B)** Three weeks later, pneumatosis also involves portions of the descending colon **(arrows)**. (Wandtke J, Skucas J, Spataro R et al: Pneumatosis intestinalis as a complication of jejunoileal bypass. AJR 129:601–604, 1977. Copyright 1977. Reproduced with permission)

linear intramural air may develop. Underlying mechanisms include the iatrogenic break in the mucosal surface due to the catheter, which extends from the jejunal lumen to the skin, and air irrigation of the catheter that may contribute to increased intraluminal pressure. Patients with this radiographic appearance have been treated conservatively with complete resolution within a few days.

Pneumatosis intestinalis in children has been associated with obstructive lesions of the colon, such as imperforate anus, Hirschsprung's disease, and the meconium plug syndrome. In these conditions, mucosal tears of a massively distended colon probably permit intestinal gas to dissect into the submucosal and subserosal layers of the bowel wall. Mucosal ischemia resulting from diminished perfusion of the overdistended colon may be a contributing factor. Once the obstruction is relieved, gas in the bowel wall spontaneously regresses.

A benign form of pneumatosis intestinalis with both cystic and linear intramural gas shadows has been reported in both children and adults with leukemia (Fig. 69-15). Although this radiographic appearance in leukemic patients may indicate irreversible intestinal gangrene, it may reflect merely a benign self-limited condition when the physical examination and the clinical course do not suggest an acute abdominal disease.

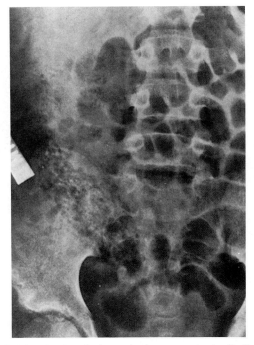

Fig. 69-15. Leukemic intestinal pneumatosis. Both cystic and linear forms of pneumatosis are present in this patient with no evidence of an acute abdomen. (Braver JM, Horrow MM, Philipps E: Leukemic intestinal pneumatosis. J Can Assoc Radiol 35:80–82, 1984)

Steroid therapy has been suggested as a possible cause of pneumatosis intestinalis. It is postulated that steroids cause severe lymphoid depletion of Peyer's patches, which is then manifested as rents in the bowel wall that allow intraluminal gas to dissect intramurally. However, since most patients receiving steroid therapy have an underlying debilitating disease that itself may predispose to the development of pneumatosis, it is unclear whether steroid therapy *per se* plays any causative role.

The epithelial destruction that occurs in graft-vs-host disease seems to predispose patients with this major complication of allogenic bone marrow transplantation to develop intramural gas that most commonly involves the cecum. The intramural air is often associated with bowel dilatation, suggesting gas dissection into the bowel wall through a damaged epithelial barrier as a pathogenic mechanism. Invasion of the bowel by gas-forming organisms would be an alternative cause, but the transient nature and benign clinical course of the pneumatosis in these patients does not support this theory.

Perforation of a jejunal diverticulum can cause subserosal dissection of gas in addition to the more common complication of pneumoperitoneum. Whipple's disease and infestation by intestinal parasites have also been reported to result in pneumatosis intestinalis.

OBSTRUCTIVE PULMONARY DISEASE

Severe obstructive pulmonary disease can be associated with the development of pneumatosis intestinalis. Partial bronchial obstruction and coughing presumably cause alveolar rupture, with gas dissecting along peribronchial and perivascular tissue planes into the mediastinum. Gas can then pass through the various hiatuses in the diaphragm to reach the retroperitoneal area, from which it dissects between the leaves of the mesentery to eventually reach subserosal and submucosal locations in the bowel wall.

CONDITIONS MIMICKING PNEUMATOSIS INTESTINALIS

An appearance that mimics pneumatosis intestinalis involving the rectum is occasionally produced by gas-filled loops of small bowel superimposed on ei-

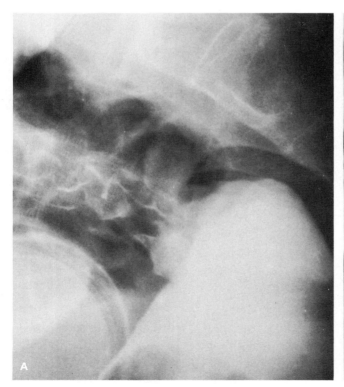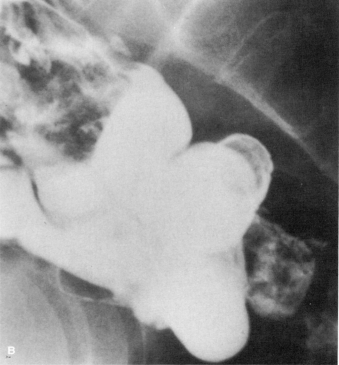

Fig. 69-16. *Pseudopneumatosis of the rectum.* **(A)** *A large amount of gas simulating pneumatosis surrounds the rectum on a postevacuation film from a barium enema examination.* **(B)** *Antegrade administration of barium demonstrates that the gas actually represented loops of small bowel that are now filled with barium.*

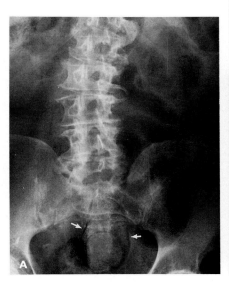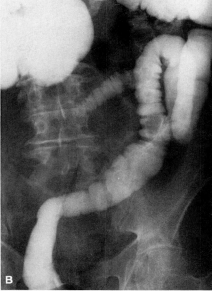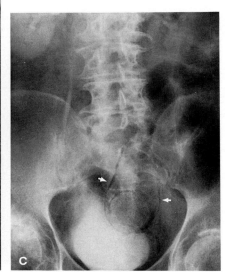

Fig. 69-17. Isolated ureteritis emphysematosa. **(A)** Supine film shows intramural gas as linear lucencies paralleling the dilated, gas-filled lumen of the left ureter. **(B)** Barium enema examination shows the sigmoid colon to be normal. **(C)** Excretory urogram shows a normal right kidney and ureter with no function on the left. The urinary bladder is indented by the dilated gas-filled left distal ureter **(arrows)**. (Imray TJ, Huberty LH: Isolated ureteritis emphysematosa simulating pneumatosis intestinalis. AJR 135:1082–1083, 1980. Copyright 1980. Reproduced with permission)

ther side of the contrast-filled rectum on barium enema examination (Fig. 69-16). Extensive gas shadows in the wall of the ureter in an extremely rare case of isolated ureteritis emphysematosa with ureteral dilatation may simulate pneumatosis intestinalis involving the descending and sigmoid colon (Fig. 69-17). Barium enema examination can demonstrate the normal colon and an extracolonic gas-lined structure.

BIBLIOGRAPHY

Berdon WE, Grossman H, Baker DH et al: Necrotizing enterocolitis in the premature infant. Radiology 83:879–887, 1964

Braver JM, Horrow MM, Philipps E: Leukemic intestinal pneumatosis. J Assoc Canad Radiol 35:80–82, 1984

Bryk D: Unusual causes of small-bowel pneumatosis: Perforated duodenal ulcer and perforated duodenal diverticula. Radiology 106:299–302, 1973

Doub HP, Shea JJ: Pneumatosis cystoides intestinalis. JAMA 172:1238–1243, 1960

Felson B: Abdominal gas: A roentgen approach. Ann NY Acad Sci 150:141–161, 1968

Freiman D, Chon HK, Bilaniuk L: Pneumatosis intestinalis in systemic lupus erythematosus. Radiology 116:563–564, 1975

Hernanz–Schulman M, Kirkpatrick J, Shwachman H et al: Pneumatosis intestinalis in cystic fibrosis. Radiology 160:497–499, 1986

Imray TJ, Huberty LH: Isolated ureteritis emphysematosa simulating pneumatosis intestinalis. AJR 135:1082–1083, 1980

Maile CW, Frick MP, Crass JR et al: The abdominal radiograph in gastrointestinal graft-vs-host disease. AJR 145:289–292, 1985

Marshak RH, Lindner AE, Maklansky D: Pneumatosis cystoides coli. Gastrointest Radiol 2:85–89, 1977

Meyers MA, Ghahremani GG, Clements JL et al: Pneumatosis intestinalis. Gastrointest Radiol 2:91–105, 1977

Miercort RD, Merril FG: Pneumatosis and pseudo-obstruction in scleroderma. Radiology 92:359–362, 1969

Mueller CF, Morehead R, Alter A et al: Pneumatosis intestinalis in collagen disorders. AJR 114:300–305, 1972

Nelson SW: Extraluminal gas collections due to diseases of the gastrointestinal tract. AJR 115:225–248, 1972

Olmsted WW, Madewell JE: Pneumatosis cystoides intestinalis: A pathophysiologic explanation of the roentgenographic signs. Gastrointest Radiol 1:177–181, 1976

Rice RP, Thompson WM, Gedgaudas RK: The diagnosis and significance of extraluminal gas in the abdomen. Radiol Clin North Am 20:819–837, 1982

Robinson AE, Grossman H, Brumely GW: Pneumatosis intestinalis in the neonate. AJR 120:333–341, 1974

Scott JR, Miller WT, Urso M et al: Acute mesenteric infarction. AJR 113:269–279, 1971

Seaman WB, Fleming RJ, Baker DH: Pneumatosis intestinalis of the small bowel. Semin Roentgenol 1:234–242, 1966

Strain JD, Rudikoff JC, Moore EE et al: Pneumatosis intestinalis associated with intracatheter jejunostomy feeding. AJR 139:107–109, 1982

Wandtke J, Skucas J, Spataro R et al: Pneumatosis intestinalis as a complication of jejunoileal bypass. AJR 129:601–604, 1977

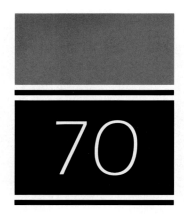

PNEUMOPERITONEUM

Disease Entities

Pneumoperitoneum *with* peritonitis
  Perforated viscus
    Peptic ulcer disease
    Colonic obstruction
    Diverticulitis
    Appendicitis
    Malignancy
  Ulcerative bowel disease
    Tuberculosis
    Typhoid fever
    Ulcerated Meckel's diverticulum
    Toxic megacolon
    Lymphogranuloma venereum
  Infection of the peritoneal cavity
  Abdominal trauma
  Delayed complication of renal
    transplantation
Pneumoperitoneum *without* peritonitis
  Iatrogenic causes
    Surgery
    Endoscopy
    Diagnostic pneumoperitoneum
  Abdominal causes
    Pneumatosis intestinalis
    Forme fruste of perforation
    Peptic ulcer
    Carcinoma of the stomach
    Crohn's disease

    Severe distention of an abdominal viscus
    Jejunal diverticulosis
    Gynecologic causes
    Rubin test for tubal patency
    Vaginal douching
    Postpartum exercises/examination
    Orogenital intercourse
  Intrathoracic causes
    Pneumomediastinum
    Ruptured emphysematous bullus

Pneumoperitoneum associated with significant abdominal pain and tenderness is often caused by perforation of a gas-containing viscus and indicates a surgical emergency. Less frequently, pneumoperitoneum results from abdominal, gynecologic, intrathoracic, or iatrogenic causes and does not require operative intervention.

RADIOGRAPHIC FINDINGS

The radiographic demonstration of free gas in the peritoneal cavity is a valuable sign in the diagnosis of perforation of the gastrointestinal tract. As little as 1 mm of free intraperitoneal gas can be identified. Free gas is best demonstrated by examination of the patient in the upright position with a horizontal beam. Because the gas ascends to the highest point in the peritoneal cavity, it accumulates beneath the domes of the diaphragm (Fig. 70-1). Free intraperitoneal gas appears as a sickle-shaped translucency that is easiest to recognize on the right side between the diaphragm and the homogeneous density of the liver. On the left, the normal gas and fluid shadows present in the fundus of the stomach can be confusing. The free gas is shown to best advantage if the patient remains in an upright (or lateral decubitus) position for 10 min before a radiograph is obtained.

If the patient is too ill to sit or stand, a lateral decubitus view (preferably with the patient on his left side) can be used (Fig. 70-2). In this position, free gas moves to the right and collects between the lateral margin of the liver and the abdominal wall. Some gas also collects in the right iliac fossa and, when large amounts are involved, can be seen along the flank down to the minor pelvis.

When the patient is in the supine position, free intraperitoneal gas accumulates between the intestinal loops and is much more difficult to demon-

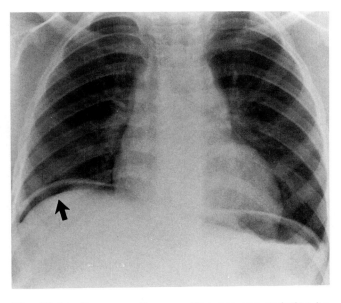

Fig. 70-1. Pneumoperitoneum. The gas accumulating beneath the dome of the right hemidiaphragm **(arrow)** appears as a sickle-shaped translucency.

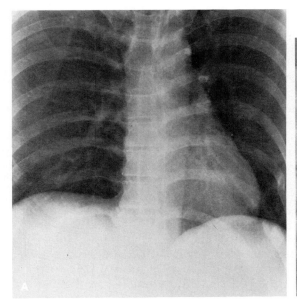 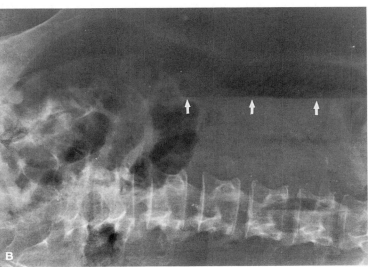

Fig. 70-2. Pneumoperitoneum. **(A)** On the semi-erect view, there is no evidence of free intraperitoneal gas beneath the domes of the diaphragm. **(B)** On the lateral decubitus view, the free intraperitoneal gas is clearly seen collecting under the right side of the abdominal wall **(arrows).** Gas can even be seen extending down the flank to the region of the pelvis.

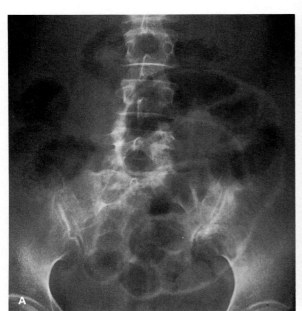
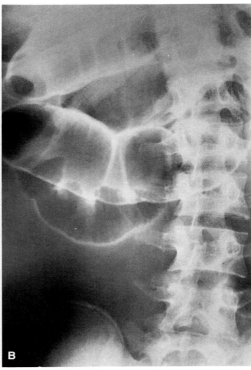

Fig. 70-3. Pneumoperitoneum demonstrated on supine view. Large quantities of free intra-peritoneal gas may be diagnosed indirectly in these two patients because the gas permits visualization of the outer margins of the intestinal wall.

strate. However, a large quantity of gas can be diagnosed indirectly, because it permits visualization of the outer margins of the intestinal wall (Fig. 70-3). The distinct demonstration of the inner and outer contours of the bowel wall is often the only sign of pneumoperitoneum in patients in such poor condition that they cannot be turned on their side or be examined upright. Air outside the bowel wall may also be recognized as small triangular collections of air between adjacent loops of bowel (triangle sign, Fig. 70-4).

In children, pneumoperitoneum can be manifest as a generalized greater-than-normal radiolucency of the entire abdomen. This radiolucency often assumes an oval configuration ("football" sign) because of the accumulation of large amounts of free gas in the uppermost (anterior) portion of the peritoneal cavity when the child is supine (Fig. 70-5). Another sign of pneumoperitoneum on the supine radiograph is demonstration of the falciform ligament. This almost-vertical, curvilinear water-density shadow in the upper abdomen to the right of the spine is outlined only when there is gas on both sides of it, as in a pneumoperitoneum (Fig. 70-6). Free gas outlining the lateral umbilical ligaments,

which contain the umbilical artery remnants, produces an inverted V in the lower abdomen as the ligaments course inferiorly and laterally from the umbilicus (Fig. 70-7). A similar pattern in adults may be created by intraperitoneal gas outlining the inferior epigastric vessels. Free intraperitoneal gas can also outline the urachus, which appears as a conical soft-tissue pelvic shadow that is widest at its junction with the urinary bladder and tapers as it courses upward (Fig. 70-8). This urachal sign of pneumoperitoneum must be differentiated from the rectangular configuration of the buttock crease that also may be seen on supine films (Fig. 70-9). Free intraperitoneal gas in the median subphrenic space beneath the central tendon of the diaphragm can appear as an arcuate collection of gas with a sharp upper margin and an ill-defined lower margin (cupola sign, Fig. 70-10). In a supine patient, free intraperitoneal gas is more likely to collect below the central tendon than below the diaphragmatic leaves, since the former is a more anteriorly located space. Confusion with air in the lesser sac is obviated if the falciform ligament is defined, because this structure lies anterior to the stomach and liver.

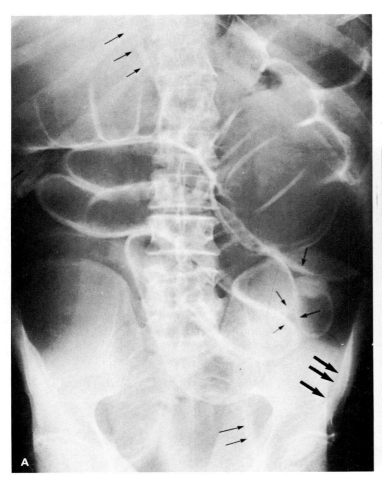

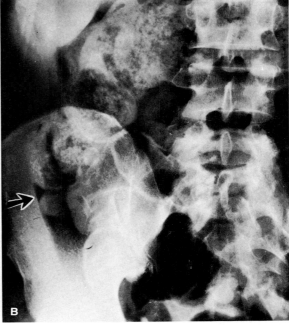

70-4

Fig. 70-4. Triangle sign of pneumoperitoneum. **(A) Arrows** in the left midabdomen point to two triangle signs between loops of bowel. Other evidence of pneumoperitoneum includes demonstration of the falciform **(top arrows)** and lateral umbilical ligaments **(lower arrows)**, the football sign **(arrows)** in the patient's left lower quadrant, and both the inner and outer walls of the large and small bowel. **(B)** In a different patient with a perforated duodenal ulcer there is a triangle sign between two fluid-filled loops of large and small bowel and the lateral abdominal wall **(arrow)**. A similar sign is seen in the right upper quadrant between the liver edge, colon, and fluid-containing small bowel. (Miller RE: The radiological evaluation of intraperitoneal gas [pneumoperitoneum]. CRC Crit Rev Diagn Imaging 4:61–85, 1973)

Fig. 70-5. Football sign of pneumoperitoneum. A massive amount of free intraperitoneal gas in an infant appears as a large oval lucency on this supine radiograph of the abdomen. The falciform ligament is seen overlying the liver and to the right of the spine. Portal venous gas can also be noted. (Wind ES, Pillare GP, Lee WJ: Lucent liver in the newborn: Roentgenographic sign of pneumoperitoneum. JAMA 237:2218–2219, 1977)

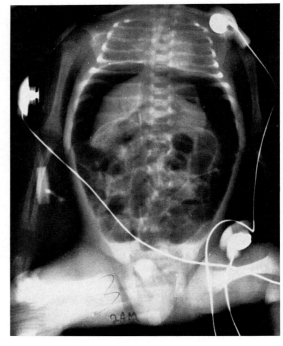

70-5

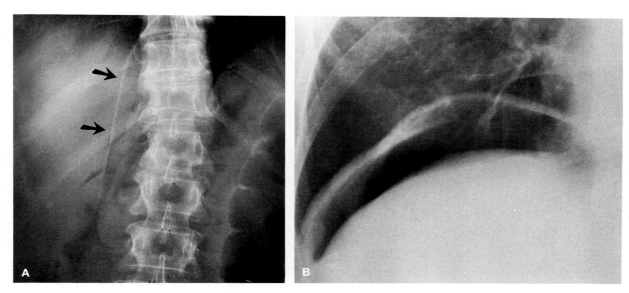

Fig. 70-6. Falciform ligament sign of pneumoperitoneum. **(A)** On the supine view, the falciform ligament appears as a curvilinear water density shadow **(arrows)** in the upper abdomen to the right of the spine. This implies that there is a pneumoperitoneum with gas on both sides of the ligament. **(B)** An upright view clearly demonstrates free gas under the right hemidiaphragm.

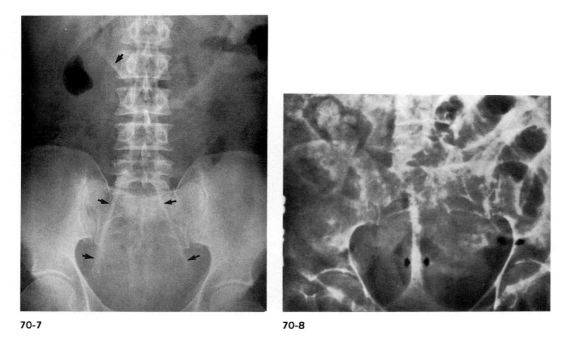

70-7   70-8

Fig. 70-7. Inverted V sign of pneumoperitoneum. Supine abdominal radiograph shows the lateral umbilical ligaments **(lower arrows)** diverging from the umbilicus, implying the presence of pneumoperitoneum. Free intraperitoneal gas also makes the falciform ligament visible **(upper arrow).** (Weiner CI, Diaconis JN, Dennis JM: The "inverted V": A new sign of pneumoperitoneum. Radiology 107:47–48, 1973)

Fig. 70-8. Urachal sign of pneumoperitoneum. Supine radiograph of the abdomen demonstrates a tapering conical soft-tissue density in the pelvis **(horizontal arrows)** representing the urachus. The outer wall of a loop of bowel in the left abdomen **(vertical arrows)** is possibly outlined by free intraperitoneal gas. (Jelaso DV, Schultz EH: The urachus: An aid to the diagnosis of pneumoperitoneum. Radiology 92:295–296, 1969)

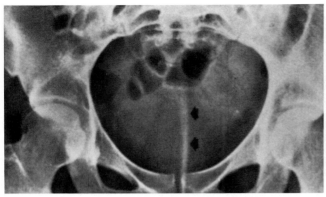

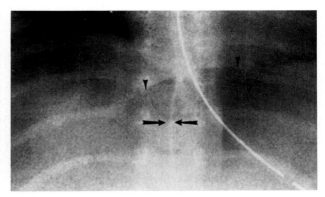

70-9   70-10

Fig. 70-9. Buttock crease. This rectangular configuration **(arrows)** on a supine film must be differentiated from the urachal sign. (Jelaso DV, Schultz EH: The urachus: An aid to the diagnosis of pneumoperitoneum. Radiology 92:295–296, 1969)

Fig. 70-10. Cupola sign of pneumoperitoneum. Air in the median subphrenic space **(arrowheads)** has a sharp upper border and poorly delineated lower margin. The falciform ligament **(arrows)** is outlined by air. (Mindelzun RE, McCort JJ: The cupola sign of pneumoperitoneum in the supine patient. Gastrointest Radiol 11:283–285, 1986)

PNEUMOPERITONEUM WITH PERITONITIS

PERFORATED VISCUS

The most frequent cause of pneumoperitoneum with peritonitis is perforation of a peptic ulcer, either gastric or duodenal (Fig. 70-11). However, in about 30% of perforated peptic ulcers, no free intraperitoneal gas can be identified. Therefore, failure to demonstrate a pneumoperitoneum is of no value in excluding the possibility of a perforated ulcer. In general, absence of gas in the stomach and the presence of gas scattered throughout the small and large bowel suggests a gastric perforation as the cause of pneumoperitoneum. Little or no colonic gas in the presence of a gastric gas–fluid level and small bowel distention makes a colonic perforation more likely. However, these radiographic findings can be difficult to discern and misleading, so that a firm diagnosis of the site of perforation often cannot be made on plain film examination and may require a contrast study using a water-soluble agent (Fig. 70-12).

Colonic perforations, especially those involving the cecum, give the most abundant quantities of free intraperitoneal gas (Fig. 70-13). Colonic perforations can be due to obstructing malignancy or severe ulcerating colitis leading to toxic megacolon.

Perforation due to diverticulitis usually results in a localized pericolic abscess. Occasionally, gas from a diverticular perforation enters the general peritoneal space and produces a pneumoperitoneum, which predominantly collects under the left hemidiaphragm. Pneumoperitoneum rarely occurs in patients with acute appendicitis.

ULCERATIVE BOWEL DISEASE

Inflammatory lesions with ulcerations in the intestinal wall can give rise to pneumoperitoneum. In the small bowel, this is most commonly seen in patients with tuberculosis or typhoid fever. Because the small bowel does not usually contain substantial amounts of gas, perforations of this organ produce relatively small amounts of free intraperitoneal gas. Ulceration within Meckel's diverticula, especially in children, can lead to perforation (Fig. 70-14), as can ulcerations in patients with chronic ulcerative colitis or lymphogranuloma venereum.

INFECTION/TRAUMA

Septic infection of the peritoneal cavity by gas-forming organisms can result in the production of a

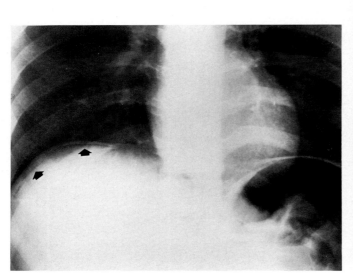

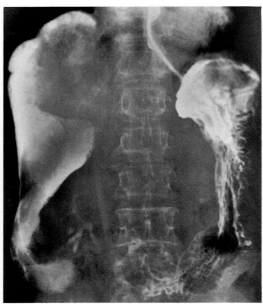

70-11   70-12

Fig. 70-11.   Pneumoperitoneum caused by a perforated duodenal ulcer.

Fig. 70-12.   Perforated duodenal ulcer. There is extensive extravasation from the upper gastrointestinal tract following the oral administration of contrast material.

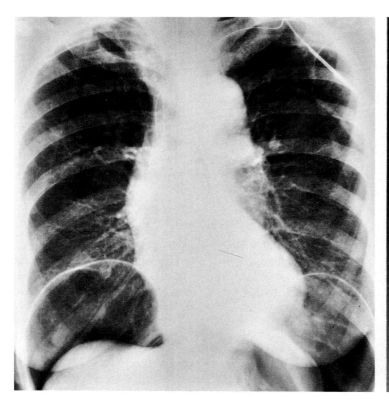

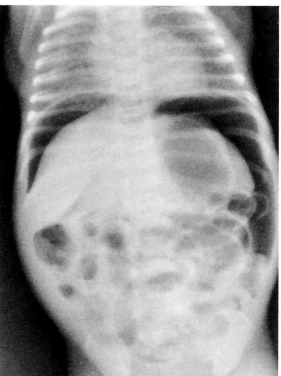

70-13   70-14

Fig. 70-13.   Extensive pneumoperitoneum following colonic perforation.

Fig. 70-14.   Pneumoperitoneum following perforation of an ulcerated Meckel's diverticulum in a child.

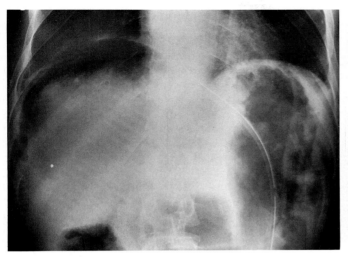

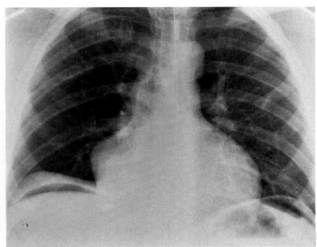

70-15   70-16

Fig. 70-15. Pneumoperitoneum that developed following trauma. Note the thickened gastric folds due to hemorrhage into the wall of the stomach.

Fig. 70-16. Pneumoperitoneum resulting from spontaneous perforation of the colon in a renal transplant patient on long-term immunosuppressive therapy.

substantial amount of gas and the radiographic appearance of pneumoperitoneum. Pneumoperitoneum can also develop following penetrating injuries of the abdominal wall and after blunt trauma causing rupture of a hollow viscus (Fig. 70-15).

DELAYED COMPLICATION OF RENAL TRANSPLANTATION

Spontaneous perforation of the colon is one of the most significant gastrointestinal complications that develop in renal transplant patients on long-term immunosuppressive therapy (Fig. 70-16). In a recent study, a majority of perforations occurred in the sigmoid colon and were related to nonocclusive ischemia. Other reports have shown that perforation is often associated with diverticular disease occurring months or years after successful transplantation and unrelated to periods of transplant rejection. Free peritoneal perforation is common with diverticular disease in transplant patients; in contrast, diverticular perforations are usually localized in nontransplant patients. Pseudomembranous colitis has also been described as a cause of colon necrosis and perforation following transplantation. In the immediate post-transplant period, perforation can be due to the development of a perinephric abscess. Colon and small bowel perforations out-

number gastroduodenal perforations more than two to one in post-transplant patients. Upper abdominal pain is the predominant clinical symptom. Clinical signs of an intra-abdominal catastrophe are infrequent or delayed, probably because of steroid or other immunosuppressive therapy. The overall mortality rate of gastrointestinal perforation in renal transplant patients is about 50% to 75%.

PNEUMOPERITONEUM WITHOUT PERITONITIS

IATROGENIC CAUSES

Iatrogenic pneumoperitoneum is generally asymptomatic and usually follows laparotomy (Fig. 70-17). In one large study, pneumoperitoneum was demonstrated in almost 60% of cases after abdominal surgery. Pneumoperitoneum usually occurs after operations on the gallbladder, stomach, or intestines, in which relatively large incisions are required. This phenomenon is seen rarely after repairs of inguinal hernias and infrequently after appendectomies. Postoperative pneumoperitoneum can be radiographically detectable for up to 3 weeks after surgery but usually can no longer be demonstrated

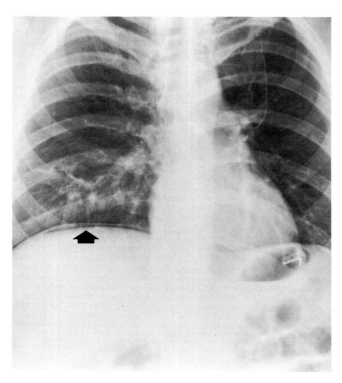

Fig. 70-17. Iatrogenic pneumoperitoneum **(arrow)** following laparotomy.

after the first postoperative week. The time required for absorption of the free intraperitoneal gas depends primarily on the volume of gas originally trapped in the abdomen (as seen on the initial postoperative radiograph). Body habitus of the patient also appears to play a major role in the incidence and rate of absorption of postoperative pneumoperitoneum. In one study, over 80% of asthenic patients showed pneumoperitoneum. Only 25% of obese patients demonstrated this finding and, in this group, the intraperitoneal gas was nearly always gone by the third postoperative day. Therefore, free intraperitoneal gas is a normal postoperative radiographic finding that, in the event of postoperative abdominal symptoms, should not enter into decisions of diagnosis or management. The major exception is in obese patients and children, in whom the presence of free intraperitoneal gas more than 3 days after surgery suggests, although it certainly does not confirm, the possibility of perforation.

An increasing amount of gas in the peritoneal cavity on serial radiographs strongly suggests a persistent abdominal abnormality and may indicate breakdown of a surgical anastomosis or other rupture of the intestinal tract. For this determination to be made, however, it is essential that all radiographs be obtained with the patient in the same position for

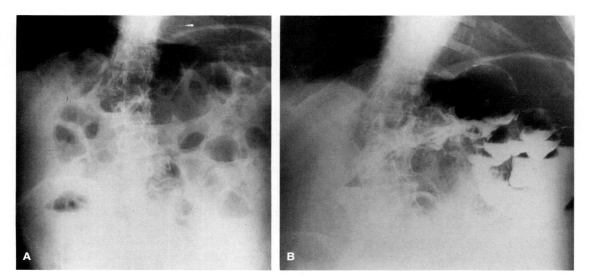

Fig. 70-18. Pneumoperitoneum associated with jejunal diverticulosis. **(A)** An erect abdominal radiograph demonstrates pneumoperitoneum as well as an unusual small bowel gas pattern from gas-filled diverticula. **(B)** An erect film taken during small bowel follow-through shows gas-barium levels in multiple large jejunal diverticula as well as the presence of the pneumoperitoneum. (Dunn V, Nelson JA: Jejunal diverticulosis and chronic pneumoperitoneum. Gastrointest Radiol 4:165–168, 1979)

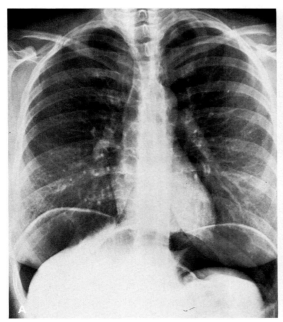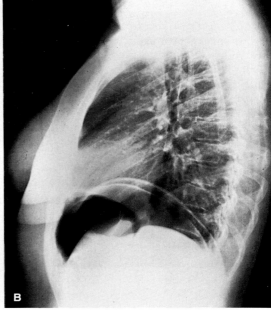

Fig. 70-19. Pneumoperitoneum following orogenital intercourse. **(A)** Frontal and **(B)** lateral chest radiographs demonstrate a large amount of free intraperitoneal gas. (Gantt CB, Daniel WW, Hallenbeck GA: Nonsurgical pneumoperitoneum. Am J Surg 134:411–414, 1977)

the same length of time and without abdominal drains.

Examples of rare iatrogenic causes of pneumoperitoneum include perforation during endoscopic procedures and the old and seldom used technique of pneumoperitoneum for diagnostic purposes. In a diagnostic pneumoperitoneum, gas is introduced into the abdominal cavity to aid in delineating the viscera, particularly the liver and spleen, to outline abdominal masses, and to demonstrate the undersurface of the diaphragm.

ABDOMINAL CAUSES

In unusual instances, free intraperitoneal gas develops without gastrointestinal perforation, infection, trauma, or recent surgery. Patients with this "spontaneous pneumoperitoneum" are only mildly ill or even totally asymptomatic. It is essential that the causes of spontaneous pneumoperitoneum be carefully considered to prevent the patient from being subjected to immediate and unwarranted laparotomy.

Pneumoperitoneum can occur as a complication of pneumatosis intestinalis following rupture of one or several of the multiple gas-filled cysts that are present in the walls of the gastrointestinal tract. Spontaneous pneumoperitoneum without peritonitis can be the result of a *forme fruste* perforation of a peptic ulcer. It is postulated that a tiny perforation,

usually missed at operation, may produce a valve-like flap that permits only gas to escape from the lumen. A similar mechanism of leakage of gas from the bowel lumen may result from lesions such as carcinoma of the stomach and Crohn's disease. There also is evidence that gas can traverse the intact wall of a severely distended viscus. Leakage through the stomach by this mechanism can be due to aerophagy, gastroscopy, excessive intake of oral sodium bicarbonate, or a misplaced oxygen tube.

Jejunal diverticulosis is one of the leading gastrointestinal causes of pneumoperitoneum without peritonitis or surgery (Fig. 70-18). In this condition, the distended diverticular mucosa may function as a semipermeable membrane allowing transmural gas equilibration. Intestinal gas enters the peritoneal cavity without gross fecal contamination.

GYNECOLOGIC CAUSES

Infrequently, gynecologic causes of pneumoperitoneum have been reported (Fig. 70-19). Gas injected into the fallopian tubes as part of the Rubin test for tubal patency can escape into the peritoneal cavity in amounts sufficient to be visualized radiographically. Ascent of air through the normal female genital tract into the peritoneal cavity has been reported following vaginal douching, knee–chest exercises and pelvic examination in the postpartum period, and orogenital intercourse.

INTRATHORACIC CAUSES

Spontaneous pneumoperitoneum may be secondary to severe pulmonary disease (chronic obstructive pulmonary disease, asthma, cavitary pneumonia), rupture of an emphysematous bleb, or ventilatory support (especially in infants with severe respiratory distress syndrome requiring high ventilator pressures). In these situations, free abdominal gas most likely arises from air that has escaped into the mediastinum from the lung and has dissected into the retroperitoneum by way of perivascular or periesophageal spaces. The gas subsequently dissects along the mesentery and ruptures into the peritoneal space. Although a pneumomediastinum or pneumothorax, or both, are almost always seen when there is an intrathoracic source of pneumoperitoneum, occasionally neither is present.

BIBLIOGRAPHY

Bray JF: The "inverted V" sign of pneumoperitoneum. Radiology 151:45–46, 1984

Dunn V, Nelson JA: Jejunal diverticulosis and chronic pneumoperitoneum. Gastrointest Radiol 4:165–168, 1979

Felson B, Wiot JF: Another look at pneumoperitoneum. Semin Roentgenol 8:437–443, 1973

Gantt CB, Daniel WW, Hallenbeck GA: Nonsurgical pneumoperitoneum. Am J Surg 134:411–414, 1977

Harrison I, Litwer H, Gerwig WH: Studies of the incidence and duration of postoperative pneumoperitoneum. Ann Surg 145:591, 1957

Jelaso DV, Schultz EH: The urachus: An aid to the diagnosis of pneumoperitoneum. Radiology 92:295–296, 1969

Madura MJ, Craig RM, Shields TW: Unusual causes of spontaneous pneumoperitoneum. Surg Gynecol Obstet 154:417–420, 1982

Menuck L, Siemers PT: Pneumoperitoneum: Importance of right upper quadrant features. AJR 127:753–756, 1976

Miller RE: The radiological evaluation of intraperitoneal gas (pneumoperitoneum). CRC Crit Rev Diag Imaging 4:61–85, 1973

Mindelzun RE, McCort JJ: The cupola sign of pneumoperitoneum in the supine patient. Gastrointest Radiol 11:283–285, 1986

Paster SB, Brogdon BG: Roentgenographic diagnosis of pneumoperitoneum. JAMA 235:1264–1267, 1976

Puglisi BS, Kauffman HM, Stewart ET et al: Colonic perforation in renal transplant patients. AJR 145:555–558, 1985

Rice RP, Thompson WM, Gedgaudas RK: The diagnosis and significance of extraluminal gas in the abdomen. Radiol Clin North Am 20:819–837, 1982

Seaman WB: The case of spontaneous pneumoperitoneum without peritonitis. Hosp Pract 12:105–108, 1977

Thompson WM, Meyers W, Seigler HF et al: Gastrointestinal complications of renal transplantation. Semin Roentgenol 13:319–328, 1978

Weiner CI, Diaconis JN, Dennis JM: The inverted "V": A new sign of pneumoperitoneum. Radiology 107:47–48, 1973

EXTRALUMINAL GAS IN THE UPPER QUADRANTS

Disease Entities

Gas not confined to a viscus
  Pneumoperitoneum
  Free retroperitoneal gas
  Subhepatic gas
Gas within an abscess
  Subphrenic
  Renal/perirenal
  Hepatic
  Splenic
  Pancreatic (abdominal fat necrosis)
  Lesser sac
Gas within the bowel wall
  Gas in the stomach wall
  Pneumatosis intestinalis
Gas in the biliary/portal system
  Biliary ductal system gas
  Emphysematous cholecystitis
  Portal vein gas
Chilaiditi's syndrome
Perforation due to a foreign body
Other causes of extraluminal gas
  Ruptured aortic aneurysm
  Postoperative renal hematoma
  Abdominal wall gas/abscess

GAS NOT CONFINED TO A VISCUS

PNEUMOPERITONEUM

Pneumoperitoneum is a major cause of extraluminal upper quadrant gas. It can be secondary to visceral perforation, surgery, or a variety of nonemergent abdominal, gynecologic, and intrathoracic causes (see Chap. 70).

FREE RETROPERITONEAL GAS

The most common cause of free retroperitoneal gas collections is perforation of the duodenum (Fig. 71-1) or rectum due to trauma, diverticulitis (Fig. 71-2), or ulcerative disease. Except for the duodenal bulb, the entire duodenum is retroperitoneal. This retroperitoneal part is fixed and therefore does not tolerate direct blows as easily as the stomach, duodenal bulb, and other more movable loops of mesenteric small bowel. Thus, the retroperitoneal parts of the duodenum are commonly ruptured in accidents that result in direct trauma to the upper part of the abdomen. In addition to causing pneumoperitoneum, pneumomediastinum or pneumatosis intestinalis (Fig. 71-3) can extend into the retroperitoneum and appear as extraluminal retroperitoneal gas. Dissection of gas into the retroperitoneal space

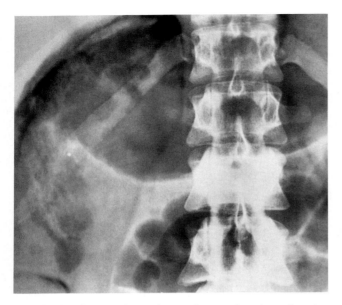

Fig. 71-1. Retroperitoneal gas after perforation of a duodenal ulcer. The gas outlines the kidney and the undersurface of the liver.

can also be a complication of an endoscopic procedure or barium enema examination. In one case, retroperitoneal gas was caused by wound irrigation with hydrogen peroxide, which resulted in dissection of molecular oxygen through retroperitoneal fascial planes (Fig. 71-4).

Retroperitoneal gas is best demonstrated on the right, where it outlines the kidney and the undersurface of the liver. Unlike intraperitoneal gas, gas in the retroperitoneum does not move freely when the patient changes position. For example, when the patient is in the left lateral decubitus position, retroperitoneal gas does not outline the lateral surface of the liver, as does a pneumoperitoneum.

SUBHEPATIC GAS

Gas can collect in the right subhepatic space above the upper pole of the right kidney. The inferior surface of the liver forms the anterior boundary of the subhepatic space; the peritoneal covering of the diaphragm and upper pole of the right kidney makes up the posterior border. Inferiorly, the subhepatic

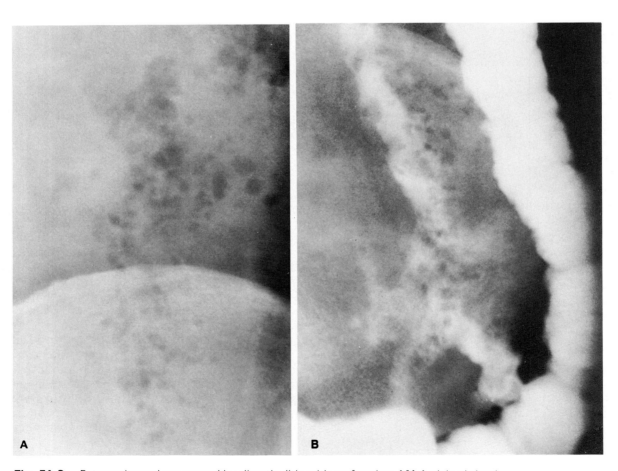

Fig. 71-2. Retroperitoneal gas caused by diverticulitis with perforation. **(A)** A plain abdominal radiograph demonstrates multiple gas bubbles along the course of the descending colon. **(B)** A contrast study demonstrates extravasation from the colon.

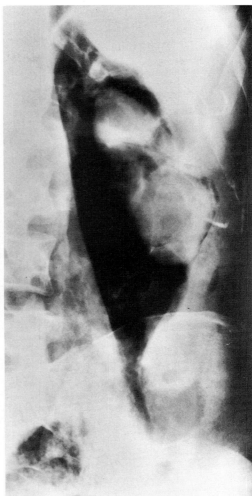

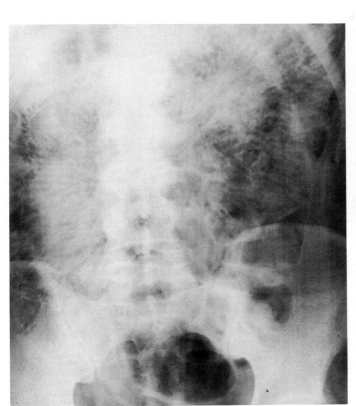

71-3   **71-4**

Fig. 71-3. Retroperitoneal gas due to extension of pneumatosis intestinalis. Gas in the retroperitoneal space is seen running horizontally, whereas that in the bowel wall is primarily seen coursing in a vertical direction.

Fig. 71-4. Retroperitoneal gas surrounding the left kidney. The gas developed following colonoscopy.

space opens into the peritoneal cavity; it is bounded superiorly by the coronary ligament.

The most common source of free gas in the right subhepatic space is perforation of a duodenal ulcer. Less common causes include perforation of the appendix (Fig. 71-5) or a sigmoid diverticulum, or leakage of a gastroenteric or ileotransverse colon anastomosis. Gas-containing abscesses in the subhepatic space can develop as complications of enteric perforation or pelvic pathology; subhepatic abscess formation in the latter instance is due to preferential flow of inflammatory exudate from the pelvis up the right gutter into the subhepatic space.

On plain abdominal radiographs, free gas in the subhepatic space usually assumes a triangular or crescent shape and overlies the right kidney inferior to the liver edge. Subhepatic abscesses are found in the same location but have a round or oval configuration, often with gas–fluid levels. Serial abdominal radiographs or films obtained with the patient in different positions are sometimes necessary to differentiate a subhepatic abscess from gas in a large duodenal bulb, duodenal diverticulum, or bowel adjacent to the liver edge.

GAS WITHIN AN ABSCESS

The majority of intra-abdominal abscesses occur postoperatively, and there is a high morbidity and

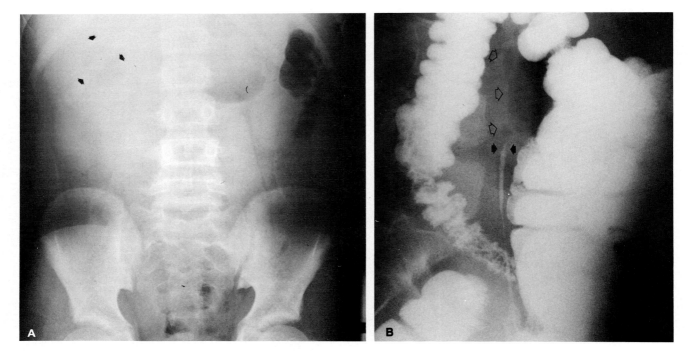

Fig. 71-5. Subhepatic gas caused by retrocecal appendicitis. **(A)** A supine abdominal radiograph reveals a gas-containing abscess in the subhepatic space **(arrows)** from a perforated retrocecal appendix. **(B)** A lateral view of a barium enema examination reveals that the retrocecal appendix has a distorted, perforated tip **(solid arrows)**. There is also a gas-containing abscess within the subhepatic space **(open arrows)**. Note that the base of the appendix is intact. (Harned RK: Retrocecal appendicitis presenting with air in the subhepatic space. AJR 126:416–418, 1976. Copyright 1976. Reproduced with permission)

mortality if the diagnosis and treatment are not accomplished expeditiously. An abscess may be difficult to diagnose clinically. Postoperative fevers may be ascribed to pulmonary or other infectious complications. Physical findings in the abdomen of a patient who has recently undergone abdominal surgery are difficult to evaluate. Various medications including antibiotics, steroids, and chemotherapeutic agents, which may be used in a variety of postoperative situations, can interfere with the clinical recognition of an abscess. Although computed tomography (CT), ultrasound, and radionuclide scans using gallium- or indium-labeled leukocytes have dramatically expanded the imaging capability of diagnosing intra-abdominal abscesses, conventional radiographic techniques still have an important role.

The radiographic appearance of gas in an abscess may be subtle and difficult to detect and differentiate from intraluminal gas, especially since many patients with an abscess have an associated ileus. The classic bubbly or mottled gas of an abscess may look like stool in the colon. Of equal importance, an abscess may contain a homogeneous collection of gas and mimic normal or dilated bowel (Fig. 71-6). It is sometimes possible to make this latter differential on plain radiographs due to the lack of any mucosal pattern in the abscess gas

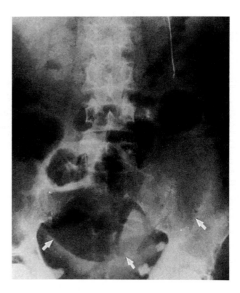

Fig. 71-6. Intra-abdominal abscess. Supine film of the abdomen shows a large homogeneous collection of gas **(arrows** outline the inferior margin) in an abscess secondary to anastomotic leak after distal ileal resection for Crohn's disease. The patient had some abdominal pain but only intermittent low-grade fever for 10 days before surgical drainage. (Rice RP, Thompson WM, Gedgaudas RK: The diagnosis and significance of extraluminal gas in the abdomen. Radiol Clin North Am 20:819–837, 1982)

(Fig. 71-7). In contrast to this, normal air-filled bowel virtually always contains some recognizable mucosal pattern. The administration of water-soluble contrast material orally or rectally may sometimes be required to determine whether a collection of gas is extraluminal or within the confines of the bowel.

It is important to remember that the presence of loculated extraluminal gas does not always indicate an abscess. Gas accumulated in necrotic tumor may be indistinguishable radiographically from abscess gas. This is especially true in patients who have undergone chemotherapy, radiation therapy, or vascular occlusion therapy in the palliative treatment of malignant neoplasms. Gas may be present in pancreatic pseudocysts after surgical or spontaneous drainage into the gastrointestinal lumen. Loculated bubbles or linear collections of gas may normally persist in the retroperitoneal space for at least 2 weeks following renal surgery. This normal gas frequently is found in the spaces lateral to the ascending and descending colon, which are common sites for abscesses, and makes the evaluation of postoperative films more difficult.

SUBPHRENIC ABSCESS

Even with the availability of broad-spectrum antibiotics and sophisticated surgical techniques, subphrenic abscesses continue to be associated with a high mortality rate (about 30%). Several decades ago, upper abdominal abscesses were often the result of intraperitoneal spread from a perforated appendix, peptic ulcer, diverticulitis, or cholecystitis. Today, most cases of upper abdominal abscesses represent complications of intra-abdominal surgery. The wide use of antibiotics often makes the clinical presentation insidious, with nonspecific symptoms such as low-grade fever, malaise, and mild pleuritic or abdominal discomfort, in contrast to the fulminant and often rapidly fatal course of upper abdominal abscesses in the past.

In one large surgical series, splenectomy was the procedure that most commonly resulted in left upper abdominal abscess formation. This was followed in descending order of frequency by gastric surgery, resection of carcinoma of the left colon, and hiatal hernia repair. Biliary tract surgery was the most common cause of a subphrenic abscess on the right side, followed by gastric and duodenal surgery and resection of carcinoma of the right colon.

Radiographic Findings

The earliest radiographic findings associated with subphrenic abscesses are elevation and restricted motion of the hemidiaphragm on the affected side (Fig. 71-8). An inflammatory pleural reaction at the base of the lung produces a nonpurulent (sympathetic) pleural effusion. Decubitus views are often necessary to demonstrate small or subpulmonic pleural fluid collections.

Extraluminal gas can be identified on plain abdominal radiographs in more than two-thirds of pa-

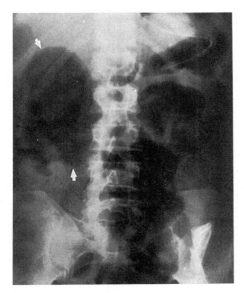

Fig. 71-7. Intra-abdominal abscess. Large homogeneous collection of gas **(arrows)** in an abscess secondary to right colostomy performed because of perforated carcinoma in the left colon. Note the absence of any mucosal pattern or haustral markings in the abscess gas compared with that of gas within the bowel. (Masters SJ, Rice RP: The homogeneous density of gas in the diagnosis of intra-abdominal abscess. Surg Gynecol Obstet 139:370–373, 1974)

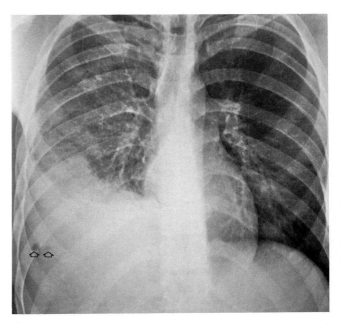

Fig. 71-8. Subphrenic abscess. Elevation of the right hemidiaphragm with pleural effusion and inflammatory reaction. Note the two tiny air bubbles **(arrows)** that indicate the presence of an underlying right upper quadrant abscess.

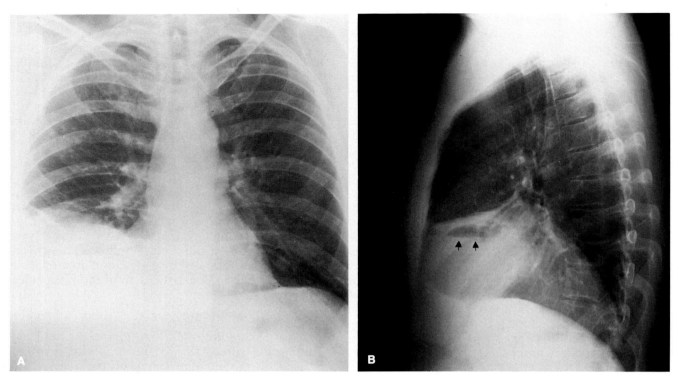

Fig. 71-9. Right subphrenic abscess. **(A)** Frontal and **(B)** right lateral views demonstrate elevation of the right hemidiaphragm, small right pleural effusion, and gas in the abscess cavity **(arrows).** (Connell TR, Stephens DH, Carlson HC et al: Upper abdominal abscess: A continuing and deadly problem. AJR 134:759–765, 1980. Copyright 1980. Reproduced with permission)

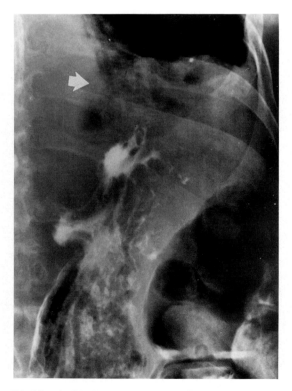

Fig. 71-10. Left subphrenic abscess. The characteristic mottled radiolucent appearance of the abscess **(arrow)**, which is located above the fundus of the stomach, is due to gas bubbles intermixed with necrotic material and pus.

tients with subphrenic abscesses (Fig. 71-9). Gas in an abscess can develop as a result of perforation of the stomach or bowel or can be related to the presence of gas-forming organisms. Regardless of the source, the interior of the abscess has a mottled radiolucent appearance caused by gas bubbles intermixed with necrotic material or pus (Fig. 71-10). On upright or decubitus views, a gas-fluid level can often be seen (Fig. 71-11). Although this appearance can be confused with gas accumulations in the bowel, the constancy of position of the gas shadows in multiple projections and on serial radiographs clearly indicates that they are outside the lumen of the bowel. Contrast studies are sometimes helpful in demonstrating the extraluminal location of the gas (Fig. 71-12); they can also identify leakage of contrast and deformity or displacement of normal structures, especially on the left side. Identification of abscesses on plain films is more difficult in the left subphrenic region than on the right, because the stomach and splenic flexure normally contain gas. Outlining of the stomach or colon with contrast material helps to differentiate intra- from extraluminal gas, as well as demonstrating a perforation or anastomotic leak.

RENAL/PERIRENAL ABSCESS

Signs of generalized peritonitis (paralytic ileus, separation of gas-filled loops of bowel, fluid in the peri-

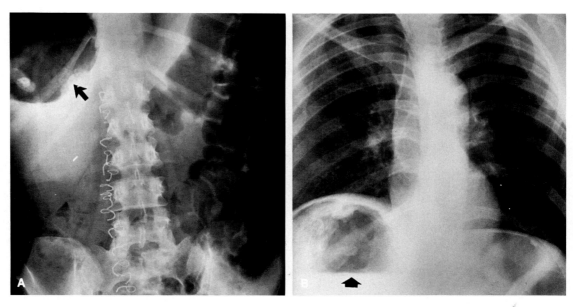

Fig. 71-11. Right subphrenic abscess. **(A)** A supine view reveals an extraluminal gas collection under the right hemidiaphragm **(arrow)**. **(B)** On the upright view, a gas-fluid level **(arrow)** can be seen in the abscess cavity.

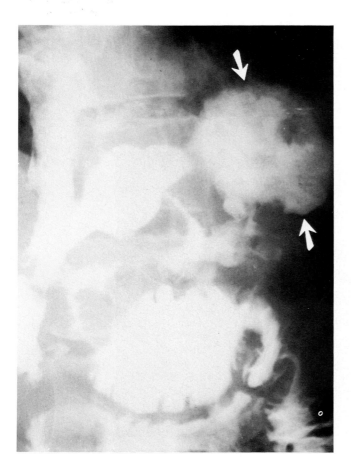

Fig. 71-12. Left subphrenic abscess. Following the oral administration of barium, contrast is seen to enter the large left subphrenic abscess **(arrows)**.

toneal cavity) can be seen in patients with abdominal abscesses. The shadow of an abscess can sometimes be confused with that of a tumor or a fluid-filled strangulated loop of bowel (pseudotumor).

Renal infection can be due to antecedent urinary tract disease (urinary tract infection, obstructive uropathy, trauma, instrumentation) or to direct or hematogenous spread of extraurinary infection. A renal abscess usually does not spread to the contralateral side, because the medial fascia surrounding the kidney is closed, and the spine and great vessels act as a natural deterrent. The inflammatory process can extend around the entire kidney, though it is usually most pronounced on the dorsal and inferior aspects, where the renal fascia is open and the surrounding tissues offer little resistance. The patient with a perirenal abscess generally complains of dysuria, chills, fever, and flank or abdominal pain. Other symptoms include flank tenderness, abdominal muscle guarding, mass, crepitation in the region of the affected kidney, and retraction of the lumbar spine from the affected side. Emphysematous pyelonephritis is a special form of acute renal inflammation affecting diabetics and patients with urinary tract obstruction.

The radiographic demonstration of extraluminal gas around or inside the kidney and in the retroperitoneal space is nearly pathognomonic of a renal or perirenal abscess (Fig. 71-13). The perirenal infection can appear to be diffuse and poorly defined, or it can be in the form of a localized mass (Fig. 71-14). Because the exudate usually localizes

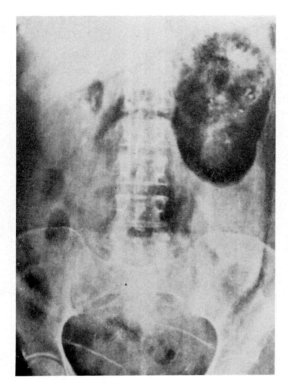

Fig. 71-13. *Perinephric abscess. A large gas collection surrounds the left kidney. The properitoneal fat line is outlined by gas in the posterior pararenal space. Nephrocalcinosis is also noted. (Love L, Baker D, Ramsey R: Gas producing perinephric abscess. AJR 119:783–792, 1973. Copyright 1973. Reproduced with permission)*

in the dorsolateral perirenal fat near the lower pole, the kidney tends to be displaced anteriorly; because of magnification, the kidney appears enlarged in the anteroposterior projection. Displacement of the descending duodenum and ascending or descending colon is common, as is obliteration of the upper half of the psoas muscle shadow.

HEPATIC ABSCESS

Gas is occasionally demonstrated in a liver abscess (Fig. 71-15). This appearance can be caused by pyogenic organisms (especially *Klebsiella*) or amebic infestation. Bubbly gas collections in the liver are characteristic of patients with gas gangrene. Although the organism that causes gas gangrene is frequently found in normal livers, it grows only in the presence of severe tissue ischemia or necrosis and thus usually develops in severely debilitated patients and persons with terminal diseases.

PANCREATIC ABSCESS

Peritoneal fat necrosis is the hallmark of acute pancreatitis and almost specific for it. This condition produces a pathognomonic mottled pattern of speckled radiolucencies, with normal fat intermingled with areas of water density that probably represent hydrolyzation products (Fig. 71-16). This "abdominal fat necrosis" sign can be differentiated from the speckled appearance of stool in the colon

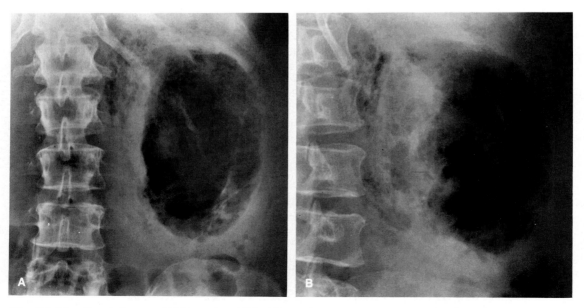

Fig. 71-14. *Renal abscess. (A) Frontal and (B) oblique views show large amounts of extraluminal gas within and around the left kidney. (Eisenberg RL: Diagnostic Imaging in Surgery. New York, McGraw–Hill, 1987)*

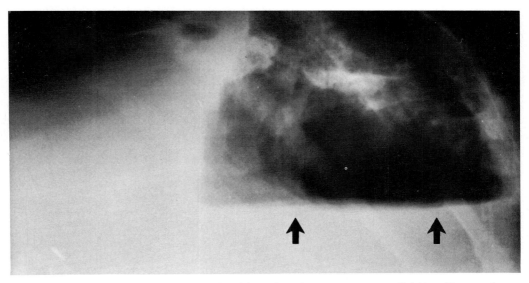

Fig. 71-15. Hepatic abscess. A lateral decubitus view demonstrates a gas-fluid level **(arrows)** in this abscess, which contains a large amount of soft-tissue necrotic debris.

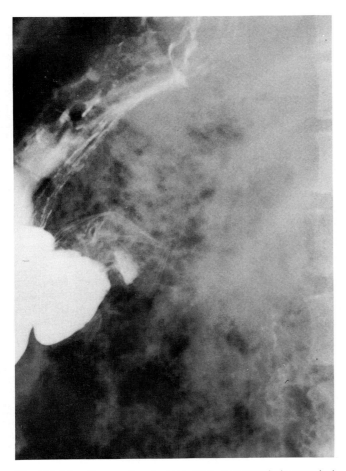

Fig. 71-16. Pancreatic abscess. The characteristic mottled pattern of speckled radiolucencies, with normal fat intermingled with areas of water density, involves much of the retroperitoneal space.

both because it does not follow the distribution of the large bowel and because the pattern does not change from day to day, as does that of stool. Although this sign is rare in relation to the frequency of acute pancreatitis, it is diagnostic of severe inflammatory disease and is associated with a high mortality rate.

LESSER SAC ABSCESS

Most lesser sac abscesses originate from disease processes in contiguous organs, especially the pancreas. The most common cause is a pancreatic abscess or an infected pseudocyst. Rarely, a lesser sac abscess can result from the spread of a more generalized process (such as peritonitis) through the foramen of Winslow. It is clinically important to differentiate an abscess in the lesser sac from one in the anterior left subphrenic space, which extends up over the liver and is thus the most superior left upper quadrant space. The lesser sac is separated from the anterior subphrenic space by the left coronary ligament, which extends from the superior dorsal aspect of the left lobe of the liver to the diaphragm.

In general, lesser sac abscesses displace the stomach anteriorly and the colon inferiorly, whereas an abscess in the left anterior subphrenic space compresses the stomach in a posterior as well as inferior and medial direction. On supine radiographs, abscesses in the lesser sac and left anterior subphrenic space may look identical, producing an epigastric collection in the left upper abdomen ex-

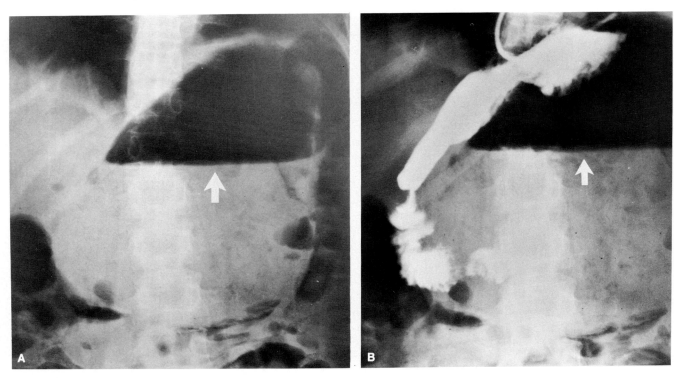

Fig. 71-17. Lesser sac abscess. **(A)** A plain abdominal radiograph and **(B)** a film from a barium study reveal a huge abscess cavity with a prominent gas-fluid level **(arrows)**.

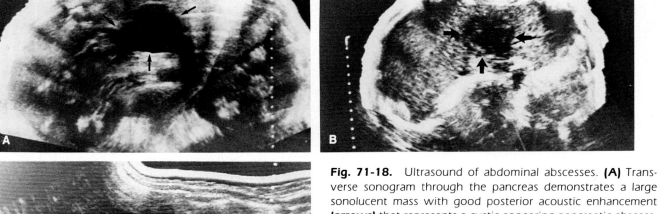

Fig. 71-18. Ultrasound of abdominal abscesses. **(A)** Transverse sonogram through the pancreas demonstrates a large sonolucent mass with good posterior acoustic enhancement **(arrows)** that represents a cystic-appearing pancreatic abscess. Note the smooth walls and the absence of internal echoes, both typical of cystic lesions. **(B)** Transverse sonogram demonstrates an amebic liver abscess **(arrows)** as an irregular mass, with extensive echoes within the lesion and poor posterior acoustic enhancement. **(C)** Parasagittal sonogram through the liver **(L)** in a patient with a liver abscess demonstrates layering of echogenic debris **(open arrows)** in the posterior portion of a large sonolucent collection. (Kressel HY, McLean GK: Abdominal abscess. In Eisenberg RL, Amberg JR (eds): Critical Diagnostic Pathways in Radiology: An Algorithmic Approach. Philadelphia, JB Lippincott, 1981)

tending slightly over the midline (Fig. 71-17). How-ever, an upright film may help differentiate ab-scesses in these two compartments. Because the anterior subphrenic space extends under the dome of the diaphragm, an abscess in this space is situated immediately beneath the central tendon of the dia-phragm. In contrast, the upper margin of a lesser sac abscess is in a more inferior position and does not reach the diaphragm.

ULTRASOUND AND CT OF ABDOMINAL ABSCESS

Although plain abdominal radiographs and contrast studies of the gastrointestinal tract may show ec-topic gas or gas–fluid levels, soft-tissue masses, pleural fluid or elevation of the diaphragm, and focal dilatation of adjacent bowel loops suggesting an intra-abdominal abscess, these findings are often nonspecific and do not permit a precise definition of the extent of the inflammatory process. The imaging of intra-abdominal abscesses has been greatly improved with the use of ultrasound and CT.

The classic ultrasound appearance of an ab-scess is a sonolucent collection surrounded by thick, irregular walls and clearly separable from the normal structures of the abdomen, pelvis, and ret-roperitoneum (Fig. 71-18*A*). In practice, however, a spectrum of patterns ranging from purely cystic to

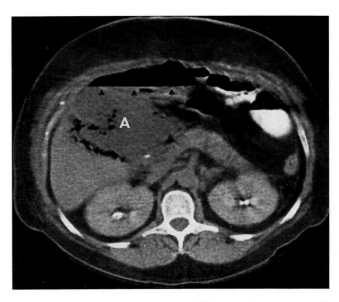

Fig. 71-20. Subhepatic abscess. CT scan shows the well-formed abscess **(A)** as a low-density mass that neither con-forms to the contour of the normal parenchymal organs nor lies within the confines of the bowel. Note the gas–fluid level within the abscess **(arrows)**. (Eisenberg RL: Diagnostic Imag-ing in Surgery. New York, McGraw–Hill, 1987)

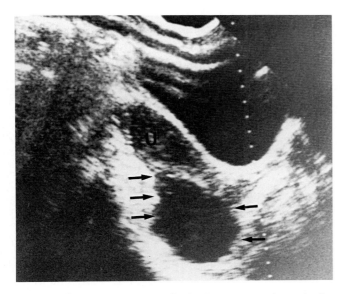

Fig. 71-19. Pelvic abscess. Sagittal sonogram through the midpelvis of a 22-year-old woman illustrates a large collection **(arrows)** posterior to the uterus **(U)**. Note the irregular walls of the collection and the good through sound transmission. Weak echoes are noted within the sonolucent region. (Kressel HY, McLean GK: Abdominal abscess. In Eisenberg RL, Amberg JR [eds]: Critical Diagnostic Pathways in Radiology: An Al-gorithmic Approach. Philadelphia, JB Lippincott, 1981)

purely solid may occur. The thick, purulent con-tents of an abscess often produce a pattern of dif-fuse, weak echoes. If there are septations or clumps of necrotic debris within the central cavity, coarse and irregular echoes are seen (Fig. 71-18*B*). The in-ternal layering of different components of an ab-scess may produce the bandlike pattern of a fluid–fluid level (Fig. 71-18*C*). Gas collections, either large or in the form of microbubbles, reflect inci-dent sound waves almost completely and cause dis-tal shadowing. Both the irregularity of the abscess walls and the nature of the abscess fluid itself result in poorer definition of the wall–fluid interface than might be expected. Similarly, the through transmis-sion of sound that is characteristic of simple cysts may not be present in abscesses. Although this wide variety of patterns may appear confusing, ultra-sound can detect more than 90% of abdominal ab-scesses. Ultrasound is especially valuable for de-tecting abscesses in the right upper quadrant or pelvis (Fig. 71-19); pancreatic abscesses and those involving the left upper quadrant may be obscured by overlying bowel gas from an accompanying ileus. Because the examination requires close contact be-tween the transducer and the skin, ultrasound may be difficult to use in postsurgical patients with re-cent incisions, wound dressings, drainage tubes, su-perficial infections, or stomas.

The CT appearance of an abdominal abscess varies with its age and maturity. Before a mature abscess cavity forms, a phlegmon may alter the nor-mal organ contours and obliterate the adjacent soft-

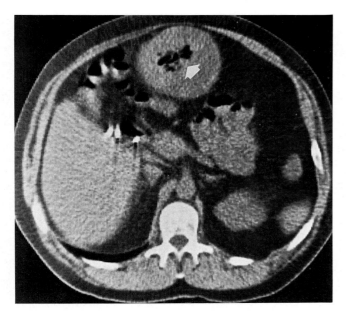

Fig. 71-21. *Abdominal abscess. There is gas within the central cavity of the abscess. (Eisenberg RL: Diagnostic Imaging in Surgery. New York, McGraw–Hill, 1987)*

tissue planes. In the appropriate clinical setting, these findings may permit the very early detection of a focal infective process. A well-formed abscess appears as a soft-tissue or low-density mass that neither conforms to the contour of the normal parenchymal organs nor lies within the confines of the bowel (Fig. 71-20). Abscesses commonly appear homogeneous, although septations and necrotic debris may present a pattern of varying attenuation values. The thick, irregular wall of a mature abscess can often be seen. The most specific CT finding of an abdominal abscess, seen in almost half of the cases, is the presence of gas within the central cavity (Fig. 71-21). Intravenous contrast agents may be used to advantage in detecting abscesses by CT. After contrast material is administered, the hypervascular wall of the abscess is enhanced, whereas the central cavity remains unchanged. The thickening of fascial planes and the abnormal density of adjacent intraperitoneal or extraperitoneal fat indicate extension of the inflammatory process. The relation of an abdominal abscess to adjacent bowel loops can be readily determined by the oral or rectal administration of dilute contrast material to opacify the gastrointestinal tract. Although CT has a high sensitivity in abscess detection, the findings are somewhat nonspecific. A similar pattern can be produced by old hematomas, tumors with central necrosis, and complicated cysts.

In selected cases, percutaneous drainage of abdominal abscesses is indicated as a safe and effective alternative to surgical intervention. The major criteria for patient selection for percutaneous

drainage of abdominal abscesses include a well-defined, unilocular abscess, a safe access route for catheter insertion, and the availability of immediate surgical backup if the procedure is not successful or if there are complications. Computed tomography is used to provide the detailed anatomic map necessary for planning the appropriate route (Fig. 71-22). Ultrasound (or CT) is then used to guide the needle into the abscess cavity. Complete resolution of the abscess can be achieved in more than 90% of cases. The complication rates of percutaneous abscess drainage are low (less than the operative morbidity) and include transient bacteremia and either perforation of a viscus or contamination of the pleural space during insertion of the catheter.

GAS WITHIN THE BOWEL WALL

Gas in the wall of the stomach can be an ominous sign of severe infection associated with phlegmonous gastritis or other necrotizing condition. It can also be a benign complication of endoscopy, gastric pneumatosis, or rupture of a pulmonary bullus into the esophageal wall.

Pneumatosis intestinalis can reflect mesenteric ischemia and necrosis in adults or necrotizing enterocolitis in children. It can also be a benign phenomenon of no clinical significance. This condition is discussed in detail in Chapter 69.

GAS IN THE BILIARY/PORTAL SYSTEM

Gas in the biliary tree is due to fistulization between the gallbladder or bile duct and the stomach or duodenum. This condition can be due to previous surgery (sphincterotomy), cholecystitis, severe peptic ulcer disease, trauma, or a tumor. Gas in the biliary tree is discussed in detail in Chapter 65.

Emphysematous cholecystitis is a rare condition in which gas-forming organisms (*Escherichia coli, Clostridium welchii*) cause collections of gas in the lumen of the gallbladder, within its wall or surrounding tissue, or in both places (Fig. 71-23). Bacterial growth in the gallbladder is facilitated by cystic duct obstruction (most often by stones), which causes stasis and ischemia in the gallbladder. Up to half of reported cases of emphysematous gastritis have been in patients with poorly controlled diabetes.

Abdominal radiographs demonstrate gas in the gallbladder lumen, in the wall of the gallbladder, or in the pericholecystic tissues (Fig. 71-24). It is postulated that gas distention of the gallbladder lumen occurs first. At this stage, the gas filling the lumen of the gallbladder can be mistaken for a normal collection of gas in the stomach or intestine. Extension of gas into the wall of the gallbladder and adjacent tissues produces the pathognomonic appearance of

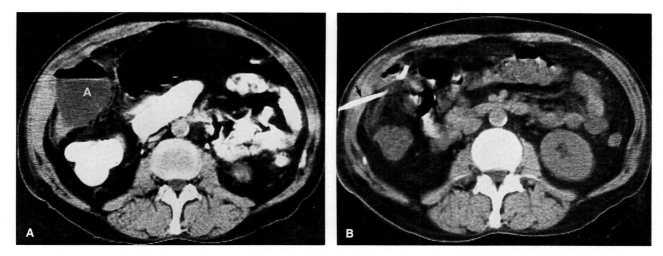

Fig. 71-22. Percutaneous drainage of abdominal abscess. **(A)** Large right pericolic gutter abscess with a gas–fluid level is secondary to a perforated duodenal ulcer. Note the swelling of the adjacent abdominal muscles. **(B)** The abscess cavity has been completely evacuated through the drainage catheter **(arrow)**. (Eisenberg RL: Diagnostic Imaging in Surgery. New York, McGraw–Hill, 1987)

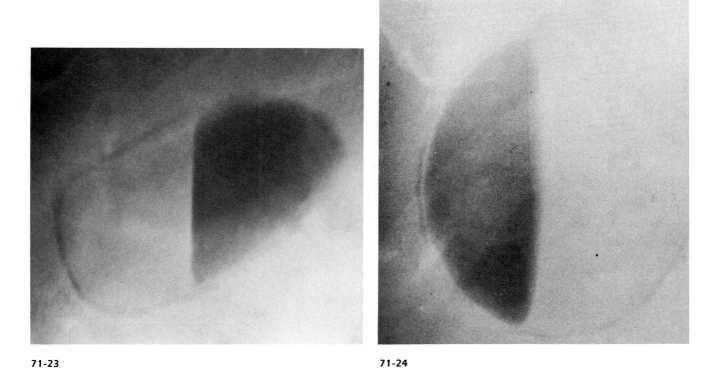

71-23   71-24

Fig. 71-23. Emphysematous cholecystitis. Gas is found within both the lumen and the wall of the gallbladder.

Fig. 71-24. Emphysematous cholecystitis. Gas is evident within the lumen and wall of the gallbladder.

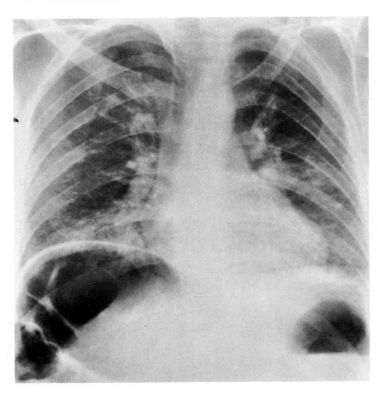

Fig. 71-25. Chilaiditi's syndrome. The transverse colon and hepatic flexure are interposed between the liver and the right hemidiaphragm.

a rim of translucent bubbles or streaks outside and roughly parallel to the gallbladder lumen. Because there is almost always obstruction of the cystic duct in emphysematous gastritis, gas is absent from the biliary ducts in the early stages of disease. If the infection spreads into the biliary tree, gas is seen in the ductal system.

At times, it may be necessary to eliminate the possibility of an internal biliary fistula as the source of the gas in the gallbladder lumen. This can be effectively done if there is no gas in the biliary ductal system.

Gas in the portal veins, discussed in detail in Chapter 66, is usually an ominous prognostic sign. It is generally related to necrotizing enterocolitis in children and mesenteric ischemia and bowel necrosis in adults. In children, a benign form of portal vein gas can be related to placement of an umbilical venous catheter.

CHILAIDITI'S SYNDROME

The transverse colon and the hepatic flexure are occasionally found interposed between the liver and the right hemidiaphragm (Chilaiditi's syn-

drome) (Fig. 71-25). This type of interposition is common, especially in mentally retarded or psychotic patients with chronic colonic enlargement. It sometimes occurs in association with chronic lung disease, postnecrotic cirrhosis, or pregnancy. This anomalous position of the colon is often transient and generally of little clinical significance. At times, however, Chilaiditi's syndrome is characterized by abdominal pain that becomes increasingly worse during the day and is often accentuated by deep breathing. Abdominal radiographs show a striking appearance of gas in the hepatic flexure interposed between the liver and diaphragm. It is essential that this pattern not be confused with free intraperitoneal gas.

PERFORATION DUE TO A FOREIGN BODY

Most ingested foreign bodies pass through the gastrointestinal tract without incident. Less than 1%, especially those that are either sharp or elongated, cause perforation and localized abscess formation. The intentional ingestion of foreign bodies is common in young children and emotionally disturbed persons. Predisposing factors in adults include decreased palatal sensitivity due to dentures, excessive

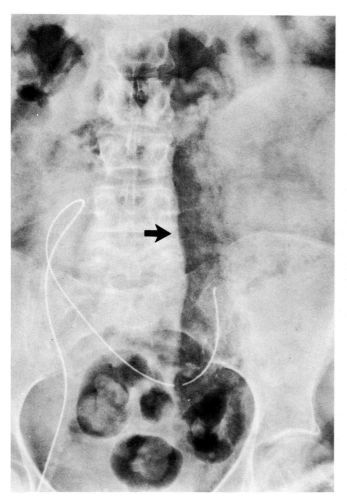

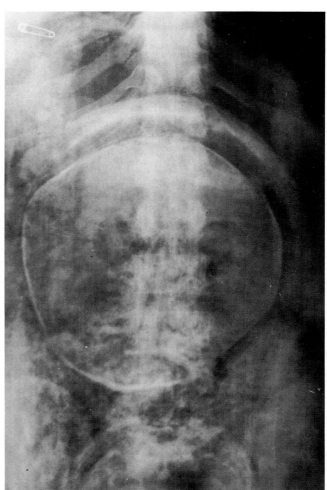

71-26   **71-27**

Fig. 71-26. Gas within a wound infection in the rectus sheath **(arrow)** following abdominal surgery.

Fig. 71-27. Gas gangrene of the uterus. Gas is evident in the wall of the uterus and in the surrounding soft tissues.

alcohol intake or drug use, ingestion of extremely cold liquids, poor vision, or rapid eating. The radiographic demonstration of the offending foreign body (*e.g.*, a chicken bone) with an associated mass or extraluminal gas collection in a patient with signs of peritonitis, mechanical bowel obstruction, or pneumoperitoneum strongly suggests this diagnosis.

OTHER CAUSES OF EXTRALUMINAL GAS

A ruptured aortic aneurysm with dissection of blood into the retroperitoneal fat can produce a mottled appearance that simulates a retroperitoneal ab-

scess. If there are no clinical signs of infection, a ruptured aortic aneurysm must be considered a possible cause of this radiographic pattern.

Postoperative perirenal hematoma can simulate a perirenal abscess. The apparent etiology of this condition is liquefaction of the hematoma, with gas entering it from the drain site.

Gas is occasionally demonstrated in the abdominal wall after surgery (Fig. 71-26). It may also be related to localized abscess formation.

Rarely, gas gangrene involves intra-abdominal structures other than the liver and gallbladder and causes the radiographic appearance of gas in the soft tissues or in the walls of abdominal organs (Fig. 71-27).

BIBLIOGRAPHY

Anschuetz SL: Extraluminal gas in the upper abdomen. Semin Roentgenol 19:255, 1984

Berenson JE, Spitz HB, Felson B: The abdominal fat necrosis sign. Radiology 100:567–571, 1971

Calenoff L, Poticha SM: Combined occurrence of retropneumoperitoneum and pneumomperitoneum. AJR 117:366–372, 1973

Connell TR, Stephens DH, Carlson HC et al: Upper abdominal abscess: A continuing and deadly problem. AJR 134:759–765, 1980

Evans JA, Meyers MA, Bosniak MA: Acute renal and perirenal infections. Semin Roentgenol 6:274–290, 1971

Fataar S, Schulman A: Subphrenic abscess: The radiologic approach. Clin Radiol 32:147–152, 1981

Fulcher WE, McLean GK: Abdominal abscess. In Eisenberg RL (ed): Diagnostic Imaging: An Algorithmic Approach. Philadelphia, JB Lippincott, 1988

Gelfand DW: Complications of gastrointestinal radiologic procedures: I. Complications of routine fluoroscopic studies. Gastrointest Radiol 5:293–315, 1980

Grainger K: Acute emphysematous cholecystitis: Report of a case. Clin Radiol 12:66–69, 1961

Halvorsen RA, Jones MA, Rice RP et al: Anterior left subphrenic abscess: Characteristic plain film and CT appearance. AJR 139:283–289, 1982

Harned RK: Retrocecal appendicitis presenting with air in the subhepatic space. AJR 126:416–418, 1976

Love L, Baker D, Ramsey R: Gas producing perinephric abscess. AJR 119:783–792, 1973

Maglinte DDT, Taylor SD, Ng AC: Gastrointestinal perforation by chicken bones. Radiology 130:597–599, 1979

Mellins HZ: Radiologic signs of disease in lesser peritoneal sac. Radiol Clin North Am 2:107–120, 1964

Nelson SW: Extraluminal gas collections due to diseases of the gastrointestinal tract. AJR 115:225–248, 1972

Older RA, Rice RP, Kelvin FM et al: Extraperitoneal gas following nephrectomy: Patterns and duration. J Urol 120:24–27, 1978

Rice RP, Thompson WM, Gedgaudas RK: The diagnosis and significance of extraluminal gas in the abdomen. Radiol Clin North Am 20:819–837, 1982

Swayne LC, Ginsberg HN, Ginsburg A: Pneumoperitoneum secondary to hydrogen peroxide wound irrigations. AJR 148:149–150, 1987

Woodard S, Kelvin FM, Rice RP et al: Pancreatic abscess: Importance of conventional radiology. AJR 136:871–878, 1981

FISTULAS INVOLVING THE SMALL OR LARGE BOWEL

72

Gastrointestinal fistulas are abnormal communications between the gastrointestinal tract and another segment of bowel (enteric–enteric fistula), another intra-abdominal organ (internal fistula), or the skin (external fistula).

CAUSES OF ENTERIC–ENTERIC FISTULAS

Crohn's disease
Diverticulitis
Malignant neoplasms (primary, metastatic)
Gastric ulcer
Radiation therapy
Ulcerative colitis
Infectious diseases
   Tuberculosis
   Pelvic inflammatory disease
   Actinomycosis
   Amebiasis
   Shigellosis
   Cytomegalovirus
Marginal ulcer (after gastric surgery)

Fistula formation is a hallmark of chronic Crohn's disease, found in at least half of all patients with this condition (Fig. 72-1). The diffuse inflammation of the serosa and mesentery in Crohn's disease causes involved loops of bowel to be firmly matted together by fibrous peritoneal and mesenteric bands (Fig. 72-2). Fistulas apparently begin as ulcerations that burrow through the bowel wall into adjacent loops of small bowel and colon (Fig. 72-3). Enteric-enteric fistulas can cause severe nutritional problems if they bypass extensive areas of intestinal absorptive surface (Fig. 72-4); the recirculation of intestinal contents and subsequent stasis can permit bacterial overgrowth and malabsorption. In addition to enteric-enteric fistulas, a characteristic finding in Crohn's disease is the appearance of fistulous tracts ending blindly in abscess cavities surrounded by dense inflammatory tissue. These abscess cavities are situated intraperitoneally, retroperitoneally, or deep within the mesentery and can produce palpable masses, persistent fever, or pain.

Fistulous communications between the colon and small bowel can be seen in about 10% of patients with diverticulitis (Fig. 72-5). These fistulas are often multiple and, when combined with a colo-vesical communication, can produce intractable perineal pain and itching, excoriation, or severe fluid and electrolyte imbalance due to loss of small bowel contents by way of the enterovesical fistula. A classic finding in this disease is dissection along the wall of the colon (double tracking; see Chap. 55). Although most commonly seen in diverticulitis and once thought to be pathognomonic of this disorder, double tracking can also develop in patients with Crohn's disease or carcinoma of the colon.

Primary or metastatic malignancy of the small bowel or colon can extend to form mesenteric or serosal deposits that draw bowel loops together to-

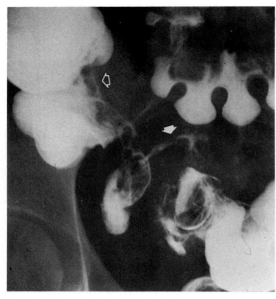
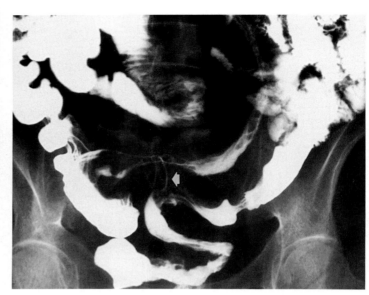

72-1   72-2

Fig. 72-1. Crohn's disease. There is fistulization between the terminal ileum and sigmoid **(solid arrow)** and double-tracking along the cecum **(open arrow)**.

Fig. 72-2. Crohn's disease. There is a fistula between the distal ileum and sigmoid **(arrow)**.

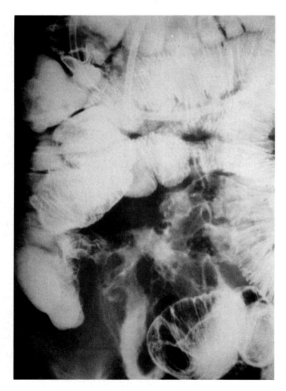

Fig. 72-3. Crohn's disease. Multiple interconnecting fistulas between distal ileal loops. (Lichtenstein JE: Radiologic–pathologic correlation of inflammatory bowel disease. Radiol Clin North Am 25:3–24, 1987)

ward a central point (Fig. 72-6). This can lead to irregular ulceration and the creation of a fistulous communication between adjacent bowel loops (Fig. 72-7).

Gastrocolic and duodenocolic fistulas can originate from primary carcinomas of the colon (Fig. 72-8) or stomach. These tumors are almost always bulky and infiltrating and are associated with a marked inflammatory reaction. The tumor apparently extends from the serosa of one viscus into the wall of another, followed by lumen-to-lumen necrosis. The presence of growing tumor and fibrous stroma within the wall of a malignant fistula accounts for the length of these tracts and the relative separation of bowel loops. A similar radiographic pattern can be caused by carcinoma of the pancreas spreading to involve both the stomach and colon (Fig. 72-9).

Malignant gastrocolic fistulas are frequently demonstrated during barium enema examination but are rarely detected on upper gastrointestinal series. This phenomenon is probably related to preferential flow from the colon to the stomach or small bowel. The higher than usual intraluminal pressure in the colon at the time of a barium enema examination may overcome resistance in the rigid, nondistensible fistula, allowing passage of barium into the stomach or small bowel. When an upper gastrointestinal series is performed under more physiologic conditions, the intraluminal pressure in the proxi-

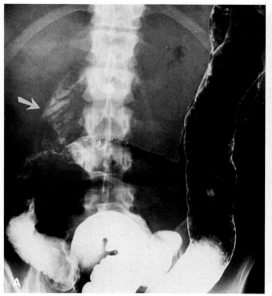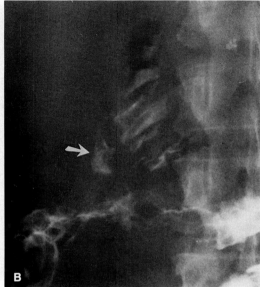

Fig. 72-4. Crohn's disease with development of a duodenocolic fistula. **(A)** A barium enema examination demonstrates retrograde filling of the fistula to the distal descending duodenum **(arrow).** There is marked irregularity of the colon with pseudopolyposis. **(B)** A delayed film from an upper gastrointestinal series demonstrates prominent duodenal folds **(arrow)** resulting from secondary reactive inflammation and not Crohn's disease. (Smith TR, Goldin RR: Radiographic and clinical sequelae of the duodenocolic anatomic relationship: Two cases of Crohn's disease with fistulization of the duodenum. Dis Colon Rectum 20:257–262, 1977)

mal gastrointestinal tract may not be sufficient to overcome this resistance.

Gastrocolic fistulas are a rare complication of benign gastric ulcer disease (Fig. 72-10). Gastric ulcers causing this condition are invariably located along the greater curvature or posterior wall of the antrum. As an ulcer penetrates posteriorly, involvement of the mesocolon permits spread of inflammation to the superior border of the transverse colon, which is almost always the site of the colonic end of the fistula (Fig. 72-11). Benign ulcer-induced gastrocolic fistulas are especially common in patients receiving steroids or aspirin, both of which have well-known ulcerogenic properties. These medications also decrease the inflammatory reaction that would ordinarily seal off a penetrating gastric ulcer. In addition, steroids can mask the severe clinical symptoms, thereby permitting a penetrating ulcer to develop into a gastrocolic fistula.

Radiation therapy, especially to the pelvic organs, can cause ischemic and inflammatory changes in the small and large bowel. In addition to mucosal ulceration and stricture formation, radiation enteritis often leads to the development of enteric-enteric fistulas.

Although enteric-enteric fistulas occur in ulcerative colitis, they are found in less than 0.5% of patients with this disease. Fistulas can also develop in other inflammatory bowel diseases, such as tu-

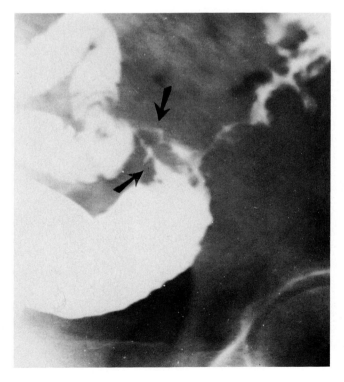

Fig. 72-5. Diverticulitis. Fistulous tracts **(arrow)** connect the sigmoid colon and ileum. (Kroening PM: Sigmoido-ileal fistulas as a complication of diverticulitis. AJR 96:323–325, 1966. Copyright 1966. Reproduced with permission)

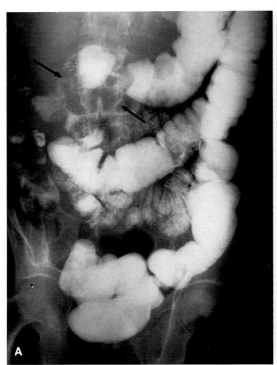
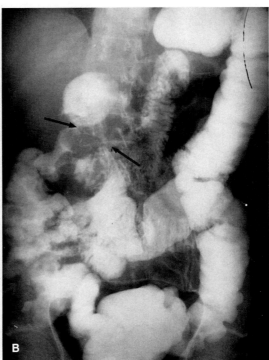

Fig. 72-6. Malignant duodenocolic fistula. **(A)** An upper gastrointestinal series demonstrates a lesion in the antrum of the stomach. There is marked deformity of the second portion of the duodenum with a duodenocolic fistula and mass deformity of the proximal transverse colon **(arrows)**. **(B)** A barium enema examination demonstrates the duodenocolic fistula, a lesion of the proximal transverse colon, and deformity of the cecum. (Vieta JO, Blanco R, Valentini GR: Malignant duodenocolic fistula: Report of two cases, each with one or more synchronous gastrointestinal cancers. Dis Colon Rectum 19:542–552, 1976)

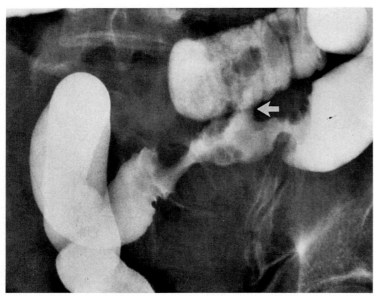

72-7

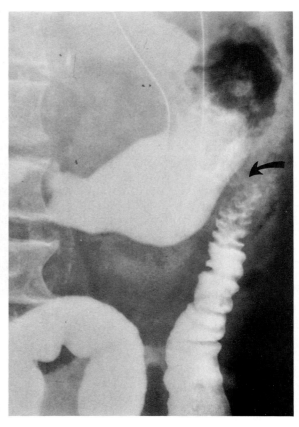

Fig. 72-7. Ileocolic fistula **(arrow)** secondary to carcinoma of the sigmoid colon.

Fig. 72-8. Gastrocolic fistula **(arrow)** caused by adenocarcinoma of the colon.

72-8

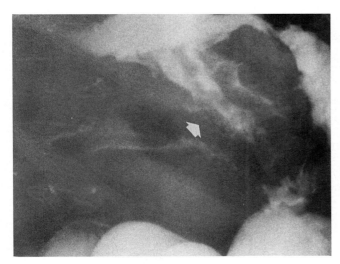

Fig. 72-9. Gastrocolic fistula due to invasive carcinoma of the tail of the pancreas. Contrast **(arrow)** appears in the stomach during a barium enema examination.

berculosis (Fig. 72-12), pelvic inflammatory disease, actinomycosis, amebiasis, shigellosis (Fig. 72-13), and cytomegalovirus infection in patients with AIDS (Fig. 72-14).

A fistulous communication between the stomach, jejunum, and colon (gastrojejunocolic fistula) or directly between the stomach and colon represents a grave complication of marginal ulceration after gastric surgery (especially gastrojejunostomy) for peptic ulcer disease (Fig. 72-15). Most patients with this condition (there is a heavy predominance in men) have diarrhea and weight loss; pain, vomiting, and bleeding occur in one-third to one-half of cases. The first evidence of the presence of such a fistula is sometimes obtained during a barium enema examination in which contrast is observed to extend directly from the transverse colon into the stomach. These postsurgical fistulas are associated with a high mortality rate, especially if recognized late.

Fig. 72-10. Gastrocolic fistula as a complication of benign gastric ulcer disease. **(A)** An upper gastrointestinal series shows contrast material entering the transverse colon through the gastrocolic fistula. **(B)** A barium enema examination demonstrates reflux of contrast material into the stomach through the gastrocolic fistula. (Smith DL, Comer TP: Gastrocolic fistula, a rare complication of benign gastric ulcer. Dis Colon Rectum 17:769–770, 1974)

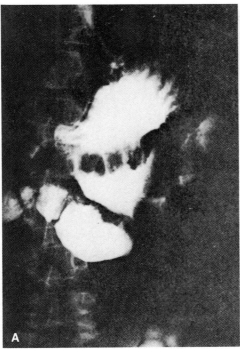

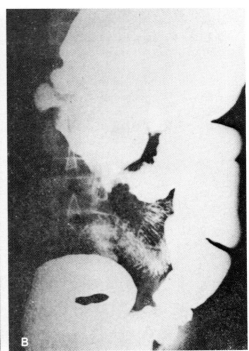

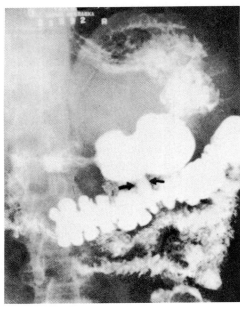

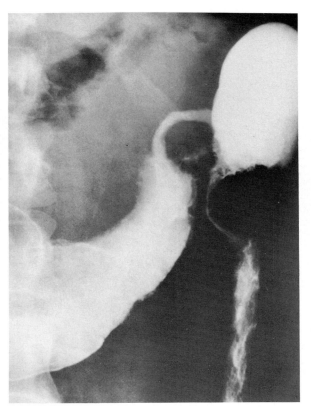

72-11   **72-12**

Fig. 72-11. Gastrocolic fistula secondary to benign ulcer disease. An upper gastrointestinal series demonstrates the fistula between the greater curvature of the stomach and the superior border of the transverse colon. (Swartz MJ, Paustian FF, Chleborad WJ: Recurrent gastric ulcer with spontaneous gastrojejunal and gastrocolic fistulas. Gastroenterology 44:527–531, 1963)

Fig. 72-12. Tuberculosis. A colocolic fistula with surrounding abscess formation is evident in the region of the splenic flexure.

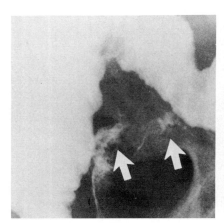

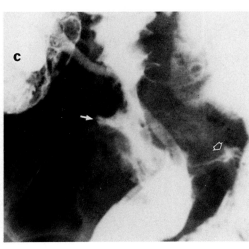

72-13   **72-14**

Fig. 72-13. Shigellosis. There is a fistulous tract between the rectum and sigmoid colon **(arrows)**.

Fig. 72-14. Cytomegalovirus. Coned view of the terminal ileum in a man with AIDS shows narrowed, spiculated, and ulcerated bowel with perforation **(closed** arrow) and fistulous tract **(open arrow)**. **C,** cecum. (Teixidor HS, Honig CL, Norsoph E et al: Cytomegalovirus infection of the alimentary canal: Radiologic findings with pathologic correlations. Radiology 163:317–323, 1987)

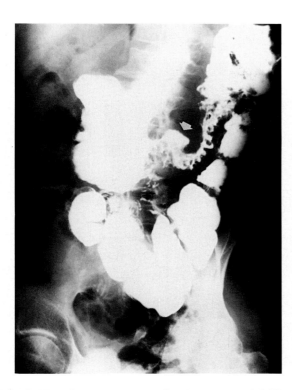

Fig. 72-15. Gastrojejunocolic fistula with partial filling of the colon seen on an upper gastrointestinal series. A large anastomotic ulcer **(arrow)** is visible near the site of a previous gastroenterostomy. (Thoeny RH, Hodgson JR, Scudamore HH: The roentgenologic diagnosis of gastrocolic and gastrojejunocolic fistulas. AJR 83:876–881, 1960. Copyright 1960. Reproduced with permission)

CAUSES OF INTERNAL FISTULAS

Diverticulitis
Ulcerative colitis
Crohn's disease
Malignant neoplasm
Radiation therapy
Pancreatitis
Prosthetic aortic graft
Gallbladder–bowel fistulas
    Acute cholecystitis
    Peptic ulcer disease
    Trauma
    Carcinoma
Duodenum–kidney fistulas
    Pyelonephritis (especially tuberculous)
    Duodenal ulcer
Entero-ovarian fistulas
Extravasation of contrast from bowel
       mimicking fistulas
    Diverticulitis
    Perforated viscus
    Trauma
    Surgery
    Abscess

Internal fistula formation is a frequent complication of diverticulitis. Colovesical fistulas (more common in men than women) account for more than 50% of all fistulas in this disease (Fig. 72-16).

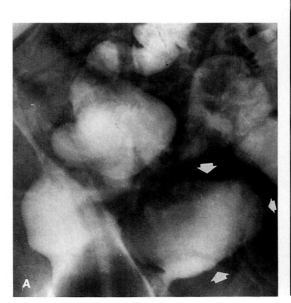
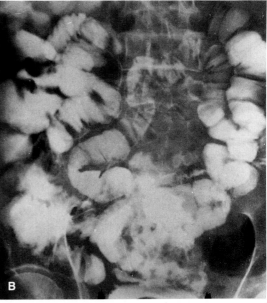

Fig. 72-16. Colovesicoenteric fistula. **(A)** A barium enema examination demonstrates barium entering the bladder **(arrows)** and small intestine by way of the sigmoid colon. **(B)** A radiograph from a cystogram shows filling of the small intestine from the bladder **(arrows)**. The presence of a colovesicoenteric fistula due to acute diverticulitis was confirmed at surgery. (Smith HJ, Berk RN, Janes JO et al: Unusual fistulae due to colonic diverticulitis. Gastrointest Radiol 2:387–392, 1978)

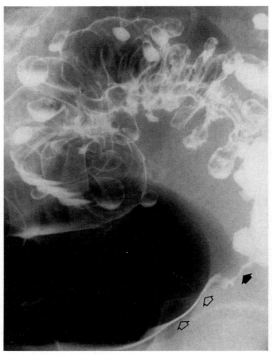

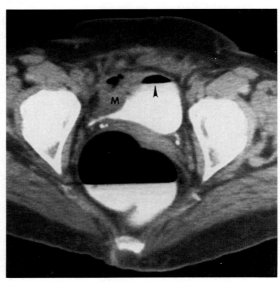

72-17   **72-18**

Fig. 72-17. Colovesical fistula (diverticulitis). A barium enema examination demonstrates barium in the fistulous tract **(solid arrow)** between the sigmoid colon and the bladder. Barium can also be seen lining the base of the gas-filled bladder **(open arrows)**.

Fig. 72-18. CT of enterovesical fistula due to appendiceal abscess. A mass **(M)** with multiple air bubbles compresses the bladder anteriorly and on the right. There is a pocket of air in the bladder **(arrowhead)**. Contrast material in the bladder is from an excretory urogram performed a day earlier. In this patient, the admitting diagnosis of "diverticulitis" was revised based on the CT findings of a right-sided abscess. (Goldman SM, Fishman EK, Gatewood OMB et al: CT in the diagnosis of enterovesical fistulae. AJR 144:1229–1233, 1985. Copyright 1985. Reproduced with permission)

They can cause recurrent urinary tract infections, chronic cystitis, pneumaturia, or fecaluria. Plain radiographs of the abdomen occasionally demonstrate gas in the bladder; excretory urography, cystography, or barium enema examinations sometime show the presence of a fistula (Fig. 72-17). Small amounts of air can be identified and correctly localized to the bladder by computed tomography (Fig. 72-18). The actual site of bladder fistulization occasionally can be identified (Fig. 72-19) or inferred by showing an area of focal thickening of the bladder wall or the wall of an adjacent loop of bowel. An associated soft-tissue mass may provide a clue to the etiology of the fistula. Cecal, appendiceal, and distal ileal fistulas affect the bladder from the right side anteriorly or laterally, whereas rectosigmoid and genitourinary (*e.g.*, prostate or uterus) inflammatory or neoplastic processes involve the bladder from the left side or posteriorly.

A radiographically undetectable colovesical fistula may be demonstrated by the Bourne test, in which radiographs are made of centrifuged urine samples obtained immediately after a nondiagnostic barium enema. The presence of radiopaque barium in the sediment gives conclusive evidence of an occult fistulous communication between the bowel and the bladder.

In women, rectovaginal fistulas can permit passage of feces or gas through the vagina (Fig. 72-20). Vaginography is far superior to a barium enema or a small bowel study for demonstrating enterovaginal fistulas (Fig. 72-21). Contrast material in the gastrointestinal tract can usually continue to traverse the bowel as a path of least resistance, whereas vaginal contrast material (after sealing the introitus) is in a confined area and thus more likely to enter a fistulous tract. In addition, although contrast material may be present in the vagina, it may be difficult to

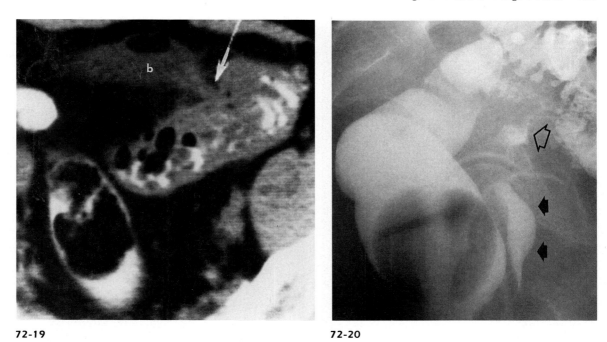

72-19   72-20

Fig. 72-19. CT of enterovesical fistula. The **arrow** points to the actual fistulous tract that clearly arises from the sigmoid colon. There is a single air bubble in the bladder **(b)** and wisps of contrast material within the fistula. (Goldman SM, Fishman EK, Gatewood OMB et al: CT in the diagnosis of enterovesical fistulae. AJR 144:1229–1233, 1985. Copyright 1985. Reproduced with permission)

Fig. 72-20. Rectovaginal fistula in diverticulitis. The **open arrow** points to the fistulous tract; the **closed arrows** point to contrast in the vagina.

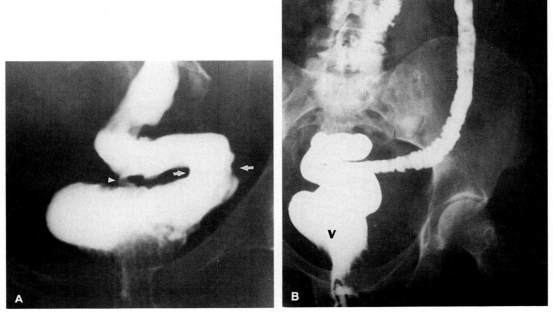

Fig. 72-21. Colovaginal fistula. **(A)** Vaginogram demonstrates a large fistula **(solid arrows)** and a second, narrower one **(arrowhead)**, both to the distal colon. **(B)** Because of the size and number of the communications, there was voluminous flow from the vagina **(v)** to the left colon. (Cooper RA: Vaginography: A presentation of new cases and subject review. Radiology 143:421–425, 1982)

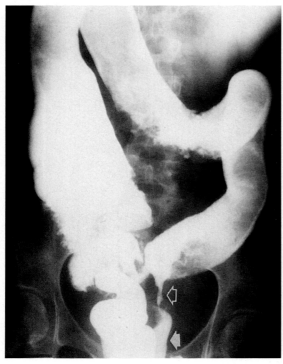
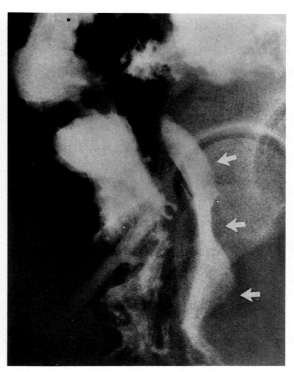

72-22   72-23

Fig. 72-22. Colovesical fistula in ulcerative colitis. The **open arrow** points to the fistula; the **closed arrow** points to contrast in the bladder.

Fig. 72-23. Rectovaginal fistula in a patient with Crohn's disease. The **arrows** point to contrast in the vagina.

recognize because of overlapping loops of rectosigmoid, whereas the detection of bowel contrast material during vaginography is relatively simple. Vaginography can also permit visualization of multiple fistulas when barium studies demonstrate only a single abnormal connection between the vagina and intestinal tract. After surgical treatment of diverticulitis, col<u>ureteral</u>, colocutaneous, or multiple internal fistulas can occur.

Rectovaginal fistulas occur in about 2% to 3% of women with ulcerative colitis. These fistulas frequently do not heal after local surgical repair; colectomy with ileostomy or a temporary diverting procedure is often required. Colovesical fistulas can also be seen in ulcerative colitis (Fig. 72-22). Although less common than enteric-enteric fistulas, internal fistulas extending from the bowel to the bladder or vagina can occur in patients with Crohn's disease (Fig. 72-23). Extension of a lower abdominal malignancy can also produce a colovesical or rectovaginal fistula (Fig. 72-24). Radiation therapy to the pelvic organs can cause fibrous inflammatory adhesions between bowel and bladder that permit the development of enteric-vesical fistulas.

Various types of internal fistula can result from severe pancreatitis or be complications of surgery for pancreatic cancer. About 2.5% of pseudocysts

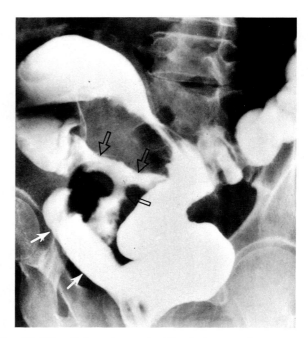

Fig. 72-24. Colovesicovaginal fistula from perforated carcinoma of the sigmoid. Note barium filling the bladder **(white arrows).** The primary tumor and fistulous tract are indicated by **black-outlined arrows**. (Skucas J, Miller RE: Colon cancer. In Taveras JM, Ferrucci JT (eds): Radiology: Diagnosis–Imaging–Intervention. Philadelphia, JB Lippincott, 1987)

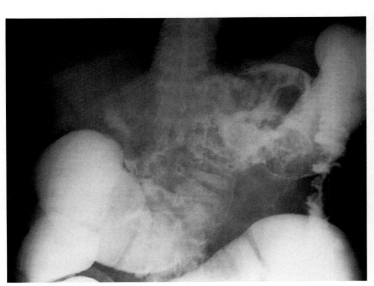

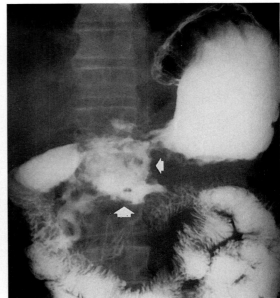

72-25   **72-26**

Fig. 72-25. Spontaneous perforation of a pancreatic pseudocyst into the colon and duodenum. (Shatney CH, Sosin H: Spontaneous perforation of a pancreatic pseudocyst into the colon and duodenum. Am J Surg 126:433–438, 1973)

Fig. 72-26. Spontaneous transenteric rupture of a pancreatic pseudocyst. Note the collection of extraluminal barium **(arrows)** in the pseudocyst cavity. Following the perforation, the patient's clinical condition improved. (Bradley EL, Clements JL: Transenteric rupture of pancreatic pseudocysts: Management of pseudocystenteric fistulas. Am J Surg 42:827–837, 1976)

rupture spontaneously into the stomach, duodenum, or colon (Fig. 72-25). Unlike free rupture into the peritoneal cavity, which is generally a catastrophic event, perforation into the gastrointestinal tract can present a variable clinical picture ranging from potentially lethal hemorrhage to substantial improvement in the patient's condition (Fig. 72-26).

Fistulas between the aorta and adjacent bowel (usually the duodenum) develop in up to 2% of patients who have undergone aortic aneurysm resection. In patients with upper or lower intestinal bleeding (often massive) occurring 3 weeks or more after aortic surgery, the possibility of a paraprosthetic-enteric fistula must be excluded. Fistula formation between the colon and venous structures can be a complication of diverticulitis (Fig. 72-27).

Fistulas between the gallbladder and bowel can be secondary to acute cholecystitis (90%) or severe peptic ulcer disease (6%). The remaining cases are the result of trauma or tumor. An acutely inflamed gallbladder can create a cholecystoenteric fistula by perforating into the lumen of an adjacent visceral organ, most commonly the duodenum (Fig. 72-28). Fistulas can extend into the hepatic flexure, stomach, or jejunum. In patients with severe peptic disease, a penetrating duodenal or gastric ulcer can perforate into the gallbladder or bile duct. Regardless of the etiology, plain abdominal radiographs

generally demonstrate gas within the biliary tree. On upper gastrointestinal series, barium usually fills the cholecystoenteric fistula.

Fistulas between the duodenum and right kidney are most often secondary to pyelonephritis, often tuberculous in origin. The pathologic mechanism is usually rupture of a perirenal abscess into the duodenum, which is best demonstrated on retrograde pyelography. On rare occasions, a duodenal ulcer penetrates into the tissues surrounding the kidney and produces a renoduodenal fistula.

Rare entero-ovarian fistulas may be due to inflammatory bowel disease, malignant neoplasm, prior radiation therapy, granulomatous disease, amebiasis, tubo-ovarian abscess (Fig. 72-29), or diverticulitis. Rupture of an ovarian dermoid cyst with fistulous formation into the bowel can be diagnosed clinically if hair, teeth, or sebaceous material are passed through the colon or radiographically if there is extravasation of barium around calcifications or teeth in the cyst (Fig. 72-30). A communication between the sigmoid colon and a tubo-ovarian abscess may produce a large rounded lucency in the lower abdomen on plain abdominal radiographs. The large air-filled cavity may be indistinguishable from a giant colonic or Meckel's diverticulum or a communicating bowel duplication or mesenteric cyst.

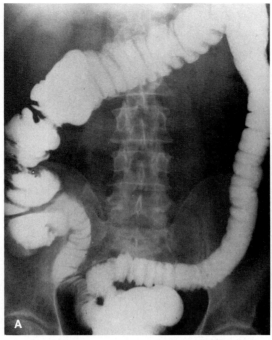

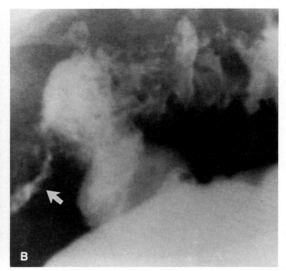

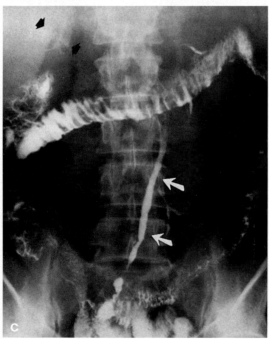

Fig. 72-27. Colovenous fistula. **(A)** A barium enema examination shows only minimal changes of spastic colon disease. **(B)** A spot film made during the barium enema examination shows narrowing of the sigmoid colon and a fistulous tract **(arrow)**. A few diverticula are present. **(C)** A post-evacuation radiograph shows barium in the inferior mesenteric vein **(white arrows)**. Barium and gas are visible in a liver abscess **(black arrows)**. The barium remained in the vein for 3 days after the examination and was gradually replaced by gas. At surgery, a small abscess was found that was due to peforation of the sigmoid colon. The patient did well for 8 days following the operation but then suddenly developed irreversible shock and died. Autopsy confirmed the presence of barium in the inferior mesenteric vein and showed thrombosis of the portal and splenic veins and multiple liver abscesses. (Smith HJ, Berk RN, Janes JO et al: Unusual fistulae due to colonic diverticulitis. Gastrointest Radiol 2:387–392, 1978)

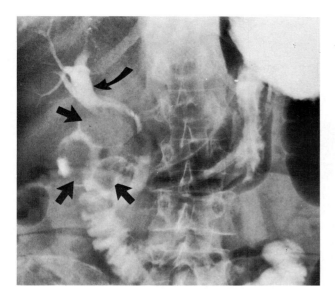

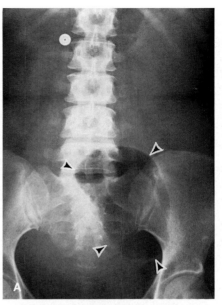

Fig. 72-28. Gallbladder–enteric fistula. There is a communication between the first portion of the duodenum and the gallbladder. At least three gallstones **(straight arrows)** are demonstrated outlined by contrast material. Contrast flows from the gallbladder lumen into the bile duct **(curved arrow)**. (Simeone JF: The gallbladder: Pathology. In Taveras JM, Ferrucci JT (eds): Radiology: Diagnosis–Imaging–Intervention. Philadelphia, JB Lippincott, 1987)

An appearance resembling fistulization can be produced by extravasation of contrast from the bowel into the retroperitoneal or peritoneal space. This can be caused by such entities as diverticulitis (Fig. 72-31), a perforated viscus (Fig. 72-32), trauma (Fig. 72-33), surgery (Fig. 72-34), or erosion by an abscess cavity (Fig. 72-35).

CAUSES OF EXTERNAL GASTROINTESTINAL FISTULAS

Postoperative fistulas
  Complication of surgery
  Intentional creation (gastrostomy, ileostomy, colostomy)
Pancreatic fistulas
  Trauma
  External drainage of pseudocyst
  Complication of surgery
Fistulas due to underlying gastrointestinal disease
  Crohn's disease
  Anorectal causes
    Malignancy
    Radiation therapy
    Tuberculosis
    Lymphogranuloma venereum
Diverticulitis
  Colocutaneous
  Colocoxal

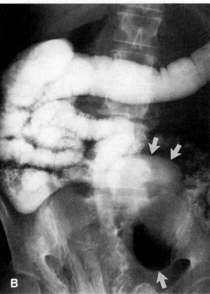

Fig. 72-29. Tubo-ovarian abscess. **(A)** Plain abdominal radiograph demonstrates a gas-filled cavity in the left lower quadrant **(arrows)** simulating a giant colonic diverticulum. **(B)** Barium enema examination shows the cavity partially filled with barium **(arrows)**; note the absence of diverticula in the colon. At surgery, the sigmoid colon was indurated, and there was a 2-cm diameter hole in its wall which communicated with a left tubo-ovarian abscess. (Telepak RJ, Huggins TJ, Bova JG: Tubo-ovarian abscess simulating giant colonic diverticulum. Gastrointest Radiol 9:369–371, 1984)

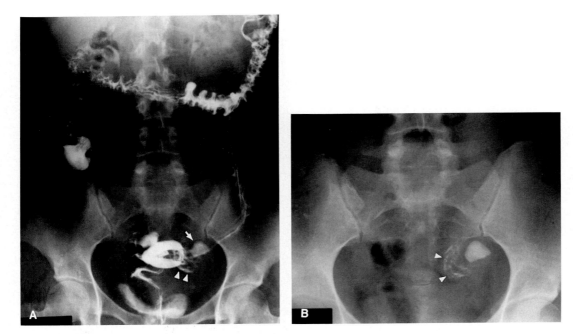

Fig. 72-30. Entero-ovarian fistula as a complication of ovarian dermoid cyst. **(A)** Postevacuation film from a barium enema examination shows a collection of contrast material **(arrowheads)** surrounding calcification within the dermoid cyst **(arrow)**. **(B)** Coned view of the pelvis taken a day after the barium enema study and following colonic lavage demonstrates persistent contrast collection **(arrowheads)** within the dermoid cyst. (Shiels WE, Dueno F, Hernandez E: Ovarian dermoid cyst complicated by an entero-ovarian fistula. Radiology 160:443–444, 1986)

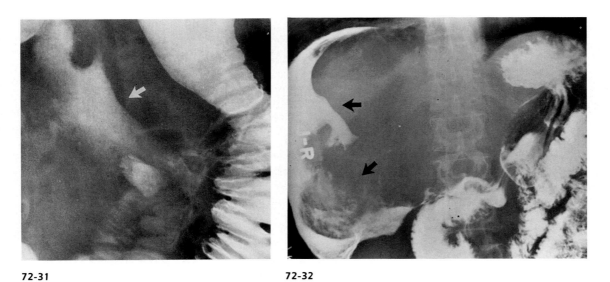

72-31   72-32

Fig. 72-31. Diverticulitis with extravasation of contrast **(arrow)** into the retroperitoneal space.

Fig. 72-32. Perforated duodenal ulcer. Extravasated contrast is seen surrounding the liver **(arrows)**.

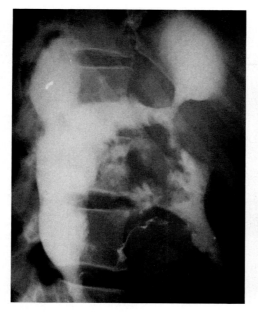 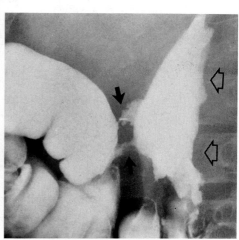

72-33 72-34

Fig. 72-33. Diffuse internal fistula formation following a gunshot wound to the abdomen.

Fig. 72-34. Fistulous communication **(solid arrows)** between the colon and a retroperitoneal abscess **(open arrows)** following nephrectomy.

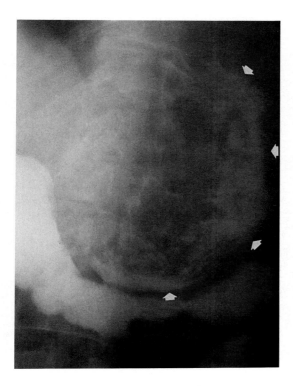

Fig. 72-35. Extravasation of contrast from the colon into the huge subphrenic abscess **(arrows)**.

The major complication of external gastrointestinal fistulas is the drainage of large amounts of electrolyte-rich fluid through them. External fistulas arising in the proximal portion of the gastrointestinal tract generally produce a large volume of fluid loss; those developing from the distal small bowel and colon are usually low-output fistulas. In addition to dehydration and electrolyte imbalance, external fistulas that bypass a large percentage of the functioning intestine often cause severe weight loss and protein-calorie malnutrition. Because intraperitoneal infections accompany many external fistulas, there are frequently abscesses along the fistulous tracts that wall off and persist if the fistulas are not adequately drained. Injection of water-soluble contrast into an external fistula usually demonstrates the source of the fistula and any communicating abscess cavities (Fig. 72-36).

The morbidity rate of external gastrointestinal fistulas is high. Even though about three-quarters of these fistulas close spontaneously if treated properly, hospitalization is frequently prolonged.

Most external gastrointestinal fistulas are complications of abdominal surgery in which an anastomosis fails to heal properly. Various factors that contribute to this lack of adequate healing include foreign bodies (*e.g.,* rubber drains) close to the su-

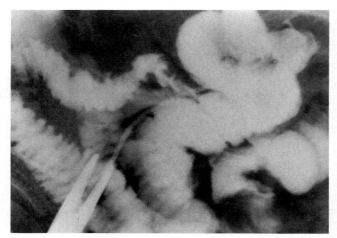

Fig. 72-36. External fistula complicating abdominal surgery. Contrast introduced through the fistulous tract fills loops of small bowel.

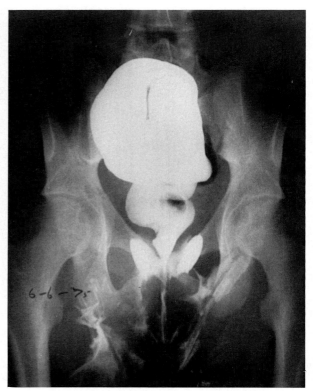

Fig. 72-37. Crohn's disease causing perirectal abscess and fistulization to the prostate.

ture line, excessive tension on the anastomosis, infection, ischemia, and radiation enteritis. Anastomosis through inadequately resected malignant tissue, surgical injury to the bowel, and intra-abdominal abscesses can also result in postoperative external gastrointestinal fistulas.

Radiographically guided percutaneous catheter drainage is now the procedure of choice for treating many abdominal abscesses and fluid collections. A vitally important technical aspect of successful catheter drainage is establishment of a safe access route enabling direct catheter insertion while simultaneously avoiding transgression of intervening vessels and bowel. Inadvertent insertion of a percutaneously placed catheter into the gut lumen may lead to peritonitis, cecal contamination of a sterile collection, or late development of an entero- or colocutaneous fistula. However, recent reports of unintentional catheter entry into the lumen of the gastrointestinal tract, as well as a growing experience with purposeful percutaneous gastrostomy, has indicated that the termination of a catheter into the bowel lumen can be managed safely and need not be considered a disastrous complication.

External gastrointestinal fistulas arising from the pancreas can occur after trauma, external drainage of a pseudocyst, or surgical procedures on the pancreas. Traumatic fistulas usually result from undetected or inadequately treated injury to the pancreatic duct. Pancreatic pseudocysts fail to obliterate after external surgical drainage in about one-third of cases, often leading to the development of pancreatic fistulas.

External gastrointestinal fistulas are commonly encountered in patients with Crohn's disease. They usually extend to the perianal area and produce chronic indurated rectal fistulas with associated fissures and perirectal abscesses (Fig. 72-37). Involvement of the skin around the umbilicus also occurs.

Anorectal fistulas are granulation-tissue-lined

tracts between the anal canal or rectum and one or more openings in the perianal skin (Fig. 72-38). These fistulas can arise from infections in the bowel wall that extend to form an abscess, which then

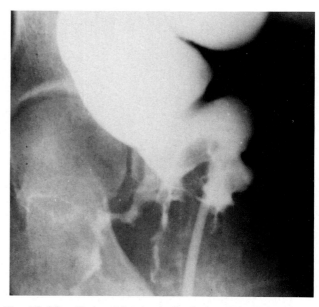

Fig. 72-38. Perianal fistulas in Crohn's colitis. These fistulas are often better delineated by obtaining coned views of the anal canal immediately after the enema tip is withdrawn. (Butch RJ: Radiology of the rectum. In Taveras JM, Ferrucci JT (eds): Radiology: Diagnosis–Imaging–Intervention. Philadelphia, JB Lippincott, 1987)

ruptures and forms a fistulous tract to the skin. Anorectal fistulas can be associated with Crohn's disease, malignancy, radiation therapy, trauma, tuberculosis, or lymphogranuloma venereum.

Colocutaneous fistulas occur in approximately 6% of patients who have received surgical treatment for diverticulitis. However, spontaneous colocutaneous fistulas are rare. A colocoxal fistula is an unusual complication of colonic diverticulitis that causes a communication between the colon (usually the sigmoid) and the hip, buttock, or thigh. This condition is characterized by emphysematous cellulitis that presents as gas between muscles and interstitial planes, in contrast to gangrene, which usually produces gas in muscle bundles. The major mechanism involved in this phenomenon is the pressure gradient between the colonic lumen and the surrounding interstitium, which allows intraluminal gas to flow into the relatively low-pressure soft tissues.

BIBLIOGRAPHY

Amendola MA, Agha FP, Dent TL et al: Detection of occult colovesical fistula by the Bourne test. AJR 142:715–717, 1984

Bradley EL, Clements JL: Transenteric rupture of pancreatic pseudocyst: Management of pseudocystenteric fistulas. Am J Surg 42:827–837, 1976

Cooper RA: Vaginography: A presentation of new cases and subject review. Radiology 143:421–425, 1982

Goldman SM, Fishman ED, Gatewood OMB et al: CT in the diagnosis of enterovesical fistula. AJR 144:1229–1233, 1985

Greenall MJ, Levine AW, Nolan DJ: Complications of diverticular disease: A review of the barium enema findings. Gastrointest Radiol 8:353–358, 1983

Korelitz BI: Colonic–duodenal fistula in Crohn's disease. Dig Dis 22:1040–1048, 1977

Laufer I, Joffe N, Stolberg H: Unusual causes of gastrocolic fistula. Gastrointest Radiol 2:21–25, 1977

Laufer I, Thornley GD, Stolberg H: Gastrocolic fistula as a complication of benign gastric ulcer. Radiology 119:7–11, 1976

Martinez LO, Manheimer LH, Casal GL et al: Malignant fistulae of the gastrointestinal tract. AJR 131:215–218, 1978

Michowitz M, Farago C, Lazarovici I et al: Choledochoduodenal fistula: A rare complication of duodenal ulcer. Am J Gastroenterol 79:416–420, 1984

Mueller PR, Ferrucci JT Jr, Butch RJ et al: Inadvertent percutaneous catheter gastroenterostomy during abscess drainage: Significance and management. AJR 145:387–391, 1985

Rosen RJ, Teplick SK, Shapiro JH: Spontaneous communication between a pancreatic pseudocyst and the colon: Unusual clinical and radiographic presentation. Gastrointest Radiol 5:353–355, 1980

Shatney CH, Sosin H: Spontaneous perforation of a pancreatic pseudocyst into the colon and duodenum. Am J Surg 126:433–438, 1973

Shiels WE, Dueno F, Hernandez E: Ovarian dermoid cyst complicated by an entero-ovarian fistula. Radiology 160:443–444, 1986

Smith DL, Comer TP: Gastrocolic fistula, a rare complication of benign gastric ulcer. Dis Colon Rectum 17:769–770, 1974

Smith DL, Dockerty MD, Black BM: Gastrocolic fistulas of malignant origin. Surg Gynecol Obstet 134:829–832, 1972

Smith HJ, Berk RN, Janes JO et al: Unusual fistulae due to colonic diverticulitis. Gastrointest Radiol 2:387–392, 1978

Smith TR, Goldin RR: Radiographic and clinical sequelae of the duodenocolic anatomic relationship: Two cases of Crohn's disease with fistulization to the duodenum. Dis Colon Rectum 20:257–262, 1977

Swartz MJ, Paustian FF, Chleborad WJ: Recurrent gastric ulcer with spontaneous gastrojejunal and gastrocolic fistulas. Gastroenterology 44:527–531, 1963

Teixidor HS, Honig CL, Norsoph E et al: Cytomegalovirus infection of the alimentary canal: Radiologic findings with pathologic correlation. Radiology 163:317–323, 1987

Telepak RJ, Huggins TJ, Bova JG: Tubo-ovarian abscess simulating giant colonic diverticulum. Gastrointest Radiol 9:369–371, 1984

Thoeny RH, Hodgson JR, Scudamore HH: The roentgenologic diagnosis of gastrocolic and gastrojejunocolic fistulas. AJR 83:876–881, 1960

Vieta JO, Blanco R, Valentini GR: Malignant duodenocolic fistula: Report of two cases, each with one or more synchronous gastrointestinal cancers. Dis Colon Rectum 19:542–552, 1976

Wills J, Oglesby JT: Percutaneous gastrostomy: Further experience. Radiology 154:71–74, 1985

Yasui K, Tsukaguchi I, Ohara S et al: Benign duodenocolic fistula due to duodenal diverticulum: Report of two cases. Radiology 130:67–70, 1979

73

ABDOMINAL CALCIFICATIONS

Calcifications can be detected on almost every plain radiograph of the abdomen in adults. Although the overwhelming majority are of little clinical significance, some calcifications indicate areas of pathology or even a precise histologic diagnosis. It is essential to determine in which of the abdominal organs the calcification is located. Some calcified lesions can be diagnosed on the basis of the appearance of the calcification, such as the number of deposits and their location, size, shape, distribution, density, and pattern. Oblique or lateral projections may be of value in differentiating chest or abdominal wall calcifications from calcifications within the intraperitoneal or retroperitoneal space. Sequential films or films taken with the patient in the upright position are helpful in distinguishing movable from fixed calcifications. Radiographic contrast studies (barium examinations, cholecystography, excretory urography) are sometimes required to determine whether a given calcification is related to a specific visceral organ. Ultrasound and computed tomography (CT) can precisely define the margins of the liver, spleen, and kidneys and can distinguish among aneurysms, tortuous vessels, and nonvascular lesions when the findings on plain radiographs are equivocal.

CALCIFICATION IN THE LIVER

Inflammatory disorders
  Tuberculosis
  Histoplasmosis
  Hydatid disease
    Echinococcus granulosus
    Echinococcus multilocularis
  Healed liver abscess
    Amebic
    Pyogenic
  Other granulomatous diseases
    Brucellosis
    Coccidioidomycosis
  Gumma (hepar lobatum)
  Other parasitic infestations
    Armillifer armillatus
    Ascaris lumbricoides
    Clonorchis sinensis
    Cysticercosis
    Filariasis
    Guinea worm
    Paragonimus westermani
    Toxoplasmosis
Neoplasms
  Carvenous hemangioma
  Hepatocellular carcinoma
  Hepatoblastoma
  Cholangiocarcinoma

Hemangioendothelioma
Metastases
    Mucinous carcinoma (breast, colon, ovary, stomach)
    Psammomatous carcinoma (ovary)
    Miscellaneous tumors (adrenal, bronchogenic, melanoma, mesothelioma, neuroblastoma, osteogenic sarcoma, pancreatic, renal, testicular, thyroid)
    Lymphoma
Nonparasitic cysts
Post-traumatic hematoma
Intrahepatic calculi
Gaucher's disease
Shock liver
Vascular calcifications
    Portal vein calcification
    Hepatic artery aneurysm
    Inferior vena cava calcification
    Atherosclerotic vessels/calcified thrombus
Capsular calcification
    Alcoholic cirrhosis
    Resolving pyogenic infection
    Pseudomyxoma peritonei
    Meconium peritonitis
    Lipoid granulomatosis
    Barium granulomatosis
Increased radiodensity without demonstrable calcification
    Alcoholic cirrhosis (contracted liver)
    Hemochromatosis
    Siderosis
    Residual Thorotrast

Intrahepatic calcifications are uncommon. When present, however, they always indicate an abnormality, though they do not necessarily define the nature or activity of the pathologic process.

The most common intrahepatic calcifications are healed foci of granulomatous disease secondary to tuberculosis (Fig. 73-1) and, more frequently, histoplasmosis (Fig. 73-2). These calcifications tend to be small (1–3 cm), multiple, dense, and discrete

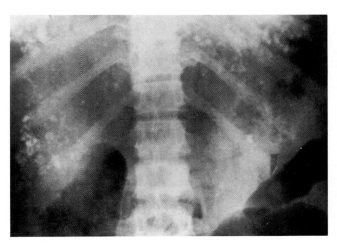

Fig. 73-1. Diffuse small calcifications in the liver and spleen representing healed foci of tuberculosis. (Darlak JJ, Moskowitz M, Kattan KR: Calcifications in the liver. Radiol Clin North Am 18:209–219, 1980)

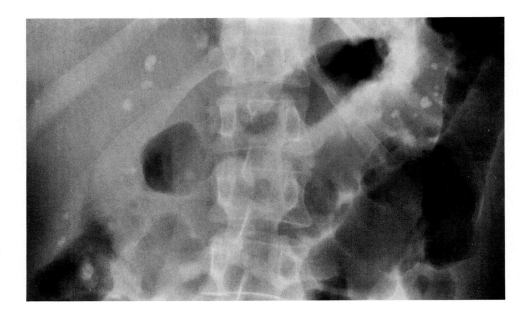

Fig. 73-2. Scattered hepatic and splenic calcifications representing healed foci of histoplasmosis.

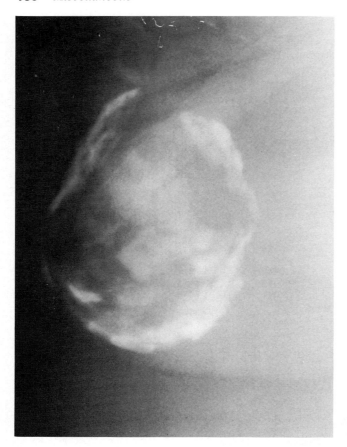

Fig. 73-3. Hydatid liver cyst (*Echinococcus granulosus*). There is complete oval calcification at the periphery of the mother cyst. Within the mother cyst are several smaller arc-like calcifications representing daughter cysts.

A rarer and more malignant form of hydatid disease is the alveolar type, due to *Echinococcus multilocularis*. Calcification occurs in about 70% of patients with this disease. The typical radiographic appearance is one of multiple small radiolucencies, measuring 2 mm to 4 mm in diameter, that are surrounded by rings of calcification, which, in turn, lie within large areas of amorphous calcifications of up to 10 cm to 12 cm in diameter (Fig. 73-4). Alveolar hydatid disease caused by *E. multilocularis* can be a fulminant, even fatal, disease, in contrast to the clinical course of *E. granulosus*, which is generally indolent.

Dense, mottled calcifications, usually solitary but occasionally multiple, can be seen in healed amebic or pyogenic liver abscesses (Fig. 73-5). In most cases, the patient is asymptomatic at the time of radiographic detection of hepatic calcification. Although usually considered a rare condition in the United States, *Entamoeba histolytica* can be found in the stools of up to 5% of the population in this country. The protozoan can spread from the colon to the liver and form an abscess. Mural calcification in a

and to be scattered throughout the liver. The combination of diffuse calcifications in the liver, spleen, and lungs is virtually diagnostic of histoplasmosis, especially in endemic areas. Calcification of the spleen secondary to tuberculosis is much less frequent. Tuberculosis and histoplasmosis sometimes present as moderately large, solidly calcified granulomas or nodular, popcornlike, or even laminated calcifications.

Hydatid cysts are the most frequent cause of hepatic calcification in endemic areas. Patients with the common *Echinococcus granulosus* typically have complete oval or circular calcification at the periphery of the mother cyst (Fig. 73-3). Within the mother cyst, there may be multiple daughter cysts with arclike calcifications. Hydatid cyst calcification generally develops 5 to 10 years after the liver has been infected and can be present in either active or inactive cysts. Extensive dense calcifications favor quiescence of the parasitic process; segmental calcification (nonhomogeneous, striped, trabeculated) suggests cystic activity and is often considered an indication for surgery.

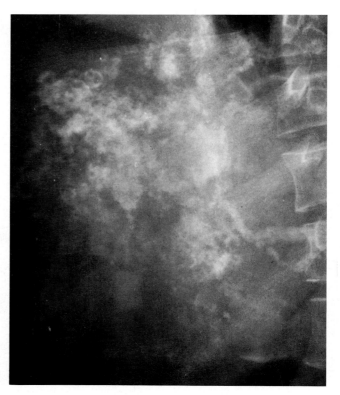

Fig. 73-4. Alveolar hydatid disease (*Echinococcus multilocularis*). Multiple small radiolucencies are surrounded by rings of calcification, which, in turn, lie within large areas of amorphous calcification. (Thompson WM, Chisholm DP, Tank R: Plain film roentgenographic findings in alveolar hydatid disease: *Echinococcus multilocularis*. AJR 116:345–358, 1972. Copyright 1972. Reproduced with permission)

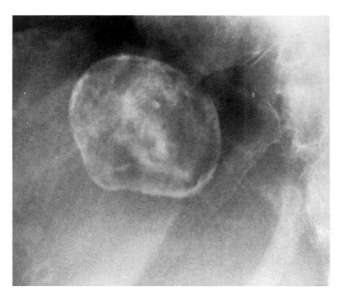

Fig. 73-5. Calcified pyogenic liver abscess.

chronic amebic abscess is often associated with secondary infection. It can also develop following cyst rupture and hemorrhage or a surgical procedure for drainage.

In brucellosis, a snowflake appearance of fluffy calcifications can be seen in the liver. Similar lesions can be found in the spleen. Hepatic calcification has also been reported in coccidioidomycosis. A very rare cause of focal parenchymal calcification is a gumma secondary to tertiary syphilis. The calcification in a gumma is dense, irregular, well defined, and often extensive.

Numerous parasitic infestations can result in hepatic calcification. Calcification of the nymphs of *Armillifer armillatus* (tongue worm) produces typical C-shaped or incomplete ring shadows (Fig. 73-6). Humans, who are the intermediate hosts of this parasite, are infected from the saliva or excreta of snakes, rats, and other wild animals. After being ingested, the larvae pass from the gut to various organs, where they can encyst and die at any stage. Necrosis of the parasite leads to the development of characteristic semilunar calcifications that can be found in the liver, lungs, pleura, peritoneum, and spleen. Guinea worm (Fig. 73-7), filariasis, toxoplasmosis, and cysticercosis can also cause calcifications in the liver. Severe infection with *Clonorchis sinensis* or *Ascaris lumbricoides* rarely produces calcifications. In these conditions, calcification is probably related to secondary infection following obstruction rather than being a manifestation of primary disease.

Calcification in liver tumors is rare in adults but somewhat more common in children. Benign cavernous hemangiomas characteristically demon-strate a sunburst pattern of spicules of calcification radiating from a central area toward the periphery of the lesion (Fig. 73-8). This is similar to the appearance of hemangiomas in such flat bones as the calvarium and sternum. These vascular tumors are usually asymptomatic and small (less than 3 cm in diameter); the vast majority are not calcified. Unlike hemangiomas of soft tissue elsewhere, calcified phleboliths are not commonly associated with hepatic hemangiomas.

Calcification in untreated hepatocellular carcinoma is unusual and is much more common in children than in adults. After treatment, it is not unusual for hepatocellular carcinoma to undergo calcification. Calcification has been reported in almost half the cases of fibrolamellar hepatocellular carcinoma, a recently recognized variant that occurs in adolescents and young adults. The calcification is central, stellate or nodular, and typically small in relation to the size of the mass (Fig. 73-9). Unlike typical hepatocellular carcinoma, patients with the fibrolamellar variant form have no predisposing risk factors (cirrhosis, hepatitis), normal levels of alpha fetoprotein, and a relatively better prognosis. In children under age 5, most calcified

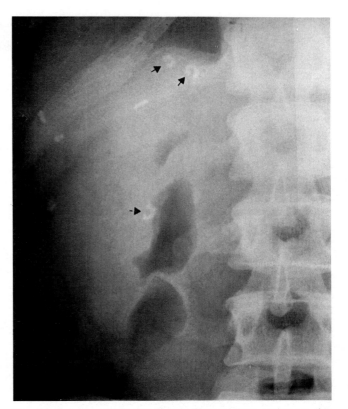

Fig. 73-6. *Armillifer armillatus.* The **arrows** point to the pathognomonic finding of C-shaped encysted larvae within the liver. (Baker SR, Elkin M: Plain Film Approach to Abdominal Calcifications. Philadelphia, WB Saunders, 1983)

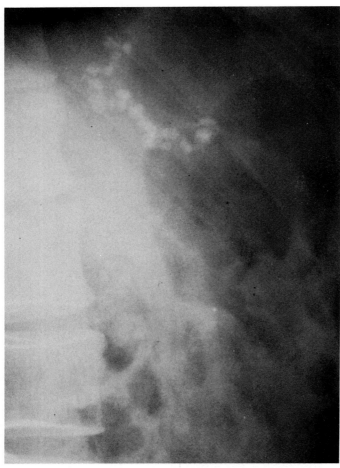

73-7

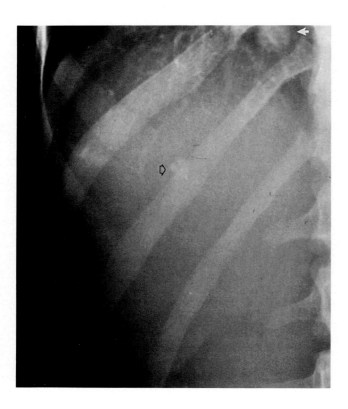

73-8

Fig. 73-7. Calcified guinea worm in the right lobe of the liver. (Darlak JJ, Moskowitz M, Kattan KR: Calcifications in the liver. Radiol Clin North Am 18:209–219, 1980)

Fig. 73-8. Cavernous hemangioma of the liver with popcornlike calcification. (Darlak JJ, Moskowitz M, Kattan KR: Calcifications in the liver. Radiol Clin North Am 18:209–219, 1980)

Fig. 73-9. Fibrolamellar hepatocellular carcinoma. Small calcification **(open arrow)** situated within a large liver mass. Note the metastasis in the right lower lobe **(closed arrow)**. (Friedman AC, Lichtenstein JE, Goodman Z et al: Fibrolamellar hepatocellular carcinoma. Radiology 157:583–587, 1985)

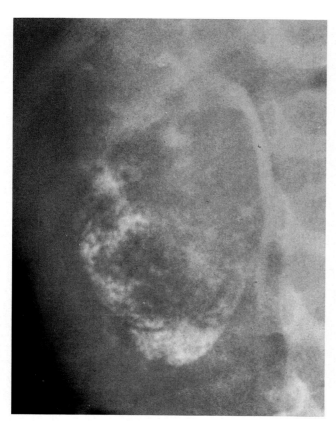

Fig. 73-10. Infantile hepatoblastoma. Extensive coarse calcification within a large mass involving the right lobe of the liver. The lesion was best seen on this excretory urogram. (Dachman AH, Pakter RL, Ros PR et al: Hepatoblastoma: Radiologic–pathologic correlation in 50 cases. (Radiology 164:15–19, 1987)

liver tumors are either hepatoblastomas or hemangioendotheliomas. A pattern of coarse or dense calcification is strongly suggestive of hepatoblastoma (Fig. 73-10) as compared with the fine granular calcifications seen in infantile hemangioendothelioma (Fig. 73-11).

Calcification in the liver has been described in association with many types of metastases, though this is a relatively infrequent finding. It is most commonly seen in metastatic colloid carcinoma of the colon or rectum, in which there may be diffuse, finely granular calcifications (2–4 mm in diameter) that have a poppy-seed appearance (Fig. 73-12). Metastases from other primary tumors usually show much larger, denser, and irregular calcifications (Fig. 73-13). Although it is impossible in most cases to determine whether hepatic calcifications are caused by a benign tumor or by a primary or metastatic malignancy, progressive increase in the size and number of calcifications and an enlarging liver make the diagnosis of a neoplasm very likely.

Rarely, calcification occurs in the wall of a congenital or acquired nonparasitic cyst of the liver, such as in polycystic disease. Calcified hematomas can be demonstrated after trauma.

Intrahepatic lithiasis is extremely rare without stones in the common duct or gallbladder. Calculi can be seen in Caroli's disease (congenital cystic dilation of the biliary radicles), though these are usually pigment stones, as opposed to cholesterol stones, and only rarely calcify.

Hepatic calcification has been described in a single patient with Gaucher's disease (Fig. 73-14), an enzymatic deficiency that results in an abnormal

Fig. 73-11. Infantile hemangioendothelioma. Fine, speckled pattern of calcification (arrows) in the left lobe of the liver. (Dachman AH, Lichtenstein JE, Friedman AC et al: Infantile hemangioendothelioma of the liver. AJR 140:1091–1096, 1983. Copyright 1983. Reproduced with permission)

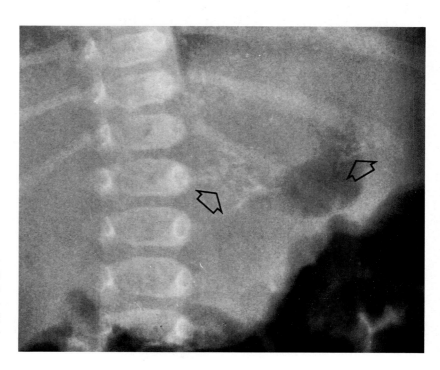

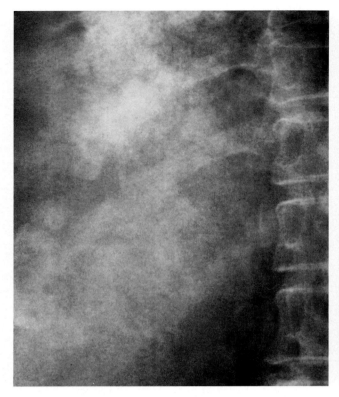

73-12

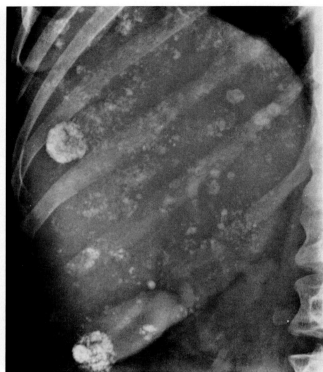

73-13

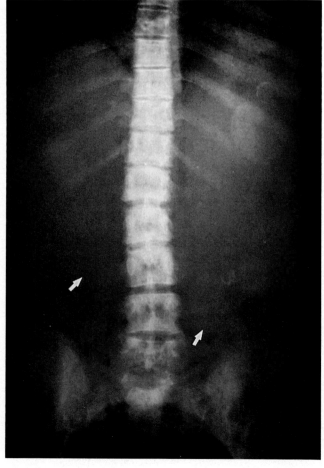

73-14

Fig. 73-12. Calcified liver metastases from colloid carcinoma of the colon producing a diffuse, finely granular pattern.

Fig. 73-13. Calcified liver metastases from thyroid carcinoma. Note that the metastases are substantially larger and more dense and discrete than in the previous figure.

Fig. 73-14. Gaucher's disease. Multiple well-circumscribed, faint nodular calcifications of varying size in a patient with hepatomegaly. The **arrows** demarcate the inferior border of the liver. (Stone R, Benson J, Tronic B et al: Hepatic calcifications in a patient with Gaucher's disease. Am J Gastroenterol 77:95–98, 1982)

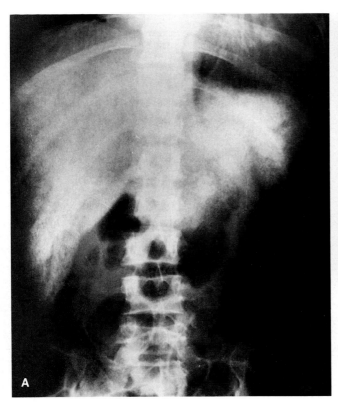

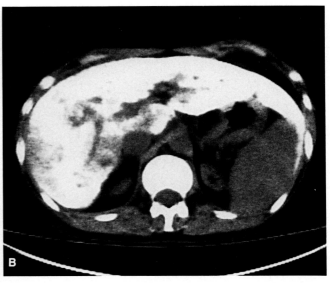

Fig. 73-15. Shock liver. **(A)** Diffuse fine calcifications throughout a markedly enlarged liver. **(B)** CT scan demonstrates hepatomegaly with increased liver density equal to that of calcium. (Shibuya A, Unuma T, Sugimoto T et al: Diffuse hepatic calcification as a sequela to shock liver. Gastroenterology 89:196–201, 1985)

accumulation of glucocerebrosides in the reticuloendothelial tissue of the bone marrow, liver, and spleen. A possible explanation for the hepatic calcification is that dense infiltration with Gaucher cells produces pressure necrosis and secondary calcification of adjacent hepatic tissue. A similar mechanism has been implicated as the basis of the anemia found in some patients with this disease who have prominent bone marrow infiltration.

In a case report, diffuse hepatic calcification developed in an area of parenchymal liver ischemia several months after an overt state of shock that lasted for 2 days (Fig. 73-15). Although the etiology of calcification in shock liver is unclear, it may be related to disturbances of intracellular calcium ion homeostasis as a result of ischemic liver injury or be related to an elevated calcium–phosphorus product in the uremic state.

Calcified clot in the portal vein is usually associated with cirrhosis and portal hypertension (Fig. 73-16). Thrombosis is occasionally the primary cause of increased portal venous pressure. When extensive, a calcified portal vein thrombus can be seen radiographically as a linear opaque density crossing the vertebral column (Fig. 73-17). The majority of hepatic artery aneurysms do not demonstrate calcification radiographically. When present, calcification has a circular pattern with a cracked-eggshell appearance indicating the saccular nature of the aneurysm. Hepatic aneurysms closely resem-

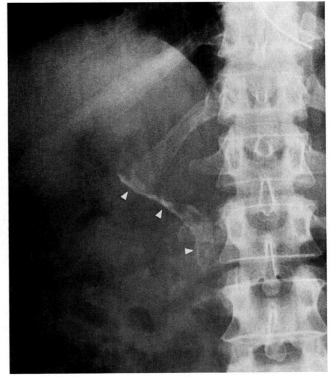

Fig. 73-16. Calcification in the portal vein. Tracklike calcification with irregular margins directed along the course of the portal vein. (Baker SR, Broker MH, Charnsangavej C et al: Calcification in the portal vein wall. Radiology 152:18, 1984)

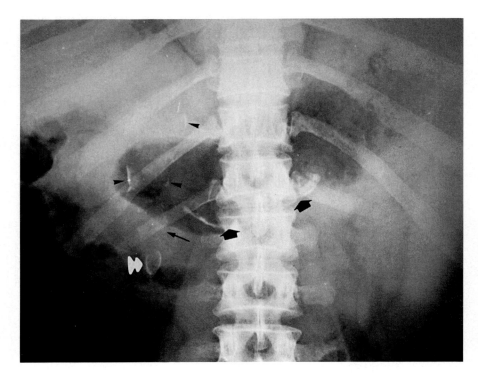

Fig. 73-17. Calcification of the portal vein. In addition to portal vein calcification **(arrowheads)**, there is also calcification in the walls of the splenic **(large black arrows)**, superior mesenteric **(small black arrow)**, and pancreaticoduodenal veins **(white arrows)**. Note the widening of the inferior mediastinum secondary to mediastinal varices. (Mata JM, Alegret X, Martinez A: Calcification in the portal and collateral veins wall: CT findings. Gastrointest Radiol 12:206–208, 1987)

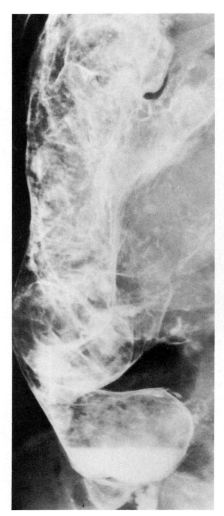

73-18

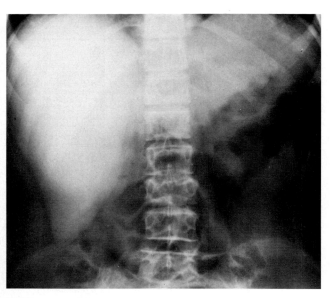

73-19

Fig. 73-18. Appearance simulating intrinsic hepatic calcification due to inadvertent intraperitoneal extravasation of barium, which produced an opaque shell around the liver.

Fig. 73-19. Hemochromatosis. An abdominal radiograph demonstrates a very dense liver shadow in the right upper quadrant caused by parenchymal deposition of iron. (Smith WL, Quattromani F: Radiodense liver in transfusion hemochromatosis. AJR 128:316–317, 1977. Copyright 1977. Reproduced with permission)

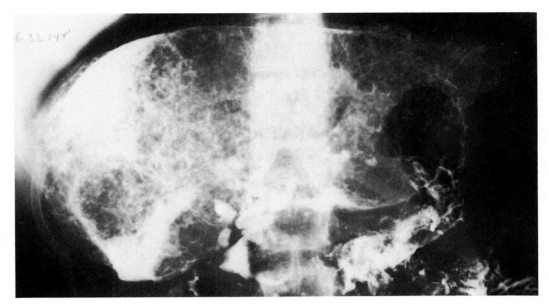

Fig. 73-20. Bubbly pattern of calcification in the liver caused by a previous injection of Thorotrast.

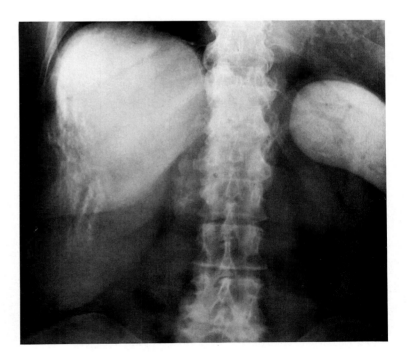

Fig. 73-21. Calcification of the liver and spleen caused by a prior injection of Thorotrast.

ble the much more common aneurysms of the splenic artery that are seen in the left upper quadrant. Calcified clots of the inferior vena cava have also been described.

Calcification of the capsule of the liver can develop in conditions such as alcoholic cirrhosis, pyogenic infection, meconium peritonitis, pseudomyxoma peritonei, and lipoid granulomatosis following intraperitoneal instillation of mineral oil. A somewhat similar pattern can be produced by the inad-

vertent introduction of barium into the peritoneal cavity through a colonic perforation (Fig. 73-18).

Several conditions can result in a generalized increase in radiodensity of the liver without demonstrable calcification. A contracted cirrhotic liver can appear to be more dense than usual, possibly because of an increase in fibrous tissue or a relative increase in density that is accentuated in relation to extraperitoneal fat. Hemochromatosis can produce a generalized increase in density of the liver (Fig.

73-19), as can a high dietary intake of iron (siderosis). A bubbly or trabeculated pattern of calcification (Fig. 73-20) can be caused by a prior injection of Thorotrast (thorium dioxide). This calcification often condenses into a dense fibrous or confluent zone that appears to involve the entire liver (Fig. 73-21). The retention of colloidal Thorotrast in the reticuloendothelial cells of the liver, spleen, and adjacent lymph nodes opacifies these organs. Although Thorotrast has not been used for many years, a few patients still demonstrate hepatic calcifications secondary to a remote injection of this contrast agent. The danger of retained thorium is that it is an alpha-emitting radionuclide that has been associated with the development of hepatobiliary carcinoma (especially the exceedingly rare angiosarcoma), leukemia, and aplastic anemia up to 30 years after the initial injection (Fig. 73-22).

CALCIFICATION IN THE SPLEEN

Disseminated calcifications
 Phleboliths
 Granulomatous disease
  Histoplasmosis
  Tuberculosis
  Brucellosis

Cysts
 Congenital
 Post-traumatic
 Echinococcal
 Dermoid
 Epidermoid
Capsular and parenchymal calcification
 Pyogenic or tuberculous abscess
 Infarction
 Hematoma
Vascular calcification
 Splenic artery calcification
 Splenic artery aneurysm
Generalized increased splenic density
 Sickle cell anemia
 Hemochromatosis
 Residual Thorotrast

Multiple small, round or ovoid calcified nodules are frequently distributed throughout the spleen. These can represent phleboliths in the splenic veins or the healed granulomas of a widely disseminated infection. In the past, most of these lesions were thought to represent calcified tuberculous nodules (see Fig. 73-1). Currently, it is believed that they more likely represent healed foci of histoplasmosis (see Fig. 73-2), especially when they are seen in patients from

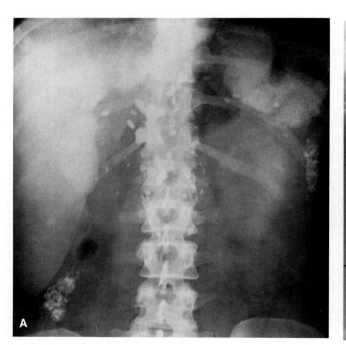
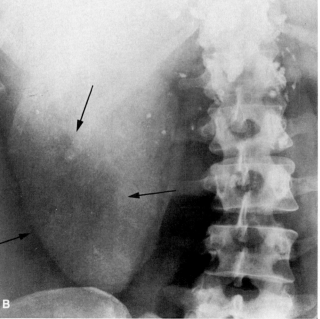

Fig. 73-22. Thorotrast-induced cholangiocarcinoma. **(A)** Initial oral cholecystogram shows striking homogeneous increased density of the liver and punctate densities in a normal-sized spleen. There are multiple dense lymph nodes. **(B)** A coned-down view obtained 2 years later shows a lucency in the right lobe of the liver **(arrow)** caused by cholangiocarcinoma. (Levy DW, Rindsberg S, Friedman AC et al: Thorotrast-induced hepatosplenic neoplasia: CT identification. AJR 146:997–1004, 1986. Copyright 1986. Reproduced with permission)

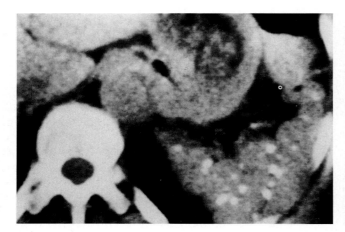

73-23

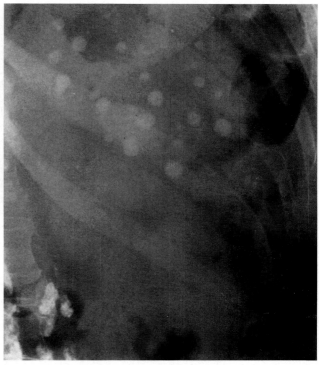

Fig. 73-23. Histoplasmosis. CT scan shows multiple small calcifications in the spleen.

Fig. 73-24. Splenic hemangioma. Multiple rounded concretions in the spleen represent calcified phleboliths, some of which have central lucencies and most of which are greater than 5-mm in diameter. (Baker SR, Elkin M: Plain Film Approach to Abdominal Calcifications. Philadelphia, WB Saunders, 1983)

73-24

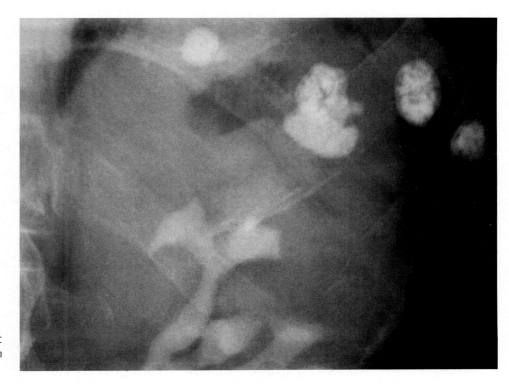

Fig. 73-25. Calcified splenic granulomas in a patient with chronic brucellosis.

endemic areas (Fig. 73-23). Similar calcifications are often distributed extensively throughout the lungs; occasionally, they are found in the liver. Multiple phleboliths may rarely be a manifestation of splenic hemangioma (Fig. 73-24).

Multiple calcified granulomas and chronic ab-

scesses of the spleen can be demonstrated in chronic brucellosis (Fig. 73-25). Unlike the lesions in histoplasmosis and tuberculosis, the lesions in chronic brucellosis tend to be still active and suppurating even in the presence of calcification. The calcified nodules in chronic brucellosis are larger (about 1–3 cm in diameter) and consist of a flocculent calcified center in a radiolucent area that is surrounded by a laminated calcified rim.

Splenic cysts calcify infrequently (Fig. 73-26). In the United States, most are of congenital origin. Occasionally, a post-traumatic hematoma becomes cystic and develops a calcified wall. In endemic areas, splenic cysts are usually due to echinococcal disease (Fig. 73-27). These hydatid cysts are often multiple and tend to have thicker and coarser rims of peripheral calcification than simple splenic cysts. Echinococcal calcification can reflect a hydatid cyst in the spleen or extension of cysts arising from neighboring organs. Dermoid and epidermoid cysts very rarely demonstrate calcification.

Plaques of calcification in a thickened and fibrotic splenic capsule (Fig. 73-28) can be found secondary to a pyogenic or tuberculous abscess, infarct, hematoma (Fig. 73-29), or hydatid cyst. Splenic infarcts calcify infrequently. Although they are usually single, multiple calcified infarcts can

occur. The calcification in a splenic infarct is often triangular or wedge-shaped, the apex of the density appearing to point toward the center of the organ. Calcified hematomas and abscesses of the spleen are rare.

Calcification within the media of the splenic artery is extremely common and produces a characteristic tortuous, corkscrew appearance (Fig. 73-30). When viewed end-on, splenic artery calcification appears as a thin-walled ring. A similar circular pattern (Fig. 73-31) or bizarre configuration (Fig. 73-32) of calcification in the left upper quadrant can be due to a saccular aneurysm of the splenic artery.

A generalized increase in splenic density is seen in up to 5% of patients with sickle cell anemia (Fig. 73-33). The spleen may appear diffusely opaque, but most often multiple punctate densities give the spleen a coarsely granular appearance. Fine miliary shadows are produced by calcification and iron deposits in the fibrotic nodules of siderosis. Contrac-

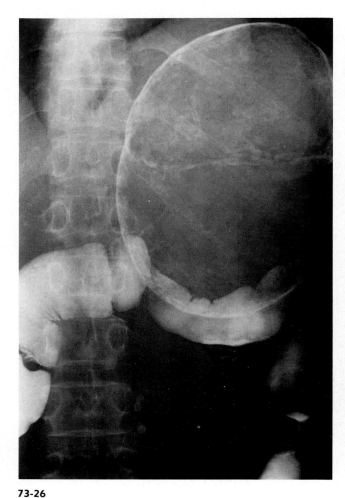

73-26

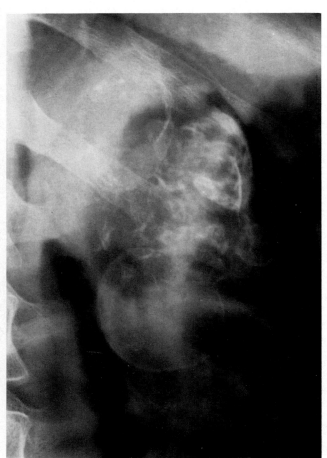

73-27

Fig. 73-26. Huge calcified splenic cyst.

Fig. 73-27. Calcified hydatid cyst of the spleen (echinococcal disease).

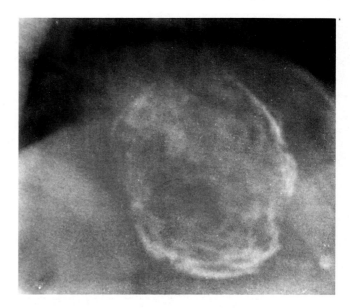

Fig. 73-28. Calcified splenic hematoma.

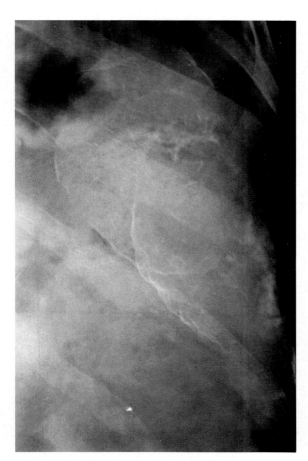

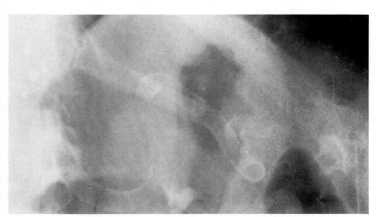

73-29   73-30

Fig. 73-29. Splenic capsule calcification. (Baker SR, Elkin M: Plain Film Approach to Abdominal Calcifications. Philadelphia, WB Saunders, 1983)

Fig. 73-30. Calcification of the splenic artery in a patient with diabetes. Note the characteristic tortuous, corkscrew appearance.

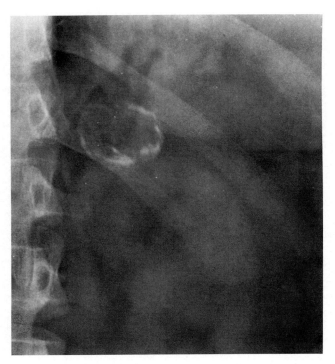

Fig. 73-31. Splenic artery aneurysm with a calcified rim.

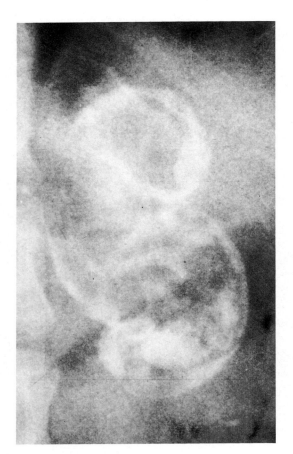

Fig. 73-32. Splenic artery aneurysm. Note the bizarre, lobulated calcification.

tion and atrophy of the spleen cause these concretions to become confluent, producing irregular areas of calcification and a diffuse increase in density. Generalized opacification of the spleen can also be demonstrated in patients with idiopathic hemochromatosis (an inherited metabolic error of iron metabolism) or excessive dietary intake of iron and in persons with abnormal iron pigment deposition related to thalassemia, Fanconi's anemia, or, rarely, multiple transfusions. Generalized increased density of the spleen (and liver) can be caused by the deposition of Thorotrast, a formerly used radiographic contrast agent that is stored in the reticuloendothelial system of the spleen, liver, and lymph nodes (see Fig. 73-21). A finely punctate pattern of opacification may also occur. Thorotrast deposits in the spleen and liver are associated with a high incidence of hepatobiliary carcinoma (especially the exceedingly rare angiosarcoma), leukemia, and aplastic anemia developing many years after the initial contrast injection (Fig. 73-34).

CALCIFICATION IN THE PANCREAS

Pancreatitis
    Alcoholic pancreatitis
    "Gallstone pancreatitis"
    Pancreatic pseudocyst
Hyperparathyroidism
Neoplasms
    Cystadenoma
    Cystadenocarcinoma
    Cavernous lymphangioma
    Solid and papillary epithelial tumor
    Insulinoma
Hereditary pancreatitis
Cystic fibrosis
Kwashiorkor (protein malnutrition)
Intraparenchymal hemorrhage
    Trauma
    Infarction
    Rupture of intrapancreatic aneurysm
Idiopathic pancreatitis

Pancreatic calcification consists almost exclusively of intraductal calculi representing calcified masses of inspissated pancreatic secretions. In most cases, the underlying pathogenic mechanism for pancreatic lithiasis appears to be relative obstruction of the pancreatic ductal system associated with stasis of pancreatic secretions. Nearly all apparently intraparenchymal calcification is found on histologic examination to represent the remains of intraductal calculi in areas of surrounding tissue necrosis.

Alcoholic pancreatitis is the most common cause of pancreatic lithiasis. Between 20% and 40% of all patients with chronic alcoholic pancreatitis develop calcific deposits in the pancreas. Conversely, almost 90% of patients with pancreatic cal-

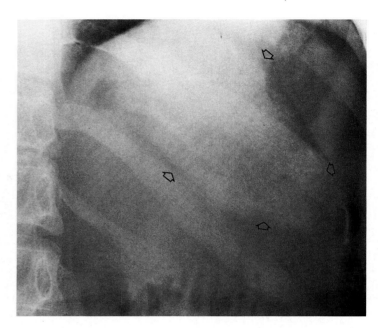

Fig. 73-33. Generalized increase in splenic density in a patient with sickle cell anemia.

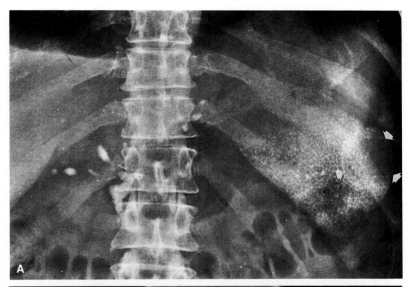

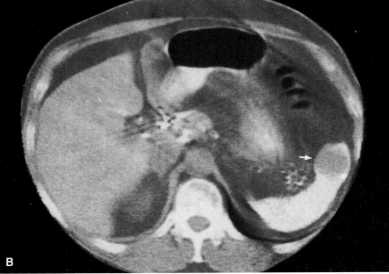

Fig. 73-34. Thorotrast-induced splenic angio-sarcoma. **(A)** Normal-sized spleen containing multiple punctate opacities. The **arrows** point to the radiolucent filling defect caused by the malignant tumor. Note the opaque lymph nodes and normal liver. **(B)** CT scan shows the solitary soft-tissue tumor mass within a nearly uniform, dense splenic background. (Levy DW, Rindsberg S, Friedman AC et al: Thorotrast-induced hepato-splenic neoplasia: CT identification. AJR 146: 997–1004, 1986. Copyright 1986. Reproduced with permission)

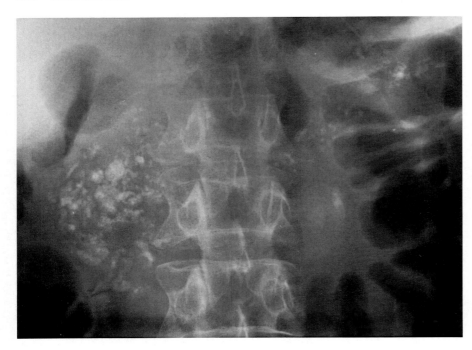

Fig. 73-35. Diffuse pancreatic calcifications in chronic alcoholic pancreatitis.

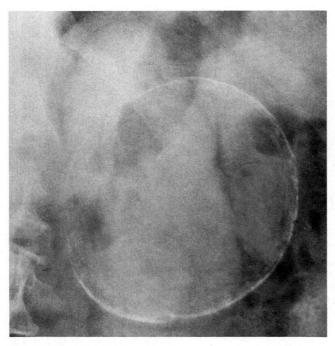

Fig. 73-36. *Calcified pancreatic pseudocyst. A rim of calcification outlines the wall of the pseudocyst.*

cification report a history of high alcohol consumption. Calcification in chronic alcoholic pancreatitis usually develops only after 5 to 10 years of episodic abdominal pain.

Pancreatic calcification secondary to alcoholic pancreatitis appears radiographically as numerous irregular, small concretions widely scattered throughout the gland (Fig. 73-35). Calcifications are limited to the head or tail of the gland in about one-quarter of cases. Solitary pancreatic calculi are rarely identified.

Pancreatic calcification occurs much less frequently in patients with pancreatitis secondary to biliary tract disease. The incidence of pancreatic lithiasis in persons with "gallstone pancreatitis" is only 2% or less. The radiographic appearance in this condition is indistinguishable from that of alcoholic pancreatitis.

Pancreatic calcification can be detected in about 20% of all patients who develop pseudocysts as a complication of chronic pancreatitis. The pattern of calcification tends to be similar to that seen in other patients with chronic pancreatitis, though a rim of calcification occasionally outlines the wall of the pseudocyst (Fig. 73-36).

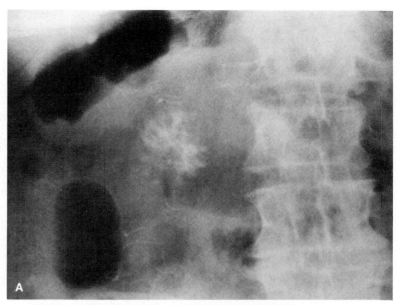

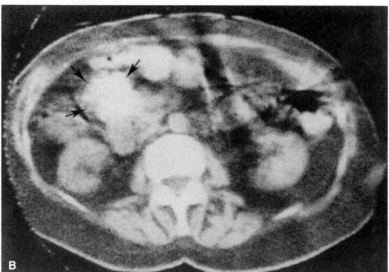

Fig. 73-37. Calcification in pancreatic insulinoma. **(A)** Plain radiograph shows "sunburst" calcification in the right upper quadrant. **(B)** CT scan without contrast shows the partially calcified mass **(arrows)** anterolateral to the pancreatic duodenal region. (Wolf EL, Sprayregan S, Frager D et al: Calcification in an insulinoma of the pancreas. Am J Gastroenterol 79:559–561, 1984)

Pancreatitis occurs in up to 20% of patients with hyperparathyroidism. Although the exact mechanism is not known, a causal relationship is suggested by numerous cases in which parathyroidectomy is followed by remission of pancreatitis. About half of the patients with pancreatitis related to hyperparathyroidism eventually develop chronic disease, and pancreatic calcification is often detected in these persons. Nephrocalcinosis and nephrolithiasis frequently complicate hyperparathyroidism, and the combination of pancreatic and renal calcification should suggest the possibility of underlying parathyroid disease. In one patient with multiple endocrine adenomatosis, nephrocalcinosis secondary to a functioning parathyroid adenoma was associated with a calcified non-beta islet cell tumor of the pancreas, which caused the Zollinger-Ellison syndrome.

The relation between pancreatic lithiasis and cancer is unclear. There is a higher than normal incidence of pancreatic cancer in patients with chronic pancreatitis. Furthermore, the incidence of pancreatic cancer in persons with pancreatic calcification is far higher than that in the general population. However, more than 95% of all patients with radiographically demonstrated pancreatic lithiasis have benign rather than malignant pancreatic disease.

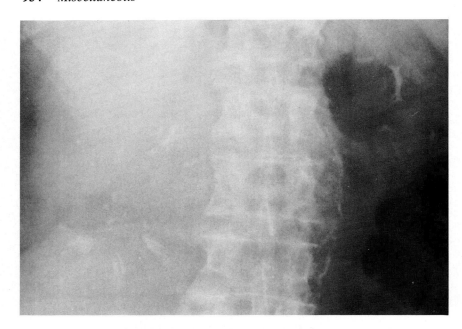

Fig. 73-38. Pancreatic calcifications in a cavernous lymphangioma.

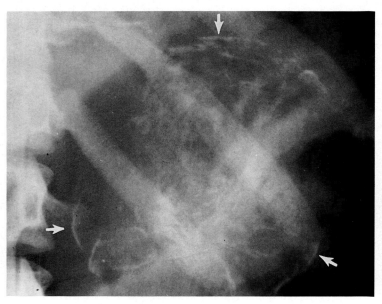

73-39

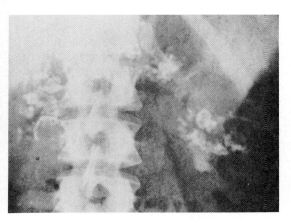

73-40

Fig. 73-39. Solid and papillary epithelial pancreatic neoplasm. Large calcified tumor **(arrows)** in the left hypochondrium. (Farman J, Chen CK, Schulze G et al: Solid and papillary epithelial pancreatic neoplasm: An unusual tumor. Gastrointest Radiol 12:31–34, 1987)

Fig. 73-40. Hereditary pancreatitis. The calcifications are rounder and larger than those usually found in other pancreatic diseases. (Ring EJ, Eaton SB, Ferrucci JT et al: Differential diagnosis of pancreatic calcification. AJR 117:446–452, 1973. Copyright 1973. Reproduced with permission)

When pancreatic cancer and lithiasis coexist, the calcium usually reflects pre-existent pancreatitis. It is diffusely present throughout the gland rather than being limited to the tumor mass. Less frequently, ductal obstruction secondary to pancreatic malignancy causes stasis of pancreatic secretions and results in lithiasis restricted to that portion of the gland that is upstream from the obstruction.

Calcification effectively does not occur in an adenocarcinoma of the pancreas. However, actual tumor calcification can be identified in about 10% of patients with cystadenoma or cystadenocarcinoma of the pancreas. Although the calcification associated with these tumors may be nonspecific, detection of the characteristic sunburst pattern is virtually pathognomonic (one case has been reported in an insulinoma of the pancreas). This appearance reflects the gross pathologic finding of cystic spaces separating spokelike stromal elements that radiate from a central nidus (Fig. 73-37). The presence of multiple phleboliths within and adjacent to the pancreas should suggest cavernous lymphangioma, a very rare pancreatic tumor (Fig. 73-38). Peripheral linear calcification may develop in the wall of a solid and papillary epithelial neoplasm of the pancreas, an uncommon low-grade malignant tumor histologically distinct from the usual ductal adenocarcinoma (Fig. 73-39). This tumor tends to occur in black women in the second or third decade of life and is amenable to cure by surgical excision. Discrete, coarse, and nodular calcification has been rarely reported as a degenerative phenomenon in insulinoma of the pancreas.

Hereditary pancreatitis and cystic fibrosis account for the great majority of pancreatic lithiasis seen in pediatric patients. Hereditary pancreatitis is an inherited disease (autosomal dominant) characterized by recurrent episodes of abdominal pain that usually begin in childhood and are refractory to medical therapy. Although patients with this condition do not appear to have any consistent anatomic abnormality of the pancreas, pancreatic ducts, or ampulla, they do have a marked propensity for developing pancreatic cancer (the cause of death in more than 20% of patients with this disease). More than half of patients with hereditary pancreatitis have radiographically visible calcifications. In children and young adults with cystic fibrosis, pancreatic calcification usually implies advanced pancreatic fibrosis associated with diabetes mellitus.

The pancreatic calcifications associated with these two pediatric diseases can usually be distinguished radiographically. The calcifications in hereditary pancreatitis are typically rounded and often larger than those found in other pancreatic diseases (Fig. 73-40). The calcification in cystic fibrosis generally has a fine granular appearance, and the individual calculi are almost invariably smaller than those in hereditary pancreatitis (Fig. 73-41).

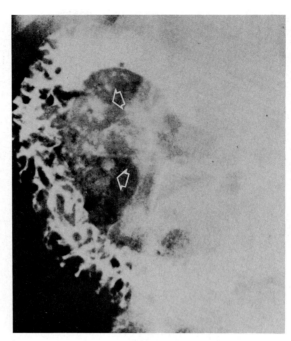

Fig. 73-41. Cystic fibrosis. These finely granular calcifications are primarily found in the head of the pancreas. (Ring EJ, Eaton SB, Ferrucci JT et al: Differential diagnosis of pancreatic calcification. AJR 117:446–452, 1973. Copyright 1973. Reproduced with permission)

Pancreatic calcification in underdeveloped countries is frequently associated with kwashiorkor. Severe protein malnutrition can lead to the development of histologic abnormalities of pancreatic acinar cells in early childhood and pancreatic lithiasis before adulthood. Complications of pancreatic disease, such as diabetes and steatorrhea, are common and tend to develop at an early age. Abdominal pain is a less prominent feature than would be expected in patients with pancreatic disease in Western countries.

True calcification of the pancreatic parenchyma can occur following intraparenchymal hemorrhage due to trauma or infarction. In patients who bleed from small intrapancreatic aneurysms secondary to pancreatitis, the resulting hematomas can subsequently calcify.

Pancreatic calcification occasionally occurs in patients who have no clinical evidence of pancreatic disease. Although the precise mechanism involved is unclear, these persons usually have nonspecific pancreatic ductal stenosis with formation of calculi upstream from the site of obstruction.

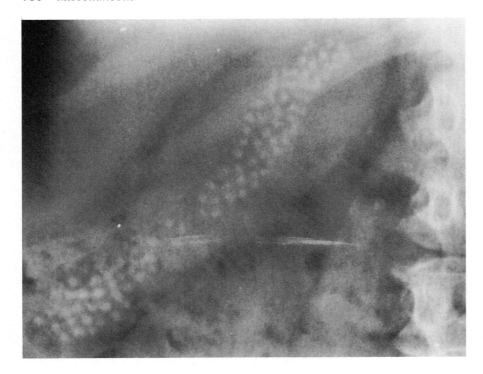

Fig. 73-42. Multiple small radiopaque stones in a large gallbladder.

CALCIFICATION IN THE GALLBLADDER/ BILE DUCT

>   Gallstone
>   Porcelain gallbladder
>   Milk of calcium bile
>   Common duct stone
>   Stone in the cystic duct remnant
>   Mucinous adenocarcinoma of the gallbladder

About 20% of gallstones contain sufficient calcium to be radiopaque (Fig. 73-42). Stones composed of pure cholesterol or a mixture of cholesterol and bile pigments are nonopaque. Although opaque gallstones vary greatly in radiographic appearance, they generally have a dense outer rim consisting of calcium bilirubinate or carbonate and a more transparent center composed of cholesterol, bile pigment, or both. Gallstones are often laminated, consisting of alternating opaque and lucent rings (Fig. 73-43). Solitary gallbladder stones are usually rounded; multiple stones are generally faceted (Fig. 73-44). In one case, calcium deposition within the fissures of biliary calculi produced dense radiating lines, the reverse appearance of the Mercedes–Benz sign (Fig. 73-45).

Several opacities in the right upper quadrant can simulate gallstones. A renal calculus can be differentiated from a gallstone overlying the renal shadow by obtaining a film in which the patient is rotated into an oblique position. A stone within a long retrocecal appendix or residual barium within a diverticulum in the hepatic flexure of the colon can mimic a radiopaque gallstone (see Fig. 73-51).

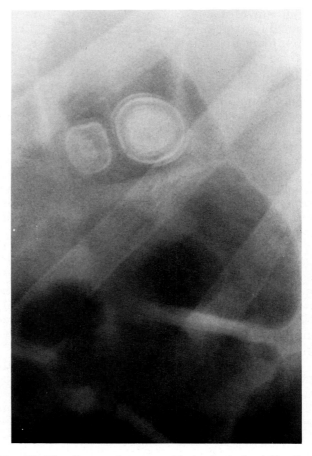

Fig. 73-43. Two gallstones with laminated calcification. (Williams SM, Harned RK: Radiology of the biliary system. In Gedgaudas–McClees RK (ed): Gastrointestinal Imaging. New York, Churchill Livingstone, 1987)

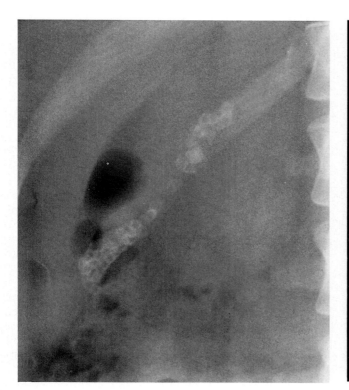

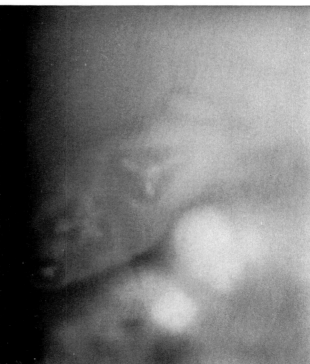

73-44

73-45

Fig. 73-44. Multiple faceted gallstones.

Fig. 73-45. Calcified gallstone fissures. Tomogram shows multiple radiolucent gallstones containing linear radiating calcifications in their centers. (Strijk SP: Calcified gallstone fissures: The reversed Mercedes–Benz sign. Gastrointest Radiol 12:152–153, 1987)

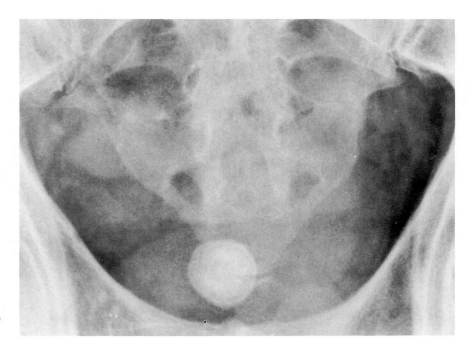

Fig. 73-46. Calcified gallstone in the rectum.

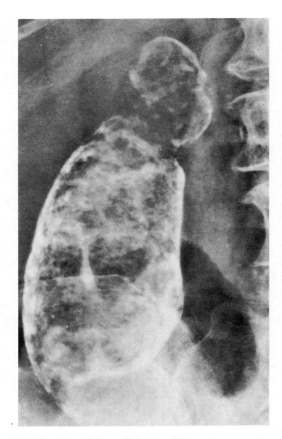

Fig. 73-47. Porcelain gallbladder. There is extensive mural calcification around the perimeter of the gallbladder.

In patients with cholecystoduodenal or other fistulas between the biliary and alimentary tracts, gallstones can be demonstrated at any point in the duodenum, small bowel, or colon (Fig. 73-46). Impaction of a gallstone in the ileum or jejunum can cause small bowel obstruction (gallstone ileus).

"Porcelain gallbladder" refers to extensive mural calcification around the perimeter of the gallbladder forming an oval density that corresponds to the size and shape of the organ (Fig. 73-47). The term reflects the blue discoloration and brittle consistency of the gallbladder wall. The calcification in a porcelain gallbladder can appear as a broad, continuous band in the muscular layers or be multiple and punctate and occur in the glandular spaces of the mucosa. Extensive gallbladder wall thickening is always accompanied by mural thickening and fibrosis secondary to chronic cholecystitis. Although a procelain gallbladder is an uncommon finding in patients with gallbladder carcinoma, there is a very high incidence of carcinoma in patients with extensive calcification of the gallbladder wall. Therefore, even if they are asymptomatic, patients with porcelain gallbladders are usually subjected to prophylactic cholecystectomy.

Milk of calcium bile is a condition in which the gallbladder becomes filled with an accumulation of bile that is rendered radiopaque because of a high concentration of calcium carbonate. The disorder is secondary to chronic cholecystitis and is accompanied by thickening of the gallbladder wall and ob-

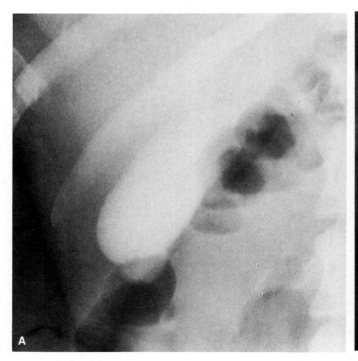

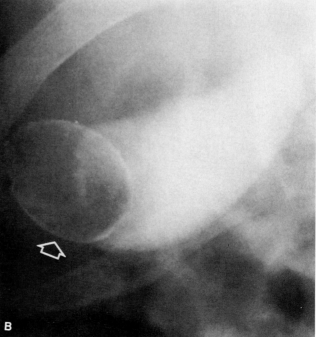

Fig. 73-48. Milk of calcium bile. **(A)** Plain abdominal radiograph demonstrates a completely opaque gallbladder in a patient who had not received any cholecystographic agent. **(B)** In this patient, a large lucent stone **(arrow)** is seen within the opaque gallbladder.

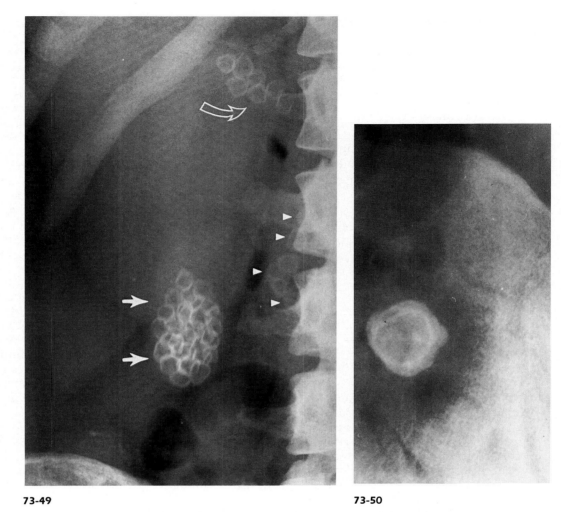

73-49   **73-50**

Fig. 73-49. Calculi in the gallbladder **(solid arrows)** and bile ducts **(open arrow)**. The **arrowheads** point to calculi in the common bile duct, some of which overlie the spine and are difficult to detect. (Baker SR, Elkin M: Plain Film Approach to Abdominal Calcifications. Philadelphia, WB Saunders, 1983)

Fig. 73-50. Laminated calcification in an appendicolith.

struction of the cystic duct. Because the increased density of bile makes the entire gallbladder opaque and simulates the appearance of a normal gallbladder filled with contrast medium (Fig. 73-48), it is necessary that a preliminary abdominal film be obtained before an oral cholecystographic contrast agent is administered to diagnose this disorder.

Calculi within the common bile duct are more difficult to diagnose on plain abdominal radiographs than are gallstones, because ductal stones are usually single and close to the spine and often overlie a transverse process (Fig. 73-49). When superimposed on the upper pole of the right kidney, common bile duct calculi can simulate renal stones; when located in the upper portion of the duct, they can be confused with calcified costal cartilage. Following cholecystectomy, opaque calculi can develop in the cystic duct remnant.

Rarely, mucinous adenocarcinoma of the gallbladder produces fine, granular, punctate flecks of calcification similar to the appearance of tumors of this same cell type in the stomach and colon.

CALCIFICATION IN THE ALIMENTARY TRACT

Enteroliths
    Appendicolith
    Meckel's stone
    Diverticular stone
    Rectal stone
Calcified mucocele of the appendix
Myxoglobulosis of the appendix
Calcified appendices epiploicae
Ingested foreign bodies
    Calcified seeds and pits
    Birdshot (from ingestion of wild game)
Mucinous carcinoma of the stomach and colon
Gastric or esophageal leiomyoma
Hemangioma
Mesenteric calcification
    Fat deposit
    Lipoma
    Cyst
Hydatid cyst
Schistosomiasis

Enteroliths are smooth, often faceted stones with radiopaque laminated calcifications. They are thought to result from stasis and are usually found proximal to an area of stricture or within diverticula. Enteroliths are not expelled with the fecal stream and can remain in place for years. They can cause mucosal ulcerations and be responsible for lower abdominal pain. Rectal enteroliths can produce fecal impaction and, if sufficiently numerous, bowel obstruction.

The most clinically important enterolith is the appendicolith. Appendicoliths are round or oval laminated stones of varying size that are found in 10% to 15% of cases of acute appendicitis (Fig. 73-50). In patients with fever, leukocytosis, and right lower quadrant pain, the radiographic demonstration of an appendicolith is highly suggestive of acute appendicitis. Surgical experience suggests that the presence of an appendicolith in combination with symptoms of acute appendicitis usually implies that the appendix is gangrenous and likely to perforate. Appendicoliths are generally situated within the lumen of the appendix but in rare instances may penetrate through the wall and lie free in the peritoneal cavity or in a periappendiceal abscess. Most appendicoliths are located in the right lower quadrant. Depending on the length and position of the appendix, an appendicolith can also be seen in the pelvis or in the right upper quadrant (in the case of a retrocecal appendix), where it can simulate a gallstone (Fig. 73-51). An appendicolith located near the midline can mimic a ureteral stone (Fig. 73-52); this is of great clinical significance, since an inflamed appendix in this region can cause hematuria and lead the physician to suspect renal colic rather than appendicitis.

Faceted stones can develop in a Meckel's diverticulum (Fig. 73-53); impaired drainage from the diverticulum leads to stasis and enterolith formation (Fig. 73-54). Complications of Meckel's stones include inflammation with perforation and peritonitis, ulceration, and hemorrhage.

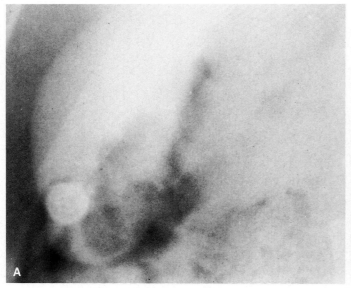
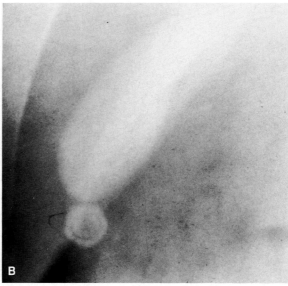

Fig. 73-51. Appendicolith in a retrocecal appendix mimicking a gallstone. **(A)** The calcified appendicolith appears to lie in the opacified gallbladder. **(B)** After a fatty meal, the appendicolith is clearly seen to lie outside the confines of the shrunken gallbladder.

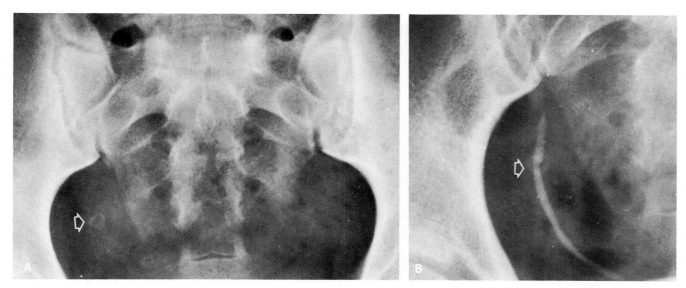

Fig. 73-52. Appendicolith mimicking a ureteral stone in a patient with hematuria. **(A)** On a plain abdominal radiograph, the appendicolith **(arrow)** is positioned in the region of the lower right ureter. **(B)** At excretory urography, the appendicolith **(arrow)** is seen to be separate from the nonobstructed right ureter.

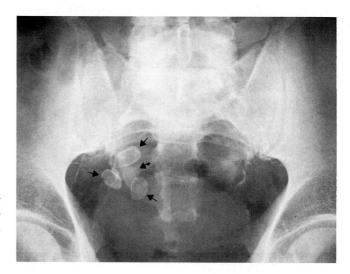

Fig. 73-53. Faceted stones in a Meckel's diverticulum. Four radiopaque calculi **(arrows)** are seen in the right side of the pelvis. (Paige ML, Ghahremani GG, Brosnan JJ: Laminated radiopaque enteroliths: Diagnostic clues to intestinal pathology. Am J Gastroenterol 82:432–437, 1987)

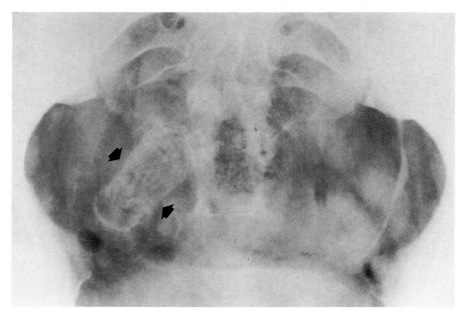

Fig. 73-54. Calcified enterolith **(arrows)** in a Meckel's diverticulum.

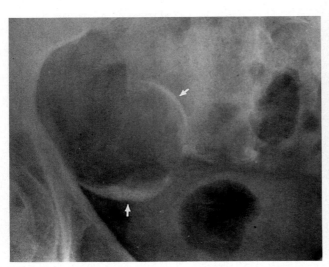

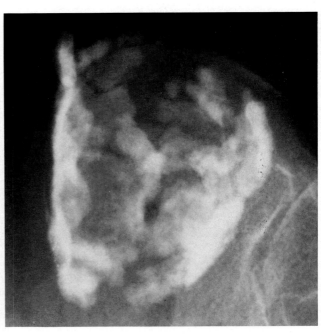

73-55   73-56

Fig. 73-55. Calcified mucocele of the appendix. Large cystic mass with an incomplete rim of calcification **(arrows)**. (Baker SR, Elkin M: Plain Film Approach to Abdominal Calcifications. Philadelphia, WB Saunders, 1983)

Fig. 73-56. Calcified mucocele of the appendix. The extensive calcification appears globular when viewed *en face*. (Dachman AH, Lichtenstein JE, Friedman AC: Mucocele of the appendix and pseudomyxoma peritonei. AJR 144:923–929, 1985. Copyright 1985. Reproduced with permission)

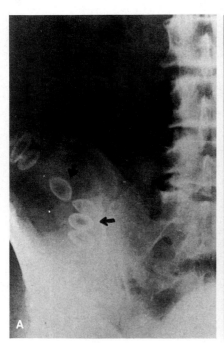

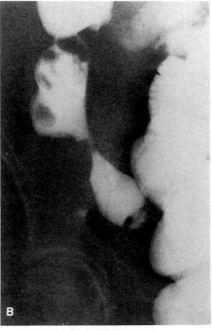

Fig. 73-57. Myxoglobulosis of the appendix. **(A)** Multiple annular and ovoid spherules in the right lower quadrant of the abdomen. **(B)** Barium enema shows a huge sac extending down from a contracted cecum and containing partially translucent ovoid bodies with thick calcified rims. (Alcalay J, Alkalay L, Lorent T: Myxoglobulosis of the appendix. Br J Radiol 58:183–184, 1985)

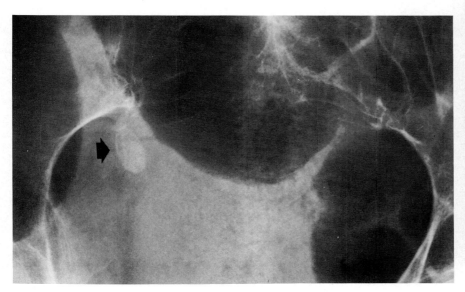

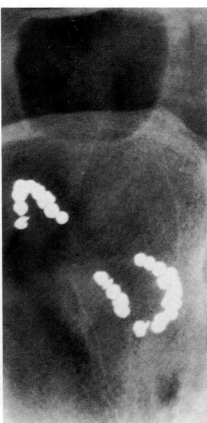

73-58

73-59

Fig. 73-58. Calcified appendix epiploica **(arrow)**. The cystlike calcific density was detached from the colon and changed position on serial films.

Fig. 73-59. Metallic foreign bodies in the appendix representing ingested birdshot in a patient who ate wild game.

A large crescent-shaped or circular calcification in the right lower quadrant is characteristic of a calcified mucocele of the appendix (Fig. 73-55). Extensive calcification may appear globular when viewed *en face* (Fig. 73-56). A mucocele is a collection of mucinous material in a dilated portion of the appendix (usually the tip). It is caused by fibrotic obstruction of the proximal lumen (*e.g.,* healed appendicitis) and an accumulation of mucus produced by the lining epithelium. A mucocele can vary in size from slight bulbous swelling to a large mass completely replacing the appendix and displacing the cecum.

Multiple annular calcifications associated with a cecal defect and usually nonfilling of the appendix is virtually pathognomonic of myxoglobulosis, a rare type of mucocele of the appendix that is composed of many round or oval translucent globules mixed with mucus (Fig. 73-57). Although the pathogenesis is unclear, it is suggested that masses of mucin are organized by ingrowth of granulation tissue from the wall of the mucocele. If a globule becomes detached from the wall, it serves as a nidus for the circumferential deposition of mucin.

Appendices epiploicae are small, pedunculated fat pads that are covered by visceral peritoneum and are located along the surface of the colon. Infarction of appendices epiploicae results in cystlike calcific densities adjacent to the gas-filled colon, most commonly the ascending portion (Fig. 73-58). These calcified appendices epiploicae can become detached from the colon and appear radiographically as small, ring-shaped calcifications that lie free in the peritoneal cavity and change position on serial films.

Ingested material (*e.g.,* seeds, pits) can become trapped in the colon within the appendix or diverticula or be found proximal to an area of stricture. The deposition of calcium on these nonopaque foreign bodies results in a characteristic ringlike appearance. In persons who have eaten wild game, ingested birdshot can present as rounded metallic densities trapped in the appendix (Fig. 73-59) or in colonic diverticula.

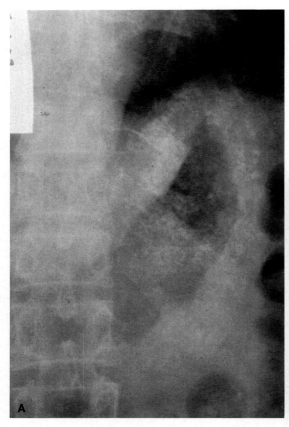
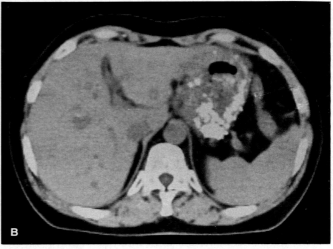

Fig. 73-60. Calcified mucinous adenocarcinoma of the stomach. **(A)** Plain abdominal radiograph after the administration of an efferverscent agent demonstrates punctate calcification within the wall of the stomach. **(B)** Unenhanced CT scan without the use of an oral contrast agent shows a thickened gastric wall with punctate calcification. No hepatic metastases are seen. (Rotondo A, Grassi R, Smaltino F et al: Calcified gastric cancer: Report of a case and review of literature. Br J Radiol 59:405–407, 1986)

Some mucinous adenocarcinomas of the stomach and colon contain small mottled or punctate deposits of calcium (Fig. 73-60). Most reported cases have been in patients under 40 years of age. The calcifications can be limited to the tumor mass or involve regional lymph nodes (Fig. 73-61), the adjacent omentum, or metastatic foci in the liver.

About 4% of leiomyomas of the stomach demonstrate some radiographic evidence of calcification. The circumscribed, stippled, or patchy calcification in these tumors simulates the pattern seen in uterine fibroids. Because the actual size of such tumors is clearly reflected by the extent of calcification, a larger, bulky lesion suggesting leiomyosarcoma may be correctly recognized. The presence of phleboliths associated with a mass in the alimentary

tract is virtually pathognomonic of hemangioma (Fig. 73-62).

Leiomyomas are the only esophageal tumors that have been reported to calcify (see Fig. 6-4). The rare calcification in these distal esophageal lesions initially presents as scattered punctate densities. This pattern progresses to the more characteristic appearance of coarse calcium deposits seen in tumors of this cell type in other sites.

Single or multiple mobile opaque nodules can reflect calcified fat deposits in the omentum. Deposition of calcium salts in omental fat can be the result of local interference with blood supply, inflammatory or traumatic pancreatic fat necrosis, or any infectious process causing caseating necrosis. More extensive concretions can develop in mesen-

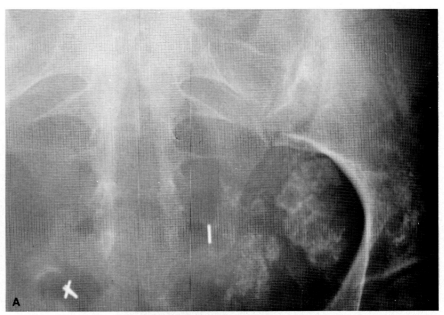

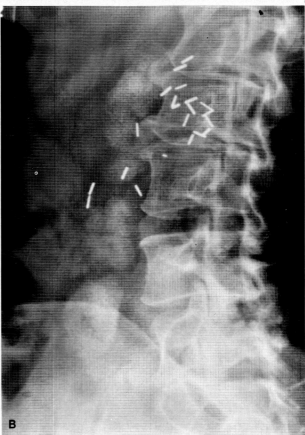

Fig. 73-61. Calcification of primary colonic carcinoma and its metastases. **(A)** Bulky tumor of the sigmoid colon with multiple calcifications in the tumor mass. **(B)** Metastases to retroperitoneal para-aortic lymph nodes with multiple fine calcifications duplicating the appearance of the primary tumor. At times, calcifications may develop in metastases without calcification of the primary tumor. (Margulis AR, Burhenne HJ (eds): Alimentary Tract Radiology. St. Louis, CV Mosby, 1983)

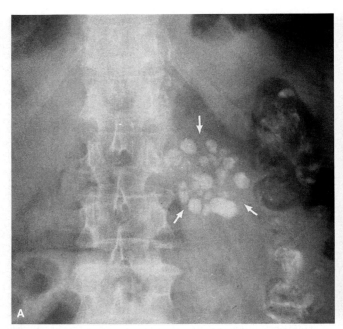 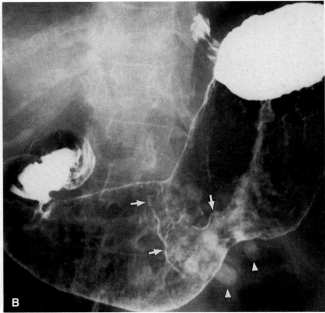

Fig. 73-62. Gastric hemangioma with phleboliths. **(A)** Plain radiograph shows clustered phleboliths **(arrows)**. **(B)** Upper gastrointestinal series shows the large gastric mass **(arrows)** with the associated rounded calcifications representing phleboliths **(arrowheads)**. (Simms SM: Gastric hemangioma associated with phleboliths. Gastrointest Radiol 10:51–53, 1985)

teric lipomas. Cysts of the mesentery or peritoneum, especially chylous cysts, can demonstrate unilocular or multilocular calcification (Fig. 73-63). Hydatid cysts, presumably forming through rupture of the primary hepatic cyst into the peritoneal cavity, can also calcify. In schistosomiasis, calcification of the rectosigmoid may produce a laminar pattern in distended bowel, a laminar or irregular amorphous density in the empty colon, and a corrugated pattern in the empty rectum (Fig. 73-64). Rectocolonic calcification is probably the most common radiographic manifestation of schistosomal infestation of the gastrointestinal tract.

CALCIFICATION IN THE KIDNEY

Calculus
Nephrocalcinosis
  Skeletal deossification
    Hyperparathyroidism
    Metastatic carcinoma to bone
    Primary carcinoma
    Severe osteoporosis
    Cushing's disease
    Steroid therapy
  Increased intestinal absorption of calcium
    Sarcoidosis

    Milk-alkali syndrome
    Hypervitaminosis D
  Renal tubular acidosis
  Medullary sponge kidney
  Hyperoxaluria
  Wilson's disease
  Renal papillary necrosis
  Tuberculosis
  Chronic pyelonephritis
Cystic disease
  Simple benign cyst
  Polycystic kidney
  Multicystic kidney
  Echinococcal cyst
Perirenal hematoma/abscess
Renal cell carcinoma
Other tumors
Xanthogranulomatous pyelonephritis
Cortical calcification
  Acute cortical necrosis
  Chronic glomerulonephritis
  Hereditary nephritis
  Dialysis therapy
Vascular calcification
  Renal artery aneurysm
  Arteriovenous malformation
Renal milk of calcium
Residual Pantopaque in a renal cyst

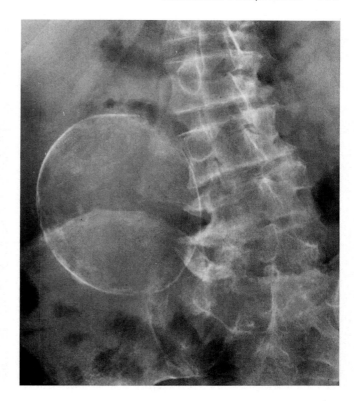

Fig. 73-63. Calcified mesenteric cyst.

Fig. 73-64. Rectocolonic calcification from schistosomiasis. Corrugated rectal calcification **(arrows)** seen through and above the bladder **(b)** filled with urine **(A)** and contrast material **(B)**. The ureters **(u)** are calcified and dilated. **(C)** The pattern of calcification changes to a laminar one when the rectum is distended with gas and feces **(arrows)**. (Fataar S, Bassiony H, Hamed MS et al: Radiographic spectrum of recto-colonic calcification from schistosomiasis. AJR 141:933–936, 1984. Copyright 1984. Reproduced with permission.)

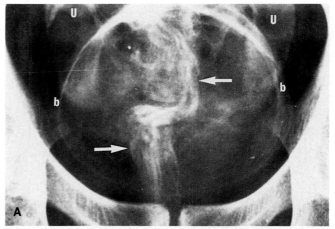

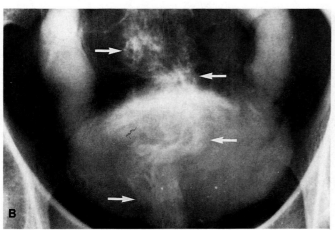

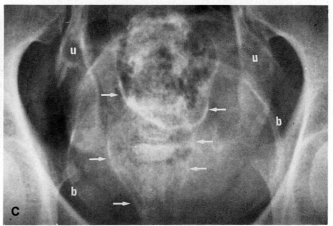

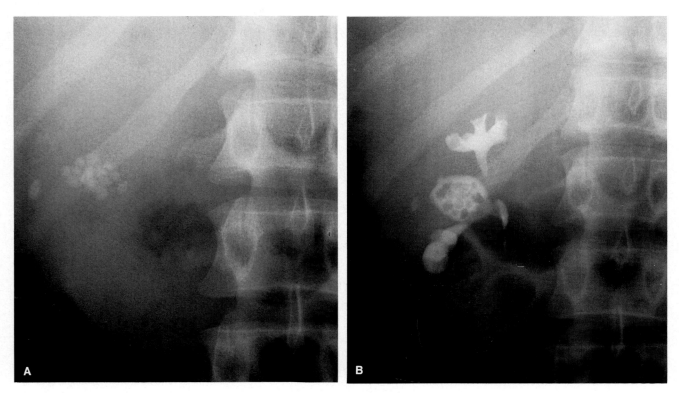

Fig. 73-65. Multiple calculi in the renal pelvis. Although the calculi are opaque on the plain abdominal radiograph **(A)**, they appear lucent on the excretory urogram **(B)** because their density is less than that of the iodinated contrast material.

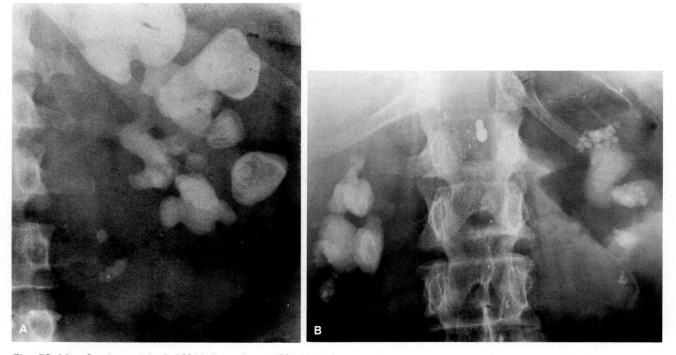

Fig. 73-66. Staghorn calculi. **(A)** Unilateral, and **(B)** bilateral.

Calculi are frequently demonstrated in the calyces and the renal pelvis (Fig. 73-65). Occasionally, almost the entire pelvocalyceal system is filled with a large staghorn calculus (Fig. 73-66). Urinary stasis and infection are important factors in promoting calculus formation. More than 80% of symptomatic renal calculi are radiopaque and detectable on plain abdominal radiographs. Calculi composed of calcium phosphate and calcium oxalate usually have uniform dense radiopacity; magnesium ammonium phosphate stones are much less radiopaque. Cystine calculi, though often considered nonopaque, are usually moderately opaque and present a frosted or ground-glass appearance. Completely radiolucent calculi contain no calcium and are composed of pure uric acid or urates, xanthine, or matrix concretions that are a combination of mucoprotein and mucopolysaccharide. These calculi usually form in the presence of *Proteus* infection. Renal calculi can be laminated as a result of deposition of alternate layers of densely radiopaque material (calcium phosphate, calcium oxalate) and material of relatively low radiodensity (magnesium ammonium phosphate, urate).

Nephrocalcinosis refers to radiographically detectable diffuse calcium deposition within the renal parenchyma, chiefly in the medullary pyramids. Histologically, calcium may be deposited in the interstitium, in tubular epithelial cells, or along basement membranes of the collecting ducts, distal convoluted tubules, or ascending limb of the loop of Henle. Calcification can also occur in the tubular lumen. Radiographically, the calcification in nephrocalcinosis varies from a few scattered punctate densities to very dense and extensive calcifications throughout both kidneys.

Nephrocalcinosis occurs in about 25% of patients with hypercalcemia due to primary hyperparathyroidism, which is caused by an adenoma or carcinoma of a single gland or diffuse hyperplasia of all the parathyroid glands. Excess secretion of parathyroid hormone increases osteoclast activity, with resulting deossification of the skeleton and hypercalcemia.

Bone destruction in patients with metastatic carcinoma leads to a release of excess amounts of calcium from osseous structures, and this can result in nephrocalcinosis. Deossification of the skeleton and subsequent nephrocalcinosis can also occur in patients with severe osteoporosis (due to immobilization, menopause, senility) or Cushing's disease and in persons receiving steroid therapy. Patients with primary carcinomas, especially of the lung or kidney, may develop a paraneoplastic syndrome with hypercalcemia and nephrocalcinosis that appears to be related to inappropriate secretion by the tumor of specific humoral factors.

Increased intestinal absorption of calcium can lead to nephrocalcinosis. In patients with sarcoidosis, an increased intestinal sensitivity to vitamin D results in excessive absorption of dietary calcium. A similar mechanism occurs in patients with hypervitaminosis D; an excess of vitamin D also promotes dissolution of calcium salts from bone. Patients with the milk–alkali syndrome have a long history of excessive calcium ingestion, usually in the form of milk and antacids containing calcium carbonate (Fig. 73-67). The large tubular load of calcium and

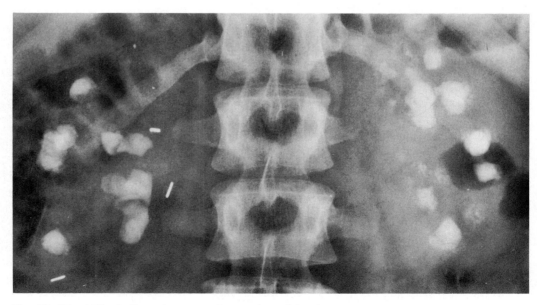

Fig. 73-67. Milk-alkali syndrome causing nephrocalcinosis.

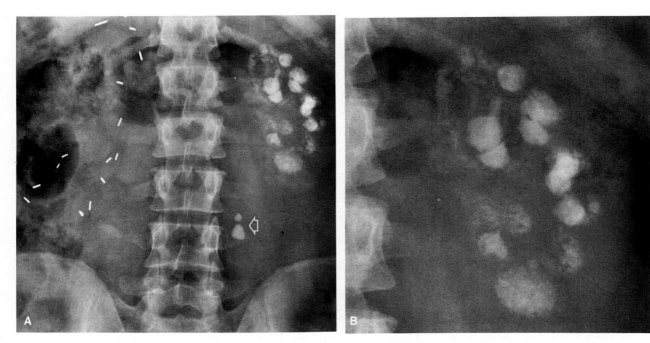

Fig. 73-68. Renal tubular acidosis causing nephrocalcinosis. **(A)** An abdominal radiograph demonstrates diffuse calcification in the medullary pyramids of the left kidney. In addition, two stones (one of which is causing an obstruction) are seen in the midportion of the left ureter **(arrow)**. The patient had previously undergone a right nephrectomy. **(B)** A close-up view of the left kidney demonstrates the intrarenal calcification.

phosphate in the presence of alkaline urine and interstitial fluid causes the development of nephrocalcinosis.

Renal tubular acidosis is a disorder in which the kidney is unable to excrete an acid urine (below *p*H 5.4) because the distal nephron cannot secrete hydrogen against a concentration gradient. In addition to nephrocalcinosis and nephrolithiasis, patients with renal tubular acidosis frequently suffer from osteomalacia. The parenchymal calcification in renal tubular acidosis is characteristically very dense and extensive, diffusely involving the medullary portion of the renal lobes (Fig. 73-68).

Calcification within cystic dilations of the distal collecting ducts is a manifestation of medullary sponge kidney (Fig. 73-69). The calculi are usually small and round, tending to cluster around the apices of the pyramids. Many patients with this disease are entirely free of urinary tract symptoms unless stone formation, urinary tract infection, or hematuria supervenes.

Hyperoxaluria produces nephrocalcinosis by interstitial deposition of calcium oxalate. The pri-

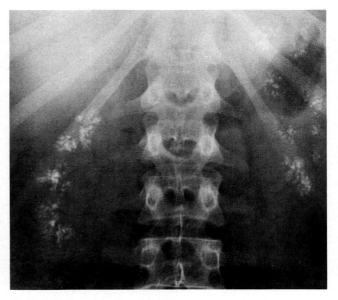

Fig. 73-69. Medullary sponge kidney. Multiple small calculi occurring in clusters and a fanlike arrangement in the papillary tips of multiple renal pyramids.

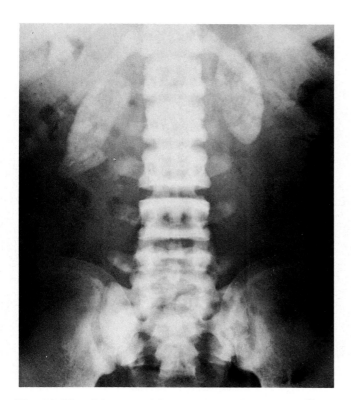

Fig. 73-70. Primary calcium oxalosis. There are diffuse, mottled renal parenchymal calcifications. Other evidence of the disease includes a "rugger-jersey" spine and sclerotic bands in the iliac crests and acetabula. (Carsen GM, Radkowski MA: Calcium oxalosis: A case report. Radiology 113:165–166, 1974)

mary form is a rare inherited metabolic disease in which symptoms of urinary tract calculi occur early in childhood (Fig. 73-70). Infection, hypertension, and obstructive uropathy usually cause a fatal outcome before the patient reaches the age of 20. Secondary oxaluria occurs in association with intestinal diseases, especially Crohn's disease (Fig. 73-71), in which increased absorption of dietary oxalate is related to the inflammatory process. Some patients with Wilson's disease develop nephrocalcinosis due to an inability to acidify the urine adequately.

Nephrocalcinosis is a common finding in patients with renal papillary necrosis (Fig. 73-72). This disease is characterized by infarction of renal papillae resulting in necrosis with sloughing of the involved tissue. Renal papillary necrosis can be secondary to analgesic abuse (*e.g.*, phenacetin), diabetes mellitus, obstruction of the urinary tract, pyelonephritis, or sickle cell anemia. The necrotic papilla can remain *in situ* and become calcified or become detached and serve as a nidus for calculus development. A characteristic radiographic finding in papillary necrosis is the "ring shadow," a triangu-

lar radiolucency surrounded by a dense opaque band representing calcification of a sloughed papilla.

Flecks of calcification in multiple tuberculous granulomas can present as nephrocalcinosis. As the disease progresses, gross amorphous and irregular calcifications can develop (Fig. 73-73). Eventually, the entire nonfunctioning renal parenchyma may be replaced by massive calcification (autonephrectomy).

Although nephrocalcinosis is commonly seen microscopically in the kidneys of patients with chronic pyelonephritis, the radiographic detection of parenchymal calcification in this condition is unusual.

Thin, curvilinear calcifications can be demonstrated in the walls of about 3% of simple renal cysts (Fig. 73-74). However, this peripheral curvilinear calcification is not pathognomonic of a benign process. In one series, 20% of patients with this pattern had adenocarcinomas of the kidney (Fig. 73-75).

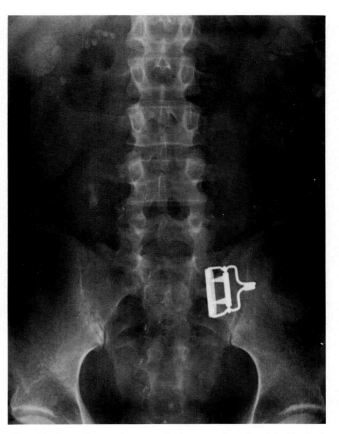

Fig. 73-71. Secondary oxaluria associated with Crohn's disease. Multiple calcifications are evident in both kidneys, both ureters, and the bladder. Calcifications are also present in the gallbladder and cystic duct. (Chikos PM, McDonald GB: Regional enteritis complicated by nephrocalcinosis and nephrolithiasis. Radiology 121:75–76, 1976)

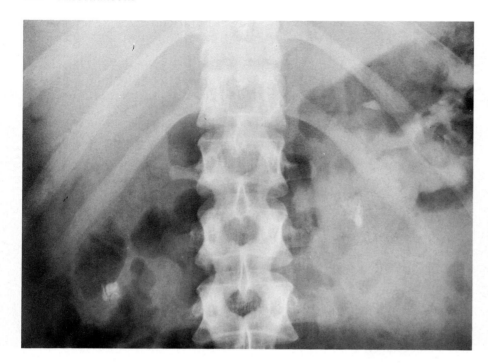

Fig. 73-72. Papillary necrosis. Ring-shaped calcifications are visible in both kidneys in a young analgesic abuser. This pattern of calcification is associated with sloughing of the entire papillary tip. (Davidson AJ: Radiologic Diagnosis of Renal Parenchymal Disease. Philadelphia, WB Saunders, 1977)

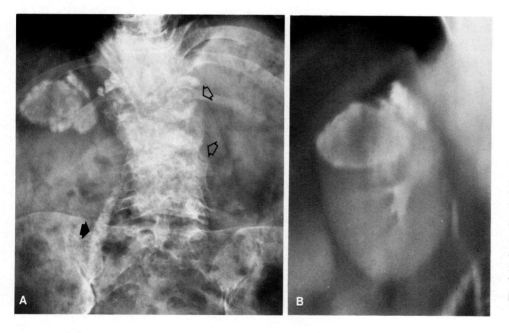

Fig. 73-73. Calcified tuberculoma. **(A)** Plain film and **(B)** nephrotomogram demonstrate a large calcified tuberculoma involving the upper pole of the right kidney. Note the diffuse destructive changes in the dorsolumbar spine **(open arrows)** and the calcified right psoas abscess **(solid arrow)**. (Tonkin AK, Witten DM: Genitourinary tuberculosis. Semin Roentgenol 14:305–318, 1979)

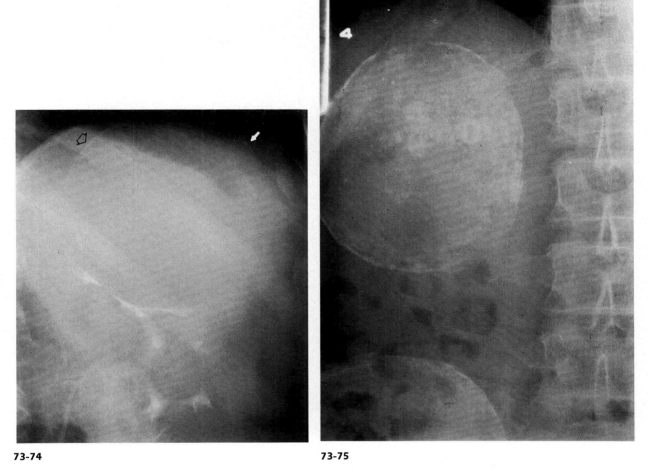

73-74   **73-75**

Fig. 73-74. Calcification in a simple renal cyst. Curvilinear, peripheral calcification outlines part of the cyst wall **(arrows)**. Smooth splaying of upper pole calyces is demonstrated on this film from an excretory urogram. (Davidson AJ: Radiologic Diagnosis of Renal Parenchymal Disease. Philadelphia, WB Saunders, 1977)

Fig. 73-75. Renal adenocarcinoma with cyst wall type of calcification. Large right upper quadrant mass with a thin, somewhat mottled rim of calcification mimicking a simple cyst. (Baker SR, Elkin M: Plain Film Approach to Abdominal Calcifications. Philadelphia, WB Saunders, 1983)

Similar peripheral calcifications can occur in persons with polycystic or multicystic disease (Fig. 73-76). About 50% to 80% of echinococcal cysts are calcified, appearing usually as complete circumferential rings (Fig. 73-77) but occasionally as scattered plaques. Large cystlike calcification can also occur following organization of a perirenal hematoma (Fig. 73-78) or old perirenal abscess.

About 10% of hypernephromas contain calcification. In most instances, the calcium is located in reactive fibrous zones about areas of tumor necrosis rather than within necrotic tissue. In the differentiation of solid tumors from fluid-filled benign cysts, the location of calcium within the mass is more important than the pattern of calcification. Of all masses containing calcium in a nonperipheral loca-

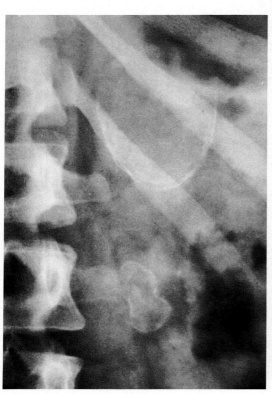

73-76

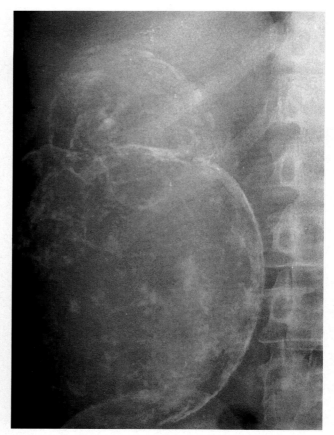

73-77

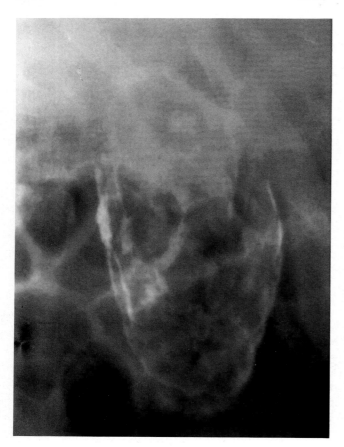

73-78

Fig. 73-76. Congenital unilateral multicystic kidney. There are three peripherally calcified masses, with no excretion of contrast medium on excretory urography. (Daniel WW, Hartman GW, Witten DM et al: Calcified renal masses: A review of ten years experience at the Mayo Clinic. Radiology 103:503–508, 1972)

Fig. 73-77. Renal echinococcal cysts. Thin curvilinear calcification in the walls of the large main cyst as well as of several daughter cysts. (Baker SR, Elkin M: Plain Film Approach to Abdominal Calcifications. Philadelphia, WB Saunders, 1983)

Fig. 73-78. Renal capsule calcification. A peel of calcification surrounds the left kidney, probably the result of an old subcapsular hematoma. (Baker SR, Elkin M: Plain Film Approach to Abdominal Calcifications. Philadelphia, WB Saunders, 1983)

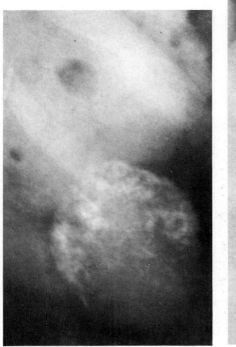

73-79

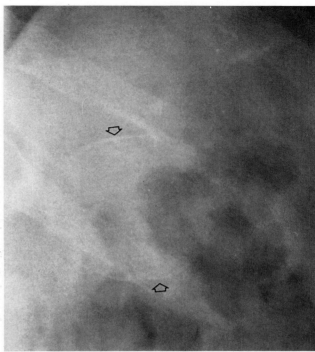

73-80

Fig. 73-79. Calcification in a renal cell carcinoma. If there is no peripheral calcification, mottled or punctate calcium that appears to be within a mass is highly indicative of a malignant lesion. (Daniel WW, Hartman GW, Witten DM et al: Calcified renal masses: A review of ten years experience at the Mayo Clinic. Radiology 103:503–508, 1972)

Fig. 73-80. Renal adenoma. Thin rim of calcification about a left upper quadrant mass. (Baker SR, Elkin M: Plain Film Approach to Abdominal Calcifications. Philadelphia, WB Saunders, 1983)

tion, almost 90% are malignant (Fig. 73-79). Although peripheral, curvilinear calcification is much more suggestive of a benign cyst, hypernephromas can have a calcified fibrous pseudocapsule that produces this radiographic appearance.

Other benign and malignant tumors may infrequently cause calcification in a renal mass. Benign neoplasms include cortical adenoma (Fig. 73-80), angiomyolipoma, dermoid, and fibroma. Among malignant tumors, osteosarcoma (Fig. 73-81), oncocytoma (Fig. 73-82), spindle cell sarcomas, transitional cell carcinoma, and metastases (thyroid, Hodgkin's disease) have been reported to produce calcification.

Diffuse parenchymal calcification can be demonstrated in patients with xanthogranulomatous pyelonephritis. This chronic inflammatory disease, which occurs predominantly in women with a long history of renal infection, is characterized by multiple inflammatory masses that frequently simulate carcinoma. In more than 70% of patients with this disorder, a large calculus is present in the renal pelvis and often causes pelvocalyceal obstruction and loss of renal function (Fig. 73-83).

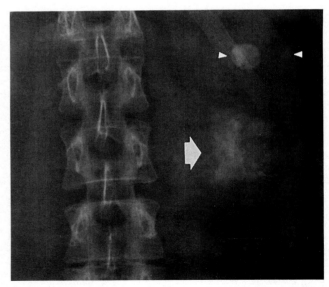

Fig. 73-81. Primary osteosarcoma of the left kidney. Characteristic sunburst appearance of the calcification **(arrow)**. The two superior calcifications represent osseous nodules in the perinephric tissues. (Mencini RA: Semin Roentgenol 17:90–91, 1982)

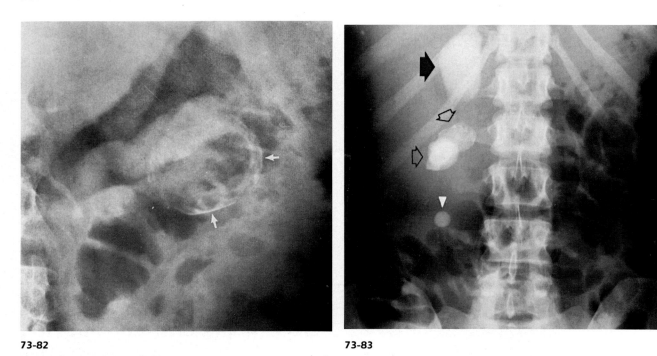

73-82   73-83

Fig. 73-82. Calcified renal oncocytoma. Thin ring-shaped calcification in the left upper quadrant. (Wasserman NF, Ewing SL: Calcified renal oncocytoma. AJR 141:747–749, 1983. Copyright 1983. Reproduced with permission)

Fig. 73-83. Xanthogranulomatous pyelonephritis. There are two large calcified calculi in the renal pelvis **(open arrows)** and another stone in the ureter **(arrowhead)**. The **closed arrow** points to contrast material in the gallbladder from an oral cholecystogram.

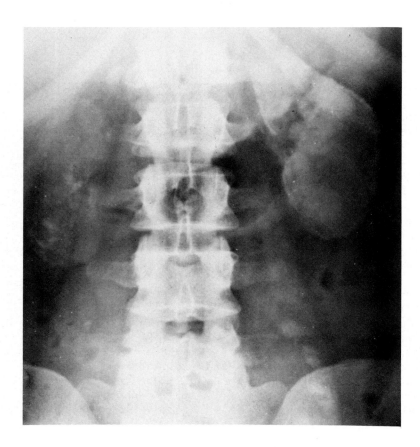

Fig. 73-84. Bilateral renal cortical necrosis.

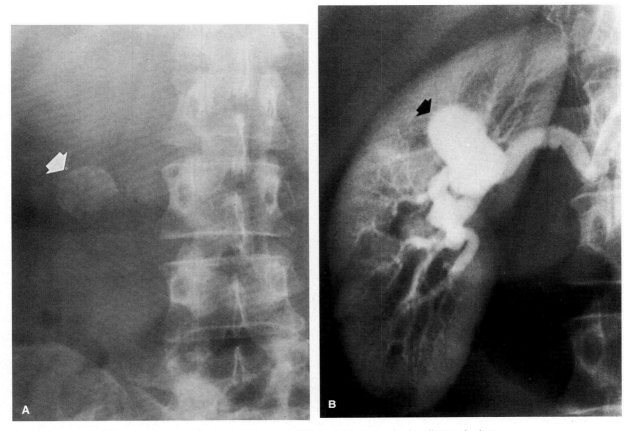

Fig. 73-85. Calcification in a renal artery aneurysm. **(A)** A plain abdominal radiograph demonstrates circular calcification with a cracked-eggshell appearance **(arrow)** at the renal hilus. **(B)** A selective right renal arteriogram shows contrast filling the saccular aneurysm **(arrow)**.

Renal calcification can be confined to the cortex of the kidney. In acute cortical necrosis (Fig. 73-84), a very uncommon form of acute renal failure in which there is death of the renal cortex and sparing of the medulla, punctate or linear ("tramline") calcification can occur within a month of the onset of the disease. Cortical calcification has also been demonstrated in patients with chronic glomerulonephritis and hereditary nephritis and in persons undergoing dialysis therapy.

About one-third of renal artery aneurysms have radiographically visible calcification (Fig. 73-85). These saccular structures have a circular cracked-eggshell appearance at the renal hilus. Calcifications can also be demonstrated in congenital or post-traumatic arteriovenous fistulas.

"Renal milk of calcium" refers to a suspension of fine sediment containing calcium that is most commonly found in a cyst or calyceal diverticulum. Less frequently, milk of calcium has been associated with obstruction of the urinary collecting system and hydronephrosis. The precise etiology of this process is unclear, but it may be related to stasis and infection. Renal milk of calcium usually is asymptomatic and an incidental finding. On plain abdominal radiographs in which the patient is supine, the appearance suggests an ordinary round or oval solid calculus (Fig. 73-86*A*). With the patient upright or sitting, however, the calcific material gravitates to the bottom of the cyst, resulting in a characteristic "half-moon" contour (Fig. 73-86*B,C*).

Residual Pantopaque from prior renal cyst puncture can appear as a confusing heavy-metal density that simulates a swallowed coin on abdominal radiographs (Fig. 73-87). Unlike water-soluble contrast, Pantopaque takes several years to be ab-

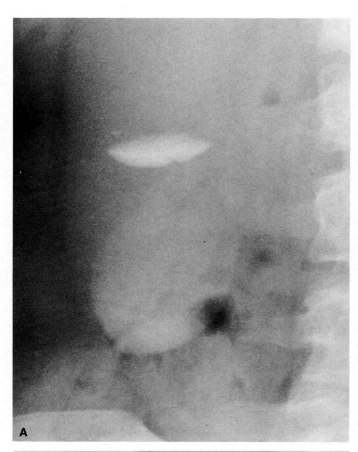

A

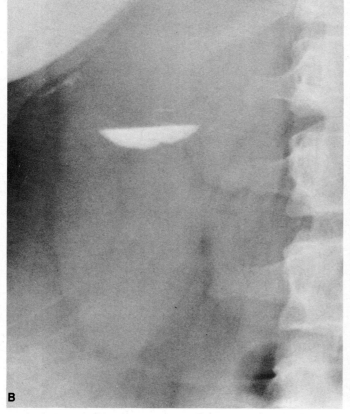

B

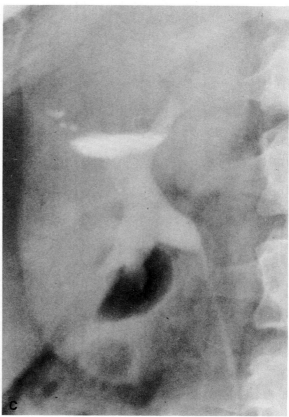

C

Fig. 73-86. Renal milk of calcium. **(A)** A supine abdominal radiograph demonstrates an oval density suggesting a renal calculus. **(B)** On the upright view, the calcium-containing sediment gravitates to the bottom of the renal cyst, resulting in the characteristic "half-moon" contour. **(C)** An excretory urogram shows that the milk of calcium is situated at the bottom of a large right upper pole renal cyst.

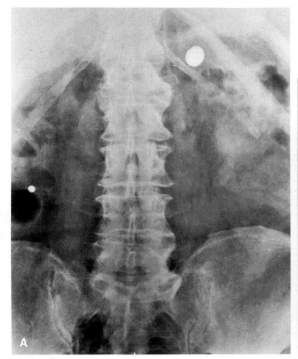

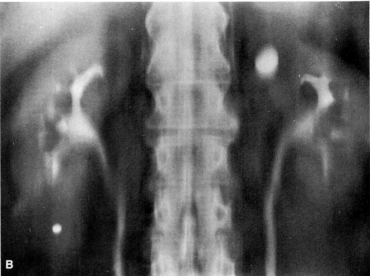

Fig. 73-87. Residual Pantopaque from prior renal cyst puncture. **(A)** A plain abdominal radiograph demonstrates two heavy-metal densities, one in the upper pole of the left kidney and the other in the lower pole of the right kidney. **(B)** Nephrotomography demonstrates that the two heavy-metal densities lie within renal cysts. (Eisenberg RL, Mani RL: Residual Pantopaque in renal cysts: An addition to the differential diagnosis of intra-abdominal heavy-metal densities. Clin Radiol 29:227–229, 1978)

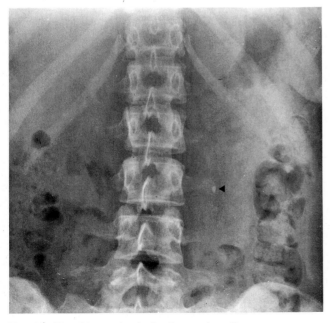

Fig. 73-88. Ureteral calculus **(arrowhead)**.

sorbed from a renal cyst and may present a diagnosis dilemma if a history of prior cyst puncture is not available.

URETERAL CALCIFICATION

> Calculus
> Schistosomiasis
> Tuberculosis

Ureteral calculi are extremely common, and their detection is clinically important (Fig. 73-88). They are usually small, irregular, and poorly calcified and are therefore easily missed on abdominal radiographs that are not of good quality. Calculi most commonly lodge in the lower portion of the ureter, especially at the ureterovesical junction and at the pelvic brim. Ureteral calculi are often oval in shape, their long axes paralleling the course of the ureter. They must be differentiated from the far more common phleboliths, which are spherical in shape and are located in the lateral portion of the pelvis below

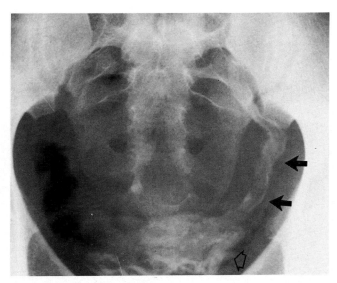

Fig. 73-89. *Schistosomiasis. There is calcification of the distal ureter* **(solid arrows)** *and bladder* **(open arrow)**.

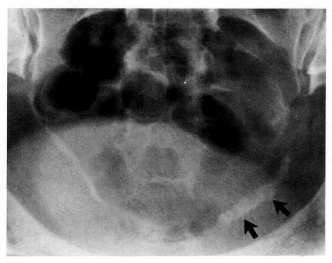

Fig. 73-90. *Tuberculosis. There is calcification of the distal ureter* **(arrows)**.

a line joining the ischial spines. In contrast, ureteral calculi are situated medially above the interspinous line.

Ureteral calcification is reported in about 15% of patients with schistosomiasis (Fig. 73-89). It appears as two roughly parallel, dense lines separated by the caliber of the ureter. Calcification is heaviest in the pelvic portion of the ureter and gradually decreases as it approaches the kidneys. Ureteral calcification is much less common than calcification of the kidney in patients with tuberculous involvement of the urinary tract (Fig. 73-90). Calcification of the bladder in tuberculosis is relatively rare.

CALCIFICATION IN THE BLADDER/ URETHRA/URACHUS

Inflammatory diseases of the bladder
  Schistosomiasis
  Tuberculosis
  Nonspecific infections (encrusted cystitis)
  Postirradiation cystitis
  Bacillary urinary tract infections
Foreign body
Bladder calculus
Urethral calculus
Urachal calculus
Bladder neoplasms
  Transitional cell carcinoma
  Squamous cell carcinoma
  Leiomyosarcoma
  Hemangioma
  Neuroblastoma
  Osteogenic sarcoma

World-wide, *Schistosoma hematobium* infestation (bilharziasis) is the most common cause of bladder wall calcification (see Fig. 73-89). In this parasitic disease, the adult female worm lays her eggs in the venules of the submucosa of lower urinary tract structures, primarily the urinary bladder. The eggs incite an intense inflammation, which causes fibrosis and subsequent calcification of the dead ova trapped in the submucosa. Calcification can also develop in the muscular and adventitial layers of the bladder wall.

About 50% of patients with schistosomiasis of the bladder have radiographically visible calcification. Initially, this calcification is most apparent and extensive at the base of the bladder, where it forms a linear opaque shadow parallel to the upper border of the pubic bone. With further calcium deposition, the linear density encircles the entire bladder. Unlike calcification in other inflammatory processes, the calcified bladder of schistosomiasis often retains a relatively normal capacity and distensibility.

Squamous cell carcinoma of the bladder is a well-known complication of schistosomiasis. This tumor alters the appearance of the calcified bladder by disrupting the continuity of the homogeneous line of calcification in the area of neoplastic infiltration.

Calcification can infrequently be demonstrated in patients with tuberculous cystitis. When visible, it appears as a faint, irregular rim of calcium outlining the wall of a markedly contracted bladder. By the time bladder wall calcification is radiographically apparent, extensive tuberculous changes are usually evident in the kidneys and ureters.

Rarely, calcium becomes deposited on mucosal erosions of the bladder due to nonspecific infections (encrusted cystitis) or appears as a consequence of postirradiation cystitis. Bladder wall calcification is extremely uncommon in patients with bacillary urinary tract infections. Bladder calcifica-

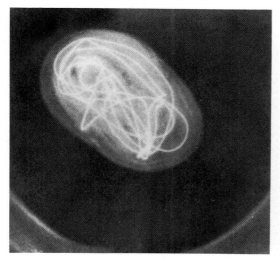

73-91

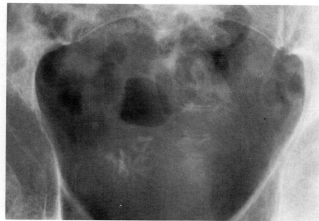

73-92

Fig. 73-91. Bladder calcification about a foreign body. A wire self-inserted into the urethra while under the influence of drugs served as the nidus of this bladder calculus. The peripheral laminations suggest a secondary infectious component. (Banner MT, Pollack HM: Urolithiasis in the lower urinary tract. Semin Roentgenol 17:140–148, 1982)

Fig. 73-92. Bladder calcification about a foreign body. Multiple serpiginous calcifications within the bladder represent incrustation of pubic hairs acting as intravesical foreign bodies. The patient was a traumatic paraplegic with reflex neurogenic bladder. (Amendola MA, Sonda LP, Diokno AC et al: Bladder calculi complicating intermittent clean catheterization. AJR 141:751–753, 1983. Copyright 1983. Reproduced with permission)

Fig. 73-93. Bladder stones.

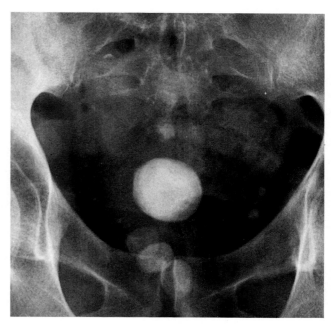

73-93

tion can develop about a foreign body, which most commonly is an object self-introduced transurethrally (Fig. 73-91). Bone fragments from a previous pelvic fracture with penetration of the bladder wall, nonabsorbable suture material used during prior pelvic surgery, prostatic chips, Foley catheter balloon fragments, and pubic hairs inadvertently introduced into the bladder during intermittent catheterization for neurogenic bladder dysfunction (Fig. 73-92) have all been reported to serve as a nidus for calcium encrustation.

Several entities simulate bladder wall calcification radiographically. Deposition of calcium salts around the balloon of an indwelling Foley catheter can mimic a calcified bladder tumor. Calcification in the prostate, a pelvic hydatid cyst, and the pelvic peritoneum (visualized after radiation therapy) have been reported to simulate bladder wall calcification.

Bladder calculi can result from upper urinary tract stones that migrate down the ureter and are occasionally retained in the bladder (migrant cal-

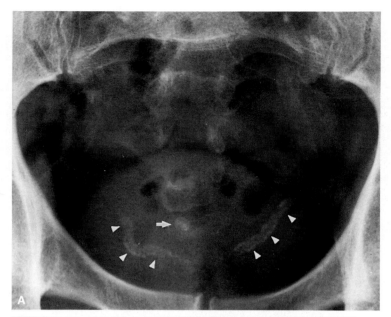

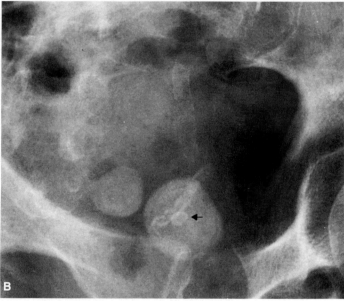

Fig. 73-94. Evolution of bladder stones. **(A)** A tiny bladder stone is evident **(arrow)**. Of incidental note is calcification in the vas deferens **(arrowheads)** in this patient who was diabetic. **(B)** A large bladder calculus has developed around the previous nidus **(arrow)**. A second bladder stone can also be seen.

culi). Stone formation in the bladder almost always occurs in elderly men with obstruction or infection of the lower urinary tract (Fig. 73-93). Frequently associated lesions include bladder outlet obstruction, urethral strictures, neurogenic bladder, bladder diverticula, and cystoceles.

Bladder calculi can be single or multiple. They vary in size from tiny concretions (Fig. 73-94), each the size of a grain of sand, to an enormous single calculus occupying the entire bladder lumen (Fig.

73-95). When located in a bladder diverticulum, calculi are occasionally identified in an unusual position close to the lateral pelvic wall.

Most bladder calculi are circular or oval in outline; however, almost any shape can be encountered. They can be amorphous, laminated, or even spiculated. One unusual type with a characteristic radiographic appearance is the hard burr or jackstone variety, which gets its name from the many irregular prongs that project from its surface (Fig.

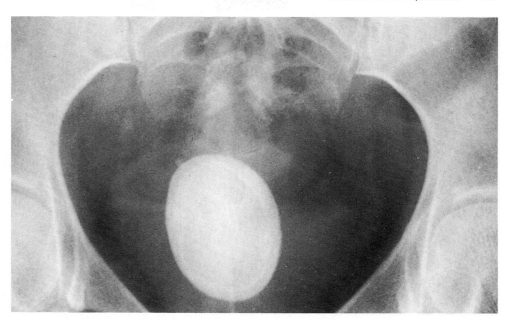

Fig. 73-95. *Single huge, laminated, calcified bladder stone.*

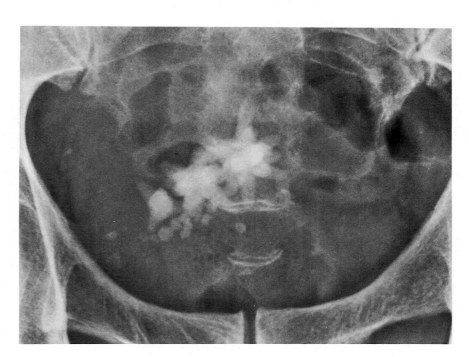

Fig. 73-96. Jackburr stone.

73-96). Dumbbell-shaped stones, with one end lodged in a diverticulum and the other projecting into the bladder, are not uncommon.

Small bladder calculi may be confused with phleboliths and thus not detected radiographically. To make this distinction, it is important to observe the radiolucent perivesical fat stripe covering much of the bladder dome on plain radiographs. If a calcific density projects within the limits of the bladder as determined from the stripe, a bladder calculus should be suspected. Oblique projections prior to bladder opacification can show whether the density in question is located anteriorly in the pelvis, as in the bladder, or posteriorly behind the bladder, as with a phlebolith. Definitive radiographic diagnosis, however, requires contrast cystography.

Urethral calculi are easily recognized because of their unique location in the subpubic angle of the

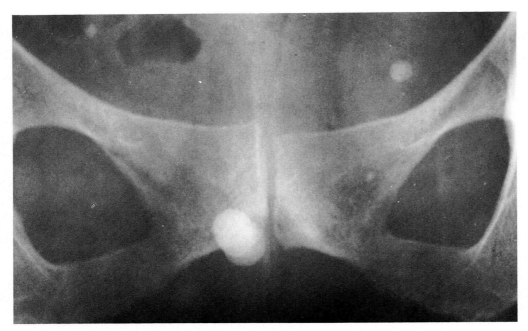

Fig. 73-97. *Calcified calculi within a urethral diverticulum. The stones are in a characteristic location in the subpubic angle of the pelvis close to the midline.*

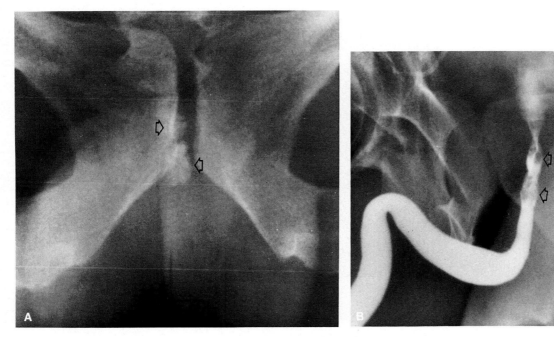

Fig. 73-98. *Urethral calculi.* **(A)** *Plain radiograph and* **(B)** *urethrogram show two stones* **(arrows)** *within the proximal urethra.*

pelvis at or close to the midline (Fig. 73-97). In men, they occur in the prostatic or bulbous urethra, usually proximal to an obstruction (Fig. 73-98). In women, urethral calculi are almost always associated with diverticula and infection (Fig. 73-99). Rarely, urethral stones may represent migrant calculi that originated in the kidney or bladder and descended into the urethra (Fig. 73-100).

A solitary urachal calculus can appear as an oval or dumbbell-shaped opacity that lies at or close to the midline of the upper pelvis and is superimposed on the sacrum. On lateral projections, a urachal calculus is readily distinguished by its extreme anterior position; on cystograms, the superior portion of the bladder is pear-shaped and points upward toward the stone.

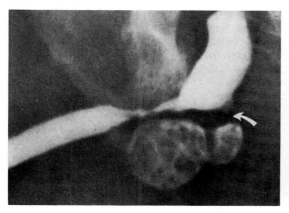

73-99

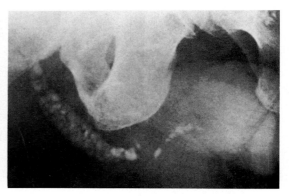

73-100

Fig. 73-99. Calculi in a urethral diverticulum. Note the narrow neck of the diverticulum **(arrow)** and the adjacent urethral narrowing, probably postinflammatory. The diverticulum may have originated as a periurethral abscess secondary to urethral stricture disease, although no corroborative history was obtained from the patient. (Banner MT, Pollack HM: Urolithiasis in the lower urinary tract. Semin Roentgenol 17:140–148, 1982)

Fig. 73-100. Urethral calculi. Multiple stones of varying size related to a bladder calculus that was crushed cystoscopically without the fragments being removed. This radiograph was obtained when the patient voided the stone fragments on the day following cystolitholapaxy. (Banner MT, Pollack HM: Urolithiasis in the lower urinary tract. Semin Roentgenol 17:140–148, 1982)

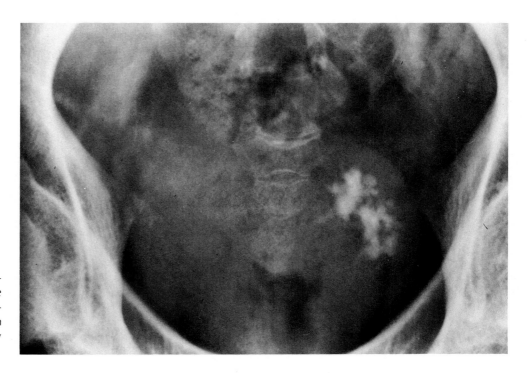

Fig. 73-101. Calcified transitional cell carcinoma of the bladder. Coarse tumor calcification was associated with an intravesical mass on excretory urography.

Although histologic calcification commonly occurs in bladder tumors, individual calcium deposits are generally too small to be appreciated radiographically. When visualized, however, calcification associated with a mass in the bladder usually indicates the presence of a bladder neoplasm (Fig. 73-101). Tumor calcification can be punctate, coarse, or linear. The calcium is usually encrusted on the surface of the tumor but occasionally lies within it. Calcification is most common in epithelial lesions (transitional cell and squamous cell carcinomas) but can also be seen in mesenchymal tumors, such as leiomyosarcoma, hemangioma, neuroblastoma, and osteogenic sarcoma.

CALCIFICATION IN THE MALE GENITAL TRACT

Vas deferens
  Diabetes mellitus
  Tuberculosis
  Degenerative change
Seminal vesicle
Prostate
  Calculi
  Tuberculosis
Scrotum
Penile implant

Calcification of the vas deferens is usually seen in male patients with diabetes mellitus (Fig. 73-102; see also Fig. 73-94). It occasionally also occurs in nondiabetics, in whom it most likely represents a degenerative phenomenon. In diabetics, calcification of the vas deferens characteristically produces bilaterally symmetric parallel tubular densities that run medially and caudally to enter the medial aspect of the seminal vesicles at the base of the prostate. The calcification is located in the muscular outer layers of the wall of the vas deferens and therefore has an appearance similar to the calcification seen in a medium-sized arteriosclerotic artery. In contrast, vas deferens calcification associated with chronic inflammatory diseases, such as tuberculosis, syphilis, and nonspecific urinary tract infec-

tion, is largely intraluminal and produces an irregular pattern of calcification.

Calcium deposition in the seminal vesicles can appear as multiple small concretions near the proximal end of the vas deferens (Fig. 73-103). These calcifications are associated with seminal vesiculitis primarily due to *Neisserian* infections, tuberculosis, or bilharziasis and can be mistaken clinically and radiographically for ureteral calculi.

Multiple small calculi of the prostate are quite common in elderly men. They appear as tiny, discrete deposits, 2 mm to 4 mm in diameter, that extend to either side of the midline overlying or directly above the level of the symphysis pubis (Fig. 73-104). The characteristic position, small size, and multiplicity of the calcifications usually cause little difficulty in differential diagnosis; however, tuberculous calcification of the prostate gland occasionally produces a radiographically indistinguishable appearance.

Radiographically detectable calcification in the scrotum is infrequent. Calcification of the ductus deferens can occur in its intrascrotal portion, and hydroceles or spermatoceles can show curvilinear mural calcification. A dense oval collection of calcification can be due to tuberculosis of the testicle or to testicular infarction secondary to torsion (Fig. 73-105). Testicular tumors rarely show calcification. Streaky or lacelike calcification has been described in an occasional Leydig cell tumor, and fine punctate calcifications have been reported in teratoma.

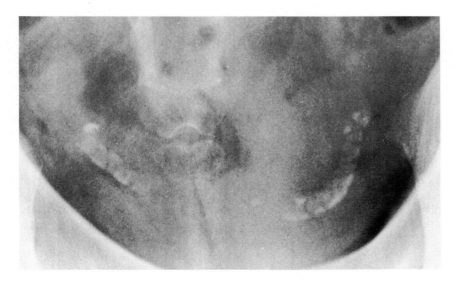

Fig. 73-102. Calcification of the vas deferens in a man with diabetes mellitus.

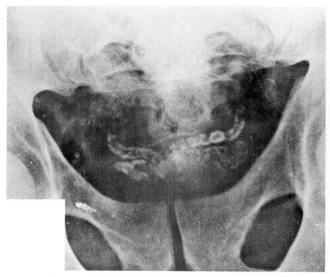

73-103

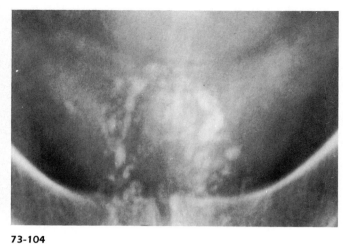

73-104

Fig. 73-103. Calcification of the seminal vesicles and vas deferens in a nondiabetic. (Ney C, Friedenberg RM: Radiographic Atlas of the Genitourinary System, 2nd ed. Philadelphia, JB Lippincott, 1981)

Fig. 73-104. Prostatic calculi.

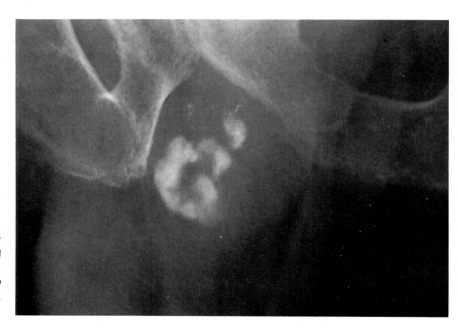

Fig. 73-105. Testicular calcification. The clumps of dense, amorphous calcification presumably developed following infarction secondary to testicular torsion. (Baker SR, Elkin M: Plain Film Approach to Abdominal Calcifications. Philadelphia, WB Saunders, 1983)

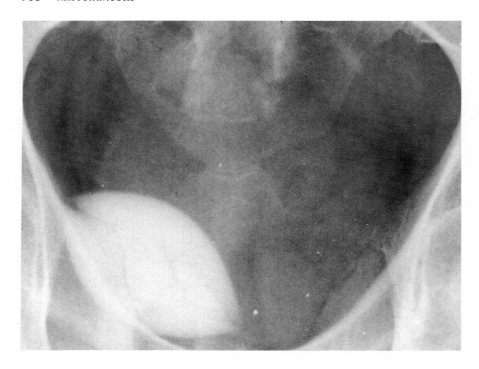

Fig. 73-106. Penile implant.

A penile implant can appear as a large opacification on a radiograph of the pelvis (Fig. 73-106).

CALCIFICATION IN THE FEMALE GENITAL TRACT

Uterine calcification
    Fibroid (leiomyoma)
Ovarian calcification
    Dermoid cyst
    Cystadenoma
    Cystadenocarcinoma (psammomatous bodies)
    Gonadoblastoma
    Spontaneous amputation of an ovary
Pseudomyxoma peritonei (pseudomucinous
      carcinoma of the ovary)
Calcification in the fallopian tubes
    Tuberculous salpingitis
    Fallopian tube occlusion rings
Placental calcification
Fetal skull/skeleton
Lithopedion
Complication of parametrial gold therapy

Uterine fibroids (leiomyomas) are by far the most common calcified lesions of the female genital tract. These frequently multiple tumors have a characteristic mottled or "mulberry" type of calcification and present as nodules with a stippled or whorled appearance (Fig. 73-107). A very large calcified fibroid occasionally occupies the entire pelvis or even extends out of the pelvis (Fig. 73-108).

About half of all ovarian dermoid cysts contain some calcification (Fig. 73-109). This is usually in the form of a partially or completely formed tooth that is extremely dense compared with other types of concretions (Fig. 73-110). Less frequently, the wall of the cyst is partially calcified. The characteristic calcification combined with the relative radiolucency of the lipid material within the lesion are pathognomonic of an ovarian dermoid cyst.

Psammomatous bodies are small calcifications that are widely distributed within papillary cystadenomas and papillary cystadenocarcinomas of the ovary. These calcareous bodies are composed of calcium carbonate and are located in the fibrous stroma. Psammomatous calcifications appear as scattered, fine amorphous shadows that are barely denser than the normal soft tissues and can therefore be easily missed unless they are extensive (Fig.

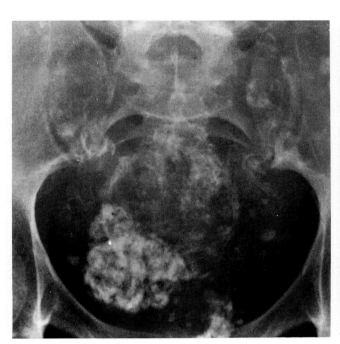

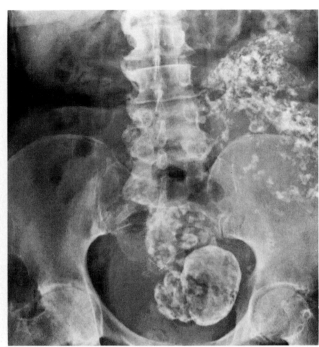

73-107

73-108

Fig. 73-107. Calcified uterine fibroid (leiomyoma). Note the characteristic stippled or whorled appearance of the calcifications.

Fig. 73-108. Calcified uterine fibroids extending far out of the confines of the pelvis.

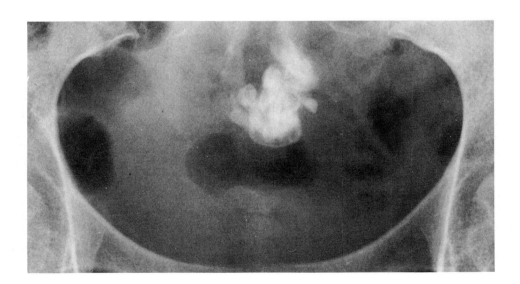

Fig. 73-109. Ovarian dermoid cyst containing a calcified mass.

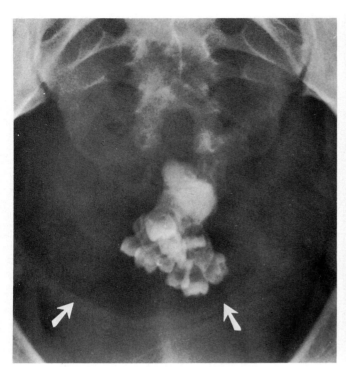

73-110

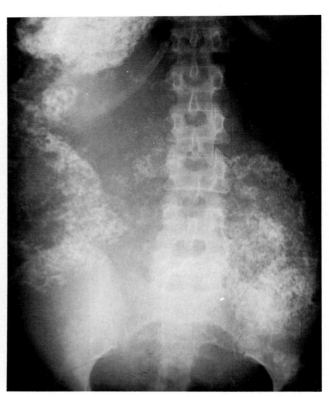

73-111

Fig. 73-110. Dermoid cyst containing multiple well-formed teeth. Note the relative lucency of the mass **(arrows)**, which is composed largely of fatty tissue.

Fig. 73-111. Psammomatous calcifications from metastatic cystadenoma of the ovary.

73-111). Infrequently, dystrophic calcification that mimics true psammomatous calcification may occur in such rare ovarian tumors as thecoma, virilizing lipid cell tumor, and Brenner tumor (Fig. 73-112).

Cystadenocarcinomas of the ovary spread widely throughout the abdomen. Their serosal and omental implants can appear as diffuse, ill-defined collections of granular amorphous calcification (Fig. 73-113). Less frequently, metastases are seen as sharply circumscribed masses of fairly homogeneous density with occasional rim calcification. Calcified metastatic deposits along the lateral abdominal wall adjacent to the peritoneal fat stripe are characteristic. Because ovarian metastases tend to be distributed along the course of the mesentery of the colon, these vague and diffuse calcifications can initially be mistaken for feces or previously ingested barium. Hemangiopericytomas, rare primary tumors of the ovary, can also demonstrate calcifications (Fig. 73-114).

Unilateral or bilateral circumscribed, mottled calcifications in the pelvis are frequently found in gonadoblastomas (Fig. 73-115). These rare, potentially malignant gonadal neoplasms are usually hormonally active and are composed of germ cells,

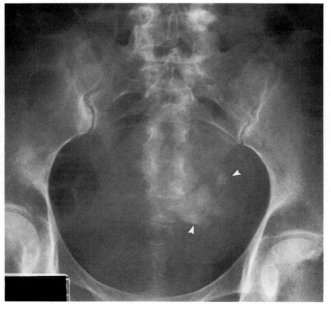

Fig. 73-112. Psammomatous calcifications in a Brenner tumor. Faint, amorphous calcification **(arrowheads)** in the left side of the pelvis (Schultz SM, Curry TS, Voet R: Psammomatous-like calcification in a Brenner tumour with a view of the ovary. Br J Radiol 59:412–414, 1986)

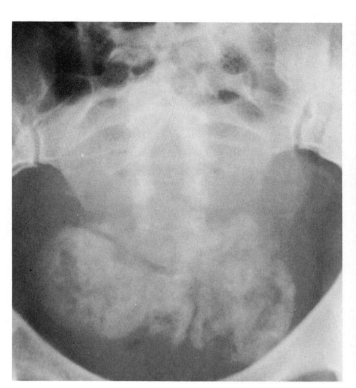

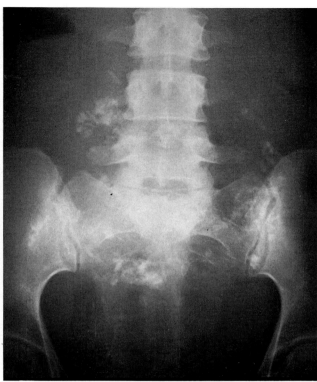

73-113   73-114

Fig. 73-113. Calcified cystadenocarcinoma of the ovary. Diffuse, ill-defined collections of granular amorphous calcification are visible.

Fig. 73-114. Calcification in a hemangiopericytoma of the ovary.

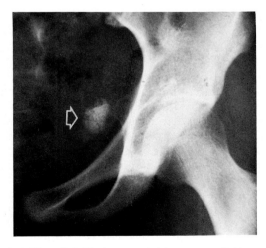

Fig. 73-115. Calcified gonadoblastoma of the ovary **(arrow)**. Note the typical circumscribed, mottled calcification in the pelvis. (Seymour EQ, Hood JB, Underwood PB et al: Gonadoblastoma: An ovarian tumor with characteristic pelvic calcifications. AJR 127:1001–1002, 1976. Copyright 1976. Reproduced with permission)

cells of sex cord origin, and, often, mesenchymal elements.

Spontaneous amputation of the ovary is presumably the result of torsion of the adnexa with subsequent infarction because of disruption of its blood supply. Although usually characterized by acute abdominal signs, subclinical spontaneous ovarian amputation can lead to the development of a small, coarsely stippled calcified mass in the pelvis that moves on serial films and when the patient's position is changed (Fig. 73-116). This typical radiographic appearance, combined with ultrasound or computed tomographic evidence of a missing ovary on one side, precludes the need for surgical confirmation.

Curvilinear calcifications may develop in the periphery of the jellylike masses that are secondary to pseudomyxoma peritonei (Fig. 73-117). This condition is a complication of spontaneous or surgical rupture of pseudomucinous carcinoma of the ovary. Deposition of tumor cells throughout the mesentery and serosa of the bowel incites a foreign-body type

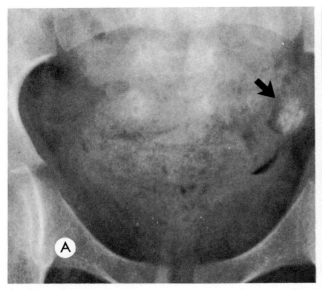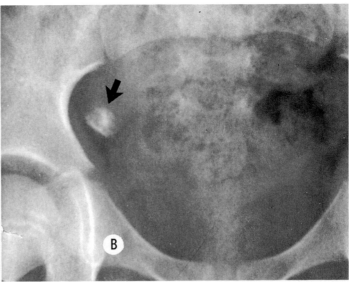

Fig. 73-116. Amputated ovary. **(A)** A plain radiograph of the pelvis shows a calcification **(arrow)** in the left lower abdomen. **(B)** A repeat film obtained 10 days later shows migration of the calcification **(arrow)** to the right. (Nixon GW, Condon VR: Amputated ovary: A cause of migratory abdominal calcification. AJR 128:1053–1057, 1977. Copyright 1977. Reproduced with permission)

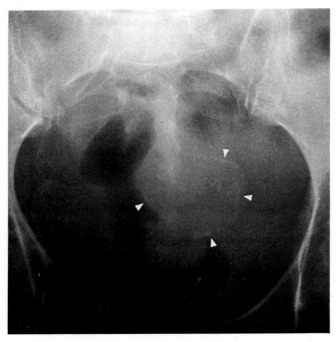

Fig. 73-117. *Pseudomyxoma peritonei. Curvilinear calcifications* **(arrowheads)** *develop at the periphery of the jellylike masses, which are a complication of spontaneous rupture of pseudomucinous carcinoma of the ovary.*

of peritonitis with thickening, fibrosis, and calcification.

Tuberculous salpingitis can produce a "string-of-pearls" calcification bilaterally within the pelvis. Tuberculous involvement causes the fallopian tubes to have an irregular contour, a small lumen, and multiple strictures.

Fallopian tube occlusion rings for sterilization may be associated with persistent or intermittent pelvic pain. The rings are coated with a barium compound and appear radiographically as circular opacifications with central lucent areas (Fig. 73-118A). Foreshortening of the ring may obscure the central lucency (Fig. 73-118B). Fallopian tube occlusion rings must be distinguished from ureteral calculi, which rarely have central lucencies and are located more laterally, and pelvic phleboliths, which often have central lucencies but infrequently have as regular contours or bilateral symmetry.

Placental calcification is a physiological phenomenon associated with involution of the placenta, which usually occurs after the 32nd week of fetal life. The calcification typically has a fine lace-like pattern, best seen in the lateral projection, that outlines the crescentic shape of the placenta and is 15 cm to 20 cm in length and about 3 cm in average thickness. Because the deposition of calcium is

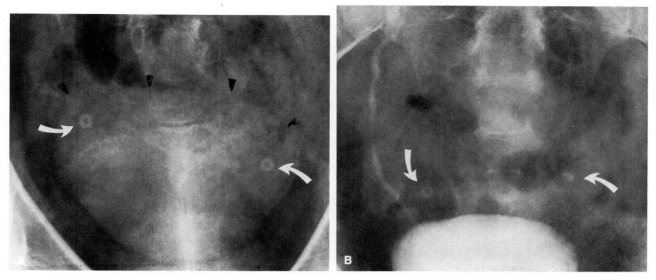

Fig. 73-118. Fallopian tube occlusion rings. **(A)** Plain film of the pelvis in a woman with recurrent urinary tract infections shows bilateral ringlike densities **(arrows)** within the true pelvis craniad to the bladder. A central pelvic mass **(arrowheads)** extends beyond these bilateral fallopian tube occlusion rings. Their densities are similar to those of phleboliths or ureteral calculi. As in this patient, recognition of occlusion rings is most often an incidental observation. **(B)** This excretory urogram of a woman with nonradiating sharp right lower quadrant pain was obtained after a radiograph showed bilateral rounded pelvic densities "possibly representing ureteral calculi." Both fallopian tube occlusion rings **(arrows)** appear medial to the ureters. The ring on the left is foreshortened, obscuring the central lucency. Recognition of the ringlike pelvic densities as occlusion rings might have precluded the need to obtain a urogram as the clinical findings were atypical for ureteral colic. (Spring DB: Fallopian tube occlusion rings: A consideration in the differential diagnosis of ureteral calculi. Radiology 145:51–52, 1982)

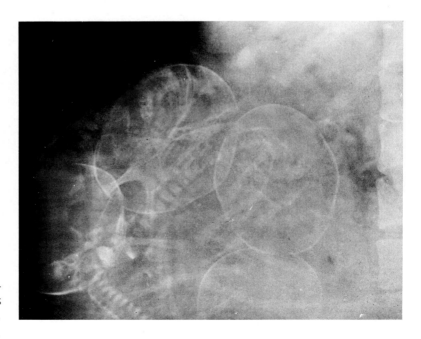

Fig. 73-119. Multiple pregnancies. Lateral abdominal radiograph of a woman with quadruplets clearly shows four separate fetal skulls and spines.

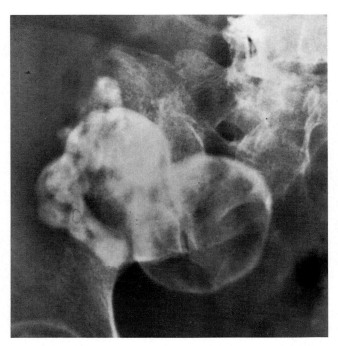

Fig. 73-120. Lithopedion. This calcified fetus was seen in a 78-year-old woman.

greatest at the periphery of the cotyledons, the outer margin of the placenta is delineated.

Plain radiographs of the abdomen in a pregnant woman may show calcification of the fetal skull and skeleton (Fig. 73-119). Although infrequently seen, a lithopedion is easily diagnosed by recognition of fetal skeletal parts in the area of calcification (Fig. 73-120). The lesion can be intrauterine, from an old missed abortion, or extrauterine, from a previous ectopic pregnancy.

Bilateral laminated calcifications that closely approximate the lateral pelvic wall have been reported as a specific complication in patients treated with parametrial injections of ^{198}Au colloid (Fig. 73-121). This radionuclide was formerly used as an adjunct to surgery and radium therapy in the treatment of the lateral parametrium and lymph node drainage of carcinoma of the cervix. Excessive complications and the introduction of supervoltage treatment forced this mode of therapy to be discontinued. The calcification in this condition appears within 5 years of treatment, is gradually progressive, and varies from thin and linear to thick and globular. Multiple short, thin metallic densities can be identified in patients treated with gold seed implants for pelvic malignancy (Fig. 73-122).

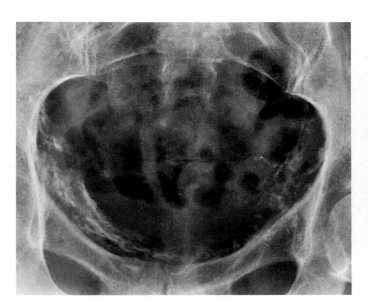

73-121

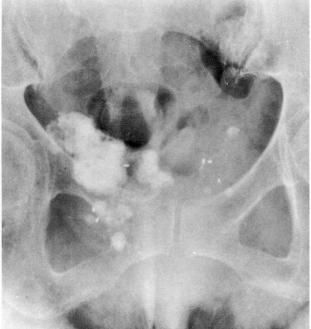

73-122

Fig. 73-121. Parametrial calcification in a patient with cervical carcinoma treated with radioactive gold. (Deeths TM, Stanley RJ: Parametrial calcification in cervical carcinoma patients treated with radioactive gold. AJR 127:511–513, 1976. Copyright 1976. Reproduced with permission)

Fig. 73-122. Gold seed implants in a patient treated for transitional carcinoma of the bladder. Note the multiple short, thin metallic densities.

ADRENAL CALCIFICATION

Neonatal hemorrhage
Tuberculosis (Addison's disease)
Adrenal cyst
Adrenal cortical carcinoma
Miscellaneous neoplasms
    Pheochromocytoma
    Adrenal cortical adenoma
    Adrenal choristoma (myelolipoma)
    Metastatic melanoma
Wolman's disease

Calcification in the adrenal gland is most commonly associated with neonatal adrenal hemorrhage. This condition often occurs in infants born to diabetic mothers and in infants with an abnormal obstetric history (prematurity, use of forceps, breech delivery). Calcification develops rapidly around the periphery of the adrenal within a few weeks of the hemorrhage (Fig. 73-123). It then contracts slowly to the size and triangular shape of the original gland. Neonatal adrenal hemorrhage can rarely produce calcification that is radiographically apparent at birth, presumably the result of severe intrauterine stress. In adults who escaped early detection of neonatal adrenal hemorrhage, the calcifications can be an incidental finding on abdominal radiographs.

About one-fourth of all patients with adrenal tuberculosis (Addison's disease) have radiographic evidence of calcification of the gland (Fig. 73-124).

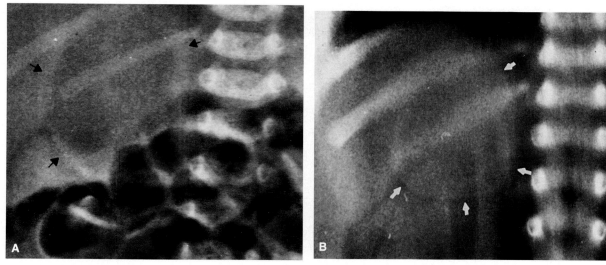

Fig. 73-123. Neonatal adrenal hemorrhage. **(A)** Excretory urogram in a 6-day-old infant demonstrates a lucent mass with a dense vascular rim, flattening and depressing the right kidney. **(B)** Three weeks later, a plain film tomogram of the right upper quadrant shows a calcified rim **(arrows)** in the identical position as the vascular rim on the previous excretory urogram. (Brill PW, Krasna IH, Aaron H: An early rim sign in neonatal adrenal hemorrhage. AJR 127:289–291, 1976. Copyright 1976. Reproduced with permission)

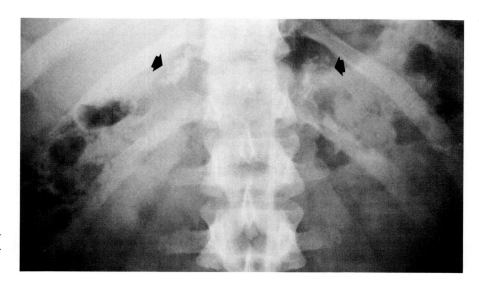

Fig. 73-124. Bilateral adrenal calcifications **(arrows)** in a patient with Addison's disease.

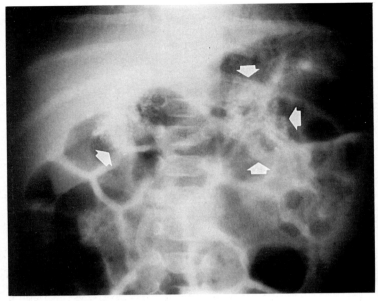

73-125

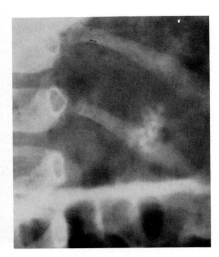

73-126

Fig. 73-125. Wolman's disease. Diffuse punctate calcifications in bilaterally enlarged adrenal glands **(arrows)**. (Eisenberg RL: Clinical Imaging: An Atlas of Differential Diagnosis. Rockville, Aspen, 1988)

Fig. 73-126. Calcification in a Wilms' tumor **(arrowheads)**.

These calcifications are typically discrete, stippled densities that often outline the entire adrenal gland. Less frequently, they present as confluent and dense calcific masses or as a homogeneous increase in density of the gland.

A thin rim of curvilinear calcification can outline the wall of an adrenal cyst. Benign adrenal cystic lesions can be serous cysts arising from lymphatic structures, pseudocysts due to necrosis and resolution of an old hemorrhage, parasitic (usually echinococcal) cysts, or cystic adenomas.

Calcification is fairly common in adrenal cortical carcinomas. These tumors usually calcify in a mottled fashion with scattered calcific densities throughout the mass, unlike adrenal cysts, which show a peripheral rim of calcification. Scattered tiny flecks of calcification are seen in a small number of pheochromocytomas. About 10% of these tumors are multiple, and a similar number arise outside the adrenal areas, primarily in retroperitoneal ganglia. Rarely, calcification can be demonstrated in benign adrenal cortical adenomas and adrenal choristomas (small masses of bone marrow elements and fat); one case has been reported of calcification in metastatic melanoma involving the adrenal. Diffuse punctate calcifications throughout enlarged, normally shaped adrenal glands are characteristic of Wolman's disease, a rare familial xanthomatosis that causes death in early infancy (Fig. 73-125).

RETROPERITONEAL CALCIFICATION

> Neoplasms
> > Wilms' tumor
> > Neuroblastoma
> > Teratoma
> > Cavernous hemangioma
> Hematoma
> Tuberculous psoas abscess
> Hydatid cyst
> Fat necrosis in pancreatitis

Wilms' tumor is the most common abdominal neoplasm of infancy and childhood. The lesion arises from embryonic renal tissue and tends to become very large. Calcification occurs in about 10% of Wilms' tumors and is usually peripheral and cystic in appearance (Fig. 73-126). Wilms' tumors often metastasize to the lungs and para-aortic lymph nodes, as well as extending locally by direct invasion, but calcification in metastases is extremely rare.

Neuroblastoma, a tumor of adrenal medullary origin, is the second most common malignancy in

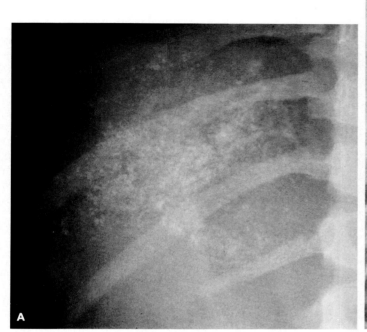
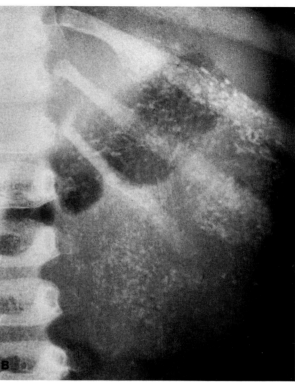

Fig. 73-127. Neuroblastoma. Diffuse amorphous calcification in large masses in the **(A)** right and **(B)** left upper quadrants.

children. About 10% arise outside of the adrenal gland, primarily in sympathetic ganglia. The tumor is highly malignant and can attain great size before detection. Calcification in a neuroblastoma is common (occurring in about 50% of all cases), in contrast to the relatively infrequent calcification in Wilms' tumor, from which a neuroblastoma must be differentiated. The calcification in a neuroblastoma has a fine granular or stippled appearance (Fig. 73-127); occasionally, there is a single mass of amorphous calcification.

Retroperitoneal teratomas are less common than either Wilms' tumor or neuroblastoma. The tumor is almost always discovered in infancy and is generally located in the upper abdomen near the midline. Most teratomas have visible calcified spicules of cartilage or bone. Teeth inclusions, pseudodigits, or pseudolimbs may be identified. Retroperitoneal cavernous hemangiomas in children can appear as large masses containing multiple phleboliths in unusual locations.

Retroperitoneal hematomas, hydatid cysts, and tuberculous psoas abscesses can calcify. However calcification in retroperitoneal tumors in adults is extremely rare. Bilateral calcification of the anterior and posterior pararenal spaces may result from extensive enzymatic fat necrosis in a patient with pancreatitis.

GENERALIZED ABDOMINAL CALCIFICATION

> Psammomatous calcification (cystadeno-
> carcinoma of the ovary)
> Pseudomyxoma peritonei
> Pseudomucinous cystadenoma of the ovary
> Mucocele of the appendix
> Undifferentiated abdominal malignancy
> Tuberculous peritonitis
> Oil granulomas
> Meconium peritonitis

Several diverse conditions can result in widespread abdominal calcifications. The granular or sandlike psammomatous calcification of ovarian cystadenocarcinoma can be confined to the primary tumor or diffusely involve metastases throughout the abdo-

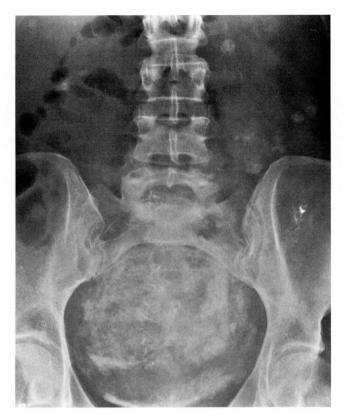

Fig. 73-128. Psammomatous calcification of ovarian cystadenocarcinoma. The granular, sandlike calcifications represent metastatic spread throughout the abdomen.

men (Fig. 73-128). Pseudomyxoma peritonei, usually caused by rupture of pseudomucinous cystadenoma of the ovary or mucocele of the appendix, can cause widespread abdominal calcifications that are annular in appearance and tend to be most numerous in the pelvis (see Fig. 73-117). Single cases have been reported of pseudomyxoma peritonei associated with carcinomas of the bowel, uterus, urachus, stomach, and pancreas, as well as mucoid omphalomesenteric cyst of the umbilicus. On CT and ultrasound, findings suggestive of pseudomyxoma peritonei are peritoneal scalloping of the liver margin and ascitic septation (Fig. 73-129). Scalloping refers to extrinsic pressure on the border of the liver by adjacent peritoneal implants without liver parenchymal metastases. Septation refers to the margins of mucinous nodules of low-attenuation material in what otherwise would appear to be ascites.

Bizarre masses of calcification that do not conform to any organ have been described in undifferentiated abdominal malignancies (Fig. 73-130). Patients with this condition have large soft-tissue masses with multiple linear or nodular calcific densities that can coalesce to form distinctive conglomerate masses.

Tuberculous peritonitis of long duration occasionally produces widespread abdominal calcifications. These calcifications are mottled and often

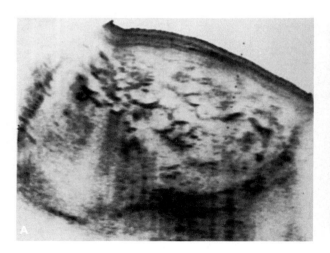
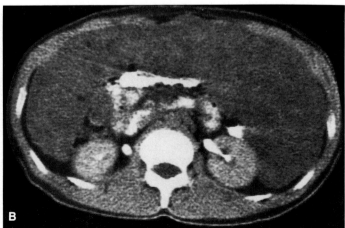

Fig. 73-129. Pseudomyxoma peritonei. **(A)** Sagittal sonogram demonstrates multiple septations throughout the peritoneal cavity. **(B)** CT scan shows diffuse epithelial implants and gelatinous ascites filling the abdomen. Note the posterior displacement of contrast-filled bowel. (Seshul MB, Coulam CM: Pseudomyxoma peritonei: Computed tomography and sonography. AJR 136:803–806, 1981. Copyright 1981. Reproduced with permission)

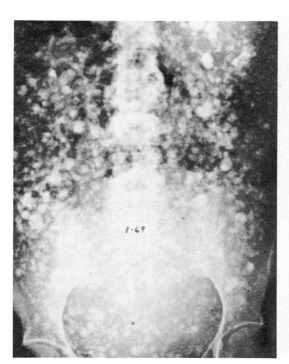

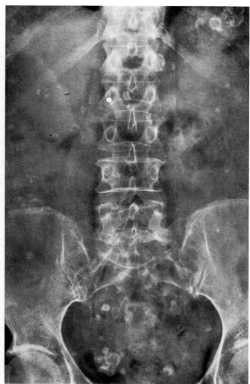

73-130   **73-131**

Fig. 73-130. Bizarre masses of calcification not conforming to any organ in a patient with an undifferentiated abdominal malignancy. (Dalinka MK, Lally JF, Azimi F et al: Calcification in undifferentiated abdominal malignancies. Clin Radiol 26:115–119, 1975)

Fig. 73-131. Intraperitoneal granulomatosis. The patient was treated with intraperitoneal mineral oil many years previously in an attempt to prevent the formation of abdominal adhesions.

simulate residual barium in the gastrointestinal tract. Thick masses of sheetlike calcification may also occur, often in association with dense calcification in mesenteric lymph nodes.

Oil granulomas, which can occur as a late effect of the instillation of liquid petrolatum into the peritoneal cavity to prevent adhesions, occasionally result in widespread annular or plaquelike deposits simulating pseudomyxoma peritonei (Fig. 73-131). The calcifications are located in masses of fibrous tissue surrounding the oil droplets. Clinically, oil granulomas can produce hard palpable masses that simulate carcinomatosis or cause intestinal obstruction.

Multiple small calcific deposits scattered widely throughout the abdomen in the newborn can represent meconium peritonitis (Fig. 73-132). This condition is a chemical inflammation of the peritoneum caused by the escape of sterile meconium into the peritoneal cavity. Meconium peritonitis usually results from perforation *in utero* secondary to a congenital stenosis or atresia of the bowel or to meconium ileus.

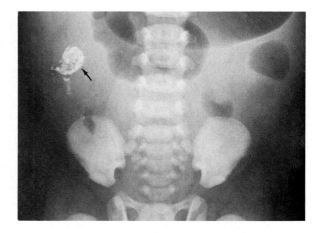

Fig. 73-132. Calcifying meconium peritonitis. Plain abdominal radiograph in an 18-day-old infant in whom signs of intestinal obstruction developed weeks after birth shows the calciferous meconium collected in a single large cluster **(arrow)** in the right side of the abdomen. The gas column in the alimentary tract is cut off in a fashion indicative of complete obstruction high in the small intestine. (Silverman SN: Caffey's Pediatric X-Ray Imaging. Chicago, Year Book, 1985)

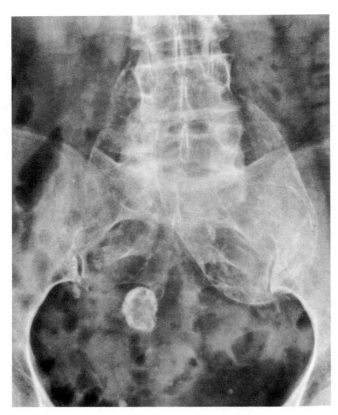

Fig. 73-133. Calcified atheromatous plaques in the walls of aneurysms of the lower abdominal aorta and both common iliac arteries.

CALCIFICATION IN VASCULAR STRUCTURES

Arteries
Veins
    Phleboliths
    Portal vein
Lymph nodes
    Chronic granulomatous disease
    Metastases
    Residual lymphographic contrast
    Silicosis
    Hemosiderin deposition

Calcification of atheromatous plaques in the walls of large abdominal arteries is a frequent observation in radiographs of middle-aged and elderly patients (Fig. 73-133). Similar calcification can also be seen in young persons, especially those suffering from diabetes. The aorta, splenic artery, and iliac artery are most frequently calcified. Arterial calcification is seen as irregular plaquelike areas that vary in size from small flecks to parallel lines several centimeters in length. The amount of visible calcification bears no relationship to the severity of vascular occlusion; complete obstruction can exist with no detectable calcification.

The calcified splenic artery typically is tortuous (see Fig. 73-30) and, when viewed end-on, appears as a thin-walled ring in the left upper quadrant.

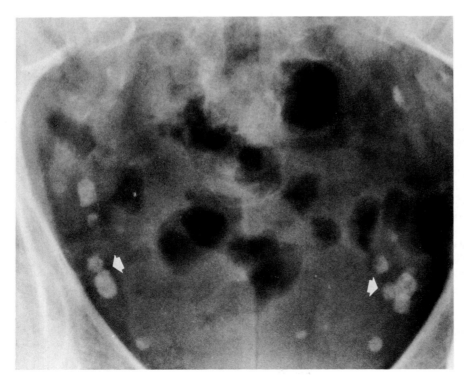

Fig. 73-134. Phleboliths. Note the characteristic position of these calcified venous thrombi **(arrows)** along the lateral walls of the pelvis.

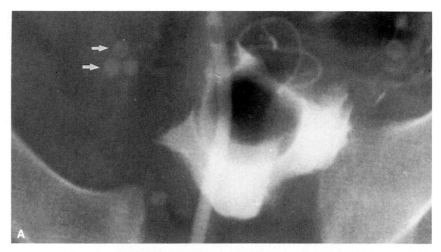

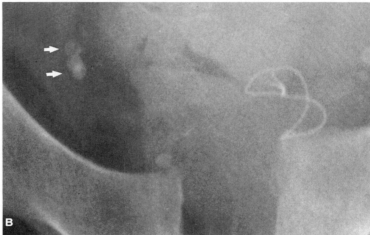

Fig. 73-135. Phlebolith displacement sign. **(A)** Three phleboliths **(arrows)** are displaced medially by a right pelvic hematoma secondary to trauma. Note the diastasis of the symphysis pubis. **(B)** Three weeks later, the hematoma is resolving, and the phleboliths have migrated laterally. In addition, the phleboliths are now arrayed linearly. (Baker SR, Elkin M: Plain Film Approach to Abdominal Calcifications. Philadelphia, WB Saunders, 1983)

Fragmentary calcification of an iliac artery just below the sacroiliac joint can be mistaken for a ureteral calculus.

A phlebolith is a calcified thrombus within a vein. Phleboliths are most frequently found along the lateral aspect of the pelvis; almost all adults have at least a few of them (Fig. 73-134). These calcifications are round or slightly oval in shape and vary in size from very tiny densities to opacifications of 0.5 cm or more in diameter. They can be of homogeneous density, be laminated, or have the characteristic ringlike appearance of a lucent center and dense periphery. The detection of many of these small, rounded rings of calcification in a localized area suggests the possibility of multiple phleboliths in a hemangioma.

Careful attention to the position of phleboliths may aid in determining the presence of a pelvic mass (Fig. 73-135). Enlargement of the bladder may cause slight inferior and lateral displacement of phleboliths situated in perivesical veins. Rectal distention may occasionally cause lateral deviation of perirectal phleboliths, whereas pelvic hematomas may displace phleboliths medially. Neoplastic masses may cause more marked phlebolith dis-

placement; indeed, the movement of phleboliths may be all that is necessary to monitor the growth or shrinkage of tumors.

In patients with symptoms of ureteral colic, a phlebolith can be confused with a calculus in the distal ureter. Unlike a smooth, rounded phlebolith, a ureteral calculus is often irregular in shape and, if elliptical, has its long axis lying parallel to that of the ureter. Ureteral calculi are seldom found below the level of the ischial spines; in contrast, phleboliths usually occupy positions below the interspinous line.

Calcification in the portal vein is a rare radiographic finding, occurring almost always in patients with portal hypertension (see Figs. 73-16, 73-17). The calcium may be deposited in a thrombus or, more rarely, in the wall of the vein. Portal vein calcification has also been described in children with multiple anomalies or sepsis and in adults with cavernous transformation of the portal vein secondary to portal thrombosis of long duration.

Calcification of mesenteric and paravascular (aorta, iliac arteries) lymph nodes represents the effects of previous infection, usually histoplasmosis but occasionally tuberculosis or other chronic

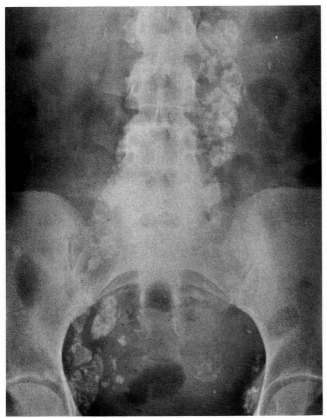

Fig. 73-136. Diffuse calcification of lymph nodes lying along the course of the aorta and iliac arteries.

granulomatous disease (Fig. 73-136). This calcification is most frequently detected in the right lower quadrant or in the lower central part of the abdomen; it can occasionally be found to the left of the midline. A calcified mesenteric lymph node appears as a mottled density seldom more than 1 cm to 1.5 cm in diameter. Clusters of two or more nodes are often seen. A characteristic feature of calcified mesenteric lymph nodes is their movement over a fairly wide area on serial radiographs and on films made with the patient in different positions (supine and upright).

Lymph node calcification may be caused by tumor infiltration (Fig. 73-137), most commonly metastatic adenocarcinoma of the colon or serous cystadenocarcinoma of the ovary. Calcified metastatic nodes tend to be larger than those involved with granulomatous disease because of enlargement of the node by tumor. Following chemotherapy or radiation therapy, calcification may develop in lymph nodes infiltrated by Hodgkin's lymphoma or cervical cancer.

Residual contrast from a prior lymphogram can be demonstrated in para-aortic and pelvic lymph nodes. Serial radiographs demonstrating displacement of the opacified nodes can be a subtle sign of an expanding or recurrent neoplasm.

Eggshell calcific deposits accompanying similar lesions in the thoracic nodes have been reported

in the lymph nodes of the para-aortic and subdiaphragmatic areas in two patients with silicosis. Increased deposition of hemosiderin can sometimes be detected on plain films as faint opacities in para-aortic nodes. Patients with thalassemia who have received multiple blood transfusions over many years may have enlarged lymph nodes that are slightly more dense than the surrounding soft tissues.

ABDOMINAL WALL CALCIFICATION

> Skin
>> Soft-tissue nodules
>> Scars
>> Tattoo markings
>> Colostomy/ileostomy stomas
> Muscle
>> Parasites
>>> Cysticercosis (pork tapeworm)
>>> Guinea worm
>> Injection sites
>>> Quinine
>>> Bismuth
>>> Calcium gluconate
>>> Calcium penicillin
>> Myositis ossificans
> Soft tissue
>> Hypercalcemic states
>> Idiopathic calcinosis

Skin lesions on the abdominal wall (papillomas, neurofibromas, melanomas, nevi) can simulate intra-abdominal calcifications (Fig. 73-138). In most cases, however, these skin lesions appear as soft-tissue rather than calcific densities. Simple inspection of the patient is sufficient to eliminate any diagnostic difficulty. Calcification or ossification of old abdominal surgical scars can produce linear densities (Fig. 73-139). Tattoo markings and colostomy and ileostomy stomas sometimes present puzzling radiographic patterns.

Although most extravisceral calcifications secondary to parasitic infestation are found in the soft tissues of the extremities, lesions in the muscles of the buttocks and anterior abdominal wall are occasionally detected on plain abdominal radiographs. In cysticercosis, the encysted larvae of the pork tapeworm (*Taenia solium*) can appear as round or slightly elongated calcified masses of varying size that are distributed throughout the muscles and tend to follow muscle planes (Fig. 73-140). The pig is the intermediate host of this worm; human infection occurs from the ingestion of raw or undercooked pork. Infestation by guinea worms (*Dracunculiasis*) can present as stringlike calcifications up to 12 cm long in the perineum and lower abdominal wall (Fig. 73-141).

Discrete rounded or irregular calcifications of varying size in the gluteal areas can follow intramus-

Text continues on page 1005

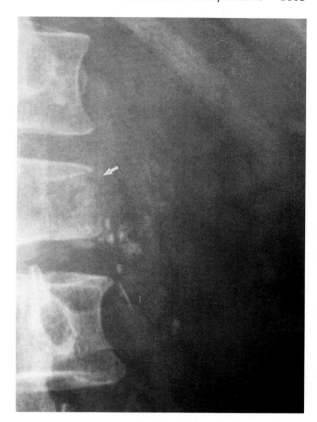

Fig. 73-137. Lymph node calcification caused by tumor infiltration. Ill-defined opacification of para-aortic lymph nodes secondary to metastases from oat cell carcinoma of the lung. Note the bone destruction **(arrow)** caused by osseous metastases. (Baker SR, Elkin M: Plain Film Approach to Abdominal Calcifications. Philadelphia, WB Saunders, 1983)

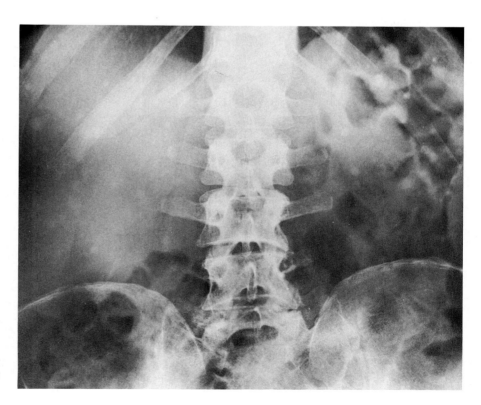

Fig. 73-138. Neurofibromatosis. The multiple nodular densities projected over the abdomen are actually skin lesions on the abdominal wall.

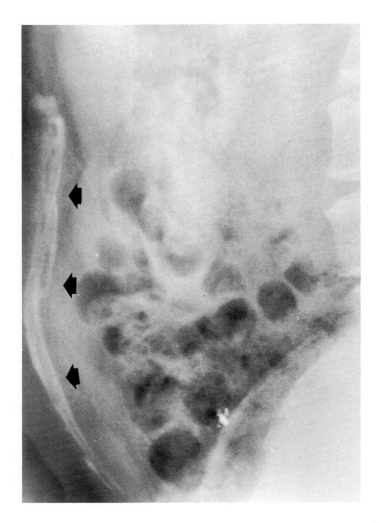

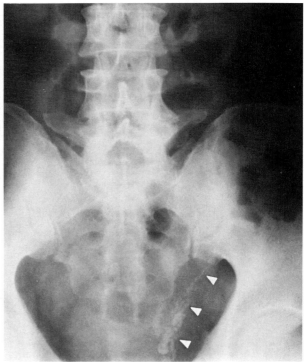

Fig. 73-139. Ossification of an old abdominal surgical scar producing a long linear density on the anterior abdominal wall **(arrows)**.

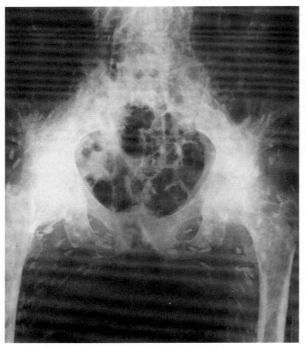

Fig. 73-140. Cysticercosis. Radiograph of the abdomen and pelvis shows multiple calcified cysticerci in the muscles of the thighs, abdomen, and gluteal regions. (Keats TE: Cysticercosis: Roentgen manifestations. Mo Med 58:457–459, 1961)

Fig. 73-141. Dracunculiasis. A long serpiginous calcified worm **(arrows)** within the pelvis. (Eisenberg RL: Diagnostic Imaging in Internal Medicine. New York, McGraw–Hill, 1987)

cular injections of quinine for malaria. Irregular calcification of the buttocks can also be a result of intramuscular injection of bismuth, calcium gluconate, or calcium penicillin.

Rarely, calcification of the skeletal muscles in myositis ossificans has been observed in the abdomen. Superficial soft-tissue calcification in the abdomen can occur in hypercalcemic states and in idiopathic calcinosis.

SKELETAL/LIGAMENTOUS CALCIFICATION

Spine
 Calcification of the nucleus pulposus/
  annular ligaments
 Tuberculosis
 Paravertebral abscess
 Neoplasm (*e.g.*, meningioma)
 Residual myelographic contrast
Costal cartilage
Ligament
 Iliolumbar calcification
 Sacrotuberous calcification
 Sacrospinous calcification

Calcification of the nucleus pulposus or annular ligaments of the lumbar spine is an extremely common degenerative lesion. Widespread spinal lesions of this type occur in ochronosis, accompanied by similar changes in the symphysis pubis (Fig. 73-142). Intraspinal tuberculous lesions or paravertebral abscesses can also become calcified. Spinal tumors, especially meningiomas, rarely become sufficiently calcified or ossified to be visible radiographically. Residual myelographic contrast in the spinal canal and occasionally extending out along nerve roots should cause no diagnostic difficulty.

Calcification of costal cartilages is common and is usually readily identified. Oblique projections demonstrate the relation of these calcifications to the anterior wall of the lower thorax. The pattern of costal cartilage calcification has been shown to be related to the patient's sex (Fig. 73-143). In men, the upper and lower borders of the cartilage become calcified first, extending directly in continuity from the ends of the bony ribs. Calcification of the central area then follows. In women, two types of calcification are described. The more common is a solid tongue of calcification extending from the rib into the adjacent cartilage. The less common pattern is

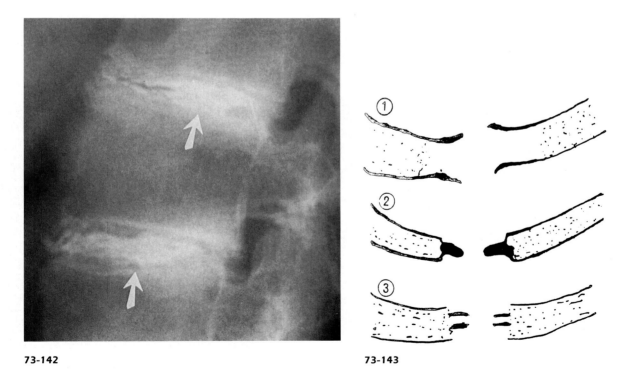

73-142
             73-143

Fig. 73-142. Ochronosis. There is calcification of the nucleus pulposus of several intervertebral disk spaces **(arrows)**.

Fig. 73-143. Costal cartilage sign. **(Top)** Male type of calcification. **(Center)** Common female type of calcification. **(Bottom)** Uncommon female type of calcification. (Sanders CF: Sexing by costal cartilage calcification. Br J Radiol 39:233–234, 1966)

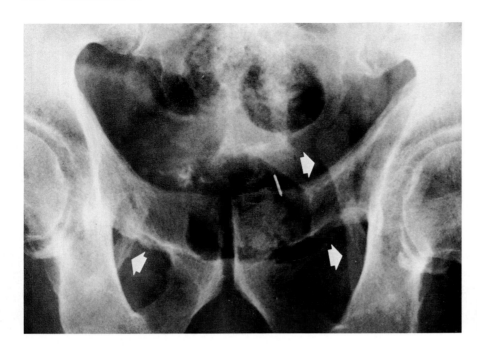

Fig. 73-144. Calcification of the sacrotuberous ligaments **(arrows)**.

two parallel lines of calcification extending from the center of the rib into the adjacent cartilage.

The lateral tip of the transverse process of a lumbar vertebra occasionally appears excessively dense. Although this pseudocalcification can resemble a ureteral calculus, close inspection should permit proper differentiation.

The iliolumbar, sacrotuberous (Fig. 73-144), and sacrospinous ligaments are sometimes calcified. Such calcification can represent a normal variant or be related to fluorosis.

MISCELLANEOUS CALCIFICATION

Ingested foreign bodies
Retained barium
Nonabsorbed cholecystographic contrast
      material
Bariolith
Suppositories
  Rectal
  Vaginal
Retained surgical sponges (gossypidoma)
Surgical gauze, drains, catheters, sutures

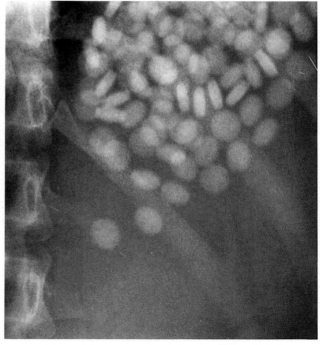

Fig. 73-145. Multiple radiopaque pills in the stomach.

A variety of miscellaneous radiopaque densities can simulate calcification on abdominal radiographs. Ingested pills (Fig. 73-145), coins (Fig. 73-146), and marbles (Fig. 73-147), as well as unusual culinary delights such as chopped razor blades (Fig. 73-148), can appear radiographically as single or multiple calcium-like densities in the gastrointestinal tract. Indeed, the variety of foreign objects that are in-

Text continues on page 1010

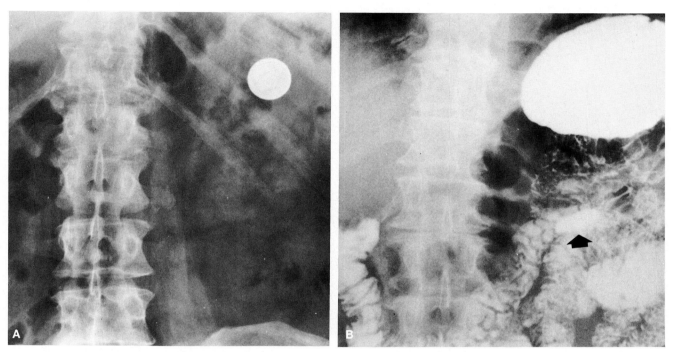

Fig. 73-146. Ingested coin (quarter) lodged in the region of the anastomosis in a patient who had undergone partial gastrectomy and gastrojejunostomy. **(A)** Plain abdominal radiograph; **(B)** upper gastrointestinal series.

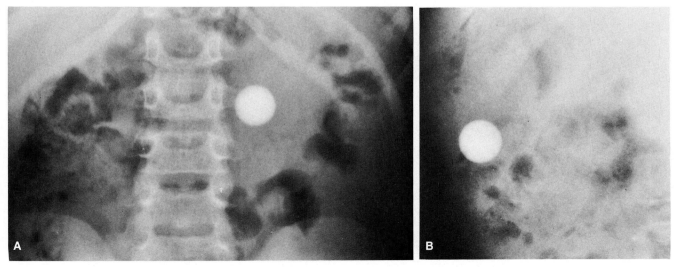

Fig. 73-147. Ingested marble. Note that the marble appears round in both **(A)** frontal and **(B)** lateral projections, thereby demonstrating that it has a spherical shape.

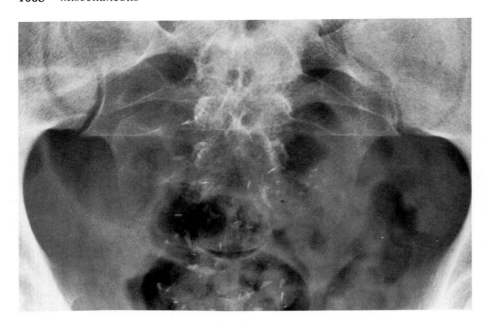

Fig. 73-148. Multiple chopped razor blades in the alimentary tract.

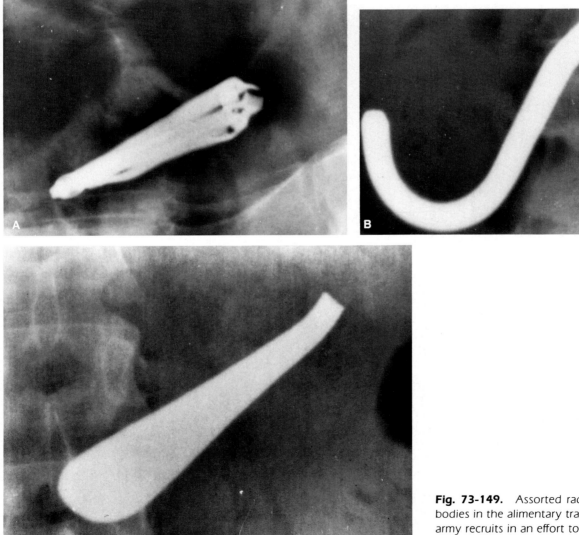

Fig. 73-149. Assorted radiopaque foreign bodies in the alimentary tract swallowed by army recruits in an effort to avoid going out on bivouac during winter. **(A)** Nail clipper; **(B)** hook from a coathanger; **(C)** shoehorn.

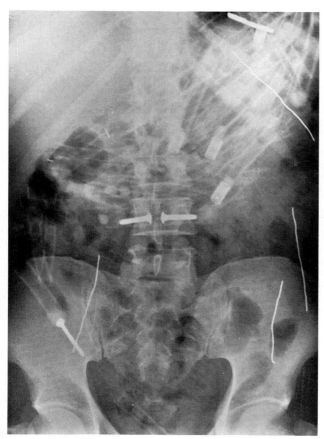

73-150

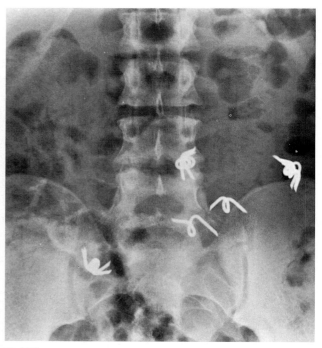

73-151

Fig. 73-150. Bizarre array of ingested foreign bodies (nails, syringes, opened paper clips, etc.) in a psychiatric patient.

Fig. 73-151. Multiple strands of barbed wire ingested by a psychotic patient.

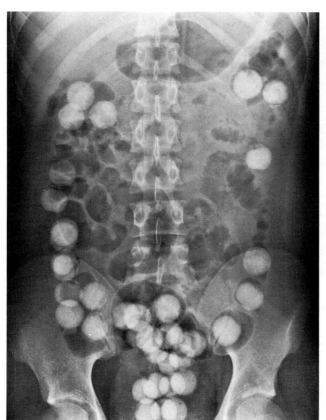

73-152

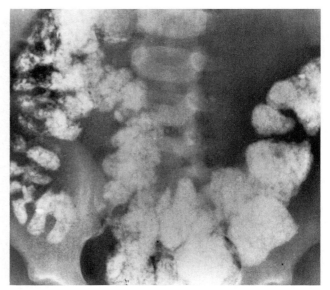

73-153

Fig. 73-152. Cocaine ''body packer.'' Plain abdominal radiograph demonstrates multiple well-defined, circular white densities. (McCarron MM, Wood JD: The cocaine ''body packer'' syndrome. JAMA 250:1417–1420, 1983)

Fig. 73-153. Pica. Ingested gravel and stones fill the colon of this child, who had received no contrast material. The mother complained that she heard a strange ''plunking'' noise whenever her child had a bowel movement.

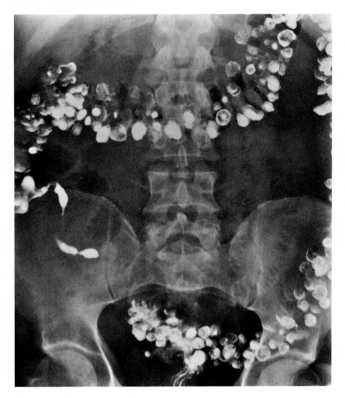

Fig. 73-154. Retained barium in multiple colonic diverticula.

gested appears to be unlimited (Figs. 73-149, 73-150, 73-151). Multiple well-defined, circular opacifications within the gastrointestinal tract may be found in cocaine "body packers," who swallow the condoms, toy balloons, or the fingers of latex gloves filled with the loose white powder in an attempt to smuggle cocaine through Customs searches (Fig. 73-152). In young children, irregular paint fragments (pica) in the gastrointestinal tract suggest lead poisoning (Fig. 73-153). Retained barium, especially in colonic diverticula (Fig. 73-154), and nonabsorbed cholecystographic contrast material (Fig. 73-155) can also appear as abdominal opacities. Infrequently, a dense opacity in the cecum may represent a retained mass of inspissated barium (bariolith) (Fig. 73-156), which can cause superficial ulceration in the adjacent cecal mucosa. Rectal suppositories containing zinc oxide and various bismuth compounds can simulate excreted urographic contrast material or stones (Fig. 73-157). Vaginal suppositories, especially those containing diiodohydroxyquinoline, can be radiopaque and mimic bladder calculi. Unusual pelvic opacifications include a pessary (Fig. 73-158) and a misplaced thermometer (Fig. 73-159). A retained surgical sponge (gossypidoma) can be easily identified on postoperative radiographs; the most commonly used types have standardized, readily recognized opaque markers (Fig. 73-160). Iodoform gauze and a variety

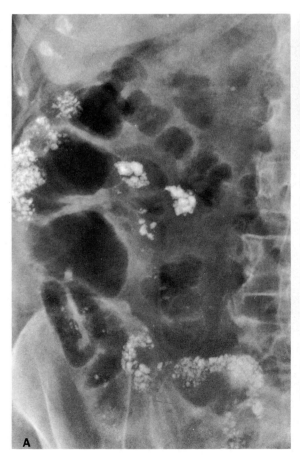

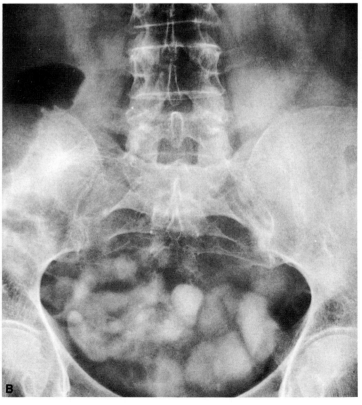

Fig. 73-155. Nonabsorbed cholecystographic contrast material. **(A)** Unconjugated Telepaque; **(B)** conjugated Telepaque.

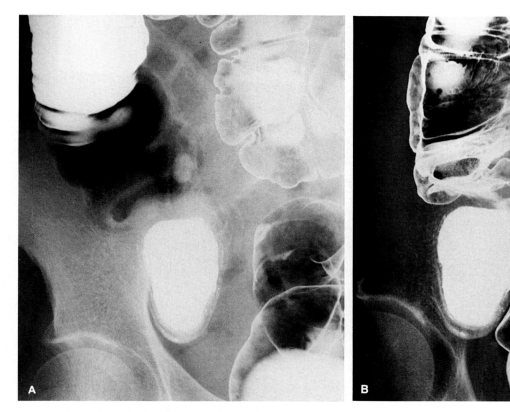

Fig. 73-156. Cecal bariolith. **(A)** Inspissated barium in the cecum seen during the course of a barium enema examination and before the barium column had reached the cecum. **(B)** After completion of the examination, barium and air have filled the colon and refluxed into the terminal ileum without filling the cecum. (Gupta SK, Fraser GM: Caecal bariolith: An unusual complication following a barium meal. Br J Radiol 58:268–269, 1985)

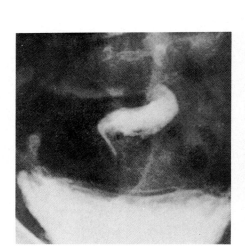

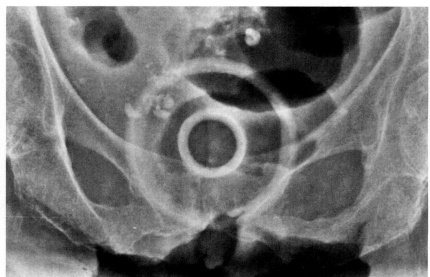

73-157   73-158

Fig. 73-157. Radiopaque rectal suppository. This 37-year-old woman was referred for urography because of urinary tract infections and was given an Anusol suppository by the nurse 45 min before this radiograph was obtained. The radiographic density of the opaque material in the rectum **(arrows)** is similar to that of the excreted urographic contrast material. (Spitzer A, Caruthers SB, Stables DP: Radiopaque suppositories. Radiology 121:71–73, 1976)

Fig. 73-158. Pessary.

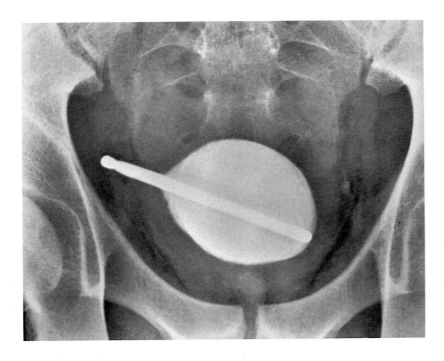

Fig. 73-159. Misplaced thermometer. The thermometer with its characteristic bulbous tip was introduced through the urethra and perforated the bladder, which is filled with contrast material on this radiograph. Note the streaks of air within adjacent pelvic soft tissues.

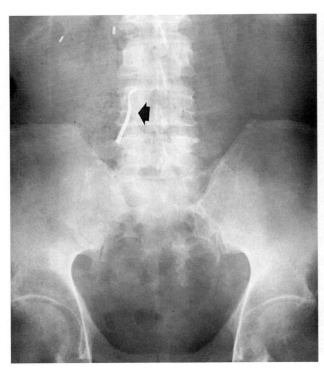

73-160

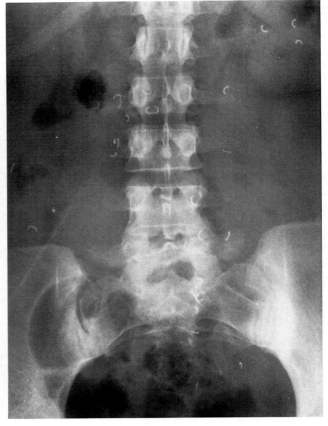

73-161

Fig. 73-160. Retained surgical sponge (gossypidoma). The radiopaque marker **(arrow)** is easily seen on a plain abdominal radiograph obtained following surgery.

Fig. 73-161. Subcutaneous acupuncture wires. (Baker SR, Elkin M: Plain Film Approach to Abdominal Calcifications. Philadelphia, WB Saunders, 1983)

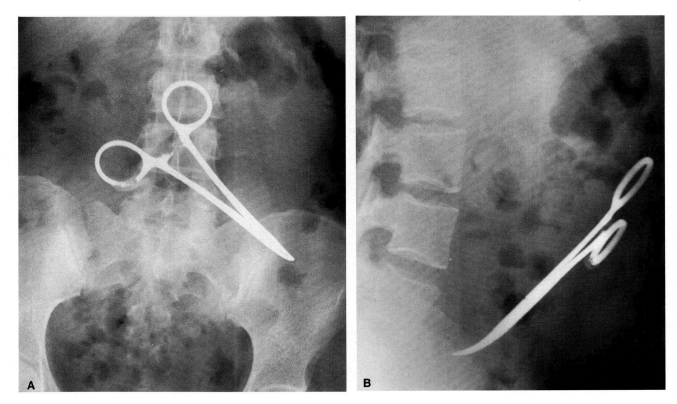

Fig. 73-162. Retained hemostat following surgery. **(A)** Frontal and **(B)** lateral abdominal radiographs demonstrate that the metallic hemostat lies in the peritoneal cavity.

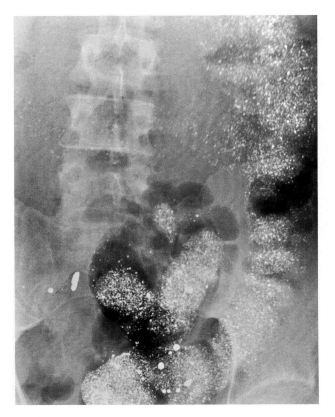

Fig. 73-163. Mercury in the bowel lumen. The patient bit off the end of a thermometer and swallowed the mercury in it.

of surgical drains, catheters, and metallic sutures occasionally present confusing opacities on abdominal radiographs. Following some forms of acupuncture, fine metallic needles passed through the skin into the subcutaneous tissues may project over the abdomen (Fig. 73-161). Unfortunate radiopaque complications of medical procedures include retained hemostats (Fig. 73-162) and globules of mercury in the bowel lumen (Fig. 73-163) from broken thermometers or rupture of a mercury bag attached to a long intestinal tube.

BIBLIOGRAPHY

General

Baker SR, Elkin M: Plain Film Approach to Abdominal Calcifications. Philadelphia, WB Saunders, 1983

McAfee JG, Donner MW: Differential diagnosis of calcifications encountered in abdominal radiographs. Am J Med Sci 243:609–650, 1962

Reeder MM, Hamilton LC: Radiologic diagnosis of tropical diseases of the gastrointestinal tract. Radiol Clin North Am 7:57–81, 1969

Liver

Bonakdarpour A: Echinococcus disease: Report of 112 cases from Iran and a review of 611 cases from the United States. AJR 99:660–667, 1967

Dachman AH, Lichtenstein JE, Friedman AC et al: Infantile hemangioendothelioma of the liver: A radiologic–pathologic clinical correlation. AJR 140:1091–1096, 1983

Dachman AH, Pakter RL, Ros PR et al: Hepatoblastoma: Radiologic–pathologic correlation in 50 cases. Radiology 164:15–19, 1987

Darlack JJ, Moskowitz M, Kattan KR: Calcifications in the liver. Radiol Clin North Am 18:209–219, 1980

Friedman AC, Lichtenstein JE, Goodman Z et al: Fibrolamellar hepatocelluar carcinoma. Radiology 157:583–587, 1985

Gelfand DW: The liver: Plain film diagnosis. Semin Roentgenol 10:177–185, 1975

Levy DW, Rindsberg S, Friedman AC et al: Thorotrast-induced hepatosplenic neoplasia: CT identification. AJR 146:997–1004, 1986

McCook TA, Putman CE, Dale JK et al: Medullary carcinoma of the thyroid: Radiographic features of a unique tumor. AJR 139:149–155, 1982

Olmstedt WW, Stocker JT: Cavernous hemangioma of liver. Radiology 117:59–62, 1975

Shibuya A, Unuma T, Sugimoto T et al: Diffuse hepatic calcification as a sequela to shock liver. Gastroenterology 89:196–201, 1985

Steinbach HL, Johnstone HG: The roentgen diagnosis of armillifer infection (porocephalus) in man. Radiology 68:234–237, 1957

Stone R, Benson J, Tronic B et al: Hepatic calcifications in a patient with Gaucher's disease. Am J Gastroenterol 77:95–98, 1982

Thompson WM, Chisholm DP, Tank R: Plain film roentgenographic findings in alveolar hydatid cyst: *Echinococcus multilocularis*. AJR 116:345–348, 1972

Spleen

Dachman AH, Ros PR, Murai PJ et al: Nonparasitic splenic cysts: A report of 52 cases with radiologic–pathologic correlation. AJR 147:537–542, 1986

Demetropoulos KC, Lindenauer SM, Rapp R et al: Target calcification of the spleen in chronic brucellosis (*Brucella suis*). J Canad Assoc Radiol 25:161–163, 1974

Seligman BR, Rosner F, Smulewicz JJ: Splenic calcifications in sickle cell anemia. Am J Med Sci 265:495–499, 1973

Pancreas

Farman J, Chen CK, Schulze G et al: Solid and papillary epithelial pancreatic neoplasm: An unusual tumor. Gastrointest Radiol 12:31–34, 1987

Friedman AC, Lichtenstein JE, Fishman EK et al: Solid and papillary epithelial neoplasm of the pancreas. Radiology 154:333–337, 1985

Jahnke RW, Gnekow W, Harell GS: Non-beta islet cell tumor calcification associated with Zollinger–Ellison syndrome and multiple endocrine adenomatosis. Gastrointest Radiol 1:345–347, 1977

Ring EJ, Eaton SB, Ferrucci JT et al: Differential diagnosis of pancreatic calcification. AJR 117:446–452, 1973

Stobbe KC, ReMine WH, Baggenstoss AH: Pancreatic lithiasis. Surg Gynecol Obstet 131:1090–1099, 1970

Wolf EL, Sprayregen S, Frager D et al: Calcification in an insulinoma of the pancreas. Am J Gastroenterol 79:559–561, 1984

Gallbladder

Oschner SF, Carrera GM: Calcification of the gallbladder ("porcelain gallbladder"). AJR 89:847–853, 1963

Parker GW, Joffe N: Calcifying primary mucus-producing adenocarcinoma of the gallbladder. Br J Radiol 45:468–469, 1972

Rogers LF, Lastra MP, Lin KT et al: Calcifying mucinous adenocarcinoma of the gallbladder. Am J Gastroenterol 59:441–445, 1973

Strijk SP: Calcified gallstone fissure: The reversed Mercedes–Benz sign. Gastrointest Radiol 12:152–153, 1987

Alimentary Tract

Alcalay J, Alkalay L, Lorent T: Myxoglobulosis of the appendix. Br J Radiol 58:183–184, 1985

Beal SL, Walton CB, Bodai BI: Enterolith ileus resulting from small bowel diverticulosis. Am J Gastroenterol 82:162–164, 1987

Borg SE, Whitehouse GH, Griffiths GJ: A mobile calcified amputated appendix epiploica. AJR 127:349–350, 1976

Crummy AB, Juhl JH: Calcified gastric leiomyoma. AJR 87:727–728, 1962

Dachman AH, Lichtenstein JE, Friedman AC: Mucocele of the appendix and pseudomyxoma peritonei. AJR 144:923–929, 1985

Fataar S, Bassiony H, Hamed MS et al: Radiographic spectrum of rectocolonic calcification from schistosomiasis. AJR 142:933–936, 1984

Ghahremani GG, Meyers MA, Port RB: Calcified primary tumors of the gastrointestinal tract. Gastrointest Radiol 2:331–339, 1978

Javors BR, Bryk D: Enterolithiasis: A report of four cases. Gastrointest Radiol 8:359–362, 1983

Paige ML, Ghahremani GG, Brosnan JJ: Laminated radiopaque enteroliths: Diagnostic clues to intestinal pathology. Am J Gastroenterol 82:432–437, 1987

Rotondo A, Grassi R, Smaltino F et al: Calcified gastric cancer. Report of a case and review of literature. Br J Radiol 59:405–407, 1986

Simms SM: Gastric hemangioma associated with phleboliths. Gastrointest Radiol 10:51–53, 1985

Kidney

Chambers AA, Carson R: Primary osteogenic sarcoma of the kidney. Br J Radiol 48:316–317, 1975

Courey WB, Pfister RC: The radiographic findings in renal tubular acidosis. Radiology 105:497–503, 1972

Daniel WW, Hartman GW, Witten DM et al: Calcified renal masses: A review of ten years experience at the Mayo Clinic. Radiology 103:503–508, 1972

Day DL, Scheinman JI, Mahan J: Radiological aspects of the primary hyperoxaluria. AJR 146:395–401, 1986

Eisenberg RL, Mani RL: Residual Pantopaque in renal cysts: An addition to the differential diagnosis of intra-abdominal heavy-metal densities. Clin Radiol 29:227–229, 1978

Fulop M, Sternlieb I, Scheinberg IH: Defective urinary acidification in Wilson's disease. Ann Intern Med 68:770–777, 1968

Jonutis AJ, Davidson AJ, Redman HC: Curvilinear calcification in four uncommon benign renal lesions. Clin Radiol 24:468–474, 1973

Lalli AF: Renal parenchymal calcifications. Semin Roentgenol 17:101–112, 1982

Margolin EG, Cohen LH: Genitourinary calcification: An overview. Semin Roentgenol 17:95–100, 1982

Mencini RA: Calcification in a renal mass. Semin Roentgenol 17:90–91, 1982

Singh EO, Malek RS: Calculus disease in the upper urinary tract. Semin Roentgenol 17:113–132, 1982

Wasserman NF, Ewing SL: Calcified renal oncocytoma. AJR 141:747–749, 1983

Ureter/Bladder

Banner MP, Pollack HM: Urolithiasis in the lower urinary tract. Semin Roentgenol 17:140–148, 1982

Pollack HM, Banner MP, Martinez LO et al: Diagnostic considerations in urinary bladder wall calcification. AJR 136:791–797, 1981

Thornbury JR, Parker TW: Ureteral calculi. Semin Roentgenol 17:133–139, 1982

Male Genital Tract

Hafiz A, Melnick JC: Calcification of the vas deferens. J Canad Assoc Radiol 19:56–60, 1968

King JC, Rosenbaum HD: Calcification of the vasa deferentia in nondiabetics. Radiology 100:603–606, 1971

Loveday BO, Price JL: Soft tissue radiography of the testes. Clin Radiol 29:685–689, 1978

Female Genital Tract

Deeths TM, Stanley RJ: Parametrial calcification in cervical carcinoma patients treated with radioactive gold. AJR 127:511–513, 1976

Moncada R, Cooper RA, Garces M et al: Calcified metastases from malignant ovarian neoplasm: A review of the literature. Radiology 113:31–35, 1974

Nixon GW, Condon VR: Amputated ovary: A cause of migratory abdominal calcification. AJR 128:1053–1055, 1977

Schultz SM, Curry TS, Voet R: Psammomatous-like calcification in a Brenner tumour of the ovary. Br J Radiol 59:412–414, 1986

Seymour EQ, Hood JB, Underwood PB et al: Gonadoblastoma: An ovarian tumor with characteristic pelvic calcifications. AJR 127:1001–1002, 1976

Spring DB: Fallopian tube occlusion rings: A consideration in the differential diagnosis of ureteral calculi. Radiology 145:51–52, 1982

Teplick JG, Haskin ME, Alavi A: Calcified intraperitoneal metastases from ovarian carcinoma. AJR 127:1003–1006, 1976

Adrenal

Naidech HJ, Chawla HS: Bilateral adrenal calcifications at birth in a neonate. AJR 140:105–106, 1983

Queloz JM, Capitanio MA, Kirkpatrick JA: Wolman's disease: Roentgen observations in three siblings. Radiology 104:357–359, 1972

Rose J, Berdon WE, Sullivan T et al: Prolonged jaundice as presenting sign of massive adrenal hemorrhage in newborn. Radiology 98:263–272, 1971

Twersky J, Levin DC: Metastatic melanoma of the adrenal: An unusual cause of adrenal calcification. Radiology 116:627–628, 1975

Retroperitoneal

Baker DE, Glazer GM: Bilateral pararenal calcifications resulting from pancreatitis. AJR 143:51–52, 1984

Generalized

Chejfec G, Rieker WJ, Jablokow VR et al: Psuedomyxoma peritonei associated with colloid carcinoma of the pancreas. Gastroenterology 90:202–205, 1986

Dalinka MK, Lally JF, Azimi F et al: Calcification in undifferentiated abdominal malignancies. Clin Radiol 26:115–119, 1975

Parsons J, Gray GF, Thorbjarnarson B: Pseudomyxoma peritonei. Arch Surg 101:545–549, 1970

Seshul MB, Coulam CM: Pseudomyxoma peritonei: Computed tomography and sonography. AJR 136:803–806, 1981

Vascular Structures

Baker SR, Broker MH, Charnsangavej C et al: Calcification in the portal vein wall. Radiology 152:18, 1984

Bertrand M, Chen JTT, Libshitz HI: Lymph node calcification in Hodgkin's disease after chemotherapy. AJR 129:1108–1110, 1977

Culver GJ, Pirson HS: Splenic artery aneurysm. Radiology 68:217–223, 1957

Fenlon JW, Augustin C: The significance of pelvic phlebolith displacement. J Urol 106:595–598, 1971

Ghahremani GG, Straus FH: Calcification of distant lymph node metastases from carcinoma of the colon. Radiology 99:65–66, 1971

Kolman MA: Radiologic soft tissues in the pelvis: Another look. AJR 130:493–498, 1977

Mata JM, Alegret X, Martinez A: Calcification in the portal and collateral veins wall: CT findings. Gastrointest Radiol 12:206–208, 1987

Mattson T: Frequency and location of pelvic phleboliths. Clin Radiol 31:115–118, 1980

Orr DP, Myerowitz RL, Herbert DL et al: Correlation of radiographic and histologic findings in arterial calcification. Invest Radiol 13:110–114, 1978

Winchester PH, Cerwin R, Dische R: Hemosiderin-laden lymph nodes. AJR 118:222–226, 1973

Abdominal Wall Calcification

Brown JS: Soft tissue calcification secondary to therapeutic quinine injection. Br J Radiol 18:183–184, 1945

Katz I, Levine M: Bone formation in laparotomy scars. AJR 84:248–261, 1960

Samuel E: Roentgenology of parasitic calcification. AJR 63:512–522, 1950

Skeletal/Ligamentous Calcification

Graves VB, Schreiber MH: Tuberculous psoas muscle abscess. J Canad Assoc Radiol 24:268–271, 1973

Sanders CF: Sexing by costal cartilage calcification. Br J Radiol 39:233–234, 1966

Miscellaneous

Gupta SK, Fraser GM: Caecal bariolith: An unusual complication following a barium meal. Br J Radiol 58:268–269, 1985

Imray TJ, Hiramatsu X: Radiographic manifestations of Japanese acupuncture. Radiology 115:625–626, 1975

McCarron MM, Wood JD: The cocaine "body packer" syndrome: Diagnosis and treatment. JAMA 250:1417–1420, 1983

Richards WO, Keramati B, Scovill WA: Fate of retained foreign bodies in the peritoneal cavity. South Med J 79:496–498, 1986

Spitzer A, Caruthers SB, Stables DP: Radiopaque suppositories. Radiology 121:71–73, 1976

Williams RG, Bragg DG, Nelson JA: Gossypiboma: The problem of the retained surgical sponge. Radiology 129:323–326, 1978

Index

An *f* following a page number indicates a figure.

Abdominal wall
  calcification of, 1002–1005,
    1003f–1004f
  herniation through, 876–878, 877f–879f
  trauma of, pneumoperitoneum in, 899,
    899f
Abetalipoproteinemia, thickening of
    small bowel mucosal folds in, 463–
    464, 464f
  irregular and distorted, 480f, 480–481
  and small bowel dilatation, 454
Abscess
  abdominal
    drainage of, 914, 915f, 934
    extraluminal gas in, 905–914,
      906f–915f
  adjacent to colon, large bowel
    obstruction in, 733
  of appendix, 554–560, 556f–559f
    colon impressions in, 681, 681f
    filling defects in, 555, 556f, 557
  duodenal and periduodenal
    filling defects in, 363, 365f, 376, 376f
    postoperative, 363, 365f
  esophageal and periesophageal
    double-barrel appearance in, 141
    impressions on esophagus in, 29
  intraperitoneal
    separation of small bowel loops in,
      526
    soap bubble appearance in, 526
  of lesser peritoneal sac, extraluminal
    gas in, 911–913, 912f
  of liver
    in amebiasis, 600
    calcification in, 938–939, 939f
    cystic dilatation of bile ducts in, 844,
      845f
    extraluminal gas in, 910, 911f
  of pancreas
    extraluminal gas in, 910–911, 911f
    gastric impressions in, 259f
  paravertebral, calcification of, 1005
  pelvic, 913, 913f
    portal vein gas in, 860
  pericholecystic, duodenal impressions
    in, 359
  presacral, retrorectal space
    enlargement in, 764f
  psoas, tuberculous, 997
  rectal and perirectal
    in Crohn's disease, 934, 934f
    retrorectal space enlargement in, 763
  renal and perirenal
    calcification in, 973
    extraluminal gas in, 908–910, 910f
  retroperitoneal, retrogastric space
    widening in, 311
  of spleen, calcification in, 948
  subhepatic, 913f
  subphrenic
    diaphragm elevation in, 156
    extraluminal gas in, 907–908,
      907f–909f
    extravasated contrast material in,
      933f
  gastric fundus displacement in, 306f,
    306–307
  tubo-ovarian, entero-ovarian fistula in,
    929, 931f
Absorption of oral cholecystographic
    agents, 773–774
  factors affecting, 774–776, 774f–776f
Acanthosis
  glycogenic, of esophagus, 143, 144f
  nigricans
    in colon carcinoma, 635
    esophageal nodules in, 145, 146f
Achalasia, 10, 11–19, 11f–19f
  carcinoma of esophagus in, 76
  cricopharyngeal, 5f, 5–8
    posterior impressions on esophagus
      in, 5, 5f, 26, 27f
  differentiation of benign and malignant
    causes, 17–19
  hyperactive, 14f, 15, 21
  in myenteric plexus disorders, 10, 11f,
    16
  narrowing of esophagus in, 93, 94f
  rat-tail or beak appearance in, 15, 15f
  tertiary contractions of esophagus in,
    14f, 15, 21, 23f
  treatment of, 19, 19f
Acid-base imbalance, nonobstructive
    gastric dilatation in, 295, 295f
Acidosis, renal tubular, nephrocalcinosis
    in, 970, 970f
Actinomycosis
  cecum in, coned shape of, 577
  of colon, 607
  enteric-enteric fistula in, 923

Actinomycosis (*continued*)
esophagorespiratory fistula in, 135
ileocecal valve in, 549
stomach narrowing in, 214
Acupuncture wires, subcutaneous,
radiographic appearance of, 1012f,
1013
Addison's disease
adrenal calcification in, 995f, 995–996
duodenal impressions in, 359, 360f
Adenocarcinoma. *See* Carcinoma
Adenoma
adrenal cortical, calcification in, 996
of bile ducts
filling defects in, 812
narrowing and obstruction in, 825
of Brunner's gland, duodenal filling
defects in, 382, 382f
of colon, villous, 671–673, 672f
bouquet of flowers appearance in,
673
signs of malignancy in, 672f, 673
single filling defect in, 672f, 673
of esophagus, filling defects in, 100, 101f
of gallbladder, 798f, 798–799
of ileocecal valve, 546–548, 547f
of kidney, calcification in, 975, 975f
of rectum, villous, 671f
of small bowel
duodenal filling defects in, 376, 377f,
382–383, 383f
solitary filling defect in, 484, 484f
of stomach
filling defects in, 246, 248f
of fundus, 299
Adenomatous polyps
of bile ducts, 814f
of cecum, 567f
of colon
differentiated from diverticula, 665,
665f
double-contrast technique in, 664f,
665
multiple filling defects in, 693, 693f,
694f
pedunculated, 666–667, 666f–667f,
668, 669f
sessile, 665f, 666, 668, 668f, 669f
single filling defect in, 663–670,
664f–669f
target sign in, 667, 667f
of esophagus, filling defects in, 100, 101f
of gallbladder, 798
of ileocecal valve, 546–548
of papilla of Vater, 850
of small bowel, filling defects in, 497
duodenal, 376, 377f
of stomach, filling defects in, 240–243,
241f
Adenomyoma, gallbladder filling defects
in, 797, 797f
Adenomyomatosis, gallbladder filling
defects in, 795, 796–798, 796f–798f
Adhesions
in colon
narrowing in, 659
obstruction in, 738, 739f

pseudotumors and filling defects in,
688f, 688–690
perigastric, narrowing of stomach in,
222, 222f
small bowel obstruction in, 419f, 420
Adrenal gland
calcification in, 995–996, 995f–996f
cyst of
calcification in, 996
retrogastric space widening in, 311f
impression on duodenum, 359, 360f
tumors of
calcification in, 996
gallbladder displacement in, 785
impression on duodenum, 359
metastatic to stomach, 299
Adriamycin therapy, esophagitis and
esophageal ulceration in, 64, 65f
Adynamic ileus, 430–440. *See also* Ileus,
adynamic
Aganglionosis
dilatation of duodenum in, 403
mosaic pattern of colon in, 735, 737f
obstruction of colon in, 734–736, 735f–
737f
pneumatosis intestinalis in, 889
Aging
esophageal impressions in, 32
gallbladder carcinoma in, 359
gallstone ileus in, 490, 504
presbyesophagus in, 10, 20, 20f
AIDS
cholangitis in, 832f, 833
colitis in, 608, 608f, 609f
coned cecum in, 580f, 581
duodenal filling defects in, 386
duodenal thickening of mucosal folds
in, 334–335
enteric-enteric fistulas in, 923, 924f
enteritis in, and separation of small
bowel loops, 517
esophagitis in, 56, 56f, 58, 58f, 60f
gastritis in
and narrowing of stomach, 215, 215f,
216f
and thickening of mucosal folds,
228, 228f
Kaposi's sarcoma in, 868. *See also*
Kaposi's sarcoma
retrorectal space enlargement in, 763,
764f
thumbprinting pattern of colon in, 751
Air bubbles
bile duct filling defects in, 810
in colon, as artifact in barium enemas,
665, 712
in duodenal atresia, double bubble
sign in, 388, 388f
in esophagus, nodular appearance in,
147
in jejunal atresia, triple bubble sign in,
427f, 427–428
sandlike lucencies of small bowel in,
512
Albumin, thickening small bowel
mucosal folds in
hypoalbuminemia, 461
and small bowel dilatation, 454f, 455

Alcohol use and alcoholism
Boerhaave's syndrome in, 134, 134f
and double-barrel appearance of
esophagus, 137, 138f
cirrhosis and liver calcification in, 945
and esophageal carcinoma, 75
esophageal ulceration in, 60, 61f
gastric erosions in, superficial, 203f, 204
gastritis in
and filling defects of stomach, 259f
and thickening of gastric mucosal
folds, 223–224, 224f, 259, 259f
Mallory-Weiss syndrome in, 139
neuropathy in, and motility disorders
of esophagus, 10
pancreatitis in, 340, 342
and calcification of pancreas,
950–952, 952f
Alimentary tract calcification, 960–966,
959f–967f
Alpha chain disease, irregular thickening
of small bowel mucosal folds in,
480
Amebiasis
bile duct narrowing and obstruction
in, 833
of cecum, 600
coned cecum in, 572, 573f, 574–576,
575f, 600
of colon
multiple filling defects in, 708–709,
709f
narrowing in, 626, 626f, 627f
obstruction in, 724
single filling defect in, 679f, 679–680
thumbprinting pattern in, 749–751,
750f
toxic megacolon in, 741, 743f
ulcerations in, 600–601, 600f–601f
enteric-enteric fistulas in, 923
of ileocecal valve, 549, 551f
liver calcification in, 938–939
retrorectal space enlargement in, 763,
763f
Amebomas, 626, 626f, 627f
multiple filling defects of colon in, 709
single filling defect of colon in, 679f,
679–680
Ampulla of Vater
biliary calculi impacted in, 834
carcinoma of. *See* Carcinoma, of
ampulla of Vater
Amputation of ovary, spontaneous, 991,
992f
Amyl nitrite test in achalasia, 18, 18f
Amyloidosis
of colon
multiple filling defects in, 720, 720f
narrowing in, 657
single filling defect in, 689f, 690
thumbprinting pattern in, 751
ulcerations in, 615
esophageal motility disorders in, 11,
12f, 16, 22f
of rectum, 689f, 690
retrorectal space enlargement in, 770
of small bowel
dilatation in, 449f, 450, 454

duodenal thickening of mucosal folds in, 337
gastric involvement in, 515, 515f
irregular thickening of mucosal folds in, 471, 472f
obstruction in, 427
pneumatosis intestinalis in, 888, 888f
regular thickening of mucosal folds in, 465, 465f
sandlike lucencies in, 510, 512f
separation of bowel loops in, 517
of stomach
  filling defects in, 269f, 270
  narrowing in, 218f, 219
  outlet obstruction in, 285
  small bowel involvement in, 515, 515f
  thickening of mucosal folds in, 235f, 236, 515, 515f
Amyotrophic lateral sclerosis, esophageal motility disorders in, 7
Anal disorders
  in condyloma acuminatum, 629, 629f
  in Crohn's disease of colon, 595, 595f
  fistulas, 934–935, 935f
  in herpes simplex infection, 607, 608
  hypertrophy of papilla, colon filling defects in, 687f, 688
  imperforate anus
    obstruction of colon in, 736–738, 737f–738f
    pneumatosis intestinalis in, 889
Analgesic drugs
  gastric erosions from, superficial, 204
  renal papillary necrosis and nephrocalcinosis from, 971, 972f
Anastomosis
  biliary-intestinal, gas in biliary system after, 853
  Billroth
    filling defects in gastric remnant in, 271, 272, 272f
    marginal ulcers in, 199f
    and pseudo-Billroth pattern in Crohn's disease, 212f, 213, 318, 318f, 513
  colon narrowing at site of, 660, 660f
  traumatic neuroma in, 493f, 674
    and small bowel filling defects, 492, 493f
Ancylostoma duodenale infection, small bowel filling defects in, 504
Anemia
  in colon carcinoma, 634f, 635
  pernicious, gallbladder visualization impaired in, 777
  sickle cell, splenic density in, 948, 951f
Aneurysm
  aortic
    bile duct narrowing and obstruction in, 836
    diaphragm elevation in, 156, 157f
    diaphragm paralysis in, 153
    duodenal impressions in, 361
    duodenal obstruction and dilatation in, 405, 406f
    duodenal sweep widening in, 356
    esophageal impressions in, 35

fistula formation after surgical repair of, 929
gastric impressions from, 267
retrogastric space widening in, 311
upper quadrant extraluminal gas in rupture of, 917
cardiac, gastric impressions in, 300, 301f
hepatic artery
  bile duct narrowing and obstruction in, 836, 836f
  calcification in, 943–945
pancreatic, calcification in, 955
renal artery, calcification in, 977, 977f
splenic artery, calcification in, 948, 950f
Angioneurotic edema
  colon thumbprinting pattern in, 751–754, 753f
  small bowel mucosal folds in, thickening of, 462–463, 463f
Angiosarcoma, splenic, Thorotrast-induced, 950, 951f
Anisakiasis
  of cecum, 578, 578f
  of ileocecal valve, 549, 551f
  of small bowel, thickening of mucosal folds in, 479, 479f
  of stomach
    filling defects in, 270
    thickening of mucosal folds in, 228, 228f
Annular carcinoma
  of colon
    narrowing in, 633–638, 633f–638f
    ulcerations in, 614
  of stomach, outlet obstruction in, 282, 283f
Annular ligaments of lumbar spine, calcification of, 1006
Annular pancreas
  duodenal impressions in, 359, 360f
  duodenal narrowing and obstruction in, 388–389, 389f
  gastric outlet obstruction in, 286
Anorectal disorders. *See* Anal disorders; Rectum
Antibiotic-associated colitis
  pseudomembranous, 609–612
  staphylococcal, 604f, 605
Anticholinergic drugs. *See also* Atropine
  esophageal motility disorders from, 10
Anticoagulant therapy, hemorrhage in
  and separation of small bowel loops, 519f
  and thickening of small bowel mucosal folds, 457f, 458, 458f
  and thumbprinting pattern of colon, 746
Anti-inflammatory agents, superficial gastric erosions from, 201, 202f, 204
Antrum, gastric
  carcinoma of
    duodenal bulb involvement in, 315, 317f, 385
    outlet obstruction in, 282, 283f
  Crohn's disease of, duodenal bulb involvement in, 315–318, 318f

diverticular of, 182, 182f
duodenal bulb involvement in disorders of, 315–319
in eosinophilic gastroenteritis, 318, 318f
gastritis of
  narrowing in, 218–219
  thickening of mucosal folds in, 225–226, 225f–227f
in hypertrophy of antral-pyloric fold, filling defects in, 261, 261f
lymphoma of, duodenal bulb involvement in, 315, 316f, 317f, 384f, 385
mucosal diaphragm of, outlet obstruction in, 285–286, 286f
mucosal folds of
  normal variations in, 223
  thickening of, 225–226, 225f–227f
pad sign in pancreatic carcinoma, 349, 349f
peptic ulcer disease of
  duodenal bulb involvement in, 315
  outlet obstruction in, 281
prolapse of mucosa, 261
  duodenal filling defects in, 370f, 370–371
  outlet obstruction in, 290
prolapse of polyp, 285, 382f
  duodenal filling defects in, 381–382, 382f
  outlet obstruction in, 285
strongyloidiasis of, duodenal bulb involvement in, 318
tuberculosis of, duodenal bulb involvement in, 318
Anus, disorders of. *See* Anal disorders
Aorta
  aneurysm of. *See* Aneurysm, aortic
  calcification of, 1000, 1000f
  coarctation of, esophageal impressions in, 35, 36f
  dissection of, compared to double-barrel esophagus, 137, 138f
  esophageal impressions from
    normal, 31f, 32
    in vascular abnormalities, 32–35, 36f, 37f
  tortuosity of
    esophageal impressions in, 35, 37f
    gastric impressions in, 267, 300
Aortic arch
  cervical, esophageal impressions from, 33–34, 34f
  double, esophageal impressions in, 34f, 34–35
  right-sided, esophageal impressions in, 32–33, 32f–33f
Aortic knob, esophageal impressions from, 32
Aortic lymph nodes, calcification of, 1001–1002, 1002f
Aorticoduodenal fistula, 327–328
  narrowing and obstruction of duodenum in, 398, 398f, 405
Aorticomesenteric angle narrowing, obstruction and dilatation of duodenum in, 403

Aphthoid ulcers
  bull's-eye lesions in, 868
  of colon, in Crohn's disease, 594, 594f
  of esophagus, in Crohn's disease, 59, 61f
  halo appearance in, 868
  of stomach, 203f, 204
Appendectomy, inverted appendiceal
    stump in, 559f–561f, 561
Appendices epiploicae, calcified, 963,
    963f
Appendicitis, 554–560, 556f, 558f
  appendicoliths in, 558f, 559, 960
  cecum in
    coiled spring appearance of, 564f, 565
    coned shape of, 576–577
    gallbladder visualization impaired in,
      776
    incomplete filling of appendix in,
      555, 556f
    pneumoperitoneum in, 897
    subhepatic gas in, 906f
Appendicoliths, 960, 959f–961f
  in appendicitis, 558f, 559, 960
  differential diagnosis of, 960, 960f, 961f
Appendix, 554–566, 556f–565f
  abscess of, 554–560, 556f–559f
    colon impressions in, 681, 681f
    filling defects in, 555, 556f, 557
  in appendicitis. See Appendicitis
  calcification of
    in mucocele, 561
    in myxoglobulosis, 563, 563f
  carcinoid tumors of, 565–566
  carcinoma of, 565f, 566
  in carcinoma of pancreas metastatic to
    cecum, 566f
  intussusception into cecum, 563–565,
    564f
  inverted stump after appendectomy,
    559f–561f, 561
  mucocele of. See Mucocele of appendix
  myxoglobulosis of, 563, 563f
    calcification in, 962f, 963
  perforation of
    retrorectal space enlargement in, 763
    subhepatic gas in, 905, 906f
  retrocecal, 554, 555f, 557
  rupture of, 557f
Apple-core appearance
  in colon carcinoma, 614, 633, 636,
    723, 725f
  in duodenal carcinoma, 397f
Areae gastricae, filling defects of stomach
    in, 238–239, 239f
Armillifer armillatus infection, liver
    calcification in, 939, 939f
Arteriovenous fistulas
  calcification of, 977
  duodenal filling defects in, 374f, 375
Arthritis
  rheumatoid
    esophageal motility disorders in, 10
    small bowel mucosal folds in,
      thickening of, 458–459
  in ulcerative colitis, 586–587
Artifacts
  bile duct filling defects in, 809–811,
    809f–811f

colon filling defects in, 665, 711–713,
    712f
  esophageal nodules in, 147
Ascariasis
  of bile ducts
    cystic dilatation in, 843–844
    filling defects in, 813, 815f
    gas in biliary system and
      pancreaticobiliary reflux in, 854,
      855
    narrowing and obstruction in, 830
  of colon, filling defects in, 681
  of gallbladder, 802
  liver calcification in, 939
  of small bowel
    multiple filling defects in, 500–503,
      503f
    solitary filling defect in, 491
Ascites
  diaphragm elevation in, 156
  ground-glass appearance in, 522, 522f
  retrogastric space widening in, 310
  small bowel loops in, separation of,
    520–523, 522f–523f
Ascorbic acid, esophageal ulceration
    from, 66
Aspirin
  gastric erosions from, superficial, 201,
    202f, 204
  gastric ulcers and gastrocolic fistulas
    from, 921
Atelectasis, elevation of diaphragm in, 157
Atherosclerosis, vascular insufficiency
    and small bowel dilatation in, 450
  thickening of mucosal folds in, 453
Atresia
  biliary, 835
  duodenal, 387–388, 388f
  ileal
    microcolon in, 428, 428f
    obstruction in, 427–428, 427f–428f
  jejunal
    obstruction in, 427f, 427–428
    triple bubble sign in, 427f, 427–428
Atrial enlargement, esophageal
    impressions in, 40, 40f, 41f
Atropine
  esophageal motility disorders from, 10
  gastric dilatation from, 293
  ileus from, adynamic, 433, 433f
  small bowel dilatation from, 442

Bacillary infections
  bladder calcification in, 981
  dysentery in
    and narrowing of colon, 626
    and toxic megacolon, 741
    and ulcerations of colon, 601–603
Backwash ileitis, 549, 550f, 576
  in ulcerative colitis, 589, 589f
Balloon catheterization
  of esophagus
    in achalasia, 19, 19f
    in carcinoma, 79–81, 80f
  intestinal, small bowel obstruction in,
    422, 423f
  rectal, portal vein gas in, 860

Bands
  adhesive, of colon, narrowing in, 659
  fibrous congenital, small bowel
    obstruction in, 420
  peritoneal congenital, duodenal
    obstruction in, 391, 391f
Banti's syndrome, 126f
Barbiturates
  ileus from, adynamic, 433
  small bowel dilatation from, 442
Barioliths, cecal, 1010, 1011f
Barium
  inadvertent intraperitoneal
    extravasation of, 944f, 945
  portal vein gas after studies with, 860
  retained, radiographic appearance of,
    1010, 1010f
Barrett's esophagus, 50–55, 53f–55f
  carcinoma in, 75f, 76, 84
  narrowing in, 84, 87f
  nodular lesions in, 144
  reticular pattern in, 52–53, 54f
  ulcerations in, 52, 53f, 84
Beak sign
  in achalasia, 15, 15f
  in sigmoid volvulus, 728, 729f
Bed rest, duodenal obstruction and
    dilatation in, 403, 403f
Behçet's syndrome
  bull's-eye lesions in, 869, 869f
  of colon
    toxic megacolon in, 741
    ulcerations in, 617, 617f
  esophagorespiratory fistula in, 135, 136f
  of esophagus
    narrowing in, 86, 89f
    ulcerations in, 60
  small bowel filling defects in, 504, 504f
Bezoars
  in colon, 289f
    filling defects in, 691
    obstruction in, 289f, 740
  drug-induced, 289f, 740
  in small bowel
    duodenal filling defects in, 364f
    multiple filling defects in, 500
    obstruction in, 422, 423f, 492
    solitary filling defect in, 492
  in stomach
    filling defects in, 261–263, 262f–263f,
      272–273, 273f
    gallbladder visualization impaired in,
      776, 776f
    outlet obstruction in, 289f, 290
    postoperative, 272–273, 273f
Bile ducts, 805–846
  adenoma of
    filling defects in, 812
    narrowing and obstruction in, 825
  atresia of, 835
  calcification of, 959, 959f
  calculi in. See Calculi, biliary
  carcinoma of
    filling defects in, 811, 811f, 812f
    narrowing and obstruction in,
      819–820, 820f–821f
    Thorotrast-induced, 946, 946f
  in Caroli's disease, 840–843, 842f–844f

cholangitis of. *See* Cholangitis
in choledochocele, 372f, 373, 840, 842f
congenital anomalies of
  cystic dilatation in, 840–843,
    842f–844f
  gas in biliary system and
    pancreaticobiliary reflux in, 856
  narrowing and obstruction in, 835f,
    835–836
cystadenoma of, 812, 814f, 826
dilatation of
  cystic, 838–846. *See also*
    Choledochal cyst
duodenal filling defects in, 372f, 373
duodenal impressions in, 358, 358f
duodenal sweep widening in, 356,
  356f
fibroma of, 812, 826
filling defects of, 805–817
impressions on duodenum, 358, 358f
metastases to
  filling defects in, 812, 813f
  narrowing and obstruction in,
    823–824, 823f–824f
in Mirizzi syndrome
  filling defects of, 807–808, 807f–808f
  narrowing and obstruction of, 807,
    834, 834f
narrowing and obstruction of, 818–837
  in calculi, 805, 807f, 807–808, 833f,
    834, 834f
  in Mirizzi syndrome, 807, 834, 834f
  postoperative pancreaticobiliary
    reflux in, 853, 853f
in Oriental cholangiohepatitis
  cystic dilatation of, 844–845, 845f
  filling defects of, 816, 816f
  narrowing and obstruction of, 828,
    828f
papilloma of
  filling defects in, 812, 843
  narrowing and obstruction in, 825,
    843
parasitic infections of. *See* Parasitic
  infections, of bile ducts
polyps of, adenomatous, 814f
strictures of, postoperative and
  traumatic, 834–835, 834f–835f
varices of, 810–811, 811f
vascular impressions on, 810, 810f, 836
Bile reflux gastritis, in postoperative
  remnant, 276–277, 277f–278f
Bile salt deficiency, gallbladder
  visualization impaired in, 776
Biliary system, 771–862
  atresia of, 835
  bile ducts in, 805–846. *See also* Bile
    ducts
  enlargement of papilla of Vater,
    847–851
  filling defects in, 787–817
  floating tumor debris in
    filling defects in, 812, 814f
    obstruction in, 825
  gallbladder in, 773–804. *See also*
    Gallbladder
  gas in, 852–862, 914–916, 915f
    in pancreaticobiliary reflux, 852–857

in portal vein, 858–862
  and pseudopneumobilia, 856, 856f
lollipop-tree appearance of, 842f, 843
tumor-induced mucus in
  filling defects in, 812, 814f
  obstruction in, 824f, 825
Billroth anastomosis
  filling defects of gastric remnant in,
    271, 272, 277f
  marginal ulcers in, 199f
  and pseudo-Billroth pattern in Crohn's
    disease, 212f, 213, 318, 318f, 513
Biopsy
  rectal, ulceration of colon after, 620,
    620f
  of small bowel, in dilatation, 450
Bird's beak appearance
  in achalasia, 15, 15f
  in volvulus of colon, 728, 729, 729f
Birth injury, paralysis of diaphragm in,
  153
Bismuth injection site, calcification of,
  1005
Bladder
  calcification of, 980–983, 980f–983f,
    985, 985f
  calculi in, 981–983, 981f–983f
  distention of, large bowel obstruction
    in, 733
  fistulas of
    colovesical, 925–926, 925f–926f, 928,
      928f
    colovesicoenteric, 925f
    colovesicovaginal, 928f
    enterovesical, 926f, 927f
  tumors of
    calcification in, 980, 985, 985f
    metastatic to rectum, retrorectal
      space enlargement in, 766
Blastomycosis, South American, coned
  cecum in, 577–578, 578f
Bleeding. *See* Hemorrhage
Blind loop syndrome, 534
Blood clots, filling defects from. *See*
  Clots, filling defects from
Blumer's shelf, in metastatic tumors of
  colon, 644, 645f
Bochdalek foramen hernia, 167–171,
  169f–170f
Body casts
  duodenal obstruction and dilatation in,
    403, 403f
  gastric dilatation in, nonobstructive,
    292
Boerhaave's syndrome, 134, 134f
  double-barrel appearance of esophagus
    in, 137, 138f
Bone carcinoma, metastatic,
  nephrocalcinosis in, 969
Bone marrow transplantation, graft-
  versus-host disease in
  and esophageal narrowing, 91, 92f
  and pneumatosis intestinalis, 890
  and separation of small bowel loops,
    527–528, 528f
Bourne test of colovesical fistula, 926
Brachial plexus block, paralysis of
  diaphragm in, 153

Brain tumors, gastric dilatation in, 293
Breast carcinoma, metastatic. *See*
  Metastases, of breast carcinoma
Brenner tumor, psammomatous
  calcification of ovary in, 990, 990f
Broad ligament hernia, 874
Bronchogenic carcinoma. *See*
  Carcinoma, of lung
Bronchus, impressions on esophagus,
  31f, 32
Brown bowel syndrome, adynamic ileus
  in, 439, 439f
Brucellosis
  liver calcification in, 939
  splenic calcification in, 947f, 947–948
Brunner's gland
  adenoma of, duodenal filling defects
    in, 382, 382f
  hyperplasia of, 329, 330f
    duodenal filling defects in, 367f,
      367–368
Buerger's disease, thickening of small
  bowel mucosal folds in, 459
Bulb, duodenal, 315–319
  gas bubble in, differentiated from
    polyp, 376, 377f, 380f
  mucosal surface pattern of, 363–367,
    366f, 367f
Bull's eye appearance, 865–870
  in melanoma, metastatic, 251, 252f,
    385, 802, 865, 866f
  of small bowel
    in flexure defect of duodenum, 363
    in metastases, 385, 500, 867f
  of stomach
    in candidiasis, 270
    in melanoma, metastatic, 251, 252f
Burkitt's lymphoma
  of cecum, 570, 571f
  of stomach, filling defects in, 251, 251f
Burns, duodenal dilatation in, 403, 403f,
  405
Buttock crease, differentiated from
  urachal sign of
  pneumoperitoneum, 894, 897f
Bypass surgery, jejunoileal, pneumatosis
  intestinalis after, 888, 889f

Calcification, 936–1015
  of abdominal wall, 1002–1005,
    1003f–1004f
  adrenal, 995–996, 995f–996f
  of alimentary tract, 960–966, 959f–967f
  of appendix
    in mucocele, 561
    in myxoglobulosis, 563, 563f
  of bile ducts, 959, 959f
  of bladder, 980–983, 980f–983f, 985,
    985f
  of costal cartilage, 1005f, 1006
  of foreign bodies, 1006–1013,
    1006f–1013f
  of gallbladder, 800, 800f, 956–959,
    956f–959f
  of gallstones, 788, 788f, 789f, 956–958,
    956f–957f
  in rectum, 957f

Calcification (*continued*)
  generalized abdominal, 997–999, 998f–999f
    of genital tract, 986–994
      in females, 988–994, 988f–994f
      in males, 986–988, 986f–988f
    of kidney, 966–979, 968f–979f
    of ligaments, 1005f, 1006f
    of liver, 936–946, 937f–946f
    of pancreas, 849, 950–955, 952f–955f
      in pancreatitis, 343, 950–952, 952f, 954f, 955
      sunburst pattern in, 953f, 955
    psammomatous of ovary, 989–990, 990f
      generalized abdominal calcification in, 997–998, 998f
    retroperitoneal, 996–997, 996f–997f
    of spine, 1005f
    of spleen, 937f, 946–950, 947f–951f
    of stomach, in carcinoma, 247, 250f
    urachal, 984
    ureteral, 979–980, 979f–980f
    urethral, 983–988, 984f–985f
    of vascular structures, 1000–1002, 1000f–1003f
      in arteriovenous fistula, 977
      in hepatic artery aneurysm, 943–945
      in portal vein, 943, 943f–944f, 1001
      in renal artery aneurysm, 977, 977f
      in splenic artery, 948, 949f, 950f, 1000
      in vena cava, inferior, 945
Calcinosis, idiopathic, abdominal wall calcification in, 1005
Calcium
  hypercalcemia
    abdominal wall calcification in, 1005
    in hyperparathyroidism, 969
  increased intestinal absorption of, nephrocalcinosis in, 969–970
  milk of
    and gallbladder calcification, 958f, 958–959
    and kidney calcification, 977, 978f
Calcium gluconate injection site, calcification of, 1005
Calculi
  biliary
    calcified, 959, 959f
    in choledochal cyst, 839, 840f
    cystic dilatation in, 843
    filling defects in, 805–808, 806f–808f
    gas in biliary system in, 853–854
    impacted in ampulla of Vater, 834
    Mirizzi syndrome in, 807–808, 807f–808f, 834, 834f
    mulberry appearance in, 805
    obstruction and narrowing in, 805, 807f, 807–808, 833f, 834, 834f
    in Oriental cholangiohepatitis, 816, 816f, 828, 828f
    papilla of Vater enlargement in, 847–848, 848f, 849, 850
    and pseudocalculi, 809–811, 809f–810f
  bladder, 981–983, 981f–983f
    jackburr, 982–983, 983f
  enteroliths, 960, 959f–961f
  gallstones. *See* Gallstones
    intrahepatic, 941
    in kidney, 968f, 969
      adynamic ileus in, 433, 434f
    pancreatic, 950, 952, 953, 955
    in prostate, 986
    urachal, 984
    ureteral, 960, 961f, 979f, 979–980
      adynamic ileus in, 433, 434f
    urethral, 983–984, 984f–985f
Campylobacter infection
  of colon
    toxic megacolon in, 741
    ulcerations in, 605–606, 605f–606f
  of small bowel, irregular thickening of mucosal folds in, 479
Candidiasis
  of colon, 607
  of esophagus, 56–58, 56f–58f
    filling defects in, 105, 106f
    motility disorders in, 11f, 21, 22f
    narrowing in, 85–86, 88f
    nodular lesions in, 143–144, 145f, 146f
    ulcerations in, 56f, 57, 57f, 58
  of stomach
    filling defects in, 270
    ulcerations in, 203f, 204
Cannon's law, 18
Cannon's point of colon, 637f
Carcinoembryonic antigen levels in colon carcinoma, 635
Carcinoid-islet cell tumors of duodenum, filling defects in, 383f, 383–385
Carcinoid tumors
  of appendix, 565–566
  of bile ducts, 812
  bull's-eye lesions in, 866
  carcinoid syndrome in, 488, 489f
  of colon, 649, 675–677, 675f, 676f
  of gallbladder, 799, 802
  of ileocecal valve, 547f, 548
  of rectum, 675, 675f, 676f
  of small bowel
    multiple filling defects in, 499, 499f
    separation of bowel loops in, 490f, 520, 521f
    solitary filling defect in, 488, 489f, 490f
  of stomach
    filling defects in, 246–247, 249f
    ulcerations in, 196, 198f, 246–247, 249f
Carcinoma
  of adrenal gland
    calcification in, 996
    duodenal impressions in, 359
  of ampulla of Vater, 385
    filling defects of bile ducts in, 811
    gas in biliary tree and pancreaticobiliary reflux in, 855
    narrowing and obstruction of bile ducts in, 821, 822f
  of appendix, 565f, 566
  of bile ducts
    filling defects in, 811, 811f, 812f
    narrowing and obstruction in, 819–820, 820f–821f
    Thorotrast-induced, 946, 946f
  of bladder, calcification in, 980, 985, 985f
  of bone, nephrocalcinosis in, 969
  of breast, metastatic. *See* Metastases, of breast carcinoma of cecum, 568f, 576f, 577, 577f
    coned cecum in, 577, 577f
  of cervix uteri
    complications of gold therapy in, 994, 994f
    metastatic. *See* Metastases, of cervical carcinoma
  cloacogenic, retrorectal space enlargement in, 765
  of colon
    achalasia in, 17f
    annular, 614, 633–638, 633f–638f
    apple-core appearance in, 614, 633, 636, 723, 725f
    calcification in, 964, 965f
    clinical presentation of, 634f, 634–635
    in Crohn's disease, 647–648
    differentiated from ameboma, 680
    differentiated from diverticula, 636, 637f, 656f, 657
    double tracking pattern in, 756, 758f, 759f
    enteric-enteric fistulas in, 920, 922f
    etiology of, 634
    impression of duodenum, 361
    internal fistula in, 928f
    ischemic colitis in, 749
    laboratory tests in, 635
    metastatic. *See* Metastases, of colon carcinoma
    multiple filling defects in, 700f, 701
    napkin-ring appearance in, 633, 723
    narrowing in, 633–649, 633f–649f
    necrotic, portal vein gas in, 860
    obstruction in, 723, 724f, 725f
    overhanging margins in, 633, 633f, 636, 636f, 641, 641f, 723
    pneumatosis intestinalis in, 886f, 887
    in polyps, 667–668, 695, 695f
    prognosis in, 635–636
    saddle appearance in, 614, 636, 669–670, 670f
    scirrhous, 639f, 639–640
    ulcerations in, 614–615, 614f–615f
    in ulcerative colitis, 588, 639–640, 647, 647f
    in ureterosigmoidostomy, 648–649, 649f
  of duodenum
    apple-core appearance in, 397f
    bile-duct narrowing and obstruction in, 823, 823f
    in extension of gastric carcinoma, 315, 317f, 385
    filling defects in, 384f, 385
    narrowing and obstruction in, 397, 397f

perivaterian, 850, 850f
postbulbar ulceration in, 325
of esophagus, 17–18
in Barrett's esophagus, 55, 55f, 84
in diverticula, 120f, 120–121
esophagorespiratory fistula in, 76, 77f, 131–133, 132f
filling defects in, 102f, 102–103, 104f, 105, 105f
granular lesions in, 144–145, 146f
narrowing in, 75–81, 75f, 77f–81f
radiation-induced, 86–90, 90f
recurrence of, 79, 79f
treatment of, 76–81, 79f–81f
ulcerations in, 62, 62f–64f, 76, 77f
varicoid, 127, 127f
of gallbladder, 799–802, 799f–802f
calcification in, 959
filling defects in, 799–802, 799f–802f
impression on duodenum, 359
narrowing and obstruction of bile ducts in, 823
nonvisualization of gallbladder in, 799
porcelain appearance in, 800, 800f
of ileocecal valve, 547f, 548, 548f
of jejunum, 421f, 520f
of kidney
calcification in, 971, 973f, 975, 975f
gallbladder displacement in, 785, 785f
laryngectomy in, esophageal impressions in, 6f, 6–7
of liver
calcification in, 939, 940f
esophageal varices in, 123
of lung
achalasia in, 17, 17f
diaphragm paralysis in, 153, 155f
esophageal impressions in, 42, 42f, 43f
esophagorespiratory fistula in, 131, 132f, 133f
metastatic. See Metastases, of lung carcinoma
of ovary
calcification in, 989, 990, 991–992, 991f–992f, 997–998, 998f
metastatic to colon, 641, 642f
pseudomucinous, 991–992, 992f
of pancreas
antral pad sign in, 349, 349f
bile duct narrowing and obstruction in, 821, 822f
calcification in, 955
duodenal filling defects in, 384f, 385
duodenal impressions in, 349–350, 359
duodenal narrowing and obstruction in, 396f, 396–397
duodenal sweep widening in, 348–352, 349f–354f
duodenal ulcerations in, 325
Frostberg sign in, 349–350, 350f
gastrocolic fistula in, 920, 923f
metastatic. See Metastases, of pancreatic carcinoma

portal hypertension and esophageal varices in, 123
retrogastric space widening in, 311
stomach filling defects in, 251, 252, 253f, 254f
stomach mucosal fold thickening in, 237
stomach narrowing in, 210, 210f
stomach ulceration in, 198f
of papilla of Vater, 850
of prostate, metastatic
colon narrowing in, 640–641, 640f–641f
colon ulceration in, 615f
retrorectal space enlargement in, 765–766, 766f
of pyloric channel, gastric outlet obstruction in, 284
of rectum, 634, 634f, 635, 635f, 636f, 637f
retrorectal space enlargement in, 765, 765f
of small bowel
bull's eye lesions in, 866
in Crohn's disease, 648, 648f
in duodenum. See Carcinoma, of duodenum
in jejunum, 421f, 520f
narrowing and obstruction in, 397, 397f, 421f
separation of bowel loops in, 517, 520f
solitary filling defect in, 486, 486f
of stomach
achalasia in, 16f, 17, 82
in adenomatous polyps, 243, 247
calcification in, 247, 250f, 964, 964f
colon narrowing in, 642f, 643, 643f
duodenal bulb involvement in, 315, 317f, 385
esophageal narrowing in, 81f, 81–82
filling defects in, 247, 249f, 250f, 273–276, 273f–276f, 297, 297f
fistulas in, enteric-enteric, 920
of fundus, 296–297, 297f–299f
gallbladder visualization impaired in, 775f
metastatic. See Metastases, of stomach carcinoma
narrowing of stomach in, 205–209, 206f–208f
outlet obstruction in, 282, 283f, 284
pneumoperitoneum in, 901
postoperative recurrence of, 276, 276f
in postoperative stump, 273–276, 273f–275f
thickening of mucosal folds in, 233f, 233–234
ulcerations in, 193–194, 193f–194f, 247, 249f
of thyroid, metastatic
esophageal narrowing in, 82, 83f
liver calcification in, 942f
Carcinomatosis, 525f
separation of small bowel loops in, 521

Carcinosarcoma of esophagus, filling defects in, 102–103, 103f
Cardia obstruction, tertiary contractions of esophagus in, 21
Carman meniscus sign, 62, 670
in gastric malignancy, 615
in gastric ulcers, 189, 189f, 190f
Caroli's disease, cystic dilatation of bile ducts in, 840–843, 842f–844f
Cartilage, costal, calcification of, 1005f, 1006
Casts, body
duodenal obstruction and dilatation in, 403, 403f
gastric dilatation in, nonobstructive, 292
Cathartics
colon narrowing from, 630–631, 631f
ileocecal valve inflammation from, 549
Catheterization
for abdominal abscess drainage, 934
balloon. See Balloon catheterization
umbilical vein, portal vein gas in, 858, 859–860, 860f
Caustic injury of colon
narrowing in, 631, 631f
ulcerations in, 613, 613f
Cecum, 541–581
amebiasis of, 572, 573f, 574–576, 575f, 600
in appendix abnormalities, 554–566, 556f–565f, 576–577
bariolith in, 1010, 1011f
Burkitt's lymphoma of, 570, 571f
carcinoma of, 568f, 576f, 577, 577f
coned cecum in, 577, 577f
coiled spring appearance in appendicitis, 564f, 565
coned, 572–581, 600
Crohn's disease of
filling defects in, 567f
narrowing in, 572, 573f
diaphragm or web of, 570–571
dilatation without perforation of, in colonic obstruction, 722, 724f
diverticula of, perforated, narrowing in, 577, 577f
diverticulitis of, 577f
ileocecal, 567–569, 569f
endometriosis of, 570, 570f
fecalith in, adherent, 569–570, 570f
filling defects of, 554–571
herniation through foramen of Winslow, 873, 873f
in ileocecal valve abnormalities, 543–553
intussusception of appendix into, 564f, 564–565
intussusception of ileum into, 553
metastases to, 566f, 566–567
mobile, 727f
obstruction of, 722
tuberculosis of
coned cecum in, 550f, 572–574, 574f
filling defects in, 567f
ulcer of, solitary benign, 569
volvulus of, 723f, 724, 727f

Celiac disease of children, 446
small bowel dilatation in, 444
Cerebrovascular disease, esophageal
motility disorders in, 8, 16
Ceroidosis, adynamic ileus in, 439, 439f
Cervical spine
herniation of intervertebral disk in,
esophageal impressions in, 28, 28f
osteophytes of, anterior marginal,
esophageal impressions in, 27f,
27–28
Cervix uteri, carcinoma of
complications of gold therapy in, 994,
994f
metastatic. *See* Metastases, of cervical
carcinoma
Chagas' disease
duodenal dilatation in, 403
esophageal motility disorders in, 10,
16, 16f
large bowel obstruction in, 724, 726f
small bowel obstruction in, 450
Chalasia of infancy, reflux esophagitis in,
47, 47f
Chemical irritation, small bowel
obstruction in, 427
Chemotherapy
esophagitis and esophageal ulceration
in, 63–64, 65f
hepatic artery infusion of
cholangitis in, 827–828, 828f
stomach narrowing in, 217f, 218
stomach ulceration in, 193, 193f
Chest wall injury, elevation of diaphragm
in, 157
Chilaiditi's syndrome, 916, 916f
Children and infants
adrenal hemorrhage and calcification
in, 995, 995f
bile duct narrowing and obstruction
in, 835f, 835–836
celiac disease of, 444, 446
chalasia of, reflux esophagitis in, 47, 47f
congenital disorders of. *See* Congenital
disorders
cystic fibrosis of, size of gallbladder in,
781, 781f
duodenal intramural hematoma in,
375, 375f, 376f, 398, 398f
duodenal narrowing and obstruction
in, 387–391, 388f–391f
in growth spurt, 403
in narrowing of aorticomesenteric
angle, 403
enterocolitis in, necrotizing, 859, 859f,
883–885, 883f–884f
esophagorespiratory fistula in, 129–131
gallbladder visualization impaired in,
777
gastric outlet obstruction in, in antral
mucosal diaphragm, 285
gastritis in, and thickening of mucosal
folds, 227
gastrophy in, hypertrophic, 230f,
231–232
hernia in, diaphragmatic, 169f, 169–171
hydrops of gallbladder in, 358

ileus in
adynamic, 439, 440f
meconium, 425, 426f
imperforate anus in, 736–738, 737f
intussusception in, 423, 424, 425, 684–
685, 732f, 733, 733f
iron intoxication in, and narrowing of
stomach, 218
liver tumors in, calcified, 939–941, 941f
lymphoid hyperplasia in
and ileocecal enlargement, 553
of small bowel, 507, 508f, 509
Meckel's diverticula in, 536
meconium plug syndrome in, 738, 889
megacolon in, psychogenic, 731f, 733
neuroblastoma in, 996–997
pancreatic calcification in, 955
pneumatosis intestinalis, 883–885,
883f–884f, 889
pneumoperitoneum in, 894, 895f
polyp of colon in
and multiple filling defects, 698,
698f, 700, 700f
and single filling defect, 671
polyposis in
colon filling defects in, 671, 698,
698f, 700, 700f
small bowel filling defects in,
496–497
portal vein gas in, 858, 859–860, 859f–
860f
pyloric stenosis in, hypertrophic, 287,
288f
small bowel dilatation in, 444
small bowel obstruction in, 420
in atresia or stenosis, 427–429, 427f–
428f
duodenal, 387–391, 388f–391f, 403
in intussusception, 423, 424, 425
in meconium ileus, 425, 426f
typhilitis in, and thumbprinting pattern
of colon, 754, 754f
Wilms' tumor in, 996
Chlamydia infection of colon, ulcerations
in, 606
Chlorpromazine, adynamic ileus from,
435f
Cholangiocarcinoma
filling defects of bile ducts in, 811, 811f
narrowing and obstruction of bile
ducts in, 819–820, 820f–821f
Thorotrast-induced, 946, 946f
Cholangiography
artifacts in, 810, 811f
in choledochocele, 372f, 373
in duodenal diverticula, 531, 531f
in floating tumor debris of biliary
system, 814f
in granular cell tumors of bile ducts,
825
in obstruction of bile ducts, 819, 819f
transhepatic, in Mirizzi syndrome, 808f
in tumor-induced mucus of biliary
system, 824f
Cholangiohepatitis, Oriental
cystic dilatation of bile ducts in,
844–845, 845f

filling defects of bile ducts in, 816, 816f
narrowing and obstruction of bile
ducts in, 828, 828f
Cholangiolitic hepatitis, 828–829, 829f
Cholangitis
AIDS-related, 832f, 833
cystic dilatation of bile ducts in, 844
in Oriental cholangiohepatitis, 816,
816f, 828, 828f, 844–845, 845f
primary sclerosing, narrowing and
obstruction of bile ducts in,
826–828, 826f–828f
Cholecystectomy, gallbladder
visualization impaired in, 777
Cholecystitis
acute, gallbladder-bowel fistula in, 929
chronic
nonvisualization of gallbladder in,
777
polyps of gallbladder in, 798
small size of gallbladder in, 781, 781f
diaphragm elevation in, 156
duodenum in
dilatation of, 405, 405f
narrowing and obstruction of, 394,
395f
thickening of mucosal folds, 333, 333f
emphysematous
biliary gas in, 855–856, 856f, 914, 915f
portal vein gas in, 860, 861f
gastric outlet obstruction in, 285
ileus in, adynamic, 434f, 435
Cholecystoduodenostomy, gas in biliary
system after, 853f
Cholecystoenteric fistulas, 929
Cholecystography
absorption and excretion of contrast
agents in, 773–774
and appearance of nonabsorbed
agents, 1010, 1010f
factors affecting, 774–776, 774f–776f
in adenoma of gallbladder, 798
in adenomyomatosis, 797
in cholesterolosis, 795f, 797
conjugated and unconjugated contrast
agents in, appearance of, 777–778,
777f–778f
in enlargement of gallbladder, 780–781
in metastases to gallbladder, 802
to Mirizzi syndrome, 808
nonvisualization of gallbladder in,
773–778
in small size of gallbladder, 781–782
Cholecystoses, hyperplastic, gallbladder
filling defects in, 795–798
Choledochal cyst, 838–840, 839f–841f
duodenal impressions in, 358
duodenal sweep widening in, 356, 356f
retrogastric space widening in, 311
Choledochele
dilatation of bile ducts in, 373, 840, 842f
filling defects of duodenum in, 372f, 373
Choledocholithiasis. *See* Calculi, biliary
Cholelithiasis. *See* Gallstones
Cholera, toxic megacolon in, 741
Cholesterolosis, gallbladder filling
defects in, 795f, 795–796

Cholesterol polyp of gallbladder, 795f, 796
Cholestyramine therapy, gallbladder visualization impaired in, 776–777
Chordomas, retrorectal space enlargement in, 766–769
Chorea, Huntington's, esophageal motility disorders in, 8
Choristomas, adrenal, calcification in, 996
Cigarette smoking, and esophageal carcinoma, 75
Cirrhosis
    ascites in, and separation of small bowel loops, 521
    bile duct narrowing and obstruction in, 836
    calcification of liver in, 945
    gallbladder visualization impaired in, 777
    portal hypertension and esophageal varices in, 123, 124
    radiodensity of liver in, 945
    small bowel mucosal folds in, thickening of, 461, 462f
Cloacogenic carcinoma, retrorectal space enlargement in, 765
Clonorchis sinesis infection
    calcification of liver in, 939
    and carcinoma of biliary system, 819
    cystic dilatation of bile ducts in, 844
    filling defects of bile ducts in, 813–815, 815f
    gas in biliary system and pancreaticobiliary reflux in, 854–855
    narrowing and obstruction of bile ducts in, 830, 831f
Clostridium difficile infection, antibiotic-associated colitis in, 610
Clots, filling defects from
    in bile ducts, 810
    in small bowel
        duodenal, 362, 363f, 364f
        multiple, 504
        solitary, 492
    in stomach, 263
Clover-leaf deformity in duodenal ulcer disease, 393, 393f
Coagulation disorders, hemorrhage in
    and separation of small bowel loops, 519f
    and thickening of small bowel mucosal folds, 461
    and thumbprinting pattern of colon, 746
Coarctation of aorta, esophageal impressions in, 35, 36f
Cobblestone appearance
    of colon, in Crohn's disease, 595, 595f, 706f, 707
    of small bowel mucosal folds
        in abetalipoproteinemia, 480f, 481
        in Crohn's disease, 473, 474f, 500
Cocaine body packers, radiographic pattern in, 1009f, 1010
Coccidioidomycosis, liver calcification in, 939
Coiled spring appearance
    of cecum, in appendicitis, 564f, 565

in duodenal intramural hematoma, 376, 376f
in intussusception, 444, 446f, 685, 686f
    of appendix into cecum, 565
    ileocolic, 732f
    of ileum into cecum, 553
    and small bowel obstruction, 424, 424f
Coin, ingested, radiographic appearance of, 1007f
Colic, ureteral, adynamic ileus in, 433, 434f, 435
Colitis. *See also* Colon
    cystica profunda
        multiple filling defects in, 714f, 714–715, 770, 770f
        retrorectal space enlargement in, 770, 770f
        single filling defect in, 690, 690f
    cystica superficialis, 715
Collar-button appearance of colon
    in Crohn's disease, 594f
    in herpes simplex infection, 607f, 608
    in shigellosis, 603
    in ulcerative colitis, 592, 592f
Collateral circulation, mesenteric arterial
    filling defects of duodenum in, 337, 375
    impression on duodenum in, 361
    simulating thickening of mucosal folds, 337–338, 338f
    widening of duodenal sweep in, 337, 356
Colocolic fistula, in tuberculosis, 924f
Colocolic intussusception, 684, 734, 734f
Colocoxal fistula, 935
Colocutaneous fistula, 935
Colon, 583–770
    adenoma of, villous, 671–673, 672f
    adhesions of
        narrowing in, 659
        obstruction in, 738, 739f
        pseudotumors and filling defects in, 688f, 688–690
    aganglionosis of. *See* Aganglionosis
    amebiasis of. *See* Amebiasis, of colon
    amyloidosis of. *See* Amyloidosis, of colon
    artifacts in barium studies of, 665, 711–713, 712f
    ascariasis of, filling defects in, 681
    bacterial infections of, 601–607, 602f–607f
    in Bechet's syndrome, 617, 617f, 741
    bezoars in, 289f
        filling defects in, 691
        obstruction in, 289f, 740
    Campylobacter infection of, 605–606, 605f–606f, 741
    carcinoid tumors of, 649, 675–677, 675f, 676f
    carcinoma of. *See* Carcinoma, of colon
    cathartic use affecting, narrowing in, 630–631, 631f
    caustic injury of
        narrowing in, 631, 631f
        ulcerations in, 613, 613f

in Chagas' disease, obstruction of, 724, 726f
Crohn's disease of. *See* Crohn's disease, of colon
cut-off sign in acute pancreatitis, 341, 342f
cytomegalovirus infection of. *See* Cytomegalovirus infection, of colon
dilatation of
    gallbladder displacement in, 783, 784f
    in Hirschsprung's disease, 734–736, 735f–737f
    in toxic megacolon, 741–745
diverticula of. *See* Diverticula, of colon
diverticulitis of. *See* Diverticulitis, of colon
diverticulosis of
    narrowing in, 650, 651–653, 652f, 653f
    thumbprinting pattern in, 751
    ulcerations in, 617, 618f
drug-induced disorders of. *See* Drug-induced disorders, of colon
in duodenocolic apposition, 361
endometriosis of. *See* Endometriosis, of colon
enterocolitis of. *See* Enterocolitis
extrinsic pressure on
    in pancreatitis, 677f
    in periappendiceal abscess, 681, 681f
in fecal impaction, obstruction of, 731f, 733
filling defects of, 662–721
    multiple, 692–721
    single, 662–691
fistulas of
    colocolic, in tuberculosis, 924f
    colocoxal, 935
    colocutaneous, 935
    colovaginal, 927f
    colovenous, 929, 930f
    colovesical, 925–926, 925f–926f, 928, 928f
    colovesicoenteric, 925f
    colovesicovaginal, 928f
    duodenocolic, 920, 921f, 922f
    gastrocolic. *See* Gastrocolic fistulas
    gastrojejunocolic, 923, 925f
    ileocolic, 922f
foreign bodies in
    differentiated from polyposis, 712f, 713
    filling defects in, 682, 686f, 687
fungal infections of
    mucormycoma in, 681, 681f
    narrowing in, 629
    ulcerations in, 607
gallstones in, 687–688
in gonorrheal proctitis
    narrowing of, 628
    ulcerations of, 603f, 604–605
granulomatous colitis of, 593
hamartomas of
    on Cowden's disease, 705, 705f

Colon, hamartomas of (*continued*)
multiple filling defects in, 697
single filling defect in, 670–671
hemangioma of
multiple filling defects in, 705
single filling defect in, 674, 674f
in hernias, obstruction of, 729, 731f
herpes zoster infection of
filling defects in, 717–718, 718f
narrowing in, 629
ulcerations in, 608
ileus of, adynamic, 435–436, 435f–436f
compared to obstruction, 436, 722
in imperforate anus, obstruction of,
736–738, 737f–738f
impression on duodenum, 361
inflammatory strictures of, 723–724
in intussusception, 732f, 733–734,
733f–735f
colocolic, 684, 734, 734f
filling defects of, 684–687, 685f, 686f
ileocolic, 567, 568f, 684, 732f, 733,
733f–735f
obstruction of, 732f, 733, 733f–735f
ischemia of. *See* Ischemia, of colon
leiomyoma of, 674, 674f
leiomyosarcoma of, 675f
narrowing in, 644f
in leukemia
multiple filling defects of, 704
thumbprinting pattern of, 754, 754f
ulcerations of, 615, 616f
lipoma of, 673f, 673–674
in lymphogranuloma venereum
narrowing of, 628, 628f, 629f
ulceration of, 606–607, 607f, 628,
628f
lymphoid follicular pattern of,
715–717, 715f–716f
lymphoid hyperplasia of, nodular, 715,
715f
lymphoma of. *See* Lymphoma, of colon
malacoplakia of, multiple filling
defects in, 719f, 719–720
meconium plug in, 738
in mercury poisoning, 617
metastases to. *See* Metastases, to colon
microcolon in ileal atresia, 428, 428f
mucormycoma of, 681, 681f
mucosal dysplasia of, 707–708, 708f
narrowing of, 622–661
neuroma of, traumatic, in ileocolic
anastomosis, 493f, 697
obstruction of, 722–740
compared to adynamic ileus, 436, 722
and pseudo-obstruction, 740
in pancreatitis. *See* Pancreatitis, colon
in
perforation of, 722
in immunosuppressive therapy, 899,
899f
pneumoperitoneum in, 897, 898f
plasmacytoma of, extramedullary, 677–
679
in pneumatosis intestinalis, 882, 882f
polyp of. *See* Polyp, of colon
polyposis of. *See* Polyposis, of colon

postoperative colitis of, 620, 620f
in diversion procedures, 620, 620f,
711
multiple filling defects in, 711
pseudomembranous, 609, 612
pseudolymphoma of, narrowing in,
660, 660f
pseudomembranous colitis of,
609–612, 611f–612f
multiple filling defects in, 711, 711f
thumbprinting pattern in, 751, 752f
toxic megacolon in, 741
pseudopolyps of. *See* Pseudopolyps, of
colon
pseudotumors of, filling defects in,
688–689, 688f–689f
radiation injury of
narrowing in, 630, 630f
ulcerations in, 612–613, 612f–613f
in retractile mesenteritis, obstruction
of, 740, 740f
sacral foramen superimposed over,
689f, 690
salmonellosis of
toxic megacolon in, 741, 743f
ulcerations in, 601–603, 602f
sarcoma of, 675f
Kaposi's 649, 702, 702f
multiple filling defects in, 702, 702f
narrowing in, 644, 644f
schistosomiasis of. *See*
Schistosomiasis, of colon
shigellosis of
toxic megacolon in, 741
ulcerations in, 601–603, 602f
sigmoid
double tracking pattern in, 756–759
herniation through mesentery of, 874
volvulus of, 728, 728f–730f
in solitary rectal ulcer syndrome
narrowing of, 632f, 633
ulceration of, 617–619, 618f
spasm of, 636–638, 637f
sphincters of, 636, 637f
spindle cell tumors of
multiple filling defects in, 704f, 704–
705
single filling defect in, 673–674,
673f–675f
splenic flexure of
carcinoma of, metastatic to stomach,
299
impression on gastric fundus, 300
strongyloidiasis of. *See*
Strongyloidiasis, of colon
submucosal edema of, 717–718,
717f–718f
thumbprinting pattern in, 754, 754f
suture granuloma of, filling defects in,
689f, 690
thumbprinting pattern of, 746–755
in cytomegalovirus infection, 608,
751, 751f
in ulcerative colitis, 598, 599f
toxic megacolon, 741–745
pneumoperitoneum in, 897

trichuriasis of, multiple filling defects
in, 710f, 710–711
tuberculosis of
filling defects in, 681
narrowing in, 626–628, 628f
ulcerations in, 603f, 603–604, 626
in typhilitis
narrowing of, 659f, 659–660
thumbprinting pattern of, 754, 754f
in typhoid fever, 741
ulcerations of, 601, 602
ulcerations of. *See* Ulcerations, of colon
ulcerative colitis of. *See* Ulcerative
colitis
varices of, multiple filling defects in,
719f, 720
viral infections of
filling defects in, 717–718, 718f
narrowing in, 629–630, 630f
ulcerations in, 607f, 608–609,
608f–610f
volvulus of, 724–726, 728–729,
728f–730f
Yersinia infection of
multiple filling defects in, 711
submucosal edema in, 718, 718f
ulcerations in, 604f, 605
Colonoscopy, complications of
pneumatosis intestinalis in, 888
portal vein gas in, 860
retroperitoneal gas in, 905f
Colostomy, radiographic patterns in, 1002
Colovaginal fistulas, 927f
Colovenous fistulas, in diverticulitis, 929,
930f
Colovesical fistulas
in diverticulitis, 925–926, 925f–926f
in ulcerative colitis, 928, 928f
Colovesicoenteric fistula in diverticulitis,
925f
Colovesicovaginal fistula in colon
carcinoma, 928f
Computed tomography
in abscess
abdominal, 913–914, 913f–914f
appendiceal, 559f, 559–560
in ascites, 523, 523f
in biliary obstruction, 819, 819f
in carcinoma
of colon, 637f, 638, 638f
esophageal, 76, 78f
of gallbladder, 800, 800f, 801f, 802f
gastric, 208f, 209
pancreatic, 352, 353f, 354f
in Caroli's disease, 843, 844f
in colitis
cytomegalovirus, 609f
ulcerative, 596, 597f
in Crohn's disease
of colon, 596, 596f, 597f, 598f
of small bowel, 475, 476f
in cysts
choledochal, 840, 841f
gastric duplication, 267, 268f
in diverticulitis
of colon, 654–656, 655f
and internal fistulas, 926, 926f, 927f

in eventration of diaphragm, 153f
in hernias
  Bochdalek, 170f
  incisional, 878, 878f
  obturator, 876, 876f
in intussusception, 424–425, 425f
in leiomyosarcoma of stomach, 254,
  256f
in lipoma
  of small bowel, 379f, 380, 497, 498f
  of stomach, 246, 247f
in lymphoma
  of small bowel, 471, 471f
  of stomach, 209f, 210
in mesenteritis, retractile, 527, 527f
in mucocele of appendix, 561–563,
  562f, 563f
in pancreatitis, 341–342, 343f, 344, 345f
in pseudocyst of pancreas, 347, 348f
in pseudomyxoma peritonei, 998, 998f
in retrorectal space enlargement, 766,
  768f
in varices of stomach, 303, 303f
Condyloma acuminatum, giant anorectal,
  629, 629f
Coned cecum, 572–578
Congenital disorders
  of bile ducts
    cystic dilatation in, 840–843,
      842f–844f
    gas in biliary system and
      pancreaticobiliary reflux in, 856
    narrowing and obstruction in, 835f,
      835–836
  duodenal narrowing and obstruction
    in, 387–391, 388f–391f
  esophageal narrowing in, 70–75
  esophagorespiratory fistulas in,
    129–131, 130f, 131f
  eventration of diaphragm in, 152
  of gallbladder, 782, 803–804
  gastric outlet obstruction in, 285–286,
    287, 288f
  hernias in
    diaphragmatic, 165, 169–171, 169f,
      171f, 173, 173f
    nondiaphragmatic, 871–880
  Hirschsprung's disease in, 734
  ileal atresia in, 427–428, 427f–428f
  jejunal atresia in, 427f, 427–428
  Meckel's diverticula in, 536
  splenic cysts in, calcified, 948
  webs or diaphragms in
    of bile ducts, 835f, 835–836
    of cecum, 570–571
    of duodenum, 389–390, 390f, 534
    of gastric antrum, 285
Connective tissue disorders
  esophageal motility disorders in, 7–10,
    8f–10f
  esophagitis in, reflux, 9, 48, 48f
  gastric dilatation in, nonobstructive,
    293–295, 294f
  pneumatosis intestinalis in, 887–888
  of small bowel
    dilatation in, 403, 404f, 446–448,
      447f, 450

    duodenum in, 403, 404f
    hide-bound sign in, 446, 447f
    pseudodiverticula in, 535, 535f
    thickening of mucosal folds in, 458–
      459
Contrast agents
  cholangiosarcoma from, 946, 946f
  cholecystographic
    absorption and excretion of,
      773–776, 774f–776f
    failure of patient to ingest,
      nonvisualization of gallbladder in,
      774
  extravasated, differentiated from
    internal fistulas, 931, 932f–933f
  residual, 1010, 1010f
    kidney calcification in, 977–979, 979f
    liver density in, 945f, 946, 946f
    lymph node calcification in, 1001
    spinal calcification in, 1005
    splenic density in, 945f, 950
  splenic angiosarcoma from, 950, 951f
Corkscrew appearance in splenic artery
  calcification, 948, 949f
Corrosive agents, ingestion of
  esophageal disorders in
    esophagorespiratory fistula in, 134,
      135f
    narrowing in, 84, 86f
    nodular lesions in, 143, 145f
    ulcerations in, 62–63, 65f
  pneumatosis intestinalis in, 886
  portal vein gas in, 860
  stomach disorders in
    gas in wall of, 312
    narrowing of, 215–217, 216f
    outlet obstruction of, 285, 285f
    thickening of mucosal folds of, 226–
      227, 227f
    ulcerations of, 191f
Costal cartilage calcification, 1005f, 1006
Courvoisier phenomenon
  in cholangiocarcinoma, 819
  duodenal impressions in, 359
  enlargement of gallbladder in, 779, 780f
Cowden's disease
  colon filling defects in, 705, 705f
  esophageal nodular lesions in, 146
  stomach filling defects in, 243f, 244
Cranial nerve disorders, esophageal
  motility disorders in, 8
Crescent sign in gastric ulcers, 182, 182f
Cricopharyngeus muscle, 3
  achalasia of, 5f, 5–8, 26, 27f
  posterior impression on esophagus, 5f,
    5–7, 6f, 26, 27f
Crohn's disease
  of appendix, 559f, 560–561
  of biliary system, pancreaticobiliary
    reflux in, 854
  of cecum
    filling defects in, 567f
    narrowing in, 572, 573f
  of colon, 586, 592–596, 593f–598f
    anal canal abnormalities in, 595, 595f
    aphthoid ulcers in, 594, 594f
    carcinoma in, 647–648

    cobblestone appearance in, 595,
      595f, 706f, 707
    collar-button ulcers in, 594f
    differentiated from diverticulitis, 756
    differentiated from ulcerative colitis,
      595, 596, 597f
    double tracking pattern in, 756, 758f
    filling defects in, 680, 680f
    ileum in, 593, 593f, 594, 595
    narrowing in, 624, 625f
    portal vein gas in, 860
    pseudopolyps in, 706f, 707, 707f
    skip lesions in, 593, 593f, 595
    thumbprinting pattern in, 749, 749f
    toxic megacolon in, 741, 742f
  differentiated from appendicitis, 557
  differentiated from tuberculosis,
    572–574, 574f
  of duodenum
    of bulb, 315–318, 318f
    narrowing and obstruction in,
      392–393, 392f–393f, 405
    postbulbar ulceration in, 327, 327f
    thickening of mucosal folds in, 334,
      334f
  of esophagus
    esophagorespiratory fistula in, 135
    filling defects in, 105–106, 107f
    narrowing in, 86, 88f
    ulceration in, 59, 61f
  fistulas in
    enteric-enteric, 919, 920f–921f
    esophagorespiratory, 135
    external, 934, 934f, 935f
    internal, 928, 928f
  gallbladder visualization impaired in,
    776
  of ileocecal valve, 548–549, 549f
  oxaluria and renal calcification in, 971,
    971f
  pneumatosis intestinalis in, 887
  pneumoperitoneum in, 901
  pseudo-Billroth pattern in, 212f, 213,
    318, 318f, 513
  retrorectal space enlargement in, 762f,
    763
  of small bowel
    carcinoma in, 648, 648f
    cobblestone appearance in, 473,
      474f, 500
    dilatation and thickening of mucosal
      folds in, 454
    in duodenum. *See* Crohn's disease,
      of duodenum
    filling defects in, 500, 502f, 510f
    in ileum, 593, 593f, 594, 595
    irregular thickening of mucosal folds
      in, 472–475, 473f–476f
    in jejunum, obstruction in, 421f
    obstruction in, 421f, 427
    pseudodiverticula in, 535, 535f
    sandlike lucencies in, 510f, 511–512
    separation of bowel loops in, 475,
      475f, 517, 518f
    skip lesions in, 474f, 475

Crohn's disease, of small bowel
  (*continued*)
    stomach involvement in, 315–318,
      318f, 513
    string sign in, 474f, 475
  of stomach
    filling defects in, 261
    narrowing in, 211f, 212f, 212–213
    outlet obstruction in, 284f, 285
    pseudo-Billroth pattern in, 212f, 213
    ram's horn sign in, 211f, 213
    small bowel involvement in,
      315–318, 318f, 513
    superficial erosions in, 203f, 204
    thickening of mucosal folds in, 234,
      513
  string sign in, 474f, 475, 572, 573f
Cronkhite-Canada syndrome
  colon polyps and multiple filling
    defects in, 698, 698f, 699f
  of small bowel
    filling defects in, 497
    sandlike lucencies in, 512
Cryptosporidiosis
  of small bowel, thickening of mucosal
    folds in
    and dilatation, 454, 454f
    in duodenum, 334–335, 335f
    irregular, 479
  of stomach, narrowing in, 215, 216f
Cupola sign of pneumoperitoneum, 894,
  897f
Cushing's disease
  nephrocalcinosis in, 969
  retrorectal space enlargement in, 770
Cyst
  adrenal
    calcification of, 996
    retrogastric space widening in, 311f
  of bile ducts, 838–846. *See also*
    Choledochal cyst
  dermoid. *See* Dermoid cysts
  developmental, retrorectal space
    enlargement in, 763–765
  duplication. *See* Duplication
  enteric, retrorectal space enlargement
    in, 763–764
  of gallbladder, intramural epithelial,
    803, 803f
  gas-filled, in pneumatosis intestinalis,
    881, 882, 882f, 883, 883f
  hydatid. *See* Hydatid cysts
  intra-abdominal, diaphragm elevation
    in, 156
  of kidney
    calcification in, 971–973, 973f–974f
    duodenal impressions in, 359, 360f
    gallbladder displacement in, 785
    residual Pantopaque in, 977–979,
      979f
  of liver
    bile duct filling defects in, 815–816,
      816f
    bile duct narrowing and obstruction
      in, 830, 831f, 833, 836
    calcification in, 938, 938f, 941
    diaphragm elevation in, 156, 156f

  duodenal impressions in, 359
  gallbladder displacement in, 784f
  gastric impressions in, 255, 258f
  mesenteric, calcification in, 964, 967f
  pericardial, compared to Morgagni
    foramen hernia, 167, 168f
  postanal, retrorectal space
    enlargement in, 763, 764
  pulmonary, esophagorespiratory fistula
    in, 136
  retroperitoneal
    duodenal sweep widening in, 356
    retrogastric space widening in, 311,
      311f
  of spleen, calcification in, 948, 948f
Cystadenocarcinoma
  of ovary
    colon narrowing in, 642f
    generalized abdominal calcification
      in, 997–998, 998f
    ovary calcification in, 989, 990, 991f
  of pancreas
    calcification in, 955
    duodenal sweep widening in, 352
Cystadenoma
  of bile ducts, 812, 814f, 826
  of gallbladder, 799
  of ovary, calcification in, 989, 990f
    generalized abdominal, 998
  of pancreas
    calcification in, 955
    duodenal sweep widening in, 352,
      354f
    retrogastric space widening in, 310
Cystic duct
  calculi in, 788, 791f
    in postoperative remnant, 959
  dilatation of, in choledochal cyst, 838,
    839f
  neurinoma of, 825
  obstruction of, gallbladder
    visualization impaired in, 777
Cysticercosis, calcification in
  of abdominal wall, 1002, 1004f
  of liver, 939
Cystic fibrosis
  colon filling defects in, 717, 717f
  duodenal fold thickening in, 338f, 338–
    339
  fecalith of cecum in, adherent,
    569–570, 570f
  gallbladder size in, 781f, 781–782
  meconium ileus in, 425
  pancreatic calcification in, 955, 955f
  sandlike lucencies of small bowel in,
    512
Cystitis, bladder calcification in, 980
Cytomegalovirus infection
  cholangitis, 832f, 833
  of colon
    narrowing in, 630, 630f
    pseudopolyps and filling defects in,
      711
    thumbprinting pattern in, 608, 751,
      751f
    ulcerations in, 608, 608f–609f, 630f

  coned cecum in, 580f, 581
    enteric-enteric fistula in, 923, 924f
    enteritis in, and separation of small
      bowel loops, 517, 519f
    esophagitis in, 58, 60f
    retrorectal space enlargement in, 763,
      764f
  of stomach
    narrowing in, 215, 215f
    superficial erosions in, 204
    thickening of mucosal folds in, 228,
      228f
Dermatomyositis
  duodenal dilatation in, 403
  esophageal motility disorders in, 7, 10
  gastric dilatation in, nonobstructive,
    295
  of small bowel
    dilatation in, 403, 446, 450
    thickening of mucosal folds in, 458–
      459
Dermoid cysts
  of ovary
    calcification in, 989, 989f, 990f
    entero-ovarian fistula in, 929, 932f
    retrorectal space enlargement in, 763
  of spleen, calcification in, 948
Developmental cysts, retrorectal space
    enlargement in, 763–765
Diabetes mellitus
  esophageal motility disorders in, 10,
    17, 21, 23f
  gallbladder enlargement in, 780, 781
  gastric dilatation in, nonobstructive,
    292f, 293, 294f, 295f
  ileus in, adynamic, 435f
  portal vein gas in, 860
  small bowel dilatation in, 448
    duodenal, 405
  splenic artery calcification in, 949f
  vas deferens calcification in, 986, 986f
Dialysis
  calcification of kidney in, 977
  thickening of duodenal mucosal folds
    in, 333–334
Diaphragm, 149–175
  elevation of, 151–158
  eventration of, 152–153, 152f–155f
  hernias of, 159–175
  paralysis of, 153–156, 155f
    sniff test in, 156
  and pseudodiaphragmatic contour in
    infrapulmonic effusion, 157f, 157–
    158
  soft-tissue space between diaphragm
    and gastric fundus, 300, 301f
Diaphragms or webs. *See* Webs
Diarrhea, gallbladder visualization
    impaired in, 774
Dienenger's sign in phlegmonous
    gastritis, 215
Dilatation
  of bile ducts, 838–846
  of colon
    gallbladder displacement in, 783,
      784f

in Hirschsprung's disease, 734–736,
735f–737f
in toxic megacolon, 741–745
of small bowel, 441–455
in duodenum, 400, 401–407, 783, 784f
in ileum of neonate, 428f, 428–429
with normal folds, 441–451
with thickened folds, 452–455
of stomach, 291–295
diaphragm elevation in, 155f
portal vein gas in, 860, 861f
Diphenoxylate therapy
adynamic ileus in, 433
small bowel dilatation in, 442
Diphtheria, esophageal motility disorders
in, 8
Diversion colitis, postoperative, 620, 620f
multiple filling defects in, 711
Diverticula
of cecum, narrowing in, 577, 577f
of colon
carcinoma differentiated from, 636,
637f
multiple filling defects in, 713f, 713–
714
narrowing in, 650–657, 650f–656f
polyps differentiated from, 665f,
665–666, 713–714
ulcerations in, 617, 618f
of duodenum, 529–531, 530f–532f
bile duct narrowing and obstruction
in, 836
differentiated from giant ulcerations,
531–533, 532f–533f
differentiated from postbulbar
ulceration, 328
distortion in pancreatic carcinoma,
350, 351f
gallbladder visualization impaired in,
775f, 776
gas-filled, filling defects in, 363, 365f
halo sign in, 398, 534, 534f
intraluminal, 390, 398, 534, 534f
obstruction in, 398
and pseudodiverticula, 533f, 533–534
epiphrenic, 119f, 120, 120f
gallbladder visualization impaired in,
776
of esophagus, 117–122
carcinoma in, 120f, 120–121
double-barrel appearance in, 141f,
141–142
esophagorespiratory fistula in, 135,
136f
lateral, 119, 119f
and pseudodiverticula, 67f, 68, 93,
94f, 121f, 121–122
pulsion, 120
traction, 118f, 119, 119f
hepatic duct, 840
of ileum, 538f, 538–539
and pseudodiverticula, 535, 539
of jejunum, 534–535, 535f
pneumatosis intestinalis in, 890
and pseudodiverticula, 535, 535f
Meckel's. *See* Meckel's diverticula
of stomach, 307, 307f

compared to benign ulcer, 182, 182f,
183f
gallbladder visualization impaired in,
776
urethral, calculi in, 984, 984f, 985f
Zenker's 5, 117–119, 118f
gallbladder visualization impaired in,
776
Diverticulitis
of cecum, 577f
of colon
differentiated from carcinoma, 636,
637f, 656f, 657
differentiated from Crohn's disease,
756
double tracking pattern in, 756, 757f
filling defects in, 681–682, 682f
narrowing in, 653–657, 653f–656f
obstruction in, 723–724, 726f
thumbprinting pattern in, 751
ulcerations in, 617, 618f
double tracking pattern in, 756, 757f,
919
extravasated contrast material in, 931,
932f
fistulas in
enteric-enteric, 919, 921f
external, 935
internal, 925–926, 925f–927f, 929,
930f
gallbladder visualization impaired in,
776
ileocecal, 567–569, 569f
jejunal, 534–535
pneumoperitoneum in, 897
portal vein gas in, 860
retroperitoneal gas in, 903, 904f
retrorectal space enlargement in, 763,
764f
Diverticulosis
of colon
narrowing in, 650, 651–653, 652f,
653f
thumbprinting pattern in, 751
ulcerations in, 617, 618f
of jejunum, 534, 535, 535f
gallbladder visualization impaired in,
776
pneumoperitoneum in, 535, 900f, 901
and pseudodiverticulosis of esophagus,
67f, 68, 121f, 121–122
narrowing in, 93, 94f
Double-barrel esophagus, 137–142
Double bubble sign in duodenal atresia,
388, 388f
Double contour effect on duodenum, in
pancreatic carcinoma, 349, 349f,
351f
Double tracking pattern
in diverticulitis, 756, 757f, 919
in pyloric stenosis, hypertrophic, 287
in sigmoid colon, 756–759
Douching, vaginal, pneumoperitoneum
after, 901
Douglas, pouch of, metastases to, 644,
645f

Doxorubicin therapy, esophagitis and
esophageal ulceration in, 64, 65f
Dracunculiasis, abdominal wall
calcification in, 1002, 1004f
Drug-induced disorders
bezoars in, 289f, 740
of colon, 620
ileus in, adynamic, 435f, 436f
narrowing in cathartic use, 630–631,
631f
pseudomembranous colitis,
postantibiotic, 609–612
staphylococcal colitis, postantibiotic,
604f, 605
thumbprinting pattern in, 746
urticaria in, 717
of esophagus
double-barrel appearance in, 141
motility disorders in, 10
reflux esophagitis in, 48
ulcerations in, 64–66, 66f
hemorrhage in
and separation of small bowel loops,
519f
and thickening of small bowel
mucosal folds, 457f, 458, 458f
and thumbprinting pattern of colon,
746
ileocecal valve inflammation in, 549
ileus in, adynamic, 433, 433f, 435f, 436f
nephrocalcinosis in, 969, 971, 972f
pneumatosis intestinalis in, 890
of small bowel
dilatation in, 442
filling defects in, 492, 500
of stomach
and appearance of radiopaque pills
in stomach, 1006f, 1007
dilatation in, 293
superficial erosions in, 201, 202f, 204
ulcerations and gastrocolic fistula in,
921
Duodenitis
filling defects in, 369, 369f
thickening of mucosal folds in,
330–333, 331f, 332f, 369f
Duodenocolic apposition, colon
impression on duodenum in, 361
Duodenocolic fistulas, 922f
in carcinoma of colon, 920
in Crohn's disease, 921f
Duodenum, 321–407
adenoma of, filling defects in, 376,
377f, 382–383, 383f
amyloidosis of, thickening of mucosal
folds in, 337
in aortic aneurysm
impressions on, 361
obstruction and dilatation of, 405,
406f
widening of sweep, 356
anomalous blood vessels of, filling
defects in, 375
atresia of, 387–388, 388f
double bubble sign in, 388, 388f
in Brunner's gland hyperplasia

Duodenum, in Brunner's gland
  hyperplasia (*continued*)
  filling defects of, 367f, 367–368
  thickening of mucosal folds, 329, 330f
 bulb of
  gas bubble in, differentiated from
    polyp, 376, 377f, 380f
  in gastric antrum disorders, 315–319
  mucosal surface pattern of, 363–367,
    366f, 367f
 carcinoma of. *See* Carcinoma, of
    duodenum
 congestion of, chronic, thickening of
    mucosal folds in, 338
 Crohn's disease of. *See* Crohn's
    disease, of duodenum
 diaphragm or web of, congenital, 389–
    390, 390f, 534
 dilatation of, 400, 401–407
  gallbladder displacement in, 783, 784f
  normal variations in, 401–403, 402f
 diverticula of. *See* Diverticula, of
    duodenum
 in duodenocolic apposition, 361
 duplication cyst of
  filling defects in, 372f, 373–374
  obstruction in, 391, 391f
 filling defects of, 362–386
 fistulas of
  aorticoduodenal, 327–328, 398, 398f,
    405
  duodenocolic, 920, 921f, 922f
  with gallbladder, 853, 854f, 929, 931f
  renoduodenal, 929
 flexure defect of, 363, 366f
 in gastroenteritis, eosinophilic, 318,
    318f
 hematoma of, intramural. *See*
    Hematoma, duodenal intramural
 hypotonic study of, normal anatomy in,
    371, 371f
 impressions on, 357–361
  in pancreatic carcinoma, 349–350
 leiomyoma of
  filling defects in, 378, 378f
  ulceration in, postbulbar, 325
 lipoma of, filling defects in, 378–380,
    378f–379f
 lymphoma of. *See* Lymphoma, of
    duodenum
 metastases to
  filling defects in, 385, 385f, 386f
  postbulbar ulceration in, 325–327
 narrowing and obstruction of, 387–400
  proximal dilatation in, 400, 401–407
 in pancreatic pseudocyst
  filling defects of, 373f, 374
  narrowing and obstruction of, 394,
    395f
  widening of sweep, 346–348,
    346f–348f
 in pancreatitis. *See* Pancreatitis,
    duodenum in
 papilla of
  enlargement of, 373
  filling defects from, 371f, 371–373
 in paraduodenal hernia, 871–872, 872f

 perforation of, retroperitoneal gas in,
    903, 904f
 peristaltic activity of, reduced,
    obstruction and dilatation in, 403–
    405, 404f
 polyps of, 371f
  filling defects in, 376, 377f, 380, 380f
 sarcoma of
  filling defects in, 385, 386
  narrowing and obstruction in, 397,
    397f
  thickening of mucosal folds in, 335
 spindle cell tumors of
  differentiated from papilla of Vater
    enlargement, 850
  postbulbar ulceration in, 325
 strongyloidiasis of
  gastric involvement in, 318
  narrowing and obstruction in, 394,
    394f, 405
  thickening of mucosal folds in, 334,
    335f
 sweep of
  normal variations in, 340
  widening of, 340–356
 thickening of mucosal folds, 329–339
 tuberculosis of. *See* Tuberculosis, of
    duodenum
 ulcerations of. *See* Ulcerations, of
    duodenum
 varices of
  filling defects in, 337, 337f, 373f,
    374–375
  impressions on duodenum in, 361
  thickening of mucosal folds in, 337,
    337f, 373f, 375
 villous tumors of, bile duct obstruction
    in, 824, 824f
 in Zollinger-Ellison syndrome
  postbulbar ulceration of, 324–325,
    326f
  thickening of mucosal folds, 324,
    326f, 330, 330f, 331f
Duplication
 of esophagus
  double barrel appearance in, 142,
    142f
  filling defects in, 106, 109f, 110f
  retrorectal space enlargement in, 763
 of small bowel
  duodenal filling defects in, 372f,
    373–374
  duodenal obstruction in, 391, 391f
  ileal, 539
  solitary filling defect in, 491
 of stomach
  filling defects in, 267, 267f–268f
  outlet obstruction in, 286
Dysautonomia, familial, esophageal
    motility disorders in, 8
Dysentery, bacillary
 narrowing of colon in, 626
 toxic megacolon in, 741
 ulceration of colon in, 601–603
Dysphagia, in esophageal carcinoma, 76
Dysplasia, mucosal, of colon, 707–708,
    708f

Dystrophy, muscular
 esophageal motility disorders in, 7, 7f,
    11
 gastric dilatation in, nonobstructive,
    295
 ileus in, adynamic, 435

Echinococcus infection
 of bile ducts
  cystic dilatation in, 846f
  filling defects in, 815–816
  narrowing and obstruction in, 830,
    831f, 833
 kidney calcification in, 973, 974f
 liver calcification in, 938, 938f
 splenic calcification in, 948, 948f
Ectopia
 of pancreas
  bull's eye lesions in, 868, 869f
  differentiated from papilla of Vater
    enlargement, 850
  differentiated from postbulbar
    ulceration of duodenum, 328
  duodenal filling defects in, 369–370,
    370f
  gallbladder filling defects in, 804,
    804f
  gastric filling defects in, 255–259,
    259f
 of sebaceous glands, nodular lesions of
    esophagus in, 146
 of stomach
  in duodenal bulb, 368f, 368–369
  in esophagus, 28–29, 29f
  gallbladder filling defects in, 804
  intussusception in, 424, 424f, 492
  in Meckel's diverticula, 536, 536f,
    538, 538f
  obstruction of small bowel in, 424,
    424f
  solitary filling defects of small bowel
    in, 491–492, 492f
Edema
 angioneurotic
  colon thumbprinting pattern in,
    751–754, 753f
  small bowel thickening of mucosal
    folds in, 462–463, 463f
 of colon, submucosal, 717–718,
    717f–718f
  thumbprinting pattern in, 754, 754f
 intestinal, thickening of small bowel
    mucosal folds in, 461–463,
    462f–463f
 of papilla of Vater, 847–850
Effusion, infrapulmonic,
    pseudodiaphragmatic contour in,
    157f, 157–158
Elderly. *See* Aging
Electrolyte imbalance
 gastric dilatation in, nonobstructive,
    295, 295f
 ileus in, adynamic, 433, 433f, 435f
Elevation of diaphragm, 151–158
Ellipse sign in gastric ulcers, 187–188,
    187f–188f

Embolism
  pulmonary, diaphragm elevation in, 157
  in ulcerative colitis, 588
Emepronium bromide, esophagitis and
    esophageal ulceration from, 66
Emesis. *See* Vomiting
Emotional stress
  duodenal dilatation in, 405
  gastric dilatation in, nonobstructive,
    295
Emphysema
  cholecystitis in
    and biliary gas, 855–856, 856f, 914,
      915f
    and portal vein gas, 860, 861f
  pneumoperitoneum in, 902
  retrogastric space widening in, 310
  of stomach, 887
    portal vein gas in, 860
    stomach wall gas in, 312, 313f, 314
Empyema, enlargement of gallbladder in,
    779–780, 780f
Endometriosis
  of cecum, 570, 570f
  of colon
    multiple filling defects in, 719, 719f
    narrowing in, 657, 657f
    obstruction in, 733
    single filling defect in, 683–684, 684f
    thumbprinting pattern in, 751
  of small bowel, solitary filling defect
    in, 491
Endoscopy
  complications of
    pneumatosis intestinalis in, 888, 888f
    pneumoperitoneum in, 901
    retroperitoneal gas in, 904
    stomach wall gas in, 314, 314f
  in gastric ulcers, role of, 188
  in retrograde
    cholangiopancreatography. *See*
    ERCP
Enema solutions, caustic injury of colon
    from
  narrowing in, 631, 631f
  ulcerations in, 613, 613f
Entamoeba histolytica infection, liver
    calcification in, 938–939
Enteric cysts, retrorectal space
    enlargement in, 763–764
Enteric-enteric fistulas, 919–925
Enteritis
  eosinophilic. *See* Eosinophilic enteritis
  infectious, dilatation and thickening of
    mucosal folds in, 454
  radiation-induced
    dilatation and thickening of mucosal
      folds in, 454
    sandlike lucencies in, 511f, 512
    separation of bowel loops in, 520,
      520f
Enterocolitis
  necrotizing
    pneumatosis intestinalis in, 883–885,
      883f–884f
    portal vein gas in, 858, 859, 859f

Yersinia
  coned cecum in, 578, 579f
  ·differentiated from appendicitis, 557
  ileocecal valve in, 549
  sandlike lucencies in, 510f, 512
Enteroliths, 960, 959f, 961f
  small bowel obstruction in, 420–422
Entero-ovarian fistulas, 929, 931f, 932f
Enteropathy, protein-losing. *See* Protein-
    losing enteropathy
Enterovesical fistula in diverticulitis,
    926f, 927f
Eosinophilic enteritis
  duodenal thickening of mucosal folds
    in, 337
  irregular thickening of small bowel
    mucosal folds in, 472, 472f
  regular thickening of small bowel
    mucosal folds in, 464–465
  sandlike lucencies of small bowel in,
    512
Eosinophilic esophagitis
  filling defects in, 106, 107f
  narrowing in, 86, 89f
  nodular and granular lesions in, 143
  ulcerations in, 60, 61f
Eosinophilic gastritis
  filling defects in, 261
  narrowing in, 214, 214f
  thickening of mucosal folds in, 234,
    235f
Eosinophilic gastroenteritis
  duodenal involvement in, 318, 318f
  thickening of mucosal folds in,
    513–514, 514f
Eosinophilic granuloma
  bull's eye lesions in, 868
  of stomach, filling defects in, 264–265,
    266f
Epidermoid cysts of spleen, calcified, 948
Epidermolysis bullosa of esophagus
  narrowing in, 90–91, 91f
  ulcerations in, 62, 62f, 91
Epiphrenic diverticula, 119f, 120, 120f
  gallbladder visualization impaired in,
    776
Epithelioma of bile ducts, cystic
    dilatation in, 843
ERCP
  in cystadenoma, 814f
  in *Echinococcus* infection and biliary
    obstruction, 831f
  in Mirizzi syndrome, 807f
  in obstruction of bile ducts, 819, 831f
  in tumor-induced mucus of biliary
    system, 814f
Erosions of stomach, superficial,
    201–204, 202f–204f
Erythroblastosis fetalis, portal vein gas
    in, 859
Escherichia coli infection, irregular
    thickening of small bowel mucosal
    folds in, 479
Esophagitis. *See* Esophagus
Esophagogastric hernia, pseudotumor of
    gastric fundus in, 300–303
Esophagogastric polyp, inflammatory,

    esophageal filling defects in, 100,
      101f
Esophagorespiratory fistulas, 129–136
  in carcinoma, 76, 77f
Esophagoscopy, complications of
  double-barrel appearance of esophagus
    in, 140, 141
  esophagorespiratory fistula in, 133, 134f
Esophagus, 1–147
  abscess of
    double-barrel appearance in, 141
    impressions on esophagus in, 29
  in achalasia, 10, 11–19, 11f–19f, 76
    narrowing of, 93, 94f
    tertiary contractions of, 15, 21, 33f
  in alcohol use and alcoholism
    carcinoma of, 75
    ulcerations of, 60, 61f
  balloon dilatation of
    in achalasia, 19, 19f
    in carcinoma, 79–81, 80f
  Barrett's. *See* Barrett's esophagus
  Behçet's syndrome of
    narrowing in, 86, 89f
    ulcerations in, 60
  candidiasis of. *See* Candidiasis, of
    esophagus
  carcinoma of. *See* Carcinoma, of
    esophagus
  cervical
    diverticula of, 117–119, 118f, 119f
    impressions on, 26–29
  corrosive injury of. *See* Corrosive
    agents, ingestion of, esophageal
    disorders in
  Crohn's disease of. *See* Crohn's
    disease, of esophagus
  cytomegalovirus infection of, 58, 60f
  diverticula of. *See* Diverticula of
    esophagus
  double-barrel appearance of, 137–142
  drug-induced disorders of. *See* Drug-
    induced disorders, of esophagus
  duplication of
    double-barrel appearance in, 142,
      142f
    filling defects in, 106, 109f, 110f
  ectopic gastric mucosa in, 28–29, 29f
  in eosinophilic esophagitis. *See*
    Eosinophilic esophagitis
  in epidermolysis bullosa
    narrowing of, 90–91, 91f
    ulcerations of, 62, 62f, 91
  in esophagogastric hernia, 300–303
  in esophagogastric polyp, 100, 101f
  feline appearance of, 49, 51f
  filling defects of, 97–116
    in varices, 106, 107f–109f, 114f, 115,
      128
  fistulas of, esophagorespiratory,
    129–136
    in carcinoma, 76, 77f
  foreign bodies in
    double-barrel appearance in, 140f,
      141
    esophagorespiratory fistula in, 133
    filling defects in, 106–113, 110f–113f

Esophagus (*continued*)
hematoma of, intramural
double-barrel appearance in,
137–141, 138f–140f
filling defects in, 113–115, 114f
herpes simplex infection of. *See*
Herpes simplex infection, of
esophagus
hirsute
filling defects in, 115
nodular lesions in, 146, 147f
histoplasmosis of
esophagorespiratory fistula in, 135
narrowing in, 86
ulcerations in, 60
leiomyoma of
calcification in, 99f, 964
filling defects in, 97–98, 98f, 99f
narrowing in, 83
lower sphincter of, 3, 4f, 11–19
reflux esophagitis in disorders of,
46–50
lymphoma of. *See* Lymphoma, of
esophagus
metastatic tumors of
filling defects in, 102, 103f
narrowing in, 82, 82f–83f
motility disorders of, 3–25
narrowing in, 93, 94f
narrowing of, 70–96
differentiation of benign and malignant
causes, 93–95, 95f
in sclerotherapy of varices, 67f, 92–93,
93f, 128
nodular lesions of, 143–147
nutcracker, 21
obstruction of, gallbladder
visualization impaired in, 774–776
peristaltic activity of, 3–4, 4f
prolapse of mucosa
filling defects of stomach in, 270
pseudotumor of stomach in, 300–303
pseudodiverticulosis of, intramural,
67f, 68, 121f, 121–122
narrowing in, 93, 94f
radiation injury of. *See* Radiation
injury, of esophagus
in reflux esophagitis. *See* Reflux
esophagitis
rings of, 73, 73f, 74f, 75f, 162, 162f
in hiatal hernia, 162, 164f
rupture of, spontaneous, 136
rupture of pulmonary bullus into,
stomach wall gas in, 314
sarcoma of, filling defects in, 102–103,
103f, 104
smooth muscle of, 3
disorders of, 8–11
spasms of, 20, 21f
narrowing in, 93
striated muscle of, 3
disorders of, 5–8
strictures of
congenital, 75
in nasogastric intubation, 85, 88f
postoperative, in hiatal hernia, 84, 88f
radiation-induced, 86, 90f

syphilis of
esophagorespiratory fistula in, 135
narrowing in, 86
tertiary contractions of, 4, 19–21,
20f–23f
in achalasia, 14f, 15, 21, 23f
in esophagitis, 10, 21, 22f
in presbyesophagus, 10, 12f, 19–20,
20f
thoracic
diverticula of, 119f, 119–120
impressions on, 30–45
tuberculosis of. *See* Tuberculosis, of
esophagus
ulcerations of. *See* Ulcerations, of
esophagus
upper sphincter of, 3
disorders of, 5–8
varices of. *See* Varices, of esophagus
webs of
impressions on esophagus in, 26–27,
27f
narrowing in, 70–73, 71f–72f
Eventration of diaphragm, 152–153,
152f–155f
Extravasated contrast material,
differentiated from internal
fistulas, 931, 932f–933f

Falciform liagment sign of
pneumoperitoneum, 894, 896f
Fallopian tubes
calcification of, 992, 993f
occlusion rings in, 992, 993f
Rubin test for patency of,
pneumoperitoneum after, 901
Fasciola hepatica infection
filling defects of bile ducts in, 813–815,
815f
narrowing and obstruction of bile
ducts in, 830
Fasting, gallbladder visualization
impaired in, 774
Fat
necrosis in pancreatitis, 910–911
calcification in, 997
retroperitoneal, loss of, duodenal
obstruction and dilatation in, 403
Fecalith
in cecum, 569–570, 570f
in colon, 732f
Fecaloma, 712, 733
Feces
as artifact in barium studies of colon,
665, 711–712, 712f
impaction of
filling defects of colon in, 683, 683f
in Hirschsprung's disease, 734, 735f
obstruction of colon in, 731f, 733
Feline appearance of esophagus, 49, 51f
Female genital tract
calcification of, 988–994, 988f–994f
and gynecologic causes of
pneumoperitoneum, 901, 901f
Femoral hernia, 874, 875
small bowel obstruction in, 420

Ferrous sulfate
esophagitis and esophageal ulceration
from, 66
stomach narrowing from, 218
Fetus, calcification of skull and skeleton,
993f, 994
Fibroadenoma of gallbladder, 799
Fibroid, uterine, calcification of, 988f,
989, 989f
Fibroid polyp of small bowel, solitary
filling defects in, 490, 492f
Fibrolipoma of esophagus, filling defects
in, 98, 99f
Fibroma
of bile ducts, 812, 826
of stomach, filling defects in, 246
Fibrosarcoma
of duodenum, narrowing in, 397f
retroperitoneal, retrorectal space
enlargement in, 768f
Fibrosis
cystic. *See* Cystic fibrosis
of liver, congenital, cystic dilatation of
bile ducts in, 842f, 843
of mesentery, thickening of small
bowel mucosal folds in, 462
pleuropulmonary, esophageal
impressions in, 45
Fibrovascular polyp of esophagus, filling
defects in, 98–100, 100f
Fibroxanthogranulomatous inflammation
of gallbladder, filling defects in,
802–803
Filariasis, liver calcification in, 939
Filiform polyps of colon, 707, 707f
Filling defects
of bile ducts, 805–817
of cecum, 554–571
of colon, 662–721
multiple, 692–721
single, 662–691
of esophagus, 97–116
in varices, 106, 107f–109f, 114f, 115,
128
of gallbladder, 787–804
of rectum, in hemorrhoids, 713, 713f
of small bowel, 482–505
in duodenum, 362–386
multiple, 495–505
solitary, in jejunum and ileum,
482–494
of stomach, 238–270
in benign ulcer, 185f
in carcinoma, 247, 249f, 250f,
273–276, 273f, 276f, 297, 297f
in postoperative remnant, 271–280
Fistulas, 919–935
anorectal, 934–935, 935f
aorticoduodenal, 327–328
narrowing and obstruction of
duodenum in, 398, 398f, 405
arteriovenous
calcification of, 977
duodenal filling defects in, 374f, 375
biliary-gastrointestinal, gallbladder
visualization impaired in, 777
colocoxal, 935

colocutaneous, 935
duodenum-kidney, 929
enteric-enteric, 919–925
entero-ovarian, 929, 931f, 932f
esophagorespiratory, 129–139
in carcinoma, 76, 77f
external, 931–935
gallbladder-bowel, 929, 931f
gas in biliary system in, 853, 854f, 929
gastrocolic. *See* Gastrocolic fistulas
internal, 925–931
differentiated from extravasated
contrast material, 931, 932f–933f
pancreatic
external, 934
internal, 928
Flexure defects of duodenum, 363, 366f
Flukes, liver
calcification of liver in, 939
and carcinoma of biliary system, 819
cystic dilatation of bile ducts in,
843–844
filling defects of bile ducts in, 813–815,
815f
gas in biliary system and
pancreaticobiliary reflux in,
854–855
narrowing and obstruction of bile
ducts in, 829–830, 831f
Food particles. *See also* Bezoars
in colon
differentiated from polyposis, 712f,
713
filling defects in, 682
in esophagus, 106, 108, 110f, 112f, 113,
113f
in small bowel, sandlike lucencies in,
512
Food poisoning, salmonellosis in,
601–603
Football sign of pneumoperitoneum, 894,
895f
Foramen
of Bochdalek, herniation through, 167–
171, 169f–170f
of Morgagni, herniation through, 166–
167, 167f–168f
retrogastric space widening in, 310
sacral, superimposed over colon, 689f,
690
of Winslow, herniation through, 420,
872–873, 873f
Foreign bodies, 1008–1010, 1007f–1009f.
See also Bezoars
alimentary tract calcification in, 963,
963f
bladder calcification in, 981, 981f
in colon
differentiated from polyposis, 712f,
713
filling defects in, 682, 686f, 687
in esophagus
double-barrel appearance in, 140f,
141
esophagorespiratory fistula in, 133
filling defects in, 106–113, 110f–113f
in rectum, 686f, 687

in small bowel
duodenal filling defects in, 362
multiple filling defects in, 500
obstruction in, 420–422
solitary filling defects in, 492
in stomach
filling defects in, 261–263, 262f–263f
outlet obstruction in, 289f, 290
upper quadrant extraluminal gas in,
916–917
Forme fruste perforation of peptic ulcer,
pneumoperitoneum in, 901
Fracture, sacral, retrorectal space
enlargement in, 770, 770f
Freezing of stomach, therapeutic
narrowing in, 218
thickening of mucosal folds in, 228–229
Frostberg sign in pancreatic carcinoma,
349–350, 350f
Fundoplication
filling defects of stomach in, 270
pseudotumor of stomach in, 303f, 304f,
305
Fundus, gastric, 296–308
Fungal infections. *See also* Candidiasis
of colon, 607
mucormycoma in, 681, 681f
narrowing in, 629
ulcerations in, 607
of esophagus, 56–58, 56f–58f

Gallbladder, 773–804
in adenomyomatosis, filling defects of,
795, 796–798, 796f–798f
alterations in size of, 779–782
anomalous position of, 776f, 777
calcification of, 800, 800f, 956–959,
956f–959f
carcinoma of. *See* Carcinoma, of
gallbladder
in cholecystitis. *See* Cholecystitis
colon displacing, 783, 784f
congenital anomalies of, 782, 803–804
Courvoisier phenomenon of, 779, 780f
in cholangiocarcinoma, 819
duodenal impressions in, 359
cyst of, intramural epithelial, 803, 803f
in cystic fibrosis, small size of, 781f,
781–782
in diabetes mellitus, enlargement of,
780
displacement or deformity of, 783–786
duodenum displacing, 783, 784f
duodenum impressions from, 358f,
358–359
filling defects in, 362, 363f
empyema of, 779–780, 780f
enlargement of, 779–781, 780f–781f
fibroxanthogranulomatous
inflammation of, 802–803
filling defects of, 787–804
fistula of, enteric, 929, 931f
gas in biliary system in, 853, 854f
folds or septa of, congenital, 803–804
gallstones in, 787–795

calcification of, 788, 788f, 789f, 956–
958, 956f–957f
in neck, 788, 791f, 792, 793f, 807
on wall, 788, 791f, 792, 793f
heterotopic gastric or pancreatic tissue
in, 804, 804f
hydrops of, 358, 779–780
liver displacing, 783–785, 784f, 785f
in metachromatic leukodystrophy, 802
metastases to, 802, 802f
nonvisualization of, in oral
cholecystography, 773–778
obstruction of neck, 777, 778
parasitic infection of, 802
Phrygian cap of, 797, 803, 803f
polyps of, 795f, 796, 798
and pseudopolyps, 803–804
porcelain appearance of, 359
calcification in, 958, 958f
in carcinoma, 800, 800f
pseudodefect in neck, 803
Rokitansky-Aschoff sinuses of, 796, 796f
compared to esophageal
pseudodiverticulosis, 67f, 68, 121
sludge in, affecting sonographic
appearance of gallstones, 792,
793f, 794f
small size of, 781f, 781–782
strawberry, 795f, 795–796
Gallstones
in adenomyomatosis, 797
calcification of, 788, 788f, 789f,
956–958, 956f–957f
calcification of
in rectum, 957f
carcinoma of gallbladder in, 799, 800
in colon, 687–688
in cystic duct, 788, 791f
density of, 788, 790f
differential diagnosis of, 956, 960f
double arcuate echo sign in, 792, 794f
filling defects of gallbladder in,
787–795, 788f–794f
fistula in, gallbladder-enteric, 931f
floating, 792, 793f
ileus in, 422, 422f, 958
biliary gas and pancreaticobiliary
reflux in, 854, 854f, 855f
small bowel obstruction and filling
defects in, 490, 491f, 504
laminated, 788, 789f, 956, 956f
layering of, 788, 790f
lucent, 788, 788f
Mercedes-Benz sign in, 788, 791f, 956,
957f
in neck of gallbladder, 788, 791f, 792,
793f, 807
and pancreatitis, 342, 342f
calcification in, 952
positioning of patient in, 788, 789f,
792, 792f
in small bowel
duodenal filling defects in, 362–363,
364f
multiple filling defects in, 504

Gallstones, in small bowel (*continued*)
  obstruction in, 417f, 420–422, 422f,
    490, 491f, 958
  solitary filling defect in, 490, 491f
  in stomach, filling defects in, 267–268
  ultrasonography in, 788–794, 792f–794f
  on wall of gallbladder, 788, 791f, 792,
    793f
Gangliocytic paraganglioma, duodenal
    filling defects in, 381, 381f
Gangrene, gas, 917, 917f
Gardner's syndrome
  colon polyposis and multiple filling
    defects in, 695–697, 695f, 696f
  small bowel filling defects in, 496, 496f
Gas
  in abdominal abscess, 905–914,
    906f–915f
  and air bubbles. *See* Air bubbles
  in biliary system, 914–916, 915f
    in pancreaticobiliary reflux, 852–857
    and pseudopneumobilia, 856, 856f
  in bowel wall, in pneumatosis
    intestinalis, 881–891
  in duodenal bulb, differentiated from
    polyp, 376, 377f, 380f
  in duodenal diverticula, filling defects
    in, 363, 365f
  in peritoneal cavity, 892–902
  in portal vein, 858–862, 916
  retroperitoneal, free, 903–904,
    904f–905f
  in small bowel obstruction, 411, 412f–
    415f, 415–416
  in stomach, in esophagorespiratory
    fistula, 129, 130, 130f, 131
  in stomach wall, 228, 312–314, 914
  subhepatic, 904–905, 906f
  in upper quadrants, 903–918
Gas gangrene, 917, 917f
Gastrectomy, partial, filling defects of
    stomach in, 271–280
Gastritis. *See* Stomach
Gastrocolic fistulas
  in colon carcinoma, 920, 922f
  gallbladder visualization impaired in,
    776
  in gastric ulcers, 921, 923f, 924f
  in pancreatic carcinoma, 920, 923f
Gastroenteritis
  eosinophilic
    duodenal involvement in, 318, 318f
    thickening of mucosal folds in, 513–
      514, 514f
    ileus in, adynamic, 432f, 433
  necrotizing, stomach wall gas in, 312
Gastroesophageal reflux, 46–50
Gastrojejunocolic fistula, postoperative,
    923, 925f
Gastropathy, pediatric hypertrophic,
    230f, 231–232
Gastroplasty procedures in obesity, 220–
    221, 220f–221f
Gastroscopy, stomach wall gas after, 312
Gastrostomy tube, duodenal filling
    defects from, 363, 364f
Gaucher's disease, liver calcification in,
    941–943, 942f

Gehrig's disease, esophageal motility
    disorders in, 7
Genital tract
  calcification of, 986–994
    in females, 988–994, 988f–994f
    in males, 986–988, 986f–988f
  and gynecologic causes of
    pneumoperitoneum, 901, 901f
Giardiasis of small bowel
  duodenal thickening of mucosal folds
    in, 334
  irregular thickening of mucosal folds
    in, 468, 468f
  lymphoid hyperplasia in, 507, 508f, 509
Glioma-polyposis syndrome, colon
    polyps and multiple filling defects
    in, 697f, 697–698
Glomerulonephritis, chronic, renal
    calcification in, 977
Glucagonoma, pancreatic, sandlike
    lucencies of small bowel in, 511f,
    512
Glue bezoar, filling defects of stomach in,
    261, 263f
Glycogenic acanthosis of esophagus, 143,
    144f
Gold therapy, parametrial, calcification
    in, 994, 994f
Gonadoblastoma of ovary, calcification
    in, 990–991, 991f
Gonorrhea, proctitis in
  and narrowing of colon, 628
  and ulceration of colon, 603f, 604–605
Good's syndrome, 507
Gossypidoma, 1010, 1012f
Graft-versus-host disease
  esophageal narrowing in, 91, 92f
  pneumatosis intestinalis in, 890
  separation of small bowel loops in,
    527–528, 528f
Granular cell tumors
  of bile ducts, 825, 825f
  of esophagus, filling defects in, 98, 100f
Granuloma
  eosinophilic
    bull's-eye lesions in, 868
    of stomach, filling defects in,
      264–265, 266f
  oil, abdominal calcification in, 999, 999f
  parasitic, of gallbladder, 802
  polypoid, of colon, filling defects in, 681
  suture
    colon filling defects in, 689f, 690
    stomach filling defects in, 270,
      271–272, 272f
Granulomatosis
  barium, 945
  lipoid, liver calcification in, 945
Granulomatous disease
  bile duct narrowing and obstruction
    in, 832, 833, 833f
  large bowel obstruction in, 724
  lymph node calcification in, 1001–1002
  of stomach, ulcerations in, 190
Growth spurt of childhood, duodenal
    compression and dilatation in, 403
Guaiac test in colon carcinoma, 635

Guinea worm infection
  abdominal wall calcification in, 1002,
    1004f
  liver calcification in, 939, 940f
Gumma of liver
  calcification of liver in, 939
  diaphragm elevation in, 156f
Gunshot wounds, abdominal, fistula
    formation in, 933f
Gynecologic causes of
    pneumoperitoneum, 901,901f

Hair growth in esophagus, postoperative
    filling defects in, 115
  nodular lesions in, 146, 147f
Halo appearance
  in aphthoid ulcers, 868
  in duodenal diverticula, intraluminal,
    398, 534, 534f
  in gastric erosions, superficial, 201, 202f
Hamartoma
  of bile ducts, 812
  of colon
    in Cowden's disease, 705, 705f
    multiple filling defects in, 697
    single filling defects in, 670–671
  of esophagus, nodular lesions in, 146
  of lung, compared to Morgagni
    foramen hernia, 167, 168f
  of small bowel
    duodenal filling defects in, 380, 380f
    multiple filling defects in, 495, 496f
    solitary filling defect in, 485f, 486
  of stomach, filling defects in, 242f,
    243f, 244
Hampton line of gastric ulcers, 181f, 182
Heart
  esophageal impressions from, 40, 40f,
    41f
  failure of
    esophageal varices in, 123
    ileus in, adynamic, 433
  gastric impressions from, 300, 301f
Heller myotomy in achalasia, 19
Hemangioendothelioma
  liver calcification in, 941, 941f
  retrorectal space enlargement in, 765
Hemangioma
  alimentary tract calcification in, 964,
    966f
  bladder calcification in, 985
  of colon
    multiple filling defects in, 705
    single filling defects in, 674, 674f
  of gallbladder, 799
  of liver, calcification in, 939, 940f
  retroperitoneal calcification in, 997
  of small bowel, filling defects in, 485,
    485f, 497, 497f
  of spleen, calcification in, 947, 947f
  of stomach, filling defects in, 246, 248f
Hemangiopericytoma of ovary,
    calcification in, 990, 991f
Hematoma
  of colon, thumbprinting pattern in, 746
  duodenal intramural
    coiled spring appearance in, 376, 376f

filling defects in, 375–376, 375f–376f
impression on duodenum in, 361
obstruction in, 398, 398f
esophageal intramural
  double-barrel appearance in,
    137–141, 138f–140f
  filling defects in, 113–115, 114f
of kidney
  calcification in, 973, 974f
  upper quadrant extraluminal gas in,
    917
liver calcification in, 941
periesophageal, impressions on
  esophagus in, 29
retroperitoneal
  calcification in, 997
  retrogastric space widening in, 311
of spleen, calcification in, 948, 949f
of stomach
  filling defects in, 263f, 307
  narrowing in, 219, 219f
Hematopoiesis, tumefactive
  extramedullary, of stomach, 268,
    269f
Hemochromatosis
  liver radiodensity in, 944f, 945
  splenic density in, 950
Hemolytic disease of newborn, portal
  vein gas in, 859
Hemolytic-uremic syndrome, colon
  thumbprinting pattern in,
    754–755, 755f
Hemophilia, hemorrhage and thickening
  of small bowel mucosal folds in,
    459–460
Hemorrhage
  adrenal neonatal, calcification in, 995,
    995f
  into bowel wall
    separation of small bowel loops in,
      517, 519f
    thickening of small bowel mucosal
      folds in, 456–461, 457f–461f
    thumbprinting pattern of colon in,
      746
  duodenal intramural
    impression on duodenum in, 361
    thickening of mucosal folds in, 338
  in esophageal varices, 124
  in pancreatitis, 341f
    duodenal sweep widening in, 341f
  rectal
    in adenomatous polyps of colon, 664
    in carcinoma of colon, 634f, 635
    retroperitoneal, adynamic ileus in, 433
Hemorrhoids, multiple rectal filling
  defects in, 713, 713f
Hemosiderin deposition, lymph node
  calcification in, 1002
Hemostat, retained, radiographic pattern
  of, 1013, 1013f
Henoch-Schönlein purpura, thickening
  of small bowel mucosal folds in,
    459, 460f
Hepatic artery
  aneurysm of

bile duct narrowing and obstruction
  in, 836, 836f
calcification in, 943–945
as biliary pseudocalculus, 810, 810f
infusion of chemotherapy in
  and cholangitis, 827–828, 828f
  and narrowing of stomach, 217f, 218
  and ulceration of stomach, 193, 193f
transcatheter embolization of, and
  cystic dilatation of bile ducts, 845,
    846f
Hepatic duct
  cyst of, 838, 839f
  diverticulum of, 840
Hepatic flexure of colon, duodenal
  impressions in carcinoma of, 361
Hepatitis
  cholangiolitic, 828–829, 829f
  gallbladder visualization impaired in,
    777
  in Oriental cholangiohepatitis, 816,
    816f, 828, 828f, 844–845, 845f
Hepatoblastoma, calcification of liver in,
  941, 941f
Hepatoma
  bile duct filling defects in, 811
  bile duct narrowing and obstruction
    in, 823
  gallbladder displacement in, 784f
Hernia
  Bochdalek foramen, 167–171,
    169f–170f
  diaphragmatic, 159–175
  esophagogastric, pseudotumor of
    stomach in, 300–303
  femoral, 874, 875
    small bowel obstruction in, 420
  gallbladder visualization impaired in,
    776
  hiatal, 159–162, 160f–164f
    Barrett's esophagus in, 52, 53, 54f
    carcinoma of esophagus in, 76
    gallbladder visualization impaired in,
      776
    pseudotumor of stomach in, 302f, 303
    reflux esophagitis in, 47, 49, 50, 50f,
      52f, 84, 85f, 159
    stricture of esophagus in,
      postoperative, 84, 88f
    ulceration of esophagus in, 159, 161f
    volvulus of stomach in, 159, 161f
  of ileum, 874f
  incisional, 876, 878, 878f, 879f
    large bowel obstruction in, 729, 731f
    small bowel obstruction in, 420
  inguinal, 874–875, 875f
    gallbladder visualization impaired in,
      776
    retrorectal space enlargement in, 770
    small bowel obstruction in, 420, 420f
  intrapericardial, 173, 173f–174f
  large bowel obstruction in, 729, 731f
  lumbar, 874
  mesentericoparietal, 871
  Morgagni foramen, 166–167, 167f–168f
    retrogastric space widening in, 310
  nondiaphragmatic, 871–880

obturator, 875–876, 875f–876f
  Howship-Romberg sign in, 876
paracecal, 874
  separation of small bowel loops in,
    527
paraduodenal, 871–872, 872f
  obstruction of small bowel in, 420
  separation of small bowel loops in,
    527, 527f
paraesophageal, 162–165, 165f–166f
  esophageal impressions in, 42–45, 44f
  gastric volvulus and outlet
    obstruction in, 286
pelvic (broad ligament), 874
retroperitoneal, separation of small
  bowel loops in, 527, 527f
scrotal, 875, 875f
sigmoid mesentery, 874
small bowel mesentery, 874, 874f
spigelian, 878–879, 880f
traumatic, 171–173, 171f–172f
umbilical, 876, 877f
  gallbladder visualization impaired in,
    776
ventral, 876, 878
  retrogastric space widening in, 310
Winslow foramen, 420, 872–873, 873f
Herniation of intervertebral disk,
  cervical, esophageal impressions
  in, 28, 28f
Herpes simplex infection
  anorectal ulcerations in, 607f, 608
  of esophagus, 58, 59f
    filling defects in, 105, 106f
    narrowing in, 86, 89f
    nodular lesions in, 144
  of stomach, superficial erosions in, 204
Herpes zoster infection of colon
  filling defects in, 717–718, 718f
  narrowing in, 629
  ulcerations in, 608
Heterotopia. *See* Ectopia
Hiatal hernia. *See* Hernia, hiatal
Hide-bound sign of small bowel folds in
  scleroderma, 446, 447f
Hirschsprung's disease
  duodenal dilatation in, 403
  mosaic pattern of colon in, 735, 737f
  obstruction of colon in, 734–736, 735f–
    737f
  pneumatosis intestinalis in, 889
Hirsute esophagus
  filling defects in, 115
  nodular lesions in, 146, 147f
Histoplasmosis
  of colon, 607
  of esophagus
    esophagorespiratory fistula in, 135
    narrowing in, 86
    ulcerations in, 60
  liver calcification in, 937f, 937–938
  of small bowel
    irregular thickening of mucosal folds
      in, 475, 476f
    sandlike lucencies in, 506–507, 507f
  spleen calcification in, 937f, 946, 947f
  stomach narrowing in, 214

Hodgkin's disease, narrowing of stomach in, 208f, 209
Hofmeister defect of stomach, postoperative, 271, 272f
Howship-Romberg sign in obturator hernia, 876
Huntington's chorea, esophageal motility disorders in, 8
Hydatid cysts
 alimentary tract calcification in, 966
 bile duct dilatation in, 845, 846f
 of liver
  calcification in, 938, 938f
  filling defects of bile ducts in, 815–816, 816f
  narrowing and obstruction of bile ducts in, 830, 831f, 833
  retroperitoneal calcification in, 997
 of spleen, calcification in, 948, 948f
Hydrogen peroxide lavage, portal vein gas after, 860
Hydronephrosis, duodenal impressions in, 359
Hydrops of gallbladder, 779–780, 781f
 duodenal impressions in, 358
Hypercalcemia
 abdominal wall calcification in, 1006
 in hyperparathyroidism, 969
Hypernephroma
 calcification of, 973–975
 duodenal impressions in, 359
 metastatic to small bowel, filling defects in, 488f
Hyperostosis, diffuse idiopathic skeletal, esophageal impressions in, 27, 42, 44f
Hyperoxaluria, nephrocalcinosis in, 970–971, 971f
Hyperparathyroidism
 nephrocalcinosis in, 969
 pancreatitis and calcification of pancreas in, 953
Hyperplasia
 of Brunner's gland, 329, 330f
  duodenal filling defects in, 367f, 367–368
 lymphoid. *See* Lymphoid hyperplasia
Hyperplastic polyps
 of colon, 663, 663f, 670
 of stomach
  filling defects in, 240, 240f, 241f, 241–243, 276–277
  in postoperative remnant, 276–277
Hypertension, portal, esophageal varices in, 123, 124, 125, 126, 126f
Hypertrophy
 of anal papilla, colon filling defects in, 687f, 688
 of antral-pyloric fold, stomach filling defects in, 261, 261f
 gastritis and thickening of mucosal folds in, 225, 225f
  in Menetrier's disease, 229–232, 229f–230f, 232f
 pyloric stenosis and gastric outlet obstruction in, 287–290, 288f–289f
Hypervitaminosis D, nephrocalcinosis in, 969

Hypoalbuminemia, thickening of small bowel mucosal folds in, 461
 and small bowel dilatation, 454f, 455
Hypofibrinogenemia, hemorrhage and thickening of small bowel mucosal folds in, 461
Hypokalemia
 ileus in, adynamic, 433, 433f, 435f
 small bowel dilatation in, 448
Hypoproteinemia
 and gastric varices in liver disease, 515
 intestinal edema in, 461
 in protein-losing enteropathy. *See* Protein-losing enteropathy
Hypoxia, pseudomembranous colitis in, 612
Hysteria, duodenal dilatation in, 405

Ileitis, backwash, 549, 550f, 576
 in ulcerative colitis, 589, 589f
Ileocecal area, diverticulitis of, 567–569, 569f
Ileocecal valve, 543–553
 competency of, in large bowel obstruction, 722, 723f
 function of, 543
 normal appearance of, 543–545, 544f
 prolapse of, 549–552, 551f–552f
 stellate or rosette pattern of, 543, 544f, 545
 tuberculosis of, 549, 550f, 576, 628, 628f
 ulceration of, 619, 619f
Ileocolic anastomosis, traumatic neuroma in, 493f, 674
Ileocolic fistula, in carcinoma of colon, 922f
Ileocolic intussusception, 567, 568f
 obstruction of colon in, 732f, 733, 733f–735f
Ileostomy, radiographic patterns in, 1002
Ileum
 atresia of
  microcolon in, 428, 428f
  obstruction in, 427–428, 427f–428f
 communicating duplication of, 539
 Crohn's disease of, 593, 593f, 594, 595
 dilatation in neonate, 428f, 428–429
 diverticula of, 538f, 538–539
 filling defects in, 482–494
 hernia of, 874f
 intussusception of
  ileocecal, 553
  ileocolic, 567, 568f, 684, 732f, 733, 733f–735f
 jejunoileal fold pattern in sprue, 444, 445f
 pneumatosis intestinalis after jejunoileal bypass surgery, 888, 889f
 prolapse of mucosa, 549–552
Ileus
 adynamic, 430–440
  of colon, 435–436, 435f–436f, 722
  compared to obstruction, 415, 430, 431f, 436–440, 437f–440f, 722
  drug-induced, 433, 433f, 435f, 436f
  gallbladder visualization impaired in, 776

gas-fluid levels in, 411, 413f
 localized, 434f, 435
 in pancreatitis, 434f, 435, 437, 437f
 pneumatosis intestinalis in, 887, 887f
 postoperative, 430, 432f, 435, 437, 776
 small bowel dilatation in, 405, 441
gallstone, 422, 422f, 958
 biliary gas and pancreaticobiliary reflux in, 854, 854f, 855f
 small bowel obstruction and filling defects in, 490, 491f, 504
 meconium, small bowel obstruction in, 425, 426f
Iliac arteriovenous fistula, duodenal filling defects in, 374f, 375
Iliac artery calcification, 1000, 1000f, 1001
Iliac lymph nodes, calcification of, 1001–1002, 1002f
Immobilization
 duodenal obstruction and dilatation in, 403, 403f
 gastric dilatation in, nonobstructive, 292
Immunodeficiency syndrome, acquired. *See* AIDS
Immunoglobulins
 IgA alpha chain disease, irregular thickening of small bowel mucosal folds in, 480
 IgM, in Waldenstrom's macroglobulinemia, 506
Immunosuppressive therapy in renal transplantation, pneumoperitoneum as complication of, 899, 899f
Impaction, fecal
 filling defects of colon in, 683, 683f
 in Hirschsprung's disease, 734, 735f
 obstruction of colon in, 731f, 733
Imperforate anus, obstruction of colon in, 736–738, 737f–738f
Incisional hernia, 876, 878, 878f, 879f
 large bowel obstruction in, 729, 731f
 small bowel obstruction in, 420
Indomethacin, superficial gastric erosions from, 202f, 204
Infants. *See* Children and infants
Infarction
 of liver, cystic dilatation of bile ducts in, 845, 846f
 mesenteric
  ileus in, adynamic, 433
  portal vein gas in, 858, 860
 myocardial, adynamic ileus in, 433
 pancreatic, calcification in, 955
 of spleen, calcification in, 948
Inguinal hernia. *See* Hernia, inguinal
Innominate lines of colon, 590f, 591
Insulinoma, pancreatic calcification in, 953f
 sunburst pattern in, 953f, 955
Intervertebral disk herniation, cervical, esophageal impressions in, 28, 28f
Intubation
 intestinal, small bowel obstruction in, 422, 423f

nasogastric
  esophageal stricture in, 85, 88f
  esophagorespiratory fistula in, 133, 133f
Intussusception
  of appendix into cecum, 563–565, 564f
  coiled-spring appearance in. *See* Coiled-spring appearance, in intussusception
  colocolic, 684, 734, 734f
  colon filling defects in, 684–687, 685f, 686f
  colon obstruction in, 732f, 733–734, 733f–735f
  duodenal filling defects in, 381–382
  in heterotopic gastric mucosa, 424f, 492
  ileocecal, 553
  ileocolic, 567, 568f, 684
    obstruction of colon in, 732f, 733, 733f–735f
  jejunogastric, stomach filling defects in, 270, 277–280, 278f–279f
  in Meckel's diverticula, 536, 536f
  reduction of, 685, 686f, 732f, 733f, 734
    dissection sign in, 734, 735f
  small bowel obstruction in, 422–425, 424f–426f
  in sprue, 444–446, 446f
Iron, ingestion of
  esophageal ulcerations in, 66
  stomach narrowing in, 218
Ischemia
  of colon
    in carcinoma, 749
    multiple filling defects in, 708, 709f, 747f
    narrowing in, 625f, 626
    pseudopolyps in, 708, 709f
    retrorectal space enlargement in, 763
    reversibility of, 748f
    submucosal edema in, 718
    thumbprinting pattern in, 598, 599f, 746–749, 747f–748f
    toxic megacolon in, 741, 742f
    ulcerations in, 596–600, 598f–599f
  mesenteric
    ileus in, adynamic, 433
    large bowel obstruction in, 724
    pneumatosis intestinalis in, 885f, 885–886
    small bowel dilatation in, 450
  of small bowel
    dilatation in, 450, 453
    obstruction in, 427
    sandlike lucencies in, 512
    thickening of mucosal folds in, 453, 458, 459f
  of stomach, stomach wall gas in, 312, 314

Jackburr calculi of bladder, 982–983, 983f
Jaundice, in bile duct narrowing and obstruction, 819, 819f
Jejunogastric intussusception, stomach filling defects in, 270, 277–280, 278f–279f

Jejunoileal bypass surgery, pneumatosis intestinalis in, 888, 889f
Jejunoileal fold pattern in sprue, 444, 445f
Jejunostomy tubes, pneumatosis intestinalis in, 888–889
Jejunum
  atresia of
    obstruction in, 427f, 427–428
    triple bubble sign in, 427f, 427–428
  carcinoma of
    obstruction in, 421f
    separation of bowel loops in, 520f
  Crohn's disease of, obstruction in, 421f
  dilatation of, with thickening of mucosal folds, 454f, 455
  diverticula of, 534–535, 535f
    pneumatosis intestinalis in, 890
    and pseudodiverticula, 535, 535f
  diverticulosis of, 534, 535, 535f
    gallbladder visualization impaired in, 776
    pneumoperitoneum in, 535, 900f, 901
  filling defects of, 482–494
  fistula of, gastrojejunocolic, 923, 925f
  lymphoma of, obstruction in, 442f
  moulage sign of, in sprue, 444, 445f
  obstruction of, 414f, 415
  in paraduodenal hernia, 872, 872f
  radiation injury of, sandlike lucencies in, 511f
Jet phenomenon in esophageal webs, 72, 72f

Kaposi's sarcoma
  bull's-eye lesions in, 866–868
  of colon, 649
    multiple filling defects in, 702, 702f
  duodenal filling defects in, 386
  duodenal thickening of mucosal folds in, 335
  esophageal filling defects in, 104
  stomach filling defects in, 255, 257f
Kidney
  abscess of
    calcification in, 973
    extraluminal gas in, 908–910, 910f
  calcification of, 966–979, 968f–979f
  calculi in, 968f, 969
    adynamic ileus in, 433, 434f
  carcinoma of
    calcification in, 971, 973f, 975, 975f
    gallbladder displacement in, 785, 785f
  chronic failure of, duodenal thickening of mucosal folds in, 333f, 333–334
  cortical necrosis of, calcification in, 976f, 977
  cysts of. *See* Cyst, of kidney
  fistula of, renoduodenal, 929
  hematoma of
    calcification in, 973, 974f
    upper quadrant extraluminal gas in, 917
  impression on duodenum, 359, 359f, 360f
  impression on stomach, 300

medullary sponge, calcification in, 970, 970f
metastatic tumors of
  in colon, 643
  in stomach, 299
nephrotic syndrome of, thickening of small bowel mucosal folds in, 461
papillary necrosis of, nephrocalcinosis in, 971, 972f
transplantation of, pneumoperitoneum as complication in, 899, 899f
Killian's dehiscence, 5
Kirklin complex in gastric ulcers, 189, 190f
Klatskin tumors, 820, 820f
Kwashiorkor, pancreatic calcification in, 955

Lactase deficiency, small bowel dilatation in, 448f, 448–449
Ladd's bands, duodenal obstruction in, 391, 391f
Laparatomy, pneumoperitoneum after, 899, 900f
Large bowel
  anal disorders of. *See* Anal disorders
  cecum, 541–581. *See also* Cecum
  colon, 583–770. *See also* Colon
  obstruction of, 722–740
    compared to adynamic ileus, 436, 722
    pneumatosis intestinalis in, 885f, 886
    pseudomembranous colitis, 609, 612
    and pseudo-obstruction, 740
    submucosal edema in, 718
  rectum. *See* Rectum
Laryngectomy, total
  cricopharyngeal impression on esophagus in, 6f, 6–7, 26
  traction diverticula of esophagus in, 118f, 119
Laser therapy in esophageal carcinoma, 81, 81f
L-Dopa therapy
  ileus in, adynamic, 433, 433f
  small bowel dilatation in, 442
Lead-pipe appearance
  in Crohn's colitis, 624
  in ulcerative colitis, 592, 623, 623f
Lead poisoning, gastric dilatation in, 295
Leather bottle stomach, 205
Leiomyoblastoma of stomach, filling defects in, 254, 257f
Leiomyoma
  of bile ducts, 826
  bull's-eye lesions in, 865, 867f
  of colon, 674, 674f
  of esophagus
    calcification in, 99f, 964
    filling defects in, 97–98, 98f, 99f
    narrowing in, 83
  of small bowel
    duodenal filling defects in, 378, 378f
    multiple filling defects in, 497

Leiomyoma, of small bowel (*continued*)
  solitary filling defect in, 483f,
    483–484
  ulceration of duodenum in, 325
  of stomach
    bull's-eye lesions in, 867f
    calcification in, 964
    filling defects in, 243f, 244f, 245,
      245f, 246f
    of fundus, 299, 300f
    retrogastric space widening in, 311
    ulcerations in, 190, 191f
  of uterus, calcification in, 988f, 989,
    989f
Leiomyosarcoma
  of bladder, calcification in, 985
  of colon, 675f
    narrowing in, 644f
  of esophagus, filling defects in, 102, 103f
  of gallbladder, 802
  of pancreas, duodenal impressions in,
    361f
  of small bowel
    separation of bowel loops in, 525f
    solitary filling defect in, 486–488,
      487f
  of stomach
    filling defects in, 252–254, 254f–256f
    of fundus, 297, 299f
    retrogastric space widening in, 311
    ulcerations in, 194, 197f, 252, 254f
Leukemia
  colon in
    multiple filling defects of, 704
    thumbprinting pattern of, 754, 754f
    ulcerations of, 615, 616f
  gastric thickening of mucosal folds in,
    233, 233f
  pneumatosis intestinalis in, 889, 889f
  small bowel thickening of mucosal
    folds in, 461
  in ulcerative colitis, 650
Leukodystrophy, metachromatic,
    gallbladder filling defects in, 802
Leukoplakia, nodular lesions of
    esophagus in, 145–146, 147f
Ligaments
  broad ligament hernia, 874
  calcification of, 1005f, 1006, 1006f
  falciform ligament sign of
    pneumoperitoneum, 894, 896f
Linitis plastica pattern, 205–222
Lipodystrophy of mesentery, 526
Lipoid granulomatosis, liver calcification
    in, 945
Lipoma
  of bile ducts, 812
  of colon, 673f, 673–674
  of esophagus, filling defects in, 98, 99f
  of ileocecal valve, 546, 546f
  mesenteric, calcification in, 966
  retrorectal space enlargement in, 765
  of small bowel
    duodenal filling defects in, 378–380,
      378f–379f
    multiple filling defects in, 497, 498f
    solitary filling defect in, 484f,
      484–485

of stomach, filling defects in, 245–246,
    246f, 247f
Lipomatosis
  of colon, filling defects in, 704f, 705
  of ileocecal valve, 544f, 545f, 545–546
  of mesentery, 526
  pelvic
    colon narrowing in, 657–659, 658f
    retrorectal space enlargement in,
      769f, 770
Liposarcoma of stomach, filling defects
    in, 254, 257f
Lithiasis. *See* Calculi
Lithopedion, 994, 994f
Liver
  abscess of. *See* Abscess, of liver
  calcification of, 936–946, 937f–946f
  calculi in, 941
  carcinoma of
    calcification in, 939, 940f
    esophageal varices in, 123
  cirrhosis of. *See* Cirrhosis
  cysts of. *See* Cyst, of liver
  disorders of
    gallbladder visualization impaired in,
      777
    thickening of small bowel mucosal
      folds in, 461, 462f
    in ulcerative colitis, 587–588
  duodenal impressions from, 359
  enlargement of
    duodenal impressions in, 359
    gallbladder displacement in, 785f
    retrogastric space widening in, 310
    stomach narrowing in, 220, 220f
  fibrosis of, congenital, cystic dilatation
    of bile ducts in, 842f, 843
  gastric impressions from, 300
  gumma of
    calcification in, 939
    diaphragm elevation in, 156f
  increased radiodensity of, without
    calcification, 945–946, 944f–946f
  infarction of, cystic dilatation of bile
    ducts in, 845, 846f
  tumors of
    calcification in, 939–941, 940f–942f
    diaphragm elevation in, 156, 156f
    gallbladder displacement in,
      783–785, 784f
    metastatic to stomach, 299
    thickening of small bowel mucosal
      folds in, 461, 462f
Liver flukes. *See* Flukes, liver
Lollipop-tree appearance of biliary
    system, 842f, 843
Loops of small bowel, separation of, 517–
    528
Lordosis, lumbar, duodenal obstruction
    and dilatation in, 405
Lucencies, sandlike, in small bowel, 506–
    512
Lumbar hernia, 874
Lumbar spine
  annular ligaments of, calcification of,
    1005
  lordosis of, duodenal obstruction and
    dilatation in, 405

Lung
  carcinoma of. *See* Carcinoma, of lung
  cyst of, esophagorespiratory fistula in,
    136
  embolism in, diaphragm elevation in,
    157
  esophageal impressions from, 31f, 32
  hamartoma of, compared to Morgagni
    formen hernia, 167, 168f
  obstructive disease of
    pneumatosis intestinalis in, 890
    pneumoperitoneum in, 902
  sequestration of, esophagorespiratory
    fistula in, 136
Lupus erythematosus
  esophageal motility disorders in, 10, 10f
  small bowel dilatation in, 449f, 450
    duodenal, 403, 404f
  small bowel thickening of mucosal
    folds in, 458–459, 459f
Lymph nodes
  calcification of, 1001–1002,
    1002f–1003f
  enlargement of
    duodenal sweep widening in, 350,
      351f, 352–356, 355f
    esophageal filling defects in, 105, 105f
    esophageal impression in, 29, 42,
      43f, 105, 105f
    esophageal ulcerations in, 62
    gastric impressions in, 299, 307
    retrogastric space widening in, 311
  metastases to. *See* Metastases, to lymph
    nodes
Lymphadenopathy, periportal, duodenal
    impressions in, 359
Lymphangiectasia, intestinal
  sandlike lucenices of small bowel in,
    509f, 509–511
  thickening of small bowel mucosal
    folds in, 463, 464f
    duodenal, 337
Lymphangiitis, radiation-induced,
    thickening of small bowel mucosal
    folds in, 461–462
Lymphangioma
  duodenal filling defects in, 381, 381f
  duodenal sweep widening in, 355f, 356
  pancreatic calcification in, 954f, 955
  separation of small bowel loops in, 524f
Lymphatic blockage, thickening of small
    bowel mucosal folds in, 461–462
Lymphogranuloma venereum
  anorectal fistulas in, 935
  of colon
    narrowing in, 628, 628f, 629f
    ulcerations in, 606–607, 607f, 628,
      628f
  pneumoperitoneum in, 897
  retrorectal space enlargement in, 763,
    763f
Lymphoid follicular pattern of colon,
    715–717, 715f–716f
Lymphoid hyperplasia
  of colon, 715, 715f
  ileocecal valve enlargement in, 553,
    553f

of small bowel
  duodenal filling defects in, 368, 368f
  multiple filling defects in, 500, 502f
  sandlike lucencies in, 507–509, 508f
Lymphoma
  bull's-eye lesions in, 865, 867f
  Burkitt's
    of cecum, 570, 571
    of stomach, filling defects in, 251, 251f
  of colon
    multiple filling defects in, 702–704, 703f, 704f
    narrowing in, 649–650, 650f
    and pseudolymphoma, 660, 660f
    single filling defect in, 677, 678f, 679f, 702
    thumbprinting pattern in, 751, 752f
    ulcerations in, 615, 616f
  diffuse intestinal
    small bowel dilatation in, 446, 450
    in sprue, 446
  of duodenum
    in bulb, 315, 316f, 317f, 384f, 385
    filling defects in, 384f, 385
    postbulbar ulceration in, 325
    thickening of mucosal folds in, 335, 336f
  of esophagus, 62
    differentiated from varices, 127, 127f
    filling defects in, 104, 104f
    narrowing in, 83, 84f
    nodular lesions in, 146
  gallbladder displacement in, 785f
  of ileocecal valve, 548, 549f
  peripancreatic, duodenal sweep widening in, 355f, 356
  of porta hepatis lymph nodes, bile duct narrowing and obstruction in, 824
  retrorectal space enlargement in, 765, 765f
  of small bowel
    dilatation and thickening of mucosal folds in, 454, 455
    in duodenum. *See* Lymphoma, of duodenum
    gastric and small bowel thickening of mucosal folds in, 513, 514f
    irregular thickening of mucosal folds in, 468–471, 469f–471f, 519f
    in jejunum, obstruction in, 442f
    multiple filling defects in, 500, 501f
    napkin-ring lesions in, 469, 469f
    pseudodiverticula in, 535
    regular thickening of mucosal folds in, 461
    separation of bowel loops in, 469f, 517, 519f
    solitary filling defect in, 486, 487f
  of stomach
    bull's-eye lesions in, 867f
    carcinoma compared to, 233–234
    duodenal involvement in, 315, 316f, 317f, 384f, 385
    esophageal narrowing in, 82–83, 83f
    filling defects in, 250f, 251, 251f, 276, 277f
    of fundus, 297, 299f

Menetrier's disease compared to, 232, 232f
  in postoperative stump, 276, 277f
  and pseudolymphoma. *See* Pseudolymphoma, of stomach
  small bowel thickening of mucosal folds in, 513, 514f
  stomach narrowing in, 208f, 209f, 209–210
  stomach thickening of mucosal folds in, 204f, 231f, 232f, 232–233, 250f, 251, 276, 277f, 513, 514f
  ulcerations in, 194, 194f–196f, 204, 204f, 250f, 251

Macroglobulinemia, Waldenstrom's, sandlike lucencies of small bowel in, 506, 507f
Malabsorption
  gallbladder visualization impaired in, 776
  small bowel dilatation in, 442–449, 450
  in sprue. *See* Sprue
Malacoplakia of colon, multiple filling defects in, 719f, 719–720
Male genital tract, calcification of, 986–988, 986f–988f
Mallory-Weiss syndrome
  double-barrel appearance of esophagus in, 137–139, 138f–139f
  narrowing of esophagus in, 93, 94f
Malnutrition
  gallbladder visualization impaired in, 774
  pancreatic calcification in, 955
Marble, ingested, radiographic appearance of, 1007, 1007f
Marginal ulcers of stomach, postoperative, 196–200, 198f–199f
Mastocytosis
  bull's-eye lesions in, 869, 869f
  sandlike lucencies of small bowel in, 506, 507f
  thickening of small bowel mucosal folds in
    duodenal, 337, 337f
    irregular, 477, 477f
Mecholyl test in achalasia, 18
Meckel's diverticula, 536–538, 536f–538f
  ectopic gastric mucosa in, 536, 536f, 538, 538f
  enteroliths in, 960, 961f
  intussusception in, 536, 536f
    and small bowel obstruction, 423–424, 424f
  pneumoperitoneum in, 897, 898f
  small bowel filling defects in, 492, 493f
  triangular plateau of mucosa in, 537–538, 537f–538f
Meconium
  ileus and small bowel obstruction from, 425, 426f
  peritonitis from, 428
    generalized abdominal calcification in, 999, 999f
    liver calcification in, 945

plug syndrome from
  colon obstruction in, 738
  pneumatosis intestinalis in, 889
Mediastinal tumors
  diaphragm paralysis in, 153
  esophageal displacement in, 30, 31f, 32, 42
  esophageal varices in, 123–124, 124f
  esophagorespiratory fistulas in, 131, 132f
  vena cava obstruction in, 123–124, 124f
Mediastinitis, chronic fibrosing, esophageal varices in, 124
Medullary sponge kidney, calcification in, 970, 970f
Megacolon
  congenital, 734
  psychogenic, 731f, 733
  toxic, 741–745
  pneumoperitoneum in, 897
Melanoma, metastatic
  to adrenal gland, calcification in, 996
  to bile ducts, 813f
  bull's-eye appearance in, 251, 252f, 385, 802, 865, 866f
  to colon, filling defects in, 701f, 702
  to duodenum, 385, 385f
    postbulbar ulceration in, 327
  esophageal, filling defects in, 103, 104f
  to gallbladder, 802, 802f
  to stomach
    bull's-eye appearance in, 251, 252f
    filling defects in, 251, 252f
    ulcerations in, 196, 197f
Menetrier's disease
  compared to lymphoma of stomach, 232, 232f
  filling defects of stomach in, 259, 260f
  thickening of gastric mucosal folds in, 229–232, 229f–230f, 232f, 259, 260f
  small bowel involvement in, 514–515
Meningioma, calcification in, 1006
Meningocele, sacral, retrorectal space enlargement in, 769
Meniscoid ulcer of colon, 614f, 615
Mercedes-Benz sign in gallstones, 788, 791f, 956, 957f
Mercury ingestion
  in broken thermometer, bowel appearance in, 1013, 1013f
  ulceration of colon in, 617
Mesenteric artery, superior, syndrome of, 400, 401–407
Mesenteritis
  radiation-induced, 520f
  retractile
    narrowing of colon in, 659, 659f
    obstruction of colon in, 740, 740f
    separation of small bowel loops in, 526–527, 526f–527f
    thumbprinting pattern of colon in, 754, 754f
Mesentericoparietal hernia, 871
Mesentery
  calcification of, 964–966, 967f
    in lymph nodes, 1001–1002
  fibrosis of, thickening of small bowel mucosal folds in, 462

Mesentery (*continued*)
  lymphangioma of, cystic, duodenal
    sweep widening in, 355f, 356
  metastatic tumors of
    dilatation of small bowel and
      thickening of mucosal folds in, 454
    obstruction of duodenum in, 405
    separation of small bowel loops in,
      524, 626f
  primary tumors of, separation of small
    bowel loops in, 524, 524f
  sigmoid, herniation through, 874
  of small bowel, herniation through,
    874, 874f
  vascular disorders of
    collateral circulation in. *See*
      Collateral circulation, mesenteric
      arterial
    dilatation of small bowel in, 450
    filling defects of duodenum in, 337,
      375
    ileus in, adynamic, 433
    impression on duodenum in, 361
    ischemic colitis in, 596
    obstruction of large bowel in, 724
    pneumatosis intestinalis in, 885f,
      885–886
    portal vein gas in, 858, 860
    separation of small bowel loops in,
      517
    simulating thickening of duodenal
      mucosal folds, 337–338, 338f
    and superior mesenteric artery
      syndrome, 400, 401–407
    widening of duodenal sweep in, 337,
      356
Mesothelioma
  bull's-eye lesions in, 867f
  esophageal narrowing in, 82, 82f
  separation of small bowel loops in,
    523f, 523–524
Metabolic disorders, adynamic ileus in,
  433
Metachromatic leukodystrophy,
  gallbladder filling defects in, 802
Metallic foreign bodies, 1007f, 1008f,
  1009f, 1012f, 1013
  in esophagus, 106–108, 111f, 113
Metastases
  achalasia in, 17, 17f
  to bile ducts
    filling defects in, 812, 813f
    narrowing and obstruction in,
      823–824, 823f–824f
  to bone, nephrocalcinosis in, 969
  of breast carcinoma
    to biliary system, 824f
    bull's-eye lesions in, 866, 867f
    to colon, hematogenous spread of,
      646, 646f
    esophageal narrowing in, 82, 82f
    to small bowel, multiple filling
      defects in, 499–500, 500f
    to stomach, 196, 197f, 210, 211f, 251,
      253f, 299, 299f, 867f
    bull's-eye lesions in, 865, 866–868,
      866f, 867f

to cecum, 566f, 566–567
of cervical carcinoma
  to colon, 641, 641f
  esophagorespiratory fistula in, 132f
  to rectum, retrorectal space
    enlargement in, 766, 766f
to colon
  direct invasion, 640–644
  hematogenous spread, 646, 646f
  intraperitoneal seeding, 644–646
  lymphangitic spread, 647
  multiple filling defects in, 701–702,
    701f–702f
  narrowing in, 640–647, 640f–646f
  single filling defect in, 676f, 677,
    677f, 678f
  striped appearance in, 646, 646f
  thumbprinting pattern in, 751
  ulcerations in, 615, 615f
of colon carcinoma
  to bile ducts, 813f
  to liver, calcification in, 941, 942f
  to lymph nodes in porta hepatis, 823f
  to stomach, 299
to esophagus
  filling defects in, 102, 103f
  narrowing in, 82, 82f–83f
to gallbladder, 802, 802f
to liver
  calcification in, 941, 942f
  thickening of small bowel mucosal
    folds in, 461, 462f
of lung carcinoma
  bull's-eye lesions in, 867f
  to lymph nodes, calcification in,
    1003f
  to mesentery and peritoneal cavity,
    525f
  to retroperitoneum, duodenal sweep
    widening in, 355f
  to small bowel, filling defects in,
    386f, 487f, 488
  stomach ulcerations in, 252f
to lymph nodes
  bile duct narrowing and obstruction
    in, 823f, 823–824
  calcification in, 1002, 1003f
  duodenal obstruction in, 397
  duodenal thickening of mucosal
    folds in, 335, 336f
  esophageal ulceration in, 62
  stomach narrowing in, 210, 210f
to mediastinum
  diaphragm paralysis in, 153
  esophagorespiratory fistula in, 131,
    132f
of melanoma. *See* Melanoma,
  metastatic
to mesentery
  dilatation of small bowel and
    thickening of mucosal folds in, 454
  obstruction of duodenum in, 405
  separation of small bowel loops in,
    524, 525f
to omentum
  colon narrowing in, 643, 643f
  of ovarian carcinoma, 211f, 677f

stomach filling defects in, 251, 253f
stomach narrowing in, 210, 211f
of ovarian tumors, 211f
  to colon, 641, 642f, 677f, 678f
  to rectum, 766
to pancreas, duodenal sweep widening
  in, 352
of pancreatic carcinoma
  to cecum, 566, 566f
  to colon, 643, 644, 644f, 676f
  to duodenum, ulcerations in, 325
  intraperitoneal seeding of, 645f
  to stomach, 299
perivaterian, gas in biliary tree and
  pancreaticobiliary reflux in, 855
of prostate carcinoma
  narrowing of colon in, 640–641,
    640f–641f
  retrorectal space enlargement in,
    765–766, 766f
  ulceration of colon in, 615f
to rectum
  of prostate carcinoma, 615f,
    640–641, 640f–641f
  retrorectal space enlargement in,
    765–766, 766f
to retroperitoneum, duodenal sweep
  widening in, 355f, 356
to small bowel
  duodenal filling defects in, 385, 385f,
    386f
  multiple filling defects in, 499–500,
    500f
  postbulbar ulceration of duodenum
    in, 325–327
  separation of bowel loops in, 523f,
    524–526, 525f
  solitary filling defect in, 487f, 488,
    488f
to stomach
  bull's-eye lesions in, 867f
  filling defects in, 251–252, 252f–254f
  in fundus, 297–299, 299f
  narrowing in, 210, 210f
  ulcerations in, 194–196, 197f, 198f,
    251, 252f–254f
of stomach carcinoma
  colon narrowing in, 642f, 643, 643f
  colon ulcerations in, 615f
  esophageal filling defects in, 102, 103f
  esophageal narrowing in, 81f, 81–82,
    83f
of thyroid carcinoma
  esophageal narrowing in, 82, 83f
  liver calcification in, 942f
Microcolon, in ileal atresia, 428, 428f
Midgut volvulus, duodenal obstruction
  in, 390f, 390–391
Milk-alkali syndrome, nephrocalcinosis
  in, 969–970
Milk of calcium
  and gallbladder calcification, 958f,
    958–959
  and kidney calcification, 977, 978f
Mirizzi syndrome
  filling defects of bile ducts in, 807–808,
    807f–808f

narrowing and obstruction of bile
ducts in, 807, 834, 834f
Mitral valve disorders, esophageal
impressions in, 40, 41f
Morgagni foramen hernia, 166–167,
167f–168f
retrogastric space widening in, 310
Morphine
ileus from, adynamic, 433
small bowel dilatation from, 442
Mosaic pattern of colon in
Hirschsprung's disease, 735, 737f
Motility disorders
of duodenum, obstruction and
dilatation in, 403–405
of esophagus, 3–25
narrowing in, 93, 94f
of large and small bowel, adynamic
ileus in, 430–440
Moulage sign in sprue, 444, 445f
Mucocele of appendix, 561–563,
561f–563f
calcification in, 561, 962f, 963
generalized abdominal, 998
myxoglobulosis in, 563, 563f
rupture of, 563, 563f
Mucormycoma of colon, 681, 681f
Mucormycosis of colon, 607
Mucosa
of colon
dysplasia of, 707–708, 708f
and submucosal edema, 717–718,
717f–718f, 754, 754f
of esophagus, prolapse of
filling defects of stomach in, 270
pseudotumor of stomach in, 300–303
of gastric antrum, outlet obstruction in
prolapse of, 290
gastric ectopic
in esophagus, 28–29, 29f
in Meckel's diverticula, 536, 536f
Mucosal folds
of small bowel, 441–481
duodenal thickening of, 329–339
gastric involvement in thickening of,
513–516
irregular thickening of, 467–481
normal appearance of, in small
bowel dilatation, 441–451
regular thickening of, 456–466
of stomach, 223–237
filling defects in thickening of,
259–261, 259f–260f
normal variations in, 223
prolapse of, esophageal filling
defects in, 115, 115f
radiation of, in ulcers, 182, 183f,
184f, 186f
small bowel involvement in
thickening of, 513–516
Mucous membrane pemphigoid,
esophageal narrowing in, 91, 91f
Mucoviscidosis. *See* Cystic fibrosis
Mucus
as artifact in barium studies of colon,
713

tumor-induced, in biliary tree
filling defects in, 812, 814f
obstruction in, 824f, 825
Mulberry stone, biliary, 805
Multicystic disease of kidney,
calcification in, 973, 974f
Multiple sclerosis, esophageal motility
disorders in, 8
Muscular dystrophy
esophageal motility disorders in, 7, 7f,
11
gastric dilatation in, nonobstructive,
295
ileus in, adynamic, 435
Myasthenia gravis, esophageal motility
disorders in, 7
Mycobacterium infections
small bowel thickening of mucosal
folds in, 454, 480f
irregular, 479–480, 480f
tuberculosis in. *See* Tuberculosis
Myeloma, multiple, hemorrhage and
small bowel thickening of mucosal
folds in, 461
Myenteric plexus disorders, esophageal
motility disorders in, 10, 16
Myoblastoma, granular cell, of bile ducts,
825
Myocardial infarction, adynamic ileus in,
433
Myopathy, esophageal motility disorders
in, 7–8
Myositis ossificans, abdominal wall
calcification in, 1005
Myotomy, Heller, in achalasia, 19
Myotonic dystrophy, esophageal motility
disorders in, 7, 7f
Myxedema, esophageal motility disorders
in, 10
Myxoglobulosis of appendix, 563, 563f
calcification in, 962f, 963

Napkin-ring appearance
in colon carcinoma, 633, 723
in small bowel lymphoma, 469, 469f
Narrowing
of bile ducts, 818–837
of colon, 622–661
of duodenum, 387–400
proximal dilatation in, 400, 401–407
of esophagus, 70–96
of stomach, 205–222
Nasogastric intubation
esophageal stricture in, 85, 88f
esophagorespiratory fistula in, 133, 133f
Necrosis
of fat, in pancreatitis, 910–911
calcification in, 997
of kidney
cortical, calcification in, 976f, 977
papillary, nephrocalcinosis in, 971,
972f
Necrotizing enterocolitis
pneumatosis intestinalis in, 883–885,
883f–884f
portal vein gas in, 858, 859, 859f

Neonates. *See* Children and infants
Neoplasms. *See also specific types and
anatomic locations of tumors*
bull's-eye lesions in, 865–868
diaphragm elevation in, 156
fistulas in
enteric-enteric, 919–920, 922f–923f
esophagorespiratory, 131–133, 132f
metastatic. *See* Metastases
retrorectal space enlargement in, 763–
769
separation of small bowel loops in,
523–526, 523f–525f
undifferentiated abdominal,
calcification in, 998, 999f
Nephritis, hereditary, renal calcification
in, 977
Nephrocalcinosis, 969–971, 969f–970f
Nephrotic syndrome, small bowel
thickening of mucosal folds in, 461
Neurinoma
of cystic duct, narrowing and
obstruction in, 825
of gallbladder, 799
Neuroblastoma
bladder calcification in, 985
retroperitoneal calcification in,
996–997, 997f
Neurocrest tumors, polyps of colon in,
698, 699f
Neurofibroma
of abdominal wall, differentiated from
calcification, 1002, 1003f
retrorectal space enlargement in, 769
of small bowel
duodenal filling defects in, 380f, 381
multiple filling defects in, 499, 499f
solitary filling defects in, 485–486
Neurofibromatosis, 246
of colon, multiple filling defects in,
704–705
of small bowel
duodenal filling defects in, 380f, 381
multiple filling defects in, 499, 499f
separation of bowel loops in, 520,
521f
Neurogenic tumors
duodenal filling defects in, 380–381,
380f–381f
retrorectal space enlargement in, 766–
769, 769f
Neurolemmonas of stomach, filling
defects in, 246, 248f
Neuroma
of bile ducts, 812
traumatic
in ileocolic anastomosis, 493f, 674
of small bowel, solitary filling defect
in, 492, 493f
Neuropathy
alcoholic, esophageal motility
disorders in, 10
central, achalasia in, 16
diabetic
duodenal dilatation in, 405
esophageal motility disorders in, 10
gastric dilatation in, 292f, 293, 294f

Nissen fundoplication, pseudotumor of
stomach in, 303f, 304f, 305
Nodular lesions of esophagus, diffuse,
143–147
Nonvisualization of gallbladder, 773–778
Nucleus pulposus calcification, 1005,
1005f
Nutcracker esophagus, 21
Nutrition
and nonvisualization of gallbladder in
fasting patients, 774
and pancreatic calcification in protein
malnutrition, 955

Obesity
diaphragm elevation in, 156
gastric restrictive surgery in, 220–221,
220f–221f
retrogastric space widening in,
309–310, 310f
Obstruction
of bile ducts, 818–837
of gastric outlet, 281–290
stomach wall gas in, 314
of large bowel, 722–740
pneumatosis intestinalis in, 885f, 886,
887
and pseudo-obstruction of intestines,
chronic idiopathic, 405, 406f, 437,
437f
small bowel dilatation in, 450, 450f
of small bowel, 411–429
in duodenum, 387–407
in jejunum, 414f, 415
Obstructive pulmonary disease
pneumatosis intestinalis in, 890
pneumoperitoneum in, 902
Obturator hernia, 875–876, 875f–876f
Howship-Romberg sign in, 876
Occlusion rings in fallopian tubes, 992,
993f
Ochronosis, nucleus pulposus
calcification in, 1005, 1005f
Oculopharyngeal myopathy, esophageal
motility disorders in, 7–8
Oil bubbles, as artifact in barium studies
of colon, 665, 713
Oil granuloma, abdominal calcification
in, 999, 999f
Omentum, metastases to. *See* Metastases,
to omentum
Omphalocele, 878, 879f
Oncocytoma of kidney, calcification of,
975, 976f
Oriental cholangiohepatitis
cystic dilatation of bile ducts in,
844–845, 845f
filling defects of bile ducts in, 816, 816f
narrowing and obstruction of bile
ducts in, 828, 828f
Osteomyelitis, spinal, esophageal
impressions in, 29
Osteophytes
cervical, esophageal impressions in,
27f, 27–28

thoracic, esophageal impressions in,
42, 44f
Osteoporosis, nephrocalcinosis in, 969
Osteosarcoma
bladder calcification in, 985
kidney calcification in, 975, 975f
Ostomy procedures
colon carcinoma in, 648–649, 649f
pneumatosis intestinalis in, 888–889
radiographic patterns in, 1002
stomach filling defects in, 271
Outlet obstruction, gastric, 281–290
stomach wall gas in, 314
Ovary
calcification of, 989–991, 989f–992f
dermoid cysts of
calcification in, 989, 989f, 990f
entero-ovarian fistula in, 929, 932f
fistulas of, entero-ovarian, 929, 931f,
932f
metastatic tumors of
in colon, 641, 642f, 677f, 678f
in rectum, retrorectal space
enlargement in, 766
psammomatous calcifications of,
989–990, 990f
generalized abdominal calcification
in, 997–998, 998f
spontaneous amputation of, 991, 992f
Oxaluria, and nephrocalcinosis in
hyperoxaluria, 970–971, 971f

Pain, gastric dilatation in, 292
Pancreas
abscess of
extraluminal gas in, 910–911, 911f
gastric impressions in, 259f
annular
duodenal impressions in, 359, 360f
duodenal narrowing and obstruction
in, 388–389, 389f
gastric outlet obstruction in, 286
calcification of, 849, 950–955,
952f–955f
in pancreatitis, 343, 950–952, 952f,
954f, 955
sunburst pattern in, 953f, 955
carcinoma of. *See* Carcinoma, of
pancreas
cystadenoma of
calcification in, 955
duodenal sweep widening in, 352,
354f
retrogastric space widening in, 310
ectopic. *See* Ectopia, of pancreas
epithelial neoplasms of, calcification
in, 954f, 955
fistulas of
external, 934
internal, 928
impression on duodenum, 359, 360f,
361f
metastatic tumors of, duodenal sweep
widening in, 352
pseudocysts of. *See* Pseudocysts of
pancreas

Pancreaticobiliary reflux, 852–857
Pancreatitis
bile duct narrowing and obstruction
in, 829, 830f
pipestem appearance of, 829, 830f
calcification in, 343, 950–952, 952f,
954f, 955
colon in
cut-off sign of, 341, 342f
impressions on, 677f
narrowing of, 657, 657f
ulcerations of, 614, 614f
duodenum in
dilatation of, 405, 405f
narrowing and obstruction of, 394,
395f, 405
thickening of mucosal folds of, 332f,
333
widening of sweep, 340–344,
341f–345f
fat necrosis in, 910–911
and calcification, 997
fistulas in, internal, 928
gallbladder visualization impaired in,
776
gallstone, calcification in, 952
hemorrhagic, portal vein gas in, 860
hereditary, calcification in, 954f, 955
ileus in, adynamic, 434f, 435, 437, 438f
papilla of Vater enlargement in,
848–849, 849f, 850
portal hypertension and esophageal
varices in, 123
retrogastric space widening in, 310, 311
stomach in
outlet obstruction of, 284f, 285
thickening of mucosal folds of, 236f,
236–237
Panniculitis, mesenteric, 526
Pantopaque, residual, kidney
calcification in, 977–979, 979f
Papilla, anal, colon filling defects in
hypertrophy of, 687f, 688
Papilla of Vater
adenomatous polyps of, 850
carcinoma of, 850
duodenal filling defects from, 371f,
371–373
edema of, 847–850
enlargement of, 373, 847–851
differential diagnosis of, 851
normal variations of, 847, 848f
in perivaterian neoplasms, 850, 850f
Papillitis, 850
Papilloma
of bile ducts
filling defects in, 812, 843
narrowing and obstruction in, 825,
843
of esophagus, filling defects in, 100, 101f
of gallbladder, 798, 798f
Papillomatosis
biliary, cystic dilatation in, 843
esophageal, nodular lesions in, 146
Paracecal hernia, 874
separation of small bowel loops in, 527

Paraduodenal hernia, 871–872, 872f
obstruction of small bowel in, 420
separation of small bowel loops in, 527, 527f
Paraesophageal hernia, 162–165, 165f–166f
esophageal impressions in, 42–45, 44f
gastric volvulus and outlet obstruction in, 286
Paraganglioma, gangliocytic, duodenal filling defects in, 381, 381f
Paralysis
of diaphragm, 153–156, 155f
sniff test in, 156
gastric dilatation in, nonobstructive, 292
Parametrial gold therapy, calcifications in, 994, 994f
Parasitic infections
abdominal wall calcification in, 1002
of bile ducts
carcinoma in, 819
cystic dilatation in, 843–844, 845, 846f
filling defects in, 813–816, 815f–816f
gas in biliary system and pancreaticobiliary reflux in, 854–855
narrowing and obstruction in, 829–833, 831f
bladder calcification in, 980, 980f
of cecum, 600
coned cecum in, 572, 573f, 574–576, 575f, 600
of colon
calcification in, 966, 967f
multiple filling defects in, 708–710, 709f–710f
narrowing in, 626, 626f, 627f
obstruction in, 724
single filling defect in, 679f, 679–680, 681
thumbprinting pattern in, 749–751, 750f
toxic megacolon in, 741, 743f
ulcerations in, 600–601, 600f–601f
of gallbladder, 802
of ileocecal valve, 549
liver calcification in, 939
pneumatosis intestinalis in, 890
rectocolonic calcification in, 966, 967f
of small bowel
duodenal thickening of mucosal folds in, 334
irregular thickening of mucosal folds in, 468, 468f
lymphoid hyperplasia in, 507, 508f, 509
multiple filling defects in, 500–504, 503f–504f
obstruction in, 427
solitary filling defect in, 491
ureteral calcification in, 980, 980f
Parathyroid gland
enlargement of, esophageal impressions in, 28
hyperparathyroidism

nephrocalcinosis in, 969
pancreatitis and calcification of pancreas in, 953
Pelvic abscess, 913, 913f
portal vein gas in, 860
Pelvic hernia, 874
Pelvic inflammatory disease, enteric-enteric fistula in, 923
Pemphigoid
benign mucous membrane, esophageal narrowing in, 91, 91f
bullous, esophageal nodules in, 146
Penicillin, calcium, calcification of injection site, 1005
Penile implant, calcification of, 988, 988f
Peptic ulcer disease, 190, 191f
in areae gastricae, 239, 239f
bull's-eye lesions in, 868, 868f
dilatation of duodenum in, 405
forme fruste perforation in, 901
gallbladder-bowel fistula in, 929
gallbladder visualization impaired in, 776
gas in stomach wall in, 312
of gastric antrum and duodenal bulb, 315
gastric outlet obstruction in, 281–282, 282f–283f
narrowing of stomach in, 211f, 212
obstruction of duodenum in, 405
pancreaticobiliary reflux in, 854, 855f
pneumatosis intestinalis in, 886–887
pneumoperitoneum in, 897, 989f, 901
in postbulbar region of duodenum, 323–324, 324f–326f
lacteral incisura appearance in, 359
postoperative marginal ulcers of stomach in, 196–200, 198f–199f
thickening of mucosal folds in
duodenal, 329, 330f
gastric, 229, 229f
Pericardium
esophageal impressions in disorders of, 40
intrapericardial diaphragmatic hernias, 173, 173f–174f
Peripheral nerve disorders, esophageal motility disorders in, 8, 16
Peristalsis
duodenal, disorders of, 403–405, 404f
esophageal
disorders of, 3–25
phases of, 3–4, 4f
Peritoneal bands, congenital, duodenal obstruction in, 391, 391f
Peritoneal sac, lesser
abscess of, extraluminal gas in, 911–913, 912f
herniation into, 872–873, 873f
Peritoneum
abscess in, separation of small bowel loops in, 526
neoplasms of, separation of small bowel loops in, 523f, 523–526, 525f
pneumoperitoneum of, 892–902

Peritonitis
adhesions and small bowel obstruction in, 420
ascites and separation of small bowel loops in, 521
gallbladder visualization impaired in, 776
gastric dilatation in, 292
ileus in, adynamic, 430–433, 432f
meconium, 428
generalized abdominal calcification in, 999, 999f
liver calcification in, 945
pneumoperitoneum in, 897–899
tuberculous, abdominal calcification in, 998–999
Pernicious anemia, gallbladder visualization impaired in, 777
Peutz-Jeghers syndrome, 486
of colon, 671, 696f, 697
multiple filling defects in, 696f, 697
single filling defect in, 671
of small bowel
duodenal filling defects in, 380, 380f
multiple filling defects in, 495, 496f
solitary filling defects in, 485f, 486
of stomach, filling defects in, 242f, 244
Pharyngeal tumors, radiation therapy and cricopharyngeal achalasia in, 7
Pharyngeal venous plexus, esophageal impressions from, 26, 27f
Pheochromocytoma, adrenal calcification in, 996
Phleboliths, 1000f, 1001, 1001f
displacement sign in, 1001, 1001f
in gastric hemangioma, 246, 248f
splenic, calcification of, 946, 947, 947f
Phlegmonous gastritis
gas in stomach wall in, 312, 313f
narrowing of stomach in, 214–215, 215f
Phrenic nerve injury, diaphragm paralysis in, 153, 156
Phrygian cap of gallbladder, 797, 803, 803f
Phytobezoars. *See also* Bezoars
gastric outlet obstruction in, 289f, 290
Pica, radiographic patterns in, 1009f, 1010
Placental calcification, 992–994
Plasmacytoma
of colon, extramedullary, 677–679
of stomach, filling defects in, 255, 258f
Pleuropulmonary disorders, esophageal impressions in, 30, 31f, 32, 45
Plummer-Vinson syndrome, 72, 76
Pneumatosis intestinalis, 881–891, 914
benign linear, 887, 887f
colon thumbprinting pattern in, 751, 753f
differential diagnosis of, 890–891, 890f–891f
pneumoperitoneum in, 901
primary, 881–883, 882f–883f
retroperitoneal gas in, 903, 905f
simulating multiple filling defects of colon, 714, 714f
small bowel thickening of mucosal folds in, 465
stomach wall gas in, 314

Pneumomediastinum,
    pneumoperitoneum in, 902
Pneumonia
  diaphragm paralysis in, 153
  ileus in, adynamic, 433
Pneumoperitoneum, 892–902
  cupola sign of, 894, 897f
  diagnostic, 901
  extraluminal upper quadrant gas in, 903
  falciform ligament sign of, 894, 896f
  football sign of, 894, 895f
  inverted V sign of, 894, 896f
  in jejunal diverticulosis, 535
  positioning of patient in, 892–894,
    893f–894f
  spontaneous, 901
  triangle sign of, 894, 895f
  urachal sign of, 894, 896f, 897f
  with peritonitis, 897–899
  without peritonitis, 899–902
Poisoning
  iron, stomach narrowing in, 218
  lead, gastric dilatation in,
    nonobstructive, 295
  mercury, colon ulceration in, 617
Poliomyelitis
  esophageal motility disorders in, 8
  gastric dilatation in, 293
Polyarteritis nodosa
  small bowel thickening of mucosal
    folds in, 458–459
  stomach narrowing in, 214, 214f
Polycystic disease
  of kidney
    calcification in, 973
    duodenal impressions in, 359, 360f
    gallbladder displacement in, 785
  of liver, gallbladder displacement in,
    784f
Polycythemia, portal hypertension and
    esophageal varices in, 123
Polymyositis
  esophageal motility disorders in, 7, 10
  gastric dilatation in, nonobstructive,
    295
Polyp
  adenomatous. *See* Adenomatous polyps
  of bile ducts, 814f
  of cecum, 567f
  of colon, 663f
    artifacts differentiated from, 665
    benign and malignant, 668–670,
      668f–670f
    carcinoma in, 667–668, 695, 695f
    in Cronkhite-Canada syndrome, 698,
      698f, 699f
    diagnostic management of, 670
    diverticula differentiated from, 665f,
      665–666, 713–714
    double-contrast technique in, 664f,
      665
    in familial polyposis, 693–695, 694f
    filiform, 707, 707f
    foreign bodies differentiated from,
      712f, 713
    in Gardner's syndrome, 695–697,
      695f, 696f

    hyperplastic, 663, 663f, 670
    juvenile, 671, 698, 698f, 700, 700f
    multiple filling defects in, 693–700
    in neurocrest tumors, 698, 699f
    pedunculated, 666–667, 666f–667f,
      668, 669f
    in Peutz–Jeghers syndrome, 671,
      696f, 697
    and pseudopolyps. *See*
      Pseudopolyps, of colon
    puckering of colon wall in, 668–669,
      669f
    in Ruvalcaba–Myhre–Smith
      syndrome, 698–700, 699f
    sessile, 665f, 666, 668, 668f, 669f
    single filling defects in, 662–670, 671
    target sign in, 667, 667f
    in Turcot syndrome, 697f, 697–698
    villoglandular, 672f, 673
  esophagogastric, filling defects of
    esophagus in, 100, 101f
  of esophagus, filling defects of
    esophagus in, 98–100, 100f, 101f
  of gallbladder, 798
    cholesterol, 795f, 796
    and pseudopolyps, 803–804
  of ileocecal valve, 546–548
  of papilla of vater, 850
  and pseudopolyps. *See* Pseudopolyps
  of small bowel
    duodenal filling defects in, 371f, 376,
      377f, 380, 380f
    multiple filling defects in, 495–497,
      496f–498f
    solitary filling defects in, 490, 492f
  of stomach
    carcinoma in, 243, 247
    in familial polyposis of colon, 242f,
      243
    filling defects in, 239–243, 240f–242f,
      265, 276–277
    inflammatory fibroid, 265
    in postoperative remnant, 276–277
    prolapse of, 285, 381–382, 382f
Polyposis
  of colon
    gastric polyps in, 242f, 243
    in juveniles, 671, 698, 698f, 700, 700f
    multiple filling defects in, 693–700,
      694f–699f
    single filling defects in, 671
  in Cronkhite–Canada syndrome, 698,
    698f, 699f
  disseminated intestinal, 697
    small bowel filling defects in, 496
  familial syndrome, 242f, 243, 693–695,
    694f
  in juveniles
    colon filling defects in, 671, 698,
      698f, 700, 700f
    small bowel filling defects in,
      496–497
Poppel's sign in pancreatitis, 848, 849f
Porcelain gallbladder, 359
  calcification in, 958, 958f
  in carcinoma, 800, 800f

Porphyria
  duodenal dilatation in, 405
  gastric dilatation in, nonobstructive,
    295
  ileus in, adynamic, 437–439, 438f
Porta hepatis
  inflammatory mass in, biliary
    obstruction in, 832f, 833
  metastases to lymph nodes in, biliary
    obstruction in, 823f, 823–824
Portal hypertension, esophageal varices
    in, 123, 124, 125, 126, 126f
Portal vein
  calcification in, 943, 943f–944f, 1001
  gas in, 858–862, 916
    compared to gas in biliary tree, 858–
      859
    prognosis in, 861
    tubular lucencies in, 858, 859f
  preduodenal, duodenal obstruction in,
    399, 399f
  thrombosis in, 943
Positioning of patient
  in achalasia, 15
  in esophageal varices, 125, 126–127
  and gallbladder displacement, 783
  in gallstones, 788, 789f, 792, 792f
  in imperforate anus, 736–738,
    737f–738f
  in pneumoperitoneum, 892–894, 893f–
    894f
  in reflux esophagitis, 48
  in toxic megacolon, 744
Postanal cysts, retrorectal space
    enlargement in, 763, 764
Postbulbar ulceration of duodenum,
    323–328
  lateral incisura appearance in, 359
  narrowing in, 392, 392f
Postcricoid impression on esophagus, 26
Potassium
  adynamic ileus in hypokalemia, 433,
    433f, 435f
  small bowel dilatation in hypokalemia,
    448
Potassium chloride tablets
  esophagitis and esophageal ulceration
    from, 66
  small bowel obstruction from, 427
Preduodenal portal vein, duodenal
    obstruction in, 399, 399f
Pregnancy
  calcification of fetal skull and skeleton
    in, 993f, 994
  diaphragm elevation in, 156
  duodenal obstruction and dilatation in,
    403
  esophagitis in, reflux, 47
  gallbladder visualization impaired in,
    777
  pneumoperitoneum after, 901
Presbyesophagus, esophageal motility
    disorders in, 10, 12f, 19–20, 20f
Probantheline bromide, in barium
    studies of esophageal varices, 125
Proctitis
  gonorrheal

narrowing of colon in, 628
ulcerations of colon in, 603f, 604–605
obliterans, 628
retrorectal space enlargement in, 763
Prostate
calcification of, 986
carcinoma of, metastatic
narrowing of colon in, 640–641,
640f–641f
retrorectal space enlargement in,
765–766, 766f
ulceration of colon in, 615f
Protein-losing enteropathy
in Menetrier's disease. *See* Menetrier's
disease
sandlike lucencies of small bowel in,
512
thickening of mucosal folds in
in small bowel, 461, 462f, 514–515
in stomach, 229–232, 229f–230f,
232f, 259f, 260f, 514–515
Protein malnutrition, pancreatic
calcification in, 955
Psammomatous calcification of ovary,
989–990, 990f
generalized abdominal calcification in,
997–998, 998f
Pseudo-Billroth pattern in Crohn's
disease, 212f, 213, 318, 318f, 513
Pseudocalculi in bile ducts, 809–811,
809f–810f
Pseudocysts of pancreas
bile duct narrowing and obstruction
in, 829
calcification of, 952, 952f
duodenum in
filling defects of, 373f, 374
narrowing and obstruction of, 394,
395f
sweep widening of, 346–348,
346f–348f
esophageal impressions in, 42, 43f
fistulas in
external, 934
internal, 928–929, 929f
gallbladder displacement in, 785
pad effect in, 346, 347f
retrogastric space widening in, 310,
310f
spontaneous rupture of, 928–929, 929f
stomach narrowing in, 220, 220f
Pseudodiaphragmatic contour in
infrapulmonic effusion, 157f, 157–
158
Pseudodiverticula
of duodenum, 533f, 533–534
of ileum, 535, 539
of jejunum, 535, 535f
Pseudodiverticulosis of esophagus,
intramural, 67f, 68, 121f, 121–122
narrowing in, 93, 94f
Pseudolymphoma
of colon, narrowing in, 660, 660f
of stomach
filling defects in, 267
narrowing in, 219, 219f

thickening of mucosal folds in, 233,
233f
ulcerations in, 192, 192f, 233, 233f
Pseudomembranous colitis, 609–612,
611f–612f
multiple filling defects in, 711, 711f
thumbprinting pattern in, 751, 752f
toxic megacolon in, 741
Pseudomyxoma peritonei
calcification in, 991–992, 992f
generalized abdominal, 998, 998f
of liver, 945
in rupture of appendiceal mucocele,
563, 563f
Pseudo-obstruction, intestinal
chronic idiopathic, 405, 406f, 437, 437f
achalasia in, 17
of small bowel, 450, 450f
of colon, 740
Pseudopolyps
of colon
in amebiasis, 709, 709f
in Crohn's disease, 706f, 707, 707f
giant, 680f, 681
in ischemic colitis, 708, 709f
multiple filling defects in, 705–711
obstruction in, 724, 726f
proximal to obstruction, 718
single filling defects in, 680f, 680–681
in ulcerative colitis, 592, 592f, 705f,
706f, 707, 726f
of gallbladder, 803–804
Pseudopneumatosis of rectum, 890f, 891
Pseudopneumobilia, 856, 856f
Pseudotumors
of colon, filling defects in, 688–690,
688f–689f
of small bowel
duodenal filling defects in, 362–363,
363f–366f
solitary filling defect in, 491
in strangulating obstruction, 418,
418f
in stomach, 244f
in fundus, 300–307, 302f–307f
Pseudoulcers of colon, 590f, 591
Psoas abscess, tuberculous, 997
Psychogenic megacolon, 731f, 733
Pulmonary artery, esophageal
impressions from, 35, 38f
Pulmonary veins, esophageal
impressions from, 31f, 32, 35, 39f
Purpura
Henoch–Schönlein, small bowel
thickening of mucosal folds in,
459, 460
thrombocytopenic, small bowel
thickening of mucosal folds in,
460, 461f
Pyelonephritis
chronic, nephrocalcinosis in, 971
duodenal-renal fistula in, 929
xanthogranulomatous, renal
calcification in, 975, 976f
Pyloric channel
carcinoma of, gastric outlet
obstruction in, 284

peptic ulcer disease of, gastric outlet
obstruction in, 281
Pyloroduodenal peptic ulcer disease,
pneumatosis intestinalis in,
886–887
Pylorus
differentiated from mass in duodenal
bulb, 363, 365f
double, filling defects of stomach in,
264, 265f
hypertrophy of antral-pyloric fold,
filling defects of stomach in, 261,
261f
stenosis of
gastric outlet obstruction in,
287–290, 288f–289f
pneumatosis intestinalis in, 886f
Pyogenic infections
liver calcification in, 945
splenic calcification in, 948

Quinidine, esophagitis and esophageal
ulceration from, 66
Quinine injection site, calcification of,
1005

Radiation injury
of bladder, cystitis and calcification in,
980
of colon
narrowing in, 630, 630f
ulcerations in, 612–613, 612f–613f
of cricopharyngeal muscle, achalasia
in, 7
of esophagus, 131, 133f
narrowing in, 86–90, 90f
nodular lesions in, 143
tertiary contractions in, 21, 22f
ulcerations in, 63–64, 65f
fistulas in
anorectal, 935
enteric-enteric, 921
esophagorespiratory, 131, 133f
internal, 928
retrorectal space enlargement in, 763,
764f, 766, 767f
of small bowel
dilatation in, 454
duodenal, 399, 399f
narrowing and obstruction in, 399,
399f, 427
of small bowel
sandlike lucencies in, 511f, 512
separation of bowel loops in, 520,
520f
thickening of mucosal folds in, 454,
461–462
of stomach
narrowing in, 216f, 217–218
thickening of mucosal folds in, 228–
229
ulcerations in, 190–192, 191f
Radiation therapy in esophageal
carcinoma, 79, 80f

Radionuclide scanning
  in Barrett's esophagus, 53, 55f
  in reflux esophagitis, 47, 47f, 49, 49f
Ram's horn sign, in Crohn's disease of
    stomach, 211f, 213
Raynaud's phenomenon, esophageal
    motility disorders in, 9f, 10
Razor blades in alimentary tract,
    radiographic appearance of, 1007,
    1008f
Rectovaginal fistulas, 926–928, 927f, 928f
Rectum
  adenoma of, villous, 671f
  amyloidosis of, 689f, 690
  balloon catheterization of, portal vein
    gas after, 860
  biopsy of, ulcerations after, 620, 620f
  calcification of, in schistosomiasis,
    966, 967f
  carcinoid tumors of, 675, 675f, 676f
  carcinoma of, 634, 634f, 635, 635f,
    636f, 637f
    retrorectal space enlargement in,
    765, 765f
  condyloma acuminatum of, giant, 629,
    629f
  Crohn's disease of, retrorectal space
    enlargement in, 762f, 763
  in enlargement of retrorectal space,
    760–770
  enteroliths in, 960
  fecal impaction in
    filling defects in, 683, 683f
    in Hirschsprung's disease, 734, 735f
    obstruction in, 731, 733f
  fistulas of
    anorectal, 934–935, 935f
    rectovaginal, 926–928, 927f, 928f
  foreign bodies in, 686f, 687
  gallstones in, calcified, 957f
  metastases to
    of prostate carcinoma, 615f,
      640–641, 640f–641f
    retrorectal space enlargement in,
      765–766, 766f
  multiple filling defects of, in
    hemorrhoids, 713, 713f
  obstruction of, 722
  perirectal abscess in Crohn's disease,
    934, 934f
  pseudopneumatosis of, 890f, 891
  suppositories affecting radiographic
    appearance of, 1010, 1011f
  ulcerations of. *See* Ulcerations, of
    rectum
Reflux
  of bile and pancreatic juices
    gas in biliary system in, 852–857
    gastritis of postoperative remnant in,
      276–277, 277f–278f
  of gastric or duodenal contents,
    esophagitis in, 46–50. *See also*
    Reflux esophagitis
Reflux esophagitis, 46–50, 47f–52f
  Barrett's esophagitis in, 52
  carcinoma in, 76
  clinical symptoms of, 48

feline appearance in, 49, 51f
filling defects in, 105
healing of, 50, 52f
and hiatal hernia, 47, 49, 50, 50f, 52f,
  84, 85f, 159
lower esophageal ring in, 73
narrowing in, 83–84, 85f
nodular lesions in, 143, 145f
predisposing conditions in, 46–48
in scleroderma, 9
ulcerations in, 49, 49f, 50, 50f, 51f
Remnant, gastric, filling defects in,
  271–280
Renal artery aneurysm, calcification of,
  977, 977f
Retractile mesenteritis. *See* Mesenteritis,
  retractile
Retrogastric space widening, 309–311
Retroperitoneum
  calcification in, 996–997, 996f–997f
  fat loss in, duodenal obstruction and
    dilatation in, 403
  gas in, free, 903–904, 904f–905f
  hernia of, separation of small bowel
    loops in, 527, 527f
  inflammatory disease of, esophageal
    varices in, 123
  neoplasms of
    calcification in, 996–997, 996f–997f
    duodenal sweep widening in, 356
    retrogastric space widening in, 311,
      311f
    retrorectal space enlargement in,
      768f
Retrorectal space
  enlargement of, 760–770
  normal variations in, 761, 761f
Rheumatoid arthritis
  esophageal motility disorders in, 10
  small bowel thickening of mucosal
    folds in, 458–459
Riley–Day syndrome, esophageal motility
    disorders in, 8
Rings, esophageal
  cartilaginous, 73, 75f
  in hiatal hernia, 162, 164f
  lower, 73, 73f, 74f, 162, 162f
Rokitansky–Aschoff sinuses of gallbladder
  in adenomyomatosis, 796, 796f
  esophageal pseudodiverticulosis
    compared to, 67f, 68, 121
Rosette pattern of ileocecal valve, 543,
  544f
Rotavirus infection of colon, 608–609,
  610f
Rubin test for tubal patency,
    pneumoperitoneum after, 901
Ruvalcaba–Myhre–Smith syndrome
  colon filling defects in, 698–700, 699f
  small bowel filling defects in, 497, 497f
  stomach filling defects in, 244

Sacrotuberous ligaments, calcification
    of, 1006, 1006f
Sacrum
  foramen of, superimposed over colon,
    689f, 690

fracture of, retrorectal space
    enlargement in, 770, 770f
  tumors of, retrorectal space
    enlargement in, 769
Saddle appearance in colon carcinoma,
  614, 636, 669–670, 670f
Salmonellosis
  toxic megacolon in, 741, 743f
  ulceration of colon in, 601–603, 602f
Salpingitis, tuberculous, 992
Sandlike lucencies in small bowel,
  506–512
Sarcoidosis
  bile duct narrowing and obstruction
    in, 833
  nephrocalcinosis in, 969
  of stomach
    filling defects in, 261
    narrowing in, 212f, 213
    outlet obstruction in, 285
    thickening of mucosal folds in, 234
Sarcoma
  bladder calcification in, 985
  botryoides, bile duct filling defects in,
    812, 813f
  bull's-eye lesions in, 866–868
  of colon, 675f
    Kaposi's, 649, 702, 702f
    multiple filling defects in, 702, 702f
    narrowing in, 644, 644f
  of esophagus, filling defects in,
    102–103, 103f, 104
  of gallbladder, 802
  Kaposi's. *See* Kaposi's sarcoma
  leiomyosarcoma. *See* Leiomyosarcoma
  osteogenic
    bladder calcification in, 985
    kidney calcification in, 975, 975f
  of pancreas, duodenal impressions in,
    361f
  retroperitoneal
    retrogastric space widening in, 311,
      311f
    retrorectal space enlargement in,
      768f
  retrorectal space enlargement in, 765,
    768f
  of small bowel
    duodenal filling defects in, 385, 386
    duodenal narrowing and obstruction
      in, 397, 397f
    duodenal thickening of mucosal
      folds in, 335
    separation of bowel loops in, 525f
    solitary filling defect in, 486–488,
      487f
  of stomach
    filling defects in, 252–255, 254f–257f
    of fundus, 297, 299f
    retrogastric space widening in, 311
    ulcerations in, 194, 197f, 252, 254f
Scars, surgical, ossification of, 1002, 1004f
Schatzki ring of esophagus, 73, 73f
  in hiatal hernia, 162, 162f
Schistosomiasis
  bile duct narrowing and obstruction
    in, 833
  bladder calcification in, 980, 980f

of colon
  calcification in, 966, 967f
  multiple filling defects in, 709–710,
    710f
  narrowing in, 626
  obstruction in, 724
  single filling defect in, 681
  thumbprinting pattern in, 751
  ulcerations in, 601
  of ileocecal valve, 549
  rectocolonic calcification in, 966, 967f
  ureteral calcification in, 980, 980f
Schwannoma of esophagus, filling
  defects in, 98, 99f
Scirrhous carcinoma
  of colon, narrowing in, 639f, 639–640
  of pyloric channel, gastric outlet
    obstruction in, 284
Scleroderma
  differentiated from sprue, 448
  of esophagus
    motility disorders in, 8f, 8–9, 9f
    reflux esophagitis in, 9, 48, 48f
  pneumatosis intestinalis in, 887
  of small bowel
    dilatation in, 403, 404f, 446–448,
      447f, 450
    in duodenum, 403, 404f
    hide-bound sign in, 446, 447f
    pseudodiverticula in, 535, 535f
  of stomach, dilatation in, 293–295, 294f
Sclerosing cholangitis, primary, bile duct
  narrowing and obstruction in,
  826–828, 826f–828f
Sclerosis
  amyotrophic lateral, esophageal
    motility disorders in, 7
  multiple, esophageal motility disorders
    in, 8
  progressive systemic. *See* Scleroderma
Sclerotherapy of esophageal varices,
  127–128
  filling defects in, 114f, 115, 128
  narrowing in, 67f, 92–93, 93f, 128
  ulcerations in, 66–68, 67f, 128
Scrotum
  calcification in, 986, 987f
  hernia of, 875, 875f
Sebaceous glands, ectopic, nodular
  lesions of esophagus in, 146
Seidlitz test in achalasia, 18–19
Seminal vesicle calcification, 986, 987f
Sentineal loop of small bowel, in
  intraperitoneal abscess, 526
Sepsis, gram-negative, adynamic ileus in,
  433
Sequestration, pulmonary,
  esophagorespiratory fistula in, 136
Sexual intercourse, orogenital,
  pneumoperitoneum after, 901, 901f
Shigellosis
  of colon
    toxic megacolon in, 741
    ulcerations in, 601–603, 602f
  enteric-enteric fistulas in, 923, 924f
  of small bowel, irregular thickening of
    mucosal folds in, 479

Shock
  ileus in, adynamic, 433
  liver calcification in, 943, 943f
Sickle cell anemia, splenic density in,
  948, 951f
Siderosis, radiodensity of liver in, 946
Sigmoid colon
  double tracking pattern in, 756–759
  herniation through mesentery of, 874
  volvulus of, 728, 728f–730f
Silicosis, lymph node calcification in,
  1002
Skip lesions in Crohn's disease
  of colon, 593, 593f, 595, 624
  of small bowel, 474f, 475
Small bowel, 409–539
  amyloidosis of. *See* Amyloidosis, of
    small bowel
  bezoars in. *See* Bezoars, in small bowel
  biopsy of, in dilatation, 450
  carcinoid tumors of
    multiple filling defects in, 499, 499f
    separation of bowel loops in, 490f,
      520, 521f
    solitary filling defect in, 488, 489f,
      490f
  carcinoma of. *See* Carcinoma, of small
    bowel
  Crohn's disease of. *See* Crohn's
    disease, of small bowel
  cryptosporidiosis of, 454, 454f, 479
    in duodenum, 334–335, 335f
  dilatation of, 441–455
    in duodenum, 400, 401–407, 783, 784f
    in ileum of neonate, 428f, 428–429
    with normal folds, 441–451
    with thickened folds, 452–455
  diverticula and pseudodiverticula of,
    529–539
  duodenum in, 321–407. *See also*
    Duodenum
  duplication of. *See* Duplication, of
    small bowel
  filling defects of, 482–505
    in duodenum, 362–386
    multiple, 495–505
    solitary, in jejunum and ileum,
      482–494
  foreign bodies in. *See* Foreign bodies,
    in small bowel
  gallstones in. *See* Gallstones, in small
    bowel
  hamartoma of
    duodenal filling defects in, 380, 380f
    multiple filling defects in, 495, 496f
    solitary filling defect in, 485f, 486
  hemorrhage into wall of
    separation of bowel loops in, 517,
      519f
    thickening of mucosal folds in, 456–
      461, 457f–461f
  herniation of
    through mesentery, 874, 874f
    through Winslow foramen, 420, 873,
      873f

histoplasmosis of
  irregular thickening of mucosal folds
    in, 475, 476f
  sandlike lucencies in, 506–507, 507f
ileum in. *See* Ileum
in ileus, adynamic, 430–440
ischemia of. *See* Ischemia, of small
  bowel
jejunum in. *See* Jejunum
leiomyoma of. *See* Leiomyoma, of
  small bowel
lipoma of
  duodenal filling defects in, 378–380,
    378f–379f
  multiple filling defects in, 497, 498f
  solitary filling defect in, 484f,
    484–485
lymphoid hyperplasia of
  duodenal filling defects in, 368, 368f
  multiple filling defects in, 500, 502f
  sandlike lucencies in, 507–509, 508f
lymphoma of. *See* Lymphoma, of small
  bowel
mastocytosis of
  sandlike lucencies in, 506, 507f
  thickening of mucosal folds in, 337,
    337f, 477, 477f
metastases to. *See* Metastases, to small
  bowel
neurofibromatosis of
  duodenal filling defects in, 380f, 381
  multiple filling defects in, 499, 499f
  separation of bowel loops in, 520,
    521f
obstruction of, 411–429
  compared to adynamic ileus, 430,
    431f, 436–440, 437f–440f
  dilatation in, 441, 442f
  in gallstones, 417f, 420–422, 422f,
    490, 491f, 958
  gas-fluid levels in, 411, 412f, 416, 416f
  pseudotumor sign in, 418, 418f
  stepladder appearance in, 415, 415f
  strangulated, 417–418, 418f
  string-of-beads appearance in, 416,
    416f
in paraduodenal hernia, 871–872, 872f
parasitic infections of. *See* Parasitic
  infections, of small bowel
polyps of
  duodenal filling defects in, 371f, 376,
    377f, 380, 380f
  multiple filling defects in, 495–497,
    496f–498f
  solitary filling defect in, 490, 492f
radiation injury of. *See* Radiation
  injury, of small bowel
sandlike lucencies in, 506–512
sarcoma of. *See* Sarcoma, of small
  bowel
scleroderma of. *See* Scleroderma, of
  small bowel
separation of loops, 517–528
strongyloidiasis of. *See*
  Strongyloidiasis, of small bowel
thickening of mucosal folds, 452–481
  and dilatation, 452–455

Small bowel, thickening of mucosal folds
  (*continued*)
 and gastric thickening of mucosal
   folds, 513–516
 irregular and distorted, 467–481
 regular, 456–466
 trauma of, thickening of mucosal folds
   in, 460
 tuberculosis of. *See* Tuberculosis, of
   small bowel
 varices of. *See* Varices, of small bowel
 Whipple's disease of
   sandlike lucencies in, 509f, 511
   separation of bowel loops in, 517, 519f
   thickening of mucosal folds in, 337,
    467, 468f, 515, 519f
Smoking, and esophageal carcinoma, 75
Smooth muscle disorders
 duodenal dilatation in, 403
 of esophagus, 8–11
South American blastomycosis, coned
  cecum in, 577–578, 578f
Sniff test, in paralysis of diaphragm, 156
Spasm
 in colon, 636–638, 637f
 esophageal, 20, 21f
   narrowing in, 93
Sphincter
 of colon, 636, 637f
 esophageal lower, 3, 4f, 11–19
   reflux esophagitis in disorders of,
    46–50
 esophageal upper, 3
   disorders of, 5–8
 of Oddi
   and filling defects of bile ducts, 809,
    809f
   and obstruction of bile ducts, 829
   and pancreaticobiliary reflux,
    852–857
Sphincterotomy, gas in biliary system
  and pancreaticobiliary reflux after,
  853
Spigelian hernia, 878–879, 880f
Spindle cell tumors. *See also specific
   tumor types*
 bull's-eye lesions in, 865, 867f
 of colon
   multiple filling defects in, 704f, 704–
    705
   single filling defect in, 673–674,
    673f–675f
 of esophagus
   calcification in, 99f, 964
   filling defects in, 97–98, 98f–100f,
    102, 104f
   narrowing in, 83
 of small bowel
   differentiated from papilla of Vater
    enlargement, 850
   duodenal filling defects in, 378–380,
    378f–379f
   multiple filling defects in, 497, 498f
   postbulbar ulceration of duodenum
    in, 325
   solitary filling defect in, 483–485,
    483f–484f

of stomach, 867f
 calcification in, 964
 filling defects in, 243f, 244–246,
  244f–248f
 of fundus, 299, 300f
 retrogastric space widening in, 311
 ulcerations in, 190, 191f
Spine
 calcification of, 1005, 1005f
 herniation of intervertebral disk,
   esophageal impressions in, 28, 28f
 lordosis of, obstruction and dilatation
   of duodenum in, 405
 neoplasms of
   esophageal impressions in, 29
   retrorectal space enlargement in, 769
 osteomyelitis of, esophageal
   impressions in, 29
 osteophytes of, esophageal impressions
   in, 27f, 27–28, 42, 44f
 sacral region of. *See* Sacrum
Splanchnic nerve disorders, duodenal
  dilatation in, 403
Spleen
 calcification of, 937f, 946–950,
   947f–951f
 impression on gastric fundus, 300,
   300f
Splenectomy, pseudotumor of stomach
  in, 304f, 305f, 305–306
Splenic artery
 calcification of, 948, 949f, 1000
   in aneurysm, 948, 950f
   corkscrew appearance in, 948, 949f
 impression on stomach, 265–267, 266f
Splenic flexure of colon
 carcinoma of, metastatic to stomach,
   299
 impression on stomach, 300
Splenic vein obstruction, 234
Splenosis, regenerated, pseudotumor of
  stomach in, 305f, 306
Spondylitis, in ulcerative colitis, 586, 587f
Sponge, surgical, retained, 1010, 1012f
Sprue, 446
 bubbly bulb pattern in, 369, 369f
 and celiac disease of children, 444, 446
 differentiated from scleroderma, 448
 dilatation of small bowel in, 442–446,
   443f–446f, 450
 filling defects of duodenum in, 369, 369f
 hypersecretion in, 443f, 444, 444f, 445f
 intussusception in, 444–446, 446f
 jejunoileal fold pattern in, 444, 445f
 lymphoma in, 446
 moulage sign in, 444, 445f
 narrowing of duodenum in, 394
 thickening of duodenal mucosal folds
   in, 335, 335f
Staghorn calculi in kidney, 968f, 969
Staphylococcal infections of colon,
  ulcerations in, 604f, 605
Starvation, gallbladder visualization
  impaired in, 774
Stellate pattern of ileocecal valve, 543,
  545

Stepladder appearance in small bowel
  obstruction, 415, 415f
Steroid therapy
 esophageal motility disorders in, 7
 gastric erosions in, superficial, 204
 gastric ulcers and gastrocolic fistulas
   in, 921
 nephrocalcinosis in, 969
 pneumatosis intestinalis in, 890
 Stierlin's sign in tuberculosis, 572, 574f
Stitch abscess of duodenum, filling
  defects in, 363, 365f
Stomach, 177–319
 air in, in esophagorespiratory fistula,
   129, 130, 130f, 131
 in alcoholic gastritis
   filling defects of, 259f
   thickening of mucosal folds of, 223–
    224, 224f, 259, 259f
 amyloidosis of. *See* Amyloidosis, of
   stomach
 antrum of. *See* Antrum, gastric
 atrophic gastritis of, chronic, 224f
 bezoars in. *See* Bezoars, in stomach
 bile reflux gastritis in postoperative
   remnant, 276–277, 277f–278f
 candidiasis of
   filling defects in, 270
   ulcerations in, 203f, 204
 carcinoid tumors of
   filling defects in, 246–247, 249f
   ulcerations in, 196, 198f, 246–247,
    249f
 carcinoma of. *See* Carcinoma, of
   stomach
 corrosive injury of. *See* Corrosive
   agents, ingestion of, stomach
   disorders in
 Crohn's disease of. *See* Crohn's
   disease, of stomach
 cytomegalovirus infection of
   narrowing in, 215, 215f
   superficial erosions in, 204
   thickening of mucosal folds in, 228,
    228f
 diaphragm or web in, outlet
   obstruction in, 285–286, 286f
 dilatation of
   diaphragm elevation in, 155f
   nonobstructive, 291–295
   portal vein gas in, 860, 861f
 diverticula of, 307, 307f
   compared to benign ulcers, 182,
    182f, 183f
   gallbladder visualization impaired in,
    776
 duodenal bulb involvement in
   disorders of, 315–319
 duplication of
   filling defects in, 267, 267f–268f
   outlet obstruction in, 286
 ectopic. *See* Ectopia, of stomach
 emphysema of, 887
   portal vein gas in, 860
   stomach wall gas in, 312, 313f, 314
 eosinophilic gastritis of
   filling defects in, 261

narrowing in, 214, 214f
thickening of mucosal folds in, 234, 235f
in esophagogastric hernia, 300–303
in esophagogastric polyp, 100, 101f
filling defects of, 238–270
in benign ulcer, 185f
in carcinoma, 247, 249f, 250f, 273–276, 273f–276f, 297, 297f
in postoperative remnant, 271–280
fistulas of
gastrocolic. *See* Gastrocolic fistulas
gastrojejunocolic, 923, 925f
foreign bodies in
filling defects in, 261–263, 262f–263f
outlet obstruction in, 289f, 290
freezing of, therapeutic
narrowing in, 218
thickening of mucosal folds in, 228–229
fundus of, 296–308
normal appearance of, 296, 297f
gallstones in, filling defects in, 267–268
gas in wall of, 228, 312–314, 914
in gastroenteritis. *See* Gastroenteritis
gastroplasty procedures in obesity, 220–221, 220f–221f
hamartoma of, filling defects in, 242f, 243f, 244
hematoma of
filling defects in, 263f, 307
narrowing in, 219, 219f
hypertrophic gastritis of, thickening of mucosal folds in, 225, 225f
in Menetrier's disease, 229–232, 229f–230f, 232f
hypertrophic gastropathy in children, 230f, 231–232
hypertrophy of antral-pyloric fold, filling defects in, 261, 261f
impressions on, 244f, 245, 255, 258f, 259f
arterial, 265–267, 266f
on fundus, 299–300, 300f–301f
intussusception of
duodenal, filling defects in, 381–382
jejunogastric, 270, 277–280, 278f–279f
leiomyoma of. *See* Leiomyoma, of stomach
leukemic infiltration of wall, 233, 233f
lymphoma of. *See* Lymphoma, of stomach
metastases to. *See* Metastases, to stomach
narrowing of (linitis plastica pattern), 205–222
neoplasms of
filling defects in, 239–255
in fundus, 296–299, 297f–300f
retrogastric space widening in, 311
outlet obstruction of, 281–290
compared to nonobstructive gastric dilatation, 292
gallbladder visualization impaired in, 774f, 774–776
gas in stomach wall in, 314

perigastric adhesions, 222, 222f
phlegmonous gastritis of
gas in stomach wall in, 312, 313f
narrowing in, 214–215, 215f
plasmacytoma of, filling defects in, 255, 258f
polyp of. *See* Polyp, of stomach
postoperative deformity of
filling defects in, 271–272, 272f
pseudotumors in, 303f, 304f, 305f, 305–306
prolapse of mucosa
duodenal filling defects in, 370f, 370–371
esophageal filling defects in, 115, 115f
outlet obstruction in, 290
pseudolymphoma of. *See* Pseudolymphoma, of stomach
pseudotumors of, 244f
in fundus, 300–307, 302f–307f
pylorus of. *See* Pylorus
radiopaque pills in, 1006f, 1007
in retrogastric space widening, 309–311
sarcoidosis of. *See* Sarcoidosis, of stomach
sarcoma of. *See* Sarcoma, of stomach
strongyloidiasis of
duodenal involvement in, 318
gas in stomach wall in, 312, 313f
narrowing in, 215
superficial erosions of, 201–204, 202f–204f
syphilis of. *See* Syphilis, of stomach
thickening of mucosal folds in, 223–237
filling defects in, 259–261, 259f–260f
in fundus, 303–305
in lymphoma, 204f, 231f, 232f, 232–233, 250f, 251, 276, 277f
small bowel involvement in, 513–516
in Zollinger-Ellison syndrome, 324, 326f
tuberculosis of. *See* Tuberculosis, of stomach
tumefactive extramedullary hematopoiesis of, filling defects in, 268, 269f
ulcerations of. *See* Ulcerations, of stomach
varices of. *See* Varices, of stomach
volvulus of. *See* Volvulus, of stomach
Strangulation, in small bowel obstruction, 417–418, 418f
Strawberry gallbladder, 795f, 795–796
Stress, emotional
duodenal dilatation in, 405
gastric dilatation in, 295
Striated muscle of esophagus, 3
disorders of, 5–8
String-of-beads appearance in small bowel obstruction, 416, 416f
String sign in Crohn's disease, 474f, 475, 572, 573f
Striped colon appearance in metastatic tumors, 646, 646f
Strongyloidiasis
of colon
multiple filling defects in, 711, 711f

narrowing in, 630
thumbprinting pattern in, 751
toxic megacolon in, 741
ulcerations in, 609, 610f, 630
gas in biliary system and pancreaticobiliary reflux in, 854
of small bowel
duodenal narrowing in, 394, 394f, 405
duodenal thickening of mucosal folds in, 334, 335f
gastric involvement in, 318
irregular thickening of mucosal folds in, 477
multiple filling defects in, 504
solitary filling defect in, 491
of stomach
duodenal involvement in, 318
gas in stomach wall in, 312, 313f
narrowing in, 215
Subclavian artery anomalies, esophageal impressions in, 33, 33f, 35, 37f
Subhepatic gas, 904–905, 906f
Submucosal edema of colon, 717–718, 717f–718f
thumbprinting pattern in, 754, 754f
Subphrenic abscess. *See* Abscess, subphrenic
Sunburst pattern in pancreatic calcification, 953f, 955
Suppositories, rectal and vaginal, radiographic patterns from, 1010, 1011f
Surgery
appendiceal stump after appendectomy, 559f–561f, 561
bezoars after, stomach filling defects in, 272–273, 273f
bile duct strictures after, 834f, 834–835
and bile reflux gastritis in postoperative remnant, 276–277, 277f–278f
colitis after, 620, 620f
in diversion procedures, 620, 620f, 711
pseudomembranous, 609, 612
colon carcinoma after, 648–649, 649f
colon narrowing after, 660, 660f
diaphragm paralysis after, 153
in esophageal carcinoma, 79, 79f
fistulas after
aorticoduodenal, 327–328
enteric-enteric, 923, 925f
esophagorespiratory, 133
external, 934, 934f, 935
internal, 929, 931, 933f
gallbladder enlargement after, 780
gallbladder visualization impaired after, 776, 777
gas in biliary system and pancreaticobiliary reflux after, 853, 853f
gas in stomach wall after, 312
gas in upper quadrants after, 907, 917, 917f
and gastric carcinoma in postoperative stump, 273–276, 273f–275f

Surgery (*continued*)
  gastric deformity after
    filling defects in, 271–272, 272f
    pseudotumors in, 303f, 304f, 305f, 305–306
  gastric dilatation after, nonobstructive, 292, 293, 293f
  and gastric lymphoma in postoperative stump, 276, 277f
  and gastric remnant filling defects, 271–280
  gastric ulcerations after
    marginal, 196–200, 198f–199f
    at suture line, 192f, 192–193
  gastroplasty procedures in obesity, 220–221, 220f–221f
  graft-versus-host disease after
    esophageal narrowing in, 91, 92f
    pneumatosis intestinalis in, 890
    separation of small bowel loops in, 527–528, 528f
  hair growth in esophagus after
    filling defects in, 115
    nodular lesions in, 146, 147f
  Heller myotomy in achalasia, 19
  ileus after, 430, 432f, 435, 437
    gallbladder visualization impaired in, 776
  incisional hernia after, 876, 878, 878f, 879f
  jejunogastric intussusception after, 277–280, 278f–279f
  materials misplaced in, radiographic patterns of, 1010, 1013, 1011f–1013f
  ossification of scars in, 1002, 1004f
  pneumatosis intestinalis after, 888, 889f, 890
  pneumoperitoneum after, 899–901, 899f–900f
  reflux esophagitis after, 48, 50f
  renal hematoma after, 917
  retrogastric space widening after, 310
  retrorectal space enlargement after, 769f, 770
  small bowel dilatation after, 441–442, 443f, 450
    duodenal, 403
  small bowel obstruction after, 419f, 420, 425, 426f, 427
    duodenal, 403
  stitch abscess of duodenum after, filling defects in, 363, 365f
  subphrenic abscess after, 907
  suture granuloma after
    colon filling defects in, 689f, 690
    stomach filling defects in, 270, 271–272, 272f
  traumatic neuroma after ileocolic anastomosis, 493f, 674
Surgical materials, misplaced, radiographic patterns of, 1010, 1013, 1012f–1013f
Suture(s), and stitch abscess of duodenum, 363, 365f
Suture granuloma
  colon filling defects in, 689f, 690

stomach filling defects in, 270, 271–272, 272f
Suture line, gastric ulcers at, 192f, 192–193
Swallowing
  in esophageal motility disorders, 5–21
  mechanism of, 3–4
Sweep of duodenum
  normal variations in, 340
  widening of, 340–356
Syphilis
  of esophagus
    esophagorespiratory fistula in, 135
    narrowing in, 86
  liver calcification in, 939
  of stomach
    narrowing in, 213f, 213–214
    outlet obstruction in, 285
    superficial erosions in, 204
    thickening of mucosal folds in, 234
Syringomyelia, esophageal motility disorders in, 8

Tabes dorsalis, gastric dilatation in, 293
Taenia infections
  abdominal wall calcification in, 1002
  small bowel filling defects in, 504, 504f
Tail gut cysts, retrorectal space enlargement in, 763, 764
Tapeworms
  abdominal wall calcification in, 1002
  small bowel filling defects in, 504, 504f
Target sign in colon polyps, 667, 667f
Tattoo markings, radiographic patterns of, 1002
Telapaque
  absorption and excretion of, 773–774
    factors affecting, 774–776, 774f–776f
  conjugated and unconjugated forms of, appearance of, 777–778, 777f–778f
Teratoma
  retroperitoneal calcification in, 997
  retrorectal space enlargement in, 769, 769f
Tertiary contractions of esophagus, 4, 19–21, 20f–23f
  in achalasia, 14f, 15, 21, 23f
  in esophagitis, 10, 21, 22f
  in presbyesophagus, 10, 12f, 19–20, 20f
Testicular calcification, 986, 987f
Tetanus, esophageal motility disorders in, 8
Tetracycline, esophagitis and esophageal ulcerations from, 66
Thermometer
  broken, mercury in bowel lumen from, 1013, 1013f
  misplaced, radiographic appearance of, 1010, 1012f
Thiamine deficiency, duodenal dilatation in, 405
Thorotrast
  cholangiocarcinoma from, 946, 946f
  residual
    liver density in, 945f, 946, 946f
    splenic density in, 945f, 950
    splenic angiosarcoma from, 950, 951f

Thromboangiitis obliterans, small bowel thickening of mucosal folds in, 459
Thrombocytopenic purpura, hemorrhage and small bowel thickening of mucosal folds in, 460, 461f
Thrombosis
  mesenteric arterial, pneumatosis intestinalis in, 885f, 886
  mesenteric vein, portal vein gas in, 860
  phleboliths in, 1000f, 1001, 1001f
  portal vein, 943
  in ulcerative colitis, 588
Thumbprinting pattern of colon, 746–755
  in cytomegalovirus infection, 608
  in ulcerative colitis, 598, 599f
Thyroid gland
  enlargement of, esophageal impressions in, 28, 28f, 42, 42f
  metastatic carcinoma of
    esophageal narrowing in, 82, 83f
    liver calcification in, 942f
  substernal, diaphragm paralysis in, 153
Torus hyperplasia, 288, 288f
Toxic megacolon, 741–745
  pneumoperitoneum in, 897
Toxoplasmosis, liver calcification in, 939
Tracheobronchial rests of esophagus, 73, 75f
Tracheoesophageal fistulas, 129–136
  in esophageal carcinoma, 76, 77f
Traction diverticula of esophagus, 118f, 119, 119f
  perforated, esophagorespiratory fistula in, 135, 136f
Transplantation
  of bone marrow, graft-versus-host disease in
    and esophageal narrowing, 91, 92f
    and pneumatosis intestinalis, 890
    and separation of small bowel loops, 527–528, 528f
  renal, pneumoperitoneum as complication of, 899, 899f
Trauma
  bile duct strictures in, 834–835, 835f
  diaphragmatic hernia in, 171–173, 171f–172f
    intrapericardial, 173, 174f
  diaphragm elevation in, 157
  diaphragm paralysis in, 153, 156
  double-barrel appearance of esophagus in, 140f, 140–141
  duodenal dilatation in, 403, 403f, 405
  fistula formation in
    esophagorespiratory, 133–134, 133f–135f
    external, 934
    internal, 929, 933f
  gallbladder visualization impaired in, 776
  gastric dilatation in, nonobstructive, 292, 293f
  hematoma formation in
    and colon thumbprinting pattern, 746
    duodenal intramural, 375, 375f, 376f, 398, 398f
    and liver calcification, 941

ileus in, adynamic, 433
in ingestion of corrosive agents. *See*
    Corrosive agents, ingestion of
neuroma formation in
    after ileocolic anastomosis, 493f, 674
    and small bowel filling defect, 492,
        493f
pancreatic calcification in, 955
pneumatosis intestinalis in, 884f, 885
pneumoperitoneum in, 899, 899f
of small bowel, thickening of mucosal
    folds in, 460
splenic cysts in, calcified, 948
of stomach, stomach wall gas in, 314
Triangle sign of pneumoperitoneum,
    894, 895f
Trichuriasis of colon, multiple filling
    defects in, 710f, 710–711
Triple bubble sign in jejunal atresia, 427f,
    427–428
Truncus arteriosus, persistent,
    esophageal impressions in, 35–40,
    39f
Trypanosomiasis, achalasia in, 16
Tuberculoma, calcified, 972f
Tuberculosis
    adrenal calcification in, 995
    bile duct narrowing and obstruction
        in, 833, 833f
    bladder calcification in, 980
    of cecum
        coned cecum in, 550f, 572–574, 574f
        filling defects in, 567f
    of colon
        filling defects in, 681
        narrowing in, 626–628, 628f
        ulcerations in, 603f, 603–604, 626
    diaphragm paralysis in, 153
    differentiated from Crohn's disease,
        572–574, 574f
    of duodenum
        gastric involvement in, 318
        narrowing and obstruction in,
            393–394, 394f, 405
        postbulbar ulceration in, 327, 327f
        thickening of mucosal folds in, 334,
            334f
    of esophagus
        esophagorespiratory fistula in, 135
        narrowing in, 86
        nodular lesions in, 144
        ulcerations in, 58–59, 60f
    fallopian tube calcification in, 992
    fistulas in
        anorectal, 935
        duodenum-kidney, 929
        enteric-enteric, 921–923, 924f
        esophagorespiratory, 135
    of ileocecal valve, 549, 550f, 576, 628,
        628f
    liver calcification in, 937f, 937–938
    nephrocalcinosis in, 971, 972f
    peritonitis in, and abdominal
        calcification, 998–999
    pleuropulmonary, esophageal
        impressions in, 45
    pneumatosis intestinalis in, 887

pneumoperitoneum in, 897
prostate calcification in, 986
psoas abscess in, 997
retrorectal space enlargement in, 763
of small bowel
    dilatation and thickening of mucosal
        folds in, 453f, 454
    in duodenum. *See* Tuberculosis, of
        duodenum
    irregular thickening of mucosal folds
        in, 475, 476f, 518f
    obstruction in, 427
    separation of bowel loops in, 517,
        518f
spinal calcification in, 1005
spleen calcification in, 937f, 946, 948
Stierlin's sign in, 572, 574f
of stomach
    duodenal involvement in, 318
    filling defects in, 261
    narrowing in, 213f, 214
    outlet obstruction in, 285
    thickening of mucosal folds in, 234
ureteral calcification in, 980, 980f
vas deferens calcification in, 986
Tubo-ovarian abscess, entero-ovarian
    fistula in, 929, 931f
Turcot syndrome, colon polyps and
    multiple filling defects in, 697f,
    697–698
Typhlitis
    coned cecum in, 580f, 581
    narrowing of colon in, 659f, 659–660
    thumbprinting pattern of colon in, 754,
        754f
Typhoid fever, 601, 602
    cecum in, coned shape of, 578, 579f
    colon in
        toxic megacolon, 741
        ulcerations of, 601, 602
    ileocecal valve in, 549
    pneumoperitoneum in, 897
    small bowel thickening of mucosal
        folds in, 477–479, 478f

Ulcerations
    aphthoid. *See* Aphthoid ulcers
    of cecum, solitary benign, 569
    of colon, 585–621
        in Crohn's disease, 594, 594f
        differentiated from innominate lines,
            590f, 591
        filling defects in, 682, 682f
        meniscoid, 614f, 615
        narrowing in, 623–633, 623f–632f
        nonspecific benign, 619f, 619–620,
            632f, 633, 682, 682f
        and pseudoulcers, 590f, 591
        in ulcerative colitis. *See* Ulcerative
            colitis
    of duodenum
        bile duct narrowing and obstruction
            in, 829
        of bulb, 315
        clover-leaf deformity in, 393, 393f
        filling defects in, 362, 363f

gastric outlet obstruction in,
    281–282, 283f
giant, differentiated from diverticula,
    531–533, 532f–533f
lateral incisura appearance in, 359
narrowing in, 392, 392f
papilla of Vater enlargement in,
    849f, 849–850
perforated, extravasation of contrast
    material in, 932f
pneumoperitoneum in, 897, 898f
in postbulbar region, 323–328, 359,
    392, 392f
renoduodenal fistula in, 929
thickening of mucosal folds in, 329,
    330f
ulcer within an ulcer appearance in,
    533, 533f
of esophagus, 46–69
    aphthoid, in Crohn's disease, 59, 61f
    in Barrett's esophagus, 84
    in epidermolysis bullosa, 62, 62f, 91
    in hiatal hernia, 159, 161f
    in sclerotherapy of varices, 66–68,
        67f, 128
of ileocecal valve, 619, 619f
in peptic ulcer disease. *See* Peptic
    ulcer disease
of rectum
    in gonorrheal proctitis, 603f, 604
    in herpes simplex infection, 607, 608f
    in lymphogranuloma venereum, 606,
        607f
    postoperative, 620, 620f
    solitary, syndrome of, 617–619, 618f,
        632f, 633, 690f, 690–691
of stomach, 179–200
    aphthoid, 203f, 204
    in areae gastricae, 239, 239f
    benign, 179–188, 180f–189f
    in carcinoid tumors, 196, 198f, 246–
        247, 249f
    in carcinoma, 193–194, 193f–194f,
        247, 249f
    Carman's meniscus sign in, 189,
        189f, 190f
    in chemotherapy, intra-arterial, 193,
        193f
    collar of, 181f, 182
    crescent sign in, 182, 182f
    duodenal involvement in, 315
    ellipse sign in, 187–188, 187f–188f
    endoscopy in, 188
    etiology of, 190–196
    false-negative and false-positive
        results of barium studies in, 179
    filling defects in, 185f, 263, 264f–265f
    gallbladder visualization impaired in,
        775f, 776
    in gastritis, 190, 191f
    gastrocolic fistula in, 921, 923f, 924f
    of greater curvature, 186f, 186–187
    Hampton line of, 181f, 182
    healing of, 188, 188f, 189f
    in leiomyosarcoma, 252, 254f
    in lymphoma, 194, 194f–196f, 204,
        204f, 250f, 251

Ulcerations, of stomach (*continued*)
  marginal, 196–200, 198f–199f
  in metastatic tumors, 194–196, 197f,
    198f, 251, 252f–254f
  mound of, 181f, 182, 184f
  narrowing in, 210–212, 211f
  penetration of, 179, 181f
  perforation of, portal vein gas in, 860
  and pseudolymphoma, 192, 192f,
    233, 233f
  radiation of mucosal folds in, 182,
    183f, 184f, 186f
  at suture line, 192f, 192–193
  thickening of mucosal folds in, 229,
    229f
Ulcerative colitis, 586–592, 587f–593f
  backwash ileitis in, 589, 589f
  carcinoma in, 588, 639–640, 647, 647f
  collar-button appearance in, 592, 592f
  coned cecum in, 575f, 576
  differentiated from Crohn's disease,
    595, 596, 597f
  filling defects in, 592, 592f, 749f
  fistulas in
    enteric-enteric, 921
    internal, 928, 928f
  of ileocecal valve, 548, 549, 550f
  lead-pipe appearance in, 592, 623, 623f
  mucosal dysplasia in, 707, 708f
  narrowing in, 623–624, 623f–624f
  obstruction in, 724, 726f
  pneumatosis intestinalis in, 887
  pneumoperitoneum in, 897
  portal vein gas in, 860
  preparation for barium studies in, 588
  pseudopolyps in, 592, 592f, 705f, 706f,
    707, 726f
  rectosigmoid, 588, 588f
  retrorectal space enlargement in, 761–
    763, 762f, 768f
  spondylitis in, 586, 587f
  thumbprinting pattern in, 749, 749f
  toxic megacolon in, 741, 742, 742f,
    743f, 744f
Ultrasonography
  in abdominal abscess, 912f, 913, 913f
  in adenomyomatosis, 797, 798f
  in appendiceal mucocele, 561–563, 562f
  in ascites, 522f, 523
  in biliary obstruction, 819, 819f
  in Caroli's disease, 843, 844f
  in choledochal cyst, 840, 841f
  in cholesterolosis, 795f, 796
  in gallbladder carcinoma, 800, 801f
  in gallstones, 788–794, 792f–794f
  in pancreatic carcinoma, 352, 352f
  in pancreatic pseudocyst, 347, 347f
  in pancreatitis, 342, 343f, 344, 345f
  in pseudomyxoma peritonei, 998, 998f
  in pyloric stenosis, hypertrophic, 288–
    290, 289f
Umbilical hernia, 876, 877f
  gallbladder visualization impaired in,
    776
Umbilical vein catheterization, portal
    vein gas in, 858, 859–860, 860f

Urachus
  calcification of, 984
  sign of pneumoperitoneum, 894, 896f,
    897f
Uremia
  colitis in, pseudomembranous, 609, 612
  duodenal thickening of mucosal folds
    in, 333–334
Ureter, calcification of, 979–980,
    979f–980f
  in calculi, 960, 961f, 979f, 979–980
  adynamic ileus in, 433, 434f
Ureteritis emphysematosa, 891f
Ureterosigmoidostomy, colon carcinoma
    in, 648–649, 649f
Urethra, calcification of, 983–988,
    984f–985f
Urine retention, adynamic ileus in, 437
Urticaria, colonic, 717, 717f
Uterus
  cervical carcinoma of
    complications of gold therapy in,
      994, 994f
    metastatic. *See* Metastases, of
      cervical carcinoma
  endometriosis of, colon narrowing in,
    657, 657f
  fibroids of, calcification of, 988f, 989,
    989f
  gas gangrene of, 917f

Vagina
  douching of, pneumoperitoneum after,
    901
  fistulas of
    colovaginal, 927f
    colovesicovaginal, 928f
    rectovaginal, 926–928, 927f, 928f
  suppositories affecting radiographic
    patterns of, 1010
Vagotomy
  esophageal motility disorders in, 8, 16–
    17
  gallbladder enlargement in, 780, 781
  gastric dilatation in, 293
  small bowel dilatation in, 441–442,
    443f, 450
  duodenal, 403
Vagus nerve disorders, duodenal
    dilatation in, 403
Varices
  bile duct, filling defects in, 810–811,
    811f
  of colon, multiple filling defects in,
    719f, 720
  of esophagus, 108f, 109f, 123–128,
    124f–127f
    disorders simulating, 127, 127f
    filling defects in, 106, 107f–109f,
      114f, 115, 128
    narrowing in, 67f, 92–93, 93f, 128
    sclerotherapy in, 66–68, 68f, 92–93,
      93f, 127–128
    ulcerations in, 66–68, 67f, 128
  of small bowel
    duodenal filling defects in, 337, 337f,
      373f, 374–375

duodenal impressions in, 361
duodenal thickening of mucosal
  folds in, 337, 337f, 373f, 375
gastric thickening of mucosal folds
  in, 515
multiple filling defects in, 504
solitary filling defect in, 492, 493f
of stomach
  filling defects in, 259, 260f, 270
  pseudotumor in, 302f, 303, 303f
  small bowel involvement in, 515
  thickening of mucosal folds in, 234,
    234f, 235f, 259, 260f, 515
Vas deferens, calcification of, 986, 986f,
  987f
Vascular structures, calcification of. *See*
  Calcification, of vascular structures
Vasculitis
  dilatation of small bowel in, 450
  thickening of small bowel mucosal
    folds in, 458–459
Vater
  ampulla of
    biliary calculi impacted in, 834
    carcinoma of. *See* Carcinoma, of
      ampulla of Vater
  papilla of. *See* Papilla of Vater
Vena cava
  inferior
    calcification of, 945
    obstruction of, retrorectal space
      enlargement in, 770
  superior, obstruction of, esophageal
    varices in, 123–124, 124f
Ventral hernia, 876, 878
Ventricular enlargement, cardiac,
  esophageal impressions in, 40, 41f
Villoglandular polyps of colon, 672f, 673
Viral infections of colon
  filling defects in, 717–718, 718f
  narrowing in, 629–630, 630f
  ulcerations in, 607f, 608–609, 608f–610f
Vitamin B$_1$ (thiamine) deficiency,
  duodenal dilatation in, 405
Vitamin C, esophagitis and esophageal
  ulceration from, 66
Vitamin D, and nephrocalcinosis, 969
Volvulus
  cecal, 723f, 726, 727f
  of colon
    bird's beak appearance in, 728, 729,
      729f
    obstruction in, 724–726
    sigmoid, 728, 728f–730f
    transverse, 729, 730f
  midgut, duodenal obstruction in, 390f,
    390–391
  small bowel obstruction in, 420
    duodenal, 390f, 390–391
  of stomach
    gas in stomach wall in, 314
    in hiatal hernia, 159, 161f
    outlet obstruction in, 286–287, 287f
    in paraesophageal hernia, 165, 165f
Vomiting
  double-barrel appearance of esophagus
    in, 137–140, 138f, 139f

esophagorespiratory fistula in, 134, 134f
gallbladder visualization impaired in, 774
in gastric outlet obstruction, 281–282, 284, 285
in gastric retention without outlet obstruction, 291
reflux esophagitis in, 47
Von Recklinghausen's disease. *See* Neurofibromatosis
V sign, inverted, in pneumoperitoneum, 894, 896f

Waldenstrom's macroglobulinemia, sandlike lucencies of small bowel in, 506, 507f
Warfarin therapy, hemorrhage in
and separation of small bowel loops, 519f
and thickening of small bowel mucosal folds, 457f, 458f
Warts, venereal giant, 629, 629f
Webs
of bile ducts, 835f, 835–836
of cecum, 570–571
of duodenum, 389–390, 390f, 534
of esophagus
impressions on esophagus in, 26–27, 27f

jet phenomenon in, 72, 72f
narrowing in, 70–73, 71f–72f
of gastric antrum, 285–286, 286f
Whipple's disease
pneumatosis intestinalis in, 890
sandlike lucencies of small bowel in, 509f, 511
separation of small bowel loops in, 517, 519f
thickening of small bowel mucosal folds in
duodenal, 337
gastric involvement in, 515
irregular, 467, 468f, 519f
Whipworms, multiple filling defects of colon in, 710f, 710–711
Wilm's tumor, calcification in, 996, 996f
Wilson's disease, nephrocalcinosis in, 971
Winslow foramen, herniation through, 420, 872–873, 873f
Wolman's disease, adrenal calcification in, 996, 996f

Xanthogranulomatous pyelonephritis, renal calcification in, 975, 976f
Xanthomatosis, small bowel thickening of mucosal folds in, 465, 465f

Yersinia infections
coned cecum in, 578, 579f
differentiated from appendicitis, 477, 557
ileocecal valve in, 549
multiple filling defects of colon in, 711
sandlike lucencies of small bowel in, 510f, 512
submucosal edema of colon in, 718, 718f
thickening of small bowel mucosal folds in, 477, 478f
ulcerations of colon in, 604f, 605

Zenker's diverticula, 5, 117–119, 118f
gallbladder visualization impaired in, 776
Zollinger–Ellison syndrome
postbulbar ulceration of duodenum in, 324–325, 326f
thickening of gastric mucosal folds in, 229, 229f, 324, 326f
small bowel involvement in, 514, 515f
thickening of small bowel mucosal folds in
and dilatation, 452–453, 453f
duodenal, 324, 326f, 330, 330f, 331f
gastric involvement in, 514, 515f

ISBN 0-397-50943-X

90000